Essential Psychiatry

Fourth Edition

Edited by

Robin M. Murray
Kenneth S. Kendler
Peter McGuffin
Simon Wessely
David J. Castle

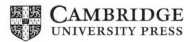
CAMBRIDGE
UNIVERSITY PRESS

CAMBRIDGE UNIVERSITY PRESS
Cambridge, New York, Melbourne, Madrid, Cape Town, Singapore, São Paulo, Delhi

Cambridge University Press
The Edinburgh Building, Cambridge CB2 8RU, UK

Published in the United States of America by Cambridge University Press, New York

www.cambridge.org
Information on this title: www.cambridge.org/9780521604086

First published 2008

Printed in the United Kingdom at the University Press, Cambridge

A catalogue record for this publication is available from the British Library
Essential psychiatry / edited by Robin Murray . . . [et al.]. – 4th ed.
       p. ; cm.
   Rev. ed. of : The essentials of postgraduate psychiatry / edited by Robin Murray,
Peter Hill, Peter McGuffin. 3rd ed. 1997.
   Includes bibliographical references and index.
   ISBN 978-0-521-60408-6 (pbk.)
   1. Psychiatry.   I. Murray, Robin, MD, M Phil, MRCP, MRC Psych.
II. Essentials of postgraduate psychiatry.
   [DNLM: 1. Mental Disorders.   2. Psychiatry.   WM 100 E7852 2008]

   RC454.E824   2008
   616.89–dc22   2008021196

ISBN 978-0-521-60408-6 paperback

The Essentials of Postgraduate Psychiatry 3rd edition – 1997 (Cambridge University Press) edited by J. L. Birley, R. Murray,
P. Hill and P. McGuffin

The Essentials of Postgraduate Psychiatry 2nd edition – 1986 (Academic Press Inc) edited by P. Hill

The Essentials of Postgraduate Psychiatry 1st edition – 1979 (Academic Press Inc) edited by P. Hill

Contents

Contributors

Katherine J. Aitchison
Senior Lecturer and Honorary Consultant Psychiatrist
MRC SGDP Centre and Division of Psychological
    Medicine and Psychiatry
Institute of Psychiatry at King's College London
London, UK

Louis Appleby
Director and Professor of Psychiatry
Centre for Suicide Prevention
Division of Psychiatry
University of Manchester
Manchester, UK

John Bancroft
Senior Research Fellow, previously Director
The Kinsey Institute for Research in Sex, Gender and
    Reproduction
Barnhurst
Horpath, Oxon, UK

Aaron T. Beck
Emeritus Professor of Psychiatry
University of Pennsylvania and Director of the Beck
    Institute
Philadelphia, Pennsylvania, USA

Sidney Bloch
Professor, Department of Psychiatry and Centre for the
    Study of Health and Society
University of Melbourne
Melbourne, Australia

Marc B. J. Blom
Department of Mood Disorders
PsyQ the Hague
The Netherlands

Roger Bloor
Senior Lecturer in Addiction Psychiatry
Keele University Medical School
Stoke-on-Trent, UK

Anne Buist
Professor of Psychiatry
Austin and Northpark
University of Melbourne
Australia

Alistair Burns
Department of Old Age Psychiatry
Education and Research Centre
Manchester, UK

E. Jane Byrne
School of Psychiatry and Behavioural Sciences
Wythenshawe Hospital
Education and Research Centre
Manchester, UK

Paul Carey
MRC Research Unit on Anxiety Disorders
Department of Psychiatry
University of Stellenbosch
Tygerberg, South Africa

David J. Castle
Chair of Psychiatry
St Vincent's Hospital and University of Melbourne
Fitzroy, Victoria, Australia

Alex Cohen
Assistant Professor
Department of Social Medicine
Harvard Medical School
Boston, Massachusetts, USA

Michael Craig
Research Fellow and Lecturer of Psychological
    Medicine
Institute of Psychiatry
London, UK

Ilana B. Crome
Professor of Addiction Psychiatry
Keele University Medical School
Stoke-on-Trent, UK

Kimberlie Dean
Clinical Lecturer and Honorary SpR in Forensic
    Psychiatry
Institute of Psychiatry
London, UK

Tom Fahy
Professor of Forensic Mental Health
Institute of Psychiatry
King's College London
London, UK

Anne E. Farmer
Social, Generic and Developmental Psychiatry Centre
Institute of Psychiatry
King's College London
London, UK

Michael Farrell
Reader in Addiction Psychiatry
National Addiction Centre
London, UK

Alan J. Flisher
Professor in Psychiatry and Mental Health, Head of the
    Division of Child and Adolescent Psychiatry and
    Director of the Adolescent Health Research Institute
University of Cape Town
South Africa
Professor II, Research Centre for Health Promotion
University of Bergen
Norway

Glen O. Gabbard
Brown Foundation Chair of Psychoanalysis and
    Professor of Psychiatry
Baylor College of Medicine
Houston, Texas, USA

Ragy R. Girgis
Resident in General Adult Psychiatry
Department of Psychiatry
College of Physicians and Surgeons
Columbia University and New York State Psychiatric
    Institute
New York, New York, USA

Sir David Goldberg
Emeritus Professor
Health Services Research Department
Institute of Psychiatry
London, UK

Ian M. Goodyer
Developmental Psychiatry Section
Department of Psychiatry
Cambridge, UK

Wayne Hall
Professor of Public Health Policy
School of Population Health
University of Queensland
Australia

Edwin Harari
Consultant Psychiatrist
Department of Psychiatry
St Vincent's Hospital
Melbourne, Australia

Anthony Holland
Section of Developmental Psychiatry
Douglas House
Cambridge, UK

Matthew Hotopf
Professor of General Hospital Psychiatry
King's College London

Department of Psychological Medicine
Institute of Psychiatry
Weston Education Centre
London, UK

Assen Jablensky
Professor of Psychiatry
Director, Centre for Clinical Research in
    Neuropsychiatry
The University of Western Australia
Perth, Australia

Navneet Kapur
Head of Research and Reader in Psychiatry
Centre for Suicide Prevention
Division of Psychiatry
University of Manchester
Manchester, UK

Shitij Kapur
Vice Dean and Professor of Schizophrenia Imaging and
    Therapeutics
Department of Psychological Medicine
Institute of Psychiatry
King's College London
London, UK

Kenneth S. Kendler
Virginia Institute for Psychiatry and Behavioral
    Genetics
Departments of Psychiatry and Human Genetics,
    Medical College of Virginia of Virginia
    Commonwealth University
Richmond, Virginia, USA

Sean Lennon
Manchester Mental Health and Social Care Trust
Wythenshawe Hospital
Manchester, UK

Jeffrey A. Lieberman
Chairman, Department of Psychiatry
Columbia University College of Physicians and
    Surgeons
New York, New York, USA

David Mamo
Assistant Professor of Psychiatry, University of Toronto
Clinician Scientist, Centre for Addiction and Mental
Health
Toronto, Canada

Peter McGuffin
Dean and Professor of Psychiatric Genetics
Institute of Psychiatry
King's College London
London, UK

Paul E. Mullen
Professor of Forensic Psychiatry, Monash University
Clinical Director, Victorian Institute of Forensic Mental
Health
Thomas Embling Hospital
Fairfield, Australia

Robin M. Murray
Professor of Psychiatry, Institute of Psychiatry
King's College London
London, UK

David Ndegwa
South London and Maudsley NHS Trust
Consultant Forensic Psychiatrist
Adult Mental Health Unit
London, UK

Jessica R. Nittler
Assistant Professor
University of Missouri – Columbia
School of Medicine
Columbia, Missouri, USA

Vikram Patel
Professor of International Mental Health and
Wellcome Trust Senior Clinical Research Fellow in
Tropical Medicine
London School of Hygiene and Tropical Medicine
London, UK

Perminder Sachdev
School of Psychiatry
University of New South Wales and Neuropsychiatric
Institute

The Prince of Wales Hospital
Sydney, Australia

Ulrike Schmidt
Professor of Eating Disorders
Section of Eating Disorders
Institute of Psychiatry
London, UK

Scott A. Schobel
Fellow in Schizophrenia Research
Department of Psychiatry
Columbia University College of Physicians and
Surgeons
New York, New York, USA

Jan Scott
Professor of Psychological Medicine, University of
Newcastle and Honorary Professor, Psychological
Treatments Research
Institute of Psychiatry
London
University Department of Psychiatry
Royal Victoria Infirmary
Newcastle upon Tyne, UK

Pak C. Sham
Department of Psychiatry and Genome Research
Centre
Li Ka Shing Faculty of Medicine,
The University of Hong Kong
Hong Kong, China

Dan J. Stein
Chair, Department of Psychiatry and Mental Health
University of Cape Town and Co-Director, MRC
Research Unit on Anxiety Disorders
University of Stellenbosch
Cape Town, South Africa

Ezra Susser
Professor and Chair
Department of Epidemiology
Mailman School of Public Health
Columbia University
New York, New York, USA

Michele Tansella
Professor of Psychiatry
Department of Medicine and Public Health
Section of Psychiatry and Clinical Psychology
University of Verona
Verona, Italy

Graham Thornicroft
Professor of Community Psychiatry
Section of Community Mental Health
Health Service and Population Research Department
Institute of Psychiatry
King's College London
London, UK

Janet Treasure
Department of Academic Psychiatry
Thomas Guy House
Guys Campus
London, UK

Evangelia M. Tsapakis
Clinical Research Fellow and Honorary Specialist
   Registrar in General Adult Psychiatry
MRC SGDP Centre and Division of Psychological
   Medicine and Psychiatry
Institute of Psychiatry at King's College
London, UK

André Tylee
Professor of Primary Care Mental Health
Section of Primary Care Mental Health
Health Services Research Department
Institute of Psychiatry
London, UK

Peter Tyrer
Department of Psychological Medicine
Imperial College
London, UK

Jim van Os
Department of Psychiatry and Neuropsychology
South Limburg Mental Health Research and Teaching
   Network
EURON, Maastricht University

Maastricht, The Netherlands
Division of Psychological Medicine, Institute of
   Psychiatry
London, UK

Elizabeth Walsh
Honorary Senior Lecturer and Consultant Forensic and
   General Adult Psychiatrist
Division of Psychological Medicine
Institute of Psychiatry
London, UK

Paul Walters
MRC Fellow
Section of Primary Care Mental Health
Health Services and Population Research Department
Institute of Psychiatry
London, UK

Myrna M. Weissman
Professor of Epidemiology in Psychiatry
College of Physicians and Surgeons
Columbia University
Chief, Division of Clinical and Genetic Epidemiology
New York State Psychiatric Institute
New York, New York, USA

Simon Wessely
Professor of Liaison and Epidemiological Psychiatry
King's College London
Department of Psychological Medicine
Institute of Psychiatry
Weston Education Centre
London, UK

Marieke Wichers
Department of Psychiatry and Neuropsychology
South Limburg Mental Health Research and Teaching
   Network
EURON, Maastricht University
Maastricht, The Netherlands

Kimberly Yonkers
Associate Professor of Psychiatry
Yale University
New Haven, Connecticut, USA

Preface to the fourth edition

Essential Psychiatry is a premium international psychiatric text with contributions from leaders in their respective fields. Whilst written essentially for the clinician, it encompasses the very latest research findings and has extensive and up-to-date referencing. It is a completely revised and updated version of *Essentials of Postgraduate Psychiatry, 3rd ed.* (eds. R. Murray, P. Hill, P. McGuffin; Cambridge University Press, 1997). Although it maintains the overall structure of that volume, it expands and extends its scope and includes cutting-edge contributions from a wide range of authors (from Europe, the Americas, Australia, Asia and Africa).

Care has been taken to ensure that, whilst chapters present contemporary research and clinical practice, they also reflect the rich historical heritage of the field of psychiatry. Both the major classification systems – the American Psychiatric Association's *Diagnostic and Statistical Manual of Mental Disorder* and the World Health Organization's *International Classification of Diseases* – are referenced throughout, with pointers to overlaps and differences between these systems.

The book is organized into sections, beginning with *The Tools of Psychiatry* and followed by *Psychiatric Disorders* (including discrete chapters on child and adolescent and old age psychiatry), *Special Topics* (e.g. social and transcultural aspects of psychiatry), *Psychiatry in Specific Settings* (e.g. psychiatry in primary care; community psychiatry) and *Treatments in Psychiatry* (covering biological, psychological and family interventions). Each chapter has supportive material, including tables and clinically focused fact boxes. The result is a book which can be read through from beginning to end, particular chapters read separately or sections read together. Each chapter, whilst standing alone, is cross-referenced to other chapters where relevant. The use of headings and subheadings and a comprehensive index make quick reference to specific topics easy.

We believe this book will be a major reference work for psychiatrists and mental health professionals across the world, as well as providing a comprehensive resource for psychiatric trainees which will endure well beyond their trainee years, and continue to be a source of knowledge and wisdom for years to come.

Robin M. Murray, Kenneth S. Kendler,
Peter McGuffin, Simon Wessely,
David J. Castle
June 2008

The Tools of Psychiatry

The mental state and states of mind

Paul E. Mullen

It is the duty, and should be the privilege of the medical examiner, to spend several days in the examination of a lunatic before they pronounce a decided opinion.

Theodric Beck (1823)

The injunction of Dr Beck may seem whimsical in these days of brief admissions and etiolated community psychiatry, but clinical psychiatry without some curiosity and concern with the mental life of the patient would be an impoverished speciality. This is as true for those psychiatrists whose primary interest is in classification and diagnosis as for those who seek first and foremost to explore the meaningful connections and mental mechanisms of their patients' internal world. The information generated by such interest, if it is to be shared, requires expression in an agreed language of sufficient clarity and precision. Putting names to things is an essential prerequisite to any meaningful discourse. Allowing definitions of such names to come to determine the supposed essence of those things is, however, the death of science and progress. Sadly this is happening not only in attempts to impose operational definitions in psychopathology but also in the classificatory approaches of both the *Diagnostic and Statistical Manual* (DSM) and *International Classification of Diseases* (ICD) systems, or at least in how these symptoms are applied in some circumstances (Mullen, 2006).

Abnormalities of mental state as symptoms

Abnormalities of mental state are frequently treated in psychiatry merely as symptoms that act as signposts pointing towards particular diagnostic conclusions. The theoretical structure underlining this approach is the familiar medical model in its most basic form.

Reservations can, however, be expressed about equating abnormalities of mental state with symptoms in a way analogous to symptoms in general medicine. In medicine itself the symptom can be seen as expressing the effect of the disease process. The pain down the left arm on exertion can reflect the physical changes accompanying cardiac ischaemia. The patient's complaint is a direct pointer to a physical lesion. The tone and quality of the patient's complaint may, in this situation, be affected by the character and culture of the individual, but still the symptom can be employed as a signpost to the disease. In psychiatry, even if one grants uncritically the claim that underlying disturbances of mental state are disorders of the brain, a straightforward expression of the disease by the symptom is less easily maintained. The so-called symptoms of psychiatric illness are virtually always disturbances of mental state. When patients give voice to their complaints, or, more often, try to express the disturbances in their experience of

Essential Psychiatry, ed. Robin M. Murray, Kenneth S. Kendler, Peter McGuffin, Simon Wessely, David J. Castle.
Published by Cambridge University Press. © Cambridge University Press 2008.

themselves and their world, there lies behind their statements the whole mental life of that particular individual. As Minkowski (1970) expressed it, "behind confusion always lies the confused person, behind melancholy the depressed, behind the syndrome of influence the influenced". Abnormalities of mental state are not necessarily to be viewed as disordered fragments but, on the contrary, can be seen as reflecting the whole personality and mental functioning of that individual. This view suggests that the syndrome in psychiatry cannot be equated so easily with a simple association of symptoms, but becomes the expression of a modification in the mental life and personality of this individual.

The clear and precise definition of clinical symptoms has manifest utility and serves the medical model of psychiatric disorder admirably. There must, however, be some disquiet over the extent to which this detracts from the exploration and delineation of the patient's actual experiences. A hallucination can be defined as a perception without an object. Employing this definition, whether or not the particular patient has had a hallucinatory experience, can be determined by asking the right questions. Having established the presence of the hallucination, the psychiatrist may feel they have exhausted this area of enquiry, but what has been defined is a symptom; what has not occurred is the elucidation of the patient's actual experience.

To take an example, hypochondriasis has been defined as painful or unpleasant worrying, specifically concentrated on the possibility of disease or malfunction that is beyond the subject's power to control and out of proportion to any actual illness or disorder that is present (Wing *et al.*, 1974). Hypochondriasis so defined may present in very different ways in the context of very different states of mind: the severely depressed patient in a state of agitated despair who complains of the decay and decomposition within her; the individual with dementia who repeats interminably a cry for help and for a cure to some ill-defined malaise; the young man who travels from physician to physician with a bizarre account of physical disorder, which he says leaves him without feeling, without will, and

unable to think of anything but his supposed malfunction; the woman who has moved from doctor to doctor for 30 years with a multiplicity of aches and pains and despite accumulating operations, vague diagnostic labels, and innumerable courses of treatment, continues to complain bitterly of being plagued by ill health. The symptom *hypochondriasis* could be used for all. The context of the hypochondriasis in these particular cases could be further placed in the context of a syndrome such as Briquet's, a psychiatric disorder such as depression or even a clinicopathologic entity such as Pick's disease. This further elaboration does not bring us much closer to understanding the state of mind which manifests in these four individuals through their worry and concern over the state of their physical health. Perhaps more importantly, if we do not recognise the qualitative differences in how the hypochondriasis is experienced and expressed, we miss an all-important sign of the nature of the disturbance of which it is a part.

If we have a real curiosity about the mental life of our patients and are not content to remain exclusively within the reductionism of the currently fashionable diagnostic labels, then the exploration of mental state must extend beyond symptom collection. Symptoms are constructs which do not exist in pure form but vary with the context, with the influence of other disturbances in mental state, with the situation in which they are experienced, with the cultural and personal background of the individual and even with the theoretical assumptions of the examiner who directs and constrains the patient's description.

Is descriptive psychopathology, then, an intellectual indulgence for mental health professionals with enough time on their hands for explorations beyond those necessary for effective care and treatment of the patient? Or is it of clinical and potential research interest? It is hoped that this chapter suggests the latter. The symptoms checklist approach is good enough most of the time, but the psychiatrist's expertise should take them beyond the limits inherent in the health professional with a clipboard. Not only will the ability to explore the mental state provide a more rounded understanding of even the most mundane clinical situation, a competent exploration will make the patient feel attended to and understood to a far greater extent than an interrogation based on a predetermined set of questions. In the more complex case, such an exploration offers protection against error and the hope of more effective management. The trajectory for much social and biological research in psychiatry in recent years has been towards the use of standardised diagnostic instruments, for very good reasons. In some areas, we are beginning to come up against the inherent limitations of this diagnostic approach which dominates both DSM-IV and ICD-10.

The carefully articulated diagnostic classifications of DSM-IV and ICD-10 are generally accepted to relate meaningfully to the world of mental disorders. Nevertheless, the increasingly obvious gaps between research findings and the definitions of mental disorders in today's diagnostic manuals is beginning to raise questions about whether validity has been sacrificed on the altar of reliability. For example, schizophrenia as a diagnostic entity is starting to fragment under the impact of genetic, neuroimaging, neuropsychological, social and other research methodologies for which findings are difficult to make sense of within anything approaching the mental models of schizophrenia. Bleuler's plurality of the schizophrenias has returned. Schizophrenia may even be in the process of regressing from disorder to syndrome. The question is once again open as to what abnormalities of mental state and behaviour best map onto the developing research database – a question which today's self-confirming and fixed diagnostic categories with their simple symptom signposts are helpless to answer (Mullen, 2006). Mental health clinicians with any critical faculties cannot but notice that the better they know a patient and the more information that is available, often the more problematic it becomes to fit them into any specific diagnostic category. This is the reverse of the situation in well-established medical specialities. The increasing use of the label *schizoaffective disorder*, for example, reflects not just sloppy practice

but genuine confusion created by attempting to read clinical reality through the categories of the diagnostic manuals.

The situation with affective disorders is even more dramatic. Following the extension of the label *depression* to cover a vast range of distress and dysphoria, we are left with supposed diagnostic entities, such as major depression, which have lost coherence from being stretched so widely. Under the tutelage of the pharmaceutical industries' favoured experts, we are seeing a similar inflation of the term *mania*. Today a diagnosis equals an indication, and an expanding indication may be worth a fortune to a pharmaceutical company. In a medical world that is increasingly commercialised, there is no innocence in psychiatric diagnostic systems. Given that they remain essentially arbitrary, at least at the all-important margins, they become the vehicles for some professors' pursuit of power and influence and for some pharmaceutical companies' pursuit of profit. The DSMs and ICDs began as attempts to create a common language by codifying what were accepted to be preliminary and tentative assumptions about diagnostic categories. Today DSM-IV and ICD-10 confront us not as hypotheses about useful ways to conceptualise disordered states of mind and behaviour, but as the very foundation of our research and clinical practice. In today's psychiatry, to be a researcher or even a mainstream clinician plunges one into the very core of the self-justifying and self-sustaining hermeneutic world of today's manuals of mental disorders. When push comes to shove, however, diagnostic entities depend on phenomenology at least until genuine clinical pathological entities emerge from the current confusion of half-truths, good intentions, and pure obscurantism.

Abnormal phenomena

In the following sections, abnormal phenomena are discussed. The emphasis is on describing mental phenomena prior to their becoming part of the formulation of particular disorders, but for convenience and coherence some common syndromes, such as mania, are used to draw together the associated phenomena. Space only allows a restricted presentation. This chapter is no more than an advert for descriptive psychopathology, which it is hoped will interest the reader to explore the area further. The best place to begin that exploration remains Karl Jaspers's (1963) *General Psychopathology*, in particular pages 55–148.

Perceptual disorders

Madmen are visionaries of the senses because they do not see things as they are and because they often see things that are not. (Malebranche, 1674/1980)

The sensory modalities are the special senses of sight, hearing, smell and taste, as well as the sensations of touch, pain, temperature, point discrimination and position. Except in peculiar circumstances we experience perceptions, not sensations. Sensations are transformed into perceptions by their origin being experienced as arising from some external object. If I experience a smell without recognition or association, it would be a simple sensation, but after it is referred to some external object – say, a rose – it forms part of a perception. In perception we usually experience ourselves in relation to an object in the world. Objects are normally perceived as particular things. This is especially true of visual perceptions in which, for example, if I look at a cube I tend to perceive it as a cube, although at most I can only immediately apprehend three of its sides, and a possibility exists, until I have examined every aspect, that it is not truly a cube. Meanings tend, therefore, to be imminent in perception. Perceived objects stand bodily before us resisting and infused with a quality of reality. In that we believe what we see, we do so usually without any verification or consideration. Traditionally, theories of perception introduce into perception itself intellectual operations and a critical examination of the evidence of the senses to which we in fact resort only when direct observation founders in ambiguity. Clearly, however, when we deal with perception rather than sensation, we are dealing not simply with the raw data itself but with a process that usually involves a knowing what as well as a sensing of. In stating that he hears a voice, the patient is recognising the type and nature of what he hears.

Disturbance in sensory function

Disturbances in the sensory modalities themselves are largely the result of organic lesions and are dealt with in standard texts of neurology. Occasionally the absence of sensation (e.g. blindness or anaesthesia), the perversion of sensation (e.g. tingling paraesthesia) or the abnormal heightening of sensation (e.g. hyperacusis) may be complained of without any obvious explanation in physical pathology. This, for example, will be seen in certain conversion symptoms of a hysterical type. In some patients with mania, all sensation may appear heightened, as they may also be in depressed individuals, although for one it is the source of pleasure and delight, in the other an additional burden and imposition. A dulling of sensations with everything experienced as lacklustre and bleak may also accompany depression.

Disturbances in perception

Agnosias
The disturbed ability to organise sensory impressions so as to allow the recognition of objects (that is, to perceive objects) is known as agnosia. Agnosias may obviously affect different sensory modalities and usually reflect cortical damage.

Micropsia and macropsia
The relative proportions of perceived objects may alter to render them enlarged (macropsia) or diminished (micropsia). Such changes may occur, for example, in severe fatigue, sleeplessness, toxic states, and temporal lobe epilepsy.

Synaesthesia
This is where perceptions in one modality, for example, hearing, are simultaneously experienced as if they were also present in another modality, for example, vision. This is encountered in some drug

intoxications. The visual effects which occur concomitantly with music in states of cannabis intoxication are often highly prized by its habitués.

False perceptions
These are actual perceptual abnormalities and imply that the experience involved is of perceiving something, not just believing something.

Hallucinations
There is a long tradition of distinguishing between illusions and hallucinations (Van Den Berg 1982). Esquirol (1833), held that

a person labours under an hallucination who has a thorough conviction of a sensation when no external object suited to excite this sensation has impressed his senses, whereas it is an illusion if the senses are deceived respecting the qualities, relations, and causes of impressions actually received and cause them to form false judgements respecting their internal and external sensations.

Hallucinations proper have the following characteristics:
- They are actual false perceptions, not distortions of real perceptions.
- They are experienced as being out there in the world and as inhabiting objective space.
- They are experienced as having the qualities and force of the corresponding normal perceptions, being just as vivid, whole and immediate.
- They are usually experienced alongside and simultaneously with normal perceptions (complex visions may be an exception).
- They are as independent of our will as is any normal perceptions, in that they cannot be conjured up or dismissed.

The hallucination may show a greater independence of our will and action than a normal perception for, although I can turn away from looking at the page before me or cease attending to the droning voice of a lecturer, my hallucinations will continue to force themselves to my attention. A hallucinated voice will usually penetrate the most efficient earmuffs, and one patient continued to be plagued by hallucinated voices even after he had destroyed his eardrums with needles thus reducing the rest of the world to silence.

Hallucinations do not yield to argument for the immediateness of the experience is that of normal perception, but the experienced reality of hallucinations can vary. On more than one occasion, I have had patients try to explain how the voices or visions differ from actual perceptions. It has been suggested that hallucinations owe as much to interpretation as perception, with patients elaborating and constructing their experiences out of more basic hallucinatory events (Horowitz, 1978). Patients frequently find no difficulty in discriminating between their hallucinations and true perceptions. Hallucinations are usually confined to a single sensory modality, and this or some other subtle difference from normal perception may make the patient aware of the false nature of the perceptions. The ease with which hallucinations are distinguished from real perceptions in some patients is illustrated by a telephonist who, despite being troubled by constant auditory hallucinations, continued to work efficiently, unerringly distinguishing them from the disembodied voices of callers. A particular patient may suffer simultaneously from hallucinations in several sensory modalities at the same time, but they will rarely be perceived as emanating from a single entity. Occasionally multimodal or scenic hallucinations are described in which a complex visual and auditory hallucination is experienced, but if a patient reports a vision that also speaks, particularly if it answers back, the most likely explanations are malingering or hysteria.

Hallucinations can be subdivided by sensory modality.

Auditory hallucinations may range from ill-defined sounds to highly organised perceptions in which, for example, a voice recognizable to the patient as that of a relative or acquaintance will be heard talking at length. One of my patients was constantly plagued with the sound of the Beatles playing "Strawberry Fields", complete with full musical accompaniment, a phenomenon that despite his fondness for popular music palled after the first few weeks. True auditory hallucinations usually have a directional quality, and the patient can describe from where they appear to be emanating. Certain modes of hearing voices were held by Kurt Schneider (1974) to be of special diagnostic importance in schizophrenia. The hearing of one's own thoughts read aloud, voices talking with one another, and voices that maintain a running commentary on the patient's thoughts and actions were considered first-rank symptoms. Occasionally tinnitus and other disturbances due to local disease of the ear may be confused with hallucinations.

Visual hallucinations may also vary from ill-defined shapes and colours through clearly recognizable objects and persons to the complex visions which may, for example, accompany ecstatic states.

Olfactory and gustatory hallucinations can occur separately or, more commonly, together. They are seen in some types of schizophrenic disorder, but may also be found in affective and epileptic disturbances. The persecuted patient may taste and smell the poisons placed in his food by his tormentors, the depressed may be assailed by the stench of his own decomposition, the oversensitive may squirm in embarrassment at what she perceives as her overpowering odour (the distinction from illusion may often be difficult in these cases).

Tactile hallucinations refer to cutaneous perceptions which vary from vague tingling or sensations of temperature change to perceptions experienced as being held, hit or caressed. In certain intoxications, typically cocaine, the patient may experience formication in which what they perceive seems like bugs crawling around, on or under the skin.

Somatic hallucinations may be difficult to distinguish from tactile hallucinations and, at the other extreme, merge into delusional beliefs about bodily change. One patient described having his semen drawn out of him by ghouls. Clearly connected with this bizarre delusional belief were tactile hallucinations involving the perceptions of being pricked with pins and tingling sensations around the base of his spine but also somatic hallucinations involving the experience of his testicles and penis shrinking into his abdomen and his spine feeling as if it were "hollow and cracking".

Somatic hallucinations may accompany epileptic activity. One patient who described strange abdominal sensations that preceded his fits perceived them as writhing movements and, in turn, interpreted that as snakes squirming around in his belly.

Disturbances of body image may occur in a variety of organic brain disorders, in some psychiatric disorders and, probably most commonly, in normal individuals under the influence of sleep deprivation, exhaustion or intoxication. The most common disturbances of body image are perceptions of changes in size and shape of parts of the body (head and hands seem most common) or of the whole body. The reported alteration in body image in anorexia nervosa would appear a more subtle phenomenon.

Illusions are distortions of real perceptions, in contrast to hallucinations that arise without external stimulus. The perceptual stimulus arises from an actual object, and the illusion is formed by the perception's transformation. The other characteristics are identical with those listed for hallucination. Illusions do, however, usually exhibit a more transient existence than hallucinations and often vanish when attention is drawn to the misperception.

A common illusion occurs in the overwrought individual whose vision on a dark night distorts the branches blowing in the wind into a perception of an attacker moving towards him. A depressed patient out driving reported being frozen in horror at the sound of a child screaming in pain, only to realise later that she had misperceived the squeaking of the brakes of her own car. It is important in this example that the patient heard distinctly a scream of pain and did not misinterpret a squealing of brakes for the squealing of a hurt child. The patient with delirium tremens is often accosted by the transformation of the articles around them into terrifying illusions.

Functional hallucinations. These hallucinations, which may be confused with illusions, are rare phenomena in which a hallucination occurs simultaneously and in association with a real perception. Thus hallucinatory voices may only be heard against the background of a running tap, and turning off the water abolishes the hallucination. The noise of running water in this example is not transformed or distorted into a hallucinatory voice nor is it misinterpreted as such, for the functional hallucination is heard alongside and separable from the accompanying real perception. A man complained that when out driving, he was assailed by insulting voices. These voices were only to be heard at traffic lights and were confined to periods when the amber signal was on. When the lights changed to red or green the voices ceased.

Pareidolia. Another common and normal phenomenon, pareidolia, are the perceptions conjured up by ill-defined sense impressions such as those that occur when staring into the dying embers of an open fire.

Phenomena related to false perceptions

Misinterpretations
These are not false perceptions, for they consist of a correct perception, the import of which is incorrectly deduced. Thus a wary prospector may mistake shiny metal for gold, the perception of glitter being correct but its interpretation overly hopeful. Misinterpretations frequently arise in paranoid patients, for example, when every creak and bang, although correctly perceived, may be misinterpreted as the approaching footsteps of the persecutor.

Pseudo-hallucinations
Pseudo hallucinations, one of the most misunderstood and undervalued of abnormal phenomena, are a form of imagery as distinct from hallucinations and illusions, which are perceptual phenomena. An image is a product of thought and a reflection on the world, unlike a perception for which there is a sensing of something external in the real world. Although an image is a cognition, it is experienced figuratively as if it were a perception. Pseudo-hallucinations are pathological images experienced as emanating from the mind; they are seen in the mind's eye and heard with the inner ear, not perceived by the actual eyes and ears. Pseudo-hallucinations inhabit subjective inner space not the outside world of objects. Pseudo-hallucinations are the patient's own thoughts, and there is a feeling of responsibility for them, although unlike the images of normal mental life, the morbid pseudo-hallucination is not under voluntary control. It confronts the patient as within the mind; it is not there at their behest, nor will it evaporate in answer to one's wishes. Inner voices are the most commonly encountered examples, often being described as voices in the head or the voice of conscience.

Thoughts experienced as being read aloud are not pseudo-hallucinations if the thoughts are alienated from the individual and become an auditory perception confronting them as part of the external reality.

A problem is created by patients who say they know the voices or visions are in their mind, thus indicating that they have insight into the morbid nature of their experience. In such a case, it is important to distinguish whether the phenomenon was experienced as a perception from objective space or was actually an image within subjective space. Pseudo-hallucinations are sometimes characterised as pathological perceptions in which the sufferer is aware of their morbid nature and does not project them into the surrounding world. It seems unwise to this author to call hallucinations pseudo-hallucinations simply because the patient has insight into their morbid nature (Fish, 1967; Hare, 1973), for this is to make the classification of a perceptual disorder dependent on the patient's judgement at the moment of being interviewed and not on the nature of the experiences themselves.

The term *pseudo-hallucination* has led to a tendency to approach the phenomenon as something to be excluded on the way to discovering "true" hallucinations. As a result it is dismissed as noise of no inherent interest – or worse, as a sign of mendacity in those who report the experience. In reality it is an abnormal experience found across a wide range of psychopathological states, from severe personality disorders to toxic confusional states. It is no more or less a real phenomenon than a hallucination, and its presence, although of little diagnostic import, is indicative of significant disturbance of mental state. Interestingly its content may be far more informative about the patient's current pre-occupations and intentions than a hallucinatory experience.

Eidetic images

Eidetic images are perfectly normal phenomena most frequently encountered in children. They are images of something once perceived, which can be conjured up with almost all the original details intact. Thus a page of a book previously read may be recalled as an image so vivid that the eidetic person can read out the text as from the original.

Perceptual disorders and pseudo-hallucinations occur in all forms of psychotic disturbance, in disturbed states of consciousness and with surprising frequency in normal individuals (Posey & Losch, 1983; Slade & Bentall, 1988). During the phase which intervenes between the waking state and sleep, many people experience illusions and hallucinations. The hallucinations on falling asleep are termed *hypnagogic,* and those on awakening *hypnopompic.* In the grief which follows a bereavement, hallucinations and pseudo-hallucinations of the lost one are a common and normal phenomenon. In situations of extreme stress, be it physical or emotional, to which high levels of general arousal pertain, perceptual disturbances tend to become more frequent, albeit fleetingly. Sensory deprivation procedures have produced a wide variety of perceptual abnormalities including organised hallucinatory experiences. A variety of organic states are associated with perceptual disturbance, and any major disruption of cerebral function can produce such phenomena usually in association with the clouded consciousness of a confusional state. Meaningful auditory and visual hallucinations are particularly associated with temporal lobe dysfunction, and it has been claimed that they may actually be produced by direct stimulation at or near the temporal lobe. Hallucinogenic drugs induce a wide range of perceptual disturbances, predominantly visual in character, the form and content of which tend to be in constant flux, unlike the hallucinatory disturbances of schizophrenia.

Tactile and somatic hallucinations require careful attention. If the patient has a tactile hallucination, such as a strange tingling, she may say it is due to rays directed at her or "as if" there were some electrical current. The sufferer from disseminated sclerosis may similarly describe a true paraesthesia as if it were an electric current (Lhermitte's sign). Care must therefore always be exercised to distinguish odd ways of expressing true sensory disturbances from the elaborations, delusional or otherwise, of false perceptions. Further, it is wise not to forget that a bizarre interpretation, particularly of a somatic sensation in schizophrenia, may mask the symptom of a physical disorder.

Feelings, emotions, affects and moods

The terminology in this area is complicated because several common usages often attach to each word. For example, *feelings* in everyday parlance can refer to sensations, beliefs, presentiments, considerations for others and may even be employed as being synonymous with the term *emotions.* Despite the wide overlap in the various terms, some rough distinction and hierarchy is worth attempting.

Feelings can be taken to be basic experiences of pleasure and displeasure. Wundt (1903) suggested that feelings vary according to their degree of pleasantness or unpleasantness, the extent to which they produce excitement and the degree of induced tension or conversely relaxation. A feeling need not be about anything per se; it is simply an account of an internal state.

Emotions can be thought of as involving a more complex state of mind than feelings, for they are usually intentional, being actively directed at something. If I am in love, it is love of someone, and it is the charms of the beloved that I am aware of, not the dissociated experience of being in love. An emotional state such as sadness could, of course, become an object for consciousness, an abstraction on which it is possible to reflect, but as soon as it becomes again the emotion of sadness, it is sadness *about* something. The distinction between feeling and emotion may be illustrated by anger.

On arriving at work, an individual discovers that the important documents they had been promised would be available without fail were not on their desk as arranged and becomes angry. They are now experiencing the emotion of anger about being let down. A few moments later, they discover the reports on top of the filing cabinet: they can no longer be angry about being let down, but the feelings accompany the emotion of anger – the sense of unpleasant arousal, palpitations and general perturbation – may continue for some time. This example also illustrates how a judgement, in this case of having been let down, is integral to an emotional experience, and with judgement comes the possibility of choice (see Solomons, 1980). It also highlights the autonomic changes which accompany the more vehement of our emotions.

Emotions often involve what Frijda (1986) referred to as *objectivity* in that they are felt to occur to one, to come unbidden and to be independent of one's conscious choices. Emotions are experienced as happening to us and often as being irrational and uncontrollable reactions. Thus although emotions are usually intentional, in the sense of being a conscious orientation towards something, they may be experienced as unintentional, in the sense of being beyond or outside of conscious control. Emotions may involve not only feelings about something but also behaviour or, more exactly, a disposition to behave in a particular manner. Thus love would be associated with a tendency to approach or behave pleasantly towards the object of that affection, just as fear would lead to a tendency to recoil or flee from what was feared. Fantasies are so intimately related to most strong emotions that they can be regarded as an integral element in the experience. Finally what gives rise to emotions, how they are expressed and possibly even how they are experienced are influenced by the social and cultural context which mould expectations (Harré, 1986; Mullen, 1991).

Romantic jealously offers an example (Mullen, 1990). It involves the experience of painful feelings associated with the fear related to loss and the anger towards the person believed to be guilty of infidelity. There is a cause in the sense of a state of affairs that has aroused suspicions and a judgement that the rights of the jealous have been infringed and disregarded. What constitutes fidelity and therefore infidelity is in part culturally determined. It has an object in that there is jealousy of someone and about something. Jealousy often brings with it vivid fantasies of the partner's supposed infidelities, sometimes described as visual images of such immediacy that it is like watching the actual event. There is a tendency to certain types of behaviour, including checking, cross-questioning and verbal or even physical aggression. The "acceptable scripts" determining jealous behaviours are culturally sanctioned.

Moods and *affects* designate more sustained and pervasive states of mind of which individual emotions may be a part. It is the prevailing tone within which the emotional life of the individual proceeds. Jaspers (1963) argued that mood comes about with prolonged emotion, but in practice it often appears as if the mood precedes and constrains the emerging emotional responses. Thus within the affective state of depression, individuals may be predisposed to experience a variety of emotions – shame, fear, anger – just as they are rendered impervious to others, such as joy. Mood and affect are more global designations than emotion and represent a more complex conceptualisation of the person's psychic experience. Mood and affect define to a significant extent our orientation to the world. The horizons of our existence can be profoundly influenced by mood; for example, depression brings with it a narrowing of possibility, a shrinkage of our sense of agency and effectiveness, as well as a general dulling of experience.

Temperament is that aspect of the individual which may be taken to be a lifelong predisposition to particular kinds and types of emotional responses and affective states.

Thus a hierarchy moving from feelings through emotions, moods, and affective state to temperament involves increasing complexity in terms of state of mind and usually to an increasing duration of that state.

Pathology of feelings and emotions

The pathology of emotions may be considered, employing the model outlined, as involving alterations in the following aspects.

1. The types and quality of events and intentions which call forth emotional responses

The alterations and pathologies involving the situations and intentions which call forth emotions are of considerable importance in psychiatry but usually receive scant attention in terms of pathology of emotion. To use love as an example, it is normally considered pathological in function of the abnormal ideas (delusions) that call it forth. Clearly, however, there are pathologies of love in which the degree of response, the types of situations invoking it and the intentions of the emotion can be grossly deviant within the accepted social and cultural norms, without any involvement of delusional beliefs about either the feelings of the beloved or one's own relationship to those feelings. Intense infatuation with unrealistic hopes for a consummation of the passion may preoccupy the individual. Except at moments when immersed in fantasy, some insight into the overly hopeful nature of the expectations may be retained, but this will not stop someone in the grip of morbid infatuation from stalking their supposed beloved to the detriment of themselves and the unfortunate target (Mullen & Pathé, 1994; Mullen *et al.*, 2000). The pathology of love could within this model be seen as occupying a wide range of disturbances, including some of the sexual perversions (Boss, 1949).

2. The characteristics, tone and strength of feelings generated

Traditionally the psychopathology of emotion has concentrated primarily on alterations in the tone and character of the feeling generated. This is in keeping with the view of emotions as occurrences that simply happen in or to us. The disturbances described in this area are as follows.

Poverty of emotional responsiveness, in which there is a loss in the intensity of feelings evoked by events, and the emotional life becomes flat and barren. This is seen in its most dramatic form in the chronic schizophrenic state and is part of the so-called negative symptomatology. The blunting of responsiveness should perhaps be distinguished from flattening, although they often seem to be used interchangeably. *Blunting* strictly refers to a loss of sensitivity or indifference to the emotional import of an event as opposed to a poverty of response (Sims, 1988). It could be described in terms of a loss of capacity for empathy, although it is not usually conceptualised in this manner. Flattening, in contrast, is illustrated by those who are aware of the potential meaning of an event and the feelings it should evoke but lack the appropriate degree of response. One articulate young woman with schizophrenia described that when with others, she would know she should be sharing their laughter, their interest and even their anger, but unlike them, she could only perform emotions, not experience them.

Anhedonia is a related phenomenon in which there is a loss of responsiveness specifically tied to the experience of pleasure, which can either be in physical experiences or the pleasures derived from social interaction.

Incongruity occurs when the emotional responses of individuals to their experiences seem inappropriate to outside observers. Marked blunting or flattening can give the impression of incongruity, although strictly the term should be restricted to situations in which the emotion expressed is totally out of keeping with the situation.

Rigidity and constriction of emotional responses occur when the patient is still capable of demonstrating emotional responses, but they tend to be limited and constricted in range and are relatively unresponsive to changes in context. Restricted affect is a term covering a similar range of phenomena. In rigidity, the response persists without altering to suit the changing situation.

Lability is when sudden, short-lived but often intense changes in feeling occur in response to minor events. This is often encountered in manic states but may be seen in depression and can be a feature of a variety of brain disorders, such as the post cerebrovascular syndromes.

Apathy is when an indifference to the individual's situation is expressed. At first glance, it may seem similar to the poverty of emotional responsiveness described, but it usually evokes a different empathic response in the interviewer. In poverty of affect, the interviewer senses a profound emptiness in emotional responses; in apathy, it is a sense of withdrawal and turning away from concern with the world rather than a loss of ability to respond. Apathy involves a giving up with a loss of the will and motivation to respond.

Ambivalence is when contradictory emotions and intentions coexist at the same instant. In its common usage, ambivalence refers to the relatively mundane experience of having a mixture of apparently contradictory emotions about someone or something that tend to alternate rapidly. The term has also been employed by Bleuler (1950) to refer to a far more fundamental split in the emotional life in which radically incompatible emotions and desires coexist at the same moment. Bleuler considered this more extreme form of ambivalence one of the fundamental symptoms of schizophrenia.

Alexithymia is employed to describe a virtual inability to recognise or verbalise emotional experiences and a paucity of associated fantasies (Sifneos, 1972). The concept has been widely, if not wisely, applied.

3. Behavioural responses and coping mechanisms employed to deal with emotions

The behaviour called forth by an emotion or affective state may be abnormal in its form and degree. In explosive reactions, there is a sudden discharge of strong emotion accompanied by ill-controlled and ill-considered behaviour. Such explosive reactions may occur in relatively normal individuals in situations of extreme emotional stress or may be called forth by mundane emotional demands in those of poorly disciplined and self-indulgent temperaments. At the other extreme strong emotion may induce an inappropriate inability to respond in which the individual "freezes" or is "paralysed" by the emotion. In shy and self-conscious individuals, the possibility of strongly desired social or sexual contact with another may induce not approaching or affectionate behaviour but rather a total inability to act, perhaps even resulting in avoidance and flight. In some individuals, the difficulty in accepting or coping with their emotions may lead to the exhibition of inappropriate behaviours: the man unable to express anger who becomes increasingly ingratiating and subservient as his internal rage mounts; the desiring woman appalled by her own erotic needs who responds with coldness, anger and condemnation towards the person she desires. There can be few of us who are so blessed as always to exhibit the behaviour appropriate to our emotions, and the vicissitudes that affect this area of function form a large part of the psychopathology of everyday life.

Pathology of affect

Depressive states

A search for a clear definition of symptoms rather than the description of phenomena dominates the discourse on depression. In part this reflects the clinical need to define a common and treatable disorder. The exploration of the experience of depression from which a phenomenology emerges may seem clinically irrelevant compared with a good diagnostic instrument on which sleep, mood, suicidal impulses and the like can be simply rated. After all, don't we know what it is like to be depressed?

Kraepelin (1921) suggested that "simple" depression could be understood as the various manifestations of an inhibition of mental life with slowed cognitions, physical activity and speech, together with an associated impaired concentration and sense of enervation and exhaustion. This psychic inhibition can culminate in depressive stupor in which one's mental life drags to a virtual stop. Kraepelin (1921) suggested that, in addition to this slowing, patients experience themselves as cut off from both their thoughts and bodies; "thinking and acting go on without the cooperation of the patient; he appears to himself to be an automatic machine" (Kraepelin, 1921, p. 75). Schneider (1959) emphasised a similar flattening of mental life in which the world becomes valueless, and the subject's own feelings are experienced as absent or alienated. Certainly in many individuals with depression there is an oppressive sense of being slowed up mentally and physically so that every movement is a struggle and every thought seems to emerge only after prolonged effort. In a smaller proportion, depression is characterised by harried and agitated excitation in which the patient, tortured by ideas of guilt or hypochondriacal fears, is in a constant state of complaining restlessness (Leonhard, 1979).

One obvious aspect of the experience of depression is the hopelessness about oneself and one's future. This involves not only a loss of optimism but a shift of horizon so that people with depression live in an interminable present for which the only prospect is the past. It is possible to regard the future as likely to be grim – or worse – without being depressed. In depression the hopelessness about the future is in large part a loss of any belief in a future. The past overwhelms the present, and it becomes a past which ceases to be a source of information and possibility for the future but a past which leads nowhere and can only be an obsessive and repeated lesson in failure and emptiness. To compound the problem is the sense of time slowing to a point at which some patients experience themselves as frozen in time or outside of time. Jaspers (1963) wrote of depressive patients feeling as if it is always the same moment, like a timeless void (p. 84). Curiously some people with depression have a sense of time as something external and separated from themselves that rushes past. Their day lasts an eternity, but the world passes by in a flash.

A sense of permanence pervades severe depression. Depression is experienced as a reality which has no end and from which there is no escape; the past is transformed into a progression of memories infused with regret and responsibility, and the future is exhausted and empty (Minkowski, 1970). There is a block on becoming, a halt in the process of self-realisation; everything is final and lost, but equally there is often a sense of finally facing up to an immutable reality. Depression is real, all else was error and self-deception.

Associated with the experience of depression are what Kraepelin (1921) referred to as *imperative ideas* focussed on wickedness, worthlessness, persecution, degeneration and death. These themes impose themselves on the depressive and become not just concerns but overwhelming experiences. The mental content of individuals with depression may be dominated by ideas of inferiority with self-accusations, self-denigration and fears of damaging others. The claims of guilt and sin can be tinged with grandiosity and hyperbole. Even mild to moderate depression may be associated with a sense of physical deterioration in both the fabric of the body and of the world. In its most flamboyant manifestations, this leads to hypochondriacal delusions and *ideas of annihilation* in which the whole world is either about to be destroyed or has already disintegrated, leaving the patient surrounded by wraiths and phantoms.

One of the many paradoxes encountered in depressed individuals is the alternation between a suicidal despair, which disclaims any interest in survival, and an anxious hypochondria, which ruminates fearfully on potentially lethal conditions. These imperative ideas often manifest both apparent depth and an overwhelming immediacy but, conversely, may have a peculiar ephemeracy. Thus one minute the agonised depressive patient grasps one's hand, contorted with grief and guilt over past indiscretions, claiming a universal responsibility for the world's evils; the next moment, the individual is complaining bitterly about the slights, lack of care and even active persecution by staff and fellow patients. No punishment is too great but, equally, no service or kindness is adequate to slake the depressive's sense of entitlement.

One aspect of the phenomenology of the depressed which is often missed or misinterpreted is the experience of persecution. Suspiciousness and persecutory ideas are to be found even in mild to moderate depression. This can become a dominant theme with complaints of being followed, talked about, deprived and disadvantaged, plotted against and even assailed by threatening voices. Sensitive ideas of reference and delusions of reference may be prominent, even obscuring the primary depressive disorder. The popularity of the diagnosis of schizoaffective disorder in part, if not in its entirety, reflects an ignorance of such basic phenomenological evidence.

The prevailing mood in depression is often described as sad. In practice the gentle quietness of sadness is rarely encountered. Gloom, active distress, dull despondency and irritable complaint are more frequent. It is also worth remembering that some socially adept depressed individuals present with a self-depreciatory irony which can disguise the underlying despair. Many great comedians have been plagued by depression, and sometimes it is in depression that the capacity to amuse others is at its height.

Central to depression are disturbances in biological processes, most particularly those concerning appetites and circadian rhythm. Sleep is disrupted. Attempts to link particular types of sleep disturbance, such as early-morning waking, to particular types of depression are often misleading. In depression there is usually a combination of difficulty initiating sleep, an unstable and restless sleep and difficulty maintaining sleep with early waking. Early waking is usually more prominent in older subjects. Interest in food along with other pleasures is attenuated or lost, and the libido shrinks to nothing.

Manic states

There is a tendency to conceive of mania as the mirror image of depression which, although useful up to a point, can miss many of the salient features. Jaspers (1963) characterised mania as "primary, unmotivated and superabundant hilarity and euphoria; as a delight in life, a lively optimism" (p. 596). Although individuals with mania may evince these charming characteristics, for all except the mildest of cases, a darker side alternates with, if not completely obscures, these elements of good cheer. Irritability manifests at the least frustration, intolerance lies imminent in the exaggerated and overbearing ambitions, and the driven physical overactivity can all too easily explode into violence.

The manic person is driven and buffeted by elevated and exaggerated emotions, desires and activities. There is an increased pace to existence, but the price of this busyness is a dislocation in the inner unity which usually directs the coherent unfolding of our ideas, intentions and activities. The fragmentation and disruption in the manic individual's activities increases with the more severe forms of mania.

The mood in mania is heightened, but with increased intensity comes an instability and lability. There can be sudden switches from jocularity to accusatory irritability, from exultation to despair. There may be an air of pompous superiority, but unlike the similar demeanour found in some delusional disorders the manic person's exaggerated self-confidence is usually a fragile and fugitive audacity.

States of *ecstasy* may occur in which the patient is transfigured by delight often remaining relatively or even completely immobile. Such patients are difficult to distract from their delighted state, accounts of which can usually only be obtained retrospectively. They may be infused with a sense of joy and contentment and may describe an "oceanic feeling" in which they experience themselves as in some kind of mystical unity with humanity, life or even the universe. Religious connotations are not surprisingly attached to such experiences. One of my patients, a philosopher previously bereft of religious sympathies, was discomforted in a manic episode by such an ecstatic experience. He felt he had to in some way integrate this into his materialist world view. Like many who have ecstatic experiences, its intensity and "realness" was too great to consign it to a symptom of illness. On recovery manic patients may have a clear insight into the fact that they have been mentally ill but still cling onto the relevance of some of their experiences and revelations.

There is a sense in most manic individuals of the tempo and profundity of their thought processes being enhanced. The speeding up is associated with difficulty sustaining attention and, in more severe states, the *flight of ideas* produces a dislocation and fragmentation sometimes termed *secondary incoherence.* The outward manifestation of pressured thinking is pressured speech and distractibility (see section in Disorders of Language).

A physical restless or *volitional excitement* in manic individuals can be impressive. One manic patient strode repeatedly around my room in a circuit which included clambering from chair to desk, across my desk and descending via the radiator. In severe mania, just as speech can disintegrate into disjointed words and phrases, so may activities descend to purposeless flapping. Even in mild mania, many tasks are initiated but few completed.

Perception is heightened in mania. The world becomes a source of colourful and intense experiences, but some patients describe a fragility and falseness to these perceptions. One young woman said it was like being on the set of some opulent stage show with everything multicoloured and gleaming but that nothing seemed to have any real substance or robustness, she said "it was as if I could reach out my finger and put it through walls, furniture, even people". Hallucinations, particularly visual and auditory, occur in more severe mania. Complex visions can accompany severe mania. One patient on emerging from an ecstatic state, described being able to see a great distance, and what she saw was a great copulation with people making love in some extended garden of carnal delights (less colourful visions are, however, more common).

A sense of physical well-being and enhanced strength is common in mania and may lead to a belief in invulnerability which can precipitate dangerous activities. One patient drove for several miles down the wrong side of a busy freeway happily bouncing his car against the sides of oncoming vehicles secure in the knowledge he was beyond injury or the law (in fact he turned out to be correct on both counts).

In even mild mania, there is a tendency to grandiosity and an exaggerated sense of personal worth. It is important to relate patients' claims and behaviour to what is usual for them. One of my patients who was employed as a lavatory attendant entertained the idea that he was a station porter, which for him was grandiose. Grandiose ideas and exaggerated expectations feed fleeting delusional notions and delusions of reference. Manic people may believe that they have immense wealth from an inheritance that had previously slipped their mind; that the latest pop song is adapted from a piece they strummed some years ago and the royalties will soon begin to flow; that they are the repository of the economic wisdom which will solve their, and everyone else's, unemployment. In mania delusions, like other mental content, usually emerge rapidly but are not sustained. This being said, states of so-called *delusional mania* occur in which the dominant feature is a fixed and often extensively elaborated delusional system, usually of religious or grandiose content, to which hallucinations and misinterpretations are often linked but in which excitement and elation are more muted. This state may have a remarkable tenacity and can create diagnostic difficulties. The elation and exaggerated sense of worth can produce fantastic claims and stories in which fantasy and fabrication combine to produce fluent confabulations. This can be difficult at first glance to distinguish from the fluent confabulations seen in association with some delusional systems, but the history of its emergence, the content and the evanescence of manic phenomena usually suffice to separate the phenomena.

In mania, heightened interest and engagement with the world go together with increased appetites of all kinds, but most obviously in the sexual area. Increased and disinhibited sexual behaviour is common. Again it is essential to relate the emergent behaviour to what is normal for the patient. A vicar's wife showed, for her, the grossest of sexual disinhibition by tiptoeing around their suburban garden in the nude, albeit in the dead of night. A lack of prudence characterises the financial as well as the sexual activities of the manic individual. Inflated self-confidence, a sense of invulnerability, and heightened acquisitiveness can combine to produce flights of financial mismanagement which are ruinous not only to the patient but to anyone over whose money they exert control.

Disturbed sleep is virtually universal, and the change in sleep pattern is often the harbinger of a manic episode. In severe mania, the sleep pattern is totally disrupted with the patient having only brief naps or micro-sleeps.

States of mania exert a fascination and attraction not only for observers but retrospectively for some patients. Although some patients fear above all else the loss of control and the driven self-damaging behaviour of mania, others hark back nostalgically to the elation, self-confidence and activity of their previous mania. Not a few patients knowingly induce a manic episode in the mistaken belief that this time they will control it rather than letting it control them. Manic states can and do lay waste our patients' lives, destroying their interpersonal, professional and economic existence.

The term *bipolar illness* incorporates into the very essence of the syndrome a polar opposition between depression and mania. This does not accord with phenomenological investigations in which states of mania and depression can merge and mix and in which, in more severe manifestations, the echoes of the alternative syndrome are often to be found. In her novel *Mrs Dalloway*, Virginia Woolf (1925/1996) projects her own experience of severe affective illness into her character Septimus Smith. This provides a vivid portrayal of the manner in which the manic and depressive elements entwine in the lived experience of melancholic madness.

Anxiety states

Anxiety plays a fundamental role in mental disorders, and we all experience it from time to time. Nevertheless, it is an experience peculiarly difficult to describe. It is relatively easy to speak of what makes us anxious, be it fear of failure, illness, crowds, snakes or otherwise. The physical concomitants of anxiety such as palpitations, muscle tensions, tremulousness, and hyperacusis are equally readily described. Attempts to capture the psychological state of being anxious often tend to produce only a list of similes such as worrying, dread, panic, terror and tension.

Anxiety occurs in response to the expectation of some approaching evil, and in essence it is the experience of some feared future possibility brought forward to plague one in the present. Anxiety is a currently experienced distress at an apprehended future threat. In straightforward fear, the arousal relates to an obvious and imminent possibility, such as the danger presented by the snake on the path or the rapidly approaching vehicle. In anxiety, a more distant and ambiguous future calamity is brought forward to vex and distress. Severe forms of anxiety usually concern a more nebulous but nevertheless overwhelming threat which seems to impinge on one's very survival. The state of being anxious creates a sense of confusion and uncertainty which disrupts the individual's capacity either to escape the dread or to form, let alone realise, any effective intentions. Anxiety often focuses on a particular threat of personal or social annihilation, such as a heart attack or exposure to overwhelming social embarrassment, but is not exhausted or coextensive with its chosen object. The fear is of the dread consequences on the heart attack or the total social ostracism consequent on the exposure of the supposed or actual transgression. Pathological anxiety brings with it an inexhaustible vision of awfulness in the face of which we stand confused, incapable of action, crying out for help in a manner which will inevitably be inadequate.

Obsessive and compulsive phenomena

The essential feature of these phenomena were described by Lewis (1967) as "the fruitless struggle against a disturbance that seems isolated from the rest of mental activity". This places the emphasis on a conscious resistance to these "home-made but disowned" impulses. A distinction is often drawn between *obsessions* as recurrent cognitions in the form of intrusive thoughts, impulses, ideas, or images and *compulsions* as repetitive seemingly purposeful stereotyped behaviours (American Psychiatric Association, 1987; Rachman & Hodgson, 1980). In practice compulsions are behavioural responses to obsessions, although not all obsessions lead to compulsions.

Central to the experience of an obsession is usually a fear or phobia. Typical fears are of death, contamination, acting violently and being blasphemous (Straus, 1948). The cognition, usually but not always a fear, is experienced in a particular manner in that the sufferer recognises to some extent that it is irrational, or at least senselessly insistent. An act of will is usually made to suppress or turn attention away from this preoccupying cognition. Occasionally the intrusive cognition will not appear to carry frightening connotations, as with an intrusive melody or an impulse to carry out some form of exercise of mental agility. Usually, however, on further elaboration these will turn out to be either performances aimed at warding off what is feared (compulsions) or displacement activities to blot out some feared cognition. One patient, referred because of increasing inability to function at work, reported an overwhelming preoccupation with mental arithmetic, which he felt impelled to carry out despite attempts to resist and return his attention to matters at hand. Only later did he acknowledge that he harboured the belief that only through the successful completion of increasingly complex arithmetical calculations could he prevent his wife's infidelity. The patent absurdity, if not of the fear of infidelity then at least of the remedy, made him believe that if he revealed this notion, he would be locked up as mad.

Not only does the fear reverberate in the sufferer's consciousness, the world itself often becomes a source of constant reminders and provocations of that fear. Cut flowers conjure up images of death and decay, the sight of a wristwatch provokes a fear that it may have a luminous dial indicating the presence of the feared radiation, the knife is a potential weapon, the spanner is a potential weapon, the glass if broken could become a potential weapon, and so on. For the obsessional individual, the sign or symbol of the feared is magically transformed into the presence of what is feared.

The compulsive element of the experience is usually secondary in that it develops to defend against the obsessing fear. Thus hand washing is a response to the preoccupying fear of contamination (which itself may be generated by a fear of bringing death or decay on oneself or others). As Lewis (1967) pointed out, the compulsions can themselves become obsessional; that is, the patient has to struggle against them and may indeed develop defensive behaviours to ward them off. Thus one patient overwhelmed by compulsive hand washing to fend off the feared contamination developed a complex set of hand movements and gyrations to defend against the impulse to keep washing.

The compulsions can become ritualised to create a magical counter-charm to the intruding obsession. It is not enough for those obsessed by contamination to wash, they have to wash in a very particular and usually increasingly complex manner. Failure to complete the precise and stereotyped ritual, or more particularly the fear of an incorrect performance, leads to a compulsion to repeat the compulsion. The perfectionism so often found in the character of the obsessional individual combines with magical thinking to produce a tangled web of obsessions, compulsions and rituals which enmesh the sufferer. In severe obsessional illness, patients can become so isolated within the multilayered obsessions and compulsions that they are overwhelmed and their consciousness of the basic irrationality of their thoughts and actions, as well as their resistance to these phenomenon, may become so attenuated as to be at times invisible. Not surprisingly some regard severe examples of these disorders as being close to, if not actually, psychotic (Insel and Akiskal, 1986).

The term *obsessional* is on occasion stretched in the current mental health literature to include obsessive concerns or behaviours which are not accompanied by any subjective resistance nor even by a consciousness of the absurdity or excessive nature of the thoughts and urges. Obsessive behaviours involving intense preoccupations associated with, for example, stalking or some forms of collecting may well be destructive to the individual and those around them (books and recorded music being excluded because their accumulation, however absorbing of time and money are so obviously central to the good life). To refer to intense preoccupations and obsessive pursuits as obsessional is to miss their central characteristic, which is a personal commitment to a goal which, far from being resisted or rejected, is most of the time enthusiastically embraced and may even form a core aspect of the individual's identity. The occasional retrospective guilt, forced renunciation or claims of inability to resist does not equate with the sense of the imposed absurdity at the centre of the obsessional experience.

Delusion

Socrates declared we do not call those mad who err in matters that lie outside the knowledge of ordinary people; madness is the name they give to errors in matters of common knowledge. . . . we don't think a slight error implies madness but just as they call strong desire love, so they name a grand delusion madness. (Xenophon, 1923)

The nature of delusional experience

Delusion involves abnormal beliefs that arise in the context of disturbed judgements and an altered experience of reality. Delusions become a source of new and false meanings. In everyday language, the term *delusion* is used simply to designate a belief considered patently false. In psychopathology, the implications of referring to someone as deluded goes far beyond merely indicating that they harbour false convictions or have made false judgements on a particular topic. Delusion has long been regarded as one of the central characteristics of madness and involves more than false and arbitrary ideas developed without adequate proof. They are the mad thoughts that mad people think.

To complicate further the description and definition of delusion, the term encompasses a variety of phenomena which may or may not be on a spectrum and may or may not constitute a number of distinct entities. Is this delusion? The question can determine not just the treatment of a patient but whether the patient is accorded the legitimacy of illness or even, in the forensic arena, anything from amelioration of punishment to removal of guilt. The question might be better phrased thus: "Is this individual experiencing any of the many and various abnormal phenomena which we traditionally label delusion?"'

Delusions usually have attributed to them the following characteristics:

- They are held with absolute conviction and are experienced as self-evident reality, not as merely opinion or belief.
- They are not amenable to reason nor modifiable by experience.
- They are experienced as being of great personal significance and usually preoccupy the person to the point of disrupting social and interpersonal functioning.
- Their content is often regarded by others as fantastic or at least inherently unlikely.
- They consist of convictions which are highly personal and idiosyncratic that are unlikely to be shared even by those of similar social and cultural backgrounds.

These characteristics are not, however, sufficient to separate delusions from nonpathological beliefs and convictions. The addition of three further characteristics assists in making such distinctions:

- They often emerge in a manner which suggests their pathological origins.
- They often extend to contaminate a wide range of patients' beliefs about themselves and their world.
- They can evoke persistent idiosyncratic behaviours which are potentially damaging to oneself and others.

These eight aspects of the delusional experience must be critically examined. The absolute conviction in the truth of one's beliefs is not confined to the deluded subject. Further, the deluded patient may on occasion paradoxically combine an apparent total certainty with, at another level, an awareness of the delusional nature of their beliefs. Patients themselves illustrate this double-entry bookkeeping when, for example, of their own volition they go to psychiatrists to tell of their divine mission rather than going to the relevant ecclesiastical body.

The imperviousness of a delusion to modification by reason or experience in no way distinguishes it from common error and opinion. Logical error is not the exclusive hallmark of delusion, nor is the failure to expose beliefs to the test of critical appraisal confined to the mad. The errors of most normal individuals are those common to their social group and take their origin from shared misconceptions. The errors of the deluded patient tend to be idiosyncratic in the extreme. Their origin is often to be sought in some as yet little understood disruption and change of mental function, which fundamentally alters the patient's knowledge of the world. The failure of deluded patients to change their opinion when faced by contrary argument should perhaps occasion no surprise. Our own mistaken, or more important, eccentric beliefs, recede before the changing structure of our environment and their gradual erosion by confrontation with the contrary opinions of our peers. The views of most of us shift more as a result of experiences wrought by the slow passage of time than they do before mere reason. Conversely, deluded individuals may on occasion shift their beliefs in response to experience and both the content, and the intensity of preoccupation in some delusional states can be modified by cognitive-behavioural therapy.

A person's delusional system is usually a private and isolating series of beliefs about the world. It forms a central and overriding series of convictions that influences, if not dominates, individuals' beliefs about themselves and their world. It is perhaps surprising that delusional systems that are nearly always pre-eminent in governing individuals' understanding of their experience are remarkably variable in the extent to which they direct actions. A study by Wessely and colleagues (1993) suggested that half of their deluded subjects had to some extent acted in a manner congruent with their morbid beliefs. Typical of the delusionally influenced behaviours were avoiding watching television, not going out socially and avoiding foods thought to be poisoned. The grandiose delusions in the sufferer with general paralysis of the insane or the extensive system of beliefs to be found in many chronic schizophrenic patients may, however, have little influence on the patient's behaviour. The delusions in affective psychoses more often call forth behaviour consistent with their beliefs. Manic individuals, for example, may well act on

their convictions, spending money they do not have, entering into impossibly ambitious projects and offering their unsolicited advice to all.

The content of delusions is often fantastic, but inherently unlikely notions are not unknown even among psychiatrists. It is not the truth or falsity of the belief that defines a delusion in psychiatry, for delusions may partake of the truth. The potentially correct delusion is most commonly encountered in morbid jealousy. One patient had the infidelity of his wife conclusively revealed to him on Christmas Eve when, returning from work, he noted that the lights on the festive tree in his front window were flashing on and off in synchrony with those of his neighbour's tree. The actual nature of the wife's relationship to this particular neighbour is not critical to the phenomenological analysis of this belief as a delusion, although it may, of course, be relevant to speculations about meaning. The way in which a belief emerges and the reasons for its acceptance are therefore part of the way we recognise delusions.

Delusions are not dependent on any defect in the patient's intelligence nor of disruption in the faculties for reason and logical thought. An intelligent and articulate individual who becomes deluded will put these abilities to the service of the delusion, and a luxuriant growth of bizarre ideas may result, which are argued and defended with all the subject's usual mental agility. An excellent example is provided by Schreber's (1955) memoirs.

Delusions can relate to the belief systems of normal individuals. False beliefs do not always indicate psychopathology. Idiosyncratic and unshared beliefs are not of necessity false, let alone morbid. Take an original concept in science. At the moment of its inception it could be confined to one individual and not shared by those of a similar social and cultural background. A concept in science would, however, be directed at a circumscribed area, would be understandable within the accepted and shared discourse of science and, although it might be of great personal significance to its instigator, that significance would be primarily in terms of what it explained about the world in general, not about the internal and intimate world of that individual. Such a belief might be termed delusional by the scientists' colleagues out of incredulity or even envy, but it is hoped that the belief would be unlikely to acquire the epithet delusional within a psychopathological framework. Religious belief, particularly sudden religious revelation, shares some of the characteristics of delusion, but again it would normally be distinguished by being recognisably part of an accepted area of religious experience and discourse. Totally private religious revelation, independent of any accepted theological context, could present considerable problems separating from a morbid phenomenon.

In distinguishing between delusion and novel scientific ideas or religious beliefs, the dimension termed *extension* by Kendler and colleagues (1983) is of value. Extension describes the extent to which a delusional belief spreads to involve various area of the individual's life. A scientific idea however fundamental is unlikely to explain why the scientist's neighbours seem unfriendly, why a colleague wears a red tie, or why their food tastes bitter. A run-of-the-mill persecutory delusion, on the other hand, can usually generate explanations for these and many other mundane events. Even religious revelations, however fervently believed, usually limit their explanatory power to spiritual, ethical and moral issues.

There is an understandable reluctance to add behaviour to the constellation of experiences which characterise delusion. This is seen as running the risk of acting as agents of social control by stripping the legitimacy from those whose behaviour and opinion are disapproved of by society. Ignoring behaviour can also lead to problems, however. For example, querulous individuals who pursue multiple complaints and claims through the courts and with agencies of accountability in the process lay waste to their lives and create administrative chaos. They may at any given moment be able to defend plausibly their quest for their particular vision of justice and be able to cloak themselves in the appearance of social reformers and whistle-blowers. The pattern of conduct which has led to their pursuing what is usually a real but inherently trivial

grievance at such terrible costs should establish for the clinician some presumption of a delusional process (Mullen & Lester, 2006). Too often we attempt to decide on whether a particular experience is delusionally based without taking into consideration the history of the patient's conduct whilst they have potentially been influenced by the delusional phenomena. It is not wise to respond to the common facile assumptions that strange and deeply offensive behaviour necessarily implies madness with the equally facile assumption that delusional experience exists in and of itself prior to and independent of the delusional person's conduct. Behaviour driven by a set of eccentric ideas which is persistently damaging to any reasonable calculation of the individual's own interests is not proof of delusion but is supportive of such an assumption in the context of other phenomena.

Classification of delusion

A number of attempts have been made to classify delusions (see reviews by Arthur, 1964; Bentall *et al.*, 2001; Garety, 1985; Maher, 2001; Oltmanns & Maher, 1987; Winters & Neale, 1993). Perhaps the simplest division that has been suggested is dependent on the degree of conviction with which the beliefs are expressed (Wing *et al.*, 1974). Partial delusions are those in which the individual is prepared to entertain the possibility of being mistaken, whereas delusions proper are held with a conviction which excludes the possibility of doubt. The problem with this division is that the way in which opinions and beliefs are expressed is largely a function of the interplay between educational and cultural background and the personality of the individual. Some of us express trivial and peripheral assumptions with force and conviction, whereas others timidly advance their most heartfelt beliefs. Should delusion supervene, this habitual method of presenting belief may mislead the observer as to the true level of adherence to the conviction. There is also considerable fluctuation in individual patients over time in how firmly they adhere to their delusional convictions.

Delusions have been divided into those judgements that arise in an understandable way from particular interactions or experiences and those that appear de novo like sudden intuitions or brain waves. Those delusions for which no connection can be comprehended between the emergence of the belief and any precursor and which confront the observer as something absolute and irreducible have been termed *primary* or *autochthonous delusions*. Jaspers (1963) observed that in these primary delusions there occurs an experience radically alien to the healthy person that comes before thought, although it becomes clear to itself only in thought. The primary delusion emerges in the context of a radical change in normal mental function and is indicative of a process at work. The primary delusion is thus assumed to be an eruption of an extraconscious process into the normal flow of intentional mental life (extraconscious in the sense of neuropathological, not emanating from any Freudian system unconscious). The primary delusion cannot be fully explained by an appeal to the meaningful connections that usually govern the stream of consciousness. On the contrary, it is an ultimately irreducible phenomenon not amenable to psychological understanding and explicable only in terms of the causal connections governing the presumed organic changes in the brain. Clearly this is an untestable hypothesis. It does not, of course, imply that the content of a primary delusion has no connection with the patient's past life or present situation; it merely claims that the emergence of the belief and part at least of its initial content will not be amendable to such an analysis. After the primary delusion is established, the further elaboration of any delusional system will in principle be open to an analysis in terms of its meaningful connections.

An example of a primary delusion is a patient who, on asking a friend for a light for his cigarette, was passed a box of matches on which appeared the slogan "the greatest match in the world". This revealed to the patient in a moment of intensely experienced insight that he was the light of the world. This delusional brain wave made sense for the patient of many of his recent experiences and much of his prior life; he realised his failures had been trials, his rejections, persecutions and sexual inadequacy part of divine inspiration. A totally new perspective on the world overthrowing most of his previous concepts came with this revelation.

Secondary delusions or *delusion-like ideas* emerge understandably from other psychic events or the individual's interaction with the world (Jaspers, 1963). Their origin can be traced to affects, drives, fears or some devastating personal experience. They are therefore amenable, at least theoretically, to analysis in terms of the meaningful connections of psychic life. A morbid alteration in a subject's mood may, for example, if it is towards elation, precede the emergence of delusions of grandeur, or, conversely, a depressive swing may be followed by delusions of poverty or guilt. The hallucinated individual's perverted senses may be the starting point of a delusional development, as may some real experience of injustice in a paranoid personality. A suspicious, prickly individual with a propensity to self-reference was exposed to a series of personal disasters, including loss of job, money, and his home following mortgage foreclosure. The events (partly self-induced) were explained by him initially as due to a generally ill-disposed world towards a man of his obvious but unrecognised talents. As he continued to ruminate on the events, a pattern became more and more obvious to him. Slowly over a period of many months, a delusional system involving a complex plot by members of his family in league with the local constabulary and public health officials emerged. This delusional system became the focal point of his life, dominating from then onwards his thoughts and actions. The slow emergence of this secondary delusional system was in the context of immense personal stress, probably associated with an unrecognised depressive mood swing occurring in a person with a suspicious and oversensitive personality structure.

There is obviously a problem in a classification that relies on as subjective a criterion as "understandability". Theoretically the division is attractive; in practice, it is often difficult and inconsistent in application (Koehler, 1979). The distinction also relies on the content of the phenomena rather than the form, which goes against the aim of classifying by form rather than content. To try to circumvent this problem to some extent, Schneider (1959) divided delusions into two major forms, *delusional perception* and *delusional notions*. Delusional perception he considered of particular significance in the diagnosis of schizophrenia. It was a two-stage phenomenon involving first a true perception of a real object and second the emergence of a delusional insight generated by the perception, this delusion having no easily comprehensible connection to the perception. This new knowledge does not derive from reflection on the perception but is imminent within it; the perceiving and the knowing are directly and immediately linked, the one contained in the other.

These classifications of delusion pay little direct attention to the extent of the restructuring of the patient's knowledge of himself and his world. The type of knowledge involved is also employed only indirectly within these classifications. Delusion involves both the elements of beliefs or knowledge about something and the interpretation or, more precisely, the misinterpretation of occurrences or objects in the surroundings. It might be helpful to construct a hierarchical model according to the degree to which patients' views differ from normal convictions in terms of how firmly they are held, how idiosyncratic they are and the extent to which they influence their views of themselves and their world. Delusion usually involves both belief and interpretation; the balance between these two elements varies, and two hierarchies are possible: those predominantly involving morbid belief and those that are morbid interpretations.

Morbid interpretations

Self-consciousness is characterised by heightened self-awareness. The individual often believes that his or her own personal preoccupations with regard to appearance, actions, and even thought will be mirrored in the attention they receive from others.

A minor facial blemish, for example, will be the centre not only of the individual's attention, but of all those whom they encounter. Their thoughts, particularly those involving sex and anger, will be embarrassingly obvious from their facial expression. Their actions will make them appear ridiculous in the eyes of all. Self-consciousness is the lot of most of us at some time or another. It is usually more marked in adolescence and when entering unfamiliar social situations. At the extreme, it can produce extensive disruption of an individual's ability to function socially.

Sensitive self-reference is a propensity to interpret habitually the words and actions of others and incidental happenings of the world as being directly concerned with oneself. It is clearly related to self-consciousness, and the two often occur together, although essentially the self-conscious individual is turned in on themself, whereas the self-referring person is painfully aware of their surroundings. In self-reference, there is not only heightened self-awareness but also a tendency to divine personal meanings in trivial and unrelated events. The world becomes centred on the individual, and the mundane words and actions of others are seen as being directed at oneself. Self-reference normally has a persecutory flavour, and thus the remarks and actions of others are invested with unpleasant and even sinister import. A couple laughing on the other side of a crowded room are laughing at the self-referring person, the overheard snatch of conversation in a bus is about them, the shrug of the shoulders of the barman is a dismissive insult rather than a mere gesture, and so on. In self-reference individuals are normally convinced at the time that the events they misinterpret were directed at them and them alone, but in retrospect they will at least entertain the possibility of error. In self-reference, the meaning attached to the action or event is not impossible nor even necessarily improbable; people could be laughing at them, passing remarks being intentionally obstructive, and so on. It is the frequency of the self-reference and its extension into every area of social and personal interaction that leads to its recognition as morbid.

Delusional mood is characterised by an altered experience of the world in which, in some intangible way, events take on an uncanny quality and tension. The events as well as the actions and words of others seem to hint at hidden meanings and are infused with a direct and personal significance. The precise nature of the meaning eludes them, and although there is often a sense that a pattern of meaning is about to emerge, it remains just out of grasp. The individual in such a state often appears perplexed or frankly fearful. This state differs from self-reference in that it involves an attribution of meaning to a far wider area of the patient's experience of the world; everything is imbued with personal meaning. On the other hand, the precise meaning of the occurrences is far less clear than in self-reference. Thus although it is a somewhat less clearly defined abnormal state of mind than self-reference, it is a more extensive and pervasive disturbance and is less easy to relate to normal experience. Delusions of reference may crystallise out of a delusional mood.

Delusions of reference have a similar structure to self-reference in that some event or aspect of the environment is taken to indicate a personal and direct meaning for the patient. The interpretation placed on the event in delusions of reference is more idiosyncratic and cannot so easily be seen as a possible, even if unlikely, interpretation. Thus a headline in a newspaper ostensibly about events in the Middle East was interpreted as a direct reference to a patient's homosexuality. The code numbers at the top of a banal communication from the tax inspector was interpreted as further evidence of a conspiracy. The colour of the tie worn by the doctor enables the patient to identify him as part of a sect dedicated to persecuting the patient. The television compere is understood as repeatedly making veiled references to the patient's sexual activity disguised as sports commentary. In delusions of reference, the meaning derived from the event is incomprehensible to others in the patient's social group. The delusion of reference remains an interpretation, thus a meaning is attributed to an event, but it is not open to doubt – it is experienced as self-evidently true. The information contained in a delusion of reference, however

bizarre, is essentially limited and restricted; it may form part of the patient's more extensive delusion system, but only a part.

Beliefs about the world

Overvalued ideas have enormous personal significance out of proportion to their overt content. They differ from the strongly held beliefs of the commonality in the degree of emotional investment and the focal part they play in the mental life of the individual. Clearly some types of convictions, particularly the religious and political, are often invested with great significance, but overvalued ideas normally concern more mundane and specifically personal matters. Despite their importance to the individual, they remain beliefs about the world, not the articulation of self-evident reality. The content, although often eccentric, is not entirely removed from what peers regard as conceivable. The overvalued idea often develops out of a conflict between a vulnerable personality and some elements in the environment (McKenna, 1984). The individual, although strongly protesting the accuracy of his or her beliefs, will entertain the possibility of error, albeit only the dimmest and most distant possibility.

The use of the term *overvalued ideas* has become problematic. Too often it is employed to dismiss the pathological significance of experiences in a manner both premature and misguided. Wide areas of traditional psychopathy around, for example, pathological jealousy, delusional claimants, and dysmorphobias have been forced by some into the overvalued ideas box. In the process the significance of these morbid phenomena has been diluted or lost. Given the choice, I would dismiss the term overvalued ideas from psychiatry; failing that, I suggest one approach its use with scepticism and start from the assumption that phenomena so described are likely to be either delusional or nonmorbid preoccupations.

Simple delusions are true delusions, in that they are absolute convictions experienced as self-evident reality that are immutable in the face of contrary argument or experiences. They are highly personal, and their content is often fantastic. They normally, however, concern a relatively limited aspect of the individual's beliefs about themselves or the world. Depressive delusions of bizarre bodily afflictions, such as one's blood drying up, heart being absent, or bowels rotting away, are typical examples. The erotomanic delusions and circumscribed persecutory delusions that attribute malevolent intent to specific individuals or groups and do not spread to affect the majority of the patient's relationships to others, are further examples. The impression given by patients with this type of morbid belief is that their beliefs about other aspects of the world are largely consonant with those of their peers, except in the particular and often narrow area occupied by the delusions. This type of delusion may fluctuate in intensity and in the extent to which it preoccupies the patient. These fluctuations are often connected to factors that appear to be related to the genesis of the delusions. Thus as the mood fluctuates, the delusions associated with an affective psychosis may wax and wane. In the persecutory delusions of some paranoid patients, interpersonal conflict may exacerbate the problem, and the removal of a source of stress may at least temporarily allow the beliefs to recede into the background.

Unsystematised delusions are those in which a number of poorly organised and unintegrated delusional notions coexist. The patient's account is often difficult to follow both because of the partial nature of the accounts provided and the frequent shifts in focus. In some cases, despite the poorly articulated nature of the beliefs, they appear to have for the patient profound significance; in others, there is a superficial and almost trivial quality to the fluctuating kaleidoscope of odd ideas and fragmented beliefs.

Systematised delusions involve a profound delusional restructuring of the patient's view of themselves and their surroundings. The delusional system contaminates wide areas of the patient's beliefs about the world. There may appear a central core to the belief system – for example, personal divinity, a plot, or some damage or injury sustained – but the delusional beliefs spread to contaminate wide

areas of the patient's understanding of his or her position and relationships. The systematised delusions may grow gradually by accretion over months or years, or they may emerge rapidly, transforming almost at a stroke the patient's mental life. Systematised delusions, perhaps because of their extended and extensive nature, change (if change they do) slowly over time rather than in obvious response to alterations in the patient or their environment. The systematised delusions offer no possibility of refutation; all new experience and information becomes incorporated within this morbid knowledge.

Systematised delusions may emerge on the basis of delusions of reference either gradually or, on occasion, as an almost immediate and extensive restructuring of the patient's view of themselves and the world. Systematised delusions are usually sustained and extended by misinterpretations, misperceptions, delusions of references and restructured, if not frankly delusional, memories.

A final point is that at the centre of many delusional systems lies an altered world view from which the details of the system spread. From the persecutory viewpoint, patients are acutely aware of the outside world and its impact on them; all occurrences are potentially threatening and destructive but, above all, meaningful and personalised. From the depressive viewpoint, patients' own internal preoccupations with guilt, loss and disintegration come to colour the world in which they live and constantly confirm and reflect their internal reality.

Delusions and reality

The relationship of patients' private delusional world to the shared reality varies (Scharfetter, 1980). In some cases, the delusion comes to dominate patients' mental life, and they withdraw completely into their private worlds. In other cases, although the delusional reality is predominant, patients continue to live to some extent within the shared social context. In some the delusional reality exists side by side with the shared reality without either seeming to affect, or contaminate, the other (Bleuler's double registration). Finally, delusional reality may be inextricably intermingled with the shared reality.

Delusions of specific content

Delusions may be classified according to content. This is usually self-explanatory (e.g. delusions of grandeur, delusions of guilt, delusions of persecution, delusions of poverty, etc.), but a few specific types require brief mention.

Nihilistic delusions involve a delusional belief that something is dead or nonexistent. This may involve a belief that some organ or part of the body has gone or rotted away or that the individual is themself dead. The term *nihilistic delusions* is often employed loosely to cover all delusional ideas about bodily dysfunction and decay in depression. When nihilistic delusions form a prominent feature within the clinical picture, the term Cotard's syndrome is occasionally employed.

Erotomanic delusions usually involve the delusional belief that someone, often a person of power and influence in the patient's life, is secretly, but passionately, in love with them. This phenomenon is sometimes known by the eponymous title of de Clerambault's syndrome which is unfortunate because this type of delusion had been well described for over a century when Clerambault (1942) wrote about passionate psychosis. The currently accepted definitions of erotomania fail to incorporate the morbid infatuations in which, although sufferers do not claim they are loved, they do have an unshakeable conviction that their love will eventually be reciprocated despite clear evidence of the continuing indifference or open hostility of their supposed love (Mullen & Pathé, 1994).

Delusions of possession are those in which patients are convinced they are possessed by some spirit or force. These tend to be found among those whose cultural background provides some basis for beliefs in possession, which can make it difficult to separate them from an overly dramatic presentation of a culturally appropriate belief. Occasionally in forensic practice, claims of being possessed are advanced to exculpate some offence. Among the possessors I have encountered are devils, holy spirits, dead relatives, warrior ancestors and the spirit of a dead rabbit (!). Beliefs in being possessed are distinct from the experience of being influenced by outside forces and the belief in being someone else. Thus one of my patients believed he was Elvis Presley and that an impostor was entombed at Graceland, whereas another believed she was on occasion possessed by the spirit of the departed rock star. In the state of possession, a tension exists between oneself and the interloping possessor, and even when the possession is welcome, as with holy spirits, it remains to some extent a separate and intruding presence.

Misidentification syndromes involve a conviction, often delusional, that the people a patient encounters are not who and what they appear or claim to be (Coleman, 1933). This can involve denying the identity of familiar individuals or claiming that strangers or chance acquaintances are in fact relatives or significant figures from the patient's past life. The misidentification may involve a belief that familiar and often closely related individuals are not really who they appear but merely have the same outward appearance, the inner psychological identity being different. This can lead to claims that the patient is being duped by doubles disguised as relatives or, as in one patient of mine, that his family's bodies had been taken over by a race of aliens. Sometimes it is a physical rather than a psychological identity which is at issue; subtle differences discernable to the individuals' appearance reveal them as impostors, or chance or subtle similarities of appearance vouchsafe identity. This phenomenon is not as uncommon in severe psychotic disturbance, as the literature sometimes suggests. It is graced by the eponym Capgras syndrome (Capgras & Reboul-Lachand, 1923; Christodoulou, 1977). Misidentifications can be bizarre when, for example, a patient seems utterly convinced that a young nurse is his dead mother or ignores the "minor issue" of gender when concluding that the man in the next bed is really his wife. More frequently, the delusional misidentification is based on some minor similarity of appearance or mannerism between the individual and who they are claimed to be by the patient. On occasion this type of misidentification is referred to as the *illusion of Fregoli,* but the term is misleading on several counts.

Delusions may come to be shared within a family, and these shared delusions may be referred to as *folie a deux, folie a trois,* and so on; as *psychosis of association;* or as *double or multiple insanity.* Several variants have been described, as follows:

- Simultaneous emergence of delusion in closely associated individuals in which the content is shared, probably as a result of shared environment, but the origin is independent
- Imposed delusions in which a dominant figure within a relationship or group imposes their delusional view on the others to such an extent that the delusional system seems eventually to be totally shared
- Communicated delusions in which two individuals living in close association, both of whom have a propensity to psychotic disturbance, come to influence and share each others delusional world

Delusional memory is a phenomenon in which a delusional insight occurs not as an intuition about the world or as a change in knowledge of or about the world but in the form of a memory. An example is provided by a patient who suddenly "remembered" that a few weeks previously she had been attacked and raped by her brother and brother-in-law in the midst of a family gathering. The conviction that this had occurred emerged de novo; the woman could point to nothing that suggested such an event. On the contrary, she was constantly surprised that everything and everybody around her were so normal and apparently unaware of the terrible happening, even those she believed to have been involved. The belief continued without seeming to alter this woman's experience of her world or even her relationship to the central figures in the memory.

Confabutory paranoia is a curious state in which fluent confabulation occurs around an often fluctuating set of delusional beliefs. When challenged or cross-questioned, individuals will launch into ever more curious accounts, often incorporating the queries and comments of the examiner. Such people are prone to be dismissed as malingerers because of the ease with which they respond to suggestion and shift their stories in response to expressions of scepticism. Sitting listening to such patients for a few hours usually dispels such scepticism.

Dysmorphophobia is an intense and unshakeable conviction on the patient's part that an aspect of their appearance or body is misshapen and conspicuously ugly. This phenomenon is associated with an intense preoccupation with the supposed deformity on which the patient ruminates at length. The actual experience and perception of the individual's own body seems altered in that the patient claims slight deviations from normal shape or size to be gross and obviously different from normal. There is often associated despondency, and this phenomenon can be secondary to depressive disorders. The narcissistic elements are usually obvious. This phenomenon can, in clinical practice, therefore partake in part at least in delusion, perceptual disturbance, obsessive ruminations, phobia and mood disturbance. The placement of body dysmorphic disorder into the categories of both delusional disorder and somatoform disorder in DSM-IV probably represent the heterogeneity of the phenomena in clinical practice and the extent to which they can be seen as forming a spectrum with varying levels of insight (Phillips, 2004).

Passivity phenomena (disturbances of ego boundary)

Passivity experiences are a group of phenomena disparate in many ways but having in common a disturbance in the experienced integrity of the self. They are sometimes referred to as disturbances of ego boundary because of this experience of the breaking down, or violation, in the unity of the self. The boundaries are breached between the patient's internal private world of thought and fantasy and the external world of objects and other people (including the internal thoughts, wishes and intentions of others). These phenomena are occasionally classified as delusions (Sims, 1988; Spitzer & Endicott, 1978) presumably on the grounds that they constitute not an experience of, for example, influence or thought broadcasting but a belief in being influenced or broadcasted. The distinction may on occasion be so subtle as to appear entirely academic but for most patients, these are direct experiences, not beliefs, although they may give rise to delusional explanations. One patient complained that a "filthy word" was repeatedly inserted into her mind. This occurred several times a day and would occasion her considerable embarrassment. She had noted that these insertions tended to occur when she was near or in sight of a tower at a Salvation Army citadel. On the basis of this observation, she had become increasingly convinced that she was being persecuted by the Salvation Army, which had a radio transmitter beaming the words into her brain. She experienced the thought insertion, but she became convinced that its origins lay in the transmitter in the tower. One is an experience, the other an explanatory belief. I have a pain in my belly. I am convinced it is an appendicitis. The experience of pain and explanatory beliefs are distinct phenomena.

These experiences are of two basic types in that they can be directed inwards or outwards. In the first there is an experience of influences or intrusion from the outside into the internal world. In the second, there is an experience of the thoughts, wishes or intentions of the individual diffusing or emanating out to influence, or become available to, others. These effects can involve the content of thoughts and fantasies, the intentions and actions and the emotions and desires of the patient.

The types of passivity experiences are now discussed under the headings of thoughts, emotions, intentions and actions.

Thoughts

Directed outwards

Thought diffusion and thought broadcasting involve a conviction on a patient's part that those around them know their innermost thoughts. It is not merely that they divine their secret thoughts from their words, actions or facial expressions but that the thoughts themselves are directly available and can be, in a real sense, read by others. There is a sense of having become transparent, making ones innermost thoughts open to direct observation. In florid form, there can be the experience of one's own thoughts being shared and participated in by everyone around them. This experience may lead to delusions of explanation. One of my patients described a complicated plot in which a neighbour, who was a BBC journalist, would nightly broadcast her every secret thought to the nation; this explained why everybody knew about them and shared them.

Thought withdrawal

This occurs when patients experience their thoughts as removed or ablated by some outside influence. This experience has been claimed to underlie the abnormality of expressive behaviour known as *thought blocking* (Fish, 1967).

Directed inwards

Thought control involves patients' experience of their innermost thoughts as falling under external influence. *Thought insertion* occurs when alien thoughts are imposed on them.

Intentions, will and actions

Directed outwards

Patients experience themselves as able to influence the apparently volitional acts of others. One patient explained to me that he could make people move and speak as he wished and pointed out from the window of the office how he was willing the people outside to walk along the street. In another case a patient described how every move or action he initiated was simultaneously mirrored in those around him because his will controlled theirs, but this disrupted his life because when, for example, he went shopping, the shops were always full of other people who, because of his influence, were on identical errands.

Directed inwards

The experience is of made impulses and made volitional acts. This can again involve the experience of the patient's intentions and will falling under outside control or of the imposition by an outside force of action upon them. An elderly and normally prim and proper lady periodically lifted her skirts and performed a brief dance. This she explained had nothing to do with her but was the result of the actions of a malevolent race of aliens she called "fantasias" who were imposing the actions upon her. Here both the control of the acts and the acts themselves were alien. More commonly, what is experienced is simply a loss of control over will and action as a result of outside influence.

Emotions

"Made" feelings and emotions occur when patients experience their emotional life as coming under outside influence, either in that they are made to feel a certain way or that alien emotions are imposed on them. Patients more frequently report being robbed of feelings or of having their emotional responses blocked by alien influence.

Depersonalisation and derealisation

Depersonalisation and derealisation refer to experiences which, although most frequently encountered in those afflicted by depressive or anxiety disorders, can occur in normal individuals when they are overtired, stressed or intoxicated. The basic disturbance involves an alteration from the usual of the experience of both the self and the world. It can manifest in such features as:

- Surroundings take on a quality of strangeness.
- A sense of unreality pervades not only the perceptions of the external world but one's own cognitions and conations.
- The experience of the passage of time is altered by a slowing or slippage.
- Spatial relationships seem altered, which can produce distortions and may even be associated with micropsia or macropsia.

- One's body image may be altered, producing not only experienced unfamiliarity in one's physical being but a nonrecognition of body parts.
- Emotions, feelings and affects lose their subjective impact, although the individual is not without emotion; on the contrary, there is usually fear and agitation consequent on the changed experiences.
- Actions appear to be carried out automatically without personal involvement or intent as if, as one patient put it, "I was trapped inside a machine which I could only watch but not control". Whatever the subjective sense of being out of control, the actions remain those of the individual, reflecting their intentions and commitments even if subsequently disowned.

Depersonalisation is to be distinguished from passivity experiences in which there is an experience not of alienation from subjective experience but of alien influence on such experiences. Depersonalisation appears in DSM-IV not as an abnormal phenomenon but as one of the currently fashionable constructions of dissociative disorders. These disorders are assumed to arise from a disruption in the functions of consciousness to create amnesia, dissociative identity disorder and depersonalisation disorder. This construction is given coherence by an unstated but implicit appeal to the reality of a system unconscious. No such archaic frippery is required for the description or recognition of the phenomena of depersonalisation provided here.

In normal mental function, there is only a tangential and passing awareness of the process of thinking or perceiving. We can by an effort of will reflect on our experience and activities, but it is neither usual nor sustainable. In depersonalisation, there is an unbidden and unwanted self-awareness in that we become conscious of our mental activities. Perceptions are disrupted by sensations being separated from the meanings usually inherent in them, and our cognitions and conations become objects of scrutiny, not lived experiences. This pervasive self-reflection totally disrupts the normal flow of psychic life and imbues it with an alien character. We no longer reach out for the pen, we become conscious of the act of reaching out for the pen; we no longer see our reflection, we become conscious of seeing a reflection which we assume must be ours. In depersonalisation, we remain conscious of our activities, and they remain accessible to normal awareness. This contrasts with the dissociations of DSM-IV in which there is assumed to be a separation or removal of selective mental events from consciousness or an emergence of previously unconscious factors into consciousness, often in a form quarantined from the rest of the individual's mental life. Depersonalisation and derealisation are a morbid exaggeration of self-awareness and self-reflection, which disrupts the sense of being part of, and at one with, one's own cognitions, conations and actions.

Volition

Pathological disturbances of action and movement largely fall within the rubric of neurology; however, certain syndromes that include characteristic disturbances of motor behaviour require brief mention (see Lohr & Wisniewski, 1987, for a thorough review).

Tics

These are repetitive stereotyped movements involving voluntary musculature. Although usually capable of brief inhibition by an act of will and to some extent responsive to mood and situation, they are for the most part outside of the patient's control. Tics cover a spectrum from minor repetitive twitches involving the small muscles of the face to complex movements, which may involve several large muscle blocks. In *Gilles de la Tourette syndrome,* motor tics are combined with repeated vocalizations, often in the form of obscenities and profanity (coprolalia).

Catatonia

First described by Kahlbaum in 1874 (1874/1973), catatonia is a syndrome which can be seen in both predominantly affective and schizophrenic disorders and may be mimicked by a number of organic disorders. It consists of disturbances in volitional movement and language. Several aspects of the syndrome seem to be polar opposites. There may be periods of uncoordinated and violent overactivity (*catatonic excitement*); at the other extreme, the patient may remain immobile for long periods, often appearing as if frozen to the spot. *Posturing* occurs when bizarre and uncomfortable poses may be held for long periods, as do reiterated *stereotyped movements,* where the same action is endlessly repeated. The normal fluidity of voluntary motor activity may be disrupted to produce an awkward and stilted quality, which is most obvious in the odd gaits encountered in this disturbance. *Automatic obedience* can be a feature with unhesitating compliance to any command or request without apparent conscious control, but so can the reverse, *negativism,* in which there is a positive effort to resist and often do the opposite or some eccentrically unrelated performance rather than what is requested or required. *Ambivalence,* in the Bleulerian sense, may effect motor action – the patient commences an act and then before completing it, reverses his or her movements and begins once more, only again to halt and reverse.

Echolalia and *echopraxia* occur where the patient repeats or imitates the words or actions of those around them. In echolalia the repetition seems to occur in an automatic fashion without any apparent understanding. Echophenomena are not confined to catatonic syndromes but occur in a range of pathological conditions (Ford, 1989). Just as the fluidity of voluntary movement is disrupted, so the usual flow of speech is disrupted to produce hesitancy with a stuttering or explosive quality. *Verbigeration,* described by Kahlbaum (1874/1973) as speech composed of oft-repeated, meaningless words and sentences, may also be present in catatonia. A characteristic disturbance of muscle tone, in which there appears to be present a *waxy flexibility* (flexibilitas cerea), can accompany posturing and immobility in the catatonic syndrome. Pouting movements of the lips are also described to accompany catatonic states *(Schnauzkrampf),* as are facial grimacing and tics. Subtle catatonic disturbances are often either not recognised or dismissed as side effects of antipsychotics.

Cataplexy

This is a sudden, partial or complete loss of tone in the voluntary musculature without disturbance of consciousness. It occurs in narcolepsy.

Stupor

This describes a syndrome in which the most prominent features are gross reductions in voluntary movement (*akinesia*) and speech (*mutism*). There is a suspension of expressive and reactive movements. Incontinence may occur. In neurology, stupor is often used rather loosely to describe a state of reduced consciousness bordering on coma. In contradistinction, attempts have been made in psychiatry to define stupor as an absence of voluntary movement in the presence of clear consciousness. This is helpful in as far as it distinguishes "functional" from "neurological" stupor, but the attribution of clear consciousness to functional stupor is clinically questionable (Berrios, 1981).

Kraepelin (1919) attempted to distinguish four types of stupor: depressive, manic, catatonic, and hysterical. In *depressive illness*, stupor usually follows a period of increasing motor retardation and withdrawal; the patient may still radiate a sense of melancholy by facial expression and by a passive turning away from proffered assistance. The refusal to eat and drink in depressive stupor may represent a total lack of interest, although one of my patients retrospectively described being convinced his insides had disappeared, so he felt anything that passed his lips would enter his abdominal cavity and kill him. In *mania*, stupor may supervene on the excited disturbances of delirious mania in which extreme restlessness, hallucinosis and some clouding of consciousness give way to a state of mute immobility. In this state, some signs of the previous gross overactivity may remain in brief outbursts of motor restlessness and in constant movements of the head and eyes. In *schizophrenia*, stupor may supervene on a catatonic picture. Retrospectively, schizophrenic patients can often provide quite detailed accounts of the happenings during the period of stupor and on occasion will give explanations of their immobility – for example, they were directed by God or under some external control. States of stupor can follow extreme stress and then can be conceptualised as dissociative states or as an extreme reaction, as if paralysed by fear. These latter may be encountered under battle conditions and following catastrophes.

Disturbance of language

Thought can never be directly observed. The attempt to study it must therefore rely on language in the form of speech, writing or other symbolic creation (Sims, 1995). The entrenched tradition of speaking of thought disorder, when actually confronted with disturbed language, rests on the assumption that language directly mirrors thought.

Speech disorder is usually separated from language and thought disorder. It is confined to disturbance in the actual articulation due to a disruption with the mechanics of speaking. Stuttering is a typical example, and the lalling speech of cerebellar dysfunction would be another. A distinction between language as a system of symbol and sign formation and thought as the content and import of those symbols and signs is occasionally made. Thus, employing this division, thought disorder would include delusions and other disturbances of the content of thought. This section is concerned with the disturbance of language.

The structure of language can be analysed in terms of semantics, which concerns itself with meaning, and of syntax, which are the rules governing the combination of words to form sentences. In most of the language disorders observed clinically by psychiatrists, the disorder is in the area of meaning, the semantics, rather than the syntax, the latter only being significantly disrupted in the most florid forms of psychotic speech. Meaning lies not only in the words used but also in the situational context of the utterances. Statements occur in particular spatiotemporal situations, which include speaker and hearer, the actions they are performing and various external objects and events. Further, a shared knowledge of what has been said earlier and its relationship to current statements is assumed. Thus what Searle (1969) termed *speech acts* consist of language in its context which communicates to the receiver. This understanding of utterances in their context is referred to as pragmatics, and it is argued that it is a derangement in this pragmatic function of language which characterises schizophrenic speech (Cutting, 1985).

In an ideal language, one word or sign would exist for one meaning. In practice, there are many synonyms for which a particular meaning is designated by several distinct words (e.g. hide, conceal, secrete) and frequent homonyms for which single words signify more than one meaning (e.g. *bank* of river, Bank of England; elephant's trunk, trunk – a piece of luggage). Words may also be used literally or metaphorically (a man's head, the head of a company; a glaring light, a glaring error). In the language disorders psychiatrists encounter, there may be semantic disruption arising from a confusion of homonym, synonym and metaphor. A patient, for example, when asked if the pills were making him better, replied, "Healed? I have no heels (glancing at the bottom of his slippers), I'm only brought to heel". The word healed is employed as a synonym for getting better, then confused with its homonym, the heel of a shoe, and in this example the metaphorical use of heel is employed to produce a nice resolution that allows the patient to comment on his resentment at being compulsorily detained. Bleuler reports a patient who when asked if anything was weighing heavily on his mind replied, "Yes, iron is heavy". A patient in a group asked if he was down, immediately left saying, "Yes, I need to lie down". This taking of the literal rather than the metaphorical use of words was referred to by Goldstein (1944) as *concrete thinking*, although whether it is truly a preference for the concrete sense or just a tendency to associate to the commonest usage of a particular word is uncertain.

A word may be chosen in language disorder not because of its relationship to the meaning of the utterance but because of an association of sound to a previous word or phrase. Thus, "I feel like going out, stout, a drink would be nice, ice, I suppose I'll stay, lay down for a while" or "everybody seems to revolve around me, involve and resolve around me" is termed a *clang association*.

Words may be invented in language disorders. These idiosyncratic words of no generally agreed significance are termed *neologisms*. They may consist of entirely new words, which even the patient may be hard pressed to explain, or be created by compressing or running together existing words. A patient referred to a "mongery ridicule", and although he could spell the word, the only definition he offered was that it "wasn't quite nice". In this example the phonetic or sound structure is acceptable for a word in English. On occasion sounds entirely foreign to English phonetics will be emitted apparently as words. An example of a word created by condensing existing terms is "a misachrist", which was used by a patient to describe a psychiatrist who misunderstood him (a mistaken psychiatrist). Jaspers (1963) suggested neologisms may arise from the patient's struggle to express unique and essentially incommunicable experiences.

Idiosyncratic similes and metaphors may be encountered. A schizophrenic patient of Bleuler (1950) announced her forthcoming pregnancy with "I hear a stork clapping in my body". A patient of mine replied to the enquiry about his religious views with "I'm for the elected by a puff of smoke from the chimney", referring obliquely to the process that heralds the election of a new pope in the Roman Catholic Church.

Words, phrases and occasionally syllables seem to recur far more frequently in the language of the schizophrenic patient than in healthy people. This is in part connected to the phenomena of *stereotopy* and *perseveration*. In the perseveration of course organic brain disease, identical words and phrases tend to be simply repeated. In those with schizophrenia, it manifests as a repeated use of similar words and phrases in different contexts. An extreme example is provided by a patient who, when asked if he understood a question, replied, "I see something like I might be wrong like, but there like the rules and I don't like the rules turned upside-down and I don't know like and I was like as though the bed turned over". A patient reported by Kraepelin (1919) would, when writing home to relatives, fill pages with similar words or phrases interminably presented in varying order. A more restricted vocabulary is also said to be found in the language-disordered schizophrenia patient than in healthy people of a similar educational and intellectual background (poverty of language). The frequent repetition involves syllables and phrases as well as words, so that the problem is more likely to stem from a tendency for the same speech elements to intrude repeatedly into the discourse rather than just a restricted repertoire of words.

The concept of *redundancy* has been borrowed from information theory and applied specifically to schizophrenic language disorder (Maher, 1972). Redundancy used in this technical sense refers to the likelihood that a particular word or letter will occur. The more predictable the word or letter is, the greater the redundancy in that it conveys less information. Normal language has a high degree of redundancy in that many of the words and phrases are predictable to a high level of certainty from the context. In the schizophrenic patient, the disruption of the context of the language and the reduced consistency and coherence within the expression of ideas leads to a decreased predictability of the words and thus to decreased redundancy. A *word salad*, for example, in which there is a total breakdown in the contextual restraint, and words follow each other apparently at random, has no redundancy, for no given word can be predicted in advance from any preceding word or phrase; each word comes as a total surprise, free of the limitations of semantics or syntax. Experiments based on the redundancy concept have demonstrated that observers provided with transcripts of normal speech and schizophrenic speech with every fifth word deleted can correctly fill in the missing word significantly more often from the normal speech, confirming the decreased redundancy in the schizophrenic utterances. In related experiments, it was suggested that speech-

disordered schizophrenia patients are themselves less able to use contextual clues and redundancy in learning written passages. The specificity of these findings has been challenged, however (Rutter, 1979).

The meaning of language depends not only on the particular words but, as has been mentioned, the context of the utterance. In normal speech, there is a tacit acceptance by speaker and hearer of all relevant conventions, beliefs and presuppositions of the common speech community. In language disorder, there may emerge in conversation or writing themes that are inappropriate to the context. Thus highly personal and idiosyncratic statements will be interposed with the more appropriate aspects of the discourse. This tends to produce in the listener a degree of confusion. The mixing in of snatches of conversation about unrelated matters into the ongoing discourse has been labelled *intermingling* (Harrow and Prosen, 1979). This appears to reflect an impairment of the subject's ability to remain within the normal social constraints on communication.

The disruption of context and the lack of sufficient connection between successive phrases is shown by a patient who wrote, "I want to leave the trees are beautiful if only the food too long low". In a single sentence, the desire for discharge, the gardens, the food, and a greeting are all combined. There is a failure to keep separate, unconnected ideas, and the patient's preoccupations are all jumbled together into a single statement. A patient replying to an enquiry as to how he felt, included the following: "it doesn't really mater if you eat refined sugar as long as you can balance it by doing something else you or using your energy expending your energy in the best manner possible and I would really like to become a DJ you know I have a high sort of ambition this is why I would like a cigarette now. That's all". There preoccupation with diet, physical fitness, job ambitions, and the desire for a cigarette become included in a response to a routine enquiry about health. This tendency was described as *overinclusion* by Cameron (1944), because the patient is unable to prevent subsidiary and peripheral thoughts from intruding and becoming included in the statement. A young librarian in the early stages of a psychotic episode was asked to reorganise the Divinity section of the library's filing system. This resulted in a total restructuring of the index with everything recatalogued under Divinity. The young man had included all topics under Divinity, not from some insight into the ubiquitous nature of God but from an inability to separate any category from any other, thus including all in one. Here overinclusion was demonstrated in action, not speech.

Thought blocking is evinced by a sudden stopping in mid-sentence, despite the subject's desire to continue speaking; after a pause, the flow of speech may recommence, perhaps on some unrelated topic. There may be a perplexed silence and a complaint that one's thoughts have been removed, stolen, or blocked or have disappeared. This phenomenon can be dramatic in some schizophrenic patients and may be accompanied by considerable subjective distress. Blocking in the context of other signs of schizophrenic speech disorder is of diagnostic importance. When it occurs as an isolated event, it is easily confused with the non-specific phenomenon of losing the train of one's thoughts, which occurs in healthy people, particularly when tired or under stress and as part of the speech retardation of depressive states. The presence of schizophrenic language disorder should not be assumed on the basis of thought blocking alone.

The clinical psychiatrist most frequently observes disturbance of language in the flight of ideas of manic and schizophrenic language disorder, often referred to as formal thought disorder. This being so, the following section continues by discussing these two specific language disturbances.

Flight of ideas

Flight of ideas is encountered in manic disturbances but is also mimicked by some organic brain syndromes and by one's more loquacious or intoxicated companions, and it can even appear in relatively pure form in some subjects, who on other criteria would undoubtedly be considered schizophrenic.

There is an accelerated tempo of speech often referred to as *pressure of talk*. In addition to the increased rate of delivery, the language employed is characterised by a wealth of associations, many of which seem to be evoked by more or less accidental connections. The relationship between statements is disrupted by this chaos of association, and the progress of speech ceases to be guided by the unfolding of a train of thought and comes under the influence of this plethora of new connections. The excited speech wanders off the point following the arbitrary connections, and the coherent progress of ideas tends to become obscured. The somewhat haphazard verbal associations become governed by sound, rhyme, associations to peripheral concepts, double entendre and so on. In classical flight of ideas, although the connections and associations are accidental or peripheral to the general sense of the statement, they are usually in themselves fairly obvious and unremarkable and would individually be acceptable in other situations. This is in stark contrast to schizophrenic language disorder in which the individual connections are often so opaque and personalised as to defy comprehension in any situation. Clang associations and puns are frequent. One manic patient I encountered attempted to speak exclusively in blank verse interspersed with long recitals from nineteenth-century poets.

In flight of ideas, a wide range of unusual connections drive on rapid speech, and the listener is often borne along by the flow and may even share in the amusement and pleasure the patient derives from the novel associations. Patients exhibiting flight of ideas often express a subjective sense of their thoughts racing and of new ideas forcing themselves on their attention.

Schizophrenic language disorder

Schizophrenic language disorder, or, as it is sometimes termed, *formal thought disorder*, is characterised by disturbance in the area of semantics, although in advanced forms the syntax may also be disrupted. Bleuler (1950) considered the disturbance of association to be a fundamental symptom of schizophrenia that led to a disruption of the threads which guide thinking. Ideas fortuitously encountered are combined in a manner dependent on incidental circumstances rather than any train of thought. When asked where she lived, one patient replied, "I come from Somerset. Somerset is a lovely place, everyone stops up that way, you know, before they go back home for the weekend. I'm home on my weekends, but I was never really satisfied with myself nor my schoolwork".

In those with schizophrenia whose language is disordered, there are found clang associations and condensations and stereotypy, evidenced by a tendency to return again and again to a single theme. The language disorder of schizophrenia can vary from a barely detectable disturbance to an almost total disorganisation of communication. Kurt Schneider (1959) considered that disjointed, fragmented, and inconsequential thought was commonly manifested in the speech of individuals with schizophrenia. However, he pointed out that milder degrees of such disturbance was not uncommon in healthy people, and this being so, however important these thought disorders might be for the theoretical definition of schizophrenia, they could not in practice hold much weight as diagnostic features. In ambiguous cases, he held that it was too difficult to pin down such phenomena as unmistakable schizophrenic symptoms, and in florid examples, other more reliable diagnostic signs would be present.

Carl Schneider, in contrast, gave considerable attention to these phenomena in his *Psychologie der Schizophrenen* (1930). He considered schizophrenic language to be characterised by (1) an interweaving or bringing together of heterogeneous elements (*fusion*), (2) a mixing and muddling up of actual definite but heterogeneous elements (*substitution*), (3) a snapping off of the chain of thought (*omission*) and (4) the disruption of the thought content with insertion of other thought contents in place of the true chain of thought (*derailment*). He described *transitory thinking* as characterised by derailments and omission in the train of thought by

which both the semantics and syntax may be disrupted and *drivelling thinking* in which there is a mixing and muddling of the thoughts (substitution) that obscures the meaning. In drivelling, the listener may obtain an initial impression that something meaningful is being said but soon realises that it is a flow of words and high-sounding phrases signifying little or nothing. A patient who talked at great length with slow, ponderous and heavily accentuated speech included the following in a monologue:

In other words you said that you were coming, and I said to myself and I dismissed it from my thoughts. I suppose it wasn't exactly forgetting that she would be appearing but no to stress this all the time that he just wanted to come home and I was foolish over money and what have you, and you see now I could talk to him about that.

The language of schizophrenic patients may be weighed down with unnecessary detail and circumstantiality in much the same way, perhaps, as writers on the subject. Complex and intricate forms of expression may serve to obscure the train of thought and platitudes and proverbs may come to totally dominate their speech.

Andreasen (1979, 1986) suggested that all the many and various terms used to describe the communication difficulties of those with schizophrenia could be reduced to 20, she claims, mutually exclusive terms. These are poverty of speech production (laconic speech), poverty in the content of speech, pressure of speech, distractible speech, tangentiality, derailment (loosening of associations), incoherence (as in *word salad*), illogicality, clanging, neologisms, word approximations (where words are used unconventionally), circumstantiality, loss of goal (where the communication drifts apparently aimlessly), perseveration, echolalia, blocking, stilted speech (ponderous and overly formal), self-referential speech (in which communications return repeatedly to the patient and their highly personal preoccupations), phonemic paraphrasis (mispronunciations because sounds or syllables have slipped out of sequence), and semantic paraphrasis (substitution of inappropriate words – malapropisms). The most frequent abnormalities she noted in her patients were derailment, loss of goal and tangentiality, although they were also found in the communications of manic subjects. Poverty of speech was the abnormality found specifically in schizophrenic rather than manic utterances. There might, one would have thought, be problems in distinguishing a number of these categories – for example, word approximations from semantic paraphrasis.

Individual patients may be aware of the disruption of their thinking even though it is not obvious to the observer. Some patients become concerned with words and the potential meanings hidden within these signs and symbols. The language disorder of one patient expressed itself in an extensive series of written productions about words, an extract of which follows:

RAYMOND = RAY-MOUND = hill of the ray = tower of the telepathic waves. Also it = RAY-MONDE, ray and world (French, Le Monde). The Germanic name which gives the modern Raymond was Regimund. Regin = strong, powerful; mund = protection. Thus my telepathy is a powerful protection. Mund = protection was often used with a word "beorg" = him to mean fortress. Regin is nearly the same word as the Anglo-Saxon Regn = rain. Thus one has Regn = rain and mund = fortress = fortress from which comes the rain, i.e. rain = telepathic waves.

This section has been concerned with language productions, but it is worth remembering that a number of reports have pointed out that in schizophrenia, abnormalities occur in the perception of speech and of short-term verbal memory. Such receptive defects could contribute to language abnormalities.

A final point that requires emphasis is that a variety of brain lesions produce dysphasic speech, which may have superficial resemblances to formal thought disorder. For excellent accounts of the organic dysphasias, see Lishman (1987) and Brain (1965).

Conclusions

Descriptive psychopathology attempts to orient the clinician towards the precise observation and description of their patient's state of mind. The descriptions can, in addition, form the basis for classification and for empirical studies. Careful observation and classification is the starting point for good clinical psychiatry, and above all it provides the best protection for the patient from being wrongfully labelled as mentally ill and treated as such or, conversely, from being denied care when in fact they need it.

REFERENCES

American Psychiatric Association (1987). *Diagnostic and Statistical Manual.* 3rd ed. (DSM-III-R). Washington, DC: American Psychiatric Association.

Andreasen, N. C. (1979). Thought, language and communication disorders. *Archives Gen Psych* **36**:1315–30.

Andreasen, N. C. (1986). Scale for the assessment of thought, language and communication. *Schizophr Bull* **12**:473–82.

Arthur, A. (1964). Theories and explanations of delusions: a review. *Am J Psychiatry* **121**:105–15.

Bentall, R. P., Corcoran, R., Howard R., *et al.* (2001). Persecutory delusions: a review and theoretical integration. *Clin Psychol Rev* **21**:1143–92.

Berrios, G. E. (1981). Stupor: A conceptual history. *Psychol Med* **11**:677–88.

Bleuler, E. (1950). *Dementia Praecox or the Group of Schizophrenias.* Translated by I. L. Abell. New York: Grune and Stratton.

Boss, M. (1949). *Meaning and Content of Sexual Perversions.* New York: Grune and Stralton.

Brain, W. R. (1965). *Speech Disorders: Aphasia, Apraxia & Agnosia.* 2nd ed. London: Butterworth.

Cameron, N. (1944). Experimental analysis of schizophrenic thinking in language and thought in schizophrenia. In J. Kasanin, ed. *Language and Thought in Schizophrenia.* Berkeley: University of California Press.

Capgras, J., & Reboul-Lachand, J. (1923). Illusion des sosies dansan défine systématisé chronique. *Bull Soc Clin Méd Mentale* **2**:6–16.

Christodoulou, G. N. (1977). The syndrome of Capgras. *Br J Psychiatry* **130**:556–64.

Coleman, S. E. (1933). Misidentification and non recognition. *J Ment Sci* **79**:42–51.

Cutting, J. (1985). *The Psychology of Schizophrenia.* London: Churchill Livingston.

De Clerambault, G. (1942). Les psychoses passionelles. *Oeuvres Psychiatriques*, pp. 315–22.

Esquirol, J. E. D. (1833). *Observations of the Illusions of the Insane*. London: Renshaw and Rush.

Fish, F. (1967). *Clinical Psychopathology*. Bristol: Wrights.

Ford, R. A. (1989). The psychopathology of echophenomena. *Psychol Med* 19:627–35.

Frijda, N. H. (1986). *The Emotions*. Cambridge: Cambridge University Press.

Garety, P. (1985). Delusions: problems in definition and measurement. *Br J Med Psychol* 58:25–34.

Goldstein, K. (1944). Methodological approach to the study of schizophrenic thought disorder. In J. Kasanin, ed. *Language and Thought in Schizophrenia*. Berkeley: University of California Press.

Hare, E. H. (1973). A short note on pseudo-hallucinations. *Br J Psychiatr* 122:469–76

Harré, R. (1986). *The Social Construction of Emotion*. London: Blackwell.

Harrow, M., & Prosen, M. (1979). Schizophrenia thought disorders; bizarre associations and intermingling. *Am J Psychiatr* 136:293–6.

Horowitz, J. M. (1970). *Image Formation and Cognition*. 2nd ed. New York: Appleton–Century–Crofts

Insel, T. R., & Akiskal, H. S. (1986). Obsessive-compulsive disorder with psychotic features: a phenomenological analysis. *Am J Psychiatr* 143:1527–1533.

Jaspers, K. (1963). *General Psychopathology*. 7th ed. Translated by J. Hoenig and M. W. Hamilton. Manchester: Manchester University Press.

Kahlbaum, K. L. (1973). *Catatonia*. Translated by G. Mora. Baltimore: Johns Hopkins University Press. Original work published 1874.

Kendler, K. S., Glazer, W. M., & Morgenstern, H. (1983). Dimensions of delusional experience. *Am J Psychiatr* 140:466–9.

Koehler, K. (1979). First rank symptoms of schizophrenia: Questions concerning clinical boundaries. *Br J Psychiatr* 134:236–48.

Kraepelin, E. (1919). *Dementia Praecox and Paraphrenia*. Translated by R. M. Barclay. Edingburg: E & S Livingstone.

Kraepelin, E. (1921). *Manic-Depressive Insanity and Paranoia*. Translated by R. M. Barclay. Edinburgh: E & S Livingstone.

Leonhard, K. (1979). *The Classification of Eudogenous Psychoses*. 5th ed. Translated by R. Berman; edited by E. Robins. New York: Wiley.

Lewis, A. (1967). *Obsessional Illness. Inquiries in Psychiatry*. London: Routledge & Kegan Paul, pp. 157–72.

Lishman, W. A. (1987). *Organic Psychiatry*. 2nd ed. London: Blackwell.

Lohr, J. B., & Wisniewski, A. A. (1987). *Movement Disorders: A Neuropsychiatric Approach*. New York: Guilford Press.

Maher, B. A. (1972). The language of schizophrenia: a review and interpretation. *Br J Psychiatry* 120:3–17.

Maher, B. A. (2001). *Delusions*. In H. E. Adams, P. B. Sutker, eds. *Handbook of Psychopathology*. New York: Plenum, pp. 309–37.

Malebranche, N. (1980). *The Search after Truth*. Translated by T. M. Lennon. Columbus: Ohio State University Press. Original work published 1674.

McKenna, P. J. (1984). Disorders with overvalued ideas. *Br J Psychiatry* 145:579–83.

Minkowski, E. (1970). *Lived Time*. Translated by N. Metzel. Evanston: Northwestern University Press.

Mullen, P. E. (1990). A phenomenology of jealousy. *Aus N Z J Psychiatry* 24:17–28.

Mullen, P. E. (1991). Jealousy: The pathology of passion. *Br J Psychiatr* 158:593–601.

Mullen, P. E. (2006). A modest proposal for another phenomenological approach to psychopathology. *Schizophr Bull* 33:113–21.

Mullen, P. E., & Lester, G. (2006). Vexatious litigants and unusually persistent complainants and petitioners: From querulous paranoia to querulous behaviour. *Behav Sci Law* 24:333–49.

Mullen, P. E., Pathé, M., & Purcell, R. (1994). The pathological extensions of love. *Br J Psychiatr* 165:614–23.

Mullen, P. E., Pathé, M., & Purcell, R. (2000). *Stalkers and Their Victims*. Cambridge: Cambridge University Press.

Oltmanns, T. F., Maher, B. A., eds. (1987). *Delusional Beliefs*. New York: John Wiley.

Phillips, K. A. (2004). Psychosis in body dysmorphic disorder. *J Psychiatr Res* 38:63–72.

Posey, T. B., & Losch, M. E. (1983). Auditory hallucinations of hearing voices in 375 normal subjects. *Imagination Cogn Person* 2:99–113.

Rachman, S. J., & Hodgson, R. J. (1980). *Obsessions and Compulsions*. Englewood Cliffs, NJ: Prentice Hall.

Rutter, D. R. (1979). The reconstruction of schizophrenic speech. *Br J Psychiatr* 134:356–9.

Scharfetter, C. (1980). *General Psychopathology. An Introduction*. Translated by H. Marshall. Cambridge: Cambridge University Press.

Schneider, C. (1930). *Psychologie der Schizophrenen*. Leipzig: Thieme.

Schneider, K. (1959). *Clinical Psychopathology.* Translated by M. Hamilton. New York: Grune and Stratton.

Schneider, K. (1974). Primary and secondary symptoms in schizophrenia. In S. Hirsch & M. Shepherd, eds. *Themes and Variations in European Psychiatry.* Bristol: Wrights.

Schreber, D. P. (1955). *Memoirs of My Nervous Illness.* Translated and edited by I. MacAlpine and R. A. Hunter. London: R. A. Dawson.

Searle, J. R. (1969). *Speech Acts: An Essay in the Philosophy of Language.* Cambridge: Cambridge University Press.

Sims, A. (1988). *Symptoms in the Mind.* London: Bailliere Tindall.

Sims, A., ed., (1995). *Speech and Language Disorders in Psychiatry.* London: Gaskell Press.

Sifneos, P. E. (1972). *Short Term Psychotherapy and Emotional Crisis.* Cambridge, MA: Harvard University Press.

Slade, P. D., & Bentall, R. P. (1988). *Sensory Deception.* London: Croom Helm.

Solomons, R. C. (1980). Emotion and choice. In A. O. Porty, ed. *Explaining Emotions.* Berkeley: University of California Press, pp. 251–81.

Spitzer, R. L., & Endicott, J. (1978). *Schedule of Affective Disorders and Schizophrenia.* 3rd ed. New York: Biomentrics Research.

Straus, E. W. (1948). *On Obsession.* Nervous and Mental Disease Monographs, No. 73.

Wessely, S., Buchanan, A., Reed, A., *et al.* (1993). Acting on delusions. *Br J Psychiatry* **163**:69–76.

Wing, J. K., Cooper, J. E., & Sartorius, N. (1974). *The Measurement and Classification of Psychiatric Symptoms.* Cambridge: Cambridge University Press.

Winters, K. C., & Neale, J. M. (1993). Delusions and delusional thinking in psychotics: A review. *Clin Psychol Rev* **3**:227–53.

Woolf, V. (1996). *Mrs Dalloway.* Hertfordshire: Wordsworth Classic. Original work published 1925.

Wundt, W. (1903). *Grundriss der Psychologie.* Stuttgart: Engelmann.

Van den Berg, J. H. (1982). On hallucinations: Critical-historical overview. In A. J. DeKoning & F. A. Jenner, eds. *Phenomenology and Psychiatry.* London: Academic Press.

Xenophon. (1923). *Memorabilia.* With an English translation by E. G. Marchant. London: Leob Classical Library.

2

Current approaches to classification

Anne E. Farmer and Assen Jablensky

Roughly once a decade, another generation of researchers and clinicians recognises the shortcomings of current methods for classifying mental disorders. This recognition may be followed by systematic reviews, attempts to compare and contrast or validate different definitions of disorder or efforts to employ multivariate statistics to devise novel definitions. However, what is humbling to those of us who have participated in such research is that the past 40 years has been full of such attempts. Although major technological advances have led to considerable progress in other aspects of psychiatric research, the issues relating to psychiatric diagnosis then, as now, are largely the same. For the clinician or trainee to understand why mental disorders are defined the way they are, it is necessary to consider some of the history of classification over the past 50 years and a literature that predates on-line search engines.

International classification of diseases and the diagnostic and statistical manual

Two international classifications currently dominate research and clinical practise; the ICD-10 (World Health Organisation [WHO], 1992) and the DSM-IV (American Psychiatric Association [APA], 1997). Both classifications provide detailed descriptions of all the main psychiatric syndromes, personality disorders and other disorders of behaviour or function. In DSM-IV, these descriptions are in an "operational" format in which the rules for applying a diagnostic category are precisely defined, whereas the ICD-10 has two versions, one of which has operational definitions (WHO, 1993) and the other, main clinical version consists of brief clinical descriptions of the main syndromes (WHO, 1992).

Achieving international consensus about the classification of mental disorders has a history that extended back to the middle of the twentieth century. This is now described.

The development of an international classification of diseases

The first comprehensive nosology covering an entire range of diseases and including a classification of mental illness was produced by the newly formed World Health Organisation in 1948. Previous attempts to list causes of death and to classify disease and injury had been unsuccessful in obtaining international use, and this revision, the sixth, although recommended for use by all the member states of WHO, also failed to gain universal acceptance. Following a large enquiry into the state of classification undertaken on behalf of WHO by Erwin Stengel (1959), a new edition was finally published in 1965, titled the 8th edition of the

Essential Psychiatry, ed. Robin M. Murray, Kenneth S. Kendler, Peter McGuffin, Simon Wessely, David J. Castle.
Published by Cambridge University Press. © Cambridge University Press 2008.

International Classification. (The 7th edition, published in 1955, had the same mental disorders section as the 6th revision.) As well as introducing a glossary of definitions for the first time, the section for all psychiatric disturbances was made self-sufficient in Section 5. For the first time, all major contributors to the psychiatric literature, with the exception of the French, were officially committed to using the same classification. The 9th revision was published in 1975 and came into use in 1978. Only minor changes were made from the 8th edition. This classification continued to be the main system in use in the United Kingdom until April 1994. However, in view of the rapid advances made in psychiatric nosology, with the introduction of operational definitions, this classification became increasingly outdated, and many psychiatrists within the United Kingdom became more familiar with the North American DSM series of classifications, in both their clinical and research practices. The publication of ICD-10 was therefore eagerly awaited.

The *International Classification of Diseases,* 10th edition: classification of mental and behavioural disorders

As just discussed, the World Health Organisation has the responsibility to produce regular revisions of the ICD for international use. In addition to providing international communications about the statistics of morbidity and mortality, the ICD classification also acts as a reference for national and other psychiatric classifications. Additional uses include scientific research, clinical work and service development and psychiatric education. Thus ICD-10's classification on mental and behavioural disorders is required to be acceptable to a wide range of users in different cultures, practical to facilitate understanding, easy to use and translate into different languages and versatile so it may be applied to various work settings and by a variety of professionals. With this in mind, Chapter F on mental and behavioural disorders consists of a family of documents. The

first of these, the "blue book" (WHO, 1992) consists of the clinical descriptions and diagnostic guidelines for service use as well as the discussion on the concepts on which the classification is based. The second part, the "green book" is the operational criteria version titled the *Diagnostic Criteria for Research*. Unlike the US national classifications, clinical guidelines are kept separate from the more narrowly prescriptive operational criteria. The third document is a shorter, simpler version of the clinical descriptions, which is used in primary care. Finally, a multi-axial system is being produced. Unlike previous international classifications, extensive consultation was undertaken with several hundred expert psychiatrists from many countries regarding the classification between 1984 and 1990. A draft version of the clinical diagnostic guidelines was circulated widely, and field trials, in which 700 clinicians took part, were undertaken in 110 clinical centres in 37 countries.

Wherever possible in Chapter F, ICD-10 is a descriptive classification, as were its predecessors ICD-9, DSM-III and DSM-III-R. However, aetiology does form some part of the organisation of the classification in some areas, particularly regarding organic brain syndromes and substance-related disorders.

ICD-10 has an alphanumeric coding scheme based on codes with a single letter followed by two numbers (e.g. A00-Z99). Further detail is provided by decimal numeric subdivisions at the four-character level. Mental and behavioural disorders are included in Chapters F00 to F99. This allows up to 100 subdivisions within mental illness, although a proportion of numbers are left unused for the time being so that the introduction of changes to the classification can be undertaken without having to redesign the entire system. The way Chapter F is subdivided is shown in Table 2.1.

The classification uses the term *disorder* to avoid difficulties in the use of terms such as *disease* and *illness*. Disorder is defined as the existence of a clinically recognised set of symptoms or behaviours,

Table 2.1 Chapter F ICD-10 list of categories

F0	Organic including symptomatic mental disorders
F1	Mental and behavioural disorders due to psychoactive substance use
F2	Schizophrenia, schizotypal states and delusional disorders
F3	Mood (affective) disorders
F4	Neurotic, stress-related and somatoform disorders
F5	Behavioural syndromes and mental disorders associated with physiological dysfunction and hormonal change
F6	Abnormalities of adult personality and behaviour
F7	Mental retardation
F8	Developmental disorders
F9	Behavioural and emotional disorders with onset usually occurring in childhood or adolescence

Table 2.2 ICD-10 Mental and behavioural disorders due to psychoactive substance use

F10	Alcohol	Acute intoxication
F11	Opioids	
F12	Cannabinoids	Harmful use
F13	Sedatives or hypnotics	
F14	Cocaine	Dependence syndrome
F15	Other stimulants (including caffeine)	
F16	Hallucinogens	
F17	Tobacco	Psychotic disorder
F18	Volatile solvents	
F19	Multiple	Amnesic syndrome
	Other	Residual or late
	Unidentified	Psychotic disorder

ICD.10 = *International Classification of Diseases*, 10th edition.

associated in most cases with distress and with interference with personal function. Terms such as *psychogenic* and *psychosomatic* have been omitted from the classification. Other terms such as *impairment, disability* and *handicap* are used according to the WHO (1980) definitions. The main innovations in ICD-10 are now discussed.

ICD-9 employed a neurotic-psychotic conceptual dichotomy, which is largely avoided in ICD-10, although the terms *neurotic* and *psychotic* are still retained as descriptive terms, for example, "Neurotic, stress related and somatoform disorders" (F40–F48); "Acute and transient psychotic disorders" (F23). In using the label "psychotic" in the latter term, no assumption is being made regarding putative psychodynamic mechanisms; it merely indicates the presence of delusions, hallucinations and some abnormalities of behaviour. Disorders in ICD-10 are arranged in groups according to major common themes or descriptive likenesses. For example, cyclothymia (F34,0) is in the affective disorder block F30–F39 rather than in F60–F69, disorders of adult personality and behaviour; and schizotypal disorder, previously regarded as a personality disorder, is included

in F26–F29 (schizophrenic illnesses) rather than in F60–F69 (disorders of adult personality and behaviour).

All disorders associated with psychoactive substance misuse are grouped together in F10–F19, regardless of severity (Table 2.2). Indeed, substance misuse is organised primarily according to substance (F10–F19), and type of disorder is shown after the decimal point (e.g. acute intoxication .0, harmful use .1, dependent syndrome .2 etc.).

F20–F29 is titled "schizophrenia, schizotypal and delusional disorders". New categories have been added such as "undifferentiated schizophrenia", "post schizophrenic depression", and "schizotypal disorder". Schizoaffective disorder is also found in this section (F25), as is an expanded section on acute, short-duration psychoses, because these are commonly seen in developing countries.

Mood disorders are categorised in F30–F39. The nomenclature "bipolar" has replaced "manic depressive", which was used in ICD-9. Much research evidence now suggests that a bipolar-unipolar dichotomy is a more appropriate way to classify mood disorders (Farmer & McGuffin, 1989). Bipolar disorder is characterised by the presence of an episode of mania within the lifetime course of the illness, whereas unipolar disorder consists of single or recurrent episodes of depression. In ICD-10, mania is subdivided by severity into hypomania and mania with or without psychotic symptoms. Similarly, depression is divided into three severity states: mild, moderate and severe. In addition, it is possible to categorise a depressive episode as being with or without somatic symptoms. Classifying a common condition such as depression according to severity as well as according to symptom profile is clinically relevant. Persistent mood disorders such as cyclothymia and dysthymia are also included in this section, as is recurrent brief depressive disorder.

F40–F49 includes anxiety disorders such as phobic disorders, panic and generalised anxiety, obsessive-compulsive disorder as well as reaction to stress, adjustment and dissociative disorders. The increasing evidence for somatoform disorders and chronic fatigue syndrome (as neurasthenia) has ensured that these disorders also have their own categories in ICD-10.

Behaviours, syndromes and mental disorders associated with physiological dysfunction and hormonal change, such as eating disorders, nonorganic sleep disorders and sexual dysfunction, are categorised in F50–F59. The greater detail included in ICD-10 compared with its predecessor is the result of the increasing importance of such disorders in liaison psychiatry.

F60–F69 includes disorders of personality as well as of adult behaviour such as pathological gambling, fire setting and stealing. Although F70–F79 covers only those disorders that are specific to childhood and adolescence (behavioural and emotional disorders with onset usually occurring in childhood and adolescence), dysfunction that can occur in persons of almost any age should be applied to children and adolescents when required; examples of such dysfunction include disorders of eating (F50), sleeping (F51) and gender identity (F64).

As described earlier, the rules of taxonomy require that each patient be restricted to the membership of a single diagnostic category. Although in theory this is highly desirable in practice, clinicians frequently encounter patients whom they consider inadequately described without using two or more categories. Thus the authors of ICD-10 recommended that clinicians should follow the general rule of recording as many diagnoses as necessary to cover the clinical picture. However, if more than one diagnosis is recorded, it is best to give one precedence over the others by specifying it as the main diagnosis and to label others as subsidiary or additional diagnoses. It is also recommended that precedence should be given to the diagnosis more relevant to the purpose for which the diagnoses are being collected. In clinical work, this is often the problem that gave rise to the consultation or contact with health services. On other occasions, e.g. in research, it may well be a main "lifetime" diagnosis. However, if there is any doubt, a useful rule is to record the diagnoses in the numerical order in which they appear in the classification, which has a built-in hierarchy (F0, organic disorders, through to F9, behavioural and emotional disorders occurring in childhood).

The development of the DSM criteria

The American Psychiatric Association was the first national body to take on the enormous tasks of producing operational definitions for clinical as well as research use and make their use central to psychiatric diagnosis for all clinical practice within the United States. Published in 1980, the third edition of the DSM (DSM-III) criteria were produced by a number of committees whose purpose was to focus on various aspects of the classification (APA, 1980). In addition, field trials of draft versions of DSM-III were held around the United States to test their applicability. In addition to producing clear operational definitions for all major psychiatric disorders, personality disorders were also operationally defined, and these main categories of DSM-III criteria were multi-axial: Axis I includes the main psychiatric syndromes, Axis II includes personality disorders; Axis III includes any concurrent physical health problems; Axis IV includes psychosocial stressors; and Axis V includes the highest level of functioning in the year before evaluation. Using all five axes allows a more holistic view of patients, and their main psychiatric problems may be placed within the context of other aspects of their health and functioning. In practice, Axes IV and V have seldom been used even in research, and most clinicians focus only on Axes I and II. The revised version of DSM-III, DSM-III-R, was published in 1987 (APA, 1987). The impact of DSM-III-R was less than its immediate predecessor, and the differences between the two manuals are not great. In 1994, DSM-IV was published, which closely resembled its predecessors.

The DSM-IV consists of a three-digit numeric code for groups of diagnoses (e.g. 295 = schizophrenia) with specific disorders or subtypes indicated by two additional numbers after a decimal point (e.g. 295.30 = paranoid schizophrenia). The codes relate to those used in ICD-9 and were first used in DSM-III. In general, this numbering schema has been kept in the three subsequent revisions. The classification starts with the dementias (290) similar to F0 in ICD 10. Acute alcohol-related problems such as intoxication and alcohol-induced psychotic disorder with hallucinations are 291 (.0 and .3, respectively). The code 292 consists of acute substance misuse, such as withdrawal (.0) or with delusions (.11). DSM-IV separates these acute problems with drugs and alcohol from the chronic difficulties of dependence and abuse that are assigned separate groups (304 and 305, respectively). Codes 293 and 294 identify mental disorders due to general medical problems including mood disorder (293.83) and dementia due to Parkinson's disease (294).

The main severe psychiatric disorders, schizophrenia and bipolar disorder, are 295 and 296, respectively. Although schizoaffective disorder is within the schizophrenia group (295.7) rather than affective disorder, schizotypal and schizoid disorders come in the personality disorder group (301).

The 295 schizophrenia group consists of the following subtypes: .10 disorganised, .20 catatonic, .30 paranoid, .4 schizophreniform, .6 residual, .7 schizoaffective and .9 undifferentiated. Delusional disorder, a psychotic illness usually occurring in later life, is in a different group, 297, and brief psychotic disorder, a different group again (298.8).

Affective disorders are characterised as single or recurrent episode of depression (296.2 and 296.3), whereas bipolar disorder is categorised as single manic episode (296.0) or according to the most recent episode, for example, bipolar disorder most recent episode hypomania (296.5) or most recent episode depressed (296.6). Similar to the ICD-10 F3 group, in mood disorders, the fifth digit is used to denote severity for major depressive, manic, and mixed episodes, namely, .01 = mild, .02 = moderate, .03 = severe without psychotic features, .04 = severe with psychotic features, .05 = in partial remission, .06 = in full remission, and .00 = unspecified.

Anxiety disorders are grouped as 300 with the suffix .2 indicating generalised anxiety disorder, .21 panic disorder with agoraphobia, and .4 dysthymia. Codes using 301 are disorders of personality, with 301.13 coding for cyclothymia and 301.7 antisocial personality disorder.

The remaining categories are for sexual dysfunctions, paedophilia and so on (302); disorders of eating and sleeping (307); acute stress reactions (308); adjustment disorders (309); disorders of impulse control such as pathological gambling (312); various disorders of childhood (e.g. 313, selective mutism); 314 (ADHD) and 315 (dyslexia).

From the above descriptions, it is clear that there are both similarities and differences between DSM-IV and ICD-10. DSM-IV has more categories than ICD-10, which may reflect the requirements of the health care system in the United States. The additional categories are necessary so that all the various conditions and problems that psychiatrists treat can be assigned a DSM code number, which is a requirement for reimbursement by health insurance companies. The ICD-10 classification does not have such a driving force. In DSM-IV, there is a clear separation of acute mental disturbance due to alcohol and drugs (292) from dependence and abuse which have separate categories (304 and 305). In ICD-10, all substance misuse disorders are found under a single group, F1. In addition, DSM-IV has two separate categories for disorders due to a general medical condition (293 and 294) such as depression or dementia, categories that are not included in ICD-10. However, the main broad groups of disorder are similar (e.g. schizophrenia F2 and 295, affective disorders F3 and 296), and the items included in the definitions needed to fulfil criteria to apply the diagnosis are also broadly similar, as are the combinatorial rules. It is hoped that the new revisions of DSM and ICD will combine into a single international classification. At the time of writing, this looks possible.

The diagnostic process

Teasing apart what is pathological from what is part of normal experience

A psychiatrist taking a history and examining the mental state is attempting to discover whether the experiences a patient describes can be considered pathological or merely part of everyday or "normal" experience. To do this requires not merely the presence of a particular complaint (which may be mild and self-limiting); the psychiatrist must also determine the intensity of the experience (how bad is it?), how long it has lasted (how much has there been of it?) and how much the experience has interfered with daily activities (how disabling has it been?). It is also recognised that groups of symptoms cluster together. For example, people who complain of feeling low also frequently complain of poor sleep, reduced appetite, lack of self-esteem, slowed thoughts and so on. Knowing which supplementary questions to ask and their significance allows

the psychiatrist to determine whether the patient's experience is pathological.

By careful cross-examination undertaken in a systematic way, the clinician builds up a picture of the patient's mental experience (Wing *et al.*, 1974). This process requires that an objective (clinical) judgement be made about the nature and severity of each symptom. Although patients can complete self-report questionnaires, these can only indicate their own subjective view, which is different from the clinician making an objective assessment about the nature and severity of individual symptoms.

Having determined which pathological features are present (and which are absent), it then becomes possible to match the symptom profile of the subject to others who belong to a particular diagnostic group. To do this, the psychiatrist uses a "mental template" acquired through clinical experience and derived from groups of individuals who share psychopathological features.

To complete the diagnostic process, it is also important that those having such symptoms are able to articulate and communicate their experiences and that the clinician is sufficiently empathic to understand and interpret their significance. This interaction between sufferer and observer also depends on what is considered pathological in the culture(s) to which they both belong, which in turn may be influenced by language, education, religious beliefs or politics.

Different schools of psychopathology

The use of systematic enquiry to establish the presence or absence of psychopathology is termed *phenomenological psychopathology*, which relates to objective descriptions of morbid mental experiences or *phenomena* and does not rely on any theories about what may have caused them. Phenomenological psychopathology was described by Jaspers (1963) as "representing, defining and classifying psychic phenomena as an independent activity".

The two other main approaches to assessment of psychopathology – namely, *psychodynamic* and *experimental* psychopathology, are described elsewhere in this book. Psychodynamic psychopathology is derived from psychoanalytical theory proposing that unconscious mental processes generate mental events. Whilst the phenomenological approach examines the details of the abnormal phenomena, the psychodynamic approach concentrates on the unconscious mechanisms assumed to have caused them. In contrast, the approach used in experimental psychopathology consists of testing hypotheses that compare normal and abnormal experiences. The approach uses a number of scientific methods, including animal models of human behaviour.

Syndromes, not diseases

As described earlier, mental disorders are defined according to the clustering together of subjective complaints (symptoms) and observable abnormalities in behaviour, cognition or speech (signs) that are considered pathological. Consequently what are described in the various categories of diagnosis are *syndromes* and not "true" disease entities. This is because the definition of disease requires the presence of demonstrable pathology, which is not yet possible for most psychiatric conditions. Because of this, the term *disorder* is preferred, rather than *disease*, and the DSM-IV and the ICD-10 are classifications of psychiatric disorders which are essentially syndromes.

Although these two classifications have international acceptance, they are only a "best guess", that is, they represent our current state of knowledge about mental disorder. As such, they must be continually reassessed and modified in the light of new understanding about the aetiology of mental states. Hence, at the time of this writing, plans are being made for the development of ICD-11 and DSM-V. We discuss both the strengths and limitations of the current system later. First, however, we consider why making a diagnosis is important.

Historical background

Current descriptions of mental disorders have their origins in French, German and British philosophical and conceptual thinking of the nineteenth century. Much of the terminology has changed its meaning over the intervening decades, and this is probably most apparent with descriptions of disordered personality (Berrios, 1993). Much subsequent effort by researchers and clinicians over the past 150 years has been to try to group these syndromal descriptions into a meaningful nosology. The most recent attempt to do this, in the 1970s, used operational approaches to define mental disorders.

Around the turn of the nineteenth century, Kraepelin (1896) delineated two main classes of psychotic illness. Individual syndromes described by Hecker (*hebephrenia* – 1871), Kahlbaum (catatonia – 1874) and Kraepelin (dementia paranoids – 1913/1919) were considered by the latter to be variants of the same disorder, which he termed *dementia praecox*. Kraepelin separated this disorder from *folie circulaire*, the name given by French psychiatrists to a group of illnesses characterised by depressive and manic mood phases (Baillarger, 1853; Falret, 1854) and which he renamed *manic depressive insanity*. Inherent in these early descriptions of the main categories of psychotic disorder was the considerable variation in clinical presentations that could occur. This phenotypic heterogeneity was implied by Bleuler (1911/1950) when he introduced the term *group of schizophrenias* for dementia praecox, a term which persists to the present day in the numerous subtypes of affective disorder and schizophrenia in modern classifications (WHO, 1992).

The term *moral insanity* was introduced by Prichard (1853) to describe individuals who were neither insane nor intellectually impaired but who behaved in a socially abnormal way. Those whose behaviour (e.g. antisocial or asocial) caused problems for others were considered to have disordered or deviant personalities. The term *psychopathic* was coined to describe such personality types (Koch, 1891). Where the socially abnormal behaviour caused distress to the individual the concept of *neurotic reaction* or *neurosis* slowly evolved.

Subsequent use of these terms, especially by the emerging psychoanalytical movement, changed their meaning and led to confusion about their definitions. For example, Kraepelin considered psychopathic personalities to be *formes frustes* of the psychoses or deviations from normal development due to genetic or organic aetiological factors. In contrast, Koch described varieties of psychopathic personality that occurred as a result of a disease process, and in psychoanalysis these terms refer to deviation from the normal line of development that has occurred in childhood.

Jaspers (1963) attempted to clarify the distinction between neurotic and psychopathic behaviour and psychosis in terms of the *understandability* of symptoms. He considered that psychopathic behaviour and neurotic symptoms were an extension of normal reactions and could therefore be "understood" by an empathic observer. Psychotic symptoms, however, could not be understood by an empathic observer. Despite these and subsequent attempts to clarify the concepts, confusion continued, and their precise meanings failed to be defined. More recently, these terms have been dropped from international classification (APA, 1994) although, in ICD-10 (WHO, 1992), the terms "psychotic" and "neurotic" have been reintroduced only to describe symptom profiles.

Another problem that bedevilled attempts to create a meaningful nosology for psychiatric disorder was the poor agreement between psychiatrists about diagnosis. In addition to confusion about the precise definitions of the terms used (noted earlier), classification was also considered less important during the 1930s and 1940s, probably because of the emerging influence of the psychoanalytic movement, especially in the United States. This was particularly noticeable for psychotic disorders. By the 1960s, huge differences in first-admission rates for schizophrenia and manic depressive illness were noted, both within the United States and between the United States and the United Kingdom. A series of studies, the US-UK diagnostic series (Shepherd, 1957; Bellak, 1958; Kramer, 1961), was undertaken to establish why this was the case. Research teams in the United States and United Kingdom were trained to use a structured interview on all new admissions to establish psychopathology. The data obtained from the interviews was scored by computer, and a "study" diagnosis was then compared with the admitting doctor's diagnosis at both sites. Whereas the standardised diagnoses in the two countries showed good agreement for the rates of various psychotic disorders, the hospital diagnoses reflected the national differences shown earlier. These studies therefore indicated that the national differences in rates of schizophrenia and manic depressive illness were due to the diagnostic practices and did not reflect true differences in incidence and prevalence of the disorders in the two sites. The studies also showed that training doctors to use standardised interview could greatly improve the reliability between them (interrater reliability; Cooper *et al.*, 1972). A computerised diagnostic programme could also assist the diagnostic process, by eliminating any personal diagnostic bias.

Subsequently, the degree to which diagnostic practice varied on a more global scale was investigated in the WHO-sponsored International Pilot Study of Schizophrenia (WHO, 1973). In addition to examining the incidence and prevalence of schizophrenia in nine countries, this study also compared local diagnostic practices. As in the US-UK diagnostic series, a structured interview, the Present State Examination, was employed by the project team to elicit current psychopathology, and cases were assigned to a single category according to the ICD-8 (WHO, 1974), using a computerised diagnostic system called CATEGO (Wing *et al.*, 1974). A total of 1,202 patients were interviewed in nine countries: the United States, the United Kingdom, the USSR, Denmark, Taiwan, Nigeria, Czechoslovakia, Columbia and India. Each patient received a clinical diagnosis from a local psychiatrist. Subsequently, the project team gathered information from 360 additional items using the Present State Examination which were then processed by the CATEGO program. The results of the study showed that for seven of the nine countries, clinical diagnoses were consistent and largely in agreement with the project diagnosis. However, in two sites, Washington, D.C. (United States) and Moscow (USSR), the local psychiatrist diagnosed schizophrenia more frequently than the project team, but for different reasons. Thus both the International Pilot Study of Schizophrenia and the US-UK diagnostic series examined the problems relating to clinical diagnoses that had been highlighted earlier. They confirmed that interrater reliability could be dramatically improved if a structured interviewing technique was used and if standardised procedure such as a computerised scoring program was adopted.

Following these studies the great impetus in psychiatric classification was to improve the reliability, as reflected in agreement between raters. The next major advance therefore was with the introduction of operational definitions of psychiatric disorder. It was originally suggested by Carl Hempel (1961) that one way to overcome the difficulties of psychiatric classification would be to adopt "operational def initions" for the various categories of illness. The term operational definition was first introduced by a physicist, Bridgman, in 1927, who defined it as fol lows: "An operational definition of a scientific term S is a stipulation to the effect that S is to apply to all and only those cases for which performance of test operation T yields the specific outcome O". To translate this for application in psychiatry, operationally defining disease S goes as follows: instead of stating that the typical features of a disease are features A, B, C, D, E and so on, an unambiguous statement is presented in the operational definition defining precisely how much of A, B, C, D and E must be present (or about) to fulfil the definition. For example, a disorder X may be diagnosed if the patient has one of the symptoms listed under A, two of the symptoms under B, one of the symptoms under C, and so on. Thus, proceeding operationally facilitates

precise, reliable, unambiguous features of disorder to be defined.

The first operational definitions to be published were the St Louis criteria (Feighner *et al.*, 1972). Interestingly the authors cited neither Bridgman nor Hempel, but the formats used were recognisably suggested by Hempel. There followed a proliferation of other authors producing operational definitions for psychiatric illness – some for a broad range of disorders and some confined to schizophrenia (Carpenter *et al.*, 1973) or its subtypes (Tsuang & Winokur, 1974). The Research Diagnostic Criteria published in 1975 (Spitzer *et al.*, 1975) together with the St Louis criteria influenced the development of the *Diagnostic and Statistical Manual*, third edition (DSM-III) of the American Psychiatric Association, which we described earlier and which was published in 1980.

As can be noted from the authors just cited, the production of operational definitions of psychiatric disorder is largely a North American phenomenon. Having demonstrated excellent reliability and proved their worth in various research studies, operational definitions of psychiatric disorders became increasingly important and virtually mandatory for researchers wishing to publish their results in reputable journals. Consequently, almost all research studies now use either the DSM IV or ICD-10 criteria to define the subjects being investigated. In addition, the operational format makes it relatively easy to produce structured or semistructured diagnostic interviews which facilitate the diagnostic process for research.

Advantages and disadvantages of operational definitions

Because of their unambiguous and precise format, operational definitions can be easily applied by clinicians. Agreement and communication between clinicians was facilitated, and this has led to an improvement in interrater agreement for diagnosis. In addition, it has been relatively straightforward to incorporate each criterion into the format for a structured interview and to devise computerised scoring programs. Indeed, structured interviews can be written in such a way that they can be administered and scored with good reliability and validity by lay interviewers who have no psychiatric training (Robins *et al.,* 1988). This can provide a highly cost-effective means to acquire information about the incidence and prevalence of psychiatric illness in general population samples in which the employment of clinicians would usually be considered far too costly. As mentioned earlier, the explicit nature of operational criteria can enhance agreement not only nationally but internationally (ICD-10). Finally, most authors of operational definitions have tried to take an aetiologically atheoretical perspective. Thus, operational definitions should be equally acceptable to behavioural, biological or psychodynamic schools of thought.

Balanced against these advantages are a number of disadvantages. First, there are many operational definitions, especially for schizophrenia and affective disorders, none of which have proven validity. As Brockington *et al.* (1978) have pointed out, the "previous state of inarticulate confusion in the diagnosis of schizophrenia has been replaced by a babble of precise but differing formulations of the same concept". In the research setting, it is possible to adopt a polydiagnostic approach and collect enough clinical information so that all operational definitions for the disorder in question can be fulfilled (Kendell, 1975). To facilitate the application of such a polydiagnostic approach for psychotic disorders, the OPCRIT computerised scoring system (McGuffin *et al.,* 1991) was devised.

Although operational definitions have been shown to be highly reliable (see Table 2.3), there is a restriction in terms of information that is used in the operational diagnostic process compared with the usual clinical situation. Previous psychiatric history, informant information, previous response to medication, as well as difficult-to-define commodities depending on "clinical impression" are

Table 2.3 Percentage agreement and kappas for five main operational criteria included in OPCRIT

	Agreement (%)	Mean kappa
DSM-III	96	0.85
DSM-III-R	90	0.74
Feighner	81	0.61
RDC	87	0.71
French	90	0.74

Three raters, 54 case vignettes. $p < 0.00001$ all definitions. DSM-III = *Diagnostic and Statistical Manual,* third edition; DSM-III-R = DMS-III, revised; RDC = Research Diagnostic Criteria.

Box 2.1 Advantages and disadvantages of operational definitions

Advantages	Disadvantages
Easily applied	Top-down and rigid
Highly reliable	Need "rag-bag" categories for individuals who do not fit precise definitions
Can construct interviews around definitions	Two-dimensional
International acceptance	Procrustean bed errors

---

usually omitted from operational definitions. Thus, there is no room for clinical hunches or intuition on the part of the doctor (see Box 2.1). In addition, there is a tendency to focus on positive symptomatology rather than less easily rated negative items, such as amotivation or anhedonia. Improved reliability has been largely brought about by the highly prescriptive "top-down" format of operational definitions in which a series of preset rules must be fulfilled before the diagnostic category can be applied. Individuals who fail to fulfil one or more items fall outside the diagnosis and end up in "not otherwise specified" or "atypical" categories. If the criteria are too narrow, the majority of subjects end up in such a category, which can then be larger than the main diagnostic groups (Farmer *et al.*, 1992). Other problems with operational definitions include the absence of standardised severity ratings in some definitions, which therefore means that both mild self-limiting and severe life-threatening disorder are included within the same diagnostic category (e.g. DSM-III major depression). The absence of an explicit diagnostic hierarchy can also be problematic for both clinicians and some types of research, such a genetic studies. Although there may be strong arguments against the introduction of such hierarchies, there is also a need for unequivocal guidance in some instances, which has so far been missing. The DSM-III, DSM-III-R and DSM-IV criteria give only limited guidance for the rater to decide, in a case with an admixture of depressive and psychotic symptoms, whether the diagnosis is one of psychotic depression or schizophrenia. In practice, this decision is left to the individual researcher or clinician's personal judgement and is therefore subject to the same potential types of prejudice and bias that the introduction of operational criteria was meant to overcome.

Diagnostic interviews

In the 1990s, for the first time in its history, the WHO supported the development of structured diagnostic interviews at the same time as it produced a new international classification. Three structured diagnostic interviews have been produced to accompany ICD-10 and DSM-IV. These are the Composite International Diagnostic Interview (CIDI; Robins *et al.*, 1988), the Schedules for the Clinical Assessment of Neuropsychiatry (SCAN; Wing *et al.*, 1990) and the International Personality Disorder Examination (IPDE; Loranger *et al.*, 1991). In addition to covering major diagnoses according to ICD-10 and DSM-IV, all three interviews have been developed for use in a variety of cultures, countries and settings. Each has been translated into all major languages and back-translated into English. Special

training in the use of each interview is required. All have computerised scoring programs, and their acceptability and reliability have been tested internationally.

The CIDI was specifically designed for epidemiological use and includes additional modules for the specific examination of individuals who misuse substances (the CIDI Substance Abuse Module). It has a highly structured format, which enables it to be used by lay interviewers who do not have any clinical background.

The SCAN interview consists of three main parts: Part 1 covers questions for nonpsychotic disorders, Part 2 for psychotic disorders and Part 3 for observations of speech, affect and the like. Clinical expertise is required for its use, and it is based on the PSE-CATEGO series of examinations and computerised scoring programmes.

The IPDE assesses the phenomena and life experiences that are relevant to the diagnoses of personality disorders in DSM-IV and ICD-10. The examination is arranged under six headings, consisting of work, interpersonal relationships, affects, reality testing, impulse control and behaviour at interview. An item-by-item scoring manual defines each criterion, and the examination is scored according to a 3-point scale. Informant information can also be used. The concurrent production of a new classification plus three structured interviews was a highly innovative move by the WHO.

Many other diagnostic interviews and rating scales are in current use. Some have been designed for specific populations (e.g. substance misusers, young people or the elderly), and others cover the main syndromes seen in adult general psychiatry, as do the SCAN and CIDI. Most require that individuals who wish to use them undergo some training to ensure that the interview or rating scale is being used consistently and with good interrater reliability. A "bird's eye view" of the history of key developments in psychiatric diagnosis and classification is provided in Box 2.2.

Box 2.2 Major historical milestones

1896–1913 Kraepelin observed his patients' symptom pattern and course over time; described "dementia praecox" and "manic depressive insanity"

1911 Bleuler described schizophrenia as a group of disorders

1927 Bridgman introduces operational definitions in physics

1939 Schneider described first-rank symptoms as diagnostic of schizophrenia (an operational definition; translated into English 1959)

1961 Kramer *et al.*: US-UK diagnostic series investigated diagnostic inconsistencies among first admission rates in New York and London; first standardised diagnostic interviews and computerised scoring systems devised

1961 Hempel recommended that an operationalised approach be used to define psychiatric disorders

1966 Spitzer introduces the Mental Status Examination, one of first diagnostic interviews

1970 Goldberg *et al.* developed the Clinical Interview Schedule, devised to evaluate milder psychopathology found in primary care

1970 Goldberg and Blackwell developed the General Health Questionnaire, a self-report inventory to screen for psychopathology in primary care settings

1972 Feighner *et al.* developed the St Louis operational definitions for psychiatric disorders

1973 World Health Organisation (WHO) undertook the International Pilot Study of Schizophrenia, extending examination of cross-national diagnostic practise

1973 Carpenter *et al.* introduced diagnostic criteria for schizophrenia

1974 Wing *et al.* published the Present State Examination (version 9; PSE9), a semistructured psychiatric interview with a glossary of definitions and computerised scoring program (CATEGO) based on systematic enquiry (the first version was developed in the 1950s)

1975 (revised in 1978) Spitzer *et al.* published the Research Diagnostic Criteria (RDC), operational definitions of major psychiatric disorders

1975 (revised in 1978) Taylor and Abrams introduced diagnostic criteria for schizophrenia

1978 Spitzer and Endicott published the Schedules for Affective Disorder and Schizophrenia (SADS) interview to accompany RDC criteria

1980 The American Psychiatric Association (APA) published the third edition of the *Diagnostic and Statistical Manual* (DSM-III) in operational format; it is the first national nosology to be entirely operationalised

1981 Robins *et al.* published the Diagnostic Interview Schedule (DIS), a highly structured interview for epidemiological use by trained lay interviewers based on DSM-III criteria

1987 APA published DSM-III-R, a revised edition of DSM-III

1988 Robins *et al.* published the Composite International Diagnostic Interview, an updated version of DIS, sponsored by the World Health Organization (WHO).

1990 Schedules for the Clinical assessment of Neuropsychiatry (SCAN) are published by WHO; an updated version of PSE (PSE10) incorporated DSM and *International Classification of Diseases* (ICD) criteria

1992 Spitzer *et al.* published the Structured Clinical Interview for Diagnoses (SCID) interview to accompany DSM-III-R criteria and improve the SADS

1992 WHO published the ICD-10 blue book of clinical guidance for psychiatric diagnosis

1993 WHO published the ICD-10 green book of operational definitions

1994 APA published DSM-IV, an updated US classification system

1994 Nurnberger *et al.* published the Diagnostic Interview for Genetic Studies (DIGS) and Family Interview for Genetic Studies (FIGS)

Future developments

As we have highlighted in this chapter, current nosologies are merely "working hypotheses" which provide the best fit for current knowledge and understanding. However, as knowledge changes, it will be necessary to revise these nosologies.

In the current run-up to DSM-V, some authors consider that a radical change is necessary, arguing that the nosology for psychiatric disorders should include dimensional diagnoses (Brown and Barlow, 2005; Helzer *et al.*, 2006) or that diagnosis should be based on what is known about aetiology, mirroring the diagnosis of physical illnesses (McHugh, 2005). Whether these approaches will be included in either DSM-V or ICD-11 is uncertain. What is known, however, is that the reviewing process will continue indefinitely until the precise aetiologies of mental disorders are found.

REFERENCES

American Psychiatric Association (1980). *Diagnostic and Statistical Manual of Mental Disorders* (DSM III), 3rd edn. Washington, DC: American Psychiatric Association.

American Psychiatric Association (1987). *Diagnostic and Statistical Manual of Mental Disorders (DSM-III-R)*, 3rd edn., revised. Washington, DC: American Psychiatric Association.

American Psychiatric Association (1994). *Diagnostic and Statistical Manual of Mental Disorders (DSM-IV)*, 4th edn. Washington, DC: American Psychiatric Association.

Baillarger, J. (1853). Note on the type of insanity with attacks characterised by two regular periods, one of depression and one of excitement. *Bull Acad Natural Med* 19:340.

Bellak, L. (1958). *Schizophrenia: A Review of the Syndrome.* New York: Logos Press.

Berrios, G. E. (1993). European views on personality disorders: a conceptual history. *Compr Psychiatry* 34:14–30.

Bleuler, E. (1950). *Dementia Praecox or the Group of Schizophrenias.* Translated by S. M. Clemens. New Haven and London: Yale University Press. Original work published 1911.

Bridgman, P. W. (1927). *The Logic of Modern Physics.* New York: Macmillan.

Brockington, J. F., Kendell, R. E., & Leff, J. P. (1978). Definitions of schizophrenia: concordance and prediction of outcome. *Psychol Med* 8:387–98.

Brown, T. A., & Barlow, D. H. (2005). Dimensional versus categorical classification of mental disorders in the fifth edition of the *Diagnostic and Statistical Manual of Mental Disorders* and beyond: comment on the special section. *J Abnormal Psychol* 114:551–6.

Carpenter, W. T., Strauss, J. S., & Bartko, J. J. (1973). Flexible system for the diagnosis of schizophrenia: a report from the WHO pilot study of schizophrenia. *Science* 182:1275–8.

Cooper, J. E., Kendell, R. E., Gurland, B. J., *et al.* (1972). *Psychiatric Diagnosis in New York and London. Maudsley Monograph.* London: Oxford University Press.

Falret, J. P. (1854), *Clinical Lectures on Clinical Medicine General Symptomatology* (in French). Paris: Bailliere.

Farmer, A. E., & McGuffin, P. (1989). The classification of the depression: contemporary confusion revisited. *Br J Psychiatry* 155:437–43.

Farmer, A. E., Wessely, S., Castle, D., & McGuffin, P. (1992). Methodological issues in using a polydiagnostic approach to define psychotic illness. *Br J Psychiatry* 161:824–30.

Feighner, J. P., Robins, E., Guze, S. B., *et al.* (1972). Diagnostic criteria for use in psychiatric research. *Arch Gen Psychiatry* 26:57–67.

Jaspers, K. (1963). *General Psychopathology.* Translated from the 7th edition by J. Hoenig and M.W. Hamilton. Manchester: Manchester University Press.

Hecker, E. (1871). Die Hebephrenie. *Virchows Archiv für Patholgische Anatomie* 52:392–449.

Helzer, J. E., Kraemer, H. C., & Krueger, R. F. (2006). The feasibility and need of dimensional psychiatric diagnoses. *Psychol Med* 36:1671–80.

Hempel, C. G. (1961). Introduction to problems of taxonomy. In J. Zubin, ed. *Field Studies in the Mental Disorders.*

Kahlbaum, K. L. (1973). *Catatonia.* Translated by G. Mora. Baltimore: Johns Hopkins University Press. Original work published 1874.

Kendell, R. E. (1975). *The Role of Diagnosis in Psychiatry.* Oxford: Blackwell Science.

Koch J. L. A. (1891). *Die Psychopatischen Minderwertigkeiten.* Ravensberg Dorn.

Kraepelin, E. (1896). Der psychologische Versuch in der Psychiatrie. *Psychologische Arbeiten* 1:1–91.

Kraepelin, E. (1919). *Psychiatrie.* Vol. 3, part 2. (Translated by R. M. Barclay as *Dementia praecox and paraphrenia.*) Edinburgh: Livingstone. Original work published 1913.

Kramer, M. (1961). Some problems for international research suggested by observations as differences in first admission rates to mental hospitals of England & Wales, and of the United States. In *Proceedings of the Third World Congress of Psychiatry*, Vol. 3, pp. 153–60.

Loranger, A. W., Sartorius, N., Andreoli, A., *et al.* (1994). The World Health Organisation/Alcohol, Drug Abuse and Mental Health Administration, international pilot study of personality disorders. *Arch Gen Psychiatry* **51**:215–24.

McGuffin, P., Farmer, A. E., & Harvey, I. (1991). A polydiagnostic application of operational criteria in studies in psychotic illness: development and reliability of OPCRIT system. *Arch Gen Psychiatry* **48**:764–70.

McHugh, P. R. (2005). Striving for coherence. Psychiatry's efforts over classification. *JAMA* **293**:2526–8.

Prichard, J. C. (1835). *Treatise on Insanity and Other Disorders Affecting the Mind*. London: Sherwood, Gilbert and Piper.

Robins, L. N., Wing, J., Wittchen, H. U., *et al.* (1988). The composite international diagnostic interview: an epidemiological instrument suitable for use in conjunction with different diagnostic systems and in different cultures. *Arch Gen Psychiatry* **45**:1069–77.

Shepherd, M. (1957). *A Study of the Major Psychoses in an English County*. Maudsley Monograph. Oxford, UK: Oxford University Press.

Spitzer, R. L., Endicott, J. R., & Robins, E. (1975). *Research Diagnostic Criteria: Instrument No. 58*. New York: New York State Psychiatric Institute.

Stengel, E. (1959). Classification of mental disorders. *Bulletin of the World Health Organization* **21**:601–63.

Tsuang, M. T., & Winokur, G. (1974). Criteria for subtyping schizophrenia. *Arch Gen Psychiatry* **31**:43–7.

Wing, J. K., Cooper, J. E., & Sartorius, N. (1974). *The Measurement and Classification of Psychiatric Symptoms*. Cambridge, UK: Cambridge University Press.

Wing, J. K., Babor, T., Brugha, T., Cooper, J., Geil, R., Jablensky, A., *et al.* (1990). SCAN: schedules for the clinical assessment in neuropsychiatry. *Arch Gen Psychiatry* **47**:589–93.

World Health Organisation (1973). *Report on International Pilot Study of Schizophrenia*, Vol. 1. Geneva: World Health Organisation.

World Health Organisation (1974). *Glossary of Mental Disorders and Guide to Their Classification*. Geneva: World Health Organisation.

World Health Organisation (1980). *International Classification of Impairments, Disabilities and Handicaps, 10th revision*. Geneva: World Health Organisation.

World Health Organisation (1992). *The ICD-10 Classification of Mental and Behavioural Disorders. Clinical Descriptions and Diagnostic Guidelines*. Geneva: World Health Organisation.

World Health Organisation (1993). *Diagnostic Criteria for Research. International Classification of Diseases, 10th revision*. Geneva: World Health Organisation.

3

Research methods in psychiatry

Marieke Wichers and Jim van Os

Psychiatric studies are often characterised by large numbers of variables, clinical outcomes that are difficult to measure ("psychometrics"), small sample sizes and conflicting results. The field, however, is developing rapidly, and a basic understanding of research methodology in psychiatry is now regarded as a necessary basic skill. Because much of this can be subsumed under the header of epidemiology, this chapter provides a succinct introduction to this basic discipline of medicine as relevant for psychiatry.

Making hypotheses

Research starts with curiosity. There is a question that requires an answer. For example:

1. What is the incidence rate of psychotic disorders in the United Kingdom?
2. Is the rate of psychotic disorders higher in those who live in urbanised areas?
3. Is the risk-increasing effect of serious life events (SLE) for major depression different for individuals with different forms of a functional polymorphism of the serotonin transporter gene?
4. Does antidepressant A works better than antidepressant B in preventing relapse after remission of a major depressive episode?

The first question is trying to determine the morbidity force of a disease in a certain population, in terms of the fraction of the population that makes the transition from a healthy state to a disease state (i.e. experiences a new onset) in a year.

The second question concerns the exploration of factors that are characterised by a specific level of morbidity force, that is, that are said to be *associated* with the disease and therefore may influence the probability of a disease outcome (risk factor). Often, findings in the realm of questions of the second type give rise to new hypotheses concerning causality: that changing the risk factor may result in changes in the morbidity force (causal risk factor). For example, differences in the rate of psychosis between urban and rural areas, with lower rates in the latter, may give rise to hypotheses about differential exposure to protective (e.g. increased social cohesion in rural areas) or toxic factors (e.g. increased rates of central nervous system [CNS] infections in urban areas) resulting in a new study elucidating aspects of causality. For the judgement of causality, however, two important conditions must be satisfied:

1. *A valid association* between the exposure (e.g. CNS infections) and the disease (psychotic disorder). Not all associations are valid. They may arise as a result of chance, bias or confounding, which are explained in more detail later;
2. *The association represents a cause-effect relationship* rather than being merely an indicator of such a relationship. For example, there may well

Essential Psychiatry, ed. Robin M. Murray, Kenneth S. Kendler, Peter McGuffin, Simon Wessely, David J. Castle.
Published by Cambridge University Press. © Cambridge University Press 2008.

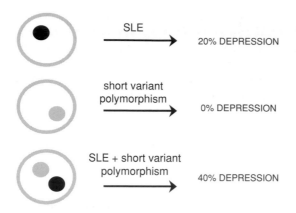

Figure 3.1. Synergistic interaction between exposure to a stressful life event (SLE) and exposure to the short variant of the 5-HTT (serotonin) transporter gene in the development of depression.

be a valid association between urbanicity and psychotic disorder, but this association can at best be only a proxy of the true causal risk factor, just as having nicotine-stained fingers is a risk indicator for lung cancer but not the cause of the disease.

The third question examines whether two exposures that separately may or may not influence the occurrence of an outcome may influence each other, in the sense that they can reinforce or antagonise each other. For example, if the rate of depression after exposure to SLE is 20% for individuals homozygous for the long variant of a length polymorphism in the gene encoding the serotonin transporter but 40% for those homozygous for the short variant of this polymorphism, the two risk factors (SLE and length polymorphism) are said to show synergistic interaction in that they reinforce the effect of each other (Figure 3.1).

The fourth question really is an extension of the second, but under special circumstances – namely, those in which certain exposures are thought to have a causal impact on outcomes – and the study takes on the form of an experiment in which individuals are randomly assigned to either the exposure condition or a control condition (experimental design).

Examining associations: hypothesis and study design

The type of hypothesis has implications for the study design. There are a number of designs, each with advantages and disadvantages. Study designs are classified along the axes of time (longitudinal or cross-sectional design), level of causal inference (descriptive or analytical design) and role of the investigator (observational or experimental).

Choice of study design

Before choosing a design, given a particular research question, it is wise first to consider which design best fits the question that needs answering and how this relates to practical possibilities and limitations. Some observational study designs are better equipped for questions of the first type (descriptive observational designs), whereas others (analytic observational design) are better equipped to handle hypotheses concerning causal inference as exemplified in the second and third question, because they not only explore the validity of an association but also characteristics that support causality – for example, a temporal or a dose-response relationship (discussed later). Experimental designs are best suited to the fourth type of question because they pay special attention to the validity of any association that may result from the study. Their use, however, is limited, because of organisational and economic, as well as legal and ethical, limits beyond which researchers cannot go. The different designs are described further later in the chapter.

Designs for observational descriptive studies

Three types of designs can be used in descriptive studies.

1. *Correlational study.* This type of study compares disease frequencies among different populations at the same time points, or in the same population at different time points. These

disease frequencies are then correlated with a certain characteristic in the population. For example, one can examine the relationship between the frequency of cannabis use *(characteristic)* in the United Kingdom, Germany and the Netherlands and, separately, the prevalence of psychosis *(disease frequency of different populations)* in the three countries to assess whether countries with higher population rates of psychosis also have higher population rates of cannabis use. The caveat to this type of study, clearly, is that an association between population cannabis use and population psychosis can be shown, but that there is no way to know whether those individuals who developed psychosis were indeed the ones who used cannabis; they may be entirely different people. In other words, the findings may be confounded: finding an association between sales of Renault cars and liver cirrhosis in European countries does not mean that Renault cars cause liver cirrhosis. Well-known and hotly debated examples of correlation studies include the association between influenza and schizophrenia, drinking-water aluminium concentration and Alzheimer's disease, prenatal famine and schizophrenia and small area deprivation and minor psychiatric disorder.

2. *Case reports and case series.* A case report is a detailed clinical report on the profile of a single patient or a series of patients. Usually a case report is written when a certain exposure or treatment has unexpected consequences in a certain patient. For example, a case report was published concerning a hepatitis C patient who was treated with interferon alpha but developed bipolar disorder during treatment (Malik & Ravasia, 2004). The case report, however, concerns only a single patient, and it therefore is not possible to draw any causal conclusions from this finding. It is possible that the development of the disease had nothing to do with the treatment and was just a coincidence. The patient in question may have had early prodromal symptoms of bipolar disorder before starting the interferon

alpha treatment. Case reports can be extended to a case series when more patients who develop the same disease under the same specific circumstances are described. Case series therefore give additional credibility to the idea that a valid association might exist because they reduce the likelihood that the association was coincidental.

3. *Cross-sectional survey.* In this type of study, the status of an individual with respect to exposure and disease is assessed at the same point in time. For example, in a population survey, one may assess, in all participating individuals, the presence of psychotic symptoms and, at the same time, personal cannabis use and other potentially important variables. The difference with the correlational study is that in the cross-sectional survey, it is possible to link exposures and outcomes to specific individuals. However, temporal relationships cannot be examined, and people with the outcome of psychotic symptoms include those who had onset of psychotic symptoms 1 week earlier, but also those with stable symptoms for a period of 10 years. The same applies to assessment of the cannabis exposure. In these types of studies, it is not possible to determine whether cannabis induced psychotic symptoms or whether psychotic symptoms gave rise to cannabis use as a form of self-medication.

Observational descriptive studies: when to use which design

In general, descriptive designs can be used to examine associations between exposures and outcomes in such a way that the results may lead to the formulation of more specific hypotheses regarding the causal implications of the exposure-disease relationship. Because of their limitations, descriptive studies are not suitable to examine causal implications. Analytic studies, however, provide better tools. They are described later.

An advantage of correlational studies is that the information needed is often already available because government and health agencies routinely

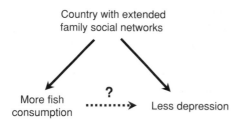

Figure 3.2. Confounding by social network of the apparent association between fish consumption and depression.

collect demographic and health data. Correlational studies therefore represent a rapid and inexpensive start in the search for possible exposure-disease relationships. Major limitations are the inability to link exposure and disease data within individuals and the resulting risk of confounding, as described earlier. For example, a study may find an association between daily fish consumption in European countries and country prevalence of major depression, suggesting a possible causal effect of poor omega-3 fatty acid status. However, this finding may simply be a reflection of the fact that people who eat more fish live in countries where extended family social networks are better developed, protecting against major depression (Figure 3.2). A correlational design cannot control for variables that provide an alternative explanation (i.e. that are confounding). A cross-sectional survey, therefore, has some advantages over the correlational study because in the cross-sectional survey, one can measure and control for additional variables that are likely to confound the hypothesised association. However, temporal relationships cannot be assessed, limiting assessment of possible causality.

Finally, case reports and case series can be useful in the recognition of new diseases and new side effects of treatments. The major disadvantage is that case reports are based on the experience of only one person. Although case series increase the likelihood of a valid association, case series cannot test the validity of the proposed association. Nevertheless, they can be used for the formulation of new hypotheses.

Designs for observational analytic studies

If the aim is to examine whether a valid association exists between a certain exposure and a disease and to reach an informed opinion about cause-effect relationships, an analytic study design is in order. There are three types of analytical studies, two observational and one experimental. Observational analytical studies are discussed first.

1. *Case-control study*. In a case-control design, subjects are selected on the basis of having a particular disease during the time that they are under study. The groups with and without a particular disease are then compared with respect to the frequency of the exposure of interest. For example, one may select a group of subjects with major depression and a healthy control group and assess whether the depressed group was more often exposed to dietary omega-3 fatty acid deficiency, resulting in poor omega-3 fatty acid status. If the depressed group shows a higher rate of dietary omega-3 fatty acid deficiency, one would conclude that there is an association between poor omega-3 fatty acid status and depression.

2. *Cohort study*. In a cohort study, groups of subjects are defined by the presence or absence of a certain exposure. Subjects are then followed over a period of time to assess how many subjects develop the outcome of interest. In a cohort study of depression and dietary omega-3 fatty acid deficiency, for example, subjects would first be classified according to their level of dietary omega-3 fatty acid deficiency and then followed for a certain period of time to compare the incidence rate of depression in exposed and nonexposed subjects. Cohort studies can be prospective or retrospective. In retrospective studies, all relevant events have already occurred (the exposure and the disease outcome) at the time of measurement, whereas in the prospective study, the disease outcome has not yet occurred, and participants are assessed at follow-up to evaluate new transitions to the outcome.

Observational analytic studies: when to use which design

Why do researchers sometimes choose a case-control study and other times opt for a cohort study? The use of case-control studies is practical when the disease is rare, because subjects are selected on the basis of having the disease, making it possible to involve specialised treatment centres to collect a sizeable group of subjects with even the rarest of disorders. A cohort study would be less practical in the case of rare disease, because a very large cohort would be necessary to yield enough disease transitions. However, in the case of a rare exposure, the cohort design is more efficient, because selection for study entry occurs on the basis of exposure status. The cohort design is also efficient in the case of studying pleiotropy – or multiple outcomes associated with the same exposure – because at follow-up more than one outcome can be measured.

The case-control design is suitable to examine aetiological heterogeneity – or different exposures resulting in the same outcome – because a range of exposures in patients and control subjects can be assessed. The major limitation of the case-control design is that both exposure and disease have already occurred when subjects enter the study. This can give rise to the phenomenon of differential selection. For example, by placing an advertisement in journals to find subjects for a study on dietary omega-3 fatty acid deficiency and depression, one risks that those with special diets who feel depressed are more likely to come forward because they hope a treatment may result from participating in the study. If an association between dietary omega-3 fatty acid deficiency and depression is subsequently found, this may have more to do with how people were selected than with a genuine relationship between the two. This problem of differential selection is a form of bias and more likely in a case-control than a cohort study. How to deal with bias is described later.

Another disadvantage of the case-control design is that it cannot distinguish any temporal relationship. The cohort study can, because it includes multiple measurements over time. However, cohort studies can be time-consuming and expensive. In addition, the validity of the results can be threatened when some subjects who participated at baseline drop out at one of the follow-ups. If dropout is differential, bias of results can also occur. Suppose that in patients with severe mental illness, exposure to case management type A is compared with case management type B in a 12-month observational prospective design, with the primary outcome of employment status at follow-up. In both groups, dropout before endpoint at 12 months was 40%. This in itself, contrary to what is often assumed, does not have to result in bias. In this case, however, dropout was differential because dropouts in the group with case management type A occurred mostly because of relapse, whereas dropout in group B occurred mostly because individuals recovered and wanted to get on with their lives rather than be in a trial. Paradoxically, trial results were in favour of case management type A rather than B, because in group A there was selective enrichment of the sample with relatively healthy people and in group B there was selective enrichment of the sample with relatively sick individuals (Figure 3.3). Thus, differential dropout with respect to disease outcome threatens the validity of the results in a cohort study.

Designs for experimental analytic studies

The distinguishing feature of any experimental design is that the investigator allocates the subjects at random to the exposure or the control condition, followed by assessment of the outcome. The experimental study is therefore always longitudinal. Experimental studies can examine between-person effects of treatments on disease outcomes (the so-called randomised controlled trial, or RCT), but, if ethical guidelines permit, individuals can also be allocated to exposures that induce a within-person change in behavioural or physiological outcomes in the individual. Examples include within-person experimental studies of the effect of intravenous delta(9)-tetrahydrocannabinol (the

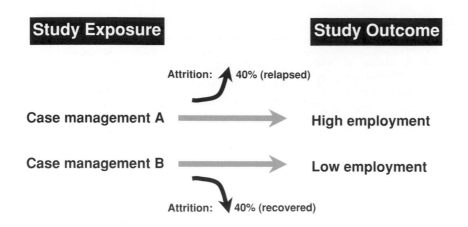

Figure 3.3. Example of differential dropout causing bias in the results.

main psychotropic component of cannabis) on cognition and psychological experiments of exposing individuals to a paranoia-inducing virtual-reality environment and measuring their behavioural responses.

Because of the randomisation of subjects, control is possible for not only known and measurable factors but also for all unknown and unmeasurable factors that may confound the association between exposure and outcome. However, such a strategy also brings ethical concerns. One cannot allocate subjects randomly to an exposure that induces health risks, and there is an ongoing debate as to what degree exposure to placebo constitutes a health risk.

Although considered the gold standard in many ways, there are numerous challenges facing experimental studies, and RCTs in particular. Outcome assessment may be contaminated by knowledge about exposure status, introducing bias. To counter this, attempts are made to keep both patients and researchers "blind" to exposure status, but blindness is often incomplete because, for example, differences in side effect profiles between experimental and control conditions exist, in particular if the control condition is an inactive placebo. RCTs also suffer from selection of particular groups, usually older and relatively treatment-refractory

patients, hampering generalisability of the results to mainstream clinical practice. RCTs, in particular those examining medication effects, are also mainly "technical", meaning they are brief, use many exclusion criteria, are registration-driven and analyse outcomes that have limited clinical relevance. The use of "pragmatic" or "simple" RCTs, using few but clinically relevant outcomes and in at least 12-month follow-up of patients that reflect the population treated in routine clinical practice, has been advocated by, for example, the Cochrane Collaboration.

Study designs: conclusion

A number of designs are available, each with its own strengths and threats to the validity of the results (see Tables 3.1 and 3.2). The choice of design thus depends on several factors, such as the type of hypothesis (causal or not), possibilities in terms of money and time, need to control for confounders and threat of bias, exposure prevalence, disease prevalence and ethical concerns. To preserve validity and the interpretation of the findings, it is important to be aware of the unique characteristics of each design. For further reading, see Hennekens and Buring (1987).

Table 3.1 Level of suitability of different research designs

	Correlational	Cross-sectional	Case-control	Cohort	Intervention
Investigation of rare disease	Medium	—	High	—	—
Investigation of rare cause	Medium	—	—	High	High
Examining multiple outcomes	Medium	Medium	—	High	High
Examining multiple exposures	Medium	Medium	High	Medium	Low
Measurement of time relationships	—	—	Low	High	High
Measurement of incidence	—	—	Low	High	High

Table 3.2 Advantages and disadvantages of several study designs

Probability of ...	Correlational	Cross-sectional	Case-control	Cohort	Intervention
Recall bias	NA	High	High	Low	Low
Loss to follow-up	NA	NA	low	high	medium
Confounding	High	Medium	Medium	Low	Low
Time required	Low	Medium	Medium	High	Medium
Cost	Low	Medium	Medium	High	Medium
Ethical concerns	Low	Low	Low	Low	High

NA — not applicable.

What to do with results

After a curiosity-driven question has been formulated and a suitable study has been conducted, it is time to think about processing the results. Medical scientific studies generally have two main interests in the examination of the results. (1) examination of the morbidity force of a disease phenotype in populations and (2) examination of associations.

Analysis of disease frequency

The morbidity force in a population can be examined by calculating measures of disease frequency. Suppose we have a group of 100 women and find that 10 subjects had developed a depressive episode within the previous 2 years. In another group of 200 men, 18 subjects had developed depression within the previous 3 years. To know in which group depression is more common, standardisation in terms of both population size and time period is necessary. Thus, it can be calculated that in the female group, 5 subjects out of every 100 develop depression over the course of a year, compared with 3 men. Thus, a frequency measure is only informative if case information about population size and time period is added.

Two measures of disease frequency are often used: prevalence and incidence. *Prevalence* describes the number of events or existing cases with disease / total population size, at a given point in time or over a given time period. For example, if we are measuring a group of 100 women at a certain moment and find 6 subjects with a depressive episode at the time of measurement, the prevalence in this group at that point in time is 6%.

Incidence quantifies the number of new events or cases that develop in a population during a specified time interval. There are two types of incidence measures: cumulative incidence or incidence

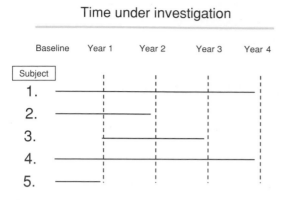

Figure 3.4. To calculate the incidence density, information about the amount of time that each subject is under investigation and without disease is necessary. In this example, persons 2, 3 and 5 develop the outcome. The incidence density is 3 divided by 15 person years $(5 + 2 + 2 + 5 + 1)$ or 0.2 per year; the 5-year cumulative incidence is 3/5 or 0.6 or 0.12 per year.

proportion (CI) and incidence density (ID). Cumulative incidence provides the risk that an individual will develop a disease during a specified period of time. If, for example, in a healthy group of 4,000 adolescents, 16 subjects develop psychosis at any time during the 4-year study period, then the CI in this population $= 16/4,000 = 0.4\%$ per 4 years or 0.1% per year.

The CI assumes that the entire population (all subjects in the study who are at risk to develop the disease) are followed from the start until the end of the study for the development of the disease under investigation. However, this is often not the case. Subjects drop out and new subjects may be included, leading to a variable time period of observation for each subject in the study (Figure 3.4). If this is the case, it is better to use the measure 'ID', which takes into account these varying time periods between subjects. Thus, ID is the number of new cases of a disease during a given time period divided by the total person-time of observation. The denominator represents the summarised measure of time that each person remained under observation and free from disease. The amount of time that subjects were in the study after they developed the

disease is excluded from the denominator because in this time period the subjects are no longer at risk to develop the disease under investigation.

For example, we wish to calculate ID for psychosis in a group of 50,000 subjects, followed up for 4 years. First, we need to count the number of new-onset cases arising during the study. Second, we count for each subject the number of years (or choose another time measure such as month or day) that he or she was under observation but free from disease. Then we summarise the number of years for all subjects. Suppose that 30 new onsets are observed, and the total summarised number of years is 166,000 (i.e. less than the 200,000 expected if all subjects had complete follow-up intervals), then the ID $= 30$ cases/166,000 person-years or 18.1 cases/10^5 person-years of observation. Had we calculated the CI instead, thus not taking into account the exact amount of person-time of observation, the rate would have been $30/50,000 = 60$ per 4 years or 15.0 per year, lower than the ID (Hennekens & Buring, 1987).

Analysis of association

Most studies examine associations between an "exposure" and an "outcome". The method for testing an association depends on the type of variable used. Dichotomous variables have only two categories such as gender (man or woman), having a disease (yes or no) or survival status (alive or dead). Continuous variables, on the other hand, are variables that can have any value along a continuum within a specified range, such as age, level of plasma serotonin or blood pressure. In case the variable that the researcher wants to predict (the *dependent* or *response* variable) is dichotomous, the association between exposure and outcome can be expressed as a measure of relative risk such as the risk ratio (RR), the odds ratio (OR) or the incidence rate ratio (IRR). However, in case the dependent variable is continuous, other measures can be used, such as testing the mean difference between exposed and nonexposed using a *t* test. These methods are explained in more detail later and are summarised in Box 3.1.

Box 3.1 Summary of tests used to examine associations between exposure and outcome∗

Test	Criteria for use	Formula
RR	– Outcome is dichotomous variable – Selection based on exposure – Proportions	$\dfrac{\%\ \text{subjects } \textbf{exposed}\ \text{who develop disease}}{\%\ \text{subjects } \textbf{nonexposed}\ \text{who develop disease}}$
IRR	– Outcome is dichotomous variable – Selection based on exposure – Incidence densities	$\dfrac{\text{Incidence density of disease in } \textbf{exposed}\ \text{subjects}}{\text{Incidence density of disease in } \textbf{nonexposed}\ \text{subjects}}$
OR	– Dichotomous variable – Selection based on disease	$\dfrac{\%\ \text{subjects } \textbf{exposed}\ \text{with disease} / \%\ \textbf{nonexposed}\ \text{without disease}}{\%\ \text{subjects } \textbf{exposed}\ \text{without disease} / \%\ \textbf{nonexposed}\ \text{with disease}}$
T-test	– Outcome is continuous variable – Sample value fit to a population mean	$\dfrac{\text{sample value} - \text{sample mean}}{\text{SE (sd} / \sqrt{n})}$
T-test	– Outcome is continuous variable – Population mean 1 fit to population mean 2	$\dfrac{\text{sample mean 1} - \text{sample mean 2}}{\text{SE (sample mean 1} - \text{mean 2})}$

∗ Only basic statistical tests are shown. If confounders must be added to the analyses, more complex statistical tests are in order:

– for models with a dichotomous outcome variable: logistic regression.

– for models with a continuous outcome variable: analysis of variance or regression analyses.

Dichotomous variables

In many studies, dichotomous variables are used both for exposure (yes or no) and disease outcome (disease, no disease). A 2 × 2 table is often used to present the counts of subjects in the study (Figure 3.5). An example is a retrospective cohort study of mothers with or without a viral exposure during pregnancy and with or without offspring with schizophrenia. If there is an association between viral exposure and development of schizophrenia in the offspring, then the rate of the disease in subjects whose mothers were prenatally exposed must be higher than the rate of disease in nonexposed subjects. This is what the risk ratio indicates: the proportion of subjects who develop disease in the exposed group divided by the proportion in the nonexposed group. A risk ratio (expressed as RR) of 1.0 indicates that the cumulative incidence of the disease in the exposed is the same as the cumulative incidence in the nonexposed subjects and thus that there is no association, whereas an RR of 3.0 indicates that exposed subjects are 3 times more likely to develop the disease. In the case of a

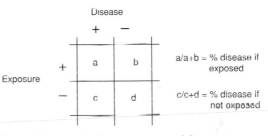

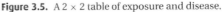

Figure 3.5. A 2 × 2 table of exposure and disease.

cohort study calculating incidence densities rather incidence proportions in exposed and nonexposed, the relative risk is expressed as the IRR, or the ratio of the incidence densities in the exposed versus nonexposed.

In the case of a case control study, in which the subjects are selected *not* on having a certain exposure, but on disease status, it is not valid to use the RR, because the proportion of subjects with the disease compared with those without is based on selection and not representative for the population. In this case, the relative risk is expressed as the OR. The OR approximates the ratio of proportions of subjects who develop the disease in a specific period of

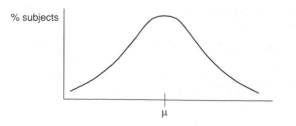

Figure 3.6. Depicted is a graph of a normally distributed trait in the population. The μ indicates the true mean value of the trait within the total population.

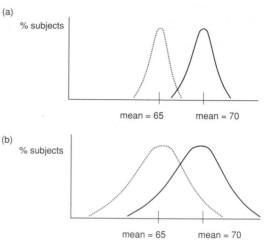

Figure 3.7. Distribution of plasma tryptophan concentrations in two samples ($n = 30$ each) of depressed (dotted line) and nondepressed (black line) subjects. (A) Low variability of plasma tryptophan concentrations. (B) High variability of plasma tryptophan concentrations.

time among exposed and nonexposed; that is, the OR approximates the RR. The estimation of the RR by the OR is not perfect but becomes nearly perfect in cases of rare diseases. The OR estimates the association by multiplying the two cells that would increase the magnitude of the association (subjects with exposure and with disease × subjects without exposure and without disease). This amount is then divided by the product of the two cells that decrease the magnitude of the association (subjects with exposure and without disease × subjects without exposure and with disease). This results in a higher ratio in case of a greater association, just like the RR (Hennekens & Buring, 1987).

Continuous variables

It is possible that the dependent variable in a study is not dichotomous but continuous – a variable that can take any value along a continuum. Such a continuous variable is often normally distributed in the population. This means that the values of the variable (at the x axis) plotted against the frequency in the population (y axis) result in a bell-shaped curve, with the mean value having the highest frequency in the population and the values at both ends of the distribution having the lowest frequency (Figure 3.6). For example, one may wish to examine the difference in plasma level of tryptophan between a group of depressed ($n = 30$) and a group of nondepressed subjects ($n = 30$) to assess whether tryptophan concentration is associated

with depression. At the end of the study, the researcher has two bell-shaped curves with two different means for depressed and nondepressed subjects (Figure 3.7) and wishes to calculate whether these two distributions of tryptophan concentrations are significantly different from each other.

The simplest, intuitive test that can be applied is to calculate the distance between the two means. For example, if depressed subjects have an average plasma tryptophan level of 65 μmol/L and nondepressed of 70 μmol/L, then the difference is 5 μmol/L. However, the importance of this difference depends as well on the variability of the values within each group. Suppose that within the nondepressed group, almost all values lie within 68 and 72 μmol/L. In this case, a mean level of 65 in depressed patients would be so extreme that there is little chance it could belong to the same distribution as the values of nondepressed subjects (Figure 3.7, *A*). However, when values in the nondepressed group range, for example, between 63 and 76, there is no a priori reason to conclude that a value of 65 μmol/L is deviant from the values within

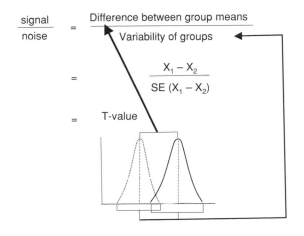

$$\frac{\text{signal}}{\text{noise}} = \frac{\text{Difference between group means}}{\text{Variability of groups}}$$

$$= \frac{X_1 - X_2}{SE\,(X_1 - X_2)}$$

$$= \text{T-value}$$

Figure 3.8. The t score can be derived by calculating the ratio of the difference between group means (signal) and the variability of the sample mean (noise).

the nondepressed group (Figure 3.7, *B*). In this case, a t test may be used to test for an association by calculating the ratio of the difference in means and a measure of variability. One can interpret this as a signal-to-noise ratio. The higher this ratio, the more relevant the difference in means (signal) compared with the variability (noise) (Figure 3.8).

It is important to understand how this measure of variability or noise can be defined because much statistical theory depends on it. The two distributions from the previous example are but small samples from the total populations they are supposed to represent (30 of all existing depressed vs. nondepressed subjects). This means that the mean values found in the study using these particular samples may deviate a little from their true population means. If we were to draw more and more samples of $n = 30$ from, for example, the population of all nondepressed subjects, the more the mean value of all these different sample means *together* will represent the true population mean. In other words, the sample mean of our sample of $n = 30$ itself is subject to variation if we were to draw many samples of $n = 30$ from the same population. The variability of the sample mean as an estimate of the true population mean is called the standard error

(SE). Thus, the SE, or the expected deviation of the sample mean from the true mean, will get smaller when sample size increases, because the larger the sample, the more representative it becomes of the true population mean. Because the same holds true for the sample of $n = 30$ from the entire population of all depressed subjects, the mean difference between the sample of 30 depressed and 30 nondepressed subjects is also subject to variation around the true population mean difference. The SE of the mean difference is therefore used as a measure of 'noise' in the t test formula and is obtained by dividing the sample standard deviation (measure of variability of values in the sample) by the square root of the sample size.

A t test thus tests the significance of the mean difference, and an arbitrary cut-off point is made for this purpose. If the mean value of plasma tryptophan in one group deviates more than 2 SE in a positive or negative direction from the other, the difference is called 'significant', because the probability that it would occur by chance is very small (less than 5%). Another way to investigate whether the mean difference in plasma tryptophan is significant is to create a so-called 95% confidence interval. The confidence interval tells us that if the study were to be repeated a 100 times in different samples of depressed and nondepressed subjects, yielding 100 estimates of the difference in mean plasma tryptophan, the confidence interval would contain the range of differences in plasma tryptophan between the two groups that would be seen 95 of the 100 times. This interval extends from the value that lies at a distance of two SEs less than the mean difference, to the value of two SEs more (Figure 3.9). If the 95% confidence interval includes the value zero, the difference is not statistically significant, because it indicates that the mean difference between the two groups is not consistently different in one direction at least 95 of a 100 times; that is, the chance of a false-positive finding is greater than 0.05. However, if the 95% confidence interval does not include zero, the mean difference is indeed statistically significant. The advantage of working with the confidence interval rather than the

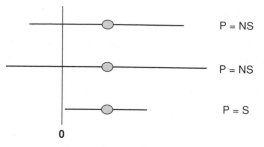

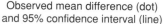

Observed mean difference (dot)
and 95% confidence interval (line)

Figure 3.9. The confidence interval extends from the value that lies at a distance of two standard errors (SEs) less than the mean difference, to the value of two SEs more. If the 95% confidence interval includes the value zero (no mean difference), the difference is not statistically significant at the 5% level ($p = $ NS). If it does not include zero, the difference is significant at the 5% level ($p = $ S).

p value alone is that a confidence interval informs the researcher about the statistical significance of the finding, but the width of the confidence interval also indicates the amount of variability inherent to the estimate. The larger the sample, the more stable the estimate and the narrower the interval.

Interpreting associations

After analysis of the results, a valid statistical association may transpire. Here, however, the scientific process does not end. Usually, much time is devoted to interpretation of any association. In addition, the process of interpretation of associations is something that should take place during the whole research process and not simply after analysis of the results. Why this is important is explained subsequently.

Validity of the association

Chance

First, the validity of the association should be considered. There are three possible threats to validity

(Hennekens & Buring, 1987; Rothman & Greenland, 1998). First is the factor "chance". The goal of research is to draw inferences about the experience of an entire population based on the evaluation of one sample. Chance may always affect such an inference because random variation exists from sample to sample (the variation that produces the SE). Further, as we have already concluded, this variation will diminish to the extent that sample sizes are larger. With a small SE, even a very small mean difference can be significant because of a very large sample size. Conversely, a larger effect may not achieve significance when examined in a small sample. To quantify the degree by which chance may play a part in the results, tests of significance are used, such as the t test, giving rise to a p value indicating the likelihood that the finding is due to chance. However, the statistical significance of an association is often misinterpreted. One should remember that the label 'significant' or 'nonsignificant' is given on the basis of an arbitrary line drawn at the p value of 0.05. Obviously, this should not become an excuse for concluding that findings with a p value of 0.06 are not important, whereas findings with a p value of 0.05 suddenly reflect important and true findings. Second, a statistically significant result does not mean that chance does not play a role, only that such an explanation is unlikely. Also, the absence of a statistical association does not simply imply that there is none. It is possible that the sample size is insufficient to exclude chance as an explanation for the association (the study has insufficient statistical power).

Bias

A second threat to validity is bias. The concept of bias was already mentioned in the section concerning the advantages and disadvantages of designs. Bias occurs when different groups of subjects are not comparable, for example, because of differential selection of subjects or differential dropout of subjects during follow-up. These are variants of selection bias. A bias may also be induced by systematic differences in the way the data is obtained between groups. For example, when information concerning an exposure, for example, childhood trauma, is asked retrospectively to subjects with and without depression, it is likely that the depressed subjects have better recollection of these events not because they experienced more, but because low mood may make them biased to recollecting negative memories and because they are searching for meaning with regard to their depressive experiences. Such a bias is an example of an observation or information bias. Although the existence of bias in the results cannot always be prevented, some efforts can be made to minimise them. This is all the more important because, contrary to the situation with confounding, bias cannot be corrected for in the analyses. Strategies to minimise bias are now described.

One strategy is to consider carefully the choice of the study population. For example, the selection of hospitalised control subjects in a case-control study will increase the comparability with the cases in terms of willingness to participate, selective factors that influence the choice of the hospital, and so forth. For cohort studies, bias due to losses to follow-up is the greatest threat. To prevent this, one can choose populations that have a better chance of being located in the future, such as subjects who are well defined with respect to occupation, place of residence or being alumni of a particular institution. A strategy to prevent observation bias is to use, for example, highly objective and clear questions, and to give standardised training to research assistants in administering questionnaires so as to ensure that the administration of questionnaires is not influenced in some way by characteristics of the subjects. Thus, thinking about the design is important in the prevention of bias. Not all bias can be prevented, however. Therefore, one should make an effort as well in the phase of interpreting the results to take into account any possible effects of bias. One can develop arguments regarding which possible biases may have played a role and in which direction a bias would have acted; that is, whether it would have caused a spurious association or, on the contrary, would have masked an existing real effect.

Confounding

A third threat to the validity of an association is confounding. Confounding exists when the association between two variables is caused by a third variable that influences both. Thus, to confound an association between an exposure and a disease, the confounder must be associated with the exposure and, independent of that, predict the disease (see Figure 3.2).

Several strategies can control for confounding, both in the design phase and in the analysis phase. Three methods can be used to control for confounding in the design: randomisation, restriction and matching. In *randomisation*, subjects are allocated randomly to the various conditions (experimental or control conditions). With a sufficient number of subjects, the advantage is that any differences in characteristics of subjects between groups are minimised. For example, the study is about the therapeutic effects of an antipsychotic treatment, and "number of previous psychotic episodes" is a possible confounder. If subjects are randomised to the experimental and control conditions, the number of psychotic episodes will not confound the results because chance predicts that both groups will have the same characteristics with respect to number of past episodes. Thus randomisation ensures that all potential confounding factors, known or unknown by the investigator, are evenly distributed among treatment groups.

In the case of *restriction*, using the previous example, the sample would have been restricted to those subjects with a similar number of previous episodes. For example, one may choose to include only subjects with a single previous episode of psychosis. In the case of *individual matching*, which is most often used in case-control studies with small numbers of subjects, each subject in the case group with a certain characteristic – say, male sex – would be matched with an individual of the same sex in the control group.

If the design allows confounding to occur, control for confounding is possible in the analysis. One simple way to do this is by conducting a

---

Box 3.2 Considerations that contribute to likelihood of a causal association

- Strength of the association
- Temporal order
- Presence of dose-response relationship
- Biological plausibility
- Consistency with other investigations

---

stratified analysis. If sex, for example, is a potential confounder, the association between exposure and disease can be estimated separately for men and for women, making confounding by sex impossible. If socioeconomic status (low, middle, high) is an additional confounder, stratification into six categories is possible: man-low, man-middle, man-high social status and woman-low, woman-middle, woman-high social status. More variables to control for will require too many stratifications. In this case, another option used is multivariate analysis. The most common way is a multiple regression model. In regression, the outcome (or dependent variable) is predicted by the exposure (independent variable). One may add other possible predicting (independent) variables, such as sex, socioeconomic status and age, to this model. The result is a prediction of the exposure on the outcome that is independent of the effects of the other (confounding) variables in the model.

Judging a cause-effect relationship

Although testing the validity of an association is something to be accomplished in the design and analysis of one's study, the question of whether the association represents a cause-effect relationship needs to be judged using information from one's own *and* other studies on a topic. Some criteria can aid in the judgement of causality (see Box 3.2).

The first of these is *strength of association*. The stronger the association, the less likely that the relationship is due to the effect of some uncontrolled, unsuspected variable. However, this does not mean that associations of small magnitude cannot be

judged to be one of cause and effect, only that in such cases it is more difficult to exclude alternative explanations. Second, *temporal order* can provide good support for a causal relationship. Prospective cohort and intervention studies are capable of demonstrating whether the exposure preceded the disease outcome or not. It is obvious that in case of causality it is necessary for the exposure to precede disease outcome.

A third factor supporting causality is the *presence of a dose-response relationship*. If all subjects, from having smoked only one joint in their life to subjects who are heavy daily users of cannabis, all show the same magnitude of association with risk for psychosis then cannabis is less likely to be a causal risk factor. However, if a dose-response relationship existed, that is, minor cannabis use shows a smaller association with risk for psychosis than heavy cannabis use, causality would be supported.

Two criteria make use of evidence available from all studies concerning the topic. The first is one about *biological plausibility*. A cause-effect relationship is more likely if a biological mechanism can be postulated to explain the effect. For example, with cannabis use, psychosis association is more likely to be causal if evidence can be invoked showing that the cannabinoid receptors in the brain interact with the dopamine system. However, the lack of a known mechanism does not mean that the association is not causal. Most brain mechanisms underlying psychiatric disorders are still unknown and have yet to be discovered. The other criterion is *consistency with other investigations*. This is perhaps the most convincing evidence available in science for cause-effect relationships: not one but several studies using different methodologies in different places and using various samples all show similar results (Hennekens & Buring, 2004; Rothman & Greenland, 1998). To support the causality of a certain association, one should collect and compare all studies available on the topic. For this purpose, meta-analyses are conducted. A *meta-analysis* is a statistical analysis of a collection of studies. Such analyses combine the results of different studies in

Box 3.3 Shortcomings of a meta-analytic approach

Overconclusiveness

Researchers conducting meta-analyses can be too eager in their conclusions when disregarding the fact that

- large numbers of subjects lead to very narrow confidence intervals for the effect estimate,
- biases may have occurred uniformly in the studies included in the analysis, and
- the statistical summary blends together results that may have unmeasured differences in validity.

Aggregation bias

Because regression methods are used in meta-analyses that regress group outcome rates on group exposure means (ecologic regression), the same problem arises as in correlational studies: the relation between group exposure and outcome may not resemble the relation between individual values of exposure and outcome.

Publication bias

If the studies included in the meta-analyses are a biased sample of studies, this may bias the conclusion of the meta-analysis. This may occur because journals more often accept more articles with positive compared with negative results. Small "positive" studies are particularly subject to publication bias. An indication that this bias is operating is a relative lack of inclusion of small studies with nonsignificant results. Some meta-analyses therefore exclude all small studies. This strategy, however, is sensible only when small studies contain a small proportion of the observed data.

Small studies

Statistical tests depend on the assumption of normality. Some studies are so small that it is unreasonable to assume normality. If a large proportion of the total weight comes from small studies like this, then statistics used in the meta-analyses may be invalid.

Bias in exclusion of studies

Exclusion of studies from the meta-analyses may induce bias if they are excluded because of a prejudice against certain methods or when decision to exclude is based on the results. Some studies, however, must be excluded because there is too little information to allow the extraction of an effect size. Meta-analyses should report all exclusions and the reasons for these.

the hope of finding consistent patterns. There are shortcomings from the meta-analytic approach, however, as detailed in Box 3.3. For further reading, see Rothman and Greenland (1998).

Thus, the judgement of causality is not something that can be concluded from only one study. Different pieces of evidence, including results from other studies, should be brought together before a judgement of causality can be made. Therefore, true scientific knowledge is not something that is produced rapidly by one researcher, but grows steadily through the combined effort of many researchers examining a hypothesis.

Conclusion

The most important aspect of all research is that the researcher must continue questioning and thinking about why the data are as they are. Dry findings alone do not mean anything. Is the discovered association a valid association? If so, is it a causal association? What, then, can one conclude from the finding in general? Or, does something in the design of the study prevent obtaining data that is representative of reality? Knowledge of epidemiology is absolutely essential to be able to engage in the thinking process demonstrated in this chapter, which is obligatory for all scientific research and, perhaps more important, for the interface between science and clinical practice.

REFERENCES

Hennekens, C. H., & Buring, J. E. (1987). *Epidemiology in Medicine*. Philadelphia: Lippincott Williams & Wilkins.

Malik, A. R., & Ravasia, S. (2004). Interferon-induced mania. *Can J Psychiatry* 49:867–8.

Rothman, K. J., & Greenland, S. (1998). *Modern Epidemiology*, 2nd edn. Philadelphia: Lippincott-Raven.

4

Imaging of brain structure and function: relevance to psychiatric disorders

David Mamo and Shitij Kapur

Psychiatry has had a chequered history that is in part attributed to the stigma associated with severe mental illness, but that is also a result of the elusive pathophysiology and diverse presentations of psychiatric disorders. In some ways, however, the attitudinal shifts in this field have come full circle over the past century, moving from a more "organic" attribution to more "functional" explanatory models, and more recently to the current refreshing lines of investigation addressing the relationship between predisposing biological factors (e.g. genetics) and psychosocial stressors (e.g. immigration) in the development and manifestations of severe mental illness. Further, pathophysiology is increasingly being understood within the context of a dysfunction of interrelated brain regions, in contrast to simplistic explanations of single neurotransmitter abnormalities. The recent re-emergence of a role for surgical interventions in the form of deep brain stimulation (Kopell *et al.*, 2004) is perhaps one of the most cogent illustrations of this exciting development in the field of psychiatry, a role that has been closely linked with our understanding of the corticostriatothalamocortical (CSTC) loops in the pathophysiology of psychiatric symptoms (Mayberg, 2003). Not surprisingly, functional brain imaging studies have played a pivotal role in our understanding of the CSTC loops, which in turn has allowed for the recent promising interventions such as deep brain stimulation in major depressive disorder (Mayberg *et al.*, 2005).

A search in the PubMed database for articles relating to "imaging" in depression, schizophrenia and dementia yields more than 12,000 articles. Clearly this has been an intensive field of scientific study. At the same time, it is not possible comprehensively to cover all the brain imaging studies of structure and function as relevant to all psychiatric disorders. Therefore, we have chosen three paradigmatic examples and have illustrated each of them in some detail to provide the reader insight as to how these methods have been applied in research studies and what may be expected of them in terms of translation to clinical practice over the next decade (Table 4.1). In particular, we have chosen studies of depression that use structural and functional imaging to examine the roles of different brain circuits and neurochemicals (in particular, serotonin) in the pathophysiology and treatment of the illness. We have reviewed data from structural and functional studies of schizophrenia with a particular focus on the impact of structural imaging studies on the neurodevelopmental hypothesis, as well as studies of the brain transmitter dopamine and its receptors and its impact in understanding psychosis and its treatment. Finally, we illustrate early clinical applications of structural and functional imaging in dementia of the Alzheimer's type, as well as the role of new positron emission tomography (PET) tracers targeting known histopathological markers of the illness.

Essential Psychiatry, ed. Robin M. Murray, Kenneth S. Kendler, Peter McGuffin, Simon Wessely, David J. Castle.
Published by Cambridge University Press. © Cambridge University Press 2008.

Table 4.1 Main imaging technologies in psychiatry and their main applications

Technology	Applications
Structural magnetic resonance imaging (MRI) In MR, hydrogen atoms are aligned in a strong magnetic field followed by a radiofrequency pulse which temporarily disrupts this alignment; realignment of the protons follows the discontinuation of the pulse, which in turn releases a radiofrequency energy signal detected by a series of coils in the scanner. The strength of this signal is related to the number of protons aligned to the magnetic field (hence greater signal in water-rich regions – CSF ¿ gray matter ¿ white matter) and the strength of the magnets inducing the proton alignment.	1. Provides good contrast between gray matter, white matter, and CSF. 2. Resolution allows for identification of gross pathology associated with neuropsychiatric manifestations (e.g. frontal lobe tumours, ischemic lesions, encephalitis, normal pressure hydrocephalus). 3. Volumetric studies or gray and white matter as well as ventricular volume 4. Allows study of association between structural lesions (e.g. white matter hyperintensities) and neuropsychological manifestations. 5. Allows co-registration of anatomical details for region of interest identification with other imaging modalities (e.g. neurochemical PET)
Functional MRI (fMRI) fMRI uses MR principles that take advantage of changes in blood oxygenation and flow during activation of brain regions in response to a cognitive task.	Measurement of changes in BOLD signal compared with baseline following a cognitive task or in the presence of neuropathology can form the basis of hypotheses regarding brain function and pathophysiology.
Magnetic resonance spectroscopy (MRS) Using MR principles, MRS is based on the fact that protons within structures are constrained by adjacent molecules to the extent that they resonate to the radiofrequency pulse. This allows for a spectrum of detected signals which forms a biochemical "signature" along the MR spectrum that can be measured in vivo.	1. Provides measurement of neuronal and glial metabolism and functional integrity (e.g. measurements of NAA in schizophrenia). 2. Provides measurement of neurotransmitters (e.g. γ aminobutyric acid). 3. Allows central quantification of drugs (e.g. lithium, SSRIs).
Diffusion tensor MRI (DTI) Noninvasive visualisation of white matter tracts using MR that is based on the preferential motion of water molecules along white matter fibres (termed "anisotropic diffusion")	1. Study of the structural integrity of white matter tracts (aka tractography) 2. Development of models of connectivity and brain function in health and disease 3. Study of structural disconnectivity between cerebral regions and the relationship to neuropsychiatric signs and symptoms
Positron emission tomography (PET) Following the administration of positron emitting radiotracers, usually through an intravenous route, the signal is detected by a PET or single photon emission computed tomography (SPECT) camera, resulting in a dynamic series of images over the scanning time period. Depending on the tracer used, the research objective, and the design, time activity curves are generated either using a hypothesis-driven approach (region of interest) or exploratory approach (voxel-based) to generate specific parameters including binding potential and volume of distribution.	Depending on the tracer used, PET and SPECT can be used to study: 1. cerebral blood flow, uptake of oxygen, and glucose metabolism in activation studies analogous to fMRI (e.g. 2-deoxy-2-[^{18}F]fluoro-D-glucose or ^{18}FDG). 2. imaging of neurochemical processes (e.g. [^{18}F]DOPA for the study of dopamine synthesis). 3. binding of radiotracer to neurotransmitter receptors to study neuroreceptor density or an indirect measure of transmitter release (e.g. [^{11}C]raclopride for D_2 receptors). 4. drug occupancy at neuroreceptors.

BOLD = blood oxygen level–dependent; CSF = cerebrospinal fluid; SSRIs = selective serotonin reuptake inhibitors.

The ultimate goals of all these research strategies are fourfold: (1) the early identification of individuals at risk of developing the respective illness, (2) the initiation and prospective testing of preventative therapeutic strategies using neuroimaging as a tool to study the progression of the pathophysiology in vivo, (3) the in vivo dissection of pathophysiology and mechanism of action of psychotropic medication used to manage the illness and (4) the development of new medication and treatment strategies. Because our goal in writing this chapter was to provide an overview of how neuroimaging research is contributing to these four domains, we have provided a selection of key references that the interested reader may wish to consider for further details.

Major depressive disorder

Major depression is one of the most common – and arguably, for most patients, one of the most treatable – major psychiatric conditions. Nonetheless, the disorder not only carries major human and economic cost, but also exhibits varying levels of response with more than half of patients showing insufficient response to first-line antidepressant treatment (Insel, 2006). As a result, a trial-and-error–based strategy of sequential and combination antidepressant, psychological and electroconvulsive therapy trials is often the norm in the management of this disorder. Moreover, its clinical presentation and triggering factors also show a large degree of variation across age, cultures and comorbid medical conditions, suggesting that a single brain region is unlikely to be responsible for this clinical syndrome. Recent evidence from neuroimaging data suggests that a disruption of a neural network including a number of cortical and subcortical structures and their associated signal transduction systems occurs in predisposed individuals, leading to the clinical manifestations of signs and symptoms of a depressive syndrome. Therapeutic strategies including antidepressant drugs and psychotherapeutic interventions would therefore be

expected to exert their therapeutic effects through modulation of these systems. A better understanding of the neural pathways involved in depression and clinical tools for predictors of response to the respective therapies are urgently needed in drug development and clinical practice, and functional imaging studies are showing promising results that are already in early stages of clinical translation.

A dysregulation in the cortical-subcortical pathways in depression is supported by early structural imaging studies in both adult and elderly patients with unipolar depression showing increased periventricular and deep white matter hyperintensities consistent with a purported disruption in white matter tracts. Furthermore, these studies have also found decreased frontal lobe and basal ganglia volumes, as well as hyperintensities in the thalamus and striatum. These findings persist after controlling for cardiovascular risk factors and occur more commonly in late-life depression, supporting a relationship with vascular disease in the elderly (Gupta *et al.*, 2004). Because depression often presents in the context of intact cognition and general physical health at least in younger adults, contributory functional studies in this disorder would be expected to demonstrate (1) increased or decreased activity in structures involved in the disrupted neural system relative to the healthy control condition, (2) a relationship between functional changes and measures of clinical severity and response and (3) restoration to the expected baseline functional maps following remission of depressive symptoms.

Results of PET and functional magnetic resonance imaging (fMRI) studies in depression have provided convergent results to support this general relationship. Functional imaging studies have demonstrated changes in metabolism in the prefrontal cortex, anterior cingulate and amygdala in depression, and these findings are at least in part reversed with antidepressant treatment and cognitive behavioural therapy (Goldapple *et al.*, 2004; Kennedy *et al.*, 2001), supporting a model of dysregulation in the cortico-limbic neural pathways. Furthermore, higher levels of prefrontal activity in depression predict better clinical response to treatment (Mayberg, 2002). In this model, hypofunction of the dorsal prefrontal cortex and cingulate gyrus would be expected to account for cognitive and psychomotor signs and symptoms of depression, whereas hyperfunction of the ventral brain regions, including the insula, hypothalamus and brainstem putatively result in neurovegetative symptoms.

The recent availability of a radio-labelled ligand for the serotonin transporter (5-HTT) has allowed the use of neurochemical PET to study the binding of antidepressant drugs in vivo. Five selective serotonin reuptake inhibitors (SSRIs) have been studied using this method (citalopram, paroxetine, fluoxetine, sertraline and venlafaxine), and at minimal therapeutic doses, these drugs were associated with at least 80% occupancy in striatal 5-HTT (Meyer et al., 2004). This similar level of occupancy was achieved notwithstanding a threefold variation in the affinity of the respective SSRIs in vitro, suggesting that in vitro analysis may not necessarily predict in vivo binding, an observation consistent with similar work using antipsychotic drugs. Using a different radiotracer for 5-HTT, another research group reported similar level of occupancy using minimum therapeutic dose of fluvoxamine, although the tricyclic clomipramine achieved 100% occupancy at subclinical doses, suggesting that this threshold may not necessarily generalise to tricyclic antidepressants (Suhara et al., 2003). In contrast to clomipramine, SSRIs do not reach higher than 90% occupancy; this finding has been taken as support for the clinical superiority of clomipramine in obsessive-compulsive disorder (Zipursky et al., 2007).

A PET radiotracer for the serotonin 5-HT$_{2A}$ receptor has also been used to study dysfunctional attitudes in depression (e.g. pessimism), and higher levels of pessimism were related to a higher 5-HT$_{2A}$ binding potential (a measure of receptor density) (Meyer et al., 2003). In light of a decrease in dysfunctional attitudes in healthy control subjects following the administration of a single-dose of d-fenfluramine (a serotoninergic agonist), the authors concluded that low levels of serotonin agonism

in the brain cortex may explain the dysfunctional attitudes associated with major depression (Meyer et al., 2003).

Recently a new PET radiotracer for the monoamine oxidase-A (MAO-A) enzyme has been developed, providing a critical tool in the study of the role of central monoamines in depression and its treatment (Ginovart et al., 2006). A recent PET study of unmedicated depressed subjects found elevated MAO-A activity across several brain regions, supporting the monoamine theory of depression (Meyer et al., 2006), which is consistent with the previous PET data showing elevated dopamine and serotonin receptor density. In this model, elevated MAO-A activity would be expected to result in decreased release of the catecholamine in the synaptic space, resulting in a number of depressive symptoms through various mechanisms (e.g. decreased dopamine associated with motor slowing and upregulation of D$_2$ receptors; decreased serotonin associated with pessimism and upregulation of 5HT$_{2A}$ receptors).

In summary, brain imaging in major depressive disorder has contributed to a better understanding of the pathophysiology of the illness from a neural system perspective as well as at the synaptic level (Table 4.2). This knowledge has in turn led to the remergence of targeted surgical approaches, as well as providing tools for the clinical development of antidepressant drugs and the finer dissection at the cellular level of the mechanisms involved in the presentation and management of the depressive syndrome. It is anticipated that in addition to contributing new knowledge in existing therapeutic strategies, these imaging tools will play an important role in the development of new antidepressant drugs and the better use of other emerging treatment modalities (e.g. Repetitive Transcranial Magnetic Stimulation or rTMS).

Schizophrenia

Brain imaging in schizophrenia has played a prominent role in re-establishing this devastating illness

Table 4.2 Salient neuroimaging findings in depression

Structural magnetic resonance imaging	1. Periventricular and deep white matter hyperintensities
	2. Decreased frontal lobe and basal ganglia volumes
	3. Hyperintensities in the thalamus and striatum
Positron emission tomography	1. Decreased metabolism and blood flow in the prefrontal cortex, anterior cingulate, and amygdala
	2. Higher levels of prefrontal metabolism predict better clinical response to treatment
	3. Minimum therapeutic doses of SSRIs associated with 80% serotonin transporter occupancy
	4. Dysfunctional attitudes associated with higher 5-HT$_{2A}$ receptor density
	5. Increased monoamine oxidase-A activity
	6. Elevated D2 receptor binding in untreated depression and associated with motor slowing

SSRIs = selective serotonin reuptake inhibitors.

as a brain disorder and decreasing the social stigma attached to severe mental illness. The most prominent and best-replicated structural findings include lateral ventricular enlargement, loss of overall gray matter and loss of temporal lobe volumes, although these changes are neither specific nor sensitive enough to allow for diagnostic use (Gupta *et al.*, 2004). Nonetheless, the findings of volume reductions in the superior temporal lobes even in prodromal and high-risk subjects laid to rest the notion that the onset of psychosis was a random insult to the brain in late adolescence and contributed to the developmental hypothesis for schizophrenia that has been arguably as influential in modern schizophrenia research as the dopamine hypothesis was a few decades ago. Volumetric changes in schizophrenia is perhaps one of the first (since the early times of pneumoencephalography) and most widely replicated findings in this field (Torrey, 2002) with studies in both unmedicated and previously medicated patients showing up to a 25% increase in lateral ventricular volume compared with control subjects. A recent meta-analysis of MRI studies in schizophrenia found that the most significant changes occur within the medial temporal lobe, an effect also noted in first-degree relatives but to a smaller extent (Boos, 2006). Functional imaging studies have shown a decrease in prefrontal blood flow and metabolism while subjects performed cognitive tasks normally associated with prefrontal

cortical activation (e.g. Tower of London task; Callicott, 2003) and magnetic resonance spectroscopy (MRS) studies have shown a decrease in N-acetyl aspartate (NAA – a measure of neuronal integrity) in the same region, which predicts negative symptomatology (Callicott *et al.*, 2000a, 2000b).

A question of great interest is how these findings change over time. Structural studies suggest that cerebral volume loss may be related to duration of illness: patients with chronic illness show more volume loss compared with patients in their first episode, although the changes in the first-episode patients is strongly correlated with the prescribed dose of antipsychotic medication, suggesting a possible selection bias – that is, severely ill patients with smaller cerebral volumes at baseline may require higher dosages of medication (Keshavan *et al.*, 2005). Further, these changes are also noted in nonaffected relatives, including unaffected co-twins and subjects considered to be at very high risk of developing schizophrenia, indicating trait- rather than state-dependent structural changes. Whether this volume loss is a consequence of early development as opposed to later adolescent changes awaits longitudinal studies. The current evidence points to an evolving loss of gray matter volume, including temporal lobe volume starting at least a few years before the clinical onset of psychosis (Job *et al.*, 2006; Pantelis *et al.*, 2003), an observation that holds promise in the prediction of emergent psychosis in high-risk individuals and the appropriate targeting of early intervention trials. Finally, the differences noted between first-episode and chronic patients may suggest an ongoing loss of cerebral volume, although it is equally plausible that patients with severe illness who later develop chronic symptoms suffer severe volume loss earlier in the illness, which then remains stable over time.

Neurochemical PET has also played an important role in our present understanding of schizophrenia and the optimal use of antipsychotic drugs. Over the past decades, a number of PET studies have focused on the occupancy of striatal dopamine receptors by antipsychotic drugs, suggesting that for most antipsychotic drugs, clinical effects are generally expected at doses resulting in more than 60% occupancy of dopamine D_2 receptors, whereas occupancy greater than 80% predicts the emergence of hyperprolactinemia and extrapyramidal side effects (Kapur & Mamo, 2003). Recently it has been demonstrated that clinically effective doses of aripiprazole result in more than 80% striatal D_2 occupancy in the absence of extrapyramidal side effects, an observation that is best explained by the drug's partial agonist profile (Mamo et al., 2006; Yokoi et al., 2002). This line of research has contributed to the identification of appropriate dosing of antipsychotic drugs in a dose range within the occupancy threshold of 60% to 80% striatal D_2 occupancy for drugs with an antagonist pharmacological profile.

The emergence of atypical antipsychotics is also largely based on the in vitro and in vivo PET findings of a higher binding to serotonin $5\text{-}HT_{2A}$ receptors compared to dopamine D_2 receptors, a pharmacological profile that was thought to be the basis of the atypical profile of the newer antipsychotic drugs. The atypical profile of amisulpride (specific D_2 profile) and the high $D_2/5HT_{2A}$ profile of aripiprazole argue against this assertion.

Finally, neurochemical PET has allowed for the possibility of a pharmacodynamic biomarker in early drug development based on the demonstration that a candidate drug in Phase I clinical development (a) crosses the blood-brain barrier and (b) binds to the neuroreceptor target. Although seemingly insignificant to the practicing physician, this is an important milestone in early drug development.

Neurochemical PET imaging has also contributed to a direct in vivo validation of the dopamine hypothesis of schizophrenia, which posits that positive symptoms of schizophrenia are associated with an increased dopamine release in the striatum, an effect that is then neutralised using the appropriate dose of an antipsychotic drug (Abi-Dargham, 2004). This line of research suggests that acute psychosis is associated with increased dopamine release in response to an amphetamine challenge (Abi-Dargham et al., 1998). Using a different paradigm, the same group showed that following synaptic endogenous dopamine depletion using α-methyl para-tyrosine (AMPT), D_2 binding was higher in patients with schizophrenia compared to healthy controls, consistent with increased baseline occupancy of D_2 receptors by dopamine in schizophrenia (Abi-Dargham et al., 2000). Furthermore, high baseline D_2 occupancy (or a state of high dopamine release) predicted response of positive symptoms to antipsychotic treatment. More recent evidence using radiolabelled DOPA as a measure of presynaptic dopamine function has suggested that, compared with healthy control subjects, dopaminergic function is elevated both in medication-free subjects in their first episode of psychosis and in nonpsychotic subjects considered at high risk of developing psychosis (Howes et al., 2006). These studies suggest that a hyperdopaminergic state is present even before the emergence of frank psychosis, and the degree of dopamine release may predict response to antipsychotic drugs – findings that have significant implications for ongoing research of predictors of response as well as for management strategies for prodromal and high-risk individuals.

In summary, as outlined in Table 4.3, neuroimaging studies in schizophrenia have firmly established the biological basis of this devastating and highly stigmatised disorder, have identified loss of cerebral

Table 4.3 Salient neuroimaging findings in schizophrenia

Structural magnetic resonance imaging (MRI)	1. Ventricular enlargement 2. Overall loss of volume of gray matter 3. Specific loss of prefrontal and medial temporal gray matter 4. Brain volume loss progressive, at least in first few years of illness
Functional MRI	Decreased activation in prefrontal cortex during specific executive tasks
Magnetic resonance spectroscopy	Decreased NAA in prefrontal cortex consistent with neuronal loss in this region and predicts negative symptoms
Diffusion tensor MRI	Widespread decreased white matter fractional anisotropy, including frontotemporal white matter and corpus callosum; changes more pronounced in chronically treated than first-episode patients, raising the possibility of progressive loss
Positron emission tomography	1. Validation of dopamine hypothesis of schizophrenia: high dopamine release is associated with acute psychosis and predicts response 2. Mechanism of action of antipsychotic drugs (binding to striatal D_2 receptors, relevance of extrastriatal binding, relevance of binding to other receptors including serotonin receptors) 3. Drug development and prediction of therapeutic dose range

volume and brain function specifically in interconnected brain areas implicated in schizophrenia (e.g. prefrontal cortex – executive deficits and negative symptoms; thalamus – impaired sensory processing and higher pain threshold; basal ganglia – spontaneous dyskinesias in untreated patients, substance abuse and increased incidence of schizophrenia; abherent salience). Furthermore, PET studies have provided in vivo evidence for a hyperdopaminergic state in psychotic disorders consistent with the dopamine hypothesis and direct evidence that antipsychotic drugs exert their therapeutic effects and neurological side effects through binding at dopamine D_2 receptors. The next major frontier in the application of these tools is relating these imaging findings with predisposing genetic polymorphisms (Egan *et al.*, 2001), as well as understanding the interaction between environmental stressors (e.g. social defeat theory and substance use) and predisposing genetic factors. This is expected to lead to the identification of a biological endophenotype – an objective "brain image" of the illness – which will be critical in our ability to predict the efficacy of targeted pharmacological, psychological and possibly even social interventions for primary psychotic disorders.

Dementia of the Alzheimer type (DAT)

Alzheimer's disease, the most common type of dementia, is a progressive neuropsychiatric disorder characterised by progressive memory and other cognitive impairments, as well as behavioural disturbance in the later stages of the illness. The disease affects up to 6% of the population over age 65 years; in light of worldwide demographic changes, it is anticipated that the prevalence of the illness will more than double over the next 2 decades. Not surprisingly, the early detection of Alzheimer's disease has advanced rapidly on the list of priorities in mental health research, largely on the basis of the expectation that it will allow for therapeutic and preventative strategies to ward off the progression of the illness. Even though more is known about the pathophysiology and genetics of Alzheimer's disease than any other major psychiatric disorder, the diagnosis is based on history and mental status examination, and treatment remains largely supportive in nature. Neuroimaging in Alzheimer's disorder is therefore discussed here within the context of an emergent public health crisis concerning an illness with a relatively well-characterised histopathology – the academic and pharmaceutical research and development process is therefore under intense pressure to identify strategies for early diagnosis and prevention of this illness that can last from 5 to 20 years and imposes a great human and economic cost on our society.

The earliest histopathological change in Alzheimer's disease is the deposition of amyloid plaques containing insoluble sheets of $A\beta$ peptides appearing first in the basal neocortex and then spreading progressively in a rostral and dorsal direction (Nordberg, 2004). Although the role of $A\beta$ in cognitive impairment and subsequent microglial and oxidative stress consequences and neuronal death remains controversial, the observation of more aggregable forms of $A\beta$ in rare forms of hereditary transmission of mutations of the amyloid precursor protein and the presenilin gene support a central role for amyloid in Alzheimer's disease. Similarly, although the total amount of amyloid deposition may not necessarily be related to clinical status in the individual patient, subjects with mild cognitive impairment (MCI) tend to have more amyloid deposition, and the amyloid load within the entorhinal cortex (thought to be involved in memory consolidation) has been related to cognitive deficits in one post-mortem study (Cummings & Cotman, 1995). The second key histopathological change associated with Alzheimer's disease is the presence of neurofibrillary tangles (NFT), consisting of hyperphosphorylated helical pairs of tau protein (an important cytoskeletal element forming microtubules). NFTs follow the same pattern of deposition as amyloid in cortical areas receiving cholinergic projections and are thought to play a critical role in mediating neuronal death.

Gross structural changes have long been established in Alzheimer's disease, and MRI is very sensitive in detecting loss of medial temporal lobe volume (Zakzanis et al., 2003), although it is neither specific to Alzheimer's disease nor are the time demands of manual volumetric analysis a practical application for routine clinical use (Gupta et al., 2004). The introduction of automated methods may lend themselves to broader clinical applications in this field, including the longitudinal monitoring of cerebral and hippocampal volume loss and its relationship to widely used clinical measures such as the Mini-Mental State Examination (MMSE). Nonetheless, at this time structural imaging is restricted to ruling out other causes of cognitive decline, including space-occupying lesions such as haematomas and tumours, hydrocephalus, infarcts and white matter changes associated with vascular dementia. Although an argument can be made for the indication of a structural scan at least once in every patient with dementia, structural imaging is definitely indicated in the presence of early-onset dementia, unusually abrupt-onset or changes in symptomatology, as well as abnormal gait or focal neurological signs. However, in the vast majority of patients with an established diagnosis of dementia, structural imaging is generally noncontributory. However, functional changes in the brain can be detected earlier, allowing for the emergence of single photon emission computed tomography (SPECT; Johnson et al., 1998) – and to a lesser degree PET, which is less widely available – as an accepted imaging technique in patients showing early insidious cognitive decline, especially in the presence of frontal lobe signs and symptoms. PET and SPECT studies in DAT show diminished blood flow in the posterior temporal and inferior parietal cortices, with temporal changes predictive of later-onset of MCI and DAT in healthy elderly individuals (Fazekas et al., 1989; Yamaguchi et al., 1997). Because similar changes can be detected with fMRI, this modality (and MRS) may in the future become the functional imaging methods of choice in the early detection of DAT.

Although impairment of brain glucose metabolism using PET has been detected many years before clinical presentation in subjects with the rare genetic mutations associated with hereditary Alzheimer's disease (Kennedy et al., 1995), as well as in patients with MCI compared with healthy control subjects (Arnaiz et al., 2001), the ability to monitor histopathological changes in vivo including amyloid beta and NFTs will be critical in the early detection and monitoring of response to novel therapeutic strategies, particularly when used in conjunction with other biomarkers (e.g. apolipoprotein E ε4 status) and structural and functional imaging – particularly in combination with ^{18}F-fluoro-deoxy-glucose PET, which already has an established role in the differential diagnosis of Alzheimer's dementia and frontotemporal lobar degeneration (Rabinovici *et al.*, 2007).

In practice, dementia remains a clinical diagnosis, and although imaging has provided an invaluable tool for challenging diagnostic situations, in the absence of neurological signs or unusual clinical presentation or course of illness, they add little to the clinical outcome for most patients. However, if our field is to have a tangible impact on the expected rise in dementia in our rapidly aging population, new drug development targeting dementia will be significantly expedited with imaging tools that would allow the monitoring of histopathological changes of the illness. Therefore, the recent advances in PET technology, particularly in the development of three PET radiotracers targeting amyloid beta protein and NFTs, may be the first and most significant step in this direction (Cai *et al.*, 2007; Nordberg, 2004; Rabinovici *et al.*, 2007). This is particularly important because the most significant novel therapeutic strategies will likely target amyloid deposition; tools for monitoring response in vivo will therefore be critical in their human testing if they are to be used as a preventative strategy or in the early and preclinical stage of cognitive decline associated with Alzheimer's disease (MCI).

Three PET tracers have been developed and tested in human subjects ([^{18}F]FDDNP, [^{11}C]PIB, and [^{11}C]SB-13), and all three tracers have shown higher retention in the cortical regions of patients with Alzheimer's disease compared with healthy control subjects (Cai *et al.*, 2007). [^{18}F]FDDNP was the first successful in vivo PET tracer in patients with AD and is thought to label both NFTs and Aβ protein (Shoghi-Jadid *et al.*, 2002) – this may prove useful in the early and preclinical detection and monitoring of the disease, but more

complicated in the monitoring of response to amyloid-specific therapeutic strategies. [^{11}C]PIB, also known as Pittsburgh Compound-B, was the second successful PET tracer showing a high degree of differentiation between AD patients and control subjects (Klunk *et al.*, 2004) and is thought to be more specific to Aβ protein. The most recent tracer to be developed is the [^{11}C]SB-13 PET tracer (Verhoeff *et al.*, 2004), which shows a similar distribution of binding and discrimination of pathology as Pittsburgh Compound-B. These tracers await further replication and validation studies in larger samples and subjects with MCI or at ultra-high risk of Alzheimer's disease, although they represent a concrete step in the application of known histopathology to imaging studies which may well translate into the first clinical application of neuroimaging in psychiatry. Table 4.4 summarises neuroimaging findings in DAT.

Conclusions

In this brief overview, we have provided a sample of how various neuroimaging modalities have contributed to our current understanding and treatment of psychiatric disorders. Without doubt the imaging approaches have increased our understanding of the neurobiological basis of mental illnesses and their treatments. What they have not readily produced is a "test" that can be used to diagnose, individualise treatment, or predict outcome. Although there are hundreds of studies showing statistically significant findings, they have not been translated into useable clinical tools. At least two realities may have slowed this translation: the first is the sample-to-sample variability across studies, such that a finding in one is either only partially replicated or sometimes even refuted in a different sample. Second, even for consistently replicated findings, the effect size tends to be relatively small. Small effect sizes yield too many false negatives and false positives (see Chapter 3) to be useful as clinical tests, limiting clinical applicability to the individual patient (as opposed to "samples" or

Table 4.4 Salient neuroimaging findings in dementia of the Alzheimer type

Structural magnetic resonance imaging (MRI)	1. Absence of space-occupying lesions, hydrocephalus and cerebral infarcts 2. Ventricular enlargement and loss of cerebral gray with earliest change being loss of temporal lobe volume
Functional MRI	Decreased activation in posterior temporal and inferior parietal lobes
Magnetic resonance spectroscopy (MRS)	Decreased NAA and increased myoinositol reflecting decreased neuronal viability and increased gliosis or metabolic dysfunction respectively; changes observed in medial temporal cortex and frontal lobes
Diffusion tensor MRI	Decreased white matter fractional anisotropy in association tracts of temporal lobe
Positron Emission Tomography	1. Decreased cerebral blood flow and metabolism in posterior temporal and inferior parietal lobes present in early stages of the illness 2. Visualisation of amyloid plaques (not diagnostic)

"groups" of patients). Nevertheless, we predict that the earliest clinical applications of neuroimaging in psychiatry will likely occur in the early recognition and treatment response strategies (e.g. predicting and/or preventing the conversion of MCI to dementia), the prediction of clinical response to pharmacological and surgical management (e.g. deep brain stimulation or DBS), and new drug development (e.g. amyloid-targeted strategies in dementia). It is therefore likely that the psychiatrists of 2020 will actually be using some of these technologies in routine clinical practice.

REFERENCES

Abi-Dargham, A. (2004). Do we still believe in the dopamine hypothesis? New data bring new evidence. *Int J Neuropsychopharmacol* 7(**Suppl 1**):S1–5.

Abi-Dargham, A., Gil, R., Krystal, J., *et al.* (1998). Increased striatal dopamine transmission in schizophrenia: confirmation in a second cohort. *Am J Psychiatry* 155:761–7.

Abi-Dargham, A., Rodenhiser, J., Printz, D., *et al.* (2000). Increased baseline occupancy of D2 receptors by dopamine in schizophrenia. *Proc Natl Acad Sci USA* 97:8104–9.

Arnaiz, E., Jelic, V., Almkvist, O., *et al.* (2001). Impaired cerebral glucose metabolism and cognitive functioning predict deterioration in mild cognitive impairment. *Neuroreport* 12:851–5.

Boos, H. B. M., Aleman, A., Cahn, W., & Kahn, R. S. (2006). Brain volumes in relatives of patients with schizophrenia: a meta-analysis. *Schizophr Res* 81:41.

Cai, L., Innis, R. B., & Pike, V. W. (2007). Radioligand development for PET imaging of beta-amyloid (Abeta) – current status. *Curr Med Chem* 14:19–52.

Callicott, J. H. (2003). An expanded role for functional neuroimaging in schizophrenia. *Curr Opin Neurobiol* 13:256–60.

Callicott, J. H., Bertolino, A., Egan, M. F., *et al.* (2000). Selective relationship between prefrontal N-acetylaspartate measures and negative symptoms in schizophrenia. *Am J Psychiatry* 157:1646–51.

Callicott, J. H., Bertolino, A., Mattay, V. S., *et al.* (2000). Physiological dysfunction of the dorsolateral prefrontal cortex in schizophrenia revisited. *Cereb Cortex* 10:1078–92.

Cummings, B. J., & Cotman, C. W. (1995). Image analysis of beta-amyloid load in Alzheimer's disease and relation to dementia severity. *Lancet* 346:1524–8.

Egan, M. F., Goldberg, T. E., Kolachana, B. S., *et al.* (2001). Effect of COMT Val108/158 Met genotype on frontal lobe function and risk for schizophrenia. *Proc Natl Acad Sci USA* 98:6917–22.

Fazekas, F., Alavi, A., Chawluk, J. B., *et al.* (1989). Comparison of CT, MR, and PET in Alzheimer's dementia and normal aging. *J Nucl Med* 30:1607–15.

Ginovart, N., Meyer, J. H., Boovariwala, A., *et al.* (2006). Positron emission tomography quantification of [(11)C]-harmine binding to monoamine oxidase-A in the human brain. *J Cereb Blood Flow Metab* 26:330–44.

Goldapple, K., Segal, Z., Garson, C., *et al.* (2004). Modulation of cortical-limbic pathways in major depression:

treatment-specific effects of cognitive behavior therapy. *Arch Gen Psychiatry* **61**:34–41.

Gupta, A., Elheis, M., & Pansari, K. (2004). Imaging in psychiatric illnesses. *Int J Clin Pract* **58**:850–8.

Howes, O., Montgomery, A. J., Asselin, M. C., *et al.* (2006). The pre-synaptic dopaminergic system before and after onset of psychosis: initial results from an from an ongoing [18F]Fluoro-DOPA PET study. *Schizophr Res* **81**:18.

Insel, T. R. (2006). Beyond efficacy: the STAR*D trial. *Am J Psychiatry* **163**:5–7.

Job, D. E., Whalley, H. C., Johnstone, E. C., & Lawrie, S. M. (2006). Structural imaging as an early diagnostic test in people at high risk of schizophrenia. *Schizophr Res* **81**:14.

Johnson, K. A., Jones, K., Holman, B. L., *et al.* (1998). Preclinical prediction of Alzheimer's disease using SPECT. *Neurology* **50**:1563–71.

Kapur, S., & Mamo, D. (2003). Half a century of antipsychotics and still a central role for dopamine D2 receptors. *Prog Neuropsychopharmacol Biol Psychiatry* **27**:1081–90.

Kennedy, S. H., Evans, K. R., Kruger, S., *et al.* (2001). Changes in regional brain glucose metabolism measured with positron emission tomography after paroxetine treatment of major depression. *Am J Psychiatry* **158**:899–905.

Kennedy, A. M., Frackowiak, R. S., Newman, S. K., *et al.* (1995). Deficits in cerebral glucose metabolism demonstrated by positron emission tomography in individuals at risk of familial Alzheimer's disease. *Neurosci Lett* **186**:1–20.

Keshavan, M. S., Berger, G., Zipursky, R. B., *et al.* (2005). Neurobiology of early psychosis. *Br J Psychiatry Suppl* **48**:s8–18.

Klunk, W. E., Engler, H., Nordberg, A., *et al.* (2004). Imaging brain amyloid in Alzheimer's disease with Pittsburgh Compound-B. *Ann Neurol* **55**:306–19.

Kopell, B. H., Greenberg, B., & Rezai, A. R. (2004). Deep brain stimulation for psychiatric disorders. *J Clin Neurophysiol* **21**:51–67.

Mamo, D., Graff A., Romeyer, F., Shammi, C. M., & Kapur S. (2006). Central D2 and 5HT2A occupancy of aripiprazole in patients with schizophrenia. *Schizophr Res* **81**:104–5.

Mayberg, H. (2002). Depression, II: localization of pathophysiology. *Am J Psychiatry* **159**:1979.

Mayberg, H. S. (2003). Modulating dysfunctional limbic-cortical circuits in depression: towards development of brain-based algorithms for diagnosis and optimised treatment. *Br Med Bull* **65**:193–207.

Mayberg, H. S., Lozano, A. M., Voon, V., *et al.* (2005). Deep brain stimulation for treatment-resistant depression. *Neuron* **45**:651–60.

Meyer, J. H., Ginovart, N., Boovariwala, A., *et al.* (2006) Elevated monoamine oxidase a levels in the brain: an explanation for the monoamine imbalance of major depression. *Arch Gen Psychiatry* **63(11)**:1209–16.

Meyer, J. H., Houle, S., Sagrati, S., *et al.* (2004a). Brain serotonin transporter binding potential measured with carbon 11-labeled DASB positron emission tomography: effects of major depressive episodes and severity of dysfunctional attitudes. *Arch Gen Psychiatry* **61**:1271–9.

Meyer, J. H., McMain, S., Kennedy, S. H., *et al.* (2003). Dysfunctional attitudes and 5-HT2 receptors during depression and self-harm. *Am J Psychiatry* **160**:90–9.

Meyer, J. H., Wilson, A. A., Sagrati, S., *et al.* (2004b). Serotonin transporter occupancy of five selective serotonin reuptake inhibitors at different doses: an [11C]DASB positron emission tomography study. *Am J Psychiatry* **161**:826–35.

Nordberg, A. (2004). PET imaging of amyloid in Alzheimer's disease. *Lancet Neurol* **3**:519–27.

Pantelis, C., Yucel, M., Wood, S. J., *et al.* (2003). Early and late neurodevelopmental disturbances in schizophrenia and their functional consequences. *Aust N Z J Psychiatry* **37**:399–406.

Rabinovici, G. D., Furst, A. J., O'Neil, J. P., *et al.* (2007). 11C-PIB PET imaging in Alzheimer disease and frontotemporal lobar degeneration. *Neurology* **68**:1205–12.

Shoghi-Jadid, K., Small, G. W., Agdeppa, E. D., *et al.* (2002). Localization of neurofibrillary tangles and beta-amyloid plaques in the brains of living patients with Alzheimer disease. *Am J Geriatr Psychiatry* **10**:24–35.

Suhara, T., Takano, A., Sudo, Y., *et al.* (2003). High levels of serotonin transporter occupancy with low-dose clomipramine in comparative occupancy study with fluvoxamine using positron emission tomography. *Arch Gen Psychiatry* **60**:386–91.

Torrey, E. F. (2002). Studies of individuals with schizophrenia never treated with antipsychotic medications: a review. *Schizophr Res* **58**:101–15.

Verhoeff, N. P., Wilson, A. A., Takeshita, S., *et al.* (2004). In-vivo imaging of Alzheimer disease beta-amyloid with [11C]SB-13 PET. *Am J Geriatr Psychiatry* **12**:584–95.

Yamaguchi, S., Meguro, K., Itoh, M., *et al.* (1997). Decreased cortical glucose metabolism correlates with hippocampal atrophy in Alzheimer's disease as shown by MRI and PET. *J Neurol Neurosurg Psychiatry* **62**: 596–600.

Yokoi, F., Grunder, G., Biziere, K., *et al.* (2002). Dopamine D2 and D3 receptor occupancy in normal humans treated with the antipsychotic drug aripiprazole (OPC 14597): a study using positron emission tomography and [11C]raclopride. *Neuropsychopharmacology* **27**:248–59.

Zakzanis, K. K., Graham, S. J., & Campbell, Z. (2003). A meta-analysis of structural and functional brain imaging in dementia of the Alzheimer's type: a neuroimaging profile. *Neuropsychol Rev* **13**:1–18.

Zipursky, R. B., Meyer, J. H., & Verhoeff, N. P. (2007). PET and SPECT imaging in psychiatric disorders. *Can J Psychiatry* **52(3)**:146–52.

5

Genetic epidemiology

Pak C. Sham and Kenneth S. Kendler

Although an inherited component in psychiatric disorders has been suspected for centuries, it was not until the early twentieth century that the gene concept was formulated and systematic genetic studies on psychiatric disorders began. The rapid development of molecular genetics in the second half of the 20th century, following the deciphering of the double helix structure of DNA, accelerated the pace of genetic research in psychiatry. In recent years, high-throughput molecular genetic technologies have enabled the sequencing of the entire human genome (International Human Genome Sequencing Consortium, 2001) and the identification of nearly all common genetic variations in major human populations. These developments in "genomics" will no doubt increase the power of psychiatric genetics to dissect out the genetic and environmental causes of mental disorders. However, all the evidence so far indicates that the majority of psychiatric disorders are complex in aetiology, suggesting that a holistic as well as reductive approach to research is required. Kendler (2005) formulated four paradigms in psychiatric genetics that have separate but interrelated goals and together provide an organizing framework to conceptualise different approaches and strategies (Box 5.1). This chapter describes the principles and methodology of psychiatric genetics using this four-paradigm framework. More detailed reviews of psychiatric genetics can be found in the textbooks *Psychiatric Genetics and Genomics*, edited by McGuffin,

Gottesman and Owen (2002), and *Psychiatric Genetics*, edited by Kendler and Eaves (2005).

Paradigm 1 – basic genetic epidemiology

The goal of *basic genetic epidemiology* is to quantify the degree to which individual differences in risk of (more technically *liability* to) illness results from familial effects (as assessed by a family study) or genetic factors (as determined by twin or adoption studies). Basic genetic epidemiology is the oldest of the four paradigms and began even before the formulation of the gene concept itself, with incidental observations by clinicians that some patients come from families with a strong history of the same disorder (Schulze *et al.*, 2004). The rediscovery of Mendel's seminal experiments on plant hybridization and the formulation and acceptance of the gene concept led to an intensification of the efforts to demonstrate genetic influences on mental disorders by the systematic study of families, twins and adoptees. It is important to point out that these studies, like the experiments of Mendel, do not require the direct measurement of genes. Rather, genetic influences are inferred indirectly through their effects of the pattern of disease among genetically related individuals. The ability to infer genetic influences without directly measuring them is similar to attempts by epidemiologists to infer the presence and nature of environmental influences by

Essential Psychiatry, ed. Robin M. Murray, Kenneth S. Kendler, Peter McGuffin, Simon Wessely, David J. Castle.
Published by Cambridge University Press. © Cambridge University Press 2008.

Box 5.1 Four major paradigms of psychiatric genetics

#	Title	Samples studied	Method of inquiry	Scientific goals
1	Basic genetic epidemiology	Family, twin and adoption studies	Statistical	To quantify the degree of familial aggregation and/or heritability
2	Advanced genetic epidemiology	Family, twin and adoption studies	Statistical	To explore the nature and mode of action of *genetic risk factors*
3	gene findingding	High-density families, trios, case-control samples	Statistical	To determine the genomic location and identify *susceptibility genes*
4	Molecular genetics	Individuals	Biological	To identify critical DNA variants and trace the biological pathways from DNA to disorder

---

studying the temporal, spatial and socioeconomic variation in disease incidence.

The presence of genetic influences on psychiatric disorders may appear self-evident to modern psychiatrists but was an issue of intense controversy in the middle of the twentieth century, when psychoanalytic theories of mental illnesses dominated. Many psychodynamic theorists assumed that any evidence that psychiatric disorders ran in families must result from familial environmental effects (Lidz *et al.*, 1965). Basic genetic epidemiology played an important role in convincingly demonstrating the presence of genetic, and hence biological, factors in mental disorders. The demonstration of substantial genetic influences on a disorder may be a rather modest goal but is nevertheless an extremely important one as it instigates further research on the nature of the genetic influences. For clinical practice, knowledge of the magnitude of genetic influences also allows clinicians to make use of family history information to inform diagnosis and risk prediction. However, the involvement of environmental factors as well as the probabilistic nature of genetic inheritance means that family history information will inevitably have limited predictive power.

Family studies

The primary aim of family studies is to demonstrate *familial aggregation* of a disease or trait. The presence of familial aggregation suggests, but does not prove, genetic aetiology because it remains possible that a range of shared environmental effects could be responsible for some or all of the observed familial aggregation. To obtain an unbiased estimate of the degree of familial aggregation and avoid overinclusion of families with multiple affected members, families must be *systematically ascertained* (Sham, 1998). The standard methodology is to adopt a two-stage sampling scheme, thus:

- In stage 1, a random sample of individuals with the disease is obtained. These affected individuals are called index cases or *probands*.
- In stage 2 the relatives of the probands are assessed for the presence or absence of the disease (as well as other related traits). Relatives found to have the disease are called *secondary cases*.

An ideal study would include a comparison group in which the probands are individuals from the same population as the index cases but differ only in that they do not have the disease. Where possible, the diagnoses of both probands and relatives should be made according to operational criteria using information obtained from personal interviews using standardised instruments (e.g. the DIGS: Diagnostic Interview for Genetic Studies).

However, some relatives may be deceased or for other reasons unavailable for direct interview. To avoid bias, it is important to obtain information on these individuals from informants (e.g. parents, siblings or children) using standardised instruments (e.g. FIGS: Family Interview for Genetic Studies). Because individuals are not always perfect historians and may seek to deny prior symptoms, the quality of information obtained in family studies can be much improved if records of prior psychiatric treatment are also available. It is also important that the assessment of relatives be blind to the affection status of the proband. Thus, ideally, when an interviewer approaches a relative in a family study, that interviewer should not know whether the respondent is related to an affected or a control proband. Family studies that incorporate a control group have been conducted on schizophrenia (Kendler & Gardner, 1997).

The risk of disease in a relative of a proband is called *morbid risk or recurrence risk*. For a disease with variable age of onset, there is the problem of "censoring", that is, some unaffected individuals of a relatively young age may yet develop the disease in later life. There are two classes of methods for making an "age-adjustment" in the calculation of morbid risk. The simpler methods, introduced by Weinberg and modified by Stromgren (Slater & Cowie, 1971), require making assumptions about the age-at-onset distribution. The more sophisticated methods use some form of survival analysis (life table or Kaplan-Meier estimators) and do not require prior assumptions to be made about the age-at-onset distribution. A measure of familial aggregation is the *relative risk ratio*, often designated as λ, defined as the ratio of morbid risk among the relatives of cases to the relatives of control subjects, for a specific class of relatives (e.g. parent, sibling, offspring).

Simple Mendelian modes of inheritance such as autosomal *dominant* and *recessive* have predictable patterns of relative risk ratios. For a rare autosomal-dominant disease, the ratios are $\frac{1}{2}$ for parents, siblings and offspring, $\frac{1}{4}$ for second-degree relatives (e.g. uncles, aunts, grandparents), and so on. For a rare recessive condition, the ratio is $\frac{1}{4}$ for siblings, and other classes of relatives are rarely affected. No classical psychiatric disorders show such simple *Mendelian ratios*. Their mode of inheritance is sometimes called non-Mendelian or complex. The complexity refers to the likely involvement of multiple genes and environmental factors, each likely to be of modest effect.

Twin studies

The task of twin studies is to estimate the proportion of variation in liability within a given population that is due to genetic differences between individuals. This proportion is called *heritability or h^2*. The statistical model that forms the basis of these calculations (the *polygenic model*) assumes a sufficiently large number of individual genetic and environmental risk factors of sufficiently small individual effect that the central limit theorem applies – that the resulting distribution of liability in the population will approximate normality. It has been shown that the assumptions of this model are rather robust and likely to be approximately met for most psychiatric conditions (Kendler & Kidd, 1986). In this chapter, we refer to "genes" identified by genetic epidemiologic methods as *genetic risk factors* to distinguish them from *susceptibility genes* identified by paradigms 3 and 4.

The existence of two types of twin pairs, *monozygotic* (MZ) and *dizygotic* (Lidz *et al.*, 1965) provides a natural experiment for untangling genetic from environmental factors. MZ twins are developed from the same fertilised ovum and therefore begin life as genetically identical individuals; DZ twins – like regular siblings – are developed from two separate fertilised ova and share on average 50% of their genes. The validity of the twin design depends on two critical assumptions (Kendler, 2001), namely:

- Twins are no different from the general population in terms of the trait in question.
- MZ and DZ twin pairs share their environments to the same extent, with respect to factors relevant to the trait in question (the *equal environment assumption*).

Although twins are clearly at increased risk for low birth weight and premature delivery – and have an associated increased risk for several congenital abnormalities – numerous studies have shown that the rates of major psychiatric disorders do not seem to differ in twins and singletons. A large literature has accumulated examining the validity of the equal environment assumption in twin studies. Most but not all studies support its validity. Although probably not perfectly valid for most studies, it seems unlikely that major biases are introduced in twin studies from violations of the equal environment assumption.

There are two main types of twin studies: those based on twin pairs ascertained through affected probands (e.g, the Maudsley Twin Register, Gottesman & Shields, 1972) and those based on population twin registers (Busjahn, 2002). The inference of a genetic component from proband-ascertained twin pairs is usually based on a difference between MZ and DZ concordance rates. The *proband-wise concordance rate* is defined as the percentage of probands who have an affected cotwin. For example, Cardno and Gottesman (2000) calculated pooled estimates for MZ and DZ concordance rates for schizophrenia and obtained values of 42% and 4% for *International Classification of Diseases* (10th edition; ICD-10) criteria, and 50% and 4% for *Diagnostic and Statistical Manual* (3rd edition, revised; DSM-III-R) criteria. An earlier measure, called the *pairwise concordance rate*, is defined as the percentage of twin pairs in which both members are affected. However, this measure cannot be interpreted without knowledge of the intensity of ascertainment and is therefore obsolete.

A variation of the twin method is the *co-twin control method*. This method studies differences in MZ twins who are discordant for a particular disorder. The ill and healthy twins are genetically identical so that these pairs can be used to study the environmental reasons why some individuals develop the disorder and others do not. Examples of this approach are the studies on neuropsychological impairment in relation to schizophrenia (Cannon et al., 2000; Goldberg et al., 1995).

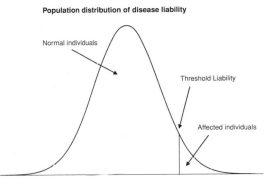

Figure 5.1 Liability-threshold model for polygenic disease.

The h^2 of a quantitative phenotype is an index of the relative contribution of genetic effects to the total phenotypic variance. In the classical twin method, Falconer's formula estimates h^2 by twice the difference in correlation between MZ twins and DZ twins. For a categorically defined trait such as schizophrenia, the estimation of heritability is based on a liability threshold model (which is an extension of the polygenic model outlined earlier; see also Figure 5.1). This model assumes that there is a continuous distribution of the underlying liability to develop the disorder in the general population. This liability is determined jointly by both genetic and environmental factors. An individual whose liability is above a certain threshold value will develop the disorder (Falconer, 1965). Under this model, concordance rates for disease can be transformed to correlations in liability, known technically as "tetrachoric correlations". These correlations can be substituted into Falconer's formula to estimate the heritability of the liability to the disorder. For example, from pooled concordance rates, Cardno and Gottesman (2000) estimated heritabilities of 88% for DSM-III-R and 83% for ICD-10 schizophrenia.

Heritability is a statistical concept that is meaningful only for populations. Indeed, the heritability of a disorder in an individual is undefined – the statistical equivalent of "one hand clapping". The heritability of a trait in a population depends not only on the nature of the genetic variants involved or on the magnitudes of their effects but also on their frequencies in the population and on the effect sizes and frequencies of environmental factors. Furthermore, the partitioning of phenotypic variance into independent genetic and environmental components is strictly valid only in the absence of correlations and interactions between the genetic and environmental factors involved. These subtleties have contributed to misunderstandings that have led to the fierce and often misinformed debates regarding the presence and implications of a genetic component in cognitive and behavioural traits such as IQ (Dickens & Flynn, 2001).

It is important to recognise that heritability is not a universal property of a trait but can vary among different populations or among different times for the same population. For example, if a new environmental risk factor for a disorder were introduced into a population, we would expect the heritability for that disorder to decrease. Furthermore, a high heritability does not necessarily mean that a trait is not subject to environmental changes. For example, height is highly heritable, but there is nevertheless a marked increase in the average height of most European populations because of improvements in general nutrition that in recent decades have benefited the entire population to about the same extent. A highly penetrant Mendelian disorder, phenylketonuria, can be treated by an extremely simple environmental manipulation – the restriction of phenylalanine from the diet.

In addition to determining the importance of genetic risk factors, twin studies also permit an estimation of the aetiological importance of shared family environment, sometimes called *common environment* or c^2. Common environment will reflect the impact of any environmental factors that tend to make members of a twin pair similar with respect to disease risk. This would include psychological factors such as parental rearing patterns, social and cultural factors such as the neighbourhood in which they were raised or the church they attended and physical factors such as diet and possible shared exposure to environmental toxins.

The genetic and environmental components of liability are valid concepts at the individual level, although their magnitudes in any individual cannot be estimated to a high level of accuracy from family data. The reason is that the amount of information contained in family data is proportional to the size of the family, and human families are typically small. Nevertheless, the extent of a patient's family history of disease may offer some indication of the relative importance of genetic and environmental factors in his or her illness (Murray *et al.*, 1985).

Adoption studies

Individuals who are adopted away at birth receive their genes from their biological parents and their rearing environment from their adoptive parents. Similarities between adoptees and their biological relatives are therefore likely to be due to shared genes, whereas similarities between adoptees and the adoptive family are likely to be due to shared environment. There are several varieties of adoption studies.

- The *adoptee's design* begins with affected biological parents who give their children up for adoption and compares the risk in those adopted-away children with those seen in adopted-away children of unaffected biological parents. An improved version of this design also incorporates the affection status of the adoptive parents, because there may be correlation between the affection status of biological and adoptive parents. If the affection status of biological parents is related to morbid risk in the adoptee, after adjusting for the affection status of adoptive parents, then genetic factors are implicated. Classic examples of the adoptees design are the studies on schizophrenia by Heston (1966) and by Rosenthal *et al.* (1971).
- The *adoptee's family design* begins with affected adoptees and examines the risk in both their adoptive and biological relatives and the adoptive and biological relatives of a matched group of control adoptees. A greater morbid risk among biological family members of affected versus unaffected adoptees would implicate genetic factors, whereas

a greater risk among the adoptive family members of the affected versus unaffected adoptee would indicate the importance of shared familial factors. A classic example of the adoptee's family design is the Danish Adoption Study by Kety *et al.* (1994).

In principle, adoption studies can be used to derive estimates of heritability, although in practice this is less often attempted compared with twin studies. Adoption studies have several potential methodological limitations. Most important are probably assortative placement and unrepresentativeness. Assortative placement occurs when adoption agencies try to match features of the biological parents with the adoptive family. If uncorrected, this could lead to biases in results. Whereas twins are generally representative of the general population, adoption families are unusual in at least two ways. Biological parents who give children up for adoption in modern Western societies now have higher rates of psychiatric illness and drug problems (although several generations ago, a more likely problem was poverty). By contrast, adoptive parents are typically mentally healthier than the general populace because adoption agencies see it as their job to select "healthy" families in which to place their adoptees. Both twin and adoption studies have potential methodological problems, so that convincing evidence for a genetic component should preferably come from both types of study design.

Paradigm 2 – advanced genetic epidemiology

The demonstration of significant heritability of a disorder raises many important questions about the nature and mode of action of the genetic and environmental risk factors. The goal of *advanced genetic epidemiology* is to answer these important questions that go far beyond the demonstration of heritability. Like basic genetic epidemiology, advanced genetic epidemiology also relies on the study of patterns of illness in families, twins

or adoptees, but the designs are more sophisticated, often involving longitudinal measurements, multiple traits and the assessment of environmental risk factors. Short of revealing the actual genes that contribute to the genetic component, advanced genetic epidemiology goes a long way in characterising the properties of the aggregate effects of these genes.

Knowledge gained from advanced genetic epidemiology has many possible uses in clinical psychiatry. For example, the demonstration of substantial shared genetic influences between apparently distinct psychiatric disorders has important implications for the classification of mental disorders. Similarly, if there is substantial interaction between the genetic component and a measurable environmental risk factor, then it would be important to reduce exposure to the environmental risk factor among genetically vulnerable individuals. Nevertheless, the utility of advanced genetic epidemiology is limited by its consideration of only the aggregate effect of genes, rather than the specific effects of individual genes.

Genetic modelling of twin data

In addition to providing an estimate of heritability, the study of twins also provides the most powerful tool for addressing the issues of advanced genetic epidemiology. Kendler (2005) listed nine questions regarding the relationship between genetic risk factors and risk of disorders that can be addressed by twin studies. These are shown in Box 5.2.

Although it is possible to address these questions using relatively simple statistical methods of analyzing the data, there are some important advantages of using a more sophisticated, model-fitting approach (Neale *et al.*, 1999; Rijsdijk & Sham, 2002). These advantages are, first, that model fitting is able to use all the relevant information contained in the data, and second, that it allows the questions to be addressed in a direct way.

Genetic model fitting was developed from path analysis and can be regarded as an application of the modern statistical methodology of structural

---

Box 5.2 Questions that can be addressed by twin studies

- Are these genetic risk factors specific to a given disorder or shared with other psychiatric or substance use disorders?
- Do these genetic risk factors have an impact on disease risk similarly in males and females?
- To what extent are the effects of these genetic risk factors mediated through *intermediate phenotypes* (or *endophenotypes*) such as personality or neuropsychological processes?
- Do these genetic risk factors moderate the impact of environmental risk factors on disease liability (genetic control of sensitivity to the environment)?
- Do these genetic risk factors have an impact on disease risk through altering the probability of exposure to environmental risk factors (genetic control of exposure to the environment)?
- Do the action of these risk factors change as a function of the developmental stage of the individual?
- Do historical experiences moderate the impact of genetic risk factors so that heritability might differ across historical cohorts?
- For disorders which have multiple stages (e.g. substantial alcohol consumption must proceed but does not always lead to alcohol dependence), what is the relationship between the genetic risk factors for these various stages?
- Does the level of heritability for a disorder differ across populations?

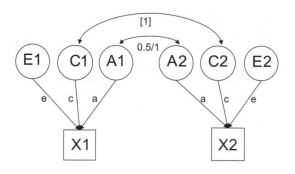

Figure 5.2 Path diagram for ACE model for twin data. A = additive genetic factors; C = common (family) environment; E = specific (individual) environment.

equation modelling. The simplest structural equation model (SEM) for twin data is the so-called ACE model, where the letters A, C and E designate additive genetic factors, common (family) environment and specific (individual) environment, respectively (Figure 5.2). In this SEM, the variables A, C and E are latent (i.e. not measured) and independent of each other, each having a direct causal influence on the phenotype (e.g. a quantitative trait or disease liability). The parameters of the model are the path coefficients a, c, and e, for the magnitudes of the causal relationships from A, C and E to the phenotype. The model also makes some additional assumptions: (1) The variances of A, C and E are fixed at 1; this is

a reasonable restriction because, being latent variables, A, C and E have entirely arbitrary units of measurement. (2) A, C and E are assumed to be independent of each other. (3) A has a correlation of 1 across MZ twins and 0.5 across DZ twins. (4) C has a correlation of 1 across both MZ and DZ twins. (5) E has a correlation of 0 across both MZ and DZ twins. Given these assumptions, a computer program such as Mx can be used to estimate the path coefficients a, c and e by minimizing a fit function that quantifies the discrepancy between the observed data and predictions from the model. The most frequently used fit function is minus twice the log-likelihood of the model, which assumes that the data follow a (multivariate) normal distribution.

This standard ACE model would be the "workhorse" of basic genetic epidemiology, producing estimates of h^2 (same as a^2) and c^2. Each of the listed questions, as examples of the advanced genetic epidemiology paradigm, requires certain modifications or elaborations of the basic ACE model. For example, the first question in the list involves adding more phenotypic variables to the model and exploring the changes in the underlying genetic and environmental components needed to account jointly for all the phenotypic variables. Similarly, the second question can be addressed by allowing the path coefficients to be different for males and females in a general model and conducting a test of this model against the restricted (null) model that the path coefficients are the same.

Genetic model fitting also has some potential disadvantages. The complexity of the methodology means that errors in the analysis can be inadvertently introduced and overlooked and that crucial assumptions may not be appreciated. It is particularly dangerous to consider only the results of model fitting, without confirming that these results are consistent with summary statistics and graphical displays derived from the raw data. Finally, these models often make causal assumptions about the associations between certain variables that might not be warranted – although such models do have one important advantage over more traditional approaches in epidemiology. We do really know that genes cause phenotypes and not the other way around!

The advanced genetic epidemiology paradigm has been used to study the relationships between neuroticism and depression (Kendler *et al.*, 2006); between anxiety and depression (Kendler *et al.*, 1992); between the syndromes of schizophrenia, schizoaffective disorder and mania (Cardno *et al.*, 2002) and between unipolar and bipolar depression (McGuffin *et al.*, 2003).

Paradigm 3 – gene finding

Whereas basic and advanced genetic epidemiological approaches are concerned with the aggregate effects of genes on disease risk, the third and fourth paradigms attempt to dissect out the overall genetic component into its constituent genes. The goal of the third paradigm, gene finding, is to determine the locations in the genome of the genes that influence liability to disorders. Gene-finding studies require the use of molecular genetic technology to detect and measure the genetic variants (or more technically *alleles*) at various chromosomal locations (or more technically *loci*). By examining the distribution of alleles, which serve as genetic markers, within families or populations, these methods (linkage and association) infer whether a locus in the genomic region under investigation contributes to disease liability. Gene-finding studies can be thought of as an extension of basic and advanced genetic epidemiological methods which involve the direct measurement of genetic variants rather than relying entirely on the patterns of disease in families to infer genetic influences.

For single-gene Mendelian diseases, finding the gene(s) on which the disease-causing mutations occur has the potential to enable accurate prenatal risk prediction and genetic counselling. For complex, polygenic disorders, simply knowing the genes involved currently has few practical uses, because of the limited predictive power of the genetic variants. For these disorders, gene finding is best regarded as an important intermediate research goal, which enables further, more detailed functional studies to be performed on the identified genes (Paradigm 4), ultimately leading to a more complete and detailed understanding of how genetic variation affects risk of disease and potentially aiding in the development of more specific preventative measures, pharmacological treatments or both.

Complex segregation analysis

If a disorder does not follow simple Mendelian patterns of inheritance, then it is natural to ask whether there is nevertheless a single gene of major importance in comparison to the others. Most attempts to address this question have been based on comparing two idealised models – the single major locus model and the polygenic model – in terms of their ability to explain empirical family data. In a *single major locus model*, the genetic component is a single gene that has a major influence on risk but is nevertheless neither necessary nor sufficient for the disease. Technically, the absence of disease among some genetically predisposed individuals is called *incomplete penetrance*, whereas individuals who are affected despite being genetically non-predisposed are called *phenocopies*.

At the other extreme, the *polygenic model* posits a very large number of genes, each of small effect. The cumulative effects of multiple genes lead to a continuous distribution, which may be related to disease through a liability-threshold model. In between these extremes are oligogenic models, in which a small number of genes are involved, and mixed models, in which a major locus is present in a background of polygenes.

Different genetic models are discriminated by an assessment of their goodness-of-fit with family data. For some psychiatric disorders (e.g. schizophrenia), morbid risk data of many classes on relatives from multiple studies have been summarised and tabulated, and such figures provide convenient data for model fitting. When raw pedigree data are available, however, a statistically more powerful approach is *complex segregation analysis*. The results of such analyses, however, are often inconsistent with some studies favouring a single major locus model and others favouring a polygenic model (Baron, 1986). It appears that the analysis of disease phenotypic data alone (without the help of molecular genetic markers) is limited in power to resolve various genetic models. Power is more favourable for quantitative traits; a locus that accounts for a substantial proportion (over a third) of the phenotypic variance is likely to be detectable by segregation analysis. However, complex segregation analysis of quantitative traits is sensitive to the frequency distribution of the trait in the population; the presence of skew and kurtosis can lead to false-positive evidence for a major locus.

Linkage studies

Linkage analysis is based on the principle that the alleles of two or more genetic loci on the same chromosome tend to segregate (i.e. be passed on) together from parent to offspring. This is because they are physically connected with each other on the same DNA molecule. The closer the two loci are together, the lower the chance of their being separated by a *recombination* event during meiosis, and the stronger the observed linkage. This phenomenon can be applied to the detection of loci for genetic diseases. If a genetic marker is close to a disease-causing gene, alleles of the marker

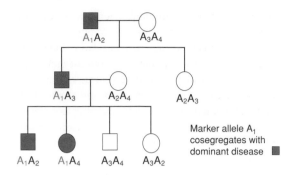

Figure 5.3 Cosegregation (linkage) between disease and genetic marker.

will tend to co-segregate with the disorder in families (Figure 5.3) or be shared between affected relatives.

Until the 1980s, the application of linkage analysis to disease gene mapping was hampered by the lack of suitable genetic markers in most regions of the genome. Then the discovery of highly polymorphic, short-sequence repeat (SSR) markers throughout the genome, and the development of high-throughput genotyping technology, made it feasible to scan the entire genome for disease-predisposing loci. Standard sets of SSR markers, evenly spaced throughout the genome, are now available for *genomewide linkage scans*. This method of mapping disease-related gene does not depend on any prior knowledge of disease pathophysiology and is therefore known as *positional cloning*.

Classical linkage analysis of Mendelian diseases is usually conducted on large, multigenerational pedigrees containing multiply affected individuals. The standard method of analysis is based on log-likelihood ratios (or *LOD scores: logarithm of the odds*) for the alternate hypotheses of linkage and nonlinkage at a particular marker or chromosomal location, assuming a specific model for the disease. The methodology involves calculating and tabulating (or plotting) the LOD scores at a series of positions, at regular intervals, for the chromosome region being examined (or for the chromosomes, in a genome scan). A LOD score of 3 or more is the standard criterion for declaring linkage, because at this level of evidence the probability of a false-positive result is less than 0.05, assuming that specified disease model is correct (Ott, 1999). A LOD score of –2 or lower is taken as evidence for *exclusion* of linkage to the marker, although exclusion is valid only if the disease model is correctly specified.

The most favourable scenario for classical linkage analysis is when a disease is clearly segregating in a Mendelian dominant fashion in a single, large, multigenerational pedigree. If the family is sufficiently large, then the disease locus can be reliably mapped to its chromosomal location, provided that the phenotype and genotype are accurate. However, when the susceptibility locus has a small effect or is involved in disease only in a proportion of families, the method has limited power to detect or exclude linkage, even when very dense marker sets are used. Nevertheless, application of the linkage approach has helped to map genes of major effect for Alzheimer's disease (Goate *et al.*, 1991), and more recently others have replicated some linkage reports on schizophrenia (Stefansson *et al.*, 2002, 2003). Nevertheless, linkage studies on complex disorders have tended to produce inconsistent results that are difficult to interpret, even though a meta-analysis of all linkage genome scans on schizophrenia has identified a number of regions with significant overall evidence for linkage (Lewis *et al.*, 2003).

An alternative strategy of linkage analysis that does not require a disease model to be specified is the affected sib pair method. This method simply uses the genetic marker data to estimate the *allele sharing* between affected sibling pairs at a particular chromosomal location and then tests whether the level of allele sharing is in excess of that expected for sibling pairs by chance alone. Like model-based LOD score methods, allele sharing linkage methods can be used to conduct whole genome scans with standard marker sets. Allele sharing methods are sometimes called *model-free* or *nonparametric* linkage and, as with model-based LOD score methods, suffer from low statistical power when the total impact of any individual gene on disease risk is modest. Sufficient power to detect susceptibility

genes of realistic effect size requires sample sizes of at least several hundred affected sibling pairs. Application of the allele-sharing linkage approach to schizophrenia has yielded disappointing results (Williams *et al.*, 2003). Allele-sharing linkage analysis has been adapted for the study of quantitative traits to detect so-called quantitative trait loci (QTL). This approach has been used in attempts to map QTLs influencing neuroticism (Fullerton *et al.*, 2003; Nash *et al.*, 2004).

A methodological limitation of linkage studies in general is that they have low resolution in the sense that the regions demonstrating linkage tend to be wide, usually extending many millions of nucleotides and containing dozens, if not hundreds, of genes.

Association studies

An association between a specific allele and a disease is defined as a greater frequency of the allele among individuals with the disease than those without. Association studies have traditionally concentrated on *candidate genes*, which are selected on the basis of their relevance to prior conceptions regarding disease aetiology. The existence of linkage disequilibrium (LD) raises the possibility of scanning chromosomal regions or the entire genome by association analysis with only a fraction of all genetic polymorphisms in the regions or in the genome. The screening of chromosomal regions by association analysis is an important strategy for following up the positive regions revealed by linkage scans.

As is well known in epidemiology, association suggests, but does not imply, causation (see Chapter 4). Aside from direct causation, an allele may be associated with a disease for two main reasons:
- Poor matching between cases and controls – either in ethnic origin (*population stratification*) or age (*selection* of longevity genes)
- The association of the allele with a causative allele through *linkage disequilibrium*

LD is the tendency for very closely linked loci to show allelic association with each other. The reason for the existence of LD is that recombination rarely occurs between very closely linked loci during meiosis, so that any allelic association introduced into the population by past mutations or population bottlenecks will be maintained for many generations. Thus a disease allele that arose through an ancestral mutation on a chromosome that happened to contain a particular combination of alleles in close proximity is expected to demonstrate association with this combination of alleles (known as a *haplotype*) for many generations after the mutational event.

From a set of single nucleotide polymorphisms (SNPs) that are in tight LD with each other, it is sufficient to select only one SNP, called the tag SNP, to act as a surrogate for the whole set. The discovery and cataloguing of millions of SNPs and the development of economic, high-throughput genotyping technologies have prepared the ground for large-scale, potentially *genomewide association studies*. An international effort, called the HapMap project, has recently characterised the whole-genome LD structure in three major human populations to identify SNP sets that are most efficient for large-scale association studies. The project obtained genotype data on 3.5 million SNPs in populations of European (Utah, United States), African (Nigeria) and Asian (Chinese and Japanese) origin (International HapMap Consortium, 2005). Data from this project show that current (and forthcoming) commercial genome-wide SNP genotyping products are able to offer nearly complete coverage of all common variations in the human genome, meaning that truly genomewide association studies are now feasible. We expect to see a number of such studies applied to major psychiatric disorders appearing in the literature in the next few years.

The most common design for association studies is the *case-control study*. Specific alleles or haplotypes are tested for differences in frequency between cases and controls, adjusting for potential confounding factors if necessary. Alternative designs that use related control subjects, usually the parents or siblings of affected individuals, have the advantage that they are robust to false-positive

association arising from hidden population stratification. Data on affected individuals and their parents are usually analysed using the *transmission/disequilibrium test* (TDT), which examines heterozygous parents to see whether some alleles are preferentially transmitted to affected offspring. Both case-control and TDT studies allow the effect of a genetic variant to be estimated by an *odds ratio*. If the frequencies of the variant and the disease are both known, then the odds ratio can be used to calculate the *population attributable fraction* of the variant.

Association studies are potentially more powerful than linkage studies for detecting susceptibility genes of small effect size. Because of this, genomewide association studies promise to detect many susceptibility loci in which effects are too small to detect by linkage scans. Nevertheless, the power of association studies is ultimately limited by the size of samples that can be realistically collected. It is therefore likely that genomewide association studies will eventually detect only the most important susceptibility loci, leaving a residue of unresolved genetic influences. However, even before whole-genome genotyping technology became feasible, association studies of candidate genes and linkage regions have yielded a number of potential susceptibility genes for psychiatric disorders. For example, the list of putative susceptibility genes for schizophrenia with positive association findings include DRD3, 5HT2a, DISC1, DISC2, COMT, ProDH, RGS4, DTNBP1 (dysbindin), NRG1 (neuregulin 1), G72 and DAAO (see also Chapter 13). However, as reviewed by O'Donovan *et al.* (2003), the results of the association studies on all of these genes have been mixed, with only a proportion of studies reporting the presence of association. Even when several studies present positive findings, the associated alleles or haplotypes are often not the same among the studies.

One major problem with gene-finding methods is that they involve many statistical tests. A genomewide linkage study might involve 300 or 400 markers. Genotyping methods now allow us to screen easily dozens of genes, and soon we will be testing hundreds of thousands of markers in a single experiment. We have little insight into the true biological causes of virtually all psychiatric disorders. Therefore, our "candidate" genes are typically based on rather weak hypotheses such as the mechanism of drugs that are used to treat the disorders. Statistical theory predicts that performing many tests, each of which has a low prior probability of being true, will produce many positive results that are due to chance alone. This has been and continues to be a major problem in interpreting the gene-finding literature in psychiatry. In general, strong scepticism is warranted for the results of any single study. Confidence should be withheld until multiple replications have been published.

Paradigm 4 – molecular genetics

The goal of the molecular genetic (or *functional genomics*) paradigm in psychiatric genetics is to trace the biological mechanisms by which DNA variation contributes to the disorder itself. The first critical goal is to identify the actual DNA sequence variation that contributes causally to increased risk and subsequently to understand how this sequence variation affects gene function, expression or both. For example, attempts have been made to interpret recent association findings in schizophrenia in terms of brain dysfunction (Harrison & Owen, 2003). A full understanding of how genetic variation leads to increased risk of disease is clearly useful for risk prediction and the formulation of preventive and treatment strategies, especially the identification of possible new drug targets. However, in comparison to single-gene Mendelian diseases, the changes in gene function that relate to complex, polygenic disorders may be subtle, and the predictive power of understanding the effect of any single gene may be limited. Nevertheless, as knowledge extends to multiple susceptibility genes involved in different parts of functional gene networks, a more complete understanding should emerge which would have greater predictive power and clinical utility.

The identification of the actual DNA sequence variation that contributes causally to increased risk may be difficult, especially if the causal variant is common, is in LD with other variants and has subtle rather than dramatic effect on gene function. The task is somewhat simpler if the variant causes a change in the amino acid sequence of the encoded protein, and the altered protein is damaging to the cell or is functionally defective. In other situations, the change of gene function may be a subtle increase, decrease or dysregulation in gene expression, and the relationship between such changes and DNA sequence variation may be difficult to establish. That is, although we are now very good at identifying the "coding regions" of genes that are transcribed into mRNA and then translated into protein, we are still substantially ignorant about the nature and location of the many levels of transcriptional control in our genome, some of which have until only recently been considered to be "junk" DNA. Thus it is not always clear even where we should be looking for the critical variants that have an impact on risk for illness.

With the increasing detail of information on human and other genomes, it may be possible to obtain clues about which variants are more likely than others to be functional. For example, sequences that are highly conserved across species are more likely to be of functional significance. Similarly, sequences that may be "recognised" by known transcription factors are sites where variations are more likely to affect gene expression and regulation.

The confounding between direct and indirect association can be untangled to some extent by statistical modelling; direct effects should remain significant even after adjustment for indirect effects, but not the other way round. Nevertheless, when confounding is strong and the underlying interrelationships complex, there may be insufficient statistical power to establish causal variants in this way. The gold standard of establishing a causal relationship is a study that involves controlled experimentation (such as a randomised clinical trial). In the context of molecular genetics, this can be achieved by creating and studying *transgenic animal models,* which have specific pieces of DNA removed from or inserted into appropriate positions of the genome. Such animals can be screened for changes in function that might be related to the disease process. However, the likely validity of animal models that could be used in such testing differs widely across psychiatric disorders. Animal models for drugs of abuse, including alcohol, and anxiety are likely to have high "face validity." Less certain is whether depression and especially psychosis can be meaningfully modelled in nonhumans.

The more complex goal of tracing the entire pathway(s) between genetic variation and disease risk is even more difficult and, in most cases, cannot be achieved by molecular genetic methods alone. The intermediate steps between genetic differences and disease may involve gene expression, cellular functions, brain development and structure, neurochemistry, neuropsychology and personality. Methodologies for studying these diverse domains are required. Furthermore, the role of the environment must not be neglected, because there may be important interactions between genetic and environmental factors. An example is the interplay between adverse life events and genetic factors in major depression (Caspi *et al.*, 2003; Kendler *et al.*, 1995).

Conclusions

Psychiatric genetics now contains at least three kinds of science. Genetic epidemiology explores the interrelationship of genetic and environmental risk factors in which "genes" are measured indirectly in ways that reflect aggregate effects "averaged" across the entire genome. Gene-finding methods use increasingly large sample sizes and advanced laboratory and statistical tools to try to localise specific genomic regions that confer risk for psychiatric conditions. Molecular genetics is an entirely laboratory-based discipline applying a range of modern methods from genomics to neuroscience to try to identify and then trace pathophysiological pathways. Each of these paradigms has

strengths and limitations, and they are in a process of dynamic interaction with each other. Genetic epidemiology has proved a reliable method to answer basic questions about the overall importance of genetic risk factors for psychiatric illness. Gene-finding methods to date have proved rather less reliable but are asking much more difficult questions. The architecture of the genetic risk for psychiatric disorders is likely to be complex, and it remains to be seen whether our ever-increasing laboratory and statistical tools are up to the task. Some progress definitely has been made, and it will be an exciting field to watch in the coming years.

REFERENCES

Baron, M. (1986). Genetics of schizophrenia 1. Familial patterns and mode of inheritance. *Biol Psychiatry* **21**:1051–66.

Busjahn, A. (2002). Twin registers across the globe: what's out there in 2002? *Twin Res* **5**:v–vi.

Cannon, T. D., Huttunen, M. O., Lonnqvist, J., *et al.* (2000). The inheritance of neuropsychological dysfunction in twins discordant for schizophrenia. *Am J Hum Genet* **67**:369–82.

Cardno, A. G., & Gottesman, I. I. (2000). Twin studies of schizophrenia: from bow-and-arrow concordances to star wars Mx and functional genomics. *Am J Med Genet* **97**:12–17.

Cardno, A. G., Rijsdijk, F. V., Sham, P. C., *et al.* (2002). A twin study of genetic relationships between psychotic symptoms. *Am J Psychiatry* **159**:539–45

Caspi, A., Sugden, K., Moffitt, T. E., *et al.* (2003). Influence of life stress on depression: moderation by a polymorphism in the 5-HTT gene. *Science* **301**:386–9.

Dickens, W. T., & Flynn, J. R. (2001). Heritability estimates versus large environmental effects: the IQ paradox resolved. *Psychol Rev* **108**:346–69.

Falconer, D. S. (1965). The inheritance of liability to certain diseases, estimated from the incidence among relatives. *Ann Hum Genet* **29**:51–76.

Fullerton, J., Cubin, M., Tiwari, H., *et al.* (2003). Linkage analysis of extremely discordant and concordant sibling pairs identifies quantitative-trait loci that influence variation in the human personality trait neuroticism. *Am J Hum Genet* **72**:879–90.

Goate, A. M., Chartier-Harlin, M. C., Mullan, M., *et al.* (1991). Segregation of a missense mutation in the amyloid precursor protein gene with familial Alzheimer's disease. *Nature* **349**:704–6.

Goldberg, T. E., Torrey, E. F., Gold, J. M., *et al.* (1995). Genetic risk of neuropsychological impairment in schizophrenia: a study of monozygotic twins discordant and concordant for the disorder. *Schizophr Res* **17**:77–84.

Gottesman, I. I., & Shields, J. (1972). *Schizophrenia and Genetics: A Twin Study Vantage Point.* New York: Academic Press.

Harrison, P. J., & Owen, M. J. (2003). Genes for schizophrenia? Recent findings and their pathophysiological implications. *Lancet* **361**:417–19.

Heston, L. L. (1966). Psychiatric disorders in foster home reared children of schizophrenic mothers. *Br J Psychiatry* **112**:819–25.

International HapMap Consortium (2005). A haplotype map of the human genome. *Nature* **437**:1299–1320.

International Human Genome Sequencing Consortium (2001). Initial sequencing and analysis of the human genome. *Nature* **409**:860–921.

Kendler, K. S. (2001). Twin studies of psychiatric illness: an update. *Arch Gen Psychiatry* **58**:1005–14.

Kendler, K. S. (2005). Psychiatric genetics: a methodologic critique. *Am J Psychiatry* **162**:3–11.

Kendler, K. S., & Eaves, L. J. (2005). *Psychiatric Genetics (Review of Psychiatry).* Washington, DC: American Psychiatric Publishing.

Kendler, K. S., & Gardner, C. O. (1997). The risk for psychiatric disorders in relatives of schizophrenic and control probands: a comparison of three independent studies. *Psychol Med* **27**:411–19.

Kendler, K. S., Gatz, M., Gardner, C. O., & Pedersen, N. L. (2006). Personality and major depression: a Swedish longitudinal, population-based twin study. *Arch Gen Psychiatry* **63**:1113–1120.

Kendler, K. S., Kessler, R. C., Walters, E. E., *et al.* (1995). Stressful life events, genetic liability, and onset of an episode of major depression in women. *Am J Psychiatry* **152**:833–42.

Kendler, K. S., & Kidd, K. K. (1986). Recurrence risks in an oligogenic threshold model: the effect of alterations in allele frequency. *Ann Hum Genet* **50**:83–91.

Kendler, K. S., Neale, M. C., Kessler, R. C., *et al.* (1992). Major depression and generalized anxiety disorder. Same genes, (partly) different environments. *Arch Gen Psychiatry* **49**:716–22.

Kety, S. S., Wender, P. H., Jacobsen, R., *et al.* (1994). Mental illness in the biological and adoptive relatives of schizophrenic adoptees: replication of the Copenhagen study in the rest of Denmark. *Arch Gen Psychiatry* **51**:442–55.

Lewis, C. M., Levinson, D. F., Wise, L. H., *et al.* (2003). Genome scan meta-analysis of schizophrenia and bipolar disorder, part II: schizophrenia. *Am J Hum Genet* **73**:34–48.

Lidz, T., Fleck, S., & Cornelison, A. R. (1965). *Schizophrenia and the Family*, 2nd edn. New York: International Universities Press.

McGuffin, P., Gottesman, I. I., & Owen, M. J. (2002). *Psychiatric Genetics and Genomics.* Oxford: Oxford University Press.

McGuffin, P., Rijsdijk, F., Andrew, M., *et al.* (2003). The heritability of bipolar affective disorder and the genetic relationship to unipolar depression. *Arch Gen Psychiatry* **60**:497–502.

Murray, R. M., Lewis, S., & Reveley, A. M. (1985). Towards an aetiological classification of schizophrenia. *Lancet* **1**:1023–6.

Nash, M. W., Huezo-Diaz, P., Williamson, R. J., *et al.* (2004). Genome-wide linkage analysis of a composite index of neuroticism and mood-related scales in extreme selected sibships. *Hum Mol Genet* **13**:2173–82.

Neale, M. C., Boker, S. M., Xie, G., & Maes, H. H. (1999). *Mx: Statistical Modeling*, 5th ed. Available from: Department of Psychiatry, Medical College of Virginia, VA Commonwealth University, Box 980126, Richmond, VA 23298

O'Donovan, M. C., Williams, N. M., & Owen, M. J. (2003). Recent advances in the genetics of schizophrenia. *Hum Mol Genet* **12**:R125–R133.

Ott, J. (1999). *Analysis of Human Genetic Linkage.* Baltimore, MD: Johns Hopkins University Press.

Rijsdijk, F. V., & Sham, P. C. (2002). Analytic approaches to twin data using structural equation models. *Brief Bioinform* **3**:119–33.

Rosenthal, D., Wender, P. H., Kety, S. S., *et al.* (1971). *The adopted-away offspring of schizophrenics. Am J Psychiatry* **128**:307–11.

Schulze, T. G., Fangerau, H., & Propping, P. (2004). From degeneration to genetic susceptibility, from eugenics to genethics, from Bezugsziffer to LOD score: the history of psychiatric genetics. *Int Rev Psychiatry* **16**:246–59.

Sham, P. C. (1998) Statistical methods in psychiatric genetics. *Stat Methods Med Res* **7**:279–300.

Slater, E., & Cowie, V. (1971). *The Genetics of Mental Disorders.* London: Oxford University Press.

Stefansson, H., Sarginson, J., Kong, A., *et al.* (2003). Association of neuregulin 1 with schizophrenia confirmed in a Scottish population. *Am J Hum Genet* **72**:83–7.

Stefansson, H., Sigurdsson, E., Steinthorsdottir, V., *et al.* (2002). Neuregulin 1 and susceptibility to schizophrenia. *Am J Hum Genet* **71**:877–92.

Williams, N. M., Norton, N., Williams, H., *et al.* (2003). A systematic genomewide linkage study in 353 sib pairs with schizophrenia. *Am J Human Genet* **73**:1355–67.

Psychiatric Disorders

6

Psychiatric disorders in childhood and adolescence

Ian M. Goodyer

This chapter concerns emotional and behavioural and developmental disorders that arise in the first 2 decades of life. It focuses on the major conditions described as "specific" to the childhood years and those that emerge in those years and may continue into adult life.

Clinical assessment

Compared with adult psychiatry diagnostic assessment, procedures and formulations in child and adolescent populations are based on information gathered from a wider inclusion of family members, parents and frequently siblings, school and peer relationships (Angold, 2003). These assessments are based on observation of behaviour both within and between individuals. Child interviews are a core feature and must be developmentally sensitive. With older children and adolescents, methods similar to those used with adults are applied to establish current mental state and personal function as well as the child's perception of current relationships, school progress and relations with friends. With children younger than 8 years, other methods, including play and the use of materials such as age-appropriate toys, are likely to be used to develop a sufficient level of trust and mutual interest with the interviewer such that content relevant to the presenting complaint, past history and the child's own perception of

current problems can be obtained. Direct questioning to elicit current mental state symptoms in younger children is invariably unsuccessful or lacks specificity.

Neurodevelopmental disorders which involve perturbations of speech, language and motor systems require careful assessment to distinguish between normal variations in general development and the presence of clinically significant impairment. Even young children are capable of reporting feelings and thoughts, including suicidal ideation. Those with marked behavioural symptoms are perhaps the least valid to interview directly because they are likely to deny antisocial acts and interpersonal difficulties.

Psychosocial assessments are key features of the examination and should, wherever possible, include an assessment of family function, marital satisfaction and sibling relationships. Family communication, problem solving, emotional warmth and care and control between family members are core features of the initial assessment phase, which often take between one and three sessions of around 1 hour each. An understanding of peer group relations and the local environment of the child are essential to appreciate the social ecology within which the child's difficulties are being expressed. An assessment of risk, maintaining protective, restitutive and resilience factors, will aid diagnostic formulation and treatment planning; these are summarised in Box 6.1.

Essential Psychiatry, ed. Robin M. Murray, Kenneth S. Kendler, Peter McGuffin, Simon Wessely, David J. Castle.
Published by Cambridge University Press. © Cambridge University Press 2008.

> **Box 6.1** Elements of Psychiatric Assessment in Childhood and Adolescence
>
> • *Risk factors* and processes are those that are judged to increase the liability for psychopathology and should be antecedent to presenting problems.
> • *Maintaining factors* are those that arise after difficulties emerge and are judged to contribute to their persistence.
> • *Restitutive factors* are those that are judged likely to facilitate improvement either through treatment compliance, enhancing treatment effects or activation of positive features in the child's life or their environment.
> • *Protective and resilience* factors refer to those features that would reduce the emergence or the impact of risk processes and, if identified, may be helpful in diminishing risk of recurrence.

Few formal tests or assessments can contribute to the clinical assessment for common behavioural and emotional disorders. Rating scales completed before the assessment may aid in the overall formulation, but invariably these instruments have been designed for epidemiological rather than diagnostic clinical purposes (Chakrabarti & Fombonne, 2005). Self-report or parental questionnaires can document change in symptom levels with over time. To date there are no physiological, biochemical or genetic assessments that can aid diagnostic evaluations or treatment for emotional or behavioural disorders.

For neurodevelopmental disorders, occupational therapy assessments for motor skills and fine motor movements, neuropsychological assessments of cognitive abilities and speech therapy assessments of speech and language all have an important place in assessment. Rating scales for hyperactivity can be an adjunct in monitoring treatment success in attention-deficit/hyperactivity disorder (ADHD). Clinical physiological assessments can also provide helpful information for neuropsychiatric disorders. The electroencephalogram (EEG) in particular can aid in those with a putative history of seizures and those at risk for seizures, such as adolescents with autism. These techniques may also be helpful in informing clinical state assessment in those with rare disorders presenting with declining cognitive function.

Causal processes in developmental psychopathology

The nature of risk for psychopathology

Risk can be defined as the degree to which the likelihood of a given adverse outcome will occur following exposure to a defined toxic agent. The relative importance of exposure is estimated by the probability of the outcome occurring in a given population compared with the level of occurrence in a nonexposed population (see Chapter 3). Risks for psychopathology occur from a variety of sources both internal and external to the child. They may be defined at the level of the individual, family or the community at large. For example, individuals may be born with genes that render them susceptible to psychiatric illness, acquire lesions such as head injury that alter their capacity for learning or become exposed to negative social environments that diminish emotional and cognitive development. Familial environmental risks might include a neglectful or hostile parenting environment, or one that is physically inadequate (such as in failure to ensure food and shelter) without being overtly emotionally negative. In addition, neighbourhood risks may occur which may be physical, such as poor housing, or functional, such as living in a violent or dangerous society.

Invariably, risks of these types are not independent of each other and determining their degree of association to each other is important. This is because it is increasingly apparent that most risk profiles for psychopathology involve multiple adverse events which may interact with each other.

Resilience

Many children and adolescents demonstrate an ability to withstand exposure to risk processes and not develop psychiatric disorders. This notion

---

Box 6.2 Dimensions of Resilience in Childhood

- Dispositional attributes (easy temperament, higher cognitive abilities and positive self-beliefs)
- Family characteristics (e.g. warmth in relations with parents, support at difficult times, good family problem-solving skills)
- Use of available external support systems (positive neighbourhood relations and friendship groups)

---

of resilience in the face of adversity refers to individuals who possess intrinsic abilities to prevent the toxic effects of risk (Luthar *et al.*, 2000). Three main dimensions of psychosocial characteristics have been identified and are shown in Box 6.2.

The presence of one or more of these protective domains is associated with better outcomes in children and adolescents within the context of risk and chronic adversities in particular. Little is currently known regarding the mechanisms of resilience within the person. Recent findings on gene-environment interactions have noted that genetic variations may confer differential levels of resilience when children are exposed to personal risks. For example, children experiencing child abuse are markedly less likely to report subsequent episodes of depression if they are homozygous for the long arm of the serotonin transporter gene (Kaufman *et al.*, 2004), suggesting a further process through which individual differences at the genetic level may increase sensitivity to social adversities. A second genotype conferring high level of monoamine oxidase A (MAOA) expression is putatively associated with reducing the risk for antisocial problems following maltreatment as a child (Caspi *et al.*, 2002).

Child maltreatment

Abusive relationships in the first two decades of life have been established as one of the most powerful adverse processes over the lifespan (Emery & Laumann-Billings, 2003; Kaplan *et al.*, 1999).

Subsequent emotional and behavioural psychopathologies are increased in those with a history of child abuse, both close to (proximal effects) and at a distance from (distal effects) the events themselves. Recent findings have demonstrated that there are likely to be epigenetic effects on brain development from early adverse experiences that are likely to determine individual differences in response to subsequent life events and difficulties (Halligan *et al.*, 2004; Weaver *et al.*, 2004). Cognitive vulnerabilities characterised by higher levels of self-criticism and lower levels of self-efficacy have been noted in experimental studies of children with even moderate histories of environmental deprivations, such as a low emotional parenting environment (Murray *et al.*, 2001). In severe recurrent abuse, effects on the self system and interpersonal relations may last through into adulthood (Jaffee *et al.*, 2002; Kaplan *et al.*, 1999).

There are no universal legal or scientific definitions of child abuse, neglect or psychological abuse. As a consequence, both research investigations and social policy development vary widely, making comparisons between studies and countries particularly difficult. One key commonality is that definitions of child maltreatment are based on social judgements and not immutable objective criteria. However, even the most parsimonious definition gives alarmingly high rates; for example, an estimate of 0.018 per 1,000 children (1,200–1,500) are killed per year in the United States by their parent or guardian (see Emery & Laumann-Billings, 2003, p. 326). Such extreme incidents comprise only a minority of abusive experiences suffered by children. Defining abuse as any act or omission that results in demonstrable harm to a child estimates that 23 to 42 per 1,000 children (i.e. between 1.5 and 2.3 million) in the United States were abused in 1993 (see Emery and Laumann-Billings, 2003, p. 326). Variations in reporting, corroborating evidence, definitions of abuse and precision of detection all contribute to the widely varying estimates and seriousness of the event(s). For example, if the social judgement of abuse is wide and includes any form of physical chastisement, then 60% of American children are sufferers (Finkelhor,

1994). If this definition is restricted to hitting anywhere but the bottom, then the rate drops to 5%. Finally, if the definition is confined to serious physical abuse such as kicking, hitting with a fist or beating up a child, the rate drops to less than 1%.

There is some evidence that, amongst economically developed societies, child abuse has increased over the past 40 years (Emery & Laumann-Billings, 2003). This seems to be because of the number of reported cases of serious abuse, which quadrupled from 1986 to 1993 (142,000 to 565,000) in the United States (Sedlak & Broadhurst, 1996). The number of cases of "grave concern" also increased in the United Kingdom (Besharov, 1996). Researchers have attributed the rise in serious abuse to greater poverty in some parts of society, illegal drugs, increases in overall violence and the disintegration of communities.

Child abuse has multiple aetiological facets (Emery & Laumann-Billings, 2003). Profiling the abuser requires a comprehensive description and understanding of the social, psychological, physiological and genetic factors within the caregiver(s); the family and neighbourhood environments; and the child. It has been suggested that abusing men (only) can be described in three rather different types:

1. generally violent antisocial with pervasive abusive behaviours across social settings and persons who are likely to abuse alcohol and have antisocial personality traits;
2. family-specific type, abusing only within family members, who are often rather dependent and jealous, feel remorse after the event and are unlikely to have a personality disorder; and
3. mood-related emotionally volatile batterers whose violence is activated during dysphoric mood only and who are more likely to have borderline personality traits, be rather socially isolated and feel inadequate about their abilities.

Child abuse represents one of the most significant long-term risk factors for psychopathology. The consequences are wide ranging and include immediate physical injury, immediate and delayed

---

> **Box 6.3** Factors Associated with Adverse Outcomes in the Context of Child Abuse
>
> - High frequency, intensity and duration of the abuse
> - Individual characteristics of the victim
> - The nature of the relationship between abuser and child
> - The response of others to abuse
> - The social and family contexts within which the abuse occurs

---

psychological distress and disorder, and in severe cases significant practical upheaval of the environment (foster homes, etc.). Factors within the abusive history that contribute to adverse outcomes are shown in Box 6.3.

The current evidence is substantially in agreement that during the childhood years emotional rather than behavioural disorders are most likely to be expressed and that maltreatment has effects independent of other environmental adversities on the liability for disorder and may of itself disrupt the normal processes of child cognitive development increasing the risk for personality difficulties and psychiatric disorders in adult life (Kim & Cicchetti, 2004; Rogosch & Cicchetti, 2004).

Treatment is dependent on a thorough evaluation of risks for psychopathology, as well as a clear assessment of the severity of the abuse. In general the more severe the abusive history in terms of frequency, intensity and duration the less successful are the interventions (Emery & Laumann-Billings, 2003). Clinicians need to identify the following:

- immediate danger to the child;
- strengths and weaknesses in the family system;
- specific parental needs in terms of parent-child training and/or relation building; and
- specific child needs such as nutrition, socialisation and quality of education.

In low-frequency, motivated families with good warmth and high care environments for the child, behavioural parenting strategies including specific skills training and cognitive restructuring of distortions of child behaviour appear to be highly effective.

Child sexual abuse is a specific form of abuse that has received increasing attention (Glazer, 2003; see also Chapter 17). Prevalence figures for sexual abuse suggest a marked distinction between contact and noncontact abuses (Finkelhor *et al.*, 2005). *Noncontact abuse* is defined as watching sexual acts, being exposed to genitalia, taking of photographs for pornographic purposes or being forced to interact sexually with each other. Between 10% and 20% of men and 40% and 60% of women will have been exposed to noncontact sexual abuse before age 16 years (Wyatt, 1985). *Contact sexual abuse* is defined as physical contact between the breasts or genitalia of a child or adult and a part of the other's body (not including accidental touch). Active abuse is often preceded by an insidious process in which the abuser befriends the child and manipulates increasing ways of them being alone together; physical violence is less frequent. Sexual intercourse is most frequent in children between ages 9 and 12 years but may occur at any age from infancy onwards. Females are 4 times more likely to be sexually abused than males. Boys are much more reluctant than girls to discuss their abusive experiences, and there is likely to be significant underreporting. In population samples, approximately 4% to 10% of women report full sexual intercourse as a child, a figure that rises to 65% in clinical samples (see Glazer, 2003, p. 342).

The majority (85%–95%) of abusers are male, but those who target prepubertal children tend to both sexes. Those who focus on adolescents tend to target females. There is no reliable and valid profile of sexual abusers. They are heterogeneous in their own developmental and psychiatric histories. A significant proportion is of low intellectual ability, many will have experienced an abusive relationship in their own childhood and some will have a history of conduct disorder as a child. There is a suggestion that for some, this is an addictive behaviour. Abusers may begin their activities at any stage in their own life-cycle.

For the child victim, there is a raised lifetime risk for emotional and behavioural disorders. In childhood and adolescence, the victim may express highly sexualised behaviour. Sexual interference with other children is a particularly difficult outcome to manage and a challenge to treatment. By adolescence, there are higher rates of depressive disorders in the abused population than the general population, and a range of problems (eating difficulties, substance misuse, early teenage pregnancy, criminal activities) can manifest. Little is known about the role of resilient and protective factors in ameliorating abusive experiences over time.

Clinical management of abuse is predicated on ensuring the safety of the child from further abusive experiences. Once achieved, treatment for psychiatric consequences can be provided (Finkelhor and Berliner, 1995). Treatment for abusers may also be offered. Reconciliation between child and the abuser, especially if a parent, is a difficult clinical and social issue that requires considerable multidisciplinary work. Outcome is related to the severity of the abusive experience more than the child's coping strategy at the time of the events. Individual and group and family treatments have all been used, and a treatment and care package should be tailored to the individual child. Little difference in overall effect has been shown between individual and group treatments (Jones & Ramchandani, 1999).

Clinical syndromes that arise during childhood and adolescence

The rest of this chapter is focussed on those clinical disorders that arise in the first two decades of life and in which the form of disorder is specific to children and adolescents. Other chapters in this volume provide detailed explanations of disorders that are uncommon in this age range but may occur sporadically. These include the major psychoses, obsessive-compulsive disorders, personality syndromes and substance misuse.

Attachment disorders

Our understanding of disorders of attachment derive from systematic observations of the emotions and behaviours of infants and children raised

Box 6.4 The Stages of Ontogeny of Attachment

- Simple orientation signals from the infant to the immediate potential caregiver with no discrimination
- Direction of these orienting signals to a specific caregiver (one or more)
- Maintenance of proximity to a discriminated figure by means of locomotion as well as signals
- The formation in the preschool years of goal-directed partnerships which accompanies the child's emerging ability to discern the caregiver's feelings and motives and is capable of attributing mental states to him or her

in institutions before and immediately after the Second World War (Bowlby, 1951, 1981). The observations gave rise to attachment theory, which has been the subject of extensive research. Curiously, the clinical phenomenology and the implications for psychopathology were largely ignored. Recent research has sought to define attachment disorders and reconnect these to advances in attachment theory (O'Connor, 2003). Attachment is a dynamic process that is viewed as biologically driven and mutually reinforcing and adaptive for the parent and the child. The process fosters care and the growth of emotional warmth within parents and children and thereby enhances reciprocal positive affiliative relationships between parent-infant dyads.

There are four broad stages in the ontogeny of attachment, as shown in Box 6.4. Contrary to earlier thinking, this process is not specific to the biological mother or father and can occur with stranger caregivers if they participate in the interpersonal processes that facilitate orienting and proximity-seeking experiences.

Although Box 6.4 refers to the ontogeny from the perspective of the child, attachment behaviour is a relational process that arises as a consequence of the contribution of behaviours from both the infant and the caregiver. This is an important principle because theoretically attachment disorders may arise as a result of a deficit or failure in relational psychology, the origins of which may reside in the caregiver or the infant.

A key clinical feature of attachment disorders within the infant is the failure to differentiate and focus on key caregivers in later infancy. Within the caregiver, a poor orienting response to infant cues to provide a positive environment (physical and/or emotional) is the key presenting feature. The implications of positive attachment are that the child is developmentally enabled to engage in further mutually reinforcing social relationships. Attachment relationships do not have deterministic lifelong prediction for a socially rewarding life; rather, they moderate the behaviours and feelings that influence the next stage of development. A related notion is that of developmental programming effects in infancy. This suggests that early environmental experiences exert permanent effects on the development of biological systems that have effects throughout the lifespan. These epigenetic processes can occur for biological systems that influence behaviour. For example, the form of maternal care can influence the tone of the hypothalamic-pituitary axis in rodents (Weaver *et al.*, 2004) and possibly in humans (Halligan *et al.*, 2004). Thus the relational processes between infant and caregiver is likely to have an organising effect on behaviours that reflects how the individual may respond to later experiences. Whether these programming effects are permanent or moderated by subsequent physiological (e.g. adrenarche and puberty), environmental (e.g. positive peer group) or both types of influence is not known.

Natural experiments charting the behavioural development of children raised in institutions and by their natural parents point to such effects as potentially likely, although the heterogeneity of the outcomes suggests the effects are not always deterministic (Rutter & O'Connor, 2004). Thus subsequent positive experiences can provide remission from undesirable behaviours within the disordered infant and restitution of some but not all abnormalities.

Disturbances in parent-child relationships in infancy (i.e. the first two years of life) significantly influence the development of psychopathology

(O'Connor, 2003). The vast majority of this work is not on attachment disorders but on children with individual differences in normative attachment behaviours. Current classification of attachment disorders has attempted to remain theory-free and focus on putative clinical characteristics.

Classification of disorder

One notable point of agreement between the *International Classification of Diseases* (10th edition; ICD-10) and *Diagnostic and Statistical Manual* (4th edition; DSM-IV) classification systems is that there are two types of attachment disorder – namely, a disinhibited and an inhibited form.

The features of *disinhibited attachment disorder* derive in the main from studies of children reared in institutions. These infants and young children show overly familiar, proximity-seeking affectionate behaviour and a rather indiscriminate manner towards strangers. They also show disturbed interactions with others (strangers), exhibiting shallow and poorly sustained relationships.

Inhibited attachment disorder (or reactive attachment disorder in ICD-10) is less well developed. It is characterised by a persistent failure to initiate or respond to social cues in most social interaction circumstances. These infants or young children will show highly ambivalent, avoidant or even aggressive behaviours.

Both subtypes onset before 5 years of age. Any child presenting with these types of behaviours but with no preschool history should be considered as likely to be suffering from a different emotional or behavioural disorder. Children who meet the age criterion must also be shown not to be suffering from neurodevelopmental delay or deficits including autistic syndromes and speech and language disorders.

Most clinical research has been on the disinhibited type of attachment disorder related to deprivation of parental care or severe maltreatment. Early severe deficits in caregiving lead to this disorder, which itself serves to increase the liability for fearfulness, general worry, poor attention and overactivity (O'Connor & Rutter, 2000). Overt aggression can occur but is not a common feature in the early phase and is more likely to occur in those children exposed to maltreatment (O'Connor, *et al.*, 2003). As yet there are no systematic studies of comorbid syndromes with disinhibited attachment subtype.

There are no reported prevalence rates for attachment disorder. A study of adoptees found 19% with severe relational disturbances by 6 years of age (O'Connor & Rutter, 2000). The degree of exposure to deprivation was an important discriminator of risk for attachment disorder. Severe disinhibited behaviour was present in 7% of those infants adopted by 6 months but in 31% of those adopted between 24 and 42 months. This suggests a complex interplay between the duration and severity of exposure to pathogenic care processes influencing the liability for restitution following fostering or adoption. Overall inattentive and quasi-autistic disturbances are more likely than emotional and conduct syndromes in severely deprived children (Rutter *et al.*, 2001). Long-term outcome studies of disinhibited attachment disorder have found that symptoms show little change over a 2-year period (O'Connor, 2003) but somewhat greater improvements over 4 years (Tizard & Hodges, 1978).

Clinical assessment requires direct observation of the child to achieve the goals shown in Box 6.5. These observations should be supported by a clinical interview of caregiver and others in a care role (e.g. nursery worker, teacher). The interview should confirm the observed behaviours and also note whether the child wanders without checking back with the caregiver, whether the behaviour is pervasive across social circumstance or specific to one environment and whether it has changed over time and with different placements.

Treatments involve improving the attachment between child and caregiver. These can modify the sensitivity of the parent or caregiver to the needs of the child and thereby improve parental responsiveness (O'Connor *et al.*, 2003).

> **Box 6.5** Goals of Observational Assessment in Attachment Disorders
>
> - Differentiation of the level of sociable behaviour directed toward the caregiver compared with a stranger
> - Detection of indiscriminate friendliness, e.g. towards different members of a multidisciplinary team
> - Assessment of the quality of friendliness (e.g. physical contact seeking, intrusive questions, disrupting the communication of others, suggesting a failure to appreciate social rules and boundaries)

Wetting and soiling

Problems of continence in childhood are common and cause a great deal of distress and difficulty to both the child and parents or caregiver. Both maturation and learning are involved in establishing competent excretion habits. Control of excreta requires integrity of the autonomic nervous innervation of the smooth muscle of the bladder and gut, together with functioning of the spinal motor and sensory nerves. In addition, children must have reached the required level of cognition to appreciate what is required and the value of continence to their caregivers. They also require a sufficient motivational state to follow the expectations of others.

Faecal incontinence

There are considerable cultural influences on the age at which a child attains bowel control. Most children in Western societies have unreliable faecal continence in the first 2 years of life; some 10% of 3 year olds are not continent, with the rate declining to around 5% by 4 years and 1.5% by 7 years. In a community survey, soiling at a frequency of once a month or more affected 1.3% of boys and 0.3% of girls (Rutter *et al.*, 1970). Only a small minority of these children are referred to child mental health services. Social expectations may be more demanding than medical ones. A young person with a learning disability may well be socially handicapped by soiling even if his or her mental age is below 4 years.

Types of faecal incontinence

Faecal incontinence is a general term for any sort of deposition of faeces. There are several patterns and a number of possible dysfunctions. Persistent leak of fluid faeces arises primarily as a physical disorder involving structural or functional difficulties (or both) in the gut and should be referred to specialist paediatric services. Leakage of semi-solid faeces into the undergarments suggests a retentive disorder, which is likely to be psychiatric in nature. The placing of fully formed stools in hidden and inappropriate places is also highly suggesting of a psychiatric disorder. *Primary incontinence* refers to any of these patterns occurring in the absence of the child being continent. *Secondary incontinence* refers to any of these patterns occurring in a child who was previously continent.

Retentive soiling

The majority of children referred to child mental health clinics for incontinence show the pattern of retentive soiling (Loening-Baucke, 1996). These children lack sensitivity to rectal sensation and distension, and a small minority show an abnormal contraction of the voluntary muscles of the pelvic floor during defecation. It is not known whether these physiological difficulties are present before symptom onset. Persistent symptoms may lead to chronic dilation of the rectum. Although there is modest evidence for a familial aggregation of retentive soiling (Bellman, 1966), it remains unclear whether there are genetic influences.

The role of variations in toilet training of toddlers as a contributory cause for retentive soiling remains uncertain. Family stressors during infancy and preschool years appear to be potential contributory processes in about half the cases presenting to clinics (Silver, 1996). Chronic constipation or retention may be a sign of sexual abuse, with the development of retentive soiling a consequence of a refusal to open bowels in fear of a further assault or because of anal injury. There are no precise estimates of the proportion of children with encopresis that results from abuse. Some cases are associated with low intelligence or more specific developmental delays of language comprehension.

Associated emotional and behavioural symptoms are significantly more likely in children with retentive soiling compared with the general population. For boys, such symptoms are 3 times more likely and for girls 8 times (Rutter *et al.*, 1970).

Treatment should be preceded by a thorough examination to rule out physical disease of the gut. Severe retention should be removed using an orally given enema wherever possible; subsequent laxative medication is preferable (Nolan *et al.*, 1991). This treatment is rather specific for this form of encopresis because it appears not to be helpful in those with nonretentive patterns of soiling (van Ginkel *et al.*, 2000). Psychological treatments are key. Basic toilet training techniques should be examined and behavioural operant techniques applied to reinforce toileting behaviours. Regular and predictable toileting (e.g. after every meal) with rewards such as star charts is particularly suitable for those with primary encopresis and can be used in secondary forms when the original training pattern was judged to be faulty.

There is evidence that some 30% of cases may persist into adolescence (Clayden *et al.*, 2003). Poor outcome is associated with comorbid risks for lower social adjustment in general. These include learning disability and difficulties, behavioural or emotional problems and noncompliance with treatment.

Urinary incontinence

Effective and efficient storage and voiding of urine is subserved by a neural system involving the pons, the sacral plexus via the cauda equine, the pudendal nerves and hypogastric plexus to innervate the bladder and the sphincter. The smooth muscle of the bladder (detrusor) is innervated by the parasympathetic postganglionic fibres, the ganglion cells of which are located in the bladder, with the preganglionic motor neurons reaching the bladder via the pudendal nerve.

Bladder control during the day is attained by age 5 years in 99% of children with normal intelligence and no health difficulties. Daytime continence is usually achieved before night. By the age 7 years, some 20% of males and 10% of females may still have nocturnal incontinence (Clayden *et al.*, 2003). By age 18 years, 1% of males and perhaps 0.5% of females are still wet at night (Butler, 1998). Daytime wetting is far less prevalent and occurs in more girls than boys (Hellstrom *et al.*, 1990). As with the night-time form the natural history is one of gradual resolution: each year some 14% of 5 to 9 year olds become dry; the corresponding rate is 10% for 10 to 18 year olds (Forsythe and Redmond, 1974).

Diagnosis of what is abnormal is not straightforward, being influenced strongly by individual differences in attaining continence that are multifactorial and include genetic, physiological, psychological, parental expectations and sociocultural factors. The decision to treat presenting cases should be based on the extent to which the child is impaired by his or her symptoms and the associated negative impact on the immediate family and social circumstances.

There are three main types of incontinence (Shaffer *et al.*, 1994). The most common is bedwetting (nocturnal enuresis) with no daytime problem. A second is that of diurnal enuresis, which has two subtypes: with or without bedwetting. In addition, it is important to establish whether the form of disorder is primary, that is, a continuing form of the normal incontinence of childhood, or secondary, starting after the child has been successfully dry.

Incontinence of urine is seldom associated with other abnormalities of micturition. For some children, the complaint will be that they are depositing urine in inappropriate places (but are otherwise continent). Inquiries should then be directed towards the motives for doing so rather than investigations of bladder function. Other sources of clinical heterogeneity include developmental delays, presence of concurrent emotional or behavioural problems, or both.

Causal pathways
Nocturnal enuresis runs in families. Of children with this form, 70% have parent or sibling who was late in becoming dry (Jarvelin *et al.*, 1991). Monozygotic

twins are almost twice as likely to suffer from nocturnal enuresis as dizygotic twins. Primary enuresis is best predicted by a positive family history and lower developmental maturity in the first 3 years of life, whereas secondary enuresis is best predicted by being late to attain bladder control and being exposed to a high rate of adverse life events (Fergusson *et al.*, 1990).

Pathophysiological mechanisms include disturbed sleep patterns (Rona *et al.*, 1997) with higher levels of reported nightmares (Moilanen *et al.*, 1998) increased levels of sodium excretion (Natochin & Kuznetsova, 2000), failing to wake from light sleep when the bladder is full (Watanabe, 1991) and with a nocturnal reduction in renal sensitivity to vasopressin (Robertson *et al.*, 1999).

There are high rates (40%–60%) of comorbid behavioural disturbance in these patients (Byrd *et al.*, 1996), being present in 40% or so of those attending child psychiatry services (Clayden *et al.*, 2003). Comorbid behavioural disorders place a higher burden of demand and difficulty on families and may lead to secondary psychological distress in parents, siblings and the probands. Children with enuresis have a lower self-percept of themselves. Children view enuresis as a highly stressful event and are often secretive. Patients often have poor peer group networks for fear of being "found out" in social circumstances.

Clinical management

Parents do not consider most wetting problems a problem and seldom seek advice. The vast majority of wetters are dealt with (quite rightly) in primary care services. Referral to child mental health services is often due to failure of response to symptomatic measures. Physical investigation should be thorough, including palpation of the abdomen and kidneys and examination of the spine and muscular systems for wasting. Urine should be sent for culture, and in rare cases diabetes may be considered. Nocturnal epilepsy or upper-airway obstruction may occasionally present with enuresis.

Family circumstances should be assessed and a mental state on the child carried out. Rigid, harsh toilet training practices or alternatively neglectful ones should be closely considered. Formal treatments should begin with education reassurance about the natural history and a review of parenting and toileting strategies. Enuresis alarms are the most successful treatment (Mellon & McGrath, 2000). The treatment is safe, and approximately three quarters of all users will achieve continence by 4 months of regular and proper use. Treatment compliance is a key feature.

Medications can reduce the incidence of night-time wetting and are useful as short-term treatment in severe cases or when there are social benefits, such as a child going on a school trip. Desmopressin, an analogue of antidiuretic hormone, produces significantly more dry nights that placebo (Skoog *et al.*, 1997). Its use is generally safe, and it can be given as a nasal spray. Tricyclic and tetracyclic antidepressants have a greater effect than placebo in reducing the frequency of wetting (Glazener & Evans, 2000). These drugs have a high risk of side effects in overdose, and treatment gains are lost when the medicine is stopped. These medications should be reserved for emergency circumstances in specialist clinics.

Attention-deficit/hyperactivity disorder

ADHD is a clinical syndrome presenting in the childhood years, generally before age 8 years, with a core set of symptoms consisting of inattention, hyperactivity and impulsivity. These terms are used in a broad clinical sense to describe a set of real-life difficulties that these children experience in school, home and social circumstances. Diagnosis is not straightforward because the core constructs are all themselves heterogeneous.

Studies using the broader-based DSM categories show the highest estimates ranging from between 5% to 10% of children between the ages of 5 and 12 years (Fergusson *et al.*, 1993; Newman *et al.*, 1996; Offord *et al.*, 1989). In the more narrowly defined

ICD types, estimates are generally between 1% and 2% for the full syndrome without comorbid features (Daenckerts & Taylor, 1995; Swanson *et al.*, 1998). There are cultural and ethnic differences in prevalence in part due to variations in the interpretation of observed behaviours.

Clinical attention difficulties include difficulties selecting a task, staying on task and finishing things, together with a high degree of switching from one task to another. *Hyperactivity* consists of motor restlessness that is not goal directed and consists of fidgetiness whilst still, overactivity whilst on the move and restlessness independent of social context, in some cases including whilst sleeping. *Impulsivity* is defined as the inability to delay a response to a stimulus, even one that carries negative consequences. The components of impulsivity are short reaction times, low inhibition and failure to learn from previous experiences leading to risk-taking behaviours. Each of these components carries a degree of impairment to the child's well-being and high symptom levels in all three areas reflects a severe disorder often requiring constant supervision in the young child.

Hyperactivity and impulsivity are more closely associated with each other than either is to attentional difficulties. In the DSM-IV classification, this has influenced the description of two forms of ADHD with three possible diagnostic implications – an inattentive type, hyperactivity type or a combined type. In contrast, ICD has a single diagnosis termed *hyperkinetic disorder* but allows the classification of attention difficulties without hyperactivity. For a diagnosis, symptoms should have begun before age 7 years and have been present for at least 6 months. The broader terminology of DSM has led to an increase in the number of children in the United States with the diagnosis of ADHD with a greater inclusion of girls, preschoolers and adults. There has also been a 50% increase in the overall prevalence within the school-age population and a marked upturn in prescribing stimulant medication (Schachar & Tannock, 2003). These increases have also occurred in other parts of the world but to a more limited extent. It may be that those countries with a bias toward the ICD classification are less likely to broaden the diagnosis or show a marked increase in prescribing medication.

ADHD invariably presents with comorbid diagnoses. In ICD, the presence of conduct disorder leads to a different diagnosis of hyperkinetic conduct disorder, whereas in DSM concurrent conduct disorder is recorded as comorbidity. More than half of ADHD cases present with comorbid diagnoses. Other comorbidities include emotional disorders and learning difficulties, and co-ordination problems and motor clumsiness are also common.

An alternative to categorical syndrome identification is a quantitative approach to the traits underlying the conditions. In this approach, it is assumed that the constituent components vary widely in the population, and it is those at the extreme ends of this distribution who are most likely to be both impaired and disordered (Fergusson *et al.*, 1991). This approach is supported by the observation that there is no bimodal distribution of scores for attention, hyperactivity or impulsivity in the child populations. Thus there is no obvious discontinuity between groups of individuals in the community with high scores and those with moderate to lower scores on any measure of hyperactivity. Dimensionally scored variables generally show a fairly consistent linear effect in that those with higher scores and therefore greater risk show more heritability and a worse outcome (Fergusson & Horwood, 1995; Levy *et al.*, 1997).

ADHD – hyperactivity type or combined type have a fivefold increased risk for adverse outcomes into adult life (McArdle *et al.*, 1997). These children show increases in disruptive behaviour disorders, substance misuse, poor academic achievement and lower status employment. Outcome is made worse by exposure to chronic psychosocial adversities and by a family history of hyperactivity (Taylor *et al.*, 1996). In the child, high symptom counts dominated by hyperactivity and/or impulsivity, comorbid conduct disorder or associated language and learning difficulties are all associated with a worsening of prognosis (Merrell & Tymms, 2001).

Aetiology

ADHD is an aetiologically heterogeneous disorder with genetic, neurochemical, affective-cognitive and social environmental adversities contributing to overall liability for disorder. Much of the available evidence points to brain-based abnormalities in executive functions in self-regulation, arousal, motivation, cognitive flexibility and working memory, arising primarily as a failure of dopaminergic neural systems to evoke normative reward systems in the developing brain (Carrasco *et al.*, 2005; Sagvolden *et al.*, 2005). Abnormalities in a distributed neural system that involves the orbital prefrontal cortex, anterior cingulate and its connections to the basal ganglia appear particularly implicated. Thus the clinical phenotypes of ADHD increasingly appear to arise from a loss of efficiency, effectiveness or across a widespread generalised dopaminergic network dysfunction and may not be easily attributable to a single basic behavioural function (Carrasco *et al.*, 2005; Doyle *et al.*, 2005).

Family, twin, adoption and molecular studies offer strong evidence for genetic susceptibility to ADHD (Cornish *et al.*, 2005; Doyle *et al.*, 2005; Reiersen, 2005; Stevenson *et al.*, 2005; Volkmar, 2005). Twin studies have reported heritability estimates of between 0.7 and 0.9, with the data favouring genetic influences on higher scores on the trait measures of hyperactivity-impulsivity. Candidate gene approaches have begun to identify markers notably in the dopamine system (DAT1 and D4 receptor gene in particular). Gene-environment interactions are likely to be important. Classical twin study analyses are particularly poor at identifying within-family environmental effects, and "pure" genetic estimates are likely to contain these interactions within their reported heritability estimates. Future studies need to include measures of the internal and the external environment of the child as well as being genetically sensitive before any firm conclusions can be reached about the relative

---

> **Box 6.6** Arms of the MTA Study
> - Medication alone (mostly methylphenidate)
> - Medication + psychosocial treatment (combined family therapy, summer camp, social skills, and classroom management)
> - Psychosocial treatment alone
> - A typical community-based intervention

contributions of genetic and epigenetic influences on ADHD traits and disorders.

Treatment

The major focus of treatment of ADHD is on reduction of hyperactivity and impulsivity, improvements on attention and, in some cases, a decrease in aggression with concomitant improvements in self-confidence and a lowering of social anxiety. In terms of medication, the most recent and largest randomised controlled trial of stimulant medication for ADHD is the MTA study outlined in Box 6.6 (Multimodal Treatment Study of Children With ADHD; Jensen *et al.*, 2007). Patients with the hyperactive type of ADHD did best on medication alone with little additional benefit from psychosocial treatments. Those who received combination treatment had equivalent improvement to medication alone but on a lower dose of medicine. The additional benefit was most apparent amongst those with comorbid anxiety disorders and a higher level of psychosocial adversities at home. Medication management resulted in better improvements in the specialist physician than the community-treated group. This was particularly true for children with comorbid anxiety symptoms. This latter finding suggests that complex cases will be better managed in specialist clinics.

Thus overall there is clear-cut evidence for medication as a first-line treatment in the hyperactive type with psychosocial interventions in an effort to maintain low-dose medication. Diagnostic uncertainty, comorbid possibilities and complex psychosocial environments are strong clinical reasons to consider referral to specialist child mental health services. The latter services should strongly consider the formation of specialist ADHD services in the light of this important treatment study.

Psychological treatments alone are not recommended for the ADHD – hyperactive-impulsive type (Kutcher *et al.*, 2004) but may be a first-line treatment of choice for the inattentive type or used as a concurrent therapy, particularly in those in whom comorbid disorders are equally dominant (Murphy, 2005).

Stimulant treatment may have a limited impact on learning and aggressive behaviour, be less effective in adolescents compared with children and, in a few children, increase social-inhibited behaviour and dysphoric feelings. There is evidence for long-term efficacy in many cases with few negative effects of comorbid disorders in stimulant responders. Psychosocial treatments should be offered to all families either because of primary behavioural difficulties in the child or secondary effects on family functions including siblings. Behavioural treatments alone have moderate to small effects in ADHD and little or no effect in the hyperactive-impulsivity type.

Most families choose multimodal treatments involving concurrent administration of psychosocial and pharmacological treatments. Indeed, child psychiatrists should work in multidisciplinary teams that are able to deliver combination treatments.

From the public health perspective, the greatest burden in schools and families is likely to arise from the ADHD – inattentive group. The treatment findings for this, the largest subtype, are equivocal, with no support for a medical intervention as a first line. Prevention strategies should be aimed at this subpopulation. In addition, preschool groups with high levels of ADHD symptoms associated with language difficulties and antisocial behaviour should be a key target for early interventions because they are most likely to develop ADHD – hyperactivity type in the school-age years (Moffitt, 1990). Current strategies are combined family-based interventions for improving parent-child relations and preschool-based behavioural programmes for managing restlessness, impulsivity and aggressive (both proactive and reactive) behaviours to peers. There is considerable optimism that treatment of the ADHD – hyperactive type will be effective. Equally there is growing sense that public health strategies in the preschool child in the community could diminish the burden of care children with these disorders may require in the school-age years.

Autism spectrum disorders

Autism spectrum disorders are characterised by the early onset of a constellation of features consisting of difficulties in social reciprocal interaction and communication and restricted and repetitive behaviours or interests. The term *autism* means withdrawal but is potentially misleading because it may be mistaken for a child withdrawing into an active internal world as a consequence of external adversities in early life. The reality is that children with autistic spectrum disorders are unable to participate in the social world due to their brain-based disorder, which leads to severe impairments in the aforementioned affective, cognitive and behavioural domains.

Autism also differs substantially from schizophrenia in its much earlier onset, greater frequency of neurological features including a high incidence of seizures in adolescence, stronger associations with mental retardation and a different pattern of cognitive deficits (Volkmar & Nelson, 1990). The classic study by Folstein and Rutter (1977) showed that autism was highly genetic in origin and that milder but related deficits are found in monozygotic twins discordant for disorder. The broader phenotype was subsequent described in first-degree relatives with milder deficits (Bolton *et al.*, 1994; Fombonne *et al.*, 1997). The notion of a spectrum disorder became accepted and encompassed the classical cases of autism and Asperger's syndrome described by Leo Kanner and Hans Asperger respectively in the late 1940s and a set of milder conditions with variable degrees of impairment. The DSM and ICD diagnostic frameworks have almost identical representation of autism spectrum disorders classified under the term *pervasive developmental disorder*. Diagnosis depends on the presence of impairments before the age of 36 months in three areas: social reciprocity, communication and restricted behaviours and interests.

The *epidemiology* of autistic spectrum disorder has shown an increase in the prevalence from 2 to 5 per 10,000 in the 1970s to around 7.5 per 10,000 in the 1990s for classical autism and 12.25 per 10,000 for atypical autism, Asperger's and other variants (Fombonne, 1999; Tidmarsh & Volkmar 2003). Precise estimates for Asperger's are not known but when included as milder variants of fautistic spectrum disorders may be as high as 60 per 10,000 (Charman, 2003). Current figures suggest about 2 cases per 1,000 individuals and are likely to be an underestimate of Asperger's and milder variants. Rates for the latter may be as high as 5 cases per 1,000 for Asperger's and related disorders and 2 per 1,000 for classical autism (Chakrabarti & Fombonne, 2005; Micali *et al.,* 2004). At least some of this increase over the past 30 years is due to a broader definition and better ascertainment. Whether there is a true rise in some of these disorders requires further study.

Clinical features

Social deficits are characterised by a profound failure in social interactions and the ability to form relationships (Tanguay *et al.,* 1998). This is substantially different from children with mental retardation and language difficulties alone who do show such interests even if they are less able to communicate. Autistic preschoolers are less likely to comfort other children, may not seek enjoyment in social events and have a limited range of direct face-to-face expressions associated with unusual eye contact. Social reciprocity can and does develop in many of these children, albeit with the retention of a rather idiosyncratic style, but they may be secondarily handicapped by their lack of opportunity to learn from normal peer group interactions.

Communication difficulties are prevalent in autistic spectrum disorders with a markedly high level of language impairments but of varying types and severity. In severe classic conditions, there is an absence of speech; however, in a small proportion of cases, there is an overproduction of speech often delivered in a rather monologue style. A further group shows directed speech delivered only rarely and invariably in a form of asking for things. Syntax and grammar may be abnormal in a variety of ways, including reversal of pronouns, delayed echolalia, stereotypical speech often borrowed from others and the making up of new words (neologisms) (Lord *et al.,* 2000).

There are also deficits in nonverbal communication, including impairments in gestures of nodding, pointing and showing. There are marked impairments in language comprehension and associated cognitive processes of imagination with consequences for social play. Autistic children have markedly restricted or absent imaginative play and noticeable severe impairments in turn taking and playing social reciprocal games such as hide and seek.

Autism is associated with severe language impairments in about 50% of cases (Volkmar *et al.,* 2005). Intensive early language work may diminish this prevalence by the school years, but the developmental trajectory of language acquisition by adolescence is about half of chronological age (Sigman & McGovern, 2005). The condition is most often associated with lower verbal than nonverbal skills.

Those children with Asperger's are distinguished by a normal onset of speech production by 36 months but a high incidence of the aforementioned abnormalities in language and cognitive processing domains (Volkmar *et al.,* 2005). About one in four will continue to show severe receptive and expressive language impairments in the first 2 decades of life, and of these there will be a noticeable subgroup with a verbal apraxia or dyspraxia that affects their articulation. These cases begin to show overlaps in their language and cognitive anomalies with children who have specific language impairments (Kjelgaard & Tager-Flusberg, 2001).

Stereotyped interests and behaviours include unusual preoccupations and circumscribed interests, compulsions and rituals, unusual hand and finger or whole-body movements, repetitive use of objects and unusual sensory reactions or interests. There is no core set of these features that occur in autistic children; rather, there are marked individual differences in presentation of these aspects. Rituals and repetitions differ from those seen in obsessive-compulsive disorder (Leckman *et al.*, 1997). In autism, they are not upsetting, and there is no resistance. The occurrence is often arbitrary and not linked to prevention of an untoward event. Autistic rituals do not contain complex tasks such as hand washing, checking or counting. In some, obsessive-compulsive disorder may develop later, and in such cases, there are typical symptoms of the latter disorder.

Stereotyped movements of the hands and fingers are also common, often but not exclusively within peripheral rather than central vision. Hand flapping, often accompanied by jumping, bouncing and rocking foot to foot, are also common. Peering at linear objects or patterns is frequently described. Until recently, stereotyped interests and behaviours were considered as secondary features, with the primary deficit being one of social communication (Tanguay *et al.*, 1998). Repetitive behaviours are not, however, secondary to an absence of social stimulation (Romanczyk, 1986). Adding a criterion of repetition to the diagnostic profile has, however, considerably improved the specificity of diagnosis (Buitelaar *et al.*, 1999).

There is a need for sameness in many but not all people with autism. Even subtle changes, such as the change of place of an ornament, in the environment can cause distress (Volkmar *et al.*, 2005). Some patients will self-harm, particularly those with learning difficulties, often hitting themselves for no apparent reason. Although there is a large proportion of patients with autism who also suffer from learning difficulties, modern community-based studies place the proportion of those with a general IQ within the normal range perhaps as high as 50% (Fombonne, 1999).

Detection and course

Autism is a brain-based disorder, and detection of difficulties by parents generally occurs in the first 2 years of life, although many parents are concerned in infancy. Parental concerns focus on low-level or absence of speech or difficulties in settling. About 25% of parents report a loss of the few words their infants have by the third year of life (Bale, 2002; Luyster *et al.*, 2005; Shinnar *et al.*, 2001). The relationship between this speech regression and later prognosis is unclear but is likely to indicate a more severe form of disorder with greater global impairments in social-cognitive function (Luyster *et al.*, 2005).

The two most powerful predictors of a better outcome are nonverbal IQ and the presence of language. The lower the nonverbal IQ, and the later the onset of speech, the worse the prognosis. Children with IQs lower than 50 and with no speech by 5 years have the poorest outcomes, but social communication, nonverbal communication and language variability all exert independent effects on outcome through into adult life, even in those with cognitive function within the normal range in childhood (Charman *et al.*, 2003; Howlin, 2003; Howlin *et al.*, 2004; Szatmari *et al.*, 2003). Other predictors of a better outcome in development by middle childhood include the presence of joint attention (a proxy of social language or relational skills; Sigman & McGovern, 2005), verbal imitation (Smith & Bryson, 1994, and social communication (Lord *et al.*, 2000).

Autistic syndromes are lifelong disorders even in those who show real improvements by young adult life (Howlin, 2003; Howlin *et al.*, 2004). Thus the likelihood of complete independence is limited. Useful employment and semi-independent living are possible, but even the most able are likely to require some help in these domains (Howlin, 2003; Howlin *et al.*, 2004). Comorbid disorders, especially depression and anxiety, are common in adults with autistic disorders (Ghaziuddin & Greden, 1998; Ghaziuddin *et al.*, 2002). These are deserving of treatment wherever possible. Their impact on prognosis into mid- and later life in autistic patients is not known.

Box 6.7   Differential Diagnosis of Autistic Spectrum Disorders

- *Receptive language disorder and semantic-pragmatic disorder:* specific developmental disorders with language delay and social communication deficits, but rarely have stereotyped interests and behaviours
- *Severe social deprivation:* usually show more social reciprocity even in the absence of speech and the presence of poor imaginative play (Rutter *et al.*, 1999)
- *Selective mutism:* associated with atypical language development (Kopp & Gillberg, 1997) but have strong social attachments to their parents, imaginative play and social reciprocity even though it may be restricted to a few persons
- *Early-onset schizophrenia:* there is a normal onset of speech and language with no idiosyncratic features
- *Rett syndrome:* a rare X-linked disorder that affects girls almost exclusively and is due to one or more mutations in the MECP2 gene (Amir *et al.*, 1999; Caballero & Hendrich, 2005); development is normal until about 12 months of age followed over the ensuing 12 months by gradual loss of speech and purposeful hand use with onset of stereotyped movements; also shows deceleration of head growth leading to acquired microcephaly
- *Childhood disintegrative disorder:* characterised by a pervasive decline in previously normal development (Volkmar & Rutter, 1995), extending well beyond language to include bowel, bladder and other neurological manifestations; some are due to metabolic disorders of the brain such as leukodystrophies, but invariably no clear cause is ever identified
- *Acquired aphasia with epilepsy (Landau-Kleffner syndrome):* may mimic autism, but the diagnosis is usually clear with a regression from normally acquired language and social communication skills associated with the onset of seizures (Deonna, 2000)

Differential diagnoses

The diagnosis is a specialist issue, and any child in whom autism is suspected should be referred to a unit with the appropriate expertise to undertake a full developmental psychiatric assessment. There are a number of other disorders to be considered, as shown in Box 6.7.

Conduct and oppositional disorders

The term *conduct disorder* refers to a persistent pattern of antisocial behaviour in which the individual repeatedly breaks social rules and carries out aggressive acts that upset others. It is the most common behavioural disorder across the world and the most frequent reason for referral to child and adolescent mental health services. Antisocial behaviour has the highest continuity into adulthood of all measured human traits, apart from intelligence. The disorder is becoming more frequent in adolescents in developed countries and places a high burden on individuals and costs on society. A high proportion of children with conduct disorders grow up to be antisocial adults, and a small but significant proportion will be classified in adult life as suffering from antisocial personality disorder.

Classification

Diagnosis is not straightforward when the core features, aggressive and defiant behaviour, are part of normal child development and context-sensitive in their expression. Determining when the behaviour is clinical and impairing is therefore complex and risks becoming arbitrary. Presenting symptoms will vary with age and gender and social context, and these factors must guide clinical assessments. The characteristic features are shown in Box 6.8.

There are two broad types of conduct disorder, an early-childhood onset and a later adolescent-onset type. *Childhood onsets* have severe symptoms starting before 7 years of age and show a sex difference with three boys for every girl. They show a high level of neuropsychological difficulties and a persistent and protracted course with a significant proportion of these developing or being reclassified as antisocial personality disorder in adult life. *Adolescent onsets* show no marked neuropsychological deficits, have an equal sex distribution and a better outcome with a markedly lower risk for antisocial personality disorder in adult life. Social factors and especially peer group deviancy play a

---

Box 6.8 Features of Conduct Disorder

Young Children
- Angry outbursts
- Temper tantrums
- Physical aggression towards peers and siblings in particular
- Destruction of property
- Arguing
- Blaming others
- General tendency to annoy and provoke others

Middle Childhood
- Swearing
- Lying about their whereabouts
- Stealing outside of the home
- Fire setting
- Cruelty to animals

Adolescence
- Violence to others
- Cruelty
- Assault
- Robbery using force
- Stealing from cars
- Running away from home
- Truanting
- Use of narcotic drugs

---

significant role in the onset of the adolescent onset form of these disorders.

The ICD and DSM systems follow each other closely for the diagnosis of conduct disorder. In ICD-10, the general clinical description requires an enduring pattern of antisocial behaviour. Details are specified for research diagnoses which are also clinically helpful. Symptoms should be present for at least 6 months and have an adverse impact on others. Symptoms are derived from four domains: aggression to people and animals, destruction of property, deceitfulness or theft and serious violation of the rules. These are most easily applied to middle childhood and adolescent patients. For younger children, the term *oppositional defiant disorder* is used, and diagnosis is made on the basis of a list of eight symptoms, of which four should be present and the individual (rather than others) should be impaired in ways that are maladaptive and inconsistent with the developmental level.

Prevalence and course

Serious oppositional behaviours in the preschool population is estimated at between 4% and 9%, and in school-age children, it is approximately 6% to 12%, with the more severe conduct disorders approximately 2% to 4%. In adolescents the estimates for oppositional disorders is as high as 15% and for severe conduct disorder between 6% and 12% (Costello *et al.*, 1996a, 1996b; Maughan *et al.*, 2004).

The early-onset group shows symptoms by 3 years of age. Symptoms continue to build and escalate. Approximately half remit or recover by age 8; the others show high levels of learning and language difficulties and callous-unemotional traits. They suffer poor parenting, are socially isolated and reach adult life with poor scholastic records, few friends and continued antisocial behaviour. They are referred to as life-course-persistent conduct disorder and are likely to receive a diagnosis of antisocial personality disorder.

The adolescent onset time-limited group do not have a child history of symptoms or neuropsychological deficits, are somewhat less antisocial and come from families with less parenting difficulties. By their 20s, patients' symptoms have frequently desisted or, at worst, remitted, and effects on them and society are negligible. Around 10% of this adolescent-onset time-limited group continue with antisocial behaviour into adult life.

Overall conduct disorders are more prevalent in urban compared with rural societies and 4 times more common in socioeconomically deprived areas where families are on low-income, state benefits or welfare. These social factors overlap considerably. These prevalence estimates and general characteristics have been confirmed in surveys from a range of Western countries including the United Kingdom, France, New Zealand and Canada. The prevalence estimates are somewhat lower in Hong Kong and South America.

There is evidence that in Western societies, conduct disorders have risen since the 1950s by as much as 20-fold.

Aetiology

Conduct disorder clusters in families and particularly in first-degree relatives of those with childhood early-onset type. Adoption studies have shown that criminal behaviour by adolescence is 2 to 3 times in the adopted-away offspring of infants from antisocial families compared with control subjects. Equally, however, those adopted into low-income families are more likely to have such histories by adolescence, indicating a key role for both genetic and environmental components to risk for conduct disorder through the first 2 decades of life.

Recent studies of molecular genetics and behaviour have confirmed a gene-environment interaction process underlying the liability for conduct disorders and antisocial personality disorder. This is most apparent for the life-course-persistent rather than the adolescent-onset group. A study of twins has shown that the most genetic components are aggressive tendencies which show continuity throughout the first 2 decades of life (Eley et al., 2003). Nonaggressive aspects of conduct disorders also show genetic influence, but the shared family environment is also highly contributory. Severe social privations, such as child maltreatment and poverty, are exerting effects of importance in conduct disorders primarily on nonsocial components such as lying, stealing and poor socialisation. As yet we do not know the precise role of social adversities in determining the potency of genetically mediated neural vulnerabilities to onset and persistence of these conditions. For example, Caspi et al. (2002) showed that maltreated children with a genotype conferring high levels of MAOA expression were less likely to develop antisocial problems. There is a powerful G $\times$ E interaction, with childhood maltreatment more likely to lead to antisocial behaviour if there is low expression of MAOA in the offspring. The combined effect leads to a greater incidence of conduct disorders and "disposition towards violence" in adult life.

Family process research has shown that coercive negative interpersonal relations between a parent and a child are important within-family moderators of the liability for conduct disorder (Conger et al., 1995; Patterson et al., 1998; Snyder et al., 2005). In families with a conduct-disordered child, negative behaviour is often reinforced by increased attention through shouting, criticism and blame. In contrast, a child's positive behaviours in such families are often ignored. Parental style is therefore an important social learning tool, and the balance of rewards and reinforcing positive behaviour is a key component in shaping positive values and diminishing antisocial behaviours in the child. It is striking that young children will show a preference for evoking negative reactions from their parents and therefore invite punishment that shows a preference for no interaction at all. This social attention rule indicates that children will behave in whatever way is required to gain parent time and proximity even when it is leading to the shaping of negative behaviours in themselves. This makes the immediate family context and the parent-child interaction patterns therein a key environmental feature of the liability for shaping the forms of behaviour within the offspring. This is a more optimistic perception than one of genetic determinism and has led to the development of effective parent-child treatments.

The gender differences in early-onset life-course-persistent conduct disorder are intriguing, and a considerable amount of research has been undertaken to identify whether there are sex-differentiated mechanisms that increase the liability for boys in the early school years to present with this severe behavioural condition.

It is crucial to distinguish between these disorders and children with moderate to severe behavioural difficulties who do not meet criteria for conduct or oppositional defiant disorder. Such children present with similar features of defiance, stubbornness and oppositional behaviours to family and friends and are often observably emotional at these times. Tears, anger and sadness frequently accompany these presentations. When highly disruptive to themselves and others, they are likely to be a significant cause for concern. These emotional-behavioural syndromes are poorly characterised but appear to have a much better outcome with no significant risk for delinquency and criminality in adult life. Although they appear somewhat more common in boys, they are poorly understood, probably consisting of a heterogeneous set of conditions.

Overall, conduct disorder is associated with erratic parenting styles in which discipline is unpredictable and accompanied by lack of warmth and by poor supervision. These parenting characteristics are not only reactions to the child's behaviour, but when they are, they contribute rather than alleviate symptoms in offspring. Persistent conduct disorder is associated with family breakdown, but even in these difficult circumstances, it is the style of parental care than predicts persistence of behavioural syndromes rather than breakdown per se.

The risks associated with poor parenting are influenced by the well-being of the parents themselves. Thus the liability for conduct disorder goes up in parents with psychiatric disorder and poor parental practices and may be attenuated in parents with poor parenting but no psychiatric disorder. It has been shown that criminality is partly brought about by a genetic predisposition, the mechanisms of which remain unknown (discussed earlier). Such an intrinsic vulnerability imparts a set of antisocial values which themselves operate to increase the liability for conduct disorders.

Child maltreatment (physical and sexual abuse) is associated with a significant increase in conduct disorders. This raised risk is somewhat nonspecific, however, because these traumatic experiences are a general vulnerability factor for emotional as well as behavioural disorders across the lifespan.

A number of nonfamilial factors may act to increase the risk of conduct disorders. These include poor school discipline with low morale amongst staff and students and high staff turnover, as well as deviant peer groups with a high incidence of antisocial behaviour. This deviant peer group factor is strongly associated with adolescent-onset disorders, whereas peer rejection is strongly associated with early-onset conduct disorder (Moffitt & Caspi, 2001; Moffitt et al., 2002). Other general risks include neighbourhood effects (Caspi et al., 2000), including poor housing, overcrowding and few amenities.

Child characteristics

A cluster of temperamental characteristics characterised by behavioural impulsivity, short attention span and motor restlessness observable in infancy are associated with aggressive problems in the preschool years. These features are highly stable and associated with antisocial behaviours in adulthood (Caspi et al., 1995). The extent to which they can be moderated by environmental features that will alter the developmental trajectory of the individual for the better is not known.

Emotional and cognitive factors include a tendency toward callous and unemotional traits, low empathy for others and a suspicious attributional style leading to a perception of hostility by others towards them. In primary school-age children, low subjective responses to emotionally arousing pictures is associated with higher scores on parent reports for deviant behaviour (Sharp et al., 2006). By adolescence, there is a low level of planning in their lives, poor social skills and low motivation for change. Recent advances in emotional psychology have noted a marked insensitivity to negative feedback and have begun to identify the neural systems that subserve these emotional and cognitive characteristics (Blair, 2001; Blair et al., 2001). Deficits in amygdala, orbitofrontal cortex and some prefrontal areas are implicated in these abnormal emotion-cognition processes in conduct-disordered youth and antisocial adults (Blair, 2004; Blair et al., 2006).

The underlying circuitry involved may vary according whether the child has high levels of callous-unemotional traits – which may be associated with a high level of neural dysfunction or is concurrently anxious – in which the underlying neural dysfunctions may be less and involve fewer of the aforementioned regions. In addition, early-onset conduct disorder is associated with a general level of intelligence some 8 to 10 points below the general population mean. This serves to act as a cognitive vulnerability which, in the presence of poor parenting, increases the liability for conduct disorders.

Finally, there is considerable evidence that autonomic underarousal is present in conduct disorders (Raine *et al.*, 1997). Compared with control subjects early-onset cases show low response and cortisol hyposecretion to emotionally arousing stimuli and low tolerance for frustration, despite self-reporting a feeling of being out of control during the tasks (van Goozen *et al.*, 1998, 2000). This dissociation between physiological and psychological parameters is marked and consistent with a central deficit in emotion processing (Blair *et al.*, 2006). These findings are not evident in those with high levels anxiety in whom responses are no different from those of control subjects (increased autonomic activity and cortisol hypersecretion). The implications of these findings for outcome and treatment remain under-investigated.

Risks as causes

Individual differences in heart rate are apparent from infancy and through the lifespan in both genders and consistently reported in association with aggressive and antisocial behaviour patterns (Pine *et al.*, 1998; Raine *et al.*, 1997; Raine, Meloy *et al.*, 1998). Lower heart rate in childhood predicts increased rates of antisocial behaviour in adult life and a higher heart rate in children with aggression predicts desistance into adult life (Raine *et al.*, 1997; Raine, Reynolds *et al.*, 1998).

The status of executive dysfunction is also being made clearer as a potential causal process. Children with no comorbid hyperactivity show low sustained attention, impaired planning, inefficient decision making, low motivation and poor problem solving independent of general IQ or memory abilities (Seguin *et al.*, 1999; Toupin *et al.*, 2000). These features correlate with clinical indices of antisocial

behaviour and may be more prevalent in adults with volumetric reductions in prefrontal cortical regions believed to subserve these executive processes (Raine *et al.*, 1998, 2000).

Long-term outcome

In the classic study by Robins (1996), nearly half of children with conduct disorders went on to develop antisocial personality disorder. These early childhood forms have become known as life-course persistent although as already noted, they may desist if the social environment is particularly emotionally positive in the preschool years. Individuals whose course begins with conflictual behaviour with parents and others are much less likely to progress to antisocial behaviour than those who have early signs of covert delinquent behaviours or cruelty and proactive aggression towards persons or animals (Loeber & Farrington 2000; Loeber *et al.*, 2000, 2001). The latter group are those most likely to show abnormalities in the prefrontal lobes and other brain regions, executive dysfunctions and impaired emotion response associated with a callous and nonempathic cognitive style (Blair, 2001, 2003; Raine *et al.*, 1998, 2000).

Treatment

For preschool and school-age subjects, treatment is largely focused on parental skills training and parent-child training. Parent management training is amongst the most successful in this age range with a focus on removing the coercive cycle of behaviour that exists in parent-child conflict situations (Webster-Stratton *et al.*, 2001a). Group parent management classes, especially for mothers with disruptive pre-schoolers, have demonstrated efficacy in the short term (Webster-Stratton *et al.*, 2001b, 2004). Improving marital dysharmony and disruptive adult behaviours and assisting adults with anger management using family-based methods and individual treatments have promise (de Kemp & Van Acker 1997; Van Acker & de Kemp 1997).

The impact of treatment on older adolescents is less clear, and there are no randomised controlled trials of psychological interventions in this age range. Similarly, it is not known whether treatment in childhood diminishes the risk for recurrence or relapse of antisocial behaviour in the long term.

Prevention

Two main preventative strategies have been employed: first, a public health approach to diminishing risk environments; second, a collective approach to improve competencies in individuals at risk for these disorders. The methods are sound, but a key variable is participation of families and ensuring treatments fit with the work-life balance of those at risk, or take up is less than satisfactory (Boyle *et al.*, 1999; Cunningham *et al.*, 2000; Hundert *et al.*, 1999).

In Canada, a comprehensive programme of nonacademic skills development was introduced for boys aged 5 to 15 years in one area and compared with another group with the same demographic features (Jones & Offord, 1989; Offord *et al.*, 1992; Sanford *et al.*, 1992). Those receiving the skills training showed a significant decrease in vandalism over the subsequent 3 years. This was not simply a result of more resources and attention paid to those youngsters because they also showed a significant increase in competence and skills. A cost analysis demonstrated that the financial savings for government far exceeded the cost of the programme. A caveat was that the improvements were limited to nonacademic areas of competence, and few gains were noted in school performance or indeed social skills. This suggests that improvements in skills are unlikely to generalise across domains of personal competencies. These latter observations point to the need for specific multimodal interventions in these children that are focused at different components of abilities to produce a realistic decline in risk reduction at the level of the individual.

With regard to learning competencies, school-based interventions have been popular for many years but have produced varying degrees of success in risk reduction. There have been many

> **Box 6.9** Elements of a Successful School Intervention for Conduct Disorder
>
> - Delivered by staff who are part of the school culture rather than perceived as "outside experts"
> - Schools are involved from the outset in designing the programme
> - Idiographic characteristics of the schools are at the centre of the programme, so that a "one size fits all" approach is not applied across widely differing student environments
> - Results are judged over time in a manner that has ecological validity for the schools

programmes in developed countries aimed at reducing risks invariably with widely different methodologies, sample sizes, population characteristics and outcome variables. Interventions in primary schools have shown that social skills and training behavioural programmes in 6 to 8 year olds can have a significant positive effect on behavioural ratings obtained from teachers and that these can endure over the primary school period (Hawkins *et al.*, 1991; Kolvin *et al.*, 1981). Cultural influences are likely to be important in the effectiveness of such programmes. A major problem identified from early studies is the key variable of efficient delivery and monitoring change in the school setting. Risk reduction policies aimed at diminishing aggressive actions between children are most likely to succeed when they accord with the principles shown in Box 6.9.

Although there is a general acceptance that risk reduction programmes should have a more powerful impact if started in vulnerable children in the preschool years, few studies have confirmed the validity of this approach. The Perry school intervention programme designed as an educational enrichment programme for 4- to 5-year-old children suggested that delinquency rates in later childhood were reduced in those who showed educational gains in the short term (Weikart & Schweinhart, 1991). This suggests that contrary to the findings described earlier for adolescents, early education programmes may have powerful generalizable effects on social and personal competencies, indicating a developmental opportunity in the younger child that may be markedly diminished by the teenage years.

In contrast to the complexities and variable outcomes from school-based programmes, home-based parent training programmes beginning in the prenatal period and extending through the first years of postnatal life have been popular. There are good reasons to be optimistic. For example, Olds and colleagues (1998) demonstrated that a long-term reduction of antisocial behaviour was most likely in adolescents who had received prenatal parenting enrichment programmes. The findings were greatest in those at the highest risk, suggesting targeting the programme at the most vulnerable may produce the best cost benefits for society at large. Infants at high risk, defined as children from low-income families with high levels of oppositional and aggressive symptoms, who received a 2-year programme of parent management training, social skills for the children and a television viewing training video for parents and children show significantly less aggressive behaviours at 3 years post-intervention than control subjects (Tremblay *et al.*, 1991; Vitaro *et al.*, 1999).

Parent training programmes alone have been shown to have a significant impact on reducing antisocial behaviour in preschool and school-age children in the community and in clinics (Scott *et al.*, 2001; Webster-Stratton *et al.*, 2004). The longer-term impact of such programmes remains unclear.

Depression

Neither DSM-IV nor ICD-10 describe a mood disorder with an onset specifically in childhood (American Psychiatric Association 1994; World Health Organisation, 1994). The ICD system contains no modifying rules for diagnoses in childhood, whereas DSM indicates that the presenting mood dysfunction in children and adolescents may be irritability rather than depression for both major depression and dysthymia. The latter diagnosis can be

made in children or adolescents with a duration of 1 year, rather than the 2 years used for diagnosis in adults. Neither system allows for children in infancy, preschool or the early school years to have a mood disorder unless they meet adult criteria. This effectively removes from clinical sight a large number of distressed children with irritable or sad mood, somatic features and social difficulties because they do not have negative cognitions. There is a significant need to undertake clinical and community-based studies in younger children to establish the nature and natural history of mood disorders in this age range. Recent studies of clinical populations clearly indicate that depressive disorders occur and can be elicited from children under age 7 (Luby *et al.*, 2004, 2006).

From the second decade onwards, there is little difference in the core characteristics of unipolar depression across the lifespan (Angold, 2003; Angold & Costello, 2001). There are some developmental effects on the pattern of symptoms in the first 2 decades of life. For example, physical symptoms are more common in children than adolescents, and negative cognitions – in particular, suicidal ideation – are more frequent in adolescents compared with children. In girls, the frequency of negative cognitions of hopelessness, helplessness and suicidal thinking increase somewhat across the adolescent age range.

Epidemiology

Major unipolar depression has an estimated 6- to 12-month prevalence of 3% in adolescence and 0.5% to 1% in children (Angold & Costello, 2001). In children, the sex ratio is about equal, but with adolescence comes an increasing rate of episodes in girls compared with boys. Dysthymia appears to be more common, with estimates around 6% for children and 10% in female adolescents. Depression is probably underestimated in the younger and particularly the preschool child (Egger & Angold, 2006). Minor depressive episodes probably occur in approximately 10% of adolescent girls and somewhat fewer boys.

Around half of depressed young people have a nondepressive comorbid disorder (Birmaher *et al.,* 1996; Costello *et al.,* 1996; Goodyer *et al.,* 1997; Lewinsohn *et al.,* 1998, 2000). Rates in clinical samples may be as a high as 80%. It is not clear, however, whether there are truly independent liabilities of co-occurrence of distinct syndromes or whether they reflect correlated liabilities thereby overinflating these rates. The natural history of depression in children and adolescence is markedly variable. The median duration of an episode is around 30 weeks but may range from a few weeks to many years. Community-ascertained cases recovery more rapidly but are just as likely to relapse as those seen in clinical settings (Dunn & Goodyer, 2006). Approximately half of clinical cases are likely to recur and may do so as long as 9 years after the initial episode (Dunn & Goodyer, 2006; Fombonne, 1995; Fombonne *et al.,* 2001; Lewinsohn *et al.,* 2000). Recurrence is associated with being female, greater severity and nondepressive comorbidity at index. In contrast, a potentially key variable for illness persisting through to adult life is being male. Onset in adolescence compared with childhood has indicated a greater probability of recurrent unipolar depression in some but not all studies. In contrast, onset of unipolar depression in childhood may indicate a greater risk for bipolar disorder in adult life (Geller *et al.,* 2000; Kovacs, 1996).

Aetiology

The aetiology of unipolar depressions is complex with evidence for genetic and environmental factors (Gregory *et al.,* 2007; Kendler *et al* , 2002; Lau *et al.,* 2007). *Behavioural genetic studies* in children and adolescents are based on level of depressive symptoms rather than disorders. In such studies, genetic influences appear to be particularly weak for child-onset disorders (Rice *et al.,* 2002). This is in contrast to the clinically based studies suggesting that child-onset unipolar cases are more likely than adolescent-onset cases to switch to bipolar disorder, which is considerably more genetic than unipolar depression. Family studies have noted a high familial density for depression with those showing at least three generations of continuity being at the most familial and perhaps the most genetic risk (Grillon *et al.,* 2005; Weissman *et al.,* 2005).

Gene-environment interactions are particularly likely at the onset of depressive episodes. Activating life events occurring relatively proximal to the onset of a depressive episode are most likely to result in major depression in those homozygous for the "s" allele of the serotonin transporter gene (Caspi *et al.,* 2003; Kendler *et al.,* 2005; Wilhelm *et al.,* 2006). Similarly child maltreatment may exert its long-standing effects on liability for depression in adolescents and young adult life most in those with homozygous for the same allelic variation in that same gene (Kaufman *et al.,* 2004).

Psychological vulnerabilities also precede the onset of depression. Negative views of the self enhance the liability for a clinical episode of depression independent of proximal life events (Alloy *et al.,* 1999, 2000; Kelvin *et al.,* 1999). Individuals with a high level of ruminative thinking style (dwelling on the negative thoughts and their meaning for the self) are amongst the most likely to experience an episode (Spasojevic & Alloy, 2001).

Early adverse experiences do not appear to cause ruminative thinking directly but are extremely likely to contribute to a developing cognitive vulnerability in the early childhood years characterised by a low self-percept, a sensitive style of feeling and little resilience in the face of competition from others or when there is a failure in problem solving (Murray *et al.,* 2001). Negative cognitions about the self may not, however, be permanent constructs resistant to change. Longitudinal studies suggest that there is a mutually active interdependent system throughout the developing years between various types of social experience, self-evaluation and social competence (Cole *et al.,* 1997, 1999).

Treatment

There is reasonable evidence that both psychological and pharmacological treatments are effective in the management of unipolar major depression in adolescents (Harrington *et al.*, 1998; March *et al.*, 2004; Whittington *et al.*, 2004). However, the more severe the depression, the greater the requirement for medication. Fluoxetine is the only selective serotonin reuptake inhibitor (SSRI) considered by the Commission of Safety on Medicines to have an acceptable balance of benefits over risks for the treatment of unipolar depressions in young people. Randomised controlled trials have shown that in moderate to severe depressions fluoxetine is superior to cognitive-behavioural therapy (CBT) alone or to placebo (March *et al.*, 2004). CBT is increasingly less effective in severe cases (Goodyer *et al.*, 2007; March *et al.*, 2004).

Current best practice for both children and adolescents is for watchful waiting together with education about the disorder for 2 to 4 weeks, followed by CBT as a first-line treatment if there is no spontaneous recovery for 6 to 12 weeks, followed by fluoxetine plus continuous CBT and family support in nonresponders to psychological treatment. Combination treatment of fluoxetine and CBT may be no more efficacious in the short term but may reduce the risk of relapse.

Parents are frequently surprised and distressed to receive a diagnosis of depression in their offspring. The disorder is often hidden from them by youngsters who fear they will be blamed for the disorder. Parents quickly become despondent that they have failed to be vigilant on behalf of their child. Family support is thus a key component of overall management. This should include siblings.

Bipolar disorder

In recent years some authorities have suggested that careful assessment of mood-related behaviours will elicit a diagnosis of childhood-onset mania (Geller *et al.*, 2004; Post *et al.*, 2004). Whether these children and young adolescents have a bipolar type disorder remains contentious (Harrington & Myatt, 2003). There is concern that in some instances, what is being measured are individual differences in the normative developmental range of emotion

---

> **Box 6.10** Contrasts between Childhood- and Adolescent-Onset Bipolar Disorder
>
> - In childhood onset, the initial episode is usually manic, compared with depressive in adolescent onset.
> - Mixed episodes and rapid cycling occur in most cases of child- compared with a minority of adolescent-onset patients.
> - Males predominate in childhood cases, whereas gender is more equal in those with adolescent onset.
> - Comorbid attention-deficit/hyperactivity disorder and/or conduct disorder occurs in more than 75% of child-onset cases, but only 10% to 20% of adolescent-onset cases.

characteristics, potentially resulting in diagnostic overinclusion.

The diagnosis debate is far less contentious with regard to postpubertal- and even peripubertal-onset mania or depression (Carlson, 2005). In this case, phenomenology more clearly resembles that of adults, regardless of the exact age after puberty that the first (manic) episode occurs. The most discordant features of prepubertal childhood and postpubertal adolescent onset forms are shown in Box 6.10.

Compared with adult onsets, clinical studies have also described child onset as characterised by an increased presence of psychosis and a poorer outcome, slower recovery times, more recurrences, greater comorbidity and a greater incidence of suicide. We do not have a precise retrospective account of the developmental psychopathology of this serious mental disorder. Recent reviews of the clinical and neurobiological characteristics of bipolar disorder suggest that overall, early- and adult-onset mania and bipolar disorder may share a common pattern of neurobiological characteristics despite developmental variations in the clinical presentation (Kyte *et al.*, 2006). In contrast, important distinctions are apparent between the child-onset syndromes of bipolar, ADHD and conduct disorders, specifically at the neural level. There is a clear-cut need to investigate more thoroughly than hitherto disorders of affect dysregulation in childhood from a neuroscientific and phenotypic perspective.

The guidelines for the treatment of bipolar disorder in children and adolescents are generally similar to those applied in adult practice (see Chapter 26). There are as yet no evidence-based data to support the use of mood stabilisers or antipsychotics in children and adolescents. Prescriptions should be limited to the most typical cases. The use of mood stabilisers or antipsychotics in the treatment of bipolar disorder in children and adolescents appears to be of limited use when a comorbid condition, such as ADHD, occurs unless aggressive behaviour is the target symptom. Pharmacological treatment should be carried out within a specialist Child and Adolescent Mental Health Service and always in conjunction with active psychosocial care.

Anxiety disorders

As outlined in Chapter 8, anxiety disorders consist of a set of syndromes ranging from very circumscribed conditions such as monophobias (e.g. a fear of spiders) to broad disorders characterised by free-floating fearfulness and general worry (e.g. general anxiety disorder). According to DSM-IV, there are two anxiety conditions that are specific to childhood: separation anxiety disorder and reactive attachment disorder. In contrast, ICD-10 notes five anxiety syndromes specific to this time of life: separation anxiety disorder, phobic anxiety, social anxiety, sibling rivalry disorder and general anxiety disorder.

Developmental appropriateness is the key feature in defining the difference between these disorders and neurotic anxiety disorders of adulthood. DSM considers that phobic, social and general anxiety disorders have similar clinical characteristics across the lifespan, and thus they are treated as a single disorder and classified only once. It is important to remember that the evidence base for both of these classification systems is modest, and expert agreement (consensual validity) is the main method for deciding on diagnostic criteria for a syndrome and

its appropriateness for inclusion as a separate disorder.

Separation anxiety disorder

The defining feature of separation anxiety disorder (SAP) is an excessive, unrealistic and persistent fear of separation from the attachment figure. This level of worry is qualitatively beyond normal. Both diagnostic systems indicate that it must be distinguished from formal thought disorder and first-rank symptoms of psychoses and schizophrenia. Although general worry is common, psychotic symptoms are rare in childhood and uncommon in adolescence.

Severe worries give rise to a typical maladaptive reaction pattern, typically involving some combination of the following:

- physiological responses, such as headaches, nausea, abdominal pain and rarely vomiting;
- behavioural symptoms, such as avoiding a feared situation, proximity seeking, tantrums; and
- extreme fearful thinking such as there may be a catastrophe, death or permanent separation that is imminent.

The diagnostic systems show relatively good agreement on the nature and characteristics of separation anxiety disorder. Both require fear of separation as the focus of anxiety and at least three symptoms of general worry from the eight possibilities shown in Box 6.11. In addition, duration of 4 weeks and the presence of personal impairment in social function must be present.

Separation anxiety disorder occurs in an estimated 2% to 4% of children and adolescents and accounts for approximately 50% of children seen for mental health anxiety disorders in this age range (Anderson et al., 1987). This syndrome is most often seen in prepubertal children, with proximity-seeking clinging behaviour being a common presenting complaint. No marked sex differences have been reported to date.

Few systematic data are available on the natural history and outcome of separation anxiety disorder. There are no longitudinal studies through adult

Box 6.11 Features of Separation Anxiety Disorder

- Harm that might befall a major attachment figure
- An event that will result in separation
- School reluctance as a result of the aforementioned fears
- Separation difficulties at night
- Reluctance to be alone
- Nightmares involving separation
- Physical symptoms involving separation
- Distress in anticipation of separations

life. During childhood, the symptoms tend to wax and wane. Normal events, such as school transitions, as well as clearly undesirable events, such as divorce or parental illness, may lead to recurrence or exacerbation. Although there has been a suggestion of continuities between panic disorder and agoraphobia in adults, longitudinal studies to date suggest any such continuities are weak (Aschenbrand *et al.*, 2003; Goodwin *et al.*, 2001; Suveg *et al.*, 2005).

School-refusal anxiety disorder

Nonattendance at school, although frequent in the general population, may result in referral to child mental health services. School phobia is uncommon and constitutes only a small proportion of school nonattenders. Social phobia, in contrast, is quite common by late adolescence consisting of two forms, a circumscribed disorder involving severe symptoms at particular times, such as performing or speaking in public, and a more generalised form involving most symptoms arising in most social interactions (Wittchen *et al.*, 1999).

Such children seek comforts at home, preferring to remain close to parental figures. They do not hide their worries from their parents and are rarely comorbid for other conditions, although mild depressive symptoms can occur. Physical symptoms similar to those found in SAD are evident. These somatic features are often limited to school mornings, reflecting the physiological consequences of intense worry about school. Invariably the physical and cognitive symptoms recede if avoidance of school is allowed.

Boys and girls are equally affected at any school age, but the transition from primary to secondary school represents a critical period of risk for this behaviour. There is no association with social class, intelligence or academic ability. The youngest in a family of several children is more likely to be affected, and parents are somewhat more likely to be older than expected. Onset tends to be gradual in the main with reluctance and difficulties increasing over weeks or months and signs and symptoms generally increasing from waking in the morning and going to school. Occasionally onset can be acute, precipitated by acute undesirable events. In such circumstances, events may be school-based and involve peer group difficulties such as bullying or, infrequently, teacher-child problems.

Severe or persistent absenteeism is generally associated with older adolescents, lower levels of fear and less active families. In such cases, the diagnosis may be truancy rather than school refusal. Truancy is associated with antisocial rather than emotional problems (Egger *et al.*, 2003). Compared with anxious school refusers, truants hide their school nonattendance from their parents. Both truancy and anxious school refusers may report concurrent depressive symptoms. Children or adolescents with both are extremely likely (>80%) to have a comorbid disorder of depression and or conduct disorder.

In *social anxiety disorder,* there is wariness of strangers and social apprehension or anxiety when encountering new, strange or socially threatening situations. The clinical characteristics are similar to those of adults (see Chapter 8), as are the rates of comorbidity with other anxious disorders.

Generalised anxiety disorder in children and adolescents shows a more limited range of symptoms than is seen in adult patients. In particular, specific symptoms of autonomic arousal are less prominent. The core features are extensive fear and general worry occurring for at least half the number of total days over at least 6 months. The worry is focussed on personal circumstances such as school performance or quality of friendships. For the diagnosis, there should be at least three other symptoms occurring concurrently, consisting of feelings of restlessness, tiredness or fatigue; poor concentration; irritability; muscular tension; or education performance. There is a nearly 80% symptom overlap with unipolar depression, and it is important to distinguish clinically between clinical mood and anxiety disorders. The presence of negative cognitions about the self rather than worries focussed on concerns that others have about oneself strongly indicates a depressive rather than an anxious diagnosis. Concurrent changes in appetite, sleep, anhedonic feelings or a combination of these are also consistent with a mood disorder. In GAD, the worries do not focus on a single theme as with SAD but are multiple and persistent rather than paroxysmal. Friendships may be less impaired than is reported in depression, perhaps because worry symptoms are more amenable to influence by important others in everyday conversation.

Aetiology

Aetiology is multifactorial and developmentally sensitive with maturational effects on the clinical phenotype. Thus, separation anxiety symptoms are more frequent in 6 to 9 year olds, death and danger fears in 10 to 13 year olds, and social anxiety symptoms as well as failure and criticism fears in 14 to 17 year olds (Abe & Masui, 1981). There is high familiality for these conditions with familial density for anxiety disorders greatest in the first-degree relatives of probands with panic disorder (Goldstein et al., 1997). Data from twins suggest that genetic and environmental factors are about equal (Hettema et al., 2001). Genetic influences may be greater in obsessional anxiety and shy/inhibited children and in early-onset cases (before age 7 years) of social and phobic disorders (Bolton et al., 2006; Eley et al., 2003). Preschool children who are cautious and shy to the unfamiliar in the preschool years are significantly more likely to develop anxiety disorders by adolescence compared with the general population

(Kagan & Snidman, 1999; Prior et al., 2000; Schwartz et al., 1999). This is particularly true for those who show shyness as trait behaviour in the early years.

Parents may foster anxiety disorders by limiting their child's exposure to fear-provoking stimuli interfering with the normative process of fear habituation and mastery. Parents need not be anxious themselves to effect such a process in their offspring. As yet there are no biological makers or concurrent pathophysiological changes associated with either the onset or outcomes of SAD or GAD in children and adolescents.

Treatment

There are few systematic treatment studies of childhood anxiety disorders. Cognitive-behavioural therapy is a treatment of choice (Kendall, 1994; Kendall et al., 1997) together with more classical behavioural therapy for monophobias and some social phobias. The evidence base is not large and confined to efficacy rather than effectiveness studies to date. Although SSRIs have been advocated and are prescribed for anxiety disorders (Brunello et al., 2000), only one randomised controlled trial in children has been reported to date (Klein & Pine, 2003). In that study, there was significant advantage for active compound over placebo which was maintained at 8 weeks. In the absence of other studies, SSRIs cannot be recommended as a first-line treatment.

Posttraumatic stress disorder

Posttraumatic stress disorder (PTSD) is classified under anxiety disorders in both the DSM and ICD classifications. There are no specific developmental features of the disorder, which may occur across the lifespan (see also Chapter 8). Until 15 years ago, it was widely assumed that children responded to acute trauma with transient brief reactions. These reports were based almost exclusively on parent reports of their offspring's emotional symptoms. Direct interviewing of children has demonstrated that parents significantly underestimated internalising symptoms, leading to underreporting of clinical syndromes (Yule, 2001). In children exposed to severe traumas (survivors of war, rape and assault; refugees) have all shown that exposure to such events is associated with a marked increase in anxious symptoms and disorders that may last years in some cases (Kaplow *et al.*, 2005; Lavi & Solomon, 2005; Saxe *et al.*, 2005; Solomon & Lavi, 2005). The most troublesome symptom appears to be visual imagery of the event, which, when intense, may result in dissociative experiences (flashbacks) and may explain social reenactment observed during the play of younger patients with the disorder. In adolescents, visual imagery is associated with increased irritable mood and sleep deprivation. Mood change of irritability and anger are often the most externally disruptive clinical features of the disorder. The personal salience of the trauma, its impact on thoughts of the future for self, others and even nationhood can all have an impact on the liability for severity and duration of symptoms.

PTSD symptoms are frequently elevated after traumatic events such as a car accident (Meiser-Stedman *et al.*, 2005; Mirza *et al.*, 1998) but usually resolve by 6 weeks although in some cases, symptoms may persist for months or even years (Bolton *et al.*, 2004). The latter are likely to have had a prior history of emotional disorder.

In terms of treatment, there are, as with other childhood anxiety disorders, few controlled studies. CBT appears to be helpful in alleviating symptoms and preventing relapse. Although critical stress debriefing soon after an event may have a limited place in some cases, this technique carries a risk for increasing adverse events including further symptoms and heightened flashbacks. There is no place for these techniques being used on large groups of children with minor symptoms.

Obsessive-compulsive disorder

Childhood obsessive-compulsive disorder (OCD) is a rather private mental disorder with parents generally underreporting symptoms compared with their offspring (Rappaport & Swedo, 2003). The disorder has been documented as early as 2 years of age,

but the typical onset period is between 8 and 16 years. Obsessive thoughts frequently centre on concerns of contamination to self or others, worries about danger and symmetry, or moral worries. Most children have a combination of rituals and obsessions, and pure obsessives are rare compared with the more frequent pure compulsives. Washing rituals are the most common compulsive acts, with hand washing somewhat more frequent than total body showering (Swedo *et al.*, 1989).

Secrecy is a hallmark of childhood-onset OCD because the child has insight recognizing the symptoms as nonsensical and wishes to avoid social embarrassment with family and friends. Overt symptoms therefore tend to reflect a severe and long-standing disorder of increasing severity and widening impairment of personal functions. There are no prospective data to determine the mean age of onset in childhood. Most retrospective reports of adults and adolescents indicate onset occurring in middle childhood around 7 years. In prepubertal retrospective reporting, males outnumber females 3:1 (Swedo *et al.*, 1989). The sex differences by adolescence are less clear-cut but appear closer to 1:1.

The natural course and history of OCD remain unclear (Rappaport & Swedo, 2003). The course in those with early-childhood onset is invariably described as poor and unremitting with increasing chronicity related to severe disorder frequently associated with tic syndromes (Bloch *et al.*, 2006; Leonard *et al.*, 1990; Snider & Swedo 2004; Swedo *et al.*, 1992). General personal impairments are also a feature arising as a consequence of OCD symptoms and high rates of comorbid illness (Valderhaug & Ivarsson, 2005). Although treatment, pharmacological and psychological, is associated with clear-cut reductions in symptoms and impairments, the longer-term prognosis appears to carry a high risk of recurrence and difficulties into adult life. Comorbidity is the rule rather than the exception with no more than one in four childhood-onset cases being "pure" OCD. Tic disorders, major depression and neurodevelopment disorders are probably the most common comorbidities. In epidemiological studies of adolescents, concurrent emotional disorders appear quite common occurring in around 30% of identified cases of OCD (regardless of the age of onset) (Heyman *et al.*, 2001; Lewinsohn *et al.*, 1993).

Treatment of the disorder in childhood and young adolescents is likely to involve both SSRIs and CBT. Clomipramine was the first antidepressant to show clear anti-obsessional effects, with subsequent studies showing a range of SSRIs (fluoxetine, sertraline and fluvoxamine) being effective in rapid reduction of obsessive and compulsive symptoms over 12 weeks. CBT has been shown to be an effective treatment for OCD in children and adolescents both as an individual treatment and used in group or family-based contexts (Barrett *et al.*, 2004; Cartwright-Hatton *et al.*, 2004; Huppert & Franklin, 2005). Combination of SSRIs and CBT may produce greater efficacy than either alone.

Conclusions

Over the past decade there have been considerable advances in the field of child and adolescent psychiatry. Longitudinal studies have been particularly powerful in denoting the pathways into and out of episodes of psychiatric disorders such as depression and anxiety, as well as in charting the course of more protracted conditions such as conduct disorders. This has made more robust the study of psychosocial risk and resilience factors involved in effecting a change in developmental trajectory.

The application of evidence-based interventions for children and adolescents with emotional or behavioural disorders is beginning to be possible as the results of randomised control trial data influence clinical guidelines and mental health policy implementation. However, relatively little is understood about antecedent risk factors within the child and adolescent that predict how they will respond to treatment. We also need a clearer understanding of how genetic factors influence the occurrence of and sensitivity to social adversities.

From the primary care perspective, an increasing interest in resilience and well-being may enable policy makers to pinpoint and highlight strengths in childhood that could be taught or disseminated to those with vulnerabilities for disorder.

Finally, child psychiatrists should continue to contribute to basic research aimed at understanding the causes of mental illness and behavioural syndromes. Technical advances in neuroimaging and genetics to pinpoint brain-based vulnerabilities and deficits that underpin psychiatric syndromes will require reliable and valid application to the child populations of interest. This cannot be achieved without the expert knowledge of the child and adolescent psychiatrist as part of a multidisciplinary research team.

REFERENCES

Abe, K., & Masui, T. (1981). Age-sex trends of phobic and anxiety symptoms in adolescents. *Br J Psychiatry* 138:297–302.

Alloy, L. B., Abramson, L. Y., Hogan, M. E., *et al.* (2000). The Temple-Wisconsin Cognitive Vulnerability to Depression Project: lifetime history of Axis I psychopathology in individuals at high and low cognitive risk for depression. *J Abnorm Psychol* 109:403–418.

Alloy, L. B., Abramson, L. Y., Whitehouse, W. G., *et al.* (1999). Depressogenic cognitive styles: predictive validity, information processing and personality characteristics, and developmental origins. *Behav Res Ther* 37:503–31.

American Psychiatric Association (1994). *Diagnostic and Statistical Manual of Mental and Behavioural Disorders.* Washington, DC: American Psychiatric Association.

Amir, R. E., Van Den Veyver, I. B., Wan, C. Q., *et al.* (1999). Rett syndrome is caused by mutations in X-linked MECP2, encoding methyl-CpG-binding protein 2. *Nat Genet* 23:185–8.

Anderson, J. C., Williams, S. McGee, R., *et al.* (1987). DSM-III disorders in preadolescent children. Prevalence in a large sample from the general population. *Arch Gen Psychiatry* 44:69–76.

Angold, A. (2003). Diagnostic interviewing with parents and children. *Child and Adolescent Psychiatry.* In M. Rutter and E. Taylor, eds. Oxford: Blackwell, pp. 32–51.

Angold, A., & Costello, E. J. (2001). The epidemiology of depression in children and adolescents. In I. Goodyer, ed. *The Depressed Child and Adolescent.* Cambridge: Cambridge University Press, pp. 143–78.

Aschenbrand, S. G., Kendall, P. C. Webb, A., *et al.* (2003). Is childhood separation anxiety disorder a predictor of adult panic disorder and agoraphobia? A seven-year longitudinal study. *J Am Acad Child Adolesc Psychiatry* **42**:1478–85.

Bale, J. F., Jr. (2002). Autistic regression: genes, environment, or both. *Am J Med Genet* **113**:229–30.

Baranek, G. T. (1999). Autism during infancy: a retrospective video analysis of sensory-motor and social behaviors at 9–12 months of age. *J Autism Dev Disord* **29**:213–24.

Barrett, P., Healy-Farrell, L. March, S., *et al.* (2004). Cognitive-behavioral family treatment of childhood obsessive-compulsive disorder: a controlled trial. *J Am Acad Child Adolesc Psychiatry* **43**:46–62.

Bellman, M. (1966). Studies on encopresis. *Acta Paediatr Scand Suppl* **170**:147–156.

Besharov, D., & Laumann-Billings, L. (1996). Child abuse reporting. In I. Garfinkel, J. Hochschild, & S. McLanahan, eds. *Social Policies for Children*. Washington, DC: Brookings Institute Press,. pp. 257–74.

Birmaher, B., Ryan, N. D. Williamson, D. E., *et al.* (1996). Childhood and adolescent depression: a review of the past 10 years. Part I. *J Am Acad Child Adolesc Psychiatry* **35**:1427–39.

Blair, R. J. (2001). Neurocognitive models of aggression, the antisocial personality disorders, and psychopathy. *J Neurol Neurosurg Psychiatry* **71**:727–31.

Blair, R. J. (2001). Neurocognitive models of aggression, the antisocial personality disorders, and psychopathy. *J Neurol Neurosurg Psychiatry* **71**:727–31.

Blair, R. J. (2003). Neurobiological basis of psychopathy. *Br J Psychiatry* **182**:5–7.

Blair, R. J. (2004). The roles of orbital frontal cortex in the modulation of antisocial behavior. *Brain Cogn* **55**:198–208.

Blair, R. J., Colledge, E. Murray, L., *et al.* (2001). A selective impairment in the processing of sad and fearful expressions in children with psychopathic tendencies. *J Abnorm Child Psychol* **29**:491–8.

Blair, R. J., Peschardt, K. S., Budhani, S., *et al.* (2006). The development of psychopathy. *J Child Psychol Psychiatry* **47**:262–76.

Bloch, M. H., & Peterson, B. S., Scahill, L., *et al.* (2006). Adulthood outcome of tic and obsessive-compulsive symptom severity in children with Tourette syndrome. *Arch Pediatr Adolesc Med* **160**:65–9.

Bolton, D., Eley, T. C., O'Connor, T. G., *et al.* (2006). Prevalence and genetic and environmental influences on anxiety disorders in 6-year-old twins. *Psychol Med* **36**:335–44.

Bolton, D., Hill, J. O'Ryan, D., *et al.* (2004). Long-term effects of psychological trauma on psychosocial functioning. *J Child Psychol Psychiatry* **45**:1007–14.

Bolton, P., Macdonald, H. Pickles, A., *et al.* (1994). A case-control family history study of autism. *J Child Psychol Psychiatry* **35**:877–900.

Bowlby, J. (1951). *Maternal Care and Mental Health*. Geneva: World Health Organisation.

Bowlby, J. (1981). *Attachment and Loss: Volume 1*. London: Pelican.

Boyle, M. H., Cunningham, C. E. Heale, J., *et al.* (1999). Helping children adjust—a Tri-Ministry Study: I. Evaluation methodology. *J Child Psychol Psychiatry* **40**: 1051–60.

Brunello, N., den Boer, J. A., Judd, L. L., *et al.* (2000). Social phobia: diagnosis and epidemiology, neurobiology and pharmacology, comorbidity and treatment. *J Affect Disord* **60**:61–74.

Buitelaar, J. K., Van Der Gaag, R. Klin, A., *et al.* (1999). Exploring the boundaries of pervasive developmental disorder not otherwise specified: analyses of data from the DSM-IV Autistic Disorder Field Trial. *J Autism Dev Disord* **29**:33–43.

Butler, R. J. (1998). Nightime wetting in children—psychological aspects. *J Child Psychology Psychiatry* **39**:453–63.

Butler, R. J., & Holland, P. (2000). The three systems: a conceptual way of understanding nocturnal enuresis. *Scand J Urol Nephrol* **34**:270–7.

Byrd, R. S., Weitzman, M. Lanphear, N. E., *et al.* (1996). Bedwetting in US children: epidemiology and related behaviour problems. *Paediatrics* **98**:414–19.

Caballero, I. M., & Hendrich, B. (2005). MeCP2 in neurons: closing in on the causes of Rett syndrome. *Hum Mol Genet* **14**(Spec No. 1): R19–26.

Carlson, G. A. (2005). Early onset bipolar disorder: clinical and research considerations. *J Clin Child Adolesc Psychol* **34**:333–43.

Carrasco, X., Lopez, V., & Aboitiz, F. (2005). Frontal and executive dysfunction is a central aspect of ADHD. *Behav Brain Sci* **28**:427–8.

Cartwright-Hatton, S., Roberts, C., Chitsabesan, P., *et al.* (2004). Systematic review of the efficacy of cognitive behaviour therapies for childhood and adolescent anxiety disorders. *Br J Clin Psychol* **43**(Pt 4):421–36.

Caspi, A., Henry, B., McGee, R. O., *et al.* (1995). Temperamental origins of child and adolescent behavior problems: from age three to age fifteen. *Child Dev* **66**: 55–68.

Caspi, A., McClay, J., Moffitt, T. E., *et al.* (2002). Role of genotype in the cycle of violence in maltreated children. *Science* 297:851–4.

Caspi, A., Sugden, K., Moffitt, T. E., *et al.* (2003). Influence of life stress on depression: moderation by a polymorphism in the 5-HTT gene. *Science* 301:386–9.

Caspi, A., Taylor, A., Moffitt, T. E., *et al.* (2000). Neighborhood deprivation affects children's mental health: environmental risks identified in a genetic design. *Psychol Sci* 11:338–42.

Chakrabarti, S., & Fombonne, E. (2005). Pervasive developmental disorders in preschool children: confirmation of high prevalence. *Am J Psychiatry* 162:1133–41.

Charman, T. (2003). Epidemiology and early identification of autism: research challenges and opportunities. *Novartis Found Symp* 251:10–9; discussion 19–25, 109–11, 281–297.

Charman, T., Baron-Cohen, S., Swettenham, J., *et al.* (2003). Predicting language outcome in infants with autism and pervasive developmental disorder. *Int J Lang Commun Disord* 38:265–85.

Clayden, G., Taylor, E., Loader, P., *et al.* (2003). Wetting and soiling in childhood. *Child and Adolescent Psychiatry*. In M. Rutter & E. Taylor. Oxford: Blackwell.

Cole, D. A., Martin, J. M., & Powers, B. (1997). A competency based model of child depression: a longitudinal study of peer, parent, teacher, and self-evaluations. *J Child Psychol Psychiatry* 38:505–14.

Cole, D. A., Peeke, L., Dolezal, S., *et al.* (1999). A longitudinal study of negative affect and self-perceived competence in young adolescents. *J Pers Soc Psychol* 77:851–62.

Conger, R. D., Patterson, G. R., Ge, X., *et al.* (1995). It takes two to replicate: a mediational model for the impact of parents' stress on adolescent adjustment. *Child Dev* 66:80–97.

Cornish, K. M., Manly, T., Savage, R., *et al.* (2005). Association of the dopamine transporter (DAT1) 10/10-repeat genotype with ADHD symptoms and response inhibition in a general population sample. *Mol Psychiatry* 10:686–98.

Costello, E. J., Angold, A., Burns, B. J., *et al.* (1996a). The Great Smoky Mountains Study of Youth. Goals, design, methods, and the prevalence of DSM-III-R disorders. *Arch Gen Psychiatry* 53:1129–36.

Costello, E. J., Angold, A., Burns, B. J., *et al.* (1996b). The Great Smoky Mountains Study of Youth. Functional impairment and serious emotional disturbance. *Arch Gen Psychiatry* 53:1137–43.

Cunningham, C. E., Boyle, M., Offord, D., *et al.* (2000). Tri-ministry study: correlates of school-based parenting course utilization. *J Consult Clin Psychol* 68:928–33.

Daenckerts, M., & Taylor, E. (1995). The epidemiology of childhood hyperactivity. In F. Verhulst & H. M. Koot, eds. *The Epidemiology of Child and Adolescent Psychopathology*. Oxford: Oxford University Press, pp. 178–209.

de Kemp, R. A., & Van Acker, J. C. (1997). Therapist-parent interaction patterns in home-based treatments: exploring family therapy process. *Fam Process* 36:281–95.

Deonna, T. (2000). Acquired epileptic aphasia or Landau-Kleffner syndrome. In D. M. V. Bishop & L. B. Leonard, eds. *Speech and Language Impairments in Children: Causes Characteristics Interventions and Outcome*. Philadelphia: Psychology Press, Taylor & Francis, pp. 261–72.

Doyle, A. E., Faraone, S. V., Seidman, L. J., *et al.* (2005). Are endophenotypes based on measures of executive functions useful for molecular genetic studies of ADHD? *J Child Psychol Psychiatry* 46:774–803.

Dunn, V., & Goodyer, I. M. (2006). Longitudinal investigation into childhood- and adolescence-onset depression: psychiatric outcome in early adulthood. *Br J Psychiatry* 188:216–22.

Egger, H. L., & Angold, A. (2006). Common emotional and behavioral disorders in preschool children: presentation, nosology, and epidemiology. *J Child Psychol Psychiatry* 47:313–37.

Egger, H. L., Costello, E. J., & Angold, A. (2003). School refusal and psychiatric disorders: a community study. *J Am Acad Child Adolesc Psychiatry* 42:797–807.

Eley, T. C., Bolton, D., O'Connor, T. G., *et al.* (2003). A twin study of anxiety-related behaviours in pre-school children. *J Child Psychol Psychiatry* 44:945–60.

Emery, R. E., & Laumann-Billings, L. (2003). Child abuse. In M. Rutter & E. Taylor, eds. *Child and Adolescent Psychiatry*. Oxford: Blackwell, pp. 325–39.

Feehan, M., McGee, R., Stanton, W., *et al.* (1990). A six year follow up of childhood enuresis: prevalence in adolescence and consequences for mental health. *Journal of Paediatrics and Child Health* 26:75–9.

Fergusson, D. M., & Horwood, L. J. (1995). Predictive validity of categorically and dimensionally scored measures of disruptive childhood behaviours. *J Am Acad Child Adolesc Psychiatry* 34:477–85.

Fergusson, D. M., Horwood, L. J., & Lloyd, M. (1991). Confirmatory factor analytic models of attention deficit and conduct disorder. *J Child Psychol Psychiatry* 32:257–74.

Fergusson, D. M., L. J. Horwood, & Lynskey, M. T. (1993). Prevalence and comorbidity of DSM-III-R diagnoses in a birth cohort of 15 year olds. *J Am Acad Child Adolesc Psychiatry* **32**:1127–34.

Finkelhor, D. (1994). Victimization of children: a developmental perspective. *Am Psychol* **49**:173–83.

Finkelhor, D., & Berliner, L. (1995). Research on the treatment of sexually abused children: a review and recommendations. *J Am Acad Child Adolesc Psychiatry* **34**:1408–23.

Finkelhor, D., Ormrod, R., Turner, H., *et al.* (2005). The victimization of children and youth: a comprehensive, national survey. *Child Maltreat* **10**:5–25.

Folstein, S. and M. Rutter (1977). Infantile Autism: a genetic study of 21 twin pairs. *J Child Psychol Psychiatry* **18**:297–321.

Fombonne, E. (1995). Depressive disorders: time trends and their possible explanatory mechanisms. In M. Rutter and D. Smith, eds. *Psychosocial Disorders in Young People*. Chichester, England: Wiley, pp. 544–615.

Fombonne, E. (1999). The epidemiology of autism: a review. *Psychol Med* **29**:769–86.

Fombonne, E., Bolton, P., Prior, J., *et al.* (1997). A family study of autism: cognitive patterns and levels in parents and siblings. *J Child Psychol Psychiatry* **38**:667–83.

Fombonne, E., Wostear, G., Cooper, V., *et al.* (2001). The Maudsley long-term follow-up of child and adolescent depression. 1. Psychiatric outcomes in adulthood. *Br J Psychiatry* **179**:210–17.

Forsythe, W. I., & A. Redmond (1974). Enuresis and spontaneous cure rate; a study of 1129 enuretics. *Arch Dis Childhood* **49**:259–63.

Franklin, M., Foa, E., March, J. S., *et al.* (2003). The pediatric obsessive-compulsive disorder treatment study: rationale, design, and methods. *J Child Adolesc Psychopharmacol* **13**(Suppl 1):S39–51.

Geller, B., Bolhofner, K., Craney, J. L., *et al.* (2000). Psychosocial functioning in a prepubertal and early adolescent bipolar disorder phenotype [in process citation]. *J Am Acad Child Adolesc Psychiatry* **39**:1543–8.

Geller, B., Tillman, R., Craney, J. L., *et al.* (2004). Four-year prospective outcome and natural history of mania in children with a prepubertal and early adolescent bipolar disorder phenotype. *Arch Gen Psychiatry* **61**:459–67.

Ghaziuddin, M., Ghaziuddin, N., *et al.* (2002). Depression in persons with autism: implications for research and clinical care. *J Autism Dev Disord* **32**:299–306.

Ghaziuddin, M., & Greden, J. (1998). Depression in children with autism/pervasive developmental disorders: a case-control family history study. *J Autism Dev Disord* **28**:111–15.

Glazener, C. M., & Evans, J. H. (2000). Tricyclic and related drugs for nocturnal enuresis in children. *Cochrane Database Syst Rev* **3**.

Glazer, D. (2003). Child sexual abuse. In M. Rutter & E. Taylor, eds. *Child and Adolescent Psychiatry*. Oxford: Blackwell.

Goldstein, R. B., Wickramaratne, P. J., Horwath, E., *et al.* (1997). Familial aggregation and phenomenology of 'early'-onset (at or before age 20 years) panic disorder. *Arch Gen Psychiatry* **54**:271–8.

Goodwin, R., Lipsitz, J. D., Chapman, T. F., *et al.* (2001). Obsessive-compulsive disorder and separation anxiety co-morbidity in early onset panic disorder. *Psychol Med* **31**:1307–10.

Goodyer, I., Dubicka, B., Wilkinson, P., *et al.* (2007). Selective serotonin reuptake inhibitors (SSRIs) and routine specialist care with and without cognitive behaviour therapy in adolescents with major depression: randomised controlled trial. *BMJ* 2007;**335**:142.

Goodyer, I. M., Herbert, J., Secher, S. M., *et al.* (1997). Short-term outcome of major depression: I. Comorbidity and severity at presentation as predictors of persistent disorder. *J Am Acad Child Adolesc Psychiatry* **36**:179–87.

Grillon, C., Warner, V., Hille, J., *et al.* (2005). Families at high and low risk for depression: a three-generation startle study. *Biol Psychiatry* **57**:953–60.

Halligan, S. L., J. Herbert, Goodyer, I., *et al.* (2004). Exposure to postnatal depression predicts elevated cortisol in adolescent offspring. *Biol Psychiatry* **55**:376–81.

Harrington, R., & Myatt, T. (2003). Is preadolescent mania the same condition as adult mania? A British perspective. *Biol Psychiatry* **53**:961–9.

Harrington, R., Whittaker, J., Shoebridge, P., *et al.* (1998). Systematic review of efficacy of cognitive behaviour therapies in childhood and adolescent depressive disorder. *BJM* **316**:1559–63.

Hawkins, J. D., Von Cleve, E., Catalano, J. F. Jr., *et al.* (1991). Reducing early childhood aggression: results of a primary prevention program. *J Am Acad Child Adolesc Psychiatry* **30**:208–17.

Hellstrom, A. L., Hanson, E., Hansson, S., *et al.* (1990). Micturition habits and incontinence in 7 year old Swedish children. *Eur J Paediatr* **149**:434–7.

Hettema, J. M., Neale, M. C., Kendler, K. S., *et al.* (2001). A review and meta-analysis of the genetic epidemiology of anxiety disorders. *Am J Psychiatry* **158**:1568–78.

Heyman, I., Fombonne, E., Simmons, H., *et al.* (2001). Prevalence of obsessive-compulsive disorder in the British nationwide survey of child mental health. *Br J Psychiatry* **179**:324–9.

Howlin, P. (2003). Outcome in high-functioning adults with autism with and without early language delays: implications for the differentiation between autism and Asperger syndrome. *J Autism Dev Disord* **33**:3–13.

Howlin, P., Goode, S., Hutton, J., *et al.* (2004). Adult outcome for children with autism. *J Child Psychol Psychiatry* **45**:212–29.

Hundert, J., Boyle, M. H., Cunningham, C. E., *et al.* (1999). Helping children adjust—a Tri-Ministry Study: II. Program effects. *J Child Psychol Psychiatry* **40**:1061–73.

Huppert, J. D., & Franklin, M. E. (2005). Cognitive behavioral therapy for obsessive-compulsive disorder: an update. *Curr Psychiatry Rep* **7**:268–73.

Jaffee, S. R., Moffitt, T. E., Caspi, A., *et al.* (2002). Differences in early childhood risk factors for juvenile-onset and adult-onset depression. *Arch Gen Psychiatry* **59**:215–22.

Jarvelin, M. R., Moilanen, I., Kangas, P., *et al.* (1991). Aetiological and precipitating factors for childhood enuresis. *Acta Paediatr Scand* **80**:361–9.

Jensen, P. S., Arnold, L. E., Swanson, J. M., *et al.* (2007). 3-year follow-up of the NIMH MTA study. *J Am Acad Child Adolesc Psychiatry* **46**:989–1002.

Jones, D. P. H., & Ramchandani, P. (1999). *Child Sexual Abuse: Informing Practise from Research*. Abingdon, England: Radcliff Medical Press.

Jones, M. B., & Offord, D. R. (1989). Reduction of antisocial behavior in poor children by nonschool skill-development. *J Child Psychol Psychiatry* **30**:737–50.

Kadesjo, B., & Gillberg, C. (1998). Attention deficits and clumsiness in Swedish 7-year old children. *Dev Med Child Neurol* **40**:796–804.

Kagan, J., & Snidman, N. (1999). Early childhood predictors of adult anxiety disorders. *Biol Psychiatry* **46**:1536–41.

Kaplan, S. J., Pelcovitz, D., Labruna, V., *et al.* (1999). Child and adolescent abuse and neglect research: a review of the past 10 years. Part I: physical and emotional abuse and neglect. *J Am Acad Child Adolesc Psychiatry* **38**:1214–22.

Kaplow, J. B., Dodge, K. A., Amaya-Jackson, L., *et al.* (2005). Pathways to PTSD, part II: sexually abused children. *Am J Psychiatry* **162**:1305–10.

Kaufman, J., Yang, B. Z., Douglas-Palumberi, H., *et al.* (2004). Social supports and serotonin transporter gene moderate depression in maltreated children. *Proc Natl Acad Sci U S A* **101**:17316–21.

Kelvin, R. G., Goodyer, I. M., Teasdale, J. D., *et al.* (1999). Latent negative self-schema and high emotionality in well adolescents at risk for psychopathology. *J Child Psychol Psychiatry* **40**:959–68.

Kendall, P. C. (1994). Treating anxiety disorders in children: results of a randomized clinical trial. *J Consult Clin Psychol* **62**:100–10.

Kendall, P. C., Flannery-Schroeder, E., Panichelli-Mindel, S. M., *et al.* (1997). Therapy for youths with anxiety disorders: a second randomized clinical trial. *J Consult Clin Psychol* **65**:366–80.

Kendler, K. S., Gardner, C. O., Prescott, C. A., *et al.* (2002). Toward a comprehensive developmental model for major depression in women. *Am J Psychiatry* **159**:1133–45.

Kendler, K. S., Kuhn, J. W., Vittum, J., *et al.* (2005). The interaction of stressful life events and a serotonin transporter polymorphism in the prediction of episodes of major depression: a replication. *Arch Gen Psychiatry* **62**:529–35.

Kim, J., & Cicchetti, D. (2004). A longitudinal study of child maltreatment, mother-child relationship quality and maladjustment: the role of self-esteem and social competence. *J Abnorm Child Psychol* **32**:341–54.

Kjelgaard, M., & Tager-Flusberg, H. (2001). An investigation of language impairment in autism: implications for genetic subgroups. *Lang Cogn Process* **16**:287–308.

Klein, G. R., & Pine, D. (2003). Anxiety disorders. In M. Rutter & E. Taylor, eds. *Child and Adolescent Psychiatry*. Oxford, Blackwell, pp. 486–509.

Kolvin, I., Garside, R. F., Nicol, A. R., *et al.* (1981). *Help Starts Here: The Maladjusted Child in Ordinary School*. London: Tavistock.

Kopp, S., & Gillberg, C. (1997). Selective mutism: a population based study: a research note. *J Child Psychol Psychiatry* **38**:257–62.

Kovacs, M. (1996). Presentation and course of major depressive disorder during childhood and later years of the life span. *J Am Acad Child Adolesc Psychiatry* **35**:705–15.

Kraemer, H. C., Kazdin, A., Offord, D. R., *et al.* (1997). Coming to terms with the terms of risk. *Arch Gen Psychiatry* **54**:337–43.

Kutcher, S., Aman, M., Brooks, S. J, *et al.* (2004). International consensus statement on attention-deficit/hyperactivity disorder (ADHD) and disruptive behaviour disorders (DBDs): clinical implications and treatment practice suggestions. *Eur Neuropsychopharmacol* 14:11–28.

Kyte, Z. A., Carlson, G. A., Goodyer, I. M., *et al.* (2006). Clinical and neuropsychological characteristics of child and adolescent bipolar disorder. *Psychol Med* 36:1–15.

Lavi, T., & Solomon, Z. (2005). Palestinian youth of the Intifada: PTSD and future orientation. *J Am Acad Child Adolesc Psychiatry* 44:1176–83.

Leckman, J. F., Grice, D. E., Boardman, J., *et al.* (1997). Symptoms of obsessive-compulsive disorder. *Am J Psychiatry* 154:911–17.

Leonard, H. L., Goldberger, E. L., Rapoport, J. L., *et al.* (1990). Childhood rituals: normal development or obsessive-compulsive symptoms? *J Am Acad Child Adolesc Psychiatry* 29:17–23.

Levy, F., Hay, D. A., McStephen, M., *et al.* (1997). Attention deficit hyperactivity disorder: a category or continuum? Genetic analysis of a large scale twin study. *J Am Acad Child Adolesc Psychiatry* 36:737–44.

Lewinsohn, P. M., Hops, H., Roberts, R. E., *et al.* (1993). Adolescent psychopathology: I. Prevalence and incidence of depression and other DSM-III-R disorders in high school students. *J Abnorm Psychol* 102:133–44.

Lewinsohn, P. M., Rohde, P., & Seeley, J. R. (1998). Major depressive disorder in older adolescents: prevalence, risk factors, and clinical implications. *Clin Psychol Review* 18:765–94.

Lewinsohn, P. M., Rohde, P., & Seeley, J. R. (2000). Natural course of adolescent major depressive disorder in a community sample: predictors of recurrence in young adults [In Process Citation]. *Am J Psychiatry* 157:1584–91.

Loeber, R., & Farrington, D. P. (2000). Young children who commit crime: epidemiology, developmental origins, risk factors, early interventions, and policy implications. *Dev Psychopathol* 12:737–62.

Loeber, R., Farrington, D. P., Stouthamer-Loeber, M., *et al.* (2001). Male mental health problems, psychopathy, and personality traits: key findings from the first 14 years of the Pittsburgh Youth Study. *Clin Child Fam Psychol Rev* 4:273–97.

Loeber, R., Green, S. M., Lahey, B. B., *et al.* (2000). Findings on disruptive behavior disorders from the first decade of the Developmental Trends Study. *Clin Child Fam Psychol Rev* 3:37–60.

Loening-Baucke, V. (1996). Encopresis and soiling. *Paediatr Clin North Am* 43:279–98.

Lord, C., Risi, S., Lambrecht, L., *et al.* (2000). The autism diagnostic observation schedule-generic: a standard measure of social and communication deficits associated with the spectrum of autism. *J Autism Dev Disord* 30:205–23.

Luby, J. L., Mrakotsky, C., Heffelfinger, A., *et al.* (2004). Characteristics of depressed preschoolers with and without anhedonia: evidence for a melancholic depressive subtype in young children. *Am J Psychiatry* 161: 1998–2004.

Luby, J. L., Sullivan, J., Belden, A., *et al.* (2006). An observational analysis of behavior in depressed preschoolers: further validation of early-onset depression. *J Am Acad Child Adolesc Psychiatry* 45:203–12.

Luthar, S. S., Cicchetti, D., Becker, B., *et al.* (2000). The construct of resilience: a critical evaluation and guidelines for future work. *Child Dev* 71:543–62.

Luyster, R., Richler, J., Risi, S., *et al.* (2005). Early regression in social communication in autism spectrum disorders: a CPEA Study. *Dev Neuropsychol* 27:311–36.

March, J., Silva, S., Petrycki, S., *et al.* (2004). Fluoxetine, cognitive-behavioral therapy, and their combination for adolescents with depression: Treatment for Adolescents With Depression Study (TADS) randomized controlled trial. *JAMA* 292:807–20.

Maughan, B., Rowe, R., Messer, J., *et al.* (2004). Conduct disorder and oppositional defiant disorder in a national sample: developmental epidemiology. *J Child Psychol Psychiatry* 45:609–21.

McArdle, P., O'Brien, G., & Kolvin, I. (1997). Is there a comorbid relationship between hyperactivity and emotional psychopathology? *Eur J Child Adolescent Psychiatry* 6:142–50.

Meiser-Stedman, R., Yule, W., Smith, P., *et al.* (2005). Acute stress disorder and posttraumatic stress disorder in children and adolescents involved in assaults or motor vehicle accidents. *Am J Psychiatry* 162: 1381–3.

Mellon, M. W., & McGrath, M. L. (2000). Empirically supported treatments in paediatric psychology: nocturnal enuresis. *J Pediatr Psychol* 25:193–214.

Merrell, C., & Tymms, P. B. (2001). Inattention, hyperactivity and impulsiveness: their impact on academic achievement and progress. *J Edu Psychol* 71:352–8.

Micali, N., Chakrabarti, S., Fombonne, E., *et al.* (2004). The broad autism phenotype: findings from an epidemiological survey. *Autism* 8:21–37.

Mirza, K. A., Bhadrinath, B. R., Goodyer, I. M., *et al.* (1998). Post-traumatic stress disorder in children and adolescents following road traffic accidents. *Br J Psychiatry* 172:443–7.

Moffitt, T. E. (1990). Juvenile delinquency and attention deficit disorder: boys developmental trajectories from age 3 to 15. *Child Development* **61**:893–910.

Moffitt, T. E., & A. Caspi (2001). Childhood predictors differentiate life-course persistent and adolescence-limited antisocial pathways among males and females. *Dev Psychopathol* **13**:355–75.

Moffitt, T. E., Caspi, A., Harrington, H., *et al.* (2002). Males on the life-course-persistent and adolescence limited antisocial pathways: follow-up at age 26 years. *Dev Psychopathol* **14**:179–207.

Moilanen, I., Tirkonnen, T., Jarvelin, M. R., *et al.* (1998). A follow up of enuresis from childhood to adolescence. *Br J Urol* **81**:94–7.

Murphy, K. (2005). Psychosocial treatments for ADHD in teens and adults: a practice-friendly review. *J Clin Psychol* **61**:607–19.

Murray, L., Woolgar, M., Cooper, P., *et al.* (2001). Cognitive vulnerability to depression in 5-year-old children of depressed mothers. *J Child Psychol Psychiatry* **42**:891–9.

Natochin, Y. V., & A. A. Kuznetsova (2000). Nocturnal enuresis. *Paediatr Clin North Am* **14**:42–7.

Newman, D. L., Moffitt, T. E., Caspi, A., *et al.* (1996). Psychiatric disorder in a birth cohort of young adults: prevalence, comorbidity, clinical significance, and new case incidence from ages 11 to 21. *J Consult Clin Psychol* **64**:552–62.

Nolan, T., Debelle, G., Oberklaid, F., *et al.* (1991). Randomised trial of laxatives in the treatment of childhood encopresis. *Lancet* **8766**:523–7.

O'Connor, T. G. (2003). Attachment disorders of infancy and childhood. In M. Rutter & E. Taylor, eds. *Child and Adolescent Psychiatry*. Oxford: Blackwell.

O'Connor, T. G., Marvin, R. S., Olrick, J. T., *et al.* (2003). Child-parent attachment following early institutional deprivation. *Dev Psychopathol* **15**:19–38.

O'Connor, T. G., & Rutter, M. (2000). Attachment disorder behavior following early severe deprivation: extension and longitudinal follow-up. English and Romanian Adoptees Study Team. *J Am Acad Child Adolesc Psychiatry* **39**:703–12.

Offord, D. R., Boyle, M. H., Racine, Y., *et al.* (1989). Ontario Child Health Study. Summary of selected results. *Can J Psychiatry* **34**:483–91.

Offord, D. R., Boyle, M. H., Racine, Y., *et al.* (1992). Outcome, prognosis, and risk in a longitudinal follow-up study. *J Am Acad Child Adolesc Psychiatry* **31**:916–23.

Olds, D., Henderson, C. R., Jr., Cole, R., *et al.* (1998). Long-term effects of nurse home visitation on children's criminal and antisocial behavior: 15-year follow-up of a randomized controlled trial. *JAMA* **280**:1238–44.

Patterson, G. R., Forgatch, M. S., Yoerger, K. L., *et al.* (1998). Variables that initiate and maintain an early-onset trajectory for juvenile offending. *Dev Psychopathol* **10**:531–47.

Pine, D. S., Wasserman, G. A., Miller, L., *et al.* (1998). Heart period variability and psychopathology in urban boys at risk for delinquency. *Psychophysiology* **35**:521–9.

Post, R. M., Chang, K. D., Findling, R. L., *et al.* (2004). Prepubertal bipolar I disorder and bipolar disorder NOS are separable from ADHD. *J Clin Psychiatry* **65**:898–902.

Prior, M., Smart, D., Sanson, A., *et al.* (2000). Does shy-inhibited temperament in childhood lead to anxiety problems in adolescence? *J Am Acad Child Adolesc Psychiatry* **39**:461–8.

Raine, A., Lencz, T., Bihrle, S., *et al.* (2000). Reduced prefrontal gray matter volume and reduced autonomic activity in antisocial personality disorder. *Arch Gen Psychiatry* **57**:119–127; discussion 128–9.

Raine, A., Meloy, J. R., Bihrle, S., *et al.* (1998). Reduced prefrontal and increased subcortical brain functioning assessed using positron emission tomography in predatory and affective murderers. *Behav Sci Law* **16**:319–32.

Raine, A., Reynolds, C., Venables, P. H., *et al.* (1998). Fearlessness, stimulation-seeking, and large body size at age 3 years as early predispositions to childhood aggression at age 11 years. *Arch Gen Psychiatry* **55**:745–51.

Raine, A., Venables, P. H., Mednick, S. A., *et al.* (1997). Low resting heart rate at age 3 years predisposes to aggression at age 11 years: evidence from the Mauritius Child Health Project. *J Am Acad Child Adolesc Psychiatry* **36**:1457–64.

Rappaport, J. L., & Swedo, S. (2003). Obsessive-compulsive disorder. In M. Rutter & E. Taylor, eds. *Child and Adolescent Psychiatry*. Oxford, Blackwell, pp. 571–92.

Reiersen, A. M. (2005). Twin study of the longitudinal course of ADHD. *J Am Acad Child Adolesc Psychiatry* **44**:625–626; author reply 626–7.

Rice, F., Harold, G., Thaper, A., *et al.* (2002). The genetic aetiology of childhood depression: a review. *J Child Psychol Psychiatry* **43**:65–79.

Robertson, G., Rittig, S., Kovacs, L., *et al.* (1999). Pathophysiology and treatment of enuresis in Adults. *Scand J Urol Nephrol Suppl* **202**:36–8.

Robins, L. N. (1996). Deviant children grown up. *Eur Child Adolesc Psychiatry* **5**(Suppl 1):44–6.

Rogosch, F. A., & Cicchetti, D. (2004). Child maltreatment and emergent personality organization: perspectives from the five-factor model. *J Abnorm Child Psychol* **32**:123–45.

Romanczyk, R. G. (1986). Self-injurious behaviour: conceptualization, assessment and treatment. *Adv Learn Behav Disabil* 5:29–56.

Rona, R. J., Li, L., Chinn, S., *et al.* (1997). Determinants of nocturnal enuresis in England and Scotland in the 90s. *Developmental Medicine and Child Neurology* **39**: 677–81.

Rueter, M. A., Scaramella, L., Wallace, L. E., *et al.* (1999). First onset of depressive or anxiety disorders predicted by the longitudinal course of internalizing symptoms and parent-adolescent disagreements. *Arch Gen Psychiatry* **56**:726–32.

Rutter, M., & O'Connor, T. G. (2004). Are there biological programming effects for psychological development? Findings from a study of Romanian adoptees. *Dev Psychol* **40**:81–94.

Rutter, M., Tizard, J., Whitmore, K., *et al.*, eds. (1970). *Education Health and Behaviour*. London: Longman.

Rutter, M. L., Kreppner, J. M., O'Connor, T. G., *et al.* (2001). Specificity and heterogeneity in children's responses to profound institutional privation. *Br J Psychiatry* **179**:97–103.

Sagvolden, T., Johansen, E. B., Aase, H., *et al.* (2005). A dynamic developmental theory of attention-deficit/hyperactivity disorder (ADHD) predominantly hyperactive/impulsive and combined subtypes. *Behav Brain Sci* **28**:397–419; discussion 419–468.

Sanford, M. N., Offord, D. R., Boyle, M. H., *et al.* (1992). Ontario child health study: social and school impairments in children aged 6 to 16 years. *J Am Acad Child Adolesc Psychiatry* **31**:60–7.

Saxe, G. N., Stoddard, F., Hall, E., *et al.* (2005). Pathways to PTSD, part I: Children with burns. *Am J Psychiatry* **162**:1299–1304.

Schachar, R., & Tannock, R. (2003). Syndromes of hyperactivity and attention deficit. In M. Rutter & E. Taylor, eds. *Child and Adolescent Psychiatry*. Oxford: Blackwell, pp. 399–418.

Schwartz, C. E., Snidman, N., Kagan, J., *et al.* (1999). Adolescent social anxiety as an outcome of inhibited temperament in childhood. *J Am Acad Child Adolesc Psychiatry* **38**:1008–15.

Scott, S., Spender, Q., Doolan, M., *et al.* (2001). Multicentre controlled trial of parenting groups for childhood antisocial behaviour in clinical practice. *BMJ* **323**:194–8.

Sedlak, A. J., & Broadhurst, D. D. (1996). Third National Incidence Study. Washington, DC: Department of Health and Human Services.

Seguin, J. R., Boulerice, B., Harden, P. W., *et al.* (1999). Executive functions and physical aggression after controlling for attention deficit hyperactivity disorder, general memory, and IQ. *J Child Psychol Psychiatry* **40**:1197–1208.

Shaffer, D. J., Gardner, A., Hedge, B., *et al.* (1994). Behaviour and bladder disturbance of enuretic children: a rational classification of a common disorder. *Dev Med Child Neurol* **26**:781–92.

Sharp, C., van Goozen, S., Goodyer, I., *et al.* (2006). Children's subjective emotional reactivity to affective pictures: gender differences and their antisocial correlates in an unselected sample of 7–11-year-olds. *J Child Psychol Psychiatry* **47**:143–50.

Shinnar, S., Rapin, I., Arnold, S., *et al.* (2001). Language regression in childhood. *Pediatr Neurol* **24**:183–9.

Sigman, M., & McGovern, C. W. (2005). Improvement in cognitive and language skills from preschool to adolescence in autism. *J Autism Dev Disord* **35**:15–23.

Silver, E. (1996). Family therapy and soiling. *J Fam Ther* **18**:415–32.

Skoog, S. J., Stokes, A., Turner, K. L., *et al.* (1997). Oral desmopressin: a randomised double blind placebo controlled study of effectiveness in children with primary nocturnal enuresis. *J Urol* **158**:1035–40.

Smith, I. M., & Bryson, S. E. (1994). Imitation and action in autism: a critical review. *Psychol Bull* **116**:259–73.

Snider, L. A., & Swedo, S. E. (2004). PANDAS: current status and directions for research. *Mol Psychiatry* **9**:900–7.

Snyder, J., Cramer, A., Afrank, J., *et al.* (2005). The contributions of ineffective discipline and parental hostile attributions of child misbehavior to the development of conduct problems at home and school. *Dev Psychol* **41**:30–41.

Solomon, Z. & Lavi, T. (2005). Israeli youth in the Second Intifada: PTSD and future orientation. *J Am Acad Child Adolesc Psychiatry* **44**:1167–75.

Spasojevic, J., & Alloy, L. B. (2001). Rumination as a common mechanism relating depressive risk factors to depression. *Emotion* **1**:25–37.

Stevenson, J., Asherson, P., Hay, D., *et al.* (2005). Characterizing the ADHD phenotype for genetic studies. *Dev Sci* **8**:115–21.

Suveg, C., Aschenbrand, S. G., Kendall, P. C., *et al.* (2005). Separation anxiety disorder, panic disorder, and school refusal. *Child Adolesc Psychiatr Clin N Am* **14**: 773–95, ix.

Swanson, J. M., Sergeant, J. A., Taylor, E., *et al.* (1998). Attention-deficit hyperactivity disorder and hyperkinetic disorder. *Lancet* **351**:429–33.

Swedo, S. E., Leonard, H. L., Rapoport, J. L., *et al.* (1992). Childhood-onset obsessive compulsive disorder. *Psychiatr Clin North Am* **15**:767–75.

Swedo, S. E., Rapoport, J. L., Leonard, H., *et al.* (1989). Obsessive-compulsive disorder in children and adolescents. Clinical phenomenology of 70 consecutive cases. *Arch Gen Psychiatry* **46**:335–41.

Szatmari, P., Bryson, S. E., Boyle, M. H., *et al.* (2003). Predictors of outcome among high functioning children with autism and Asperger syndrome. *J Child Psychol Psychiatry* **44**:520–8.

Tanguay, P. E., Robertson, J., Derrick, A., *et al.* (1998). A dimensional classification of autism spectrum disorder by social communication domains. *J Am Acad Child Adolesc Psychiatry* **37**:271–7.

Taylor, E., Chadwick, O., Heptinstall, E., *et al.* (1996). Hyperactivity and conduct problems as risk factors for adolescent development. *J Am Acad Child Adolesc Psychiatry* **35**:1213–26.

Tidmarsh, L., & Volkmar, F. R. (2003). Diagnosis and epidemiology of autism spectrum disorders. *Can J Psychiatry* **48**:517–25.

Tizard, J., & Hodges, J. (1978). The effect of early institutional rearing on the development of 8 year old children. *J Child Psychol Psychiatry* **19**:99–118.

Toupin, J., Dery, M., Pauze, R., *et al.* (2000). Cognitive and familial contributions to conduct disorder in children. *J Child Psychol Psychiatry* **41**:333–44.

Tremblay, R. E., McCord, J., Bolleau, H., *et al.* (1991). Can disruptive boys be helped to become competent. *Psychiatry* **54**:148–61.

Valderhaug, R., & Ivarsson, T. (2005). Functional impairment in clinical samples of Norwegian and Swedish children and adolescents with obsessive compulsive disorder. *Eur Child Adolesc Psychiatry* **14**:164–73.

Van Acker, J. C., & R. A. de Kemp (1997). The Family Project Approach. *J Adolesc* **20**:419–30.

van Ginkel, R., Benninga, M. A., Blommaart, P. J., *et al.* (2000). Lack of benefit of laxatives as an adjunctive therapy for functional non-retentive fecal soiling in children. *J Paediatr* **137**:808–13.

van Goozen, S. H., Matthys, W., Cohen-Kettenis, P. T., *et al.* (2000). Hypothalamic-pituitary-adrenal axis and autonomic nervous system activity in disruptive children and matched controls. *J Am Acad Child Adolesc Psychiatry* **39**:1438–45.

van Goozen, S. H., Matthys, W., Cohen-Kettenis, P. T., *et al.* (1998). Salivary cortisol and cardiovascular activity during stress in oppositional-defiant disorder boys and normal controls. *Biol Psychiatry* **43**:531–9.

Vitaro, F., Brendgen, M., Tremblay, R. E., *et al.* (1999). Prevention of school dropout through reduction of disruptive behaviours and school failure in elementary school. *J School Psychol* **37**:205–26.

Volkmar, F. (2005). Toward understanding the basis of ADHD. *Am J Psychiatry* **162**:1043–4.

Volkmar, F., Chawarska, K., Klin, A., *et al.* (2005). Autism in infancy and early childhood. *Annu Rev Psychol* **56**:315–36.

Volkmar, F., & Nelson, S. (1990). Seizure disorder in autism. *J Am Acad Child Adolesc Psychiatry* **29**:127–9.

Volkmar, F. R., & Rutter, M. (1995). Childhood disintegrative disorder: results of the DSM-IV autism field trial. *J Am Acad Child Adolesc Psychiatry* **34**:1092–5.

Watanabe, H. (1991). Nocturnal enuresis in children. *Scand J Urol Nephrol Suppl* **173**:55–6.

Weaver, I. C., Cervoni, N., Champagne, F. A., *et al.* (2004). Epigenetic programming by maternal behavior. *Nat Neurosci* **7**:847–54.

Webster-Stratton, C., Reid, M. J. Hammond, M., *et al.* (2001a). Preventing conduct problems, promoting social competence: a parent and teacher training partnership in head start. *J Clin Child Psychol* **30**:283–302.

Webster-Stratton, C., Reid, M. J., Hammond, M., *et al.* (2001b). Social skills and problem-solving training for children with early-onset conduct problems: who benefits? *J Child Psychol Psychiatry* **42**:943–52.

Webster-Stratton, C., Reid, M. J., Hammond, M., *et al* (2004). Treating children with early-onset conduct problems: intervention outcomes for parent, child, and teacher training. *J Clin Child Adolesc Psychol* **33**:105–24.

Weikart, D. P., & Schweinhart, L. J. (1991). Disadvantaged children and curriculum effects. *New Dir Child Dev* **Fall** (53):57–64.

Weissman, M. M., Wickramaratne, P., Nomura, Y., *et al.* (2005). Families at high and low risk for depression: a 3-generation study. *Arch Gen Psychiatry* **62**:29–36.

Whittington, C. J., Kendall, T., Fonagy, P., *et al.* (2004). Selective serotonin reuptake inhibitors in childhood depression: systematic review of published versus unpublished data. *Lancet* **363**: 1341–5.

World Health Organisation (1994). *ICD-10 Classification of Mental and Behavioural disorders.* Geneva: World Health Organisation.

Wilhelm, K., Mitchell, P. B., Niven, H., *et al.* (2006). Life events, first depression onset and the serotonin transporter gene. *Br J Psychiatry* **188**:210–15.

Wittchen, H. U., Stein, M. B., & Kessle, R. C. (1999). Social fears and social phobia in a community sample of adolescents and young adults: prevalence, risk factors and co-morbidity. *Psychol Med* **29**:309–23.

Wyatt, G. (1985). The sexual abuse of Afro-American and White-American women in childhood. *Child Abuse Neglect* **9**:507–19.

Yule, W. (2001). Posttraumatic stress disorder in the general population and in children. *J Clin Psychiatry* **62**(Suppl 17):23–8.

7

Personality disorder

Peter Tyrer

Personality disorder has for many years been in the parentheses of psychiatric classification, a group of disorders that one almost had to apologise before mentioning. We have commented that personality disorder has many of the same attributes as body odour, it is "indubitably affected by constitution and environment, a source of distress to both sufferer and society, yet imbued with ideas of degeneracy and inferiority" (Tyrer & Ferguson, 1988, p. 11). This illustrates its stigmatising, alienating and negative attributes but also emphasises its ubiquity. All of us have personalities and in varying ways are proud of them, but a small group are alleged to have their personality in the form of a disorder. The personality attributes of those with disorder are viewed universally as negative and undesirable. Those unfortunate enough to suffer from personality disorder, like those with body odour, have the propensity to offend by exhibiting more of something that everyone already possesses to some degree.

The paradox of embracing personality as a general concept, and labelling negatively a small group at the extreme is not confined to personality disorder; it is certainly much more prominent in this group of conditions than in others, however. It has unfortunately had a negative influence on the way personality disorder has been described in the psychiatric literature and used in clinical practise. I still consider it amazing, after many years of using the term, that so many clinicians never mention it to their patients

and often only to their colleagues when they are emotionally aroused.

Times are changing, and a great deal has happened in the past 20 years. Not surprisingly, at a time of frequent change, some of the issues discussed in this chapter will be likely to be incorporated into the core of learning about these conditions, whereas others may well be abandoned.

Classification

Classification by category

There are five common ways of classifying personality disorder, and although they can be combined to some extent, they are worth discussing separately. Classification is one of the areas in which there is currently a great deal of activity and a general feeling of dissatisfaction with current practice.

In Table 7.1, the standard (official) classifications of *International Classification of Disease* (ICD) and the *Diagnostic and Statistical Manual of Mental Disorders* (DSM) are listed. However, there is an earlier stage in the classification of personality disorder that is often forgotten. The assessor is asked to decide whether the patient satisfies the criteria for the general diagnosis of personality disorder. These are "characteristic and enduring patterns of inner experience and behaviour that deviate markedly from the culturally expected and accepted

Essential Psychiatry, ed. Robin M. Murray, Kenneth S. Kendler, Peter McGuffin, Simon Wessely, David J. Castle. Published by Cambridge University Press. © Cambridge University Press 2008.

Table 7.1 Summary of ICD-10 and DSM-IV classifications of personality disorder

ICD-10		DSM-IV	
Code	Disorder	Disorder	Code
F 60.0	Paranoid – excessive sensitivity, suspiciousness, preoccupation with conspiratorial explanation of events, persistent tendency to self-reference	Paranoid – interpretation of people's actions as deliberately demeaning or threatening	301.0
F 60.1	Schizoid – emotional coldness, detachment, lack of interest in other people, eccentricity, introspective fantasy	Schizoid – indifference to social relationships and restricted range of emotional experience and expression	301.20
	No equivalent	Schizotypal – deficit in interpersonal relatedness with peculiarities of ideation, odd beliefs and thinking, unusual appearance and behaviour	301.22

The above three conditions constitute Cluster A (inhibited, withdrawn and schizoid personalities)

F 60.2	Dissocial – callous unconcern for others, with irresponsibility, irritability and aggression, incapacity to maintain enduring relationships	Antisocial – pervasive pattern of disregard for and violation of the rights of others occurring since age 15	301.7
F 60.4	Histrionic – self-dramatisation, shallow mood, egocentricity and craving for excitement with persistent manipulative behaviour	Histrionic – excessive emotionality and attention seeking, suggestibility, superficiality	301.50
F 60.30	Impulsive – inability to control anger, to plan ahead or to think before acts, with unpredictable mood and quarrelsome behaviour	No equivalent	
F 60.31	Borderline – pervasive instability of mood, interpersonal relationships and self-image associated with marked impulsivity, fear of abandonment, identity disturbance and recurrent suicidal behaviour	Borderline – impulsivity with uncertainty over self-image, liability to become involved in intense and unstable relationships, recurrent threats of self-harm	301.83
	No equivalent	Narcissistic – pervasive grandiosity, lack of empathy, arrogance, requirement for excessive admiration	301.81

The above five conditions constitute Cluster B (erratic, flamboyant and dramatic personalities)

F 60.5	Anankastic – indecisiveness, doubt, excessive caution, pedantry, rigidity and need to plan in immaculate detail	Obsessive-compulsive – preoccupation with orderliness, perfectionism and inflexibility that leads to inefficiency	301.4
F 60.6	Anxious – persistent tension, self-consciousness, exaggeration of risks and dangers, hypersensitivity to rejection, restricted lifestyle because of insecurity	Avoidant – pervasive social discomfort, fear of negative evaluation and timidity, with feelings of inadequacy in social situations	301.82

(*cont.*)

Table 7.1 (*cont.*)

ICD-10		DSM-IV	
Code	Disorder	Disorder	Code
F 60.7	Dependent – failure to take responsibility for actions, with subordination of personal needs to those of others, excessive dependence with need for constant reassurance and feelings of helplessness when a close relationship ends	Dependent – persistent dependent and submissive behaviour	301.60

The above three conditions constitute Cluster C (anxious, fearful and dependent personalities); The anankastic/obsessive-compulsive personality group can sometimes be analysed separately because it is a separate factor in the structure (see Table 7.2)

DSM-IV = *Diagnostic and Statistical Manual of Mental Disorders,* 4th edition (American Psychiatric Association, 1994); ICD-10 = *International Classification of Diseases,* 10th edition (World Health Organisation, 1992).

range" with regard to cognition, affectivity, impulse control and ways of relating to others, inflexibility of behaviour "across a broad range of personal and social situations", accompanied by "personal distress or adverse impact on the social environment", onset in late childhood or adolescence and not explicable in terms of other mental disorder (World Health Organisation, 1992). The clinician, at least in theory, is then meant to go through each of the individual categories of personality disorder and decide which of those apply to the patient.

In many years of assessing, and helping others to assess, personality disorder I have yet to see one person who actually goes through this process in the way expected by the classification. This is probably because of the immense pulling power of the different categories in ICD and DSM. This was originally given to us by Kurt Schneider (1923) who, in a brilliant exposition, gave telling descriptions of most of the major personality disorder categories honed entirely from clinical experience. Each of these he described as *psychopathic personalities,* and in some ways it is curious that the adjective *psychopathic* has been abstracted from his descriptions and given to a completely

different group of callous, glib, antisocial personalities, written about in similar compelling language by Henderson (1939) and Cleckley (1941).

The major problem with classifying personality disorder into categories is that, apart from the obvious exceptions that are in the original writings, most people with personality disorder qualify for more than one category. Indeed, with some individuals in forensic institutions, it is possible to score positively for every single one of the categories

Classification by cluster

The recognition that many people could score for several personality disorders was embarrassing for the classification (not least because it gave a confusing second meaning to the term *multiple personality disorder*). However, it was noticed that some personality disorders tended to congregate more closely together than others. The three-cluster model (Reich & Thompson, 1987) arose from this:

• Cluster A (odd eccentric cluster) represented by paranoid and schizoid personality disorders, with schizotypal personality disorder in the DSM classification;

Table 7.2 Dimensions of normal and abnormal personality identified from factor and cluster analysis (using the Five-Factor Model as a base)

Authors	Factor 1 – neuroticism/ emotional stability	Factor 2 – extraversion/ withdrawal	Factor 3 – agreeableness/ psychopathy	Factor 4 – conscientious/ easygoing	Factor 5 – openness to experience/ closed attitudes
Costa & McCrae, 1992	Divided into anxiety, hostility, depression, self-consciousness, impulsivity, vulnerability	Divided into warmth, gregariousness, assertiveness, activity, excitement seeking, positive emotions	Divided into trust, straightforwardness, altruism, compliance, modesty, tender-mindedness	Divided into competence, order, dutifulness, achievement striving, self-discipline, deliberation	Divided into fantasy, aesthetics, feelings, actions, values
Walton & Presly, 1973	Submissiveness	Schizoid	Hysterical, sociopathic	Obsessional	?
Tyrer & Alexander, 1979	Passive-dependent	Schizoid	Sociopathic	Anankastic	?
Clark, 1990	Negative affectivity	Schizoid	Antisocial	Obsessive-compulsive	?
Livesley & Jackson, 2002	Emotional dysregulation	Inhibitedness	Dissocial behaviour	Compulsivity	?

Note that there are personality disorder equivalents to all but the "openness to experience" factor from the Five-Factor Model.

- Cluster B (flamboyant, erratic or dramatic personalities) including compulsive, borderline, antisocial, histrionic and narcissistic personality disorders; and
- Cluster C (the anxious/fearful group) represented by anxious (avoidant), dependent and anankastic (obsessive-compulsive) personality disorders.

This cluster model simplifies description but is not entirely satisfactory. There really should be a fourth cluster, the obsessional one which allows Cluster C to be separated into two and which fits factor analytical studies that identify four areas of difference in both normal and abnormal personality functioning (Clark, 1993; Schroeder *et al.*, 1992; Tyrer & Alexander, 1979). The fifth factor of what is called commonly called the Big Five (Costa & McCrae, 1992; Costa & Widiger, 1990) is called *openness to experience* and is not really identifiable

as a separate grouping in those with personality disorder (Table 7.2). Although the Big Five is currently the most prominent model in the field, it is not without its critics, and its appropriateness for the classification of abnormal personality is open to question (Reynolds & Clark, 2001).

Classification by severity

A good diagnosis should demonstrate what Kendell (1975) called a "point of rarity" between it and other conditions. In practice, virtually no psychiatric diagnoses achieve this distinction and represent the extremes of a dimensional continuum. In the case of personality disorder, this makes the arbitrary distinction between "no personality disorder" and "personality disorder" much more difficult to accept. This argument has been reinforced

Table 7.3 Dimensional system of classifying personality disorders

Level of severity	Description	Definition by categorical system
0	No personality disorder	Does not meet actual or subthreshold criteria for any personality disorder
1	Personality difficulty	Meets sub-threshold criteria for one or several personality disorders
2	Simple personality disorder	Meets actual criteria for one or more personality disorders within the same cluster
3	Complex (diffuse) personality disorder	Meets actual criteria for one or more personality disorders within more than one cluster
4	Severe personality disorder	Meets criteria for creation of severe disruption to both individual and to many in society

After Tyrer, 2000, pp. 129–301; Tyrer & Johnson, 1996.

by a great deal of empirical research demonstrating that the most parsimonious explanation of personality pathology is a dimensional trait one (Clark, 1992; Livesley *et al.*, 1992). This states that normal personality and personality disorder are all on the same continuum and that the variation in normal personality is exactly the same as that reflected in disorder.

There are currently no internationally accepted ways of classifying severity of personality disturbance but I have argued – not surprisingly because it is a personal investment – that one approach (Tyrer & Johnson, 1996) should be an apposite one. This uses both the notion of personality difficulty as a measure of subthreshold scores for personality disorder using standard interviews and the evidence that those with the most severe personality disorders demonstrate a "ripple effect" of personality disturbance across the whole range of the disorders shown in Table 7.1. Because the cluster model derived from Table 7.1 is the nearest to the four-factor dimensional model, severity is linked to this. Thus in addition to subthreshold (personality difficulty) and single cluster (simple personality disorder), this also derives complex or diffuse personality disorder (two or more clusters of personality disorder present) and can also derive severe personality disorder for those of greatest risk (Table 7.3).

There are several advantages to classifying personality disorder by severity. The first is that it not only allows for but also takes advantage of the tendency for personality disorders to be comorbid with each other. The second is that it represents the influence of personality disorder on clinical outcome more satisfactorily than the simple dichotomous system of no personality versus personality disorder.

This is illustrated in Table 7.4 in which the outcome of several studies that recorded personality status at baseline are separated by levels of severity of personality disturbance. These figures show that more information is gleaned from the separation into four groupings than in the dichotomous classification.

The third advantage is that this system accommodates the new, and to some highly suspect, diagnosis of severe personality disorder, particularly "dangerous and severe personality disorder" (DSPD). Although severity is not normally taken into account when classifying mental illness, its importance has been illustrated by its almost universal adoption by planners of mental health services, such that nosologists, almost against their will, have been drawn into defining which disorders constitute severe mental illness and which do not (Ruggeri *et al.*, 2000). The same applies to personality disorder. Politicians and the public both want to know who comprise the most dangerous group, which only amounts to about 700 people who constitute a significant danger to the public; the remaining

Table 7.4 Examples of severity model of recording personality abnormality in predicting the effect of personality abnormality in the presence of other symptoms and behaviour

Clinical population	Specific outcome	Authors	No personality disorder	Personality difficulty	Simple personality disorder	(Complex) (diffuse) personality disorder	*p* Value
Anxiety and depressive disorders (outcome after 12 years)	Global outcome (NDOS)	Tyrer *et al.*, 2004b	1.7	2.1	2.3	3.7	<0.001
	Social function	Seivewright *et al.*, 2004	6.3	7.9	9.2	12.1	<0.001
Recurrent psychotic illness	Mean police contacts over 1 year	Gandhi *et al.*, 2001	0.05	0.13	0.34	0.39	<0.001
Psychosis (UK700 study)	Duration of in-patient treatment (median)	Tyrer & Seivewright, 2000	8m	8m	10m	13.5m	0.002
	Quality of life (LQOL)	Tyrer & Seivewright, 2000	4.72	4.51	4.45	4.45	0.002
Recurrent self-harm	% with self-harm over 1 yr	Tyrer *et al.*, 2004a	20.5	37.6	51.3	55.1	<0.001

*NDOS (Neurotic Disorders Outcome Scale)

4 million who have personality disorder in epidemiological studies but pose no danger are completely ignored. It is unlikely that the diagnosis of DSPD (discussed later) will remain the same after it has been subjected to closer scrutiny, but I suspect that it will be retained in some form. A severity system will allow it to take place.

Classification by impact on social functioning

This is a relatively neglected subject that is not yet formalised in a classification structure. However, personality disorder was nicely, if not quite accurately, defined succinctly by Schneider as "such abnormal personalities who suffer through their abnormalities or through whose abnormalities society suffers" and this, in the absence of a measure of suffering (even though one has now recently become available; see Buchi *et al.*, 2000) is regarded as equivalent to social functioning. Rutter (1987) suggested that personality disorder was so much associated with the problems of interactions with others and social functioning that there was little point in sub the condition further. The Personality Assessment Schedule (Tyrer & Alexander, 1979; Tyrer *et al.*, 1979) also gives social function priority in creating a hierarchy in which the personality disorder creating the greater social dysfunction is given primacy over others in a subsequent description of personality disorder.

Social function is affected by many other aspects of mental functioning apart from that of personality. However, whenever there is persistently impaired social functioning in conditions in which it would normally not be expected, the evidence suggests that this is more likely to be created by personality abnormality than by other clinical variables (Nur *et al.*, 2004; Seivewright *et al.*, 2004).

Classification by attribution

Some may find it surprising that personality disorders are generally common in the community, yet only a small proportion present for treatment, although many others who present for treatment with mental health problems also have a concurrent personality disorder. One reason is that many who have a personality disorder do not recognise any abnormality and defend valiantly their continued occupancy of their personality role. This group have been termed the *Type R*, or treatment-resisting personality disorders, as opposed to the *Type S* or treatment-seeking ones, who are keen on altering their personality disorders and sometimes clamour for treatment. Preliminary evidence suggests that Type R exceeds Type S personalities by a ratio of around 3:1 (Tyrer, Mitchard *et al.*, 2003).

Synthesis of views

There is general agreement among personality disorder researchers that a fundamental change in the classification of personality disorder must occur. The changes that I would like to see are those I have outlined in this section.

Aetiology

There is also much debate over the aetiology of personality disorder. The continued arguments over the relative roles of nature (genetics) and nurture (environment) have been a battleground for proponents of each viewpoint. This has been further complicated by a suggestion that temperament and character could be separated from personality and have different genetic loadings. The Temperament and Character Inventory (TCI) of Cloninger and his colleagues (1993) has stimulated this split, because the notion that temperament could be linked directly to neurobiological mechanisms that were genetically determined might contrast with the more heterogeneous mix of personality disorders in which environmental factors may play a major part.

The (unsurprising) judgement of research is more prosaic. Environmental and genetic factors interweave to influence personality development almost equally, and many genes interact to create different trait groupings. In the words of Livesley *et al.* (1998) "the residual heritability of the lower-order traits (of personality) suggests that the personality phenotypes are based on a large number of specific genetic components". This clashes to some extent with the views of those who argue that some personality abnormalities (particularly borderline personality disorder) are a consequence of childhood abuse and trauma (e.g. Herman *et al.*, 1989), but there is no clear evidence that borderline personality disorder is influenced to a greater extent by environment than are other personality disorders. Recent evidence of reduced hippocampal volumes in those with borderline personality disorder (Driessen *et al.*, 2000) is a productive area of enquiry that will help in the developmental understanding of this and related conditions.

Treatment of personality disorder

Diagnostic entities in psychiatry attract little attention from clinicians until effective treatments are available. Much of the current interest in personality disorder has come from the perception that effective treatments are, or should be, available to people with this diagnosis. This is an interesting shift, because the whole history of the condition has implied untreatability and persistence (as indicated in this chapter when describing the definition of personality disorder). The interest in treatability has come from two quarters.

The first is from the criminal justice system. It has been recognised for many years that one group of the original Schneiderian psychopaths, now described variously as antisocial, dissocial or core psychopathic (Hare, 1991), contains a few individuals who are especially dangerous. In many countries, these individuals are regarded as outside the healthcare system and are treated as criminals rather than patients. However, in the United Kingdom (or, more accurately, in England and Wales because Scotland has gone its own way) those with DSPD have been designated separately for a special programme of psychiatric care, and specific criteria are now available for detecting these individuals (Maden & Tyrer, 2003). At one level, this policy is understandable because some with certain personality disorders create major problems in the community (e.g. Gandhi *et al.*, 2001), but to many this provision is viewed as draconian. At the time of writing, a draft bill has been formulated which suggests that such individuals can be detained compulsorily if clinically appropriate treatment is available for them. It is not absolutely clear whether "clinically appropriate" includes all forms of management or treatment designed to alleviate the symptoms, behaviour, personality abnormality or all three. What is clear, however, is that if individuals are to be detained for long periods and not given treatment, this would amount to an abuse of human rights and would be likely to be successfully challenged in the courts.

The second stimulus to treatment has been increasing evidence that personality is not stable over time and, particularly in those attending for treatment, that significant improvement in functioning, behaviour and even personality pathology, can occur. It is to the credit of psychodynamic psychiatry that practitioners in this subject continued treating personality disorder when others had almost abandoned it, and much of the stimulus for treatment research was originally generated in settings in which personality disorder, mainly borderline and narcissistic groups, were being treated with

different forms of dynamic psychotherapy over the long term (Higgitt & Fonagy, 1992).

The main treatments with at least some measurable evidence of efficacy are shown in Table 7.5. The field is expanding rapidly and interested readers may like to examine the Web site of the British and Irish Group for the Study of Personality Disorders (BIGSPD) (http://www.bigspd.net), which gives a regular update of all treatment studies.

The main treatments are, as for all mental disorders, psychological, drug and alternative or complementary treatments. The omission of a treatment from the list that follows does not mean that it is ineffective in the treatment of personality disorders; it has just not been tested adequately according to the tenets of evidence-based medicine.

Psychotherapy

In this section are included all those treatments which (1) are psychological in nature in that they primarily involve verbal interaction between therapist and patient, (2) are defined in a way that allows them to be replicable and (3) are structured in such a way that allows fidelity of the treatment to be tested. There is currently a great deal of activity in this area, but most is focused on the treatment of borderline personality disorder. In those randomised trials that have demonstrated efficacy, the control treatment has usually been "treatment as usual" (TAU). Because this varies greatly, other control treatments may have to be chosen in future. It will also become necessary to test different types of active treatment in a controlled fashion; one such study is in progress (Clarkin *et al.*, 2004).

No specific preferences are given in Table 7.5, but the evidence is summarised and, although absence of evidence is not evidence of absence, there is clearly much that needs to be done before clear recommendations can be given for many of the treatments.

Drug treatments

Drug treatments are somewhat easier to test than psychological treatments, but in studies related to

Table 7.5 Treatment trials in people with personality disorders

Type of treatment	Main studies	Results	Recommendation
Psychodynamic treatment linked to day hospital and mentalisation-based treatment	Bateman & Fonagy, 1999, 2001, 2003, 2004 (same study carried out with patients with borderline personality disorder)	Small randomised controlled trial with excellent results for symptoms, self-harm, hospitalisation and costs of care	Needs replication, but results at this stage sufficient to suggest that day hospitals could well refocus on this group using this approach in principle
Dialectical behaviour therapy (DBT)	Linehan et al., 1991; Verheul et al., 2003 (all studies in borderline personality disorder, some exclusively with women)	Series of small randomised trials showing definite advantages of DBT over treatment as usual for self-harming behaviour, with other symptoms equivocal and some loss of effect over time	Now an established treatment although the evidence base is still somewhat slim, particularly for men
Cognitive-behavioural therapy (CBT) and problem-solving therapy	Evans et al., 1999; Tyrer et al., 2003, 2004 (treatment in self-harm population but 42% had personality disorders, and 91% had personality disturbance of some type)	One small trial suggesting efficacy; second showing less effect but cost-effective in brief form In large trial (n = 480). Problem-solving psychotherapy effective in preventing self-harm recurrence (Guthrie et al., 2001)	Detailed analysis suggests CBT in brief form only suited for non-borderline patients with limited self-harming behaviour (further studies with longer treatment in progress)
Cognitive analytical therapy	Ryle, 1997, 2004 (treatment specifically for borderline personality disorder)	No randomised trials; keen group of enthusiasts	More evidence awaited
Therapeutic communities	Chiesa & Fonagy, 2000 (one of the best controlled studies but not able to reach randomised allocation)	No randomised controlled trials except of "concept" communities for substance misuse which have attendant coercion	Although the most established treatment in the United Kingdom for personality disorder, it is beginning to be supplanted by newer psychological therapies; forms adapted to day and home support seem to have best evidence of cost-effectiveness
Transference-focused psychotherapy	Clarkin et al., 1999, 2004 (Otto Kernberg's treatment for borderline personality disorder applied in formal research form)	Randomised trial in progress at present	Well-established treatment awaiting evidence
Nidotherapy	Tyrer, 2002; Tyrer & Bajaj, 2004; Tyrer et al., 2003; (treatment suited for Type R personality disorders)	Randomised trial currently in progress	Early stage of new approach focusing on environment

(*cont.*)

Table 7.5 (*cont.*)

Type of treatment	Main studies	Results	Recommendation
Haloperidol and other typical antipsychotics in low dosage	Cornelius *et al.*, 1993; Soloff *et al.*, 1986 (mainly borderline personality disorders)	Contrasting results with very positive effects of haloperidol (7 mg/day) in first study but not replicated	No clear evidence of benefit despite widespread use in Cluster B personality disorders; adherence to treatment may explain contrasting results
Fluoxetine, paroxetine and other selective serotonin reuptake inhibitors (SSRIs)	Coccaro & Kavoussi, 1997; Salzman *et al.*, 1995; Verkes *et al.*, 1998	Benefit of SSRIs in reducing self-harm and aggression – better evidence than most other treatments because of large trials, but some doubt over generalisability	Evidence only sufficient to regard both SSRIs and antipsychotic drugs as "adjunctive" treatments in borderline personality disorder (American Psychiatric Association, 2001)
Other drugs, including mood stabilisers, atypical antipsychotic drugs, omega-3 fatty acids and monoamine oxidase inhibitors	Summarised in Newton-Howes & Tyrer, 2003; Tyrer & Bateman, 2004	Some evidence of benefit from small randomised trials, but these are too small to yield clear evidence	No clear guidelines about use of these compounds, but there is likely to be a strong drive to use atypical antipsychotic drugs in some personality disorders

personality disorders, there has been a tendency toward small sample sizes (often less than 10 in each treatment arm), and this is of no value except for feasibility purposes. From Table 7.5, it can be seen that only SSRIs and, to a much lesser extent, antipsychotic drugs in relatively low dosage can be recommended for treatment of personality disorders, mainly for borderline personality. The only treatment available for Type R personality disorders currently is nidotherapy (nest therapy; Tyrer *et al.*, 2003), in which the focus is on changing the environment rather than the person, and for someone who has no desire to change, this can be an attractive option. However, much more evidence of the value of this approach is necessary.

Conclusions

Our understanding of personality disorders has come of age since the mid-1990s. We have better knowledge of their nature and course and are beginning to find ways to alter their core features. Despite this, this is a very young discipline, and many of our attractive ways forward are likely to turn out to be dead ends.

REFERENCES

American Psychiatric Association (1994). *Diagnostic and Statistical Manual of Mental Disorders*, 4th edn. (DSM-IV). Washington, DC: American Psychiatric Association.

American Psychiatric Association (2001). Practice guideline for the treatment of patients with borderline personality disorder. *Am J Psychiatry* **158(Suppl)**:1–52.

Bateman, A., & Fonagy, P. (1999). Effectiveness of partial hospitalisation in the treatment of borderline personality disorder: a randomised controlled trial. *Am J Psychiatry* **156**:1563–9.

Bateman, A., & Fonagy, P. (2001). Treatment of borderline personality disorder with psychoanalytically oriented partial hospitalization: an 18-month follow-up. *Am J Psychiatry* **158**:36–42.

Bateman, A., & Fonagy, P. (2003). Health service utilization costs for borderline personality disorder patients treated with psychoanalytically oriented partial hospitalization versus general psychiatric care. *Am J Psychiatry* **160**:169–71.

Bateman, A. W., & Tyrer, P. (2004). Psychological treatment for personality disorders. *Adv Psychiatr Treat* **10**:378–88.

Buchi, S., Sensky, T., Sharpe, L., & Timberlake, N. (1998). Graphic representation of illness: a novel method of measuring patients' perceptions of the impact of illness. *Psychother Psychosom* **67**:222–5.

Chiesa, M., & Fonagy, P. (2000). Cassel Personality Disorder Study: methodology and treatment effects. *Br J Psychiatry* **176**:485–91.

Clark, L. A. (1992). Resolving taxonomic issues in personality disorders. *J Person Disord* **6**:360–76.

Clark, L.A. (1993). *Manual for the Schedule for Non-Adaptive and Adaptive Personality*. Minneapolis: University of Minnesota Press.

Clarkin, J. F., Levy, K. N., Lenzenweger, M. F., & Kernberg, O. (2004). The Personality Disorders Institute/Borderline Research Foundation randomised controlled trial for borderline personality disorder: rationale, treatment methods, and patient characteristics. *J Person Disord* **18**:52–72.

Clarkin, J. F., Yeomans, F., & Kernberg, O. (1999). *Psychotherapy of Borderline Personality*. New York: Wiley.

Cleckley, H. (1941). *The Mask of Sanity*. London: Henry Kimpton.

Cloninger, C. R., Svrakic, D. M., & Pryzbeck, T. R. (1993). A psychobiological model of temperament and character. *Arch Gen Psychiatry* **50**:975–90.

Coccaro, E. F., & Kavoussi, R. J. (1997). Fluoxetine and impulsive aggressive behavior in personality-disordered subjects. *Arch Gen Psychiatry* **54**.1081–8.

Cornelius, J. R., Soloff, P. H., Perel, J. M., *et al.* (1993). Continuation pharmacotherapy of borderline personality disorder with haloperidol and phenelzine. *Am J Psychiatry* **150**:1843–8.

Costa, P. T., & McCrae, R. R. (1992). *Revised NEO Personality Inventory (NEO-PI-R) and the NEO Five-Factor Inventory (NEO-FFI) professional manual*. Odessa, FL: Psychological Assessment Resources.

Costa, P. T., & Widiger, T. A., eds. (1990). *Personality Disorders and the Five-Factor Model of Personality*. Washington, DC: American Psychological Association.

Driessen, M., Herrmann, J., Stahl, K., *et al.* (2000). Magnetic resonance imaging volumes of the hippocampus and the amygdala in women with borderline personality disorder and early traumatization. *Arch Gen Psychiatry* **57**:1115–22.

Evans, K., Tyrer, P., Catalan, J., *et al.* (1999). Manual-assisted cognitive-behaviour therapy (MACT): a randomised controlled trial of a brief intervention with bibliotherapy in the treatment of recurrent deliberate self-harm. *Psychol Med* **29**:19–25.

Gandhi, N., Tyrer, P., Evans, K., *et al.* (2001). A randomised controlled trial of community-oriented and hospital oriented care for discharged psychiatric patients: influence of personality disorder on police contacts. *J Person Disord* **15**:94–102.

Guthrie, E., Kapur, N., Mackway-Jones, K., *et al.* (2001). Randomised controlled trial of brief psychological intervention after deliberate self poisoning. *BMJ* **323**:135–8.

Hare, R. D. (1991). *The Hare Psychopathy Checklist – Revised*. Toronto: Multi-Health Systems.

Henderson, D. K. (1939). *Psychopathic States*. New York: Norton.

Herman, J. L., Perry, J. C., & Van Der Kolk, B. A. (1989). Childhood trauma in personality disorder. *Am J Psychiatry* **146**:490–5.

Higgitt, A., & Fonagy, P. (1992). Psychotherapy in borderline and narcissistic personality disorder. *Br J Psychiatry* **161**:23–43.

Kendell, R. E. (1975). The concept of disease and its implications for psychiatry. *Br J Psychiatry* **127**:305–15.

Linehan, M. M., Armstrong, H. E., Suarez, A., *et al.* (1991). Cognitive-behavioural treatment of chronically para suicidal borderline patients. *Arch Gen Psychiatry* **48**:1060–4.

Livesley, W. J., & Jackson, D. N. (2002). *Manual for the Dimensional Assessment of Personality Pathology*. Port Huron, Minnesota: Sigma Press.

Livesley, W. J., Jackson, D. N. & Schroeder, M. L. (1992). Factorial structure of traits delineating personality disorders in clinical and general population samples. *J Abnorm Psychol* **101**:432–40.

Livesley, W. J., Jang, K. L., & Vernon, P. A. (1998). Phenotypic and genetic structure of traits delineating personality disorder. *Arch Gen Psychiatry* **55**:941–8.

Maden, T., & Tyrer, P. (2003). Dangerous and severe personality disorders: a new personality concept from the United Kingdom. *J Person Disord* **17**:489–96.

Nur, U., Tyrer, P., Merson, S., & Johnson, T. (2004). Relationship between clinical symptoms, personality disturbance, and social function: a statistical enquiry. *Irish J Psychol Med* **21**:19–22.

Reich, J., & Thompson, W. D. (1987). DSM-III personality disorder clusters in three generations. *Br J Psychiatry* **150**:471–5.

Reynolds, S. K., & Clark, L. A. (2001). Predicting dimensions of personality disorder from domains and facets of the Five-Factor Model. *J Person* **69**:199–222.

Ruggeri, M., Leese, M., Thornicroft, G., *et al.* (2000). Definition and prevalence of severe and persistent mental illness. *Br J Psychiatry* **177**:149–55.

Rutter, M. (1987). Temperament, personality and personality disorder. *Br J Psychiatry* **150**:443–58.

Ryle, A. (1997). *Cognitive Analytical Therapy and Borderline Personality Disorder: The Model and the Method*. Chichester, England: Wiley.

Ryle, A. (2004). The contribution of cognitive analytical therapy to the treatment of borderline personality disorder. *J Person Disord* **18**:3–35.

Salzman, C., Wolfson, A. N., Schatzberg, A., *et al.* (1995). Effect of fluoxetine on anger in symptomatic volunteers with borderline personality disorder. *J Clin Psychopharmacol* **15**:23–9.

Schneider, K. (1923). *Die Psychopathischen Persönlichkeiten*. Berlin: Springer.

Schroeder, M. L., Wormworth, J. A., & Livesley, W. J. (1992). Dimensions of personality disorder and their relationships to the Big Five dimensions of personality. *Psychol Assess* **4**:47–53.

Seivewright, H., Tyrer, P., & Johnson, T. (2004). Persistent social dysfunction in anxious and depressed patients with personality disorder. *Acta Psychiatr Scand* **109**:104–9.

Soloff, P. H., George, A., Nathan, R. S. *et al.* (1986). Progress in pharmacotherapy of borderline disorders: a double blind study of amitriptyline, haloperidol and placebo. *Arch Gen Psychiatry* **43**:691–7.

Tyrer, P. (2000). Challenges for the future. In P. Tyrer, ed. *Personality Disorders: Diagnosis, Management and Course*, 2nd edn. London: Arnold, pp. 126–32.

Tyrer, P. (2002). Nidotherapy: a new approach to the treatment of personality disorder. *Acta Psychiatr Scand* **105**:469–71.

Tyrer, P., & Alexander, J. (1979). Classification of personality disorder. *Br J Psychiatry* **135**: 163–7.

Tyrer, P., Alexander, M. S., Cicchetti, D., *et al.* (1979). Reliability of a schedule for rating personality disorders. *Br J Psychiatry* **135**:168–74.

Tyrer, P., & Bajaj, P. (2005). Nidotherapy: letting the environment do the therapeutic work. *Adv Psychiatr Treat.* **11**:232–8.

Tyrer, P., & Bateman, A. W. (2004). Drug treatment for personality disorders. *Adv Psychiat Treatment* **10**:389–98.

Tyrer, P., & Ferguson, B. (1988). Development of the concept of abnormal personality. In P Tyrer, ed. *Personality Disorders: Diagnosis, Management and Course*. London: Butterworth/Wright, pp. 1–11.

Tyrer, P., & Johnson, T. (1996). Establishing the severity of personality disorder. *Am J Psychiatry* **153**:1593–7.

Tyrer, P., Mitchard, S., Methuen, C., & Ranger, M. (2003). Treatment-rejecting and treatment-seeking personality disorders: Type R and Type S. *J Person Disord* **17**: 265–70.

Tyrer, P., & Seivewright, H. (2000). Studies of outcome. In P. Tyrer, ed. *Personality Disorders: Diagnosis, Management and Course*, 2nd edn. Oxford: Butterworth/Heinemann, pp. 105–25.

Tyrer, P., Seivewright, H., & Johnson, T. (2004). The Nottingham Study of Neurotic Disorder: predictors of 12 year outcome of dysthymic, panic and generalised anxiety disorder. *Psychol Med* **34**:1385–94.

Tyrer, P., Thompson, S., Schmidt, U., *et al.* (2003). Randomised controlled trial of brief cognitive behaviour therapy versus treatment as usual in recurrent deliberate self-harm: the POPMACT study. *Psychol Med* **33**: 969–76.

Tyrer, P., Tom, B., Byford, S., *et al.* (2004). Differential effects of manual assisted cognitive behavior therapy in the treatment of recurrent deliberate self-harm and personality disturbance: the POPMACT study. *J Pers Disorders* **18**:82–96.

Verkes, R. J., Van Der Mast, R. C., Hengeveld, M. W. *et al.* (1998). Reduction by paroxetine of suicidal behavior in patients with repeated suicide attempts but not major depression. *Am J Psychiatry* **155**:543–7.

Walton, H. J., & Presly, A. S. (1973). Use of a category system in the diagnosis of abnormal personality. *Br J Psychiatry* **122**:259–68.

World Health Organisation (1980). *International Classification of Impairments, Disabilities and Handicaps*, 10th revision. Geneva: World Health Organisation.

8

Anxiety disorders

Paul Carey, David J. Castle and Dan J. Stein

Anxiety is arguably an emotion that predates the evolution of man. Its ubiquity in humans, and its presence in a range of anxiety disorders, makes it an important clinical focus. Developments in nosology, epidemiology and psychobiology have significantly advanced our understanding of the anxiety disorders in recent years. Advances in pharmacotherapy and psychotherapy of these disorders have brought realistic hope for relief of symptoms and improvement in functioning to patients.

The anxiety disorders are the most prevalent of the psychiatric disorders in both the developed and developing world (Demyttenaere et al., 2004; Kessler, Berglund, et al., 2005). A chronic course with high levels of comorbidity (Kessler et al., 1994), significant disability, and impaired quality of life are typical features (Alonso et al., 2004; Lochner et al., 2003). The economic burden of anxiety disorders to healthcare funds and society in general is considerable (Greenberg et al., 1999). Nevertheless, these disorders remain underdiagnosed and undertreated in most settings (Demyttenaere et al., 2004).

The word *anxiety* is derived from the Latin *anxietas* (to choke, throttle, trouble, upset) and encompasses the behavioural, affective and cognitive responses to the perception of danger. Such responses are fundamental to the survival of species. In lower animals, the behavioural response to danger is hardwired and may be characterised by flight or freezing. In higher organisms, memory and other cognitive-affective processes play a more important role. Laboratory and animal studies of anxiety provide useful models for advancing our understanding of the mechanisms that may underlie the persistence of responses to fear and danger in humans.

Anxiety is a normal phenomenon, and some degree of anxiety/arousal is vital for optimal performance in situations which require it. Too little or too much anxiety/arousal leads to suboptimal performance, as governed by the Yerkes-Dodson curve (Yerkes & Dodson, 1908). When a person's anxiety is out of proportion to the particular situation, causes distress and impairs overall functioning, it can be considered that the individual has an anxiety disorder. The anxiety disorders are conventionally subdivided into: generalised anxiety disorder (GAD), panic disorder (PD), social phobia (social anxiety disorder – SAD), posttraumatic stress disorder (PTSD) and obsessive-compulsive disorder (OCD). Note that panic attacks (discrete episodes of severe anxiety) are pathognomonic for none of these disorders and can occur in people without anxiety disorders as well as in association with a number of other psychiatric and medical conditions. The characteristics of a panic attack are shown in Table 8.1.

It is also important to stress that "general medical" factors can precipitate or perpetuate anxiety symptomatology and need to be investigated and treated in their own right. Box 8.1 provides an overview of these medical factors.

Essential Psychiatry, ed. Robin M. Murray, Kenneth S. Kendler, Peter McGuffin, Simon Wessely, David J. Castle.
Published by Cambridge University Press. © Cambridge University Press 2008.

Table 8.1 DSM-IV-TR criteria for a panic attack

A discrete period of intense fear or discomfort in which four (or more) of the following symptoms developed abruptly and reached a peak within 10 minutes:

- palpitations, pounding heart, or accelerated heart rate
- sweating
- trembling or shaking
- sensations of shortness of breath or smothering
- feeling of choking
- chest pain or discomfort
- nausea or abdominal distress
- feeling dizzy, unsteady, lightheaded or faint
- derealization (feelings of unreality) or depersonalization (being detached from oneself)
- fear of losing control or going crazy
- fear of dying
- paresthesias (numbness or tingling sensations)
- chills or hot flushes

Reprinted with permission from the *Diagnostic and Statistical Manual of Mental Disorders*, 4th edn., text revision. © 2000 American Psychiatric Association.

The classification of the anxiety disorders

The current edition of the *Diagnostic and Statistical Manual of Mental Disorders*, the DSM-IV-TR (American Psychiatric Association, 2000) lists 12 anxiety disorders, with broadly similar categories listed in the *International Classification of Impairments, Disabilities and Handicaps*, 10th revision (ICD-10; World Health Organisation, 2006). These systems reflect the advances in our conceptualization of anxiety disorders in recent decades and provide clinicians and researchers with a reliable descriptive terminology. The approaches are compared and contrasted in Table 8.2.

The current nomenclatures have also received significant criticism from those who believe a dimensional approach is more appropriate to clinical realities. For instance, the phenomenology of fear/anxiety and adaptive/avoidant responses cuts across the major anxiety disorders. Similarly, there is significant overlap in the psychobiology and treatment of these conditions. High rates of

Box 8.1 Summary of more common general medical causes of anxiety

Cardiovascular and respiratory
Anaemia, arrhythmias, heart failure, mitral valve prolapse bronchospasm (asthma), chronic obstructive airway disease, hypoxia, pneumonia, pneumothorax, pulmonary embolism

Neurological
Seizure disorders, post-concussion syndrome, vestibular disease, delirium, cerebrovascular disease, mass lesions, pain

Endocrinological
Thyroid disease, hypoglycaemia, parathyroid disease, pheochromocytoma, adrenal dysfunction, premenstrual syndrome, pituitary disease

Metabolic
Porphyria, electrolyte disturbance, acidosis, hypothermia, vitamin B_{12} deficiency

Substance/medication induced
Intoxication, withdrawal (caffeine, benzodiazepines, clonidine, selective serotonin reuptake inhibitors, opiates, amphetamines, phencyclidine, cocaine, inhalants)

Toxicological
Carbon monoxide, carbon dioxide, heavy metals, organophosphates

comorbidity between anxiety and depressive disorders may reflect a common aetiology and pathogenesis. There are perhaps advantages to both categorical and dimensional approaches, with the former being useful in clinical diagnosis and the later more useful when considering fundamental questions of psychobiology.

In this chapter, we follow the current DSM-IV classification, but it is as well to note that this approach is being challenged and changes might be seen in further iterations of the major classification systems. OCD, for instance, is increasingly being seen as different from the other disorders with which it is currently classified, and it has been predicted that it might be better classified with a group of related disorders on a putative obsessive-compulsive spectrum (see Castle & Phillips, 2006; Stein & Hollander, 1993).

Table 8.2 Comparison of ICD-10 and DSM-IV-TR classifications of the anxiety disorders

DSM-IV-TR – Anxiety Disorders		ICD-10 Neurotic and stress-related disorders	
293.89	Anxiety disorder due to general medical condition	F06.4	Organic anxiety disorder
292.89	Substance-induced anxiety disorder (amphetamine, caffeine, cannabis, cocaine, hallucinogen, inhalant, phencyclidine, sedative, other [or unknown])	F10–19 (.8)	Other mental and behavioural disorders due to psychoactive substance use
300.00	Anxiety disorder NOS	F41.9	Anxiety disorder, unspecified
300.02	Generalized anxiety disorder	F41.1	Generalized anxiety disorder
300.01	Panic disorder without agoraphobia	F41.0	Panic disorder
300.21	Panic disorder with agoraphobia		
300.22	Agoraphobia without history of panic disorder	F40.0	Agoraphobia
300.23	Social phobia	F40.1	Social phobias
300.29	Specific phobia	F40.2	Specific (isolated) phobias
		F40.9	Phobic anxiety disorder, unspecified
300.3	Obsessive-compulsive disorder	F42	Obsessive-compulsive disorder
308.3	Acute stress disorder	F43.0	Acute stress reaction
309.81	Posttraumatic stress disorder	F43.1	Posttraumatic stress disorder
		F41.2	Mixed anxiety and depressive disorder
		F41.8	Other specified anxiety disorders – anxiety hysteria

DSM-IV TR = *Diagnostic and Statistical Manual of Mental Disorders*, 4th edition, text revision (American Psychiatric Association, 2006); ICD-10 = *International Classification of Diseases*, 10th edition (World Health Organisation, 2006); NOS = not otherwise specified.

Generalised anxiety disorder

GAD is characterised by persistent, uncontrollable worry and anxiety. A range of physical symptoms invariably accompanies psychic anxiety and includes restlessness, fatigability, poor concentration, irritability, muscle tension and sleep disturbances. GAD is the most common anxiety disorder seen in primary care with a lifetime prevalence of around 3% to 4% in community samples and has a higher prevalence in women (2:1; Maier *et al.*, 2000). GAD is often chronic, with onset in the teenage years and increasing linearly until the fourth decade. Until its introduction into the third edition of the DSM (DSM-III) as an independent disorder, GAD was considered a residual disorder. Today our understanding has been refined considerably,

and, although not without controversy, there is growing acceptance of GAD as an independent condition (Kessler, 2000; Kessler, Brandenburg, *et al.*, 2005).

Diagnosis

Core symptoms required for diagnosis of GAD are uncontrollable worry and anxiety that should be present for more days than not for 6 months or longer. In addition, three or more physical symptoms of anxiety and tension need to accompany the psychic symptoms. Since the introduction of GAD as an independent disorder in DSM-III (1980), the diagnostic criteria have changed considerably. There continues to be debate about the current criteria, and empirical studies suggest that additional changes may be useful to emphasise that GAD is often characterised by "double anxiety" – that is, a chronic underlying level of tension, with shorter periods of exacerbation of anxiety symptoms (Kessler, Brandenburg, *et al.*, 2005).

In primary care settings, GAD most frequently presents with a range of physical symptoms. Also, numerous medical conditions, physical treatments and illicit substances can mimic symptoms of GAD. Thus, a comprehensive approach must be taken to the diagnosis and evaluation of GAD-like symptoms. Symptoms should also be distinguished from health-related concerns that may be the focus of hypochondriasis (see also Chapter 23). Also, everyday worries should be differentiated from nonadaptive or pathological worry; evaluation of the intensity and appropriateness of the worry rather than the specific content may be helpful in making this distinction.

High rates of comorbidity with mood and other anxiety disorders in GAD is the rule (although such comorbidity is not necessarily higher in GAD than in disorders such as major depression). This comorbidity suggests that screening for the full range of anxiety, mood and substance-related disorders should form part of the routine assessment of patients in the clinic with suspected GAD.

Failure to identify and treat GAD results in unnecessary chronicity of symptoms and social and occupational impairment. Physicians should caution against minimizing symptoms and underestimating the degree of functional impairment in GAD. Standardised rating scales such as the Hamilton Anxiety Rating Scale (HAS) (Hamilton, 1959) may be helpful in assessing symptom severity and in monitoring changes with treatment.

Pathogenesis

Both biological and psychosocial factors have been posited to be important determinants of GAD onset and perpetuation. Genetic studies suggest that GAD and depression may share a genetic vulnerability, but the disorders appear to have differing predisposing environmental factors (Kendler, 1996; Torgersen, 1990). Trait anxiety may also be influenced by genetic variation in components of neurochemical systems believed to be involved in GAD, such as the serotonin transporter protein (Lesch, 2001).

An expanding body of brain imaging findings in GAD have demonstrated increased amygdala volumes (Schweizer *et al.*, 1995a), reduced benzodiazepine receptor binding in the anterior temporal lobe (Tiihonen, Kuikka, Rasanen, *et al.*, 1997). Functional imaging findings have been mixed (Gur *et al.*, 1987; Wu *et al.*, 1991) but in general support the involvement of limbic prefrontal regions, as well as basal ganglia and occipital regions in GAD.

Neurochemistry investigations have focused primarily on the serotonergic, noradrenergic and GABA systems in GAD. Serotonergic neurons are widely projected from the brainstem raphe to regions implicated in mediating anxiety and conditioning to fear-provoking cues. Specific serotonergic involvement has been suggested through findings of increased serotonin turnover in GAD (Garvey *et al.*, 1995) as well as increased anxiety in response to a serotonin agonist, m-chlorophenylpiperazine (mCPP; Germine *et al.*, 1992). Nevertheless, not all data are consistent, and additional work in this area is needed (Iny *et al.*, 1994).

Involvement of the noradrenergic (NA) system in GAD has been suggested with findings of increased NA turnover, consistent with α_2-adrenergic receptor downregulation and lower sensitivity (Cameron *et al.*, 2004; Sevy *et al.*, 1989). Corticotrophin releasing hormone (CRF), also crucial in mediating stress responsivity, interacts with NA and 5-HT to mediate anxious behaviour in the temporolimbic regions of animals (Sullivan *et al.*, 1999). Again, not all findings are consistent, so that additional work is necessary to delineate fully the role of NA in GAD.

The inhibitory neurotransmitter GABA is implicated indirectly in GAD through the efficacy of GABA-A receptor agonists, benzodiazepines, in treating GAD (Schweizer *et al.*, 1995b). More direct evidence of GABA involvement comes from imaging studies mentioned earlier with changes in GABA receptor density in temporal regions (Tiihonen,

Kuikka, Rasanen, *et al.*, 1997) and lower GABA platelet binding (anxiety) (Weizman *et al.*, 1987). Effective treatment also appears to normalise patterns of receptor binding (Cameron *et al.*, 1990).

Neurochemistry and brain imaging studies have influenced the development of theoretical models of GAD. For instance, a cognitive-affective model of GAD suggests that prefrontal brain regions are likely to mediate the characteristic anticipatory symptoms. Responses to internally or externally generated affective representations of the environment are co-ordinated through prefrontal limbic connections with generally activated basic fear circuitry in which the amygdala and anterior temporal pole are central. Additional limbic and paralimbic connections to the brainstem and the stria terminalis may be involved in mediating somatic and free-floating anxiety, respectively.

Developmental studies have found that adults with GAD report having experienced their parents as controlling and overinvolved, implying that overprotection of children conveys ideas of the world being dangerous (Rapee, 1997). Nurturing of this kind may facilitate the development of cognitive schemas that result in young people developing exaggerated, catastrophic thoughts and attentional bias to potentially threatening stimuli and consequently a higher vulnerability to subsequent stressors (Clark, 1988). Some authors suggest that GAD constitutes a constellation of maladaptive personality traits which include high levels of anxiety. Although these traits may not manifest as anxiety in childhood, their impact on cognitive development and later stress responsivity is likely to be significant (Rapee, 1985). A genetic influence on trait anxiety (mentioned earlier) is one indication that a fuller understanding of the pathogenesis of GAD will in future need to integrate genetic findings with regional neural circuitry and aspects of psychosocial development.

Management

Following diagnosis, psychoeducation is a helpful first step in the management of GAD. Patients should be informed about risks and benefits of the variety of available treatment options, the proposed duration of these treatments, risk of relapse, as well as long-term prognosis and outcomes of GAD. It is important for clinicians to develop an understanding of patients' interpretation of their symptoms, with particular attention being paid to differences in expression of distress by individual patients. The potential stigma associated with a psychiatric diagnosis should be considered in all cases.

Pharmacotherapy

Psychotropic agents with varied mechanisms of action (anxiolytic, antidepressant, anticonvulsant) have proved effective in the treatment of GAD. Efficacy must always be weighed against the risk of side effects. On this basis, the antidepressants and, in particular, the selective serotonin reuptake inhibitors (SSRIs) are presently recommended as the reasonable first-line pharmacotherapy option in GAD (Baldwin & Polkinghorn, 2005).

Most medications effective for depression are effective for anxiety. Early studies in GAD demonstrated the superior efficacy of the tricyclic antidepressants (TCAs) compared with benzodiazepines for anxious patients with subsyndromal depression (Rickels *et al.*, 1993). Subsequently a number of studies have shown efficacy for various SSRIs. The superior tolerability of the SSRIs now makes them the preferred choice over the older TCAs (Masand & Gupta, 2003; Schmitt *et al.*, 2005). Recent studies have also indicated benefits in acute and long-term treatment with the serotonin and norepinephrine reuptake inhibitor (SNRI), venlafaxine (Liebowitz *et al.*, 2005) and the anticonvulsant pregabalin (Rickels *et al.*, 2005).

Benzodiazepines remain the most widely prescribed treatment for GAD (Vasile *et al.*, 2005). Although reasonable evidence supports their use in the short term, concerns remain about their adverse event profile, including withdrawal symptoms.

Buspirone, a partial serotonin 1A receptor agonist, has some evidence to support its efficacy in short- and long-term treatment of GAD (Cohn &

Rickels, 1989). This agent has similar rates of efficacy but longer time to onset of action than benzodiazepines and a more favourable safety profile in respect to rebound anxiety.

Hydroxyzine, a histamine-1 receptor antagonist, has shown symptom relief that is sustained over time and upon abrupt withdrawal. Efficacy appears similar to benzodiazepines, with fewer cognitive effects reported (Gale & Oakley-Browne, 2004; Lader & Scotto, 1998).

Psychotherapy

Evidence supports the efficacy of a number of psychotherapeutic techniques when compared with no treatment in GAD. The strongest evidence is for cognitive-behavioural therapy (CBT), but there are also data for supportive-expressive psychodynamic therapy (Crits-Chritoph *et al.*, 1996; Durham *et al.*, 1994).

Patients are encouraged to endure symptoms through a variety of exposure techniques, thereby attenuating the provoked anxiety and limiting the motivation for avoidance. Cognitive-behavioural techniques may include "structuring" of "worry times" during the day with deferment of worrying to this allotted time. Relaxation exercises also have an initial role in treatment. Cognitive restructuring is focused on identifying automatic thoughts that have an irrational basis and confronting or challenging these ideas.

Long-term follow-up of some early CBT studies suggests that treatment gains may continue after therapy is discontinued and that these gains can be maintained for years after the intervention (White, 1998a, 1998b).

Panic disorder

Panic disorder (PD) is a chronic and frequently disabling disorder characterised by episodic panic attacks (see Table 8.1) that typically occur unexpectedly and are followed at some time during the course of the disorder by at least a month of fearful or phobic anticipation or fear of subsequent panic attacks.

Phenomenology and diagnosis

Panic attacks in panic disorder are typically discrete, intense and have an abrupt onset with symptoms (minimum of four) peaking in intensity within minutes of onset. These symptoms are frequently accompanied by feelings of terror and a fear of dying. The focus in DSM-IV on the fearful anticipation/fear of future attacks removes any previous reference to specified frequency of panic attacks, which may vary considerably between similarly impaired people. This change follows evidence that some people with panic disorder avoid all situations that are likely to precipitate a panic attack and so experience few panic attacks.

The majority of people with panic disorder will experience comorbid agoraphobia (Goodwin *et al.*, 2005), a fearful anticipation of a variety of situations from which they would find withdrawal or escape difficult. Varying degrees of avoidance may result as a consequence. There is ongoing debate on the validity of agoraphobia as an independent entity when there is no history of panic disorder. This evolution is reflected in the differences seen in the DSM-IV and the ICD-10 (Schmidt *et al.*, 2005).

The current debate is informed by equivocal data from epidemiology studies which suggest that in the general population, agoraphobia has a higher prevalence than panic disorder and that previous panic attacks may not be essential for diagnosis. Despite these findings, clinical studies suggest that agoraphobia seldom occurs without a history of panic attacks. Further, the association of agoraphobia with early onset, increased severity and chronicity of panic disorder has led some authors to speculate on the question of whether panic with agoraphobia is in fact a severe form of the core disorder which incorporates both clusters of symptoms.

The introduction of panic disorder as a separate entity in the DSM-III (1980) has lead to a number of epidemiological studies which have found lifetime prevalence of panic attacks to range from 7% to 15%, and 1.5 to 3.5% for panic disorder (Demyttenaere et al., 2004; Kessler et al., 1994; Kessler, Berglund, et al., 2005).

People with panic disorder experience high levels of functional impairment with levels approaching, and in some cases exceeding, those with chronic medical conditions (Kennedy et al., 2002; Mogotsi et al., 2000; Rodriguez et al., 2005). PD is frequently complicated by comorbidity with other psychiatric conditions, most notably other anxiety disorders, depression and alcohol abuse. High rates of comorbidity may complicate diagnosis. In differentiating panic disorder from other anxiety disorders, clinicians should focus on the fact that in PD, anxiety or anticipation is for the panic attack itself.

Panic attacks may mimic a wide range of medical conditions (see Box 8.1). Many of these conditions (cardiac, respiratory, substance/medication induced and endocrine) will have associated signs and symptoms that will alert clinicians to the underlying disease and assist in accurate differentiation of panic disorder. For the minority of patients for whom this is not true, clinicians should maintain a high index of suspicion at initial evaluation. During follow-up, patients who fail to respond as expected to treatment should also be carefully screened for underlying medical conditions.

Pathogenesis

Our current understanding of PD is based on a number of clear and plausible biological models that draw together a range of supporting neurochemical and neuroanatomical evidence.

Current neuroanatomical models of panic disorder draw on the understanding of the functional neuroanatomy of fear conditioning in animals. These models propose a central role for the amygdala in processing the emotional aspects of fear. In particular, the central nucleus of the amygdala is responsible for co-coordinating the stress response and assigning valence to particular emotional cues (internal or external). These signals interact with afferent connections from the hypothalamus relaying sensory information that mediates the fight-or-flight response. The hypothalamic lateral nucleus regulates autonomic discharge, while the paraventricular nucleus regulates adrenocorticoid release. The result is activation within brainstem regions that include the dorsal motor nucleus (heart rate), parabrachial nucleus (breathing rate), periaqueductal grey (fight-and-flight or defensive and freezing behaviours) and pontine reticular formation (startle reaction). Neuronal and neurochemical communication between these regions is largely mediated through serotonergic and noradrenergic fibres originating in the raphe nuclei and locus coeruleus, respectively (Gorman et al., 2000). These two crucial systems release CRF and growth hormone (GH), now known to be important neuroendocrine mediators of anxiety.

The importance of the amygdala to the neuroanatomical model of PD is supported by findings that lesions of the amygdala render people unable to recognise fearful faces, a crucial aspect of fear responsivity (Davis, 1986; Morris et al., 1996; Vuilleumier et al., 2004; Weiskrantz, 1956). In close anatomic proximity to the amygdala lies the hippocampus, which processes contextual and spatial aspects of fear conditioning and as such feasibly mediates avoidant behaviours in PD (Fendt et al., 2005). The hippocampus is richly connected through limbic connections with prefrontal limbic regions that are believed to mediate the "conscious" cognitive responses to fear-provoking situations.

Neurochemical studies in PD have been guided by observations that drugs affecting the noradrenergic, serotonergic and GABA systems modulate anxiety and panic frequency (Maron & Shlik, 2005; Versiani et al., 2002; Zwanzger & Rupprecht, 2005). The noradrenergic system contributes to hypothalamic-pituitary-adrenal (HPA) axis activation in PD. A blunted GH response to the α_2-agonist clonidine (Graeff et al., 2005) and high 3-methoxy-4-hydroxyphenylglycol (MHPG) volatility in PD compared with control subjects provides evidence of such noradrenergic mediation of PD.

The serotonergic system has also been implicated in PD, with some evidence of increased sensitivity to serotonin activation. Serotonin system subreceptors such as the 5-HT receptor, densely distributed in the hippocampus, mediate aspects of anxiety and potentially modulate resilience. Other possible characteristics of PD include upregulation of postsynaptic serotonin receptors, as well as receptor supersensitivity to serotonergic challenge (Deakin, 1991; Maron & Shlik, 2005).

Clinical evidence for the anxiolytic effects of the benzodiazepines through action on benzodiazepine (BZ) receptors of the GABA-A receptor complex also implicates this system in PD. BZ receptors, widely distributed in the brain, are most dense in the amygdala and hippocampus. Lower GABA concentrations (Goddard *et al.*, 2001) and BZ receptor binding in PD in these regions further underscore the involvement of the BZ system.

Prominence of autonomic symptoms in PD has led some to speculate on the role brainstem function may have in mediating PD. Observations that lactate infusion is panicogenic in PD (Otte *et al.*, 2002; Reiman *et al.*, 1989) led Klein to hypothesise that (1) higher preinfusion HPA axis activity evidenced by higher cortisol levels and (2) hyperventilation-induced respiratory alkalosis in PD are the result of an abnormally sensitive suffocation alarm. This lead to the formulation of the false suffocation alarm model for panic (Klein, 1993).

Management

Advances in treatment for PD now make remission an attainable goal (Kjernisted & Bleau, 2004). Interventions focus on reducing the frequency and intensity of panic attacks and limiting avoidant behaviours that are the consequence of fearful anticipation of future panic attacks (Lader, 2005; Roy-Byrne, Wagner, *et al.*, 2005). Cognitive distortions that invariably accompany this chronic and disabling condition may require specific attention in cognitive-behavioural interventions. The available treatment options are likely to benefit 50% to 70% of PD sufferers substantially.

As with initial management of all the anxiety disorders, psychoeducation should be provided. This is aimed at eliminating misconceptions related to

medical well-being and perceived danger of panic attacks. Information on treatment options and their efficacy is imperative if patients are to make informed treatment choices. Misconceptions may be responsible for unnecessary delays in diagnosis and treatment. The value of a strong doctor/therapist relationship in treatment adherence and outcome cannot be overstated.

Pharmacotherapy

A number of factors need to be considered when selecting treatments for PD. These include the assessment of coexisting psychiatric and medical conditions as both may significantly impact on treatment outcome. Although older TCAs are effective in PD, the SSRIs are equally effective and have superior tolerability with fewer patients discontinuing treatment due to side effects. Consequently current guidelines recommend the use of SSRIs as first-line pharmacotherapy for panic disorder. Signs of response can be expected within 4 to 6 weeks of initiating treatment. Increasingly experts recommend long-term treatment for 12 to 24 months in the majority of patients. In long-term treatment, the added difficulty of persistent side effects such weight gain, sexual dysfunction and insomnia and how they affect patients' willingness to stay on treatment long term should be addressed (Pollack *et al.*, 2003; Roy-Byrne, Wagner, *et al.*, 2005). Poor response to treatment in a sizeable proportion of patients remains a challenge to clinicians (Denys & de Geus, 2005; Rickels & Schweizer, 1998b; Roy-Byrne, Stein, *et al.*, 2005).

A number of benzodiazepines have demonstrated efficacy over placebo in PD (Kasper & Resinger, 2001b). Despite concerns with cognitive side effects and withdrawal difficulties, benzodiazepines remain accepted by many patients, due in part to their more rapid onset of action. Interestingly, patients do not appear to develop tolerance to the antipanic effects. However, there are some indications of an increased risk of emergent depression with long-term benzodiazepine use. Despite current guidelines, benzodiazepines remain widely

> **Box 8.2** Symptoms of benzodiazepine withdrawal
>
> **Psycho/Behavioural**
> - anxiety/tension
> - panic attacks
> - depression
> - irritability
> - insomnia
> - aggression
>
> **Somatic**
> - headache
> - tremor
> - confusion
> - altered level of consciousness with or without diurnal fluctuation (delirium)
> - seizures
> - arrhythmias

used. This fact means that most clinicians will be confronted with the challenge of managing discontinuation. This should be approached once a mutual understanding of the process has been attained and should be slow enough to avoid the emergence of physical withdrawal symptoms and panic attacks (Chouinard, 2004; Kasper & Resinger, 2001a; Verster & Volkerts, 2004). Box 8.2 outlines features of benzodiazepine withdrawal.

Efficacy for the monoamine oxidase inhibitors (MAOIs) has been demonstrated in PD, but more widespread use is limited by poor tolerability and the need for dietary restrictions. These limitations are of lesser concern with the newer reversible MAOI, moclobemide (Rickels & Schweizer, 1998a). The anticonvulsants (valproic acid and gabapentin) have some uncontrolled evidence suggesting they may be helpful. To date, despite widespread use in the general population as well as in people with PD, herbal treatments lack any supportive empirical evidence in PD. Clinicians should be aware that their concomitant use with conventional pharmacological treatments may be complicated. This should prompt clinicians to enquire about their use in all assessments.

Psychotherapy

A range of psychotherapeutic approaches in PD have supporting empirical evidence. Strongest evidence is for cognitive and behavioural therapies which have demonstrated greater effect sizes when compared with pharmacological treatments (Butler *et al.*, 2005). The superior benefit of the combination shown in some studies may, however, be lost over time. As such, the benefit of the combination still needs to be weighed against the cost. Taken together, it is reasonable to consider both CBT and pharmacotherapy with SSRIs as equally viable first-line treatments in PD.

The psychotherapies in PD with supportive evidence include panic control therapy, cognitive therapy alone and computer-assisted or manualised self-directed CBT. Attempts to uncover the likely "active" ingredient in CBT seem to point to the most substantial clinical benefit coming from behavioural therapy techniques such as in vivo or interoceptive exposure (Landon & Barlow, 2004; Otto & Deveney, 2005).

Exposure therapy most commonly utilises techniques of systematic desensitization, beginning by drawing up a list of feared or avoided situations in ascending order of propensity to cause fear and anxiety. With exposure to sequential situations that provoke escalating anxiety responses, the intense and automatic responses are attenuated and become tolerable with time. Previously, exposure through flooding was a treatment option, but it is used less frequently because of high rates of noncompletion and consequently poorer outcomes (Chambless, 1990; Hafner & Marks, 1976).

Relaxation therapies in the form of progressive muscle relaxation (PMR) are generally considered weak treatments in PD. More recently, applied relaxation therapy has been described. Here subjects are taught to apply PMR rapidly in the face of mounting panic. Studies suggest that this technique is as effective as cognitive therapy and imipramine for acute treatment, although to date evidence suggests the effect is not sustained in the long term (Barlow *et al.*, 1989).

Social anxiety disorder (social phobia)

Social anxiety disorder (SAD; or social phobia [SP]) is characterised by persistent fear of social interaction or performance. People fear that they will act in a way that will humiliate or embarrass them or attract undue scrutiny. SAD is second only to specific phobia as the most common anxiety disorder in population-based community studies, and prevalence ranges from 3% to 16% (Eaton *et al.*, 1994; Kessler, Berglund, *et al.*, 2005; Kessler, Demler, 2005; Lee *et al.*, 2005). The wide range is probably due to variability in diagnostic criteria employed and study methodology. Overall, gender distribution is equal. Onset is in the mid-teenage years and extends into the middle of the third decade. Onset beyond this age is relatively uncommon (Schneier *et al.*, 1992; Turk *et al.*, 1998).

As with many other anxiety disorders, SAD also has a relatively brief history in the DSM, having first been introduced in DSM-III (1980) as an independent disorder. A subsequent evolution in diagnostic criteria has seen the current DSM-IV-TR criteria allowing for differentiation of generalised (in which most performance and interpersonal social situations are feared and avoided) and non-generalised subtypes (involving one particular performance-related situation, e.g. public speaking). Since the introduction of the DSM-IV (1994), the diagnosis of SAD has also been possible in children in whom a diagnosis of avoidant and overanxious disorder was previously made.

Diagnosis

The core clinical feature of SAD is the fear of embarrassment or humiliation in social or performance situations. This fear may present with either psychic or somatic anxiety symptoms and in some cases may escalate into a full panic attack. Typical triggering situations include social interaction (e.g. talking in small groups, dating, telephoning unknown people) and performance (e.g. speaking or eating in front of others). In those who develop regular panic attacks in the course of SAD, clinical differentiation is on the basis of the primary focus of the fear. In SAD this is of the actual performance or social situation and not the panic attack itself. Other features including blushing, tremor and avoidance of eye contact are commonly seen in patients with SAD. These symptoms result in fearful anticipation of a range of social situations and consequent behavioural adjustments such as avoidance. In other patients, situations are endured with considerable distress.

Given the frequent onset of SAD in the midteens and early 20s, the impact on psychosocial development at this crucial time may be significant. As a consequence, people with SAD are more likely to remain unmarried, to drop out of school or university and to earn less than those without SAD.

As with most of the anxiety disorders, the wide range of clinical symptoms that may present as part of SAD can make diagnosis a challenge. This is not helped by the reality that many people are unaware that their symptoms constitute a treatable condition. People frequently accept symptoms as being on a continuum with an avoidant disposition believed to be enduring and not amenable to treatment. For this and other reasons, most people in whom SAD is eventually diagnosed have experienced symptoms for many years.

There is considerable clinical overlap between SAD and avoidant personality disorder (APD). Attempts to distinguish them in practice are compounded by the fact that they co-occur in between 22% and 89% of sufferers (Fahlen, 1995). These data underline the difficulty inherent in holding to the view that these are in fact distinct disorders. Some view APD as the most severe form of an SAD spectrum. The other extreme of the spectrum is represented by shyness or mild forms of behavioural inhibition (Muller *et al.*, 2005).

Comorbid anxiety and depressive disorders occur frequently in SAD and may negatively affect treatment outcomes. SAD usually predates the onset of comorbid conditions (Kessler *et al.*, 1999) and also increases the risk of subsequent depressive episodes (Stein *et al.*, 2001).

Table 8.3 Developmental models of social anxiety disorder

Cognitive model (Clark & Wells, 1995)	This model attempts to explain how phobic avoidance/anticipation is maintained. It suggests assumptions are made by an individual and that performance or social interaction will be inept in some way and will have dire consequences.
Behavioural model (Kagan *et al.*, 1988)	This model is based on the theory that behavioural inhibition is a stable temperament characteristic. The excess of similar traits in parents of behaviourally inhibited children has an impact on social behaviour of the child.
Conditioning model (Barlow, 1988)	This model suggests that behavioural consequences of aversive situations can result in phobic anticipation and avoidance behaviours following previous sensitization/exposure.
Ethological model (Mineka & Zinbarg, 2005; Ohman, 1986; Stein & Bouwer, 1997)	This model emphasises the apparent role of shyness in evolution and suggests that avoidance of gaze and behavioural inhibition may be linked. Increased arousal and fear in social situations may represent a heritable familial trait.
Personality model (Bruch & Cheek, 1995)	This model suggests that shyness is a personality trait with a heritable component that differentiates in early life into fearful and self-conscious subtypes, with the former akin to social anxiety disorder.

Pathogenesis

Modern investigative tools have advanced our understanding of the neurobiological underpinnings of SAD in recent years. Advances in many cases continue to be influenced by a range of developmental models of which a number have been proposed in SAD. These are outlined in Table 8.3.

Some of these developmental models hypothesize that heritability of behaviour related to SAD may be an important determinant risk for developing the disorder. This is supported in family studies, particularly for the generalised subtype of SAD (Fyer, 1993; Stein *et al.*, 1998). Available twin studies and genetic linkage analyses to date, however, remain inconclusive (Kendler *et al.*, 1992; Skre *et al.*, 1993).

Brain-imaging studies have suggested that SAD is mediated by anatomical regions (Allison *et al.*, 2000). Lesions of the amygdala, as in the case of Klüver-Bucy syndrome, typically lead to loss of social fear. Particular involvement of striatal neurocircuitry is suggested with preferential loss of putamen volume. Reduced choline and creatinine signal-to-noise ratios in subcortical and thalamic regions using magnetic resonance spectroscopy, as well as decreased N-acetyl-aspartate (NAA) levels and a lower ratio of NAA to other metabolites in cortical and subcortical regions implicate a complex array of brain regions. Disorder-relevant cues may provoke frontal and dorsolateral prefrontal regional activation implicating prefrontal aspects of the limbic cortex (Adolphs *et al.*, 2001; Davidson, Krishnan, *et al.*, 1993; Nutt *et al.*, 1998; Potts *et al.*, 1994; Tupler *et al.*, 1997).

Chemical activation studies using pentagastrin, a cholecystokinin agonist (van Vliet *et al.*, 1997), and CO_2 inhalation (Holt & Andrews, 1998) have been able to distinguish patients with SAD from those with other anxiety disorders and from control subjects. The anxiety these agents induce is qualitatively different from that experienced in the course of SAD.

To date, studies of potential peripheral markers for SAD have been preliminary. Beta-receptor density on lymphocytes (Stein *et al.*, 1993), platelet serotonin transporters (Stein *et al.*, 1995), G-protein subunit density on platelets and leucocytes (Stein *et al.*,

1996) and BZ receptor density on platelets in SAD (Johnson *et al.*, 1998) have all been shown to be lower in people with SAD compared with healthy control subjects.

Similar to the other major anxiety disorders, the first-choice use of SSRIs in the treatment of SAD indirectly supports serotonergic involvement in its pathogenesis. Some evidence suggests that functional changes in SAD are possibly restored to something approaching that of asymptomatic control subjects following treatment. Regions most affected during treatment include the amygdala, hippocampus and areas of the prefrontal cortex (Furmark *et al.*, 2002; van der Linden *et al.*, 2000).

Evidence for the involvement of subcortical structures in SAD also suggests that the dopaminergic system may be involved. Lower dopamine levels correlate with greater timidity, whereas reduced striatal D_2 receptor binding is associated with lower status in nonhuman primates. Similarly, in humans, lower striatal D_2 receptor density and lower dopamine transporter density at the presynaptic reuptake site has been shown in SAD (Tiihonen, Kuikka, Bergstrom, *et al.*, 1997).

Significant strides have been made in our understanding of SAD in recent years. Despite advances in our understanding of SAD in recent years, the reliability with which investigations are able to distinguish biochemical and brain functional patterns from other anxiety disorders remains a challenge. Further advances may depend on broadening our conceptualization and understanding of potentially related social behaviours such as socially submissive and appeasing behaviours of avoidance (including gaze avoidance) and blushing. These behaviours are a feature of normal development and in many people may be appeasing and function to maintain control of overly sensitive fear-mediated alarm systems that are variably responsive to environmental social cues.

Management

Possibly the greatest challenge to the management of SAD remains its effective identification and diagnosis in primary care settings. To this end, increasing community and healthcare-centre efforts to raise awareness of available treatment options should be promoted. After a definitive diagnosis is made, treatment should begin with psychoeducation addressing the understanding of the disorder, its amenability to treatment, patient treatment expectations, and available options.

Pharmacotherapy

Evidence to support of the use of SSRIs as first-line treatments in SAD (limited and generalised types) is now widely accepted (Blanco *et al.*, 2003; Stein *et al.*, 2001; Van Ameringen *et al.*, 2003). Although the efficacy in SAD of the MAOIs, and more recently the reversible inhibitors of monamine oxidase (of RIMAs), has been known for some time, they have been surpassed as the agents of choice by the SSRIs. An adequate trial of treatment should probably extend to 12 weeks, with most experts agreeing that a minimum of 6 to 8 weeks at highest tolerated doses should be administered before considering a switch to an alternative.

The use of benzodiazepines in SAD is supported by a number of open-label studies. Results from double-blind placebo-controlled studies have been positive (Davidson, Potts, *et al.*, 1993; Gelernter *et al.*, 1991). In general, relapse rates appear to be high, in part related to possible withdrawal effects. Nevertheless, add-on, short-term use of benzodiazepines has proved helpful in severely anxious subjects during the early phases of treatment. A role for benzodiazepines in isolated performance anxiety is partially supported but in turn limited by the potential for sedation and consequent impairment of performance.

The use of beta-adrenergic antagonists in generalised SAD has not been established. However, there is an abundance of anecdotal evidence for their successful use in circumscribed performance related anxiety. The greatest benefit accrues to those with high levels of autonomic arousal and symptoms such a tremor, palpitations and sweating.

There is presently only limited controlled data for treatments of SAD in children. Venlafaxine recently demonstrated efficacy (March, Entusah *et al.*, 2007). The benzodiazepine alprazolam was ineffective in a sample of children with overanxious disorder (Simeon & Ferguson, 1987). There is growing evidence that SSRIs may be effective in some children. Some suggest that considerable overlap exists between SAD and selective mutism in children and a small controlled study of fluoxetine in selective mutism has demonstrated efficacy (Black & Uhde, 1994).

Psychotherapy

Evidence for the effectiveness of psychotherapy interventions in SAD has accumulated in recent years. Evidence of variable strength supports conventional cognitive therapies, cognitive restructuring, cognitive group therapies, behavioural therapies such as exposure, social skills training and relaxation training.

Meta-analyses consistently show lasting benefits for CBT in SAD (Butler *et al.*, 2005; Feske & Chambless, 1995). However, efforts to distinguish the relative efficacy of different techniques within CBT have been inconclusive. It seems likely that the distinction of behavioural and cognitive interventions may be somewhat artificial because of significant overlap. Exposure and cognitive restructuring appear to be particularly important features in addressing social fears and performance related anxiety. Patients who show improvement with CBT appear to maintain the clinical response.

Exposure seeks to habituate automatic anxious responses to the feared stimuli while minimizing the reinforcing effects of non-fear-based behaviours. Cognitive therapies focus on the potential to learn new and corrective/rational thoughts in feared situations, with consequent changes to irrational behaviours (Ellis, 1962) or the negative and selective bias in information processing typical of SAD (Beck, 1976; DiGiuseppe *et al.*, 1990). Efficacy has also been shown for a combination therapy devised by Kendall *et al.* (1997) that incorporates cognitive,

exposure and educational aspects into treatment of children and adolescents with SAD, formally termed avoidant disorders. Evidence also exists for interventions that incorporate a family anxiety management component (Barrett *et al.*, 1996).

The comparative efficacy of psychotherapies and psychopharmacological treatments in meta-analyses have been mixed. In arguably the most helpful study on the relative efficacy of treatments to date, the MAOI phenelzine was compared with cognitive-behavioural group therapy (CBGT) against pill placebo and educational-supportive group therapy. Results suggested more rapid and robust responses for phenelzine with no differences on completion of the 12-week treatment phase (Gelernter *et al.*, 1991). At follow-up, those who received CBGT were significantly less likely than those treated with phenelzine to have relapsed.

Recent findings from a functional imaging study suggest that changes in brain function that accompany clinical improvement from either pharmacotherapy or psychotherapy overlap considerably (Furmark *et al.*, 2002). Because very little empirical data exist to support the appealing combination of pharmacotherapy and CBT, it seems reasonable to consider pharmacotherapy as first-line treatment in patients who are unable to tolerate the anxiety caused by exposure therapy, and equally reasonable to recommend CBT to those who are either averse to taking medication or are intolerant of it.

Finally, the question of treatment of SAD that is refractory to conventional approaches has received only limited attention in the literature to date. Standard principles of evaluating failure to respond to treatment (compliance, medical and substance use disorders) should always be followed. Given the strength of evidence for the MAOIs, it seems reasonable to consider this group of agents after failure of trials with SSRIs (Ipser, Carey *et al.*, 2006).

Posttraumatic stress disorder

Posttraumatic stress disorder (PTSD) is unique among the anxiety disorders in that it is the only disorder that requires a specific triggering event before the onset of symptoms. The emotional and behavioural effects of severe trauma have been well described since the start of the twentieth century. However, it was not until the burden of symptoms on returning US servicemen from Vietnam in the 1970s that formulation of clinical criteria for PTSD occurred, and this culminated in its inclusion in the DSM-III (1980).

Epidemiology

Of the substantial proportion of the general population who experience trauma in their lifetime, only a minority of 1% to 12% will actually develop PTSD (Davidson *et al.*, 1991; Helzer *et al.*, 1987; Kessler *et al.*, 1995). Women, who experience higher rates of sexual and intimate partner trauma, are more likely than men, who have higher rates of combat-related and interpersonal violence, to develop PTSD (Nemeroff *et al.*, 2005). Although trauma type and severity determine some of the risk for developing PTSD, additional gender-specific factors are also likely to play a role in mediating greater vulnerability to developing PTSD in women (Breslau *et al.*, 1998; Seedat, Stein, *et al.*, 2005).

Diagnosis and phenomenology

Traumatic events able to cause PTSD vary considerably, but the core symptom domains remain remarkably consistent across populations. Changes to the clinical criteria, and in particular the trauma criterion, for PTSD have run parallel with advances in our understanding of this disorder. In DSM-III, only traumas that were severe enough to be regarded as outside the range of normal human experience met this criterion. We now know that trauma severe enough to cause PTSD occurs during the lifetime of up to 50% of people in the general population with only a small minority going on to develop PTSD. As a consequence, the trauma criterion was revised in DSM-IV. So in addition to (1) experiencing, witnessing or being confronted with a trauma that involves actual or threatened death/serious injury/threat to integrity of self or others, the individual should (2) experience emotions of intense fear, helplessness or horror in direct response to the trauma for the incident to qualify as a triggering event.

To make a DSM-IV-TR diagnosis of PTSD, a prescribed number of symptoms are required from each of the three key symptom domains, and these have to have been present for a minimum of 1 month. The minimum number of symptoms from each domain includes one or more reexperiencing symptoms (Criterion B, 1–5), three or more symptoms of avoidance of trauma-related stimuli and numbing of emotional responsiveness (Criterion C, 1–7) and two or more symptoms indicating a state of persistently increased arousal (Criterion D, 1–5). Box 8.3 summarises the symptom clusters for PTSD.

When symptoms suggestive of PTSD present in the acute aftermath of the traumatic event, DSM-IV-TR permits a separate diagnosis of acute stress disorder (ASD). In this instance, the clinical picture may be dominated by dissociative symptoms. This difference from otherwise standard PTSD criteria is reflected in the requirement of three or more symptoms from a dissociative cluster including numbing or detachment in emotional responsivity, reduced awareness of surroundings, derealization, depersonalisation and dissociative amnesia.

Course

The majority of trauma survivors who are likely to develop PTSD will do so within the first 3 months of the trauma. For those who develop ASD, some 20% to 40% of cases are likely to persist beyond 1 month (Shalev *et al.*, 1997). Established PTSD will persist beyond 2 years in around 50% of patients (Perkonigg *et al.*, 2005). Course specifiers in DSM-IV-TR designate either acute (lasting up to 3 months) or chronic (4 months or longer) PTSD. After chronic symptoms are established, spontaneous recovery becomes unlikely. In a minority of cases, PTSD may also have a delayed onset (longer than 6 months after the traumatic event).

Box 8.3 Symptom clusters in posttraumatic stress disorder (based on *Diagnostic and Statistical Manual of Mental Disorders,* 4th edn., text revision [DSM-IV-TR] criteria)

Re-experiencing (DSM-IV-TR Criterion Set B)

(1) recurrent and intrusive distressing recollections of the event, including images, thoughts or perceptions

(2) recurrent distressing dreams of the event

(3) acting or feeling as if the traumatic event were recurring (includes a sense of reliving the experience, illusions, hallucinations and flashbacks)

(4) intense psychological distress at exposure to internal or external cues that symbolize or resemble an aspect of the traumatic event

(5) physiological reactivity on exposure to internal or external cues that symbolize or resemble an aspect of the traumatic event

Avoidance/numbing (DSM-IV-TR Criterion Set C)

(1) efforts to avoid thoughts, feelings or conversations associated with the trauma

(2) efforts to avoid activities, places or people that arouse recollections of the trauma

(3) inability to recall an important aspect of the trauma

(4) markedly diminished interest or participation in significant activities

(5) feeling of detachment or estrangement from others

(6) restricted range of affect (e.g. unable to have loving feelings)

(7) sense of a foreshortened future (e.g. does not expect to have a career, marriage, children or a normal lifespan)

Increased arousal (DSM-IV-TR Criterion Set D)

(1) difficulty falling or staying asleep

(2) irritability or outbursts of anger

(3) difficulty concentrating

(4) hypervigilance

(5) exaggerated startle response

Psychiatric comorbidity in PTSD is the rule. Depression, substance abuse and other anxiety disorders (most notably panic disorder in women) are the most prevalent (Perkonigg *et al.*, 2000). Disorders that coexist with PTSD have the effect of prolonging the course of symptoms and may impact treatment responsivity. The effect of personality factors on vulnerability to develop PTSD following trauma on the one hand and the effect of trauma in causing enduring personality changes on the other remains a topic of debate. Central to this debate is the role of trauma in precipitating and perpetuating complex disorders of dissociation and constructs such as borderline personality disorder (see Chapter 7), which some authors suggest represent an enduring and maladaptive response to severe and repetitive trauma (Goodwin, 2005).

Pathogenesis

A large literature now supports the conceptualisation of PTSD as a psychobiological disorder. Considerable advances in our understanding of the psychobehavioural changes in PTSD have been made in recent years. However, despite the amenability of neuroendocrine, neurocognitive and structural/functional brain systems to investigation, specific pathogenic mechanisms of PTSD remain to be uncovered.

An understanding of risk for PTSD after trauma is crucial given the apparent window of opportunity for secondary preventative interventions before the onset of PTSD symptoms. Considerable work on this has shown repeatedly that female gender, trauma severity, previous history of trauma, previous psychiatric history and poor peri-traumatic psychosocial support are among the most robust indicators of higher risk for developing PTSD following trauma (Brewin *et al.*, 2000).

In established PTSD, studies investigating HPA axis function have demonstrated a number of replicable findings. For example, decreased cortisol release, as well as increased sensitivity of the hypothalamus to negative feedback and hypersecretion of CRF, are relatively consistent findings (Bremner *et al.*, 1993; Yehuda, 1998; Yehuda *et al.*, 1998). Hypersensitivity of CRF receptors in receptor-rich regions of the amygdalo-hippocampal complex has led to speculation about how CRF receptors function to mediate vulnerability to developing and perpetuating symptoms of PTSD.

Structural brain imaging studies in PTSD support the involvement of the medial temporal regions through near consistent demonstration of reduced hippocampal volumes (Smith, 2005). Functional imaging of limbic and paralimbic regions as well as the visual cortex (visual re-experiencing) and speech areas (processing verbally traumatic memories) are implicated in studies of PTSD patients in whom symptoms are provoked with a variety of emotional cues (Nutt & Malizia, 2004). Hypothesised dysfunction within medial prefrontal cortex (MPFC) and hippocampus is also supported by preliminary evidence of abnormal neuronal integrity and glial proliferation measured with magnetic resonance spectroscopy (Mahmutyazicioglu *et al.*, 2005; Seedat, Videen, *et al.*, 2005).

A number of neurotransmitter systems have been studied in PTSD. Receptor imaging of the benzodiazepine system has demonstrated lower receptor density in PTSD, but the specificity of these findings is unclear given similar findings in other anxiety disorders (Bremner, Innis, *et al.*, 2000; Fujita *et al.*, 2004). The noradrenergic system is implicated through findings of lower levels of circulating catecholamines and changes in alpha-adrenergic receptor density.

Neuroanatomical models of PTSD overlap to some extent with those of basic fear-mediating circuitry. The amygdalo-hippocampal complex in the medial temporal brain regions are responsible for attributing emotional valence and contextual memory to traumatic/fear inducing experiences in animals. Neurochemical and neurocognitive responses to acute stressors appear to interact with medial prefrontal brain regions in a way that impairs normal attenuation of the initial fear response. A failure of normal "top-down" regulation of the fear response within MPFC is hypothesised. This is supported by findings of abnormally activated fear circuitry through activation of amygdala in subjects with PTSD relative to controls (Nutt & Malizia, 2004). The abnormal response to or recovery from stress is likely to have an impact on cognitive responses to trauma and trauma cues. This response in turn may suggest the value of therapeutic interventions that eventually restore "top-down control" of the abnormally activated fear response.

Management

A common goal of all treatments for PTSD should be to (1) reduce the frequency and intensity of intrusive trauma memories, (2) restore social and occupational functioning and (3) enhance resilience against future traumatic life events. Although a number of treatments for PTSD have been available for some time, in recent years a focus on pharmacotherapy and cognitive-behavioural techniques aimed at secondary (after the trauma) prevention of PTSD has emerged.

Prevention

The emergence of ASD as a strong predictor of progression to PTSD has attracted attention to this as an opportunity for secondary prevention. Predominantly open-label treatments of ASD suggest a range of interventions may be effective. Initial reports suggested benefit in using beta-blockers, but in a controlled study, improvements in autonomic reactivity did not translate to additional benefits for reducing the likelihood of developing PTSD (Pitman *et al.*, 2002). Preliminary data from studies in children with severe burns and adults with septic shock suggest some benefit for imipramine and high-dose hydrocortisone respectively (Schelling *et al.*, 2001, 2004). Studies using benzodiazepines are noteworthy in that they suggest that their use may in fact increase the risk of PTSD (Gelpin *et al.*, 1996; Mellman *et al.*, 2002; Shalev *et al.*, 1998) The results of ongoing investigations using the second generation (atypical) antipsychotics and anticonvulsants are awaited.

Accumulating evidence now supports the use of a range of psychotherapies in secondary prevention of PTSD. Short-course CBT is one such example. This stands in contrast to negative results from meta-analyses of single-session debriefing techniques (van Emmerik *et al.*, 2002). Despite widespread use of these techniques, at best they appear to confer a neutral effect on PTSD outcome and in some instances may even be negative. It remains a challenge as to how to disentangle the effects of good psychosocial support and the specific effects of brief CBT interventions in the aftermath of trauma.

Pharmacotherapy

From the available trial data, it seems safe to conclude that SSRIs, TCAs and MAOIs are effective for treating PTSD. When considering safety, tolerability and convenience of use, SSRIs should probably be considered first choice for both acute and chronic treatment of PTSD (Stein *et al.*, 2000; Tucker *et al.*, 2001).

A number of open-label and controlled studies using mood stabilisers (lithium, carbamazepine, valproate and lamotrigine) in PTSD have been conducted with positive results. The use of the second-generation antipsychotics has also received attention on the basis of their action on serotonin 2a receptors, which have been linked to trauma-induced changes in medial temporal brain regions. Preliminary open-label data suggest that quetiapine, risperidone and olanzapine may be beneficial in PTSD (Butterfield *et al.*, 2001; David *et al.*, 2004; Hamner *et al.*, 2003).

After symptoms have responded to initial treatment, the question of how long to continue treatment is not clear. There are emerging data from clinical, cognitive and brain volumetric studies suggesting that improvements in all of these measures may continue with longer term treatment. Future studies should attempt to redress gender imbalances that have characterised studies to date (Seedat, Stein, *et al.*, 2005). Nevertheless, there are relatively few long-term pharmacotherapy studies.

Psychotherapy

Evidence now attests to the value of cognitive-behavioural psychotherapy in the acute management of PTSD. In general, there is considerable overlap between the principles of CBT as applied to PTSD and certain psychodynamic psychotherapies. The complexity of symptoms and the degree to which they affect patients' ability to engage in

---

> **Box 8.4** A phased approach to treating PTSD
>
> 1. Facilitate the patient's taking control over the dominance of intrusive and disruptive memories of the trauma
> 2. Provide psychoeducation with which acceptance of the impact of the trauma goes hand in hand
> 3. Assist patient in establishing mastery over feelings including fear of symptoms and somatic responses to them
> 4. Assist patient to be specifically mobilised to use available social supports to facilitate stabilization

---

therapy means that a phased approach may be necessary; an outline is shown in Box 8.4.

In addition, being able to tell "the story" in a safe, controlled environment may facilitate the integration of implicit somatic and explicit verbal memories into new or re-established cognitive constructs of the traumatic event.

A number of techniques that fall within the general ambit of CBT have also been tested in PTSD. Some evidence supports a role for stress inoculation therapy, as well as prolonged exposure therapy.

Obsessive-compulsive disorder

OCD is characterised by obsessions and compulsions. Obsessions are repetitive, intrusive thoughts, impulses or mental images that are frequently distressing, anxiety provoking and difficult to control. Compulsions, by contrast, are repetitive physical or mental acts performed as a response to an obsession and aimed at avoiding the supposed outcome or reducing the distress it causes.

Epidemiology

OCD was the 4th most prevalent psychiatric disorder in the Epidemiological Catchment Area Survey (ECA; Robins *et al.*, 1984) and the 10th most disabling of all medical disorders in an early burden of disease study (Murray & Lopez, 1996; World Health

> **Box 8.5** Obsessive-compulsive disorder: common subtypes
>
> 1. Contamination/washing – with or without fears of harm
> 2. Harm avoidance/checking and ordering
> 3. Pure obsessions (without overt compulsive behaviours)
> 4. Hoarding

Organization, 2001). An estimated lifetime prevalence of OCD of approximately 1% to 4% has been reported relatively consistently across epidemiological studies in the United States and elsewhere. However, the precise diagnostic criteria applied can have a marked impact on prevalence rates, and more restrictive DSM-IV criteria result in a rate of around 0.7% (Crino *et al.*, 2005). The average age of onset is somewhat later in females (22 years vs. 19 years in males), but the overall sex distribution is equal.

Phenomenology and diagnosis

The content of obsessions and the nature of the related compulsions is remarkably consistent across time and nationalities. The most prevalent obsessions involve contamination, pathological doubt or uncertainty, somatic obsessions and a need for symmetry in descending order of prevalence (Eisen & Rasmussen, 2002). Checking followed in turn by washing, counting and needing to confess are the most prevalent compulsions. A number of studies have now converged in delineating a set of specific symptom dimensions in OCD (see Box 8.5). Within individuals, symptoms may vary in nature and fluctuate in intensity over time.

In refining the diagnosis of OCD, DSM now permits subtyping OCD in terms of whether or not there is poor insight. This follows the description of a sizeable proportion of patients with OCD who are at best unsure about whether resisting compulsions would bring them harm (Eisen & Rasmussen, 1993). In DSM-IV field trials, approximately 29% of subjects were either sure or mostly sure that their obsessions were reasonable (Foa *et al.*, 1995).

Symptom severity is an important determinant of treatment outcome. In this regard, standardised ratings of symptom severity using scales such as the Yale Brown Obsessive-Compulsive Symptom checklist (Goodman *et al.*, 1989) facilitate more objective monitoring of treatment progress.

The obsessive compulsive spectrum

The notion that a number of disorders that share features of obsessions and compulsions or repetitive behaviours ("habits") can be grouped together has gained some currency, and the case for an obsessive-compulsive spectrum (OCS) of disorders has been articulated (see Figure 8.1). Membership of the spectrum is usefully grouped into three "clusters". Lending some support to the construct of OCS is the fact that a number of members of the putative spectrum share a response to the same treatments (notably serotonergic antidepressants), some (but by no means all) aggregate in families and some have similarities in domains such as age at onset and longitudinal course. However, membership of the spectrum cannot at this stage be well supported for a number of disorders currently subsumed within it, and the proof of the validity and utility of this approach requires considerable further work (see Castle & Phillips, 2006).

Course and comorbidity

The majority of people with OCD report depressive symptoms at some point in the course of their disorder. In the majority of cases, depressive features manifest after the onset of OCD and are conceptualised as being secondary to the OCD (Eisen & Rasmussen, 2002). In the clinic, the distinction of primary and secondary depression may be challenging. Indeed it seems reasonable that depression-like reactions are probable in those with chronic and frequently unremitting symptoms. Other anxiety disorders also co-occur with OCD, but substantially less frequently than depression.

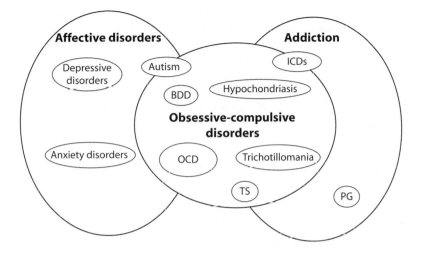

Figure 8.1 Summary view of the obsessive-compulsive spectrum.

Much has been written on the comorbidity of OCD with tics and Tourette's disorder. People with a lifetime history of tics tend to have an earlier onset of illness and are more likely to have a family history of OCD. Some 30% to 40% of adults with OCD report tic symptoms through the course of their illness (Leckman *et al.*, 1993). The high rates of coexistence of tics and OCD have advanced speculation on the possibility of a shared aetiology and genetic diathesis. In particular, dopaminergic involvement in OCD with tics may be crucial. This hypothesis emerged with the knowledge of the relatively selective nature of the response of tic-related disorders to dopamine receptor antagonists (Leckman *et al.*, 2003).

A number of studies have investigated the intriguing and as yet unresolved association of OCD and schizophrenia (see Pokos & Castle, 2006). The prevalence of OCD amongst people diagnosed with schizophrenia ranges from 0% to 40%. Psychotic symptoms in people with OCD are heterogeneous and include a spectrum of diagnoses from coexisting schizophrenia to delusional disorder unrelated to OCD and finally OCD with poor insight mentioned above (Rasmussen & Eisen, 1992). Only limited evidence that argues for an increased

or even shared risk for developing OCD and schizophrenia.

Comorbidity of DSM-IV Cluster C personality disorders such as obsessive-compulsive personality disorder (OCPD) is frequently assumed to be high. In recent years, this association has become more tenuous, with some studies suggesting low levels of comorbidity. It may be that OCPD represents a response to obsessions and compulsions in OCD. Comorbidity with a range of personality disorders including borderline, schizotypal and paranoid personality types do occur with OCD, and their presence appears to affect treatment outcome adversely.

A sizeable minority of patients with OCD will have a chronic course suffering significant fluctuations in symptom severity over time (Rasmussen & Eisen, 1994; Thomsen, 1995).

Pathogenesis

There is now widespread support for a biological basis for OCD. A network of functionally integrated brain regions quite distinct from other anxiety disorders appears to interact with neurochemical and genetic factors to mediate OCD. Although the specific pathogenic mechanisms of OCD have yet to be uncovered, animal and clinical research has advanced our understanding considerably in recent years. Increasingly OCD is conceptualised on a spectrum with a range of potentially related conditions, and this may in time help uncover the distinct underlying neural mechanisms.

Genetics

Family and twin studies provided initial indications of a genetic contribution to the vulnerability to develop OCD with concordance rates as high as 80%. Heritability, however, does not appear to be consistent in all people with OCD. For instance, OCD and tic-related disorders with early onset appear to be associated with a stronger heritable component in first-degree relatives (Hemmings *et al.*, 2004; Nestadt *et al.*, 2000; Pauls *et al.*, 1995). Conversely, OCD with later onset may be a less heritable form. Another less heritable group develops OCD as a consequence of infective, metabolic, autoimmune and traumatic insults to the brain. Evidence of heritability has focussed efforts to uncover genetic associations and candidate genes for OCD. A number of promising lines of evidence for genes encoding for functional aspects of the serotonergic and dopaminergic systems have emerged. In the main, however, these have failed the test of replication, and many of those candidate genes have been uncovered.

Neurocircuitry

Some of the earliest indications of the biological basis for OCD come from evidence that people with encephalitis lethargica and parkinsonian features had higher rates of obsessive-compulsive symptoms and tics. These appear to have been associated with focal disruption involving basal ganglia regions (Cheyette & Cummings, 1995). Similarly, recognition of the presence of OC symptoms and tics in some children with post–streptococcal infection autoimmunity, the so-called paediatric autoimmune neuropsychiatric disorders associated with

Streptococcus (PANDAS; Swedo *et al.*, 1998) also implicated striatal brain regions. Soft neurological signs with subtle changes in motor function, coordination and planning in OCD also point to the involvement of corticostriatal regions. A range of other central nervous system insults have resulted in OC symptoms (e.g. head injuries, manganese poisoning).

Brian imaging data provide perhaps the most compelling evidence to support a functional neuroanatomical model of OCD. Structural imaging studies point primarily to the involvement of cortico-striatal structures in OCD. Often there has been evidence of striatal shrinking although in PANDAs there may be volume increase. This suggests that apparently different mechanisms may operate to precipitate the same disorder. Functional imaging studies at baseline in OCD demonstrate hyperactivity in the orbitofrontal cortex, anterior cingulate and caudate nucleus that is increased following symptom provocation and approaches the activity levels of normal controls following treatment response (Baxter, 1992).

Neurochemistry

Current neurochemical hypotheses to some extent complement the functional anatomic models in OCD in that serotonergic and dopaminergic systems are primarily responsible for communication between the regions implicated in this model. The selective response of OCD to serotonergic agents and more recent indications that dopaminergic agents may hold some advantages for treatment of more refractory cases lends indirect support to a role for these systems in OCD.

Animal studies of the 5-HT1B terminal autoreceptor suggest desensitization follows SSRI administration. This has the effect of increasing serotonergic tone and may take up to 8 weeks to occur. This runs parallel with the generally longer time to clinical response to SSRIs in OCD, as well as the need for longer treatment trials and higher doses. Despite SSRIs being the treatment of choice in OCD, the fact that not all patients respond predictably to serotonergic challenges and SSRI treatment raises the possibility that abnormalities in this system may be relatively minor and that modulating treatments may simply effect changes to downstream dysfunction in a range of systems with which the richly interconnected serotonin system communicates.

Striatal brain regions are richly innervated by the dopamine system. Dopamine agonists increase levels of stereotypic behaviour in animals and obsessive-compulsive symptoms and tics in humans (Goodman *et al.*, 1990). Dopamine antagonists, on the other hand, ameliorate tics and probably OC symptoms in humans who have failed to respond to SSRIs (Denys *et al.*, 2004; McDougle *et al.*, 1994).

A neuroevolutionary approach to understanding OCD posits that brain regions fail to inhibit or regulate a range of procedural strategies from intruding into consciousness. Recent factor analytical approaches seem to support a relatively limited range of symptom domains (pathological doubt, contamination, somatic and symmetry), and there are some indications of their evolutionary importance from activation of phylogenetically older regions of the brain during implicit cognitive processing (Rauch *et al.*, 1997). In examining procedural response strategies possibly relevant to OCD such as contamination and grooming in animals, responses to pharmacotherapy akin to humans with OCD suggest some evolutionary link with the prominence of these behaviours (Rapaport *et al.*, 1992; Stein & Young, 1992).

The refinement of OCD models has raised questions as to whether it should continue to be classified as an anxiety disorder. As we have seen, OCD-mediated distress through cortico-striatal-thalamo-cortical (CSTC) circuitry differs fundamentally from other anxiety disorders in which fear is a central emotion and mediated by temporal brain structures (hippocampus and amygdala). The notion that the primary emotion of disgust mediated by the CSTC circuit is conceivably involved in somatic, contamination, grooming and doubting domains of OCD seems to lend support both to the evolutionary perspectives on OCD and to its distinction from other anxiety disorders.

Management

Psychoeducation following diagnosis may facilitate patients' understanding of their symptoms. It may also correct broad misconceptions relating to prevalence and the impact of OCD on function. Treatment alternatives and the anticipated course and outcome are other important areas on which to focus.

Pharmacotherapy

Pharmacotherapy should be considered an important constituent in the treatment of OCD. In view of the superior tolerability of the SSRIs, these agents should probably be considered as a first option. The serotonergic TCA clomipramine should probably be reserved for second-line use in more refractory subjects. Patients should be informed of the anticipated time to onset of action, which is typically longer for OCD than for depression. Clinicians should be aware that generally higher doses than are used for depression may be required. The duration of an adequate trial of acute treatment for OCD should not be shorter than 12 weeks at a maximum tolerated dose of a particular agent (Greist *et al.*, 2003; Kaplan & Hollander, 2003). Treatment of OCD in adolescents with pharmacotherapy is also supported (Thomsen, 2001).

Evidence for the value of long-term treatment of OCD is not yet comprehensive. Relapse rates following abrupt discontinuation of treatment are high. Some studies indicate that following a treatment response, the clinical efficacy can be maintained at lower doses, but not all data are consistent.

One of the biggest challenges in the pharmacotherapy of OCD is the high rate of inadequate treatment response to SSRIs alone (approximately 40% to 60% of patients respond). In general, the adequacy of the dose of the first-line agent needs to be maximised. Although combination strategies may be helpful, there is only limited controlled evidence to support such approaches. Interventions have included tryptophan, fenfluramine, lithium, buspirone, clonazepam, trazodone, pindolol, another SSRI and behavioural therapy. Increasingly, evidence supports the use of conventional or second-generation antipsychotic agents for augmenting SSRIs in refractory OCD (Keuneman *et al.*, 2005). Initial findings of a preferential benefit for those with comorbid tics have not been consistently replicated. Finally, in the most refractory and impaired group of patients, some evidence supports the use of stereotactic surgery (cingulotomy, capsulotomy, limbic leucotomy) after all other alternatives have been exhausted (Hollander *et al.*, 2002). Deep brain stimulation techniques are being explored as an alternative to psychosurgery in severe OCD.

Psychotherapy

First-line psychotherapy of OCD is behavioural therapy involving exposure and response prevention (EXRP). A number of studies have now confirmed the efficacy of exposure (in vivo greater than imaginal exposure, and the combination of the two is more effective than in vivo alone) for obsessions and response (ritual) prevention for compulsions (de Araujo *et al.*, 1995; Foa *et al.*, 2005; Franklin *et al.*, 2000; Ito *et al.*, 1995). Symptom reduction is robust with in excess of 90% of subjects experiencing at least a 30% reduction in symptoms in a large effectiveness study (Foa *et al.*, 1985). Treatment effect is also sustained in the medium term (Foa & Kozak, 1996). There are some indications that treatment effects for behavioural therapy may be larger than for trials with SSRIs (van Balkom *et al.*, 1994, 1998). Some authors promote the addition of a cognitive component to EXRP in treating OCD, but the additional benefit of the cognitive element has not been shown, probably reflecting the fact that most patients do recognise their obsessional concerns to be excessive. Having said that, some patients seem particularly amenable to challenging irrational cognitive processes, and it can be

useful in such individuals. Controlled evidence also supports a role for CBT in children with OCD (Wever & Rey, 1997). Few controlled studies have examined the relative efficacy of EXRP and pharmacological treatments, but a number of open-label and a few controlled studies support the use of a combination of CBT and SSRI therapy.

EXRP in OCD requires the therapist to facilitate a process through which a patient comes to an understanding of the triggers for obsessions and compulsions. Education helps the therapist and patient develop realistic and shared goals for therapy with a plan for the number and length of sessions. Exposure varies in duration and progressively moves subjects through a hierarchy of increasing intensity of distress and anxiety. Careful attention needs to be paid to containing anxiety in situations where ritual comforting is now also prevented. As therapy progresses, patients grow in confidence as they achieve success. The possibility that symptoms may change in nature and severity over time should be anticipated and contingency plans be put in place so that the patient does not view these as failure.

Many experts agree that both pharmacotherapy and psychotherapy have a role in the treatment of OCD. For reasons of severity, poor insight and secondary depression, engagement in behavioural therapy may be impossible. Some patients may, however, prefer psychotherapy over medication for reasons of stigma related to taking of psychotropic medication. Alternatively, previous intolerance of pharmacotherapy may be an important determinant of patient preference.

Conclusion

The relatively recent history of OCD has moved it from being conceptualised as a rare and obscure disorder to a not uncommon malady with a clear anatomical and chemical basis. This has contributed to the development and establishment of a range of effective treatments with sustained efficacy. Despite this, many clinicians fail to acknowledge symptoms and diagnose patients in a timely fashion. The result is that many patients lose the opportunity to try effective treatments for this often chronic and debilitating disorder.

Specific phobia

Specific phobia (SP) is a common anxiety disorder characterised by marked persistent, excessive and unreasonable fear cued by anticipation or exposure to a feared object or situation. Phobic objects or situations are either avoided or endured with distress, resulting in impairment in functioning. Particular types of SP that occur more frequently include animal phobias (notably spiders and snakes); phobias related to the environment (height, weather, etc.); injection, blood and injury–type phobias; and situational phobias (airplane, lifts, enclosed spaces).

Onset is typically in the teenage years, with considerable variability between types of SP. Women are twice as likely as men to have SP and also to have multiple phobias. Clinical differentiation from other anxiety disorders, with which there are high levels of comorbidity, is on the basis of the focus of the anxiety/fearful anticipation and reasons for avoidance.

Developmental models include behavioural (associative) conditioning in response to previous exposure and nonassociative behavioural (innate, without previous exposure) theories in SP. Cognitive theories on the maintenance of phobias have also emerged. Early indications of a biological basis for SP are found in family studies with higher rates in offspring of sufferers, particularly for blood and injury phobia (Fyer *et al.*, 1990).

Few people spontaneously seek treatment for SP. For those in treatment, systematic desensitisation and in vivo exposure is generally effective. There is some evidence from a small crossover trial that SSRIs are effective in SP.

Mixed anxiety and depressive disorder

Coexisting depressive and anxiety symptoms that do not meet criteria for individual disorders are frequently seen in primary care. This clinical reality is reflected in the ICD-10 with this condition enjoying status as an independent subsyndromal disorder. ICD-10 requires the presence of distinct mood and anxiety symptoms that are not of sufficient intensity to warrant the diagnosis of separate disorders. The DSM-IV-TR criteria continue to subsume mixed anxiety-depressive disorder in the category of anxiety disorders not otherwise specified. DSM-IV-TR criteria require dysphoric mood and a combination of cognitive/psychic and autonomic symptoms of anxiety for this diagnosis.

A number of lines of evidence in mood and anxiety disorders, including neuroendocrine findings in cortisol and growth hormone responses to alpha-2-agonists, frequently converge. For instance, neuroendocrine findings in cortisol and growth hormone responses to alpha-2 agonists are often similar. Family studies suggest some overlap in the heritability of mood and anxiety disorders, and first-line treatment for most of the disorders in these categories are the SSRIs.

To fulfil diagnostic criteria, both mood and anxiety symptoms may not meet threshold criteria for any other independent anxiety disorder. Nonetheless, they must result in significant functional impairment. Intensity of symptoms in each of the domains may vary within the individual over time. Treatment recommendations in the absence of well-controlled evidence are that treatments with established efficacy in mood and anxiety disorders are reasonable options. Similarly, there are no published controlled or case series data on the effectiveness of psychological treatments in patients with this disorder.

Anxiety disorders in pregnancy

Anxiety disorders that present or require treatment during pregnancy pose a particular challenge to clinicians (see Yonkers *et al.*, 2006). The psychobiological impact of pregnancy can have a range of effects on maternal emotional well-being. If left unchecked, the anxiety symptoms can have significant negative consequences for maternal and infant well-being postpartum. Rates of new onset anxiety disorders in pregnancy are not known. The course of preexisting anxiety in pregnancy is mixed, with no evidence to suggest that pregnancy has any protective effect. The postpartum period, as with a range of mood disorders, may represent a particularly vulnerable time for exacerbations of anxiety symptoms (Rubinchik *et al.*, 2005).

In deciding who and when to treat, a few matters are important to consider. Most psychotropic medications readily cross the placenta, and as a consequence the risks and benefits of treatment must be carefully weighed. Cognitive and behavioural therapies should be attempted as first line wherever possible. If clinically indicated, treatment with an antidepressant can be considered. Despite widespread use of antidepressants in pregnancy, only limited data are available on their safety, including their risk to the unborn foetus. Emerging evidence of teratogenicity and long-term consequences of in utero exposure to SSRIs and TCAs is available (Bérard *et al.*, 2007). Concerns with use of benzodiazepines in pregnancy and a higher incidence of cleft palate than the general population have been raised. When treating pregnant mothers, clinicians should be aware of the changes that occur in all aspects of drug pharmacokinetics and pharmacodynamics. Although target doses may not vary from nonpregnant patients, dose and side effects may vary within and between individuals, requiring detailed monitoring. A summary of treatment issues for anxiety disorders in pregnancy and postpartum is provided by Dodd and colleagues (2006).

Anxiety disorders in the medical setting

There are a wide range of medical conditions that can cause and perpetuate symptoms of anxiety. The DSM-IV category of an anxiety disorder secondary to a general medical condition is possible to diagnose in the context of most of the major anxiety disorders. The presentation is typical in respect to the core symptoms of the disorder in question but differs in that a temporal relationship to the onset,

continuation or resolution of the medical disorder is shown.

If an anxiety disorder is felt to be a direct result of a medical condition, treatment is primarily aimed at the underlying medical condition. Treatment in line with standard treatment for individual anxiety disorders can in most cases be initiated concurrently. Careful monitoring of clinical response is essential, and combination treatments (medical and psychological/psychopharmacological) may be necessary to limit the impact of continuing anxiety symptoms on compliance and disability.

Substance-induced anxiety disorder

The propensity for a range of illicit, recreational and prescription drugs to cause anxiety symptoms and indeed a wide range of psychiatric symptoms is well known. These symptoms may occur during normal use of prescription drugs, intoxication (either deliberate or accidental) and during withdrawal. The full range of anxiety symptoms has been described in the context of substance use. Diagnosis requires establishing a clear relationship between the use of the substance and the onset or exacerbation of anxiety symptoms. In general, stopping the drug long term will resolve the anxiety. If, however, the drug is a prescribed one, exposure should be limited when possible and alternatives sought. Failing this, specific treatment for the anxiety in line with general guidelines is preferred.

Conclusions

Despite considerable advances in our understanding of anxiety disorders in recent decades, much still needs to be done to explain fully and ultimately treat this range of chronic and disabling conditions. Nevertheless, advances in our treatment armamentarium continue to make anxiety disorders some of the most rewarding of psychiatric conditions to manage. With persistently high levels of stigmatisation and misunderstanding of the value of treatments for this group of disorders, it remains incumbent on all mental health practitioners to educate local populations about the availability and effectiveness of treatments for these disorders through the use of accessible and destigmatising programmes.

REFERENCES

Adolphs, R., Jansari, A., & Tranel, D. (2001). Hemispheric perception of emotional valence from facial expressions. *Neuropsychology* 15:516–24.

Allison, T., Puce, A., & McCarthy, G. (2000). Social perception from visual cues: role of the STS region. *Trends Cogn Sci* 4:267–78.

Alonso, J., Angermeyer, M. C., Bernert, S., *et al.* (2004). Disability and quality of life impact of mental disorders in Europe: results from the European Study of the Epidemiology of Mental Disorders (ESEMeD) project. *Acta Psychiatr Scand Suppl* 38–46.

American Psychiatric Association (2000). *Diagnostic and Statistical Manual of Mental Disorders*, 4th edn., text revision (DSMIV-TR). Washington, DC: American Psychiatric Association.

Baldwin, D. S., & Polkinghorn, C. (2005). Evidence-based pharmacotherapy of generalized anxiety disorder. *Int J Neuropsychopharmacol* 8:293–302.

Barlow, D. (1988). Anxiety and its disorders. In *The Nature and Treatment of Anxiety and Panic*. New York: Guilford Press.

Barlow, D. H., Craske, M. G., & Cerny, J. A. (1989). Behavioural treatment of panic disoder. *Behav Ther* 20:261–82.

Barrett, P. M., Dadds, M. R., & Rapee, R. M. (1996). Family treatment of childhood anxiety: a controlled trial. *J Consult Clin Psychol* 64:333–42.

Baxter, L. R. (1992). Neuroimaging studies of obsessive compulsive disorder. *Psychiatr Clin North Am* 15:871–84.

Beck, A. T. (1976). *Cognitive Therapy and the Emotional Disorders*. New York: International Universities Press.

Beck, J. S. (1995). *Cognitive Therapy: Basics and Beyond*. New York, Guilford Press.

Bérard, A., Ramos, E., Rev, E., *et al.* (2007). First trimester exposure to paroxetine and risk of cardiac malformations in infants: the importance of dosage. *Birth Defects Res B Dev Reprod Toxicol* 80:18–27.

Black, B., & Uhde, T. W. (1994). Treatment of elective mutism with fluoxetine: a double-blind, placebo-controlled study. *J Am Acad Child Adolesc Psychiatry* 33:1000–6.

Blanco, C., Schneier, F. R., Schmidt, A., *et al.* (2003). Pharmacological treatment of social anxiety disorder: a meta-analysis. *Depress Anxiety* 18:29–40.

Bremner, J. D., Innis, R. B., Southwick, S. M., *et al.* (2000). Decreased benzodiazepine receptor binding in prefrontal cortex in combat-related posttraumatic stress disorder. *Am J Psychiatry* 157:1120–6.

Bremner, J. D., Innis, R. B., White, T., *et al.* (2000). SPECT [I–123]iomazenil measurement of the benzodiazepine receptor in panic disorder. *Biol. Psychiatry*, 47:96–106.

Bremner, J. D., Southwick, S. M., Johnson, D. R., *et al.* (1993). Childhood physical abuse and combat-related posttraumatic stress disorder in Vietnam veterans. *Am. J Psychiatry*, 150:235–9.

Breslau, N., Kessler, R. C., Chilcoat, H. D., *et al.* (1998). Trauma and posttraumatic stress disorder in the community: the 1996 Detroit Area Survey of Trauma. *Arch Gen Psychiatry* 55:626–32.

Brewin, C. R., Andrews, B., & Valentine, J. D. (2000). Meta-analysis of risk factors for posttraumatic stress disorder in trauma-exposed adults. *J Consult Clin Psychol* 68:748–66.

Bruch, M. A., & Cheek, J. M. (1995). Developmental factors in childhood and adolescent shyness. In R. G. Heimberg, M. R. Liebowitz, & D. A. Hope, eds. *Social Phobia: Diagnosis, Assessment, and Treatment*. New York: Guilford Press, pp. 163–82.

Butler, A. C., Chapman, J. E., Forman, E. M., *et al.* (2005). The empirical status of cognitive-behavioral therapy: a review of meta-analyses. *Clin Psychol Rev*

Butterfield, M. I., Becker, M. E., Connor, K. M., *et al.* (2001). Olanzapine in the treatment of post-traumatic stress disorder: a pilot study. *Int Clin Psychopharmacol* 16:197–203.

Cameron, O. G., Abelson, J. L., & Young, E. A. (2004). Anxious and depressive disorders and their comorbidity: effect on central nervous system noradrenergic function. *Biol Psychiatry* 56:875–83.

Cameron, O. G., Smith, C. B., Lee, M. A., *et al.* (1990). Adrenergic status in anxiety disorders: platelet alpha 2-adrenergic receptor binding, blood pressure, pulse, and plasma catecholamines in panic and generalized anxiety disorder patients and in normal subjects. *Biol Psychiatry* 28:3–20.

Castle, D. J., & Phillips, K. A. (2006). Obsessive-compulsive spectrum of disorders: a defensible construct? [Review]. *Aust N Z J Psychiatry* **40(2):**114–20.

Chambless, D. L. (1990). Spacing of exposure sessions in the treatment of agoraphobia and simple phobia. *Behav Ther* 21:217–29.

Cheyette, S. R., & Cummings, J. L. (1995). Encephalitis lethargica: lessons for contemporary neuropsychiatry. *J Neuropsych Clin Neurosci* 7:125–35.

Chouinard, G. (2004). Issues in the clinical use of benzodiazepines: potency, withdrawal, and rebound. *J Clin Psychiatry* **65**(Suppl 5):7–12.

Clark, D. M. (1988). A cognitive model of panic. In S. Rachman & J. Maser, eds. *Panic: Psychological Perspectives*. Hillsdale, NJ: Lawrence Erlbaum, pp. 71–89.

Clark, D. M., & Wells, A. (1995). A cognitive model of social phobia. In *Social Phobia: Diagnosis, Assessment, and Treatment*. New York: Guilford Press, pp. 69–93.

Cohn, J. B., & Rickels, K. (1989). A pooled, double-blind comparison of the effects of buspirone, diazepam and placebo in women with chronic anxiety. *Curr Med Res Opin* 11:304–20.

Coplan, J. D., Pine, D. S., Papp, L. A., *et al.* (1997). A view on noradrenergic, hypothalamic-pituitary-adrenal axis and extrahypothalamic corticotrophin-releasing factor function in anxiety and affective disorders: the reduced growth hormone response to clonidine. *Psychopharmacol Bull* **33**:193–204.

Crino, R., Slade, T., & Andrews, G. (2005). The changing prevalence and severity of obsessive-compulsive disorder criteria from DSM-III to DSM-IV. *Am J Psychiatry* **162**:876–82.

Crits-Chritoph, P. C., Connolly, M. B., & Azarian, K. (1996). An open trial of brief supportive-expressive psychotherapy in the treatment of generalised anxiety disorder. *Psychotherapy* **33**:418–30.

David, D., De, F. L., Lapeyra, O., *et al.* (2004). Adjunctive risperidone treatment in combat veterans with chronic PTSD. *J Clin Psychopharmacol* **24**:556–9.

Davidson, J. R., Hughes, D., Blazer, D. G., *et al.* (1991). Post-traumatic stress disorder in the community: an epidemiological study. *Psychol Med* 21:713–21.

Davidson, J. R., Krishnan, K. R., Charles, H. C., *et al.* (1993). Magnetic resonance spectroscopy in social phobia: preliminary findings. *J Clin Psychiatry* 54(Suppl):19–25.

Davidson, J. R., Potts, N., Richichi, E., *et al.* (1993). Treatment of social phobia with clonazepam and placebo. *J Clin Psychopharmacol* 13:423–8.

Davis, M. (1986). Pharmacological and anatomical analysis of fear conditioning using the fear-potentiated startle paradigm. *Behav Neurosci* 100:814–24.

de Araujo, L. A., Ito, L. M., Marks, I. M., *et al.* (1995). Does imagined exposure to the consequences of not ritualising enhance live exposure for OCD? A controlled study. I. Main outcome. *Br J Psychiatry* **167**:65–70.

Deakin, J. F. (1991). Depression and 5HT. *Int Clin Psychopharmacol* 6(Suppl 3):23–28; discussion 29–31.

Demyttenaere, K., Bruffaerts, R., Posada-Villa, J., *et al.* (2004). Prevalence, severity, and unmet need for treatment of mental disorders in the World Health Organization World Mental Health Surveys. *JAMA* **291**:2581–90.

Denys, D., de Geus, F., van Megen, H., *et al.* (2004). A double-blind, randomized, placebo-controlled trial of quetiapine addition in patients with obsessive-compulsive disorder refractory to serotonin reuptake inhibitors. *J Clin Psychiatry* **65**:1040–8.

Denys, D., & de, G. F. (2005). Predictors of pharmacotherapy response in anxiety disorders. *Curr Psychiatry Rep* 7:252–7.

DiGiuseppe, R., McGowan, L., Sutton-Simon, K., *et al.* (1990). A comparative outcome study of four cognitive therapies in the treatment of social anxiety disorder. *Cogn Behav Ther* 129–46.

Dodd, S., Opie, J., & Berk, M. (2006). Pharmacological treatment of anxiety and depression in pregnancy and lactation. In D. J. Castle, J. Kulkarni, K. M. Abel, eds. *Mood and Anxiety Disorders in Women*. Cambridge: Cambridge University Press, pp. 163–84.

Durham, R. C., Murphy, T., Allan, T., *et al.* (1994). Cognitive therapy, analytic psychotherapy and anxiety management training for generalised anxiety disorder. *Br J Psychiatry* **165**:315–23.

Eaton, W. W., Kessler, R. C., Wittchen, H. U., *et al.* (1994). Panic and panic disorder in the United States. *Am J Psychiatry* **151**:413–20.

Eisen, J. L., & Rasmussen, S. A. (1993). Obsessive compulsive disorder with psychotic features. *J Clin Psychiatry*, **54**:373–9.

Eisen, J. L., Rasmussen, S. A. (2002). Phenomenology of obsessive-compulsive disorder. In *Textbook of Anxiety Disorders*, D. J. Stein & E. Hollander (eds.). The American Psychiatric Publishing, pp. 173–90.

Ellis, A. (1962). *Reason and Emotion in Psychotherapy*. New York: Lyle Stuart.

Fahlen, T. (1995). Personality traits in social phobia, I: Comparisons with healthy controls. *J Clin Psychiatry* **56**:560–8.

Fendt, M., Fanselow, M. S., & Koch, M. (2005). Lesions of the dorsal hippocampus block trace fear conditioned potentiation of startle. *Behav Neurosci* 119:834–8.

Feske, U., & Chambless, D. L. (1995). Cognitive-behavioural versus exposure treatment for social phobia: a meta-analysis. *Behav Ther* 695–720.

Foa, E. B., & Kozak, M. J. (1996). Psychological treatment for obsessive-compulsive disorder. In *Long-Term Treatment for Anxiety Disorders*. Washington, DC: American Psychiatric Press, pp. 285–309.

Foa, E. B., Kozak, M. J., Goodman, W. K., *et al.* (1995). DSM-IV field trial: obsessive-compulsive disorder. *Am J Psychiatry* 152:90–6.

Foa, E. B., Liebowitz, M. R., Kozak, M. J., *et al.* (2005). Randomized, placebo-controlled trial of exposure and ritual prevention, clomipramine, and their combination in the treatment of obsessive-compulsive disorder. *Am J Psychiatry* 162:151–61.

Foa, E. B., Steketee, G., Ozarow, B. J. (1985). Behavior therapy with obsessive-compulsives: from theory to treatment. In M. R. Mavissakalian, S. M. Turner, & L. Michelson, eds. *Obsessive-Compulsive Disorder: Psychological and Pharmacological Treatment*. New York: Plenum, pp. 49–129.

Franklin, M. E., Abramowitz, J. S., Kozak, M. J., *et al.* (2000). Effectiveness of exposure and ritual prevention for obsessive-compulsive disorder: randomized compared with nonrandomized samples. *J Consult Clin Psychol* 68:594–602.

Fujita, M., Southwick, S. M., Denucci, C. C., *et al.* (2004). Central type benzodiazepine receptors in Gulf War veterans with posttraumatic stress disorder. *Biol Psychiatry* 56:95–100.

Furmark, T., Tillfors, M., Marteinsdottir, I., *et al.* (2002). Common changes in cerebral blood flow in patients with social phobia treated with citalopram or cognitive-behavioral therapy. *Arch Gen Psychiatry* 59:425–33.

Fyer, A. J. (1993). Heritability of social anxiety: a brief review. *J Clin Psychiatry* 54(Suppl):10–2.

Fyer, A. J., Mannuzza, S., Gallops, M. S., *et al.* (1990). Familial transmission of simple phobias and fears. A preliminary report. *Arch Gen Psychiatry* 47:252–6.

Gale, C., & Oakley-Browne, M. (2004). Generalised anxiety disorder. *Clin Evid* 1437–59.

Garvey, M. J., Noyes, R., Jr., Woodman, C., *et al.* (1995). Relationship of generalized anxiety symptoms to urinary 5-hydroxyindoleacetic acid and vanillylmandelic acid. *Psychiatry Res* 57:1–5.

Gelernter, C. S., Uhde, T. W., Cimbolic, P., *et al.* (1991). Cognitive-behavioral and pharmacological treatments of social phobia. A controlled study. *Arch Gen Psychiatry* 48:938–45.

Gelpin, E., Bonne, O., Peri, T., *et al.* (1996). Treatment of recent trauma survivors with benzodiazepines: a prospective study. *J Clin Psychiatry* 57:390–4.

Germine, M., Goddard, A. W., Woods, S. W., *et al.* (1992). Anger and anxiety responses to m-chlorophenyl-piperazine in generalized anxiety disorder. *Biol Psychiatry* 32:457–61.

Goddard, A. W., Mason, G. F., Almai, A., *et al.* (2001). Reductions in occipital cortex GABA levels in panic disorder detected with 1h-magnetic resonance spectroscopy. *Arch Gen Psychiatry* 58:556–61.

Goodman, W. K., McDougle, C. J., & Price, L. H. (1990). Beyond the serotonin hypothesis: a role for dopamine in some forms of obsessive-compulsive disorder. *J Clin Psychiatry* 51(Suppl):36–43.

Goodman, W. K., Price, L. H., Rasmussen, S. A., *et al.* (1989). The Yale-Brown Obsessive Compulsive Scale. I. Development, use, and reliability. *Arch Gen Psychiatry* 46:1006–11.

Goodwin, J. M. (2005). Redefining borderline syndromes as posttraumatic and rediscovering emotional containment as a first stage in treatment. *J Interpers Violence* 20:20–5.

Goodwin, R. D., Faravelli, C., Rosi, S., *et al.* (2005). The epidemiology of panic disorder and agoraphobia in Europe. *Eur Neuropsychopharmacol* 15:435–43.

Gorman, J. M. (2003). Does the brain noradrenaline network mediate the effects of the CO_2 challenge? *J Psychopharmacol* 17:265–6.

Gorman, J. M., Kent, J. M., Sullivan, G. M., *et al.* (2000). Neuroanatomical hypothesis of panic disorder, revised. *Am J Psychiatry*, 157:493–505.

Graeff, F. G., Garcia-Leal, C., Del-Ben, C. M., *et al.* (2005). Does the panic attack activate the hypothalamic-pituitary-adrenal axis? *An Acad Bras Cienc* 77:477–91.

Greenberg, P. E., Sisitsky, T., Kessler, R. C., *et al.* (1999). The economic burden of the anxiety disorders in the 1990s. *J Clin Psychiatry* 60(7):427–35.

Greist, J. H., Bandelow, B., Hollander, E., *et al.* (2003). WCA recommendations for the long-term treatment of obsessive-compulsive disorder in adults. *CNS Spectr* 8:7–16.

Gur, R. C., Gur, R. E., Resnick, S. M., *et al.* (1987). The effect of anxiety on cortical cerebral blood flow and metabolism. *J Cereb Blood Flow Metab* 7:173–7.

Hafner, J., & Marks, I. (1976). Exposure in vivo of agoraphobics: contributions of diazepam, group exposure, and anxiety evocation. *Psychol Med* 71–88.

Hamilton, M. (1959). The assessment of anxiety states by rating. *Br J Med Psychol* **32**:50–5.

Hamner, M. B., Deitsch, S. E., Brodrick, P. S., *et al.* (2003). Quetiapine treatment in patients with posttraumatic stress disorder: an open trial of adjunctive therapy. *J Clin Psychopharmacol* **23**:15–20.

Helzer, J. E., Robins, L. N., & McEvoy, L. (1987). Posttraumatic stress disorder in the general population. Findings of the epidemiologic catchment area survey. *N Engl J Med* **317**:1630–4.

Hemmings, S. M., Kinnear, C. J., Lochner, C., *et al.* (2004). Early- versus late-onset obsessive-compulsive disorder: investigating genetic and clinical correlates. *Psychiatry Res* **128**:175–82.

Hollander, E. (ed.) (1993). *Obsessive-Compulsive Related Disorders*. Washington DC: American Psychiatric Press.

Hollander, E. (ed.) (1993). The spectrum of obsessive-compulsive related disorders. In *Obsessive-Compulsive Related Disorders*. Washington, DC: American Psychiatric Press.

Holt, P. E., & Andrews, G. (1998). Hyperventialation and anxiety in panic disorder,social phobia, GAD and normal controls. *Behav Res Ther* **27**:453–60.

Iny, L. J., Pecknold, J., Suranyi-Cadotte, B. E., *et al.* (1994). Studies of a neurochemical link between depression, anxiety, and stress from [3H]imipramine and [3H]paroxetine binding on human platelets. *Biol Psychiatry* **36**:281–91.

Ipser, J. C., Carey, P., Dhansay, Y., *et al.* (2006). Pharmacotherapy augmentation strategies in treatment-resistant anxiety disorders. *Cochrane Database Syst Rev* **4**:CD005473.

Ito, L. M., Marks, I. M., de Araujo, L. A., *et al.* (1995). Does imagined exposure to the consequences of not ritualising enhance live exposure for OCD? A controlled study. II. Effect on behavioural v. subjective concordance of improvement. *Br J Psychiatry* **167**:71–5.

Johnson, M. R., Marazziti, D., Brawman-Mintzer, O., *et al.* (1998). Abnormal peripheral benzodiazepine receptor density associated with generalized social phobia. *Biol Psychiatry* **43**:306–9.

Kagan, J., Reznick, J. S., & Snidman, N. (1988). Biological bases of childhood shyness. *Science* **240**:167–71.

Kaplan, A., & Hollander, E. (2003). A review of pharmacologic treatments for obsessive-compulsive disorder. *Psychiatr Serv* **54**:1111–18.

Kasper, S., & Resinger, E. (2001a). Panic disorder: the place of benzodiazepines and selective serotonin reuptake inhibitors. *Eur Neuropsychopharmacol* **11**:307–21.

Kasper, S., & Resinger, E. (2001b). Panic disorder: the place of benzodiazepines and selective serotonin reuptake inhibitors. *Eur Neuropsychopharmacol* **11**:307–21.

Kendall, P. C., Flannery-Schroeder, E., Panichelli-Mindel, S. M., *et al.* (1997). Therapy for youths with anxiety disorders: a second randomized clinical trial. *J Consult Clin Psychol* **65**:366–80.

Kendler, K. S. (1996). Major depression and generalised anxiety disorder. Same genes, (partly) different environments–revisited. *Br J Psychiatry Suppl* (30):68–75.

Kendler, K. S., Neale, M. C., Kessler, R. C., *et al.* (1992). The genetic epidemiology of phobias in women. The interrelationship of agoraphobia, social phobia, situational phobia, and simple phobia. *Arch Gen Psychiatry* **49**:273–81.

Kennedy, B. L., Lin, Y., & Schwab, J. J. (2002). Work, social, and family disabilities of subjects with anxiety and depression. *South Med J* **95**:1424–7.

Kessler, R. C., McGonagle, K. C., Zhao, S., *et al.* (1994). Lifetime and 12-month prevalence of DSM-III-R psychiatric disorders in the United States: Results from the National Comorbidity Survey. *Arch Gen Psychiatry* **51**:8–19.

Kessler, R. C. (2000). The epidemiology of pure and comorbid generalized anxiety disorder: a review and evaluation of recent research. *Acta Psychiatr Scand Suppl* (**406**):7–13.

Kessler, R. C., Berglund, P., Demler, O., *et al.* (2005). Lifetime prevalence and age-of-onset distributions of DSM-IV disorders in the National Comorbidity Survey Replication. *Arch Gen Psychiatry* **62**:593–602.

Kessler, R. C., Brandenburg, N., Lane, M., *et al.* (2005). Rethinking the duration requirement for generalized anxiety disorder: evidence from the National Comorbidity Survey Replication. *Psychol Med* **35**:1073–82.

Kessler, R. C., Demler, O., Frank, R. G., *et al.* (2005). Prevalence and treatment of mental disorders, 1990 to 2003. *N Engl J Med* **352**:2515–23.

Kessler, R. C., Sonnega, A., Bromet, E., *et al.* (1995). Posttraumatic stress disorder in the National Comorbidity Survey. *Arch Gen Psychiatry* **52**:1048–60.

Kessler, R. C., Stang, P., Wittchen, H. U., *et al.* (1999). Lifetime co-morbidities between social phobia and mood disorders in the US National Comorbidity Survey *Psychol Med* **29**:555–67.

Keuneman, R. J., Pokos, V., Weerasundera, R., & Castle, D. J. 2005. Antipsychotic treatment in obsessive-compulsive disorder: a literature review. *Aust N Z J Psychiatry* **39**(5):336–43.

Kjernisted, K. D., & Bleau, P. (2004). Long-term goals in the management of acute and chronic anxiety disorders. *Can J Psychiatry* **49**:51S–63S.

Klein, D. F. (1993). False suffocation alarms, spontaneous panic, and related conditions. an integrative hypothesis. *Arch Gen Psychiatry.* **50**:306–17.

Lader, M. (2005). Management of panic disorder. *Expert Rev Neurother* **5**:259–66.

Lader, M., & Scotto, J. C. (1998). A multicentre double-blind comparison of hydroxyzine, buspirone and placebo in patients with generalized anxiety disorder. *Psychopharmacology (Berl)* **139**:402–6.

Landon, T. M., & Barlow, D. H. (2004). Cognitive-behavioral treatment for panic disorder: current status. *J Psychiatr Pract* **10**:211–26.

Leckman, J. F., de Lotbiniere, A. J., Marek, K., *et al.* (1993). Severe disturbances in speech, swallowing, and gait following stereotactic infrathalamic lesions in Gilles de la Tourette's syndrome. *Neurology* **43**:890–4.

Leckman, J. F., Pauls, D. L., Zhang, H., *et al.* (2003) Obsessive-compulsive symptom dimensions in affected sibling pairs diagnosed with Gilles de la Tourette syndrome. *Am J Med Genet B Neuropsychiatr Genet* **116**:60–8.

Lee, S., Lee, M. T., & Kwok, K. (2005). A community-based telephone survey of social anxiety disorder in Hong Kong. *J Affect Disord* **88**:183–6.

Lesch, K. P. (2001). Serotonergic gene expression and depression: implications for developing novel antidepressants. *J Affect Disord* **62**:57–76.

Liebowitz, M. R., Mangano, R. M., Bradwejn, J., *et al.* (2005). A randomized controlled trial of venlafaxine extended release in generalized social anxiety disorder. *J Clin Psychiatry* **66**:238–47.

Lochner, C., Mogotsi, M., du Toit, P. L., *et al.* (2003). Quality of life in the anxiety disorders: a comparison of obsessive-compulsive disorder, social anxiety disorder, and panic disorder. *Psychopathology* **36**:255–62.

Mahmutyazicioglu, K., Konuk, N., Ozdemir, H., *et al.* (2005). Evaluation of the hippocampus and the anterior cingulate gyrus by proton MR spectroscopy in patients with post-traumatic stress disorder. *Diagn Interv Radiol* **11**:125–9.

Maier, W., Gansicke, M., Freyberger, H. J., *et al.* (2000). Generalized anxiety disorder (ICD-10) in primary care from a cross-cultural perspective: a valid diagnostic entity? *Acta Psychiatr Scand* **101**:29–36.

March, J. S., Entusah, Q. R., Albano, A. M., & Tourian, K.A. (2007). A randomized controlled trial of venlafaxine ER versus placebo in pediatric social anxiety disorder. *Biol Psychiatry.* **62**:1149–54. Epub 2007 Jun 5.

Maron, E., & Shlik, J. (2006). Serotonin function in panic disorder: important, but why? *Neuropsychopharmacology* **31**:1–11.

Masand, P. S., & Gupta, S. (2003). The safety of SSRIs in generalised anxiety disorder: any reason to be anxious? *Expert Opin Drug Saf* **2**:485–93.

Mataix-Cols, D., Rauch, S. L., Baer, L., Eisen, J. L., *et al.* (2002). Symptom stability in adult obsessive-compulsive disorder: data from a naturalistic two-year follow-up study. *Am J Psychiatry* **159**:263–8.

McDougle, C. J., Goodman, W. K., Leckman, J. F., *et al.* (1994). Haloperidol addition in fluvoxamine-refractory obsessive-compulsive disorder. A double-blind, placebo-controlled study in patients with and without tics. *Arch Gen Psychiatry* **51**:302–8.

Mellman, T. A., Bustamante, V., David, D., *et al.* (2002). Hypnotic medication in the aftermath of trauma. *J Clin Psychiatry* **63**:1183–4.

Mineka, S., Zinbarg, R. (2005). Conditioning and ethological models of social phobia. In R. G. Heimberg, M. R. Liebowitz, & D. A. Hope, eds. *Social Phobia: Diagnosis, Assessment, and Treatment.* New York: Guilford Press, pp. 134–62.

Mogotsi, M., Kaminer, D., & Stein, D. J. (2000). Quality of life in the anxiety disorders. *Harv Rev Psychiatry* **8**:273–82.

Morris, J. S., Frith, C. D., Perrett, D. I., *et al.* (1996). A differential neural response in the human amygdala to fearful and happy facial expressions. *Nature* **383**:812–15.

Muller, J. E., Koen, L., Seedat, S., *et al.* (2005). Social anxiety disorder: current treatment recommendations. *CNS Drugs* **19**:377–91.

Murray, C. J. L., Lopez, A. D. (1996). *Global burden of disease: a comprehensive assessment of mortality from diseases injuries and risk factors in 1990 and projected to 2020.* Cambridge, Massachusetts: Harvard University Press.

Nemeroff, C. B., Bremner, J. D., Foa, E. B., *et al.* (2006). Post-traumatic stress disorder: a state-of-the-science review. *J Psychiatr Res* **40**:1–21.

Nestadt, G., Samuels, J., Riddle, M., *et al.* (2000). A family study of obsessive-compulsive disorder. *Arch Gen Psychiatry* **57**:358–63.

Nutt, D. J., Bell, C. J., & Malizia, A. L. (1998). Brain mechanisms of social anxiety disorder. *J Clin Psychiatry* **59**(Suppl 17):4–11.

Nutt, D. J., & Malizia, A. L. (2004). Structural and functional brain changes in posttraumatic stress disorder. *J Clin Psychiatry* **65**(Suppl 1):11–17.

Ohman, A. (1986). Face the beast and fear the face: animal and social fears as prototypes for evolutionary analyses of emotion. *Psychophysiology* **23**:123–45.

Otte, C., Kellner, M., Arlt, J., *et al.* (2002). Prolactin but not ACTH increases during sodium lactate-induced panic attacks. *Psychiatry Res* **109**:201–5.

Otto, M. W., & Deveney, C. (2005). Cognitive-behavioral therapy and the treatment of panic disorder: efficacy and strategies. *J Clin Psychiatry* **66**(Suppl 4):28–32.

Pauls, D. L., Alsobrook, J. P., Goodman, W., *et al.* (1995). A family study of obsessive-compulsive disorder. *Am J Psychiatry* **152**:76–84.

Perkonigg, A., Kessler, R. C., Storz, S., *et al.* (2000). Traumatic events and post-traumatic stress disorder in the community: prevalence, risk factors and comorbidity 12. *Acta Psychiatr Scand* **101**:46–59.

Perkonigg, A., Pfister, H., Stein, M. B., *et al.* (2005). Longitudinal course of posttraumatic stress disorder and posttraumatic stress disorder symptoms in a community sample of adolescents and young adults. *Am J Psychiatry* **162**:1320–7.

Perna, G., Bertani, A., Arancio, C., *et al.* (1995). Laboratory response of patients with panic and obsessive-compulsive disorders to 35% CO_2 challenges. *Am J Psychiatry* **152**:85–9.

Pitman, R. K., Sanders, K. M., Zusman, R. M., *et al.* (2002). Pilot study of secondary prevention of posttraumatic stress disorder with propranolol. *Biol Psychiatry* **51**:189–92.

Pokos, V., & Castle, D. J. (2006). Prevalence of comorbid anxiety disorders in schizophrenia spectrum disorders: a literature review. *Current Psychiatry Reviews* **2**:285–307.

Pollack, M. H., Allgulander, C., Bandelow, B., *et al.* (2003). WCA recommendations for the long-term treatment of panic disorder. *CNS Spectr* **8**:17–30.

Potts, N. L., Davidson, J. R., Krishnan, K. R., *et al.* (1994). Magnetic resonance imaging in social phobia. *Psychiatry Res* **52**:35–42.

Rapaport, J. L., Ryland, D. H., & Kriete, M. (1992). Drug treatment of canine acral lick. *Arch Gen Psychiatry* 517–21.

Rapee, R. M. (1985). Distinctions between panic disorder and generalised anxiety disorder: clinical presentation. *Aust N Z J Psychiatry* **19**:227–32.

Rapee, R. M. (1997). Potential role of childrearing practices in the development of anxiety and depression. *Clin Psychol Rev* **17**:47–67.

Rasmussen, S. A., & Eisen, J. L. (1992). The epidemiology and clinical features of obsessive compulsive disorder. *Psychiatr Clin North Am* **15**:743–58.

Rasmussen, S. A., & Eisen, J. L. (1994). The epidemiology and differential diagnosis of obsessive compulsive disorder. *J Clin Psychiatry* **55**(Suppl):5–10; discussion 11–4.

Rauch, S. L., Savage, C. R., Alpert, N. M., Fischman, A. J., & Jenike, M. A. (1997). The functional neuroanatomy of anxiety: a study of three disorders using positron emission tomography and symptom provocation. *Biol Psychiatry* **42**(6):446–52.

Reiman, E. M., Raichle, M. E., Robins, E., *et al.* (1989). Neuroanatomical correlates of a lactate-induced anxiety attack. *Arch Gen Psychiatry* **46**:493–500.

Rickels, K., Downing, R., Schweizer, E., *et al.* (1993). Antidepressants for the treatment of generalized anxiety disorder. A placebo-controlled comparison of imipramine, trazodone, and diazepam. *Arch Gen Psychiatry* **50**:884–95.

Rickels, K., Pollack, M. H., & Feltner, D. E. (2005). Pregabalin for treatment of generalized anxiety disorder: a 4-week, multicenter, double-blind, placebo-controlled trial of pregabalin and alprazolam. *Arch Gen Psychiatry* **62**:1022–30.

Rickels, K., & Schweizer, E. (1998). Panic disorder: long-term pharmacotherapy and discontinuation. *J Clin Psychopharmacol* **18**:12S–18S.

Robins, L. N., Helzer, J. E., Weissman, M. M., *et al.* (1984). Lifetime prevalence of specific psychiatric disorders in three sites. *Arch Gen Psychiatry* **41**:949–58.

Rodriguez, B. F., Bruce, S. E., Pagano, M. E., *et al.* (2005). Relationships among psychosocial functioning, diagnostic comorbidity, and the recurrence of generalized anxiety disorder, panic disorder, and major depression. *J Anxiety Disord* **19**:752–66.

Roy-Byrne, P., Stein, M. B., Russo, J., *et al.* (2005). Medical illness and response to treatment in primary care panic disorder. *Gen Hosp Psychiatry* **27**:237–43.

Roy-Byrne, P. P., Wagner, A. W., & Schraufnagel, T. J. (2005). Understanding and treating panic disorder in the primary care setting. *J Clin Psychiatry* **66**(Suppl 4):16–22.

Rubinchik, S. M., Kablinger, A. S., & Gardner, J. S. (2005). Medications for panic disorder and generalized anxiety disorder during pregnancy. *Prim Care Companion J Clin Psychiatry* **7**:100–5.

Schelling, G., Briegel, J., Roozendaal, B., *et al.* (2001). The effect of stress doses of hydrocortisone during septic shock on posttraumatic stress disorder in survivors. *Biol Psychiatry* **50**:978–85.

Schelling, G., Kilger, E., Roozendaal, B., *et al.* (2004). Stress doses of hydrocortisone, traumatic memories, and symptoms of posttraumatic stress disorder in patients after cardiac surgery: a randomized study 13. *Biol Psychiatry* **55**:627–33.

Schmidt, N. B., Salas, D., Bernert, R., *et al.* (2005). Diagnosing agoraphobia in the context of panic disorder: examining the effect of DSM-IV criteria on diagnostic decision-making. *Behav Res Ther* **43**:1219–29.

Schmitt, R., Gazalle, F. K., Lima, M. S., *et al.* (2005). The efficacy of antidepressants for generalized anxiety disorder: a systematic review and meta-analysis. *Rev Bras Psiquiatr* **27**:18–24.

Schneier, F. R., Johnson, J., Hornig, C. D., *et al.* (1992). Social phobia. Comorbidity and morbidity in an epidemiologic sample. *Arch Gen Psychiatry* **49**:282–8.

Schweizer, E., Rickels, K., Uhlenhuth, E. H. (1995a). Issues in pediatric generalized anxiety disorder. In F. E. Bloom & D. J. Kupfer, eds. *Psychopharmacology: The Fourth Generation of Progress.* New York: Raven, pp. 51 7.

Schweizer, E., Rickels, K., Uhlenhuth, E. H. (1995b). Issues in the longterm treatment of anxiety disorders. In F. E. Bloom & D. J. Kupfer, eds. *Psychopharmacology: The Fourth Generation of Progress.* New York: Raven, pp. 1349–59.

Seedat, S., Videen, J. S., Kennedy, C. M., *et al.* (2005). Single voxel proton magnetic resonance spectroscopy in women with and without intimate partner violence-related posttraumatic stress disorder. *Psychiatry Res* **139**:249–58.

Sevy, S., Papadimitriou, G. N., Surmont, D. W., *et al.* (1989). Noradrenergic function in generalized anxiety disorder, major depressive disorder, and healthy subjects. *Biol Psychiatry* **25**:141–52.

Shalev, A. Y., Bloch, M., Peri, T., *et al.* (1998). Alprazolam reduces response to loud tones in panic disorder but not in posttraumatic stress disorder. *Biol Psychiatry* **44**:64–8.

Shalev, A. Y., Freedman, S., Peri, T., *et al.* (1997). Predicting PTSD in trauma survivors: prospective evaluation of self-report and clinician-administered instruments. *Br J Psychiatry* **170**:558–64.

Simeon, J. G., & Ferguson, H. B. (1987). Alprazolam effects in children with anxiety disorders. *Can J Psychiatry* **32**:570–4.

Skre, I., Onstad, S., Torgersen, S., *et al.* (1993). A twin study of DSM-III-R anxiety disorders. *Acta Psychiatr Scand* **88**:85–92.

Smith, M. E. (2005). Bilateral hippocampal volume reduction in adults with post-traumatic stress disorder: a meta-analysis of structural MRI studies. *Hippocampus* **15**:798–807.

Stein, D. J., & Bouwer, C. (1997). Blushing and social phobia: a neuroethological speculation. *Med Hypoth* **49**:101–8.

Stein, D. J., & Hollander, E. (1993). The spectrum of obsessive-compulsive related disorders. In E. Hollander, ed. *Obsessive-Compulsive Related Disorders.* Washington, DC: American Psychiatric Press.

Stein, D. J., Ipser, J. C., & Balkom, A. J. (2004). Pharmacotherapy for social phobia. *Cochrane Database Syst Rev* **18**:CD001206. Review.

Stein, D. J., Seedat, S., van der Linden, G. J., *et al.* (2000). Selective serotonin reuptake inhibitors in the treatment of post-traumatic stress disorder: a meta-analysis of randomized controlled trials. *Int Clin Psychopharmacol* **15**(Suppl 2):S31–S39.

Stein, D. J., Young, J. E. (1992). *Cognitive Science and Clinical Disorders.* San Diego, California: Academic Press.

Stein, M. B., Chartier, M. J., Hazen, A. L., *et al.* (1998). A direct-interview family study of generalized social phobia. *Am J Psychiatry* **155**:90–7.

Stein, M. B., Chen, G., Potter, W. Z., *et al.* (1996). G-protein level quantification in platelets and leukocytes from patients with panic disorder. *Neuropsychopharmacology* **15**:180–6.

Stein, M. B., Delaney, S. M., Chartier, M. J., *et al.* (1995). [3H]paroxetine binding to platelets of patients with social phobia: comparison to patients with panic disorder and healthy volunteers. *Biol Psychiatry* **37**:224–8.

Stein, M. B., Fuetsch, M., Muller, N., *et al.* (2001). Social anxiety disorder and the risk of depression: a prospective community study of adolescents and young adults. *Arch Gen Psychiatry* **58**:251–6.

Stein, M. B., Huzel, L. L., & Delaney, S. M. (1993). Lymphocyte beta-adrenoceptors in social phobia. *Biol Psychiatry* **34**:45–50.

Sullivan, G. M., Coplan, J. D., Kent, J. M., *et al.* (1999). The noradrenergic system in pathological anxiety: a focus on panic with relevance to generalized anxiety and phobias. *Biol Psychiatry* **46**:1205–18.

Swedo, S. E., Leonard, H. L., Garvey, M., *et al.* (1998). Pediatric autoimmune neuropsychiatric disorders associated with streptococcal infections: clinical description of the first 50 cases. *Am J Psychiatry*, 155:264–71.

Thomsen, H. (2001). [Pharmacological treatment of children and adolescents with OCD]. *Ugeskr Laeger* 163:3763–8.

Thomsen, P. H. (1995). Obsessive-compulsive disorder in children and adolescents: predictors in childhood for long-term phenomenological course. *Acta Psychiatr Scand* 92:255–9.

Tiihonen, J., Kuikka, J., Bergstrom, K., *et al.* (1997). Dopamine reuptake site densities in patients with social phobia. *Am J Psychiatry* 154:239–42.

Tiihonen, J., Kuikka, J., Rasanen, P., *et al.* (1997). Cerebral benzodiazepine receptor binding and distribution in generalized anxiety disorder: a fractal analysis. *Mol Psychiatry* 2:463–71.

Torgersen, S. (1990). Comorbidity of major depression and anxiety disorders in twin pairs. *Am J Psychiatry*, 147:1199–1202.

Tucker, P., Zaninelli, R., Yehuda, R., *et al.* (2001). Paroxetine in the treatment of chronic posttraumatic stress disorder: results of a placebo-controlled, flexible-dosage trial. *J Clin Psychiatry* 62:860–8.

Tupler, L. A., Davidson, J. R., Smith, R. D., *et al.* (1997). A repeat proton magnetic resonance spectroscopy study in social phobia. *Biol Psychiatry* 42:419–24.

Turk, C. L., Heimberg, R. G., Orsillo, S. M., *et al.* (1998). An investigation of gender differences in social phobia. *J Anxiety Disord* 12:209–23.

Van Ameringen, M., Allgulander, C., Bandelow, B., *et al.* (2003). WCA recommendations for the long-term treatment of social phobia 22. *CNS Spectr* 8:40–52.

van Balkom, A. J., de, H. E., van, O. P., *et al.* (1998). Cognitive and behavioral therapies alone versus in combination with fluvoxamine in the treatment of obsessive compulsive disorder. *J Nerv Ment Dis* 186:492–9.

van Balkom, A. J., van Oppen, P., & Vermeulen, A. W. (1994). A meta-analysis on the treatment of obsessive-compulsive disorder: a comparison of antidepressants, behaior, and cognitive therapy. *Clin Psychol Rev* 14:359–81.

Van Der Linden, G. J., van Heerden, B., Warwick, J., *et al.* (2000). Functional brain imaging and pharmacotherapy in social phobia: single photon emission computed tomography before and after treatment with the selective serotonin reuptake inhibitor citalopram. *Prog Neuropsychopharmacol Biol Psychiatry* 24:419–38.

Van der Wee, N. J., van Veen, J. F., Stevens, H., *et al.* (2008). Increased Serotonin and Dopamine Transporter Binding in Psychotropic Medication-Naive Patients with Generalized Social Anxiety Disorder Shown by 1231-{beta}-(4-Iodophenyl)-Tropane SPECT. *J Nucl Med* 49:757–63.

van Emmerik, A. A., Kamphuis, J. H., Hulsbosch, A. M., *et al.* (2002). Single session debriefing after psychological trauma: a meta-analysis. *Lancet* 360:766–71.

van Vliet, I., Westenberg, H. G., Slaap, B. R., *et al.* (1997). Anxiogenic effects of pentagastrin in patients with social phobia and healthy controls. *Biol Psychiatry* 42:76–8.

Vasile, R. G., Bruce, S. E., Goisman, R. M., *et al.* (2005). Results of a naturalistic longitudinal study of benzodiazepine and SSRI use in the treatment of generalized anxiety disorder and social phobia. *Depress Anxiety* 22:59–67.

Versiani, M., Cassano, G., Perugi, G., *et al.* (2002). Reboxetine, a selective norepinephrine reuptake inhibitor, is an effective and well-tolerated treatment for panic disorder. *J Clin Psychiatry* 63:31–7.

Verster, J. C., & Volkerts, E. R. (2004). Clinical pharmacology, clinical efficacy, and behavioral toxicity of alprazolam: a review of the literature. *CNS Drug Rev* 10:45–76.

Vuilleumier, P., Richardson, M. P., Armony, J. L., *et al.* (2004). Distant influences of amygdala lesion on visual cortical activation during emotional face processing. *Nat Neurosci* 7:1271–8.

Weiskrantz, L. (1956). Behavioural changes associated with ablation of the amygdaloid complex in monkeys. *J Comp Physiol Psychol* 49:381–91.

Weizman, R., Tanne, Z., Granek, M., *et al.* (1987). Peripheral benzodiazepine binding sites on platelet membranes are increased during diazepam treatment of anxious patients. *Eur J Pharmacol* 138:289–92.

Wever, C., & Rey, J. M. (1997). Juvenile obsessive-compulsive disorder. *Aust N Z J Psychiatry* 31:105–13.

White, J. (1998a). "Stress control" large group therapy for generalized anxiety disorder: two year follow-up. *Behav Cogn Psychother* 26:237–46.

White, J. (1998b). Stresspac: three year follow-up of a controlled trial of a self-help package for the anxiety disorders. *Behav Cogn Psychother* 26:133–41.

World Health Organization (2001). *The World Health Report 2001: Mental Health: New Understanding, New Hope.* Geneva: World Health Organization.

World Health Organization (2006). International Statistical Classification of Diseases and Related Health Problems, 10th revision version for 2006. Geneva: World Health Organization.

Wu, J. C., Buchsbaum, M. S., Hershey, T. G., *et al.* (1991). PET in generalized anxiety disorder. *Biol Psychiatry* **29**:1181–99.

Wu, J. C., Tanne, Z., Granek, M., *et al.* (1987). PET in generalized anxiety disorder. *Biol Psychiatry* **29**:289–92.

Yehuda, R. (1998). Psychoneuroendocrinology of post-traumatic stress disorder. *Psychiatr Clin North Am* **21**:359–79.

Yehuda, R., McFarlane, A. C., & Shalev, A. Y. (1998). Predicting the development of posttraumatic stress disorder from the acute response to a traumatic event. *Biol Psychiatry* **44**:1305–13.

Yerkes, R. M., & Dodson, J. D. (1908). The relation of strength of stimulus to rapidity of habit-formation. *J Compar Neurol Psychol* **18**:459–82.

Yonkers, K. A., Holthausen, G. A., Poschman, K., & Howell, H. B. (2006). Symptom-onset treatment for women with premenstrual dysphoric disorder. *J Clin Psychopharmacol* **26**(2):198–202.

Zwanzger, P., & Rupprecht, R. (2005). Selective GABAergic treatment for panic? Investigations in experimental panic induction and panic disorder. *J Psychiatry Neurosci* **30**:167–75.

9

Eating disorders

Janet Treasure and Ulrike Schmidt

Eating disorders predominately have their onset in adolescence and can disrupt maturation during this critical developmental phase. These disorders have a major impact on both physical and psychological health. Guidelines for the management of these disorders have been produced in several countries; however, many of the recommendations are not firmly evidence based.

There is a degree of fluidity in the classification of the eating disorders. Therefore in this chapter for some concepts such as classification and epidemiology, we have grouped the disorders together, whereas in other areas in which the specific diagnosis is of more relevance (such as comorbidity, aetiology, and management) we have used anorexia nervosa, bulimia nervosa and binge eating categories.

History

The framing of eating disorders has been a subject of debate. The various names given over time have reflected beliefs about aetiology and psychopathology. A psychological conceptualization with the recognition of gender-related aspects was first apparent in the nineteenth century in Gull's description of "apepsia hysterica" (Gull, 1868). He changed the name later to anorexia nervosa to reflect his view of the central origin of the disorder (Gull, 1874).

Eating disorders expanded from the historical accounts, which were of restricting anorexia nervosa to include a variety of disorders typified by the chaotic pattern of eating of the binge-eating disorders. Gerald Russell (1979) described bulimia nervosa as a condition which included periodic overeating coupled with excessive concerns about weight and shape, leading to behaviours to compensate for the effects of eating. He considered bulimia nervosa to be an "ominous variant" of anorexia nervosa. However, although there is movement across the diagnoses, this does not follow an inevitable pattern, and the majority of cases of bulimia nervosa are not preceded by an episode of anorexia nervosa. Binge eating disorder has been added as an additional syndrome for further study in the fourth edition of the *Diagnostic and Statistical Manual of Mental Disorders* (DSM-IV). In this disorder, the concerns and behaviours related to shape and weight are less extreme.

Classification

The classification systems of eating disorders according to DSM-IV and the 10th revision of the *International Classification of Diseases* (ICD10) are shown in Table 9.1. Binge-eating disorder is not yet considered as a separate category in the DSM-IV criteria. Eating disorder not otherwise specified (EDNOS) is a large catch-all category. It can include people in the entry or resolving phase of the illness (especially for anorexia nervosa in which change

Essential Psychiatry, ed. Robin M. Murray, Kenneth S. Kendler, Peter McGuffin, Simon Wessely, David J. Castle. Published by Cambridge University Press. © Cambridge University Press 2008.

Table 9.1 Anorexia nervosa and Bulimia nervosa according to DSM-IV and ICD-10

DSM-IV-R (307.1)	ICD 10 (F50.0)

Anorexia Nervosa	
Refusal to maintain body weight over a minimal norm, leading to body weight less than 85% of that expected or failure to make expected weight gain during a period of growth	Body weight is maintained at least 15% below that expected (either lost or never achieved) or Quetelet's body mass index 17.5 kg/m^2); prepubertal patients may show failure to make the expected weight gain during the period of growth
Intense fear of gaining weight or becoming fat	Weight loss is self-induced by avoiding fattening foods; one or more of the following may also be present (a) vomiting (b) purging (c) excessive exercise (d) appetite suppressants (e) diuretics
Disturbance in the way in which one's body weight, size or shape is experienced (e.g. "feeling fat" [denial of seriousness of underweight or undue influence of body weight and shape on self-evaluation])	Body image distortion in the form of a specific psychopathology whereby a dread of fatness persists as an intrusive overvalued idea and the patient imposes a low weight threshold on self
In postmenarchal females, amenorrhoea (i.e absence of at least 3 consecutive menstrual cycles)	Widespread endocrine disorder (a) amenorrhoea or, in men, loss of sexual interest and potency (b) raised growth hormone (c) raised cortisol (d) reduced T3 If onset is prepubertal, the sequence of pubertal events is delayed or arrested

Bulimia Nervosa	
DSM-IV-R Bulimia nervosa (307.51)	ICD 10 (F50.2)
Recurrent episodes of binge eating	A persistent preoccupation with eating and an irresistible craving for food; patient succumbs to episodes of overeating in which large amounts of food are consumed in a short time
Recurrent inappropriate compensatory behaviour to prevent weight gain such as vomiting, misuse of laxatives, diuretics, enemas or other medications, fasting or excessive exercise	The patient attempts to counteract the fattening effects of food by one or more of the following: (a) vomiting; (b) purging; (c) alternating periods of starvation; (d) appetite suppressants, diuretics, thyroid preparations When bulimia occurs in diabetic patients, they may choose to neglect their insulin treatment
The binge eating and inappropriate compensatory behaviors both occur on average at least twice a week for 3 months.	The psychopathology consists of a morbid dread of fatness, and the patient imposes a low weight threshold on herself well below the premorbid weight that constitutes the optimum or healthy weight
Self-evaluation is unduly influenced by body shape and weight	
The disturbance does not occur exclusively during episodes of anorexia nervosa	

occurs slowly). It also includes disorders which cause clinical impairment but do not meet the frequency, severity or duration criteria to be classified as full syndromes. In DSM-IV, anorexia nervosa is subclassified into restricting and binge-purge subtypes. The binge-purge subtype of anorexia nervosa shares many aetiological elements with the bulimic disorders. A third of cases anorexia nervosa transform into a bulimic disorder within 5 years. Movement from bulimia nervosa to anorexia nervosa occurs less commonly.

Low weight and the physiological markers of starvation are of key diagnostic importance in anorexia nervosa. Weight loss (or, in a developing child or adolescent, failure to gain weight) to below 85% of that expected for height, or below a body mass index (BMI) of 17.5, is considered significant.

The boundaries among purging disorder, bulimia nervosa, nonpurging subtype of bulimia nervosa, binge-eating disorder, EDNOS and overeating in obesity are somewhat indistinct. A time-limited binge can be difficult to separate from a protracted pattern of overeating. Compensatory methods other than vomiting and purging are more difficult to define. The intensity of symptoms and the duration that are required to define a "case" have varied over time. Approximately one quarter of cases can dip into anorexia nervosa, binge purge subtype, within 5 years of the onset, especially in the group with low novelty seeking.

Spitzer *et al.* (1991) suggested that an additional category of "binge eating disorder" could be defined from within the "eating disorder not otherwise specified" category. This condition is in DSM-IV (Table 9.1) as a proposed category pending further research. People with binge-eating disorder have episodes of bingeing as defined by bulimia nervosa, but they do not compensate for this with extreme behaviours such as vomiting or taking laxatives, fasting or the use of excessive exercise, which occur in bulimia; their absence is the main diagnostic distinction from bulimia. Thus these people are often obese. The levels of psychopathology observed in individuals with binge-eating disorder fall between the high levels seen in bulimia nervosa and the low levels seen in simple obesity. Emotional and personality difficulties are common, and there may be impaired work and social functioning.

Epidemiology

Van Hoeken and colleagues (2003) reviewed the epidemiological literature and found an average prevalence rate for anorexia nervosa of 0.3% in young females and an overall incidence of at least 8 per 100,000 person-years. For bulimia nervosa, the same authors suggested an average prevalence rate in young females of 1% and incidence of 12 per 100,000 person-years. The ratio of females to males is around 10:1 for both conditions. The peak age of onset for anorexia nervosa (15–19 years) is younger than for bulimia nervosa (20–24 years). Hay (1998) found a point prevalence of 1% for binge-eating disorder. The prevalence of EDNOS varies between 2% and 10%. There is considerable comorbidity in eating-disorder cases detected by community screening (Jacobi, Wittchen, *et al.*, 2004).

Bulimia nervosa was rare in women born before the 1950s, and the incidence increased in the 1990s (Jacobi, Wittchen, *et al.*, 2004). There is a suggestion, however, that the incidence in the twenty-first century is decreasing (Currin *et al.*, 2005; Jacobi, Wittchen *et al.*, 2004). Some of this variability represents changes in detection and presentation to services (many cases of bulimia nervosa in the community are undetected). A systematic review of the epidemiology of eating disorders concluded that the prevalence of bulimic disorders varies according to time and place – that is, it is a culture-bound syndrome (Keel & Klump, 2003). Furthermore, some of the diagnostic criteria may be culture bound: for example, in China, Lee and colleagues (1993) identified a large proportion of cases of anorexia nervosa that lacked fear of fatness.

The rapid increase in bulimia nervosa in the last half of the twentieth century may have resulted from some degree of contagion or social transmission of the values and behaviours that underpin the disorder. Food and appearance are of importance in

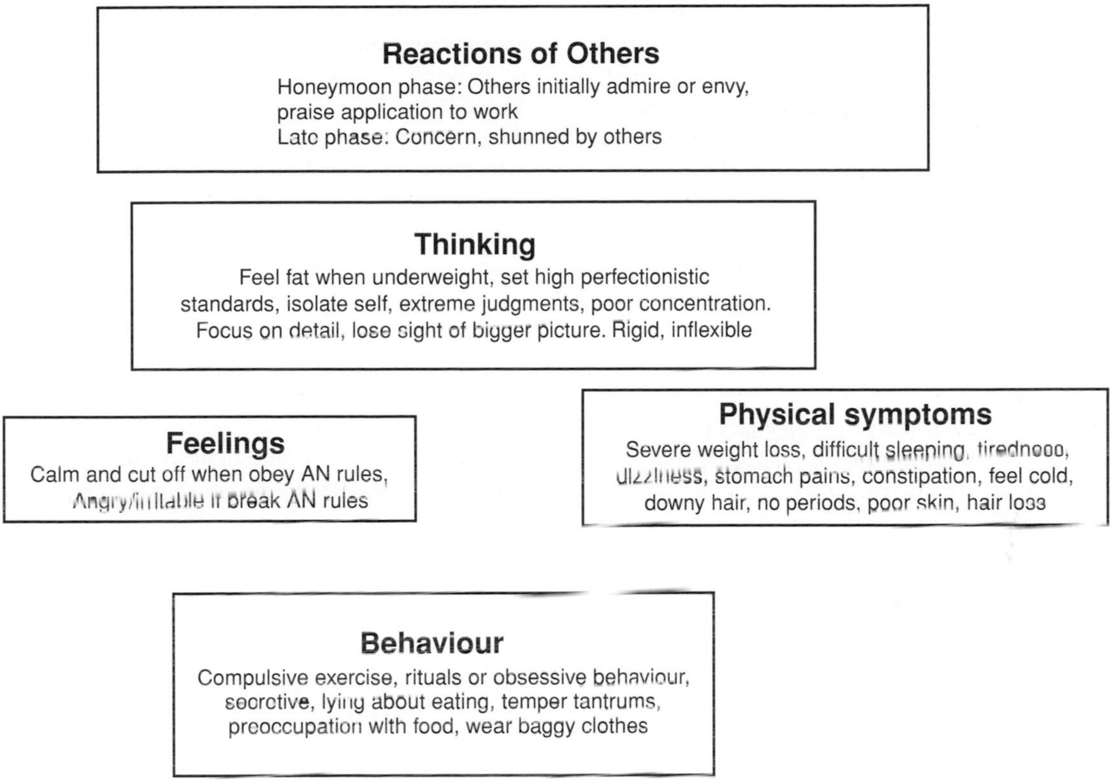

Reactions of Others
Honeymoon phase: Others initially admire or envy,
praise application to work
Late phase: Concern, shunned by others

Thinking
Feel fat when underweight, set high perfectionistic
standards, isolate self, extreme judgments, poor concentration.
Focus on detail, lose sight of bigger picture. Rigid, inflexible

---

Feelings
Calm and cut off when obey AN rules,
Angry/irritable if break AN rules

Physical symptoms
Severe weight loss, difficult sleeping, tiredness,
dizziness, stomach pains, constipation, feel cold,
downy hair, no periods, poor skin, hair loss

Behaviour
Compulsive exercise, rituals or obsessive behaviour,
secretive, lying about eating, temper tantrums,
preoccupation with food, wear baggy clothes

Figure 9.1 The clinical picture of anorexia nervosa

women's lives. The internalisation of the thin ideal varies across time and geography. Dieting to attain this idealised form can trigger the erratic pattern of eating, especially if it used in combination with extreme behaviours that compensate for overeating. Rates of bulimia nervosa are higher in urban populations.

Anorexia nervosa

The clinical features of anorexia nervosa and the reactions of other people are shown in Figure 9.1.

Comorbidity

Figure 9.2 illustrates the comorbidity which is common across the spectrum of eating disorders.

Anorexia nervosa normally clusters with other internalising disorders. High levels of comorbidity with depression have been reported, perhaps as a secondary effect of starvation. Anorexia nervosa has also been linked to the obsessive-compulsive (OC) spectrum of disorders. OC personality traits manifest early in development (Anderluh *et al.*, 2003), present after recovery (Bastiani *et al.*, 1995; Matsunaga *et al.*, 2000; Srinivasagam *et al.*, 1995) and affect outcome (Lock *et al.*, 2005). Gillberg and colleagues (1996) suggested that there may also be a link with the autistic spectrum of disorders. OC personality traits are common features of the OC and autistic clusters of disorders and of eating disorders. The reader is referred to Chapter 8 for a more detailed discussion about the putative OC spectrum of disorders.

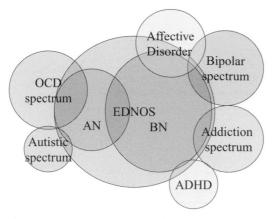

Figure 9.2 The comorbidity of eating disorders

Aetiology

The quality of evidence from risk-factor studies is generally weak for anorexia nervosa because most data have been ascertained from cross-sectional studies in which biases and uncertainty about temporal precedence limit interpretation. However, Jacobi, Hayward, *et al.* (2004) have performed a systematic review of all work in progress. Figure 9.3 represents an adaptation of Jacobi's model separating environmental and intrinsic vulnerabilities.

Intrinsic vulnerability

In most animal models of anorexia nervosa, females are most vulnerable to the stress (nutritional or otherwise) that triggers the expression of these behaviours (Connan & Treasure, 1998; Owen, 1998). Furthermore, certain genetic strains of animal are particularly vulnerable.

Research into the biology of the genetic aspects of eating disorders is an area of rapid growth. Eating disorders aggregate in families. Strober and colleagues (2000) found that the relative risk for anorexia nervosa in female relatives of anorexic subjects was 11.3. Bulimia nervosa was also more common in the families of people with anorexia nervosa (relative risk: 4.2) and bulimia nervosa (relative risk: 4.4). Partial syndromes (EDNOS) were also

more common than in control families. Twin studies estimate the heritability of eating disorders to lie between 33% and 84% for anorexia nervosa, 28% and 83% for bulimia nervosa and 31% and 50% for binge eating disorder (Bulik, 2005).

In terms of specific genes, linkage to chromosome 1 has been reported in families with restricting anorexia nervosa (Grice *et al.*, 2002). A meta-analysis of the results from candidate gene studies implicated anomalies in the 5-HT system (Gorwood *et al.*, 2003). However, the effect size found from candidate gene studies is small, and the confidence in any finding is as yet uncertain. It remains to be determined how many of the anxiety and obsessive-compulsive traits which are comorbid with anorexia nervosa are linked to the genetic vulnerability.

Extrinsic vulnerability

A variety of environmental factors increase the risk of developing an eating disorder. These include adversities in pregnancy, birth-related complications (Favaro *et al.*, 2006) and high-concern parenting (in which the parents appear to have high levels of anxiety; Shoebridge & Gowers, 2000). Triggering factors include nutritional stress (caused by levels of exercise, dieting behaviour, or both) in combination with hassles or life events occurring in the context of the developmental changes linked to puberty and early adolescence (including the biological maturation of the brain and social development; Southgate *et al.*, 2005). Cultural factors related to body image probably play less of a role in the causation of anorexia nervosa than bulimia nervosa and are therefore considered later.

Clinical conceptualisations

A variety of clinical conceptualisations are used for the foundations of various treatment approaches, but most are not based on strong empirical evidence nor do they have proven procedures of change associated with treatment efficacy. Bruch (1973) developed a psychodynamic hypothesis centred on insecure attachment and the lack of attunement

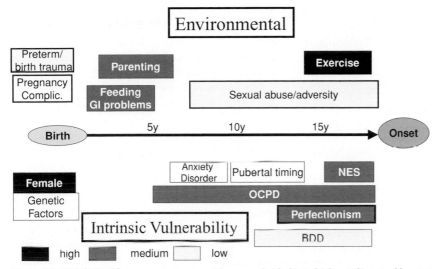

Figure 9.3 Risk factors for anorexia nervosa: These are divided into high, medium and low potency factors. Adapted from Jacobi *et al.*, 2004.

between the infant and the caretaker. Family models emphasise either causal or maintaining factors risk (Eisler & Asen, 2003). The Maudsley model is a manualised form of family treatment (Lock *et al.*, 2005) evolving from the evidence implicating expressed emotion as a key factor in maintenance. Cognitive behavioural formulations for anorexia nervosa have also been described (Fairburn *et al.*, 1999; Waller & Kennerley, 2003). Neurodevelopmental models (Connan *et al.*, 2003; Southgate *et al.*, 2005) have also been translated into treatment models including trait management (Treasure *et al.*, 2005).

Assessment and management

A characteristic feature of anorexia nervosa is patients' denial of their illness and their resistance to seeking help. This has implications for engagement. Often a nonmedical friend or relative makes a spot diagnosis and recommends a medical assessment. However, given the ambivalence about the process of diagnosis and treatment, it can be helpful to start the assessment broadly enquiring about functioning in the psychosocial domains shown in Box 9.1.

Box 9.1 Domains of assessment in anorexia nervosa

General
- Family (their concerns and the consequences on them)
- Disadvantage in career and education (poor attention etc.)
- Impaired social functioning/interactions
- Difficulties in interpersonal and intimate relationships
- General psychopathology (depression, anxiety, obsessionality, rituals, preoccupation with food, etc.).

Physical consequences of starvation
- Loss of stamina and strength
- Altered sleep cycle
- Sensitivity to cold
- Dry skin (with altered hair distribution)
- Dizziness
- Dental problems
- Sore throat
- Abdominal symptoms (constipation, fullness after eating)
- Amenorrhea (if not taking an oral contraceptive)
- Circulatory problems – poor capillary flow
- Gastrointestinal-tract problems secondary to purging

The specific features of the eating disorder are more usefully addressed when some trust has been developed. The features to look out for include the following:

- Severely restricted food intake (interspersed with binging in the binge-purge subtype)
- Overexercise
- Self-induced vomiting
- Misuse of laxatives or diuretics
- Premorbid personality: obsessive-compulsive features, low self-esteem.

The meaning of the food restriction is variable and has transcultural implications (Lee *et al.*, 2001). However, the common aspects related to the motivated food restriction are (1) preoccupation with the detail about food issues, (2) fear of normal body weight, (3) lack of concern about low weight and (4) judging self solely in terms of weight and shape.

The context: family and other carers

As previously discussed, the visible nature of ill health in anorexia nervosa draws in others to intervene. It is therefore usual and helpful for family members to be included in the first assessment. It is good practice to include carers in the process (1) to provide a multiperspective conceptualization and (2) for information sharing, which allows them knowledge and skills about how to avoid participating in any of the maintaining mechanisms.

Caring for someone with an eating disorder is difficult, and carers themselves may benefit from a needs assessment because many are distressed and overwhelmed by their role. A lack of information is commonly cited as a difficulty, and sources of information are available on the Internet and in numerous self-help books.

Interventions to give family members the skills and knowledge to help their loved one are under investigation. A variety of ways to include the family in treatment such as the use of separated family work (differential input to parents and individual) or multifamily groups have been used.

> **Box 9.2** Internet sites with information about eating disorders
>
> www.eatingresearch.com
> www.rcpsych.ac.uk
> http://www.b-eat.co.uk/
> www.nhsdirect.nhs.uk

Issues of confidentiality can cause confusion. For a start, such a highly visible illness can never be kept confidential between doctor and patient. Second, starvation affects capacity and decision making, and combined with the high risk associated with severe starvation, this has legal implications. Thus it is good practice to balance the need for confidentiality with the need to practise safely, which includes information sharing with both professional and nonprofessional carers.

The assessment and management of risk

A diagram illustrating the assessment of risk is shown in Figure 9.4. Fuller details about measuring risk can be attained from published guidelines (American Psychiatric Association, 2000; Beumont *et al.*, 2004; National Collaborating Centre, 2004) or from Internet sites in Box 9.2.

If there are markers suggesting that the nutritional risk is high, increasing intake is of highest priority. This is best done orally, starting with 50 kcal/kg/day and gradually increasing to about 3,000 kcal/day. A normal soft diet is recommended, but in some cases liquid food is better tolerated. This should be supplemented with micronutrient replacement (a standard dose of vitamins and minerals). For further information about nutritional management, refer to the Royal College of Psychiatrists Guidelines (http://www.rcpsych.ac.uk/publications/collegereports/cr/cr130.aspx).

A disturbance in fluid and electrolyte balance usually occurs as a consequence of purging but in some cases results from deliberate self-imposed fluid restriction. Again, this is best managed

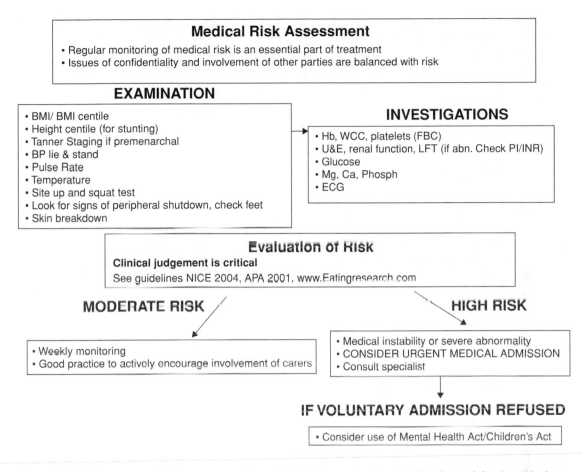

Medical Risk Assessment

- Regular monitoring of medical risk is an essential part of treatment
- Issues of confidentiality and involvement of other parties are balanced with risk

EXAMINATION

- BMI/ BMI centile
- Height centile (for stunting)
- Tanner Staging if premenarchal
- BP lie & stand
- Pulse Rate
- Temperature
- Site up and squat test
- Look for signs of peripheral shutdown, check feet
- Skin breakdown

INVESTIGATIONS

- Hb, WCC, platelets (FBC)
- U&E, renal function, LFT (if abn. Check PI/INR)
- Glucose
- Mg, Ca, Phosph
- ECG

Evaluation of Risk

Clinical judgement is critical

See guidelines NICE 2004, APA 2001, www.Eatingresearch.com

MODERATE RISK

- Weekly monitoring
- Good practice to actively encourage involvement of carers

HIGH RISK

- Medical instability or severe abnormality
- CONSIDER URGENT MEDICAL ADMISSION
- Consult specialist

IF VOLUNTARY ADMISSION REFUSED

- Consider use of Mental Health Act/Children's Act

Figure 9.4 This figure summarises the processes of examining risk in people with eating disorders and the plan of further management.

conservatively with oral electrolyte replacement solutions or oral potassium and should be closely monitored, avoiding intravenous replacement whenever possible.

The context in which this acute risk is managed can vary depending on prognostic factors detailed subsequently and in the available resources. For example, people with a good prognosis (young cases with a short duration) can be managed with home support. Others may need a period of inpatient care in a setting where nurses have skills in managing this problem. Patience, perseverance and

kindness are of more value than technology in this procedure.

The assessment of prognosis

Good outcome is associated with minimal weight loss (BMI >17 kg/m^2), absence of medical complications, strong motivation to change behaviour and supportive family and friends who do not condone the abnormal behaviour. Poor outcome is indicated by vomiting in very emaciated patients, onset in adulthood, coexisting psychiatric or personality

> **Box 9.3** Factors associated with a prolonged course in anorexia nervosa
>
> - The reactions of close others exemplified by the features of high expressed emotion (overprotection and criticism)
> - Compulsive traits, rigidity and perfectionism
> - High anxiety and avoidance
> - A prolonged period of starvation with the cascade of biological, psychological and psychosocial consequences

disorder, disturbed family relationships and a long duration of illness (Steinhausen, 2002). In general, the morbidity risk (one of the highest within psychiatry) is estimated to be approximately 0.5% per year of follow-up (Nielsen *et al.*, 1998).

In most case series, anorexia nervosa has a prolonged course (the median duration of illness is 6 years). Schmidt and Treasure (2005) reviewed the features that contribute to the maintenance of anorexia nervosa. These are shown in Box 9.3.

The aim of treatment is to interrupt these maintaining factors. For example, early, effective intervention can produce a good outcome for 60% of cases in the first year progressing to 90% recovery by 5 years (Eisler *et al.*, 1997). The family approaches given the highest rating of evidence contain procedures designed to reduce expressed emotion within the family (Lock *et al.*, 2001).

The therapeutic relationship

The key issue in the treatment of anorexic patients is engagement in the therapeutic relationship. Most people with anorexia nervosa are not ready to change. Using the terminology of the transtheoretical model of change, most patients are in the precontemplation stage. The strategies of motivational interviewing can facilitate movement into action by increasing the importance and confidence that an improvement in nutritional health is necessary. Thus the first phase of motivational interviewing starts with open questions meant to explore the overall quality of the patient's life (the

domains outlined earlier are salient cues) and help the patient to hear herself talk about her problems. The clinician should have a compassionate, empathetic stance. Confrontation is unhelpful.

Planning treatment

Planning treatment for someone with anorexia nervosa is not a simple issue solved by entering in the appropriate key words and searching the literature for systematic reviews of evidence-based treatments. Guidelines are available but have to be interpreted judiciously (American Psychiatric Association, 2000; Beumont *et al.*, 2004; National Collaborating Centre, 2004). The first question is what stage and type of anorexia nervosa is it? The next considerations are the level of medical and psychiatric risk and the age of the patient. Treatment will be tailored to match patient needs as well as available resources.

A variety of service models – inpatient, day patient and outpatient settings – and various forms of clinical conceptualizations (discussed earlier) have been used, including psychotherapy and medication. The broad conclusion is that specialist expertise combining a focus on medical risk, diet and weight and linking this to interpersonal and psychological issues is most acceptable to people with anorexia nervosa. Surprisingly, nonspecific manualised supportive clinical management given by a specialist produced a better clinical outcome than cognitive-behavioural therapy or interpersonal psychotherapy in a mild subgroup (McIntosh *et al.*, 2005); replication of this finding is needed in a more representative population. There appears to be little difference amongst family, focal dynamic and cognitive analytical therapies, although all of these were more effective than general, nonspecialised psychiatric management (Dare *et al.*, 2001).

Medication

A recent Cochrane systematic review concluded that there was little to support the use of antidepressants

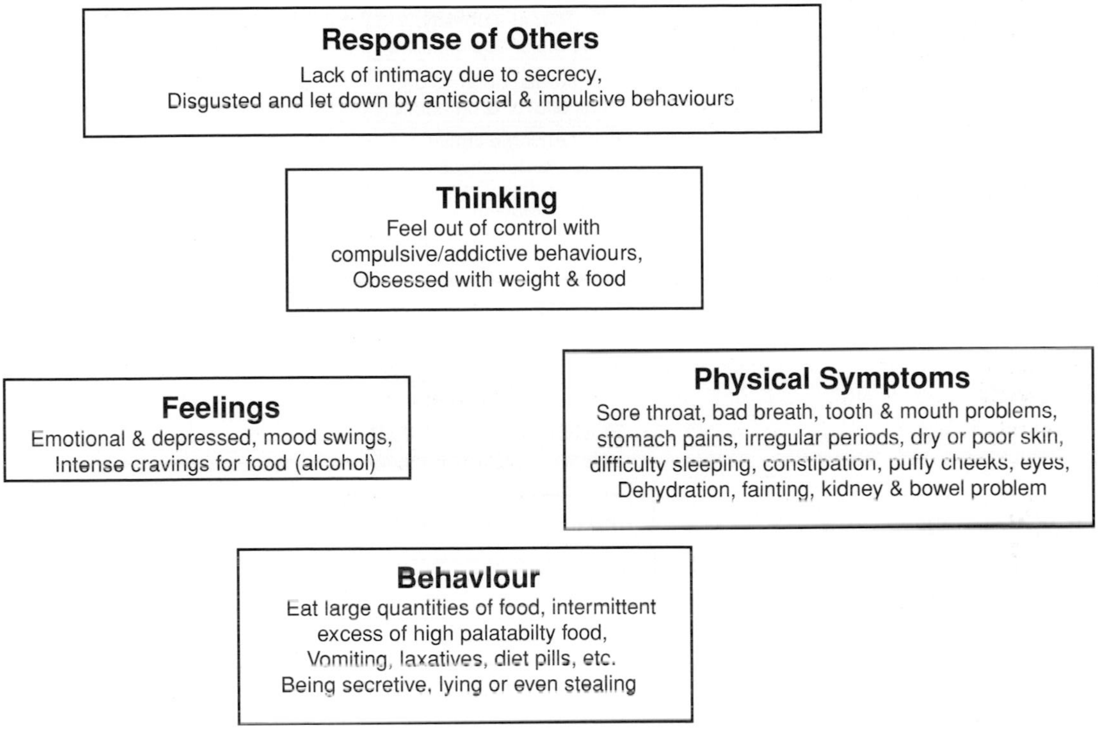

Response of Others
Lack of intimacy due to secrecy,
Disgusted and let down by antisocial & impulsive behaviours

Thinking
Feel out of control with
compulsive/addictive behaviours,
Obsessed with weight & food

Feelings
Emotional & depressed, mood swings,
Intense cravings for food (alcohol)

Physical Symptoms
Sore throat, bad breath, tooth & mouth problems,
stomach pains, irregular periods, dry or poor skin,
difficulty sleeping, constipation, puffy cheeks, eyes,
Dehydration, fainting, kidney & bowel problem

Behaviour
Eat large quantities of food, intermittent
excess of high palatabilty food,
Vomiting, laxatives, diet pills, etc.
Being secretive, lying or even stealing

Figure 9.5 The clinical picture of bulimia nervosa

in the management of anorexia nervosa either in the acute or relapse prevention phase The National Institute for Health and Clinical Excellence (NICE) guidelines also found no evidence to support the use of other medication. Nevertheless, there is interest in atypical antipsychotics for severe cases, and tranquilisers such as promazine are often used in this context.

Conclusion

The UK NICE guidelines recommend that outpatient treatment should be the preferred initial approach if medical risk allows. They also recommend the inclusion of members of the family especially for adolescent cases. Treatment manuals are available (Lock *et al.*, 2001). Early effective

intervention is critical (Currin & Schmidt, 2005; Treasure & Schmidt, 2005).

Bulimia nervosa

The clinical features of bulimia nervosa are shown in Figure 9.5.

Comorbidity

As illustrated in Figure 9.2, the comorbidities of the bulimic disorders differ from those of anorexia nervosa in that there is more association with the affective disorders and personalities in which affective dysregulation plays a key role. There has been a particular interest in the link with bipolar disorder. There are also associations with conditions

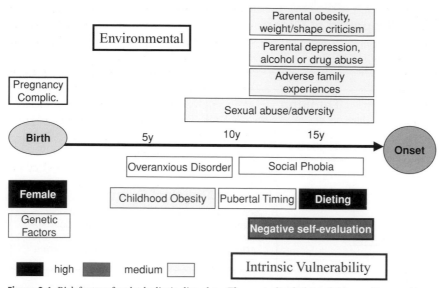

Figure 9.6 Risk factors for the bulimic disorders: These are divided into high, medium and low potency factors. Adapted from Jacobi *et al.*, 2004.

in which impulsiveness is a core feature, such as the addictions. Yet another subgroup has obsessive-compulsive traits and behavioural inhibition, merging more with anorexia nervosa.

Aetiology

There is more confidence about the risk factors for bulimia nervosa than for anorexia nervosa because there is higher quality evidence within the systematic reviews of literature (Jacobi, Hayward, *et al.*, 2004; Stice, 2002)). An outline of the core features is shown in Figure 9.6 in which intrinsic and environmental features have been separated.

Intrinsic mechanisms

Genetic mechanisms account for more than 50% of the variance in the risk for developing bulimia nervosa, and linkage to chromosome 10 has been reported. As in anorexia nervosa, for a subgroup of bulimia patients, perfectionism, anxiety and low self-esteem are developmental dispositions that increase the risk of developing bulimia. However, in

contrast to anorexia nervosa, there is also a pattern of impulsivity and overeating with associated obesity in childhood.

Environmental mechanisms

Parental problems are also more marked than in anorexia nervosa and include alcoholism, depression and drug abuse. Adverse experiences such as sexual abuse and physical neglect are also seen. The proximal risk factors for bulimia nervosa include dieting, early puberty, low self-esteem and stress in the context of body dissatisfaction, thin ideal internalisation and negative affect (Stice, 2002).

Clinical conceptualisations

The original cognitive-behavioural model of bulimia nervosa in which overvalued ideas about weight and shape played a key role underpinned the procedures involved in the model of cognitive-ural therapy that has been successfully used in the treatment of bulimia nervosa (Fairburn, 1983). This model has limitations, however, and

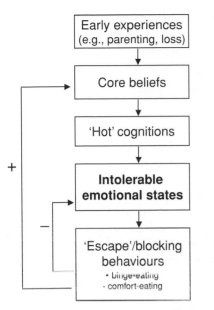

Figure 9.7 Models of maintenance of bulimia nervosa. Adapted from Waller & Kennerley, 2003.

therefore additional features have been added (see Figure 9.7). Fairburn and colleagues (2003) developed a transdiagnostic model which is purportedly applicable to the treatment of all forms of eating disorders. Waller and Kennerley (2003) place emotional dysregulation more centrally.

Assessment

The assessment of bulimia nervosa is in essence similar to that for anorexia nervosa. The issue of engagement is usually less problematic because people with bulimia nervosa are generally more ready to change at least their binging behaviour (reducing the overevaluation of weight and shape and strict dietary restriction is more of a challenge). Eating pathology and the methods of weight control they have adopted need to be fully assessed. It is important to ascertain during history taking whether there are any significant medical consequences. The enquiry should cover teeth and salivary glands, as well as gastrointestinal (bleeding, regurgitation), kidney and endocrine function. A physical examination and a screen for electrolyte abnormalities are also required. The clinical examination should focus on the specific problems that result from purging behaviour.

Other forms of weight control (e.g. insulin purging whereby people with diabetes mellitus forgo their insulin) can have specific adverse consequences. In the case of diabetes, the mortality and rate of physical complications is markedly increased (Peveler *et al.*, 2005). People with bulimia nervosa are also more likely than those with anorexia to have children, and this can be associated with the transmission of abnormal attitudes to food and shape (Patel *et al.*, 2002).

Treatment

As noted earlier, the quality and quantity of research into the treatment of bulimia nervosa is much greater than that in anorexia nervosa. Thus a more evidence-based approach is possible. The clinical presentation is less diverse, and the context of treatment is more uniform (i.e. typically these patients are treated in outpatient settings). Research into the treatment of bulimia nervosa has been summarised in systematic reviews in the Cochrane library series (Bacaltchuk *et al.*, 1999, 2000; Hay & Bacaltchuk, 2000). This systematic search was updated and reanalysed as part of the process of constructing the NICE guidelines (National Collaborating Centre for Mental Health, 2004).

Psychotherapy

The NICE guidelines were able to give a grade A recommendation for cognitive-behavioural treatment for bulimia nervosa, and a meta-analysis found that the number needed to treat to gain benefit was four (National Collaborating Centre for Mental Health, 2004). A manual describing the standard CBT treatment adopted in treatment studies for bulimia nervosa is available (Fairburn *et al.*, 1993). This approach is at least moderately effective in approximately 70% of cases (Agras *et al.*, 2000), and those who do respond generally do so in the first weeks of therapy.

The first phase of treatment includes an explanation about the cognitive model of bulimia nervosa and the vicious circle of bingeing. One of the basic maintaining cycles is that the overconsumption of food leads to regret and anxiety about having broken strict dietary rules. This then leads to reversing behaviours (fasting, vomiting, laxatives, etc.). These in turn exacerbate feelings of starvation, which leads to more craving and a predisposition to overeat and the cycle starts again (see the core features in Figure 9.7).

There is also evidence supporting the use of interpersonal therapy in bulimia nervosa (see Chapter 29); however, this appears to be associated with a slower rate of change.

Medication

The NICE guidelines concluded that drugs alone are less effective than psychotherapy in bulimia nervosa, with the number needed to treat being nine (National Collaborating Centre for Mental Health, 2004). There is also scant information about the long-term outcome from pharmacological treatment. It was therefore suggested that antidepressants might be used as an alternative or additional first step in the management of bulimia nervosa. The combination of medication and psychological treatment seems to be more effective than either treatment on its own, but it also has higher dropout rates.

Clinical practice

Many centres now adopt a stepped-care approach starting with the least intensive, least costly and least invasive intervention. The first step is guided self-care treatment using cognitive-behavioural therapy delivered from books (Cooper, 1993; Schmidt & Treasure, 1993; Fairburn, 1995). Computer- or web-based treatments have also been successfully used (Bara-Carril *et al.,* 2004; Carrard *et al.,* 2005). It remains to be seen whether

the new models such as Fairburn's transdiagnostic model produce better outcomes for the more treatment-resistant group.

Prognosis and outcome

Follow-up studies on people with bulimia nervosa after treatment show that after 10 years, approximately 10% continue to have the full syndrome (Keel *et al.,* 1999). The natural course of cases ascertained from a community study showed marked initial improvement, with only a minority continuing to meet full diagnostic criteria for bulimia nervosa, although up to two thirds had some subclinical form of eating disorder. There are few consistent predictors of longer-term outcome, but several studies have found that a shorter illness duration and reduced comorbidity are associated with a better outcome.

Binge-eating disorder

Binge-eating disorders is a proposed new category for DSM-IV. It is an area in which there is a rapid growth of knowledge. The clinical features of binge eating disorder are shown in Figure 9.8.

Aetiology

Many of the risk factors for bulimia nervosa are shared by people with binge-eating disorder although they may be less intense. Sexual and physical abuse is common, as is abuse from peers in the form of bullying, often related to fatness.

Treatment

Psychotherapy

Most of the treatments applied in bulimia nervosa (e.g. self-help approaches using CBT manuals or the computer-based packages) have been adopted for people with binge-eating disorder. Efficacy in terms of reduction in binge eating is good, although there

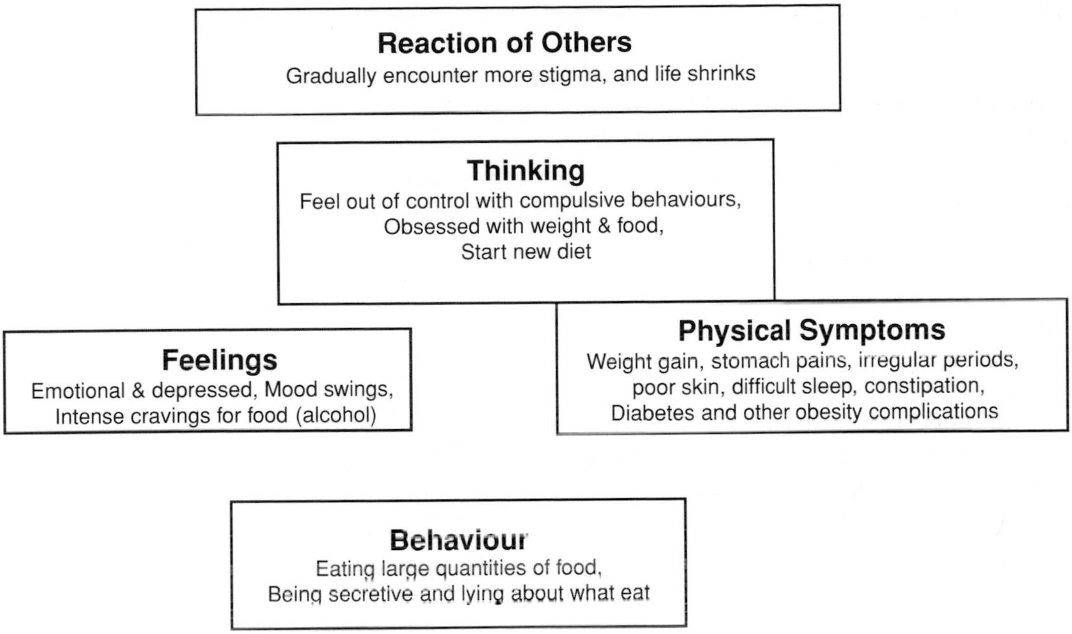

```
┌─────────────────────────────────────────────────────┐
│              Reaction of Others                     │
│   Gradually encounter more stigma, and life shrinks │
└─────────────────────────────────────────────────────┘

      ┌─────────────────────────────────────────────┐
      │                 Thinking                    │
      │  Feel out of control with compulsive        │
      │            behaviours,                      │
      │        Obsessed with weight & food,         │
      │              Start new diet                 │
      └─────────────────────────────────────────────┘

┌──────────────────────────────┐  ┌──────────────────────────────────┐
│          Feelings            │  │      Physical Symptoms           │
│  Emotional & depressed,      │  │  Weight gain, stomach pains,     │
│      Mood swings,            │  │    irregular periods,            │
│  Intense cravings for food   │  │  poor skin, difficult sleep,     │
│         (alcohol)            │  │      constipation,               │
│                              │  │  Diabetes and other obesity      │
│                              │  │      complications               │
└──────────────────────────────┘  └──────────────────────────────────┘

      ┌─────────────────────────────────────────┐
      │              Behaviour                  │
      │     Eating large quantities of food,    │
      │  Being secretive and lying about what   │
      │                eat                      │
      └─────────────────────────────────────────┘
```

Figure 9.8 The clinical picture of binge eating disorder.

is usually little success in terms of weight loss for those who are obese. Combinations of psychotherapy to manage binge eating and weight control are now frequently used.

Medication

Antidepressants or antiobesity drugs are being evaluated and are effective in reducing weight. Antidepressants (selective serotonin reuptake inhibitors) produce greater levels of remission than placebo (Arnold *et al.*, 2002; Hudson *et al.*, 1998; McElroy *et al.*, 2000) as does topiramate (McElroy *et al.*, 2003, 2004). Sibutramine, a specific noradrenaline and serotonin reuptake inhibitor, has been used in the treatment of obese patients with binge eating disorder and has been found to reduce both weight and binge frequency (Appolinario *et al.*, 2003).

Prognosis

The outcome of community ascertained binge eating disorder in terms of abnormal eating behaviour

is better than that reported for bulimia nervosa. Thus, by five years, fewer than one in five patients have any form of clinical eating disorder. However, obesity is a common outcome.

Obesity

Obesity is a condition which was embedded within psychiatric disorders in the middle of the twentieth century, when psychoanalytical methods dominated, but was not included in the initial psychiatric classification manuals. Nevertheless now that binge-eating disorder has been defined, this subtype of obesity (3%–20%) may now be included. However, the majority of cases of obesity in our current culture probably do not fulfil the necessary criteria for inclusion as a mental disorder (a clinically significant behavioural or psychological syndrome or pattern which causes distress or disability).

Obesity is caused by both genetic and environmental influences. The ready access to highly palatable and cheap food in the context of an environment in which the need for energy expenditure for activity and thermoregulation is limited have combined to produce the epidemic of obesity that is seen in many cultures. Although there are a few autosomal-dominant causes of obesity, the majority of cases are caused by multiple genes of small effect. This is a rapidly changing field, and up-to-date information is available on http://obesitygene.pbrc.edu/.

Psychiatric comorbidity

There is an increase in psychological comorbidity particularly in clinical samples (van der Merwe, 2007). Obesity is not merely considered to be a disturbance in metabolic regulation but a disturbance in reward and emotional regulation centres may account for the rapid increase in obesity in our changing environment (Zhang & Bartould, 2007).

Treatment

Behavioural and pharmacological treatments for obesity produce low to moderate initial results, and these are poorly sustained. The most effective treatments for massive obesity are surgical. There is no evidence that these procedures are contraindicated in the groups with psychiatric comorbidity. In the short term, bariatric procedures eliminate the problem of binge eating, but in the longer term, these patients may have more weight regain.

Conclusions

The history, breadth and scope of eating disorders remain in a state of flux. The clinical features of anorexia nervosa are well defined, but there are as yet few evidence-based treatments for it. The clinical features of the bulimic group of disorders are less certain, but there are high-quality clinical treatment trials, and so treatment is more certain. These are common problems of young women and can be associated with prolonged disability. Early assessment and engagement into effective treatment is essential.

REFERENCES

Agras, W. S., Walsh, T., Fairburn, C. G., *et al.* (2000). A multicenter comparison of cognitive-behavioral therapy and interpersonal psychotherapy for bulimia nervosa. *Arch Gen Psychiatry* **57**:459–66.

American Psychiatric Association. (2000). Practice guideline for the treatment of patients with eating disorders (revision). American Psychiatric Association Work Group on Eating Disorders. *Am J Psychiatry* **157**:1–39.

Anderluh, M. B., Tchanturia, K., Rabe-Hesketh, S., & Treasure, J. (2003). Childhood obsessive-compulsive personality traits in adult women with eating disorders: defining a broader eating disorder phenotype. *Am J Psychiatry* **160**:242–7.

Appolinario, J. C., Bacaltchuk, J., Sichieri, R., *et al.* (2003). A randomized, double-blind, placebo-controlled study of sibutramine in the treatment of binge-eating disorder. *Arch Gen Psychiatry* **60**:1109–16.

Arnold, L. M., McElroy, S. L., Hudson, J. I., *et al.* (2002). A placebo-controlled, randomized trial of fluoxetine in the treatment of binge-eating disorder. *J Clin Psychiatry* **63**:1028–33.

Bacaltchuk, J., Hay, P., & Mari, J. J. (2000). Antidepressants versus placebo for the treatment of bulimia nervosa: a systematic review. *Aust N Z J Psychiatry* **34**:310–17.

Bacaltchuk, J., Trefiglio, R. P., de Oliveira, I. R., *et al.* (1999). Antidepressants versus psychotherapy for bulimia nervosa: a systematic review. *J Clin Pharm Ther* **24**: 23–31.

Bacaltchuk, J., Trefiglio, R. P., Oliveira, I. R., *et al.* (2000). Combination of antidepressants and psychological treatments for bulimia nervosa: a systematic review. *Acta Psychiatr Scand* **101**:256–64.

Bara-Carril, N., Williams, C. J., Pombo-Carril, M. G., *et al.* (2004). A preliminary investigation into the feasibility and efficacy of a CD-ROM-based cognitive-behavioral self-help intervention for bulimia nervosa. *Int J Eat Disord* **35**:538–48.

Bastiani, A. M., Rao, R., Weltzin, T., & Kaye, W. H. (1995). Perfectionism in anorexia nervosa. *Int J Eat Disord* **17**:147–52.

Beumont, P., Hay, P., Beumont, D., *et al.* (2004). Australian and New Zealand clinical practice guidelines for the treatment of anorexia nervosa. *Aust N Z J Psychiatry* **38**:659–70.

Bruch, H. (1973). *Eating Disorders: Obesity, Anorexia Nervosa and the Person Within*. New York: Basic Books.

Bulik, C. M., Devlin, B., Bacanu, S. A., *et al.* (2003). Significant linkage on chromosome 10p in families with bulimia nervosa. *Am J Hum Genet* **72**:200–7.

Bulik, C. M. (2005). Exploring the gene-environment nexus in eating disorders. *J Psychiatry Neurosci* **30**(5):335–9.

Carrard, I., Rouget, P., Fernandez-Aranda, F., *et al.* (2005). Evaluation and deployment of evidence based patient self-management support program for bulimia nervosa. *Int J Med Inform* **75**:101–9.

Connan, F., & & Treasure, J. L. (1998). Stress, eating and neurobiology. In H. Hoek, J. Treasure, & & M. Katzman, eds *Neurobiology in the Treatment of Eating Disorders* London: Wiley.

Connan, F., Campbell, I. C., Katzman, M., *et al.* (2003). A neurodevelopmental model for anorexia nervosa. *Physiol Behav* **79**:13–24.

Cooper, P. (1993). *Bulimia Nervosa and Binge Eating*. London: Robinson.

Currin, L., & Schmidt, U. (2005). A critical analysis of the utility of an early intervention approach in eating disorders. *J Mental Health* **14**:611–24.

Currin, L., Schmidt, U., Treasure, J., & Jick, H. (2005). Time trends in eating disorder incidence. *Br J Psychiatry* **186**:132–5.

Dare, C., Eisler, I., Russell, G., *et al.* (2001). Psychological therapies for adults with anorexia nervosa: randomised controlled trial of out-patient treatments. *Br J Psychiatry* **178**:216–221.

Eisler, I, Le Grange, D., & Asen E (2003). Family interventions. In J. Treasure, U. Schmidt & E. Van Furth (Eds.), *Handbook of Eating Disorders*, 2nd edn. Chichester, UK: Wiley, pp. 311–25.

Eisler, I., Dare, C., Russell, G. F., *et al.* (1997). Family and individual therapy in anorexia nervosa. A 5-year follow-up. *Arch Gen Psychiatry* **54**:1025–30.

Fairburn, C. G. (1995). *Overcoming Binge Eating*. New York: Guilford Press.

Fairburn, C. G., Marcus, M. D., & Wilson G. T. (1993). Cognitive-behavioral therapy for binge eating and bulimia nervosa: a comprehensive treatment manual. In C. G. Fairburn & G. T. Wilson, eds. *Binge Eating: Nature,*

Assessment, and Treatment. New York: Guilford Press, pp. 361–404.

Fairburn, C. G. (1983). Bulimia nervosa. *Br J Hosp Med* **29**:537–42.

Fairburn, C. G., Cooper, Z., & Shafran, R. (2003). Cognitive behaviour therapy for eating disorders: a "transdiagnostic" theory and treatment. *Behav Res Ther* **41**:509–28.

Fairburn, C. G., Shafran, R., & Cooper, Z. (1999). A cognitive behavioural theory of anorexia nervosa. *Behav Res Ther* **37**:1–13.

Favaro, A., Tenconi, E., & Santonastaso, P. (2006). Perinatal factors and the risk of developing anorexia nervosa and bulimia nervosa. *Arch Gen Psychiatry* **63**:82–8.

Gillberg, I. C., Gillberg, C., Rastam, M., & Johansson, M. (1996). The cognitive profile of anorexia nervosa: a comparative study including a community-based sample. *Compr Psychiatry* **37**:23–30.

Gorwood, P., Kipman, A., & Foulon, C. (2003). The human genetics of anorexia nervosa. *Eur J Pharmacol* **480**:163–70.

Grice, D. E., Halmi, K. A., Fichter, M. M., *et al.* (2002). Evidence for a susceptibility gene for anorexia nervosa on chromosome 1. *Am J Hum Genet* **70**:787–92.

Gull, W. W. (1868). The address in medicine to the Annual Meeting of the British Medical Association at Oxford. *Lancet* **2**:171–6.

Gull, W. W. (1874). Transactions of the clinical Society of London. *Lancet* **7**.

Hay, P. (1998). The epidemiology of eating disorder behaviors: An Australian community-based survey. *Int J Eat Disord* **23**(4):371–82.

Hay, P. J., & Bacaltchuk, J. (2000). Psychotherapy for bulimia nervosa and binging (Cochrane Review). *Cochrane Database Syst Rev* **4**:CD000562.

Hudson, J. I., McElroy, S. L., Raymond, N. C., *et al.* (1998). Fluvoxamine in the treatment of binge-eating disorder: a multicenter placebo-controlled, double-blind trial. *Am J Psychiatry* **155**:1756–62.

Jacobi, C., Hayward, C., de Zwaan, M., *et al.* (2004). Coming to terms with risk factors for eating disorders: application of risk terminology and suggestions for a general taxonomy. *Psychol Bull* **130**:19–65.

Jacobi, F., Wittchen, H. U., Holting, C., *et al.* (2004). Prevalence, co-morbidity and correlates of mental disorders in the general population: results from the German Health Interview and Examination Survey (GHS). *Psychol Med* **34**:597–611.

Keel, P. K., & Klump, K. L. (2003). Are eating disorders culture-bound syndromes? Implications for conceptualizing their etiology. *Psychol Bull* **129**:747–69.

Keel, P. K., Mitchell, J. E., Miller, K. B. *et al.* (1999). Long-term outcome of bulimia nervosa. *Arch Gen Psychiatry* **56**:63–9.

Lee, S., Ho, T. P., Hsu, L. K. (1993). Fat phobic and non-fat phobic anorexia nervosa: a comparative study of 70 Chinese patients in Hong Kong. *Psychol Med* **23**(4):999–1017.

Lee, S., Lee, A. M., Ngai, E., Lee, D. T., Wing, Y. K. (2001). Rationales for food refusal in Chinese patients with anorexia nervosa. *Int J Eat Disord* **29**(2):224–9.

Lock, J., Le Grange, D., Agras, W. S., & Dare, C. (2001). *Treatment Manual for Anorexia Nervosa. A Family Based Approach.* New York: Guilford Press.

Lock, J., Agras, W. S., Bryson, S., & Kraemer, H. C. (2005). A comparison of short- and long-term family therapy for adolescent anorexia nervosa. *J Am Acad Child Adolesc Psychiatry* **44**:632–9.

Matsunaga, H., Kaye, W. H., McConaha, C., *et al.* (2000). Personality disorders among subjects recovered from eating disorders. *Int J Eat Disord* **27**:353–7.

McElroy, S. L., Arnold, L. M., Shapira, N. A., *et al.* (2003). Topiramate in the treatment of binge eating disorder associated with obesity: a randomized, placebo-controlled trial. *Am J Psychiatry* **160**:255–61.

McElroy, S. L., Casuto, L. S., Nelson, E. B., *et al.* (2000). Placebo-controlled trial of sertraline in the treatment of binge eating disorder. *Am J Psychiatry* **157**:1004–6.

McElroy, S. L., Shapira, N. A., Arnold, L. M., *et al.* (2004). Topiramate in the long-term treatment of binge-eating disorder associated with obesity. *J Clin Psychiatry* **65**:1463–9.

McIntosh, V. V., Jordan, J., Carter, F. A., *et al.* (2005). Three psychotherapies for anorexia nervosa: a randomized, controlled trial. *Am J Psychiatry* **162**:741–7.

National Collaborating Centre for Mental Health (2004). National Clinical Practice Guideline: Eating disorders: core interventions in the treatment and management of anorexia nervosa, bulimia nervosa, and related eating disorders. National Institute for Clinical Excellence [online]. Available at http://www.nice.org.uk.

Nielsen, S., Moller-Madsen, S., Isager, T., *et al.* (1998). Standardized mortality in eating disorders—a quantitative summary of previously published and new evidence. *J Psychosom Res* **44**:413–34.

Owen, J. B. (1998). Models of eating disturbances in animals. In H. W. Hoek, J. L. Treasure, & M. A. Katzman, eds. *Neurobiology in the Treatment of Eating Disorders.* Chichester, UK: Wiley, pp. 169–94.

Patel, P., Wheatcroft, R., Park, R. J., & Stein, A. (2002). The children of mothers with eating disorders. *Clin Child Fam Psychol Rev* **5**:1–19.

Peveler, R. C., Bryden, K. S., Neil, H. A., *et al.* (2005). The relationship of disordered eating habits and attitudes to clinical outcomes in young adult females with type 1 diabetes. *Diabetes Care* **28**:84–8.

Russell, G. (1979). Bulimia nervosa: an ominous variant of anorexia nervosa. *Psychol Med* **3**:429–48.

Schmidt, U., & Treasure, J. (2006). Anorexia nervosa: valued and visible. A cognitive-interpersonal maintenance model and its implications for research and practice. *Br J Clin Psychol* **45**:343–66.

Schmidt, U., & Treasure, J. (1993). *Getting Better Bit(e) by Bit(e). A Survival Kit for Sufferers of Bulimia Nervosa and Binge Eating Disorder.* Hove, UK: Brunner-Routledge.

Shoebridge, P., & Gowers, S. G. (2000). Parental high concern and adolescent-onset anorexia nervosa. A case-control study to investigate direction of causality. *Br J Psychiatry* **176**:132–7.

Southgate, L., Tchanturia, K., & Treasure, J. (2005). Building a model of the aetiology of eating disorders by translating experimental neuroscience into clinical practice. *J Mental Health* **14**:553–66.

Spitzer, R. L., Devlin, B., Walsh, A., *et al.* (1991). Binge eating disorder: to be or not to be in DSMIV. *Int J Eat Disord* **10**:627–9.

Srinivasagam, N. M., Kaye, W. H., Plotnicov, K. H., *et al.* (1995). Persistent perfectionism, symmetry, and exactness after long-term recovery from anorexia nervosa. *Am J Psychiatry* **152**:1630–4.

Steinhausen, H. C. (2002). The outcome of anorexia nervosa in the 20th century. *Am J Psychiatry* **159**:1284–93.

Stice, E. (2002). Risk and maintenance factors for eating pathology: a meta-analytic review. *Psychol Bull* **128**:825–48.

Strober, M., Freeman, R., Lampert, C., Diamond, J., Kaye, W. (2000). Controlled family study of anorexia nervosa and bulimia nervosa: evidence of shared liability and transmission of partial syndromes. *Am J Psychiatry* **157**(3):393–401.

Treasure, J., & Schmidt, U. (2005). The early phase of eating disorders. *J Mental Health* **14**:535–38.

Treasure, J., Tchanturia, K., & Schmidt, U. (2005). Developing a model of the treatment for eating disorder: using neuroscience research to examine the how rather than the what of change. *Counsel Psychother Res* **5**:187–90.

Van Der Merwe, M. T. (2007). Psychological correlates of obesity in women. *Int J Obes* (Lond) **2**:S14–S18.

Van Hoeken D., Seidell, J. C., Hoek, H. W. (2003). Epidemiology. In J. Treasure, E. F. van Furth, & U. Schmidt, eds. *Handbook of Eating Disorders*, 2nd edn. Chichester, UK: Wiley, pp. 11–34.

Waller, G., & Kennerley, H. (2003). Cognitive-behavioral treatments. In J. Treasure, E. Van Furth, & U. Schmidt, eds. *Handbook of Eating Disorders*, 2nd edn. Chichester, UK: Wiley, pp. 233–52.

Zheng, H., & Berthoud, H. R. (2007). Eating for pleasure or calories. *Curr Opin Pharmacol* **7**(6):607–12.

10

Alcohol problems

Ilana B. Crome and Roger Bloor

This chapter outlines the historical background, current classificatory systems for diagnosis, psychological and physical related disorders, the epidemiology of alcohol disorders, the "drivers" of drinking behaviour as we currently conceptualise them and a range of approaches as well as treatment assessment, management and cost-effectiveness.

Historical background

The term *alcoholism* was coined by the Swede Magnus Huss (1849) to describe "those disease manifestations which without any direct connection with organic changes of the nervous system take on a chronic form in persons who, over long periods, have partaken of large quantities of brandy" (Crome, 1995). Physicians in America (Rush, 1785) and Britain (Trotter, 1804) made graphic descriptions, but sound contributions, which have stood the test of time. They recognised and diagnosed the vast array of clinical presentations.

Jellinek (1946) described the evolution of drinking behaviour and, in a summary of a series of his lectures (World Health Organisation [WHO], 1952), recognised the heterogeneity of the condition and described five species of alcoholism:

alpha: representing a purely psychological continued dependence without loss of control or inability to abstain

beta: physical complications without physical or psychological dependence

gamma: acquired tissue tolerance, adaptive cell metabolism, physical dependence and loss of control

delta: shares the first three features of gamma, but inability to abstain replaces loss of control

epsilon: dipsomania or periodic alcoholism

In 1955, the World Health Organisation made the distinction between the physical and psychological basis of alcohol-seeking behaviour. Craving was considered an appropriate construct for people who were drinking for the effect of alcohol – that is, to control withdrawal symptoms or physical dependence. Jellinek did not view craving as a marker of psychosocial dependence – that is, during abstinence with no withdrawal symptoms. Jellinek also proposed that, when physically dependent, one drink would reinstate craving. This was in keeping with the disease concept of alcoholism.

A number of studies questioned this view that "one drink led to one drunk", because loss of control was not demonstrated to be an inevitable outcome of one drink or some drinks (Gottheil *et al.,* 1972; Mello & Mendelson, 1965; Paredes *et al.,* 1973). This research reinforced the notion of a psychological dimension to "craving", as well as a physical one.

Essential Psychiatry, ed. Robin M. Murray, Kenneth S. Kendler, Peter McGuffin, Simon Wessely, David J. Castle.
Published by Cambridge University Press. © Cambridge University Press 2008.

The alcohol dependence syndrome

Edwards and Gross (1976) described and included as essential the following components of the alcohol dependence syndrome:

- a subjective awareness of compulsion to drink,
- increased tolerance to alcohol,
- repeated withdrawal symptoms, and
- relief or avoidance of withdrawal symptoms by further drinking.

This provisional description of a syndrome considered complex issues, for example, decreased tolerance, the possibility of tolerance without dependence, the sequencing of withdrawal symptoms over years, the unresolved association between withdrawal and increased intake and the dual cues of withdrawal relief *and* avoidance, as well as the nuances of craving, loss of control and compulsion to drink. The *dependence syndrome* concept is useful in that it provides an agreed set of clinical criteria or constellation of symptomatology from which a diagnosis can be made, thus improving communication not only between health professionals but also for researchers. Further, over time this capacity to differentiate the more from the less severely dependent individual has been demonstrated to have some predictive power (Edwards *et al.*, 2003). One practical result has been the development of numerous questionnaires for assessment and to measure severity of dependence (see Table 10.1).

Classification

There have been a number of revisions of both the American Psychiatric Association's *Diagnostic and Statistical Manual* (DSM) and the World Health Organisation's *International Classification of Diseases* (ICD). Despite this, Rounsaville and colleagues (1993) and others (Hasin *et al.*, 1988; Kosten *et al.*, 1987) have found high agreement for the dependence syndrome construct across the three diagnostic systems DSM-III-R (the third revised edition), DSM-IV (the fourth edition; APA, 1994) and ICD-10 (10th revision; WHO 1992).

The ICD-10 includes a strong desire or sense of compulsion to use substances, impaired capacity to control substance use, a physiological withdrawal state with withdrawal relief and avoidance, tolerance, a preoccupation with substance use and persistent substance use despite clear evidence of harmful consequences. DSM-IV includes tolerance, withdrawal, a persistent desire for or unsuccessful effort to control substance use, substances taken in larger amounts or over longer periods than intended, time spent in obtaining substances, reduction in obligations and activities and continued use despite knowledge about harmful consequences. DSM-IV does not include craving or compulsion to take substances but concedes that "craving" (a strong subjective desire to use the substance) is likely to be experienced by most (if not all) individuals with substance dependence. DSM-IV also specifies characteristics of the withdrawal syndrome and goes on to state that "withdrawal is usually but not always associated with substance dependence" and that "most (perhaps all) individuals with the withdrawal state have a craving to re administer the substance to reduce the symptoms". Only three criteria need be present to diagnose a substance use disorder. Withdrawal symptoms and withdrawal relief, and compulsion to take the substance (in ICD-10 only), need not be present to diagnose dependence in either set of criteria (see Table 10.2).

Epidemiology

In the United Kingdom, a unit is 8 grams of pure alcohol, equivalent to half a pint of ordinary beer, a small glass of wine (9% strength), or one measure of spirits. In the Interim Analytical Report the following definitions were used (The Prime Minister's Strategy Unit, 2003):

Binge drinking: Over twice the daily guidelines in one day (8 units for men, 6 units for women).

Low to moderate: Weekly, drinking up to 14 units for women and 21 units for men.

Table 10.1 Questionnaires for the assessment of alcohol problems and to determine their severity

Test	Description
ADS (Alcohol Dependence Scale; Skinner & Allen, 1982, 1983; Skinner & Horn, 1984)	The 25-item ADS takes approximately 10 minutes to complete and measures severity of dependence.
APQ (Alcohol Problems Questionnaire; Drummond, 1990)	This is a 44-item self-report instrument, which covers physical, psychological and social problems associated with substance use.
ASI (Addiction Severity Index; McLellan *et al.*, 1980)	This is a 161-item clinical and research instrument delivered by face-to-face structured interview.
AUDIT (Alcohol Use Disorders Identification Test; Saunders *et al.*, 1993)	This is a 10-item questionnaire, covering quantity, frequency, inability to control drinking, withdrawal relief, loss of memory, injury and concern by others. A score of 8 or more indicates that the person is drinking to a degree that is harmful or hazardous, whereas a score of 13 or more in women and 15 or more in men is indicative of dependent drinking. It is a very useful and widely used scale.
CAGE (Ewing, 1984)	The CAGE questionnaire is a simple, easily administered instrument, which has only four items: 1. Have you ever felt like **c**utting down on your drinking? 2. Have people **a**nnoyed or criticized you for drinking? 3. Have you ever felt bad or **g**uilty about your drinking? 4. Have you ever had a drink first thing in the morning to steady your nerves or to get rid of a hangover (**e**ye opener)? A positive answer should raise suspicion of an alcohol problem, and a score of 2 is highly suggestive of one. The instrument takes 30 seconds to administer
CIWA-Ar (Clinical Institute Withdrawal Assessment for Alcohol; Sullivan *et al.*, 1989)	Health professionals use this scale to rate the severity of alcohol withdrawal. It consists of 10 items, 9 of which can be scored on a range of 0–7 and one on a range of 0–4 (total of 67). It can be used regularly throughout the day and night to assess the extent of withdrawal and the impact of treatment. It covers nausea; tremor; paroxysmal sweating; anxiety; agitation; auditory, visual and tactile disturbances; headache and orientation.
LDQ (Leeds Dependence Questionnaire; Raistrick *et al.*, 1994)	Ten items, concentrating on the psychological aspects of dependence.
MAST (Michigan Alcohol Screening Test; Selzer, 1971)	This is a simple, self-report, 25-item test, which has yes/no answers. A score of 3–5 is an early indicator of a problem drinker, whereas someone who scores 6 or more is highly likely to be a problem drinker. There are variants on this test, e.g. the Brief MAST, which can discriminate problem drinkers from nonproblem drinkers on the basis of 10 items only. There are also a G-MAST and a Brief G-MAST for older people, which have a slightly different phraseology to capture the problems that may lead to or reflect older people who drink too much.

(cont.)

Table 10.1 (*cont.*)

Test	Description
SADQ (Severity of Alcohol Dependence Questionnaire; Stockwell *et al.*, 1979, 1983)	A short, self-administered, 20-item questionnaire designed to measure severity of dependence on alcohol.
SAPC (Substance Abuse Problem Checklist; Carroll, 1984)	This focuses on both drug and alcohol problems.
SADD (Short Alcohol Dependence Data; Davidson & Raistrick, 1986; Raistrick *et al.*, 1983)	This was designed as a brief (15-item) self-report measure of alcohol dependence and assesses behavioural, subjective and psychobiological changes associated with alcohol dependence. It is for the use of both clinicians and researchers and is aimed at the mildly to moderately dependent general adult population. It can be completed in 2–5 minutes.

Heavy to moderate: Weekly, drinking 14–35 units for women and 21–50 units for men.

Very heavy drinking: Weekly consumption of 35 units or more for women, and 50 units or more for men.

Chronic: Sustained drinking, which is causing or is likely to cause harm.

At present, it is estimated that 4.7 million of the UK population are abstainers, 6.4 million are drinking up to 35 units (women) or 50 units (men), while 1.8 million drink at the 35/50 level or over. Moreover, the per capita consumption in 2001 was 8.6 litres of pure alcohol – an increase of 121% since 1951, and between 1970 and 2000, consumption increased 5 times over. In comparison to other countries, UK consumption is rising, especially in women and young people, although UK adults are not among the heaviest consumers in Europe. British teenagers, however, are amongst the heaviest consumers in Europe (Hibbell *et al.*, 2000).

When considering the overall population impact, it is quantity of alcohol and pattern of drinking, as well as the harm accrued and the development of dependence, that need to be taken into account. "Binge drinking" in young people has become a particular source of concern in some countries. Although it is postulated that this behaviour does not necessarily persist into adult life, there are concerns that harms accrued during this period

may be damaging in the long term. There is considerable interest around the "risk" of harm, for example, heavy alcohol intake may lead to cirrhosis, but "moderate" consumption may reduce the risk of coronary artery disease.

Younger drinkers are more likely to suffer accidents, assaults and acute intoxication. It is estimated that 30,000 hospital admissions per year are due to alcohol dependence syndrome, and 150,000 are related to alcohol misuse, while 20,000 alcohol misusers die prematurely. At a conservative estimate, this costs the National Health Service £1.9 bn, and this excludes the cost to families and communities, partly due to alcohol-related crime and public order offences. In this context, there are 1.2 million incidents of alcohol-related violence, 80,000 arrests for drunk and disorderly behaviour, 360,000 arrests for domestic violence, and 80,000 drink driving cases per year. These crimes include fatalities (approximately 500) and 17,000 injuries. The cost is calculated at £7.3 bn, and the emotional cost is inestimable. Unemployment and decreased productivity are additional consequences and costs. The wider, and more difficult to quantify, social harms cannot be ignored. Family relationships, stability and income diminish, with an estimated 1 million children affected by alcohol misuse in the family. Alcohol dependence is associated with homelessness and "rough sleepers".

Table 10.2 Comparison of Edwards and Gross' Alcohol Dependence Syndrome, DSM-IV and ICD-10 criteria for alcohol dependence (Heather *et al.*, 2001)

Alcohol Dependence Syndrome	DSM-IV (American Psychiatric Association, 1994)	ICD-10 (World Health Organisation, 1992)
	A. A maladaptive pattern of substance use, leading to clinically significant impairment or distress as manifested by three or more of the following occurring at any time in the same 12-month period:	A. Three or more of the following have been experienced at some time over the previous year:
(3) Increased tolerance to alcohol	(1) Tolerance, as defined by either of the following: (a) Need for markedly increased amounts of a substance to achieve intoxication or desired effect (b) Markedly diminished effect with continued use of the same amount of the substance.	(d) Evidence of tolerance, such that increased dosages are required to achieve effects originally produced by lower dosage
(4) Repeated withdrawal symptoms (5) Relief or avoidance of withdrawal by further drinking (2) Salience of drink-seeking behaviour	(2) Withdrawal, as manifested by either of the following: (a) characteristic withdrawal syndrome for the substance, or (b) the same (or a closely related substance is taken to relieve or avoid) withdrawal symptoms. (3) The substance is often taken in larger amounts or over a longer period than was intended (4) There is a persistent desire or unsuccessful efforts to cut down or control substance use (5) A great deal of time is spent in activities necessary to obtain the substance, use the substance, or recover from its effects	(c) A physiological withdrawal state when substance use has ceased or been reduced evidenced by: characteristic withdrawal syndrome, or use of the same (or a closely related) substance with the intention of relieving or avoiding withdrawal symptoms (b) Difficulties in controlling substance-taking behaviour in terms of its onset, termination, or levels of use
(1) Narrowing of the drinking repertoire	(6) Important social, occupational or recreational activities are given up or reduced because of substance use (7) The substance use is continued despite knowledge of having a persistent or recurrent physical or psychological problem that is likely to have been caused or exacerbated by the substance.	(e) Progressive neglect of alternative pleasures or interests because of substance use, increased amount of time necessary to obtain or take the substance or to recover from its effects (f) Persisting with substance use despite clear evidence of overtly harmful consequences, such as harm to the liver through excessive drinking, depressive mood states consequent to heavy substance use, or drug-related impairment of cognitive functioning. Efforts should be made to determine that the user was actually, or could be expected to be, aware of the nature and extent of the harm.

Table 10.2 (*cont.*)

Alcohol Dependence Syndrome	DSM-IV (American Psychiatric Association, 1994)	ICD-10 (World Health Organisation, 1992)
	Specifiers • With physiological dependence (1) or (2) • Without physiological dependence	
	Course specifiers: • Early Full Remission • Early Partial Remission • Sustained Full Remission • Sustained Partial Remission • On Agonist Therapy • In a Controlled Environment	
(7) Rapid reinstatement of symptoms after a period abstinence		
(6) Subjective awareness of compulsion to drink		(a) A strong desire or sense of compulsion to take the substance

DSM IV = *Diagnostic and Statistical Manual of Mental Disorders*, 4th edn.; ICD-10; *International Classification of Diseases*, 10th revision.

There are a host of "reasons" people drink and which factors, or what interaction of factors, may influence their decisions. These may include increasing availability, low price, promotion of drinks aimed at a particular group, peer pressure, a culture which encourages "drinking to get drunk", early onset of drinking, parental divorce, poor parental supervision, parental drinking, age, sex, region of the country, genetic predisposition and personality type. Associations or correlations between some of these so-called risk factors do not equate to causality, so decreasing or eliminating one or more should not result in the expected reduction. There are as many potential preventive and treatment "interventions", which include political, social, medical, psychiatric and economic measures. Some may be implemented before the drinker ever experiences a "problem", in many different settings; some may be at crisis point. Currently it is acknowledged that those drinkers who access the health system are the more severely affected, whilst binge drinkers may be subject to criminal justice measures; whereas the entire population could benefit from educational interventions and market forces, for example, supply and pricing. Thus any policy needs to be sustainable, coherent, long-term and pragmatic.

"Dual diagnosis" or coexisting substance problems and psychological disorder

The terms *comorbidity*, *dual diagnosis* and *coexisting/ co-occurring substance problems and psychological disorder* are used interchangeably (Crawford *et al.*, 2003). Other terms which cover this are *mental illness and chemical abuse, chemical addiction and mental illness* and *co-occurring addictive and mental disorders*.

Comorbidity may present itself in a range of combinations and permutations, including the following:

- Substance use – even one dose – may lead to psychological symptoms or psychiatric syndromes.
- Harmful use may produce psychiatric symptoms.
- Dependence may produce psychological symptoms.
- Intoxication by a substance may produce psychological symptoms.
- Withdrawal from substances may produce psychological symptoms.
- Withdrawal from substances may produce psychiatric syndromes.
- Substance use may exacerbate a preexisting psychiatric disorder.
- Psychological morbidity not amounting to a "disorder" may precipitate substance use.
- Primary psychiatric disorder may lead to substance use disorder.
- Primary psychiatric disorder may precipitate substance use disorder, which may in turn lead to psychiatric disorder (Crome, 1999).

In the Epidemological Catchment Area study in the United States (Regier *et al.*, 1990), 47% of people misused substances: 37% misused alcohol. Schuckit *et al.* (1997) highlighted that two thirds of alcohol-dependent patients entering treatment had anxiety, sadness, manic conditions or severe and pervasive antisocial behaviours.

Similarly, the COGA (genetics of alcoholism) study (Bierut *et al.*, 2002) demonstrated that the alcohol-dependent group had a significantly higher lifetime rate of independent disorders than the control subjects. Nearly 10% of alcohol-dependent subjects had at least one of four independent major anxiety disorders, compared with 3.7% among control subjects. In almost 80% of those who were alcohol dependent, onset of the anxiety disorder predated alcohol dependence. In subjects with independent major depressive disorder, manic depression, social phobia and agoraphobia, a significantly higher rate of similar independent psychiatric disorder among first-degree relatives was found than in those of control subjects. It should be noted that there was a higher rate of concurrent – but not independent – depressive disorder in those patients with alcohol dependence. Of interest, however, is that, in the relatives of those labelled "concurrent",

a higher rate of "independent" depression was found.

Bipolar affective disorder poses a particular risk of alcohol misuse (Brady & Sonne, 1995; Feinman & Dunner, 1996; Goldberg *et al.*, 1999), as does schizophrenia, which is associated with patients being three times more likely to abuse alcohol than those without it (Ries *et al.*, 2000).

In the most recent national comorbidity study in the United Kingdom (Coulthard *et al.*, 2002), 12% of men and 3% of women were dependent on alcohol. This behaviour was likely to be associated with more frequent visits to their general practitioners, receiving treatment or accessing mental health services. In general, this dovetails with other findings which demonstrate that comorbidity leads to more frequent recurrence of mental disorder, greater time spent in hospital and increased violence, homelessness and family disintegration.

Some important clinical issues to emerge from these findings include that often substance use or misuse is not limited to one substance. Also, the distinction as to whether a psychiatric disorder preceded or is the result of substance use disorder can be difficult to make. It is important to be cognisant of the role of early childhood psychiatric disorder, and the likelihood that this might predispose to substance misuse in later life.

Physical consequences of alcohol misuse

The physical complications of alcohol use are numerous. The level of risk globally is equivalent to that of malaria, tuberculosis and measles and is far greater then the risks from tobacco or illegal drugs (Jernigan *et al.*, 2000). The health risks relate to the pharmacological effects of alcohol, withdrawal, toxicity and deficiency syndromes as a result of chronic abuse and from secondary effects such as domestic violence and injury resulting from drunk-driving offences. Some studies have demonstrated a protective effect of low levels of alcohol intake for some diseases, but this needs to be balanced against the clear evidence of harm from excessive or prolonged heavy consumption (Gaziano *et al.*, 2000).

Central nervous system

There is no absolute threshold for blood alcohol concentrations below which there is no impairment of complex psychomotor skills (Ogden & Moskowitz, 2004). At blood alcohol concentrations (BAC) of 25 mg%, euphoria is apparent, lack of co-ordination occurs at levels of 50 to 100 mg% and unsteadiness, ataxia, poor judgement and labile mood are observed at 100 to 200 mg%. At 200 to 400 mg%, the drinker may be in a stage 1 anaesthetic state, with periods of amnesia. Intoxication can lead to death from coma and respiratory depression at 400 to 700 mg%. Acute intoxication with alcohol may result in coma or death resulting from CNS depression, leading to respiratory depression and cardiovascular collapse. Intoxicated patients are at an increased risk for other traumatic and medical pathologies that may precipitate or be exacerbated by head injury, infection or hypoglycaemia, which must be ruled out or appropriately treated. Toxicology analysis is thus mandatory in such cases, and the expertise of physicians is essential. The effects of raised alcohol levels are modified by age, sex and degree of alcohol dependence; a high level of tolerance is indicated by high alcohol levels associated with low levels of apparent impairment.

Alcohol withdrawal syndromes

These may be precipitated by a variety of circumstances, including lack of money to purchase alcohol, acute illness or injury, nausea and vomiting or a decision to stop drinking. Alcohol withdrawal syndromes (AWS) can be classified by severity into mild, moderate or severe (see Box 10.1). In clinical practice, severity is often seen to present along a continuum from mild tremor through to delirium and convulsions. It is probable that the components of this continuum comprise a series of symptom clusters related to the specific neurochemical system which is involved (Raistrick, 2001).

Seizures, hallucinations and delirium tremens (DT) are considered major phenomena. Seizures can occur with any severity level of withdrawal but are normally seen 12 to 48 hours after stopping

---

Box 10.1 Alcohol withdrawal severity

Mild alcohol withdrawal

Occurs less than 24 hours after stopping or decreasing alcohol intake. It may include tremulousness, anxiety, nausea, vomiting, sweating, hyperreflexia and minor autonomic hyperactivity.

Moderate alcohol withdrawal

An intermediate position along the continuum with the hallmark of hallucinosis but an otherwise clear sensorium

Severe Alcohol Withdrawal

Occurs more than 24 hours and up to 5 days after stopping or decreasing alcohol intake. It is characterized by disorientation, agitation, hallucinations and severe autonomic derangement.

---

alcohol (Lishman, 1987). Seizures may also be secondary to intoxication or trauma or as a toxic effect of alcohol.

DT has a mortality of about 5%, the severity generally being related to a previous history of delirium tremens, heavy alcohol consumption and the presence of physical illness. The condition begins 2 to 3 days after stopping or decreasing alcohol intake and peaks within about a week (Chick, 1989).

A quantitative score system enables more objective monitoring and evaluation of interventions. The Clinical Institute Withdrawal Assessment for Alcohol (CIWA-Ar) scale (Sullivan et al., 1989) is a short 10-item scale for clinical measurement of the severity of the alcohol withdrawal syndrome which can be completed in a few minutes by nursing staff. Points are assigned for categories of symptoms and signs including sweating, anxiety, tremor, agitation, hallucinations, nausea and vomiting, headache, orientation and impaired consciousness.

Neurological nutritional deficiency syndromes

These must be considered in alcohol abusers (Lishman, 1990). The initial presentation of nutritional deficiency may be of peripheral neuropathy and cardiovascular disorder, for example, hypotension or high-output cardiac failure (e.g. beriberi) in combination with oral inflammation, and this is the result of thiamine deficiency. Peripheral neuropathy may be caused by toxicity and vitamin deficiency and may be mild peripheral or a severe incapacitating sensorimotor neuropathy. Lower limbs are affected more than upper, but foot and wrist drop, distal muscle weakness and wasting may be noted. Pellagra (niacin and protein deficiency) and scurvy (vitamin C deficiency) are less common (Cook *et al.*, 1998).

The most important presentation of nutritional deficiency is the Wernicke-Korsakoff syndrome (WKS), which is consequent on thiamine deficiency. Wernicke's encephalopathy (WE) and Korsakoff's psychosis (KP) are both part of this syndrome. WE is a potentially reversible neurological condition which, if untreated, is fatal in 17% of cases, with permanent brain damage occurring in 85% of patients who are inappropriately managed. Postmortem findings indicate that the diagnosis of WE is missed in up to 90% of patients (Thomson *et al.*, 2002). In its classic form, it is characterised by the triad of ocular abnormalities, ataxia and a global confusional state. This classic triad is found in only 16% of patients (Harper *et al.*, 1986), and the onset of the syndrome may be acute or gradual, evolving over several days.

KP presents as lack of insight, apathy and antegrade and retrograde amnesia with confabulation. Although originally seen as a distinct syndrome, it is now viewed as part of the progression of WKS and has been shown to share an underlying causation and a common neuropathological basis. Findings from postmortem studies have shown that the most common abnormalities in WKS are in the areas surrounding the cerebral aqueduct and the third and fourth ventricles. The thalamus, mammillary bodies and the cerebellum are also affected (Harper *et al.*, 2003).

A variety of brain lesions related to alcohol have been defined (Charness, 1993; Viola *et al.*, 2001). Alcohol toxicity, probably causing neuronal loss, results in cerebral dementia. Initially this may come to light only following psychological testing or the observation of dilated ventricles and cortical atrophy on magnetic resonance imaging or computed tomography scans. Reversibility can occur with abstinence. Alcoholic cerebellar degeneration presents as gross ataxia, and the pathology is that of cell loss. It may respond to thiamine in the early stages. Central pontine myelinolysis, a rare condition, results from demyelination, presents with pseudo-bulbar palsy and may be fatal. Extrapontine myelinolysis in chronic alcoholism results in Marchiafava-Bignami syndrome due to demyelination of the corpus callosum (Gabriel *et al.*, 1999).

Liver disease and gastrointestinal disorder

Alcoholic liver disease is a very common cause of morbidity and mortality in the developed world (Tome & Lucey, 2004), and there is a dose-dependent increase in relative risk of developing alcohol-induced liver disease for both men and women, with the steepest increase among women (Becker *et al.*, 1996).

The spectrum of liver disease is not uniform but can be described under three main headings: fatty liver, alcoholic hepatitis and cirrhosis. In reality, there is considerable overlap in the clinical setting (Baptista *et al.*, 1981; see Box 10.2).

Alcoholic fatty liver results from the inhibition of oxidation of fatty acids combined with an increased ingeneration of triglycerides. The effects can be reversed within a few weeks of abstinence from alcohol. Fatty liver is generally asymptomatic and may in the early stages produce no changes in liver function tests other than those related to the direct effect of the alcohol on liver function. It may, however, present with right abdominal pain, nausea and vomiting, which resolve on abstinence.

Alcoholic hepatitis and cirrhosis result from chronic alcohol abuse. *Alcoholic hepatitis* produces liver cell necrosis and inflammation and can raise AST, ALT and bilirubin levels. AST activity is higher than that of ALT in alcoholic hepatitis and Reye syndrome, in contrast to most other types of liver disease in which ALT is higher (Dufour *et al.*, 2000). The clinical presentation is with jaundice, pyrexia, right

Box 10.2 Management of disorders associated with alcoholic liver disease

- Ascites is treated with diuretics and sodium restriction and possibly paracentesis.
- Encephalopathy is treated by protein restriction and lactilol or lactulose.
- Variceal haemorrhage is treated by transfusion, reduction of portal venous pressure with vasoactive drugs, oesophageal tamponade and sclerosis of the varices.
- Propylthiouracil has been used to treat chronic alcoholic liver disease. A recent Cochrane review concluded that there is no evidence for using propylthiouracil for alcoholic liver disease outside randomised clinical trials (Rambaldi & Gluud, 2002). Adapted from Klatsky, 2000.

abdominal pain, ascites and possible encephalopathy. In patients with poor liver function and a prothrombin time prolonged to a degree which precludes liver biopsy, the prognosis is poor, with a third of patients dying in the acute episode (Finlayson *et al.*, 2000). Severe acute alcoholic hepatitis has a poor outcome with standard supportive management. The reported mortality rate of patients with severe alcoholic hepatitis is between 35% and 46% (Tome & Lucey, 2004).

Cirrhosis involves a permanent loss of liver cells, which are replaced by fibrosis with loss of the normal liver architecture. It may be asymptomatic or present with gastrointestinal symptoms, ascites, encephalopathy and oesophageal varices, which may cause haemorrhage. Liver function tests may be normal until the process is advanced and diagnosis is confirmed by biopsy. Obviously, abstinence and good nutrition are mandatory. Prognosis is poor unless alcohol intake ceases; overall only 25% of patients with cirrhosis survive 5 years from diagnosis (Finlayson *et al.*, 2000).

Acute and chronic pancreatitis and gastritis and peptic ulcer are other gastrointestinal consequences of alcohol abuse. More than 70% of cases of chronic pancreatitis are caused by long-term heavy alcohol abuse which may in addition result in severe weight loss, diabetes and malabsorption syndrome.

Cancer

Chronic alcohol consumption is a strong risk factor for cancer in the oral cavity, pharynx, hypopharynx, larynx and oesophagus and is also a major aetiological factor in hepatocarcinogenesis. Alcohol also increases the risk for cancer of the colorectum and the breast (Poschl *et al.*, 2004). The exact mechanism underlying this association is not understood, but acetaldehyde, a potent mutagen and carcinogen, is seen as the possible link (Poschl & Seitz, 2004).

Heavy drinkers are more likely to be heavy smokers, and the increased risk from each substance problem appears to be potentiated by the combination; men who both smoke and drink are nearly 38 times more likely to develop head and neck cancers than men who do neither (Romberger & Grant, 2004). The risk of developing cancer of the oesophagus is 50 times greater in heavy drinkers and heavy smokers than in those who abstain. It has been estimated that 25% to 68% of upper aerodigestive tract cancers are attributable to alcohol and that up to 80% of these tumours could be prevented by abstaining from alcohol and smoking (Poschl & Seitz, 2004).

Cardiovascular disease

The effects of alcohol on the cardiovascular system are well documented and range from the protective effects of light drinking for ischemeic stroke and coronary disease through to the increased risk from heavy drinking for haemorragic stroke, cardiomyopathy, hypertension and cardiac arythmias.

Reviews of studies of the balance of risk versus protection from alcohol have concluded that the balance of harm and benefit does not support recommendations to the public to increase consumption to prevent coronary heart disease. Whether the benefits for cardiovascular disease persist at heavier drinking levels or are attenuated is not relevant in terms of health policy, because harm in terms of overall mortality from high levels of intake outweighs any benefits in the reduction of cardiovascular disease (Sesso, 2001; see Table 10.3).

Table 10.3 Risk and protective factors of alcohol for cardiovascular disease

Disease	Low alcohol intake	High alcohol intake
Cardiomyopathy	No relationship	Causal
Hypertension	No relationship	Causal
Coronary disease	Protective	Possibly protective
Arrhythmia	No relationship	Causal
Haemorrhagic stroke	Possible increased risk	Increased risk
Ischaemic stroke	Protective	Possibly protective

Other alcohol-related disorders

Muscle disease

- Alcohol-related skeletal muscle myopathy is more common than any other alcohol-induced disease (Preedy *et al.,* 2003). The acute clinical symptoms include muscle pain, progressive weakness, reduced mobility and frequent falls. In its chronic form, it may present with progressive painless wasting and reduced power in all limbs.

Bone disease

- Alcohol-related fractures are common in chronic alcohol misuse and are associated with reduced bone mass and a higher incidence of osteoporosis. Poor nutrition and associated smoking habits contribute to the risks of fracture.
- Reviews of the effects of alcohol on bone have concluded that there is a detrimental effect of chronic alcohol abuse on the skeleton of men and a neutral or beneficial effect of light to moderate alcohol consumption, especially in older women (Turner, 2000).
- The protective effect of oestrogen levels on women has also been confirmed in a study of bone density in women who drink modest amounts of alcohol (Turner & Sibonga, 2001).

Skin disease

- In a study of 100 patients with alcohol dependence, more than 80% had significant skin lesions, including acne, folliculitis, seborrheic dermatitis, tinea pedis, xerosis and rosacea (Parish & Fine, 1985).
- The common skin stigmata in alcohol-dependent patients are often related to chronic alcoholic liver disease (Higgins & du Vivier, 1999). The skin may, however, be affected as an early feature of alcohol misuse. In particular, psoriasis, discoid eczema and superficial infections are found to be more common in heavy drinkers (Higgins & du Vivier, 1992).

Reproductive disorders

- In premenopausal female alcoholics, there is an increase in the frequency of menstrual disturbances, abortions and miscarriages and infertility. These effects may be seen before severe liver dysfunction has appeared (Becker, 1993).
- Regular consumption of alcohol during pregnancy may affect the foetus. The abnormalities range from growth retardation to foetal alcohol syndrome. There is no evidence on which to base a recommendation of a safe level of alcohol intake in pregnancy (Eustace *et al.,* 2003).
- Uncontrolled studies of male alcoholics have reported that alcohol consumption may affect spermatogenesis and spermiogenesis and cause reduced sperm counts (Kucheria *et al.,* 1985). This effect has also been demonstrated in animal studies (Anderson *et al.,* 1983).
- A review of the literature on alcohol, smoking and male fertility has identified methodological problems in previous studies. There is only a modest weight of evidence for an adverse effect of alcohol on sperm counts in the absence of smoking. There is, however, an apparent protective effect of moderate alcohol drinking on sperm parameters (Marinelli *et al.,* 2004).
- Gonadal atrophy as a direct result of toxicity and suppression of the hypothalamic pituitary

axis is associated with impotence and diminished fertility.

Aetiology

A variety of research methodologies have been adopted to examine the relative contribution of genetic and environmental factors to alcohol dependence (see Box 10.3) (Ball, 2004).

Family studies

In a review of family studies Cotton (1979) demonstrated that parental alcoholism was 6 times more likely in alcoholics, although 47% to 82% of alcoholics did not come from families with parental alcoholism. In a study of 8,296 relatives of alcoholic probands and 1654 control subjects, Nurnberger and colleagues (2004) reported that the risk of alcohol dependence in relatives of probands was increased about twofold. Lifetime risk rates were reported at 28.8% and 14.4% for DSM-IV alcohol dependence in relatives of probands and control subjects, respectively (37.0% and 20.5% for the less stringent DSM-III-R alcohol dependence). Risks increase with the number and proximity of affected relatives. Family studies using direct interviews with probands and first-degree relatives, standardised diagnostic criteria and inclusion of a control group have demonstrated that first-degree relatives of alcoholics are, on average, 7 times more likely to develop this disorder than relatives of nonalcoholics (Conway *et al.*, 2003).

Family studies do not, however, enable the separation of genetic from environmental aetiological factors, and other methodologies are more effective at achieving this.

Twin studies

A number of studies in the United Kingdom and United States have reported concordance rates for mono (MZ)- and dizygotic (DZ) twins for alcohol

---

Box 10.3 The evidence on genetics and alcohol dependence (Ball, 2004)

Family studies
- Alcohol dependence clusters in families.
- Rates are increased in relatives.
- Risks increase with the number and proximity of affected relatives.
- Evidence is consistent with a genetic influence but is not proof.

Adoption studies
- Adoptees with an affected biological parent are at higher risk.
- Risk is the same as being reared by an affected parent.

Twin studies
- Heritability is 50% for males.
- Heritability is 25% for females.
- This emphasises the importance of environmental influences particularly for females.

Molecular genetics
- **Linkage studies**
  - A number of chromosome regions have been implicated on chromosomes 1, 2, 4, 7 and 11.
  - These findings are not robust, and the effects of the individual genes approaches the limitations of linkage methods.
- **Association studies**
  - The dopamine D2 receptor (DRD2) was identified as having a role in alcohol dependence but replication of the finding was not successful and this finding may be a false positive.
  - A coding error in the ALDH2 gene is responsible for the Japanese flushing reaction to alcohol.
  - There is evidence that polymorphisms in the ADH 1–7 genes produce up to 40-fold variations in the rate of removal of acetaldehyde.

---

problems. The results of these studies are summarised in Table 10.4.

In summary, male MZ twins show significantly more concordance for alcohol problems than do DZ twins. Thus genetic variability accounts for 50% to 80% of the variation in risk for alcoholism in males, whereas the evidence for females is not so strong (Prescott, 2003).

Table 10.4 Concordance rates in twin studies

Study	Sex	Criteria	Concordance %		MZ/DZ ratio
			MZ	DZ	
Kaij, 1960	M	Drinking behaviour	53.5	28.3	1.9
	M	Chronic alcoholism	71.4	32.3	2.2
Hbrec & Ommen, 1981	M	Alcoholism	26.3	11.9	2.2
Kendler, 1985	M	Alcoholism	64.7	8.5	7.6
Gurling, Clifford, *et al.* 1981	M & F	Alcohol dependency	21	25	0.8
	M	Alcohol dependency	33	30	1.1
	F	Alcohol dependency	8	13	0.6
Koskenvuo, Langinvainio, *et al.*, 1984	M	Alcohol abuse and/or dependency	23.1	10.8	2.1
Pickens, Svikis, *et al.* 1991	M	Alcohol abuse and/or dependency	76	61	1.2
	F	Alcohol abuse and/or dependency	36	25	1.4
	M	Alcohol dependence	59	36	1.6
	F	Alcohol dependence	25	5	5
Caldwell & Gottesman, 1991	M	Alcohol abuse	68	46	1.5
	M	Alcohol dependence	40	13	3.1
	F	Alcohol abuse	47	42	1.1
	F	Alcohol dependence	29	25	1.2
Kendler, Heath, *et al.* 1992	F	Alcoholism with tolerance or dependence	26.3	11.9	2.2
	F	Alcoholism with or without tolerance-dependence or problem drinking	46.9	31.5	1.5

DZ = dizygotic; F = female; M = male; MZ = monozygotic.

Although alcohol dependence and levels of alcohol consumption are related, the causes of variation in the patterns of alcohol intake and in those of susceptibility to alcohol dependence are not necessarily the same. Twin studies of the amount of alcohol consumed and frequency of alcohol use have reported that variations in alcohol intake are genetically determined, in contrast to lack of control and social problems which were subject to environmental factors. In a review of the data from Australian twin studies of alcohol consumption, Whitfield and colleagues (2004) reported that nearly all variation in alcohol intake is due to genetic effects. This suggests that the genes affecting intake also affect

dependence risk but that there are other genes that affect dependence alone.

The value of the classic twin method in studying alcohol dependence has been questioned (Cook & Gurling, 1990; Joseph, 2002). The twin method is based on an "equal environment assumption", which assumes that there are no differences in the family environments of twins. It is clear, however, that not all children (including twins) within a family are treated in exactly the same way by both parents. Studies of normal drinking have reported that concordance rates were greater in twins living together than in those living apart, pointing to how different environmental conditions affect

---

Box 10.4 Types of alcoholism

- Type 1 alcoholism (milieu limited)
  - Age of onset over 25 years
  - No criminality or treatment for alcohol problems in the biological parents
  - Loss of control (or psychological dependence)
  - Guilt and fear about dependence
  - Harm avoidance
  - Reward dependence
- Type 2 alcoholism (male limited)
  - Teenage age of onset (under 25 years)
  - Alcohol abuse, criminality and treatment are extensive in the biological father
  - Inability to abstain
  - Aggressive behaviour
  - Novelty-seeking personality traits (Sigvardsson *et al.*, 1996)

---

consumption (Clifford *et al.*, 1994). The interpretation of twin studies is therefore complicated by factors such as the differential shared environment of MZ versus DZ twins or the effect of living with a heavy drinking twin.

Adoption studies

Adoption studies have been widely used in research to separate genetic and environmental influences on the risks of developing psychiatric illness. The adoption method has been criticised on a series of points:

- Adoptive parents may be selected because of background similarity to the biological parents, thus producing a correlation between the environment in the adoptive family and that in the biological family (Cook & Gurling, 1990).
- Parents who offer children for adoption are not typical of the general population (Cook & Gurling, 1990).
- Adoptees are not typical of the general population (Slap *et al.*, 2001).
- Studies of children adopted by alcoholic and non-alcoholic adoptive parents show that being raised with an alcoholic adoptive parent increases the

risk for alcohol-related problems in the adopted child (Newlin *et al.*, 2000).

Despite such potential weaknesses, adoption studies on alcohol-related problems do support a genetic contribution to the development of alcoholism. Three main research groups have identified a genetic contribution to the development of alcohol problems using adoption studies:

The Iowa Adoption Studies: A review of a series of adoption studies undertaken at the University of Iowa, using private and public adoption agencies within the state of Iowa from 1974 to 1995, reported on four main studies (Cadoret *et al.*, 1994).

- Study 1 demonstrated significant genetic as well as environmental effects in the aetiology of alcoholism.
- Study 2 had similar findings to study 1.
- Study 3 failed to show a genetic effect.
- Study 4 used adoptees from four agencies – two agencies showed a genetic effect and two showed no effect.

The Copenhagen Studies (Goodwin *et al.*, 1973, 1974) have concluded that:

- Sons of alcoholic biological parents adopted at birth are 4 times more likely to become alcoholics than sons of normal control fathers.
- Alcohol problems experienced by adopted sons included early onset of heavy drinking, loss of control, hallucinations and treatment for drinking.

The Swedish Temperance Board Studies: A large adoption study of more than 2,000 children placed in adoptive homes before the age of 3 (Bohman, 1978) reported the following:

- There was a threefold increase in alcohol abuse in adopted-away sons of alcoholic parents.
- Males who had lived with their biological mother for more than 6 months had 1.5 times the risk of others.
- No genetic effects were found in females.
- A reanalysis of the Bohman study (Cloninger *et al.*, 1981) identified two types of alcoholism: milieu limited (Type 1) and male limited (Type 2) (see Box 10.4).

- A replication of the Swedish study (Sigvardsson *et al.*, 1996) produced evidence to confirm the Type 1–Type 2 model.

Molecular genetics of alcohol dependence

Molecular genetic studies seek to determine not only whether alcohol dependence has a genetic component but also the location of the gene or genes. Two main methods have been employed: linkage studies and association studies.

Linkage studies

The largest published linkage study is the Collaborative Study on the Genetics of Alcoholism (COGA) (Bierut *et al.*, 2002), involving more than 1,000 alcoholic subjects and their families. A number of phenotypes were investigated:

- Alcohol dependence using defined criteria
- Low level of response to alcohol (Schuckit & Smith, 2001)
- Presence of alcohol dependence or depression
- Using alcohol but not dependent
- Maximum number of drinks in 24 hours
- Electrophysiological measures, such as electroencephalograms and event-related potentials (ERPs)

The study showed evidence for loci on chromosomes 1 and 7, possible evidence of a locus on chromosome 2 and evidence of a protective locus on chromosome 4. However, a review of linkage studies (Ball, 2004) concluded that these findings are not robust and that the size of the effects in alcoholism are approaching the limits of linkage techniques.

Association studies

Candidate genes which have been studied include the following:

The DRD2 – dopamine D2 receptor gene
- DRD2 was initially reported as a firm association gene for alcoholism (Blum *et al.*, 1990).

- A review of the evidence in 1996 (Noble, 1996) concluded that DRD2 could represent one of the most prominent single-gene determinants of susceptibility to severe substance abuse.
- More robust association studies have, however, failed to confirm the original reports, and the most recent review (Ball, 2004) concludes that the DRD2 gene evidence is probably a false positive.

ALDH2 – aldehyde dehydrogenase 2 gene
- The unpleasant flushing reaction in some Japanese people after alcohol consumption is thought to be responsible for the low prevalence of alcoholism in this population. This is explained by the fact that ALDH2 (aldehyde dehydrogenase), the enzyme responsible for the majority of aldehyde oxidation, exists in two forms, one of which is inactive, ALDH2-2 (Yoshida *et al.*, 1984). As a result of the inactive ALDH2-2, acetaldehyde levels increase in the blood after alcohol consumption. Drinking leads to the accumulation of acetaldehyde, which results in a disulfiram-like reaction (i.e. flushing, nausea, palpitations).
- Shibuya and Yoshida (1988) genotyped individuals with a diagnosis of alcohol-related liver disease and compared them with control subjects. The allele frequency for the low-activity enzyme was higher (0.35) in the control group than the experimental group (0.07).
- Studies of alcohol intake in Thai males have shown that possession of the mutant ALDH2-2 allele prevents high alcohol consumption because of the flushing reaction and thus reduces the risk of development of alcohol dependence (Assanangkornchai *et al.*, 2003).
- The ALDH2*2 studies provide the most robust evidence of a single gene effect which influences the patterns of alcohol intake and the incidence of alcohol dependence in those with the mutant allele.

Alcohol dehydrogenase (ADH)
- There are seven known alcohol dehydrogenase (ADH) genes on the long arm of chromosome 4,

which encode enzymes that catalyse the conversion of alcohols to aldehydes (Osier *et al.*, 2002).

- Variants occur in ADH2 and ADH3 that affect the rate of conversion of alcohol to acetaldehyde.
- High activity variants are decreased in subjects with alcohol dependency, indicating a protective effect of faster production of acetaldehyde from alcohol (Ball, 2004).

A meta-analysis of genetic research on alcohol abuse (Walters, 2002) concluded that the heritability of alcohol misuse is stronger in males and in studies employing stricter definitions of abuse. The meta-analysis showed that there is evidence of an effect of genes on alcohol misuse, but that evidence for the effect of the environment in modifying genetic expression is also strong.

Environmental risk factors

Environmental factors that play a part in the aetiology of drinking behaviour may be divided into those factors that influence the availability of alcohol and those that render the individual vulnerable to the use and abuse of alcohol. In a comparison of risk and protective factors for adolescent substance use between the United States and Australia, common risk and protective factors for the use of alcohol were identified as (Beyers *et al.*, 2004):

Risks

- Community norms favourable toward alcohol use
- Perceived availability of alcohol
- Poor family management
- Family history of substance use
- Parental attitudes favourable to alcohol use
- Favourable attitudes toward antisocial behaviour
- Favourable attitudes toward alcohol use
- Friends' alcohol use
- Sensation seeking
- Antisocial behaviour

Protective factors

- Social skills
- Belief in the moral order

Family interaction

Positive parental attitudes to alcohol and drug use have a major influence in shaping use in children. Where one or both parents abuse alcohol, families manifest higher levels of conflict, disruption, economic difficulties, breakdown and impaired mother-child attachment (Velleman & Orford, 1993). In addition, problem drinking by parents may lead to inconsistent and unpredictable parenting behaviours and contribute to poorer monitoring of adolescent behaviours (Windle, 1977). A history of unfair, inconsistent and harsh discipline by parents predicts both alcohol and depressive disorders (Holmes & Robins, 1987).

Peer affiliation

Adolescents with alcohol- and drug-using friends are more likely to use the same substances themselves (Barnow *et al.*, 2002; Hawkins *et al.*, 1992; Hill & Yuan, 1999). A study of US college students found that drinking behaviour is positively related not to the perception of typical students' drinking but to perceptions of actual male friends' drinking, for both male and female students (Campo *et al.*, 2003). Some adolescents may self-select into high-risk groups because of high levels of risk-taking and novelty-seeking behaviour.

Employment

Certain occupations carry a higher risk of alcohol-related problems. These include being a publican, where there is easy access to alcohol, and in professions such as law, where income and social pressure facilitate drinking (Brooke *et al.*, 1991; Plant, 1979).

The level of stress in a work environment may also contribute to risks for high alcohol intake (Head *et al.*, 2004). Working during adolescence, expressly more than 10 hours a week, has also been related to heavy alcohol use (Paschall *et al.*, 2004). This effect is thought to be due to associated variables such as age, personal income and peer group associations.

Unemployment

Unemployment itself has been suggested as a causative factor for heavy drinking. The relationship between unemployment and level of alcohol intake appears to vary with length of unemployment, such that recent unemployment decreases alcohol use, whereas longer unemployment increases it (Khan *et al.,* 2002). Population studies of alcohol sales during periods of economic stress, however, report that problem drinkers decrease their intake because of reduced income, although overall this is balanced by an increase in light drinking (Dee, 2001; Ruhm & Black, 2002).

Culture

Social and cultural factors associated with increased risk of alcohol problems include permissive alcohol legislation such as lower age of legal drinking, greater availability of alcohol and greater socioeconomic deprivation. The acceptance or otherwise of drunken behaviour by societies shows great variation. In a study of alcoholism in the United States (Vaillant, 1983), Irish subjects demonstrated high rates of alcoholism, drank in pubs and familial alcoholism did not influence the later development of dependence. In other ethnic groups, drunkenness was considered unacceptable, drinking was more frequent in the family setting and alcohol dependence occurred more frequently if they had alcoholic relatives. Cultural differences in the form and acceptability of intoxicated behaviour have been described (MacAndrew & Edgerton, 1969). These variations are culture-bound, but there are historical examples of cultures in which changes in the behaviours that are seen as acceptable have occurred over time (Room, 2001).

Explanatory models of alcohol use

Explanatory models for age and sex differences in adolescent drug use can be derived from a variety of theories, including social learning theory and social control theory (Svensson, 2003). *Social theories* encompass the following:

- *Social control theory* concentrates on controlling factors which restrain deviant activity, the family being seen as one of the key controlling factors. It involves both actual and virtual parental monitoring (Hirschi, 1969).
- *Social learning theory*, in contrast, suggests that drug use is influenced by role models and normative beliefs and that deviant behaviour is learned by association with a deviant peer group (Kandel, 1985).
- *The social development model* is an integrated theory that combines elements from several main theories to develop a framework, which overcomes some of the limitations of the single models. It incorporates elements of control theory and social learning theory into a developmental framework (Catalano & Hawkins, 1996).
- *Expectancy theory* is based on a social learning perspective and seeks to explain motivation to drink and motivation to restrain from drinking in terms of a person's expectations of the outcomes of their behaviour.

In contrast, *conditioning theories* include the following:

- *Classical conditioning* proposes that cues associated with previous experiences with alcohol are conditioned stimuli, which become associated with the unconditioned effects of alcohol (Lowman *et al.,* 2000). Re-exposure to the cues then evokes a conditioned response (Drummond, 2000). The model provides a possible explanation for cues to induce tolerance during drinking and withdrawal in the absence of alcohol.
- *Operant conditioning* proposes that an individual learns through repeated exposure to alcohol that the process involves both pleasant and negative experiences. Positive reinforcement of drinking behaviour is associated with the euphoria or relaxation which results from drinking. The negative reinforcing effect of alcohol is associated with relief of boredom, withdrawal symptoms or anxiety and anger.

- *Cue reactivity* has been used in the study of alcohol dependence and centres on the observations of a reactivity to alcohol-related cues, using a series of types of cues and reactions to cues. Cues have been observed to elicit a range of reactions (Drummond, 2000):
  - ○ Expressive reactivity, such as craving or pleasure
  - ○ Physiological reactivity, such as changes in heart rate
  - ○ Behavioural reactivity, such as drink-seeking behaviour

The biopsychosocial model

The biopsychosocial model of addiction is a comprehensive model which starts from an assumption of multifactorial causality of addiction, including biological, genetic, psychological and sociocultural factors. The model proposes that there are a series of subpopulations in which specific factors may play a more important role in causation than in other groups and may thus explain the number of cases of coexisting psychiatric and alcohol problems (Zimberg, 1993).

The self-medication hypothesis (Khantzian, 1990) suggests that the specific pharmacological properties of addictive substances are used to control the symptoms of psychiatric illness. However, although this view has clinical and empirical support, it has not as yet been supported by consistent research evidence (Khantzian, 1997). A factor which may have contributed to the lack of clear support for this hypothesis is that attribution of a self-medicating effect by the user may not align with the actual result of using the medication (Carrigan & Randall, 2003).

In summary, alcohol use and abuse is best viewed through the framework of a multifactorial biopsychosocial model, which acknowledges the interplay of genetic, familial, physiological, psychological and social factors. Age, role, sex, social group and peer pressure, the family, community and occupational environment, as well as overall cultural values and controls on alcohol use, will act upon drinking behaviour. The individual's genetic makeup, personality, sense of control and efficacy, degree of dependence, the presence of brain damage or psychiatric problems, reaction to internal and external cues or stimuli, financial state and the values of a treatment programme will all affect attempts to change drinking behaviour.

Assessment and intervention

The key to appropriate management is a thorough history (Crome, 2004; see Table 10.5). This general protocol is adapted from that developed for nicotine dependence and is a useful way to formulate the assessment process, because it translates into specific management plans (Raw *et al.*, 1998). Important aspects from the alcohol use misuse perspective are as follows.

Phase 1 – Ask

- Ask all patients about alcohol and other substance misuse, including prescribed and over-the-counter medications.
- Differentiate between alcohol use, harmful use and dependence.
- Conceptualise assessment as ongoing and not necessarily "one-off" and record the information.
- Recognise that the manner and style in which this is done can be a powerful determinant of both the extent to which relevant information is elicited and engagement with the therapeutic process.
- Be aware of, and sensitive to, the ambivalence alcohol-misusing patients may feel.
- Be nonjudgemental and act in a nonconfrontational way.

Phase 2 – Assess

- Assess the degree of dependence.
- Use the assessment process to educate patients about the effects of alcohol.
- Inform about withdrawal symptoms.
- Make some assessment of the level of motivation or "stage of change" at which the patient may be.

Table 10.5 Protocol for history taking (Crome, Ghodse, *et al.*, 2004)

Components of history	Specific details
Demographic characteristics	Age
	Gender
	School, college, employment or retirement
	Nationality and religious affiliation
	Living arrangements, e.g. with parent(s), partners, relatives, friends, homeless, institutional care
	General environment, e.g. deprivation, affluence, violence
Presenting complaint(s)	May or may not be a substance problem
Each substance should be discussed separately:	Age of initiation "first tried"
	Age of onset of weekend use
Alcohol	Age of onset of weekly use
Amphetamines	Age of onset of daily use
Benzodiazepines	Pattern of use during each day
Cannabis	Route of use, e.g. oral, smoking, snorting, intramuscular, intravenous
Cocaine	Age of onset of specific withdrawal symptoms and dependence syndrome features
Ecstasy	Current use over previous day, week, month
Heroin and other opiates	Current cost of use
Methadone	Maximum use ever
Nicotine	How is the substance use being funded?
Over-the-counter medication	Periods of abstinence
Prescribed medication	Triggers to relapse
General	Preferred substance(s) and reasons
Treatment episodes for substance problems	Dates, service, practitioner details, treatment interventions, success or otherwise
Family history	Parents, siblings, grandparents, uncles, aunts
	History of substance misuse and related problems
	History of psychiatric problems, e.g. suicide, deliberate self-harm, depression, anxiety, psychotic illness
	History of physical illness
	Separation, divorce, death
	Family relationships, conflict, support
	Occupational history
Medical history	Episodes of acute or chronic illnesses: respiratory, infective, HIV, hepatitis
	Admission to hospital, dates, problems, treatment and outcome
Psychiatric history	Assessment by general practitioner for any "minor" complaints, e.g. anxiety, depression
	Treatment by general practitioner with any psychoactive drugs
	Referral to psychiatric services: dates, diagnosis, treatment and outcome
Personal history	Developmental milestones
Educational background	Age started and left school
	School reports
	Educational psychology reports
	Achievements and aspirations
	Truancy
	Special educational needs
	Suspension and exclusion

(cont.)

Table 10.5 (*cont.*)

Components of history	Specific details
Training and occupational activities	Ongoing activities and plans
Criminal activities	Involvement in criminal activities preceding or directly related to substance problems
	Cautions, charges, convictions
	Probation service involvement
	Shoplifting, violence, prostitution, imprisonment
Social services	Child protection history
	Child abuse and neglect
Social environment	Level of community support
Social activities	Sports, hobbies, community work, religious affiliation and activities
Financial situation	Debt to finance substance problems
Useful information	Current address
	Phone number including mobile phone
	General practitioner's name, address and phone number
	Details of other professionals involved
Investigations	Biochemical, haematological, urinary
	Special investigations, e.g. brain scan, and psychometric testing
Collateral information	Family and friends
	School
	Social services
	Criminal justice agencies
	Health services
	Voluntary agencies
Consent and confidentiality	

- In this context, aim to provide advice or suggestions as to what the "goals" for a particular patient at a particular stage may be (e.g. abstinence or harm reduction).
- Discuss and negotiate treatment choices and appropriateness (e.g. pharmacological interventions, the need for admission to specialist services).
- Be aware of the possibility that clinical manifestations of the condition may impair the history-taking process (e.g. neurocognitive dysfunction).
- Follow an assessment schedule.

Phase 3 – Advise

- Continue the assessment within a brief 5- to 10-minute "motivational interviewing" framework.

- Provide the patient with the opportunity to express anxieties and concerns.
- Offer personalised feedback about clinical findings, including physical examination and biochemical and haematological tests.
- Discuss and outline the personal benefits and risks of continued drinking and safe levels of drinking.
- Provide self-help materials (e.g. manuals).

Phase 4 – Assist

- Provide support and encouragement and instil positive expectations of success.
- Acknowledge that previous attempts may have engendered loss of confidence and self-esteem.
- Suggest that if the goal is abstinence, a "quit date" is set, so the patient can plan accordingly (e.g. get

rid of any alcohol in the house) and safely (is it safe to stop drinking abruptly or not?).

- Work through a range of alternative coping strategies, including the identification of cues that might help distract the patient.

Phase 5 – Arrange

- Be prepared to refer or organise admission to a specialist or appropriate unit if the patient
  – is in severe withdrawal, including delirium tremens;
  – is experiencing unstable social circumstances;
  – is likely to develop serious withdrawal due to a severe degree of dependence or a previous episode of severe withdrawal, including delirium tremens;
  – is severely dependent;
  – has a severe comorbid physical illness;
  – has comorbid mental illness, including suicidal ideation;
  – is using multiple substances;
  – has a history of frequent relapse.

During all phases, close attention should be paid to the appropriateness of various options for the particular individual – "tailor-made" where possible.

Treatment of alcohol problems

Psychological approaches

Alcohol misusers vary in their suitability for psychological treatments, and it may be more or less appropriate in individual cases due to age, cognitive ability or dysfunction, education, willingness and capability or capacity to view problems as psychological. However, psychological treatments are pivotal to treatment effectiveness, even when pharmacological treatments are administered.

Standardisation of approaches and outcome measures is complex. Treatment philosophies, environments and settings may differ greatly (e.g. primary care, accident and emergency, prisons).

Additional resources for treatment (e.g. support by other agencies such as housing, education, probation) may vary. Some groups may be discriminated against across a variety of services, because of general stigmas around substance misuse (Crisp *et al.*, 2000), poorly trained staff (Crome & Shaikh, 2004), and lack of resources or due to old age, female sex or ethnic minority status.

Stages of change

The process by which change occurs has been formulated as a series of stages – preconception, contemplation, preparation, action and maintenance (Prochaska & DiClemente, 1984). This theory has been influential in treatment and research.

There is considerable evidence from other health and social care fields that provision of information, in itself, may be of help. Information needs to be accurate and up to date and provide advice – not only on the negative effects of substance use but also on any potential benefits. Responses to situations in which overdose might have occurred, physical consequences and psychological problems are a useful baseline from which to start.

Counselling is a widely used term which can be imprecise and embody various theoretical models (e.g. psychodynamics, cognitive, behavioural). In practice, however, counselling may have one or more objectives (e.g. problem solving, acquisition of social skills, cognitive change, behavioural change, systems change). The term may be used to describe therapies that are supportive, directive or motivational for individuals, groups or families.

Behavioural therapies have become the mainstay of treatment over the past decade and encompass social skills and self-control training, motivational counselling (which includes motivational interviewing and motivational enhancement therapies), marital therapy, stress management, contingency management, community reinforcement and cognitive therapies (Heather & Robertson, 1997). Pivotal studies are shown in Box 10.5.

Box 10.5 Pivotal intervention studies for alcohol dependence

Mesa Grande Project (Miller & Wilbourne, 2002)

This project assessed controlled studies on an ongoing basis (see Table 10.6). The "top ten" are brief interventions, motivational enhancement, acamprosate, naltrexone, social skills training, community reinforcement, behavioural contracting, behavioural marital therapy, case management and self-monitoring.

Project MATCH

A multisite trial in the United States, costing $20 million, this study incorporated three treatment interventions, i.e. cognitive-behavioural therapy (CBT), motivational enhancement therapy (MET) and 12-step facilitation or a procedure based on Alcoholics Anonymous. This study has demonstrated that each intervention is beneficial and that this continues at 3-year follow-up. Outcome measures were days abstinent and drinks per drinking day. Although the main objective of the project was to evaluate whether "matching" patients to particular treatments had any effect, in general this was not shown to be the case. MET was delivered in fewer sessions than the other therapies. This had cost implications. That 12-step facilitation was equally effective was interesting from the perspective that good evidence on Alcoholics Anonymous became available.

United Kingdom Alcohol Treatment Trial (UKATT)

This study was the largest multisite study trial in the United Kingdom: 742 patients were treated with MET or social behavioural network therapy (SBNT). SBNT is an amalgam of therapies (community reinforcement, social skills training, family therapy and relapse prevention). There was no difference in outcome at 1 year or in cost-effectiveness. Alcohol dependence, problems and consumption, as well as quality of life, improved.

Reviews have been conducted in Scotland (Slattery *et al.*, 2003), Sweden (Berglund *et al.*, 2003) and Australia (Shand *et al.*, 2003). The Health Technology Board and the Australian researchers concluded that behavioural self-control training, coping skills and marital/family therapy have similar benefits. In keeping with these findings, the Swedish study demonstrated the value of cognitive-behavioural therapy, 12-step approaches and motivational approaches. In addition, structured interactional therapy with a psychodynamic reference framework and partner/family therapy show similar benefits.

Brief interventions have been identified as
- Opportunistic
- Occurring in nonspecialist settings
- Bringing about a reduction in drinking
- Delivered by a nonspecialist
- More appropriate for nondependent drinkers
- Focused on motivation to change
- Self-directed

A great deal of information on this has been published since the early work of Thom and Tellez (1986), especially in primary care (Miller *et al.*, 1995; Moyer *et al.*, 2002; Wilk *et al.*, 1997) but also in medical and psychiatric care (Hulse & Tait, 2003), and to some extent in accident and emergency departments (Saitz *et al.*, 2005). There is also new evidence regarding the use of this technique for insomnia in alcoholism (Currie *et al.*, 2004).

Pharmacotherapy

Although it is imperative that pharmacological treatment is administered safely, it is equally important to see it as one part of a phased treatment management process. In other words, "prescribing" is nested within the overall treatment package, which includes psychosocial components that have been negotiated, whether community or hospital based.

The basis for the guidance that follows is drawn from the consensus statement produced by the British Association for Psychopharmacology, because it is the most up-to-date evidence available (Lingford-Hughes *et al.*, 2004). The objective of this group was to produce "helpful and useable" guidelines for clinicians, especially in psychiatric and primary care settings, as well to identify gaps or "key uncertainties". Its focus was on adults rather than adolescents or the ageing population.

Pharmacological treatments are usually reserved for patients who have dependence (as discussed

Table 10.6 Mesa Grande results: a selection from review where there were three or more studies available (Lingford-Hughes *et al.,* 2004)

Rank	Treatment modality	CES	No. of studies	Rank	Treatment modality	CES	No. of studies
1	Brief intervention	280	31	11	Cognitive therapy	21	10
2	Motivational enhancement	173	17	12.5	Client-centred counselling	20	7
3	Acamprosate	116	5	12.5	Disulfiram	20	24
4	Opiate antagonist	100	6	16.5	Acupuncture	14	3
5	Social skills training	85	25	18	Self-help	11	5
6	Community reinforcement	80	4	23	Family therapy	−5	3
7	Behaviour contracting	64	5	24.5	12-step facilitation	−13	3
8	Behaviour marital therapy	60	8	30	Hypnosis	−41	4
9	Case management	33	6	35	Relapse prevention	−87	20
10	Self-monitoring	25	6	39.5	Alcoholics Anonymous	−108	7

CES = Cumulative Evidence Score: MQS (Methodological Quality Scores) × OLS (Outcome Logic Scores) such that a high score indicates a predominance of evidence that the treatment modality exerts some benefit on drinking outcomes. The top 10 ranked treatments are listed, followed by other commonly used treatments. The ranking reflects cumulative evidence and not necessarily relative efficacies (Miller & Wilbourne, 2002).

earlier) and are available to treat withdrawal syndromes, to maintain abstinence, to prevent complications (including vitamin replacement) and to treat psychological and physical disorders.

Management of alcohol withdrawal and detoxification

Note: This section does not describe treatment regimes in detail. Readers are referred to Lingford-Hughes *et al.* (2004).

Benzodiazepines

There is Category Ia evidence that different benzodiazepines are equally efficacious. For uncomplicated withdrawal, 20 mg qds (four times a day) for 7 days, supplemented by additional treatment for symptom suppression is "typical", although age, degree of severity of dependence and the need for seizure prevention should be taken into account. A longer-acting drug may prevent seizures and delirium but could lead to accumulation. Each patient should be assessed, treated and monitored regularly. Other methods of administering benzodiazepines are

"front-loading" (i.e. until light sedation is achieved, at which point no further medication is given) or "symptom-triggered" (as opposed to a fixed regime). Both these regimes require skilled staff.

Chlormethiazole

Although demonstrated at Category Ia level to be superior to placebo, there are concerns due to respiratory depression, addictive potential and "street value". It has a place in specialist inpatient units for severe withdrawal.

Carbamazepine

Carbamazepine may be a first-line alternative to benzodiazepines in that it reduces alcohol withdrawal symptoms and is not contraindicated for liver failure. However, carbamazepine has not been evaluated in treating delirium, and evidence is limited in treating seizures.

Seizure prevention and treatment

Category Ia evidence has been generated and indicates that both benzodiazepines and anticonvulsants are equally effective in reducing seizure rate

33333333333

from about 8% to 3% (especially those with a longer half-life) but that there is no advantage to combining them. However, phenytoin is ineffective in the prevention of a secondary seizure in the same withdrawal episode; thus, continuation with an anticonvulsant, if it has been used to treat an alcohol-related seizure, is not recommended.

Delirium

Category Ia evidence has accrued on the use of benzodiazepines in the prevention and treatment of delirium.

Other complications of alcohol withdrawal

It is suggested that a beta-blocker could be used to treat hypertension and that in patients with hypoglycaemia and in psychiatric patients, a "slower" regime be administered. Recent Category Ib evidence exists which shows no advantage in adding lofexidine to chlordiazepoxide. Similarly, magnesium and a benzodiazepine did not improve withdrawal. Category Ia evidence for antipsychotics shows that they reduce withdrawal, but not seizures or delirium. Indeed, they may increase seizure risk and therefore should be used with caution.

Vitamin replacement: thiamine

Wernicke's encephalopathy (WE)

Despite the commonness of vitamin deficiency, the quality of evidence for the prevention and treatment of WE is weak. Thus it was stated that the confidence with which recommendations can be made is low and the strength of recommendations is "D".

In healthy, uncomplicated alcohol dependence, or "heavy drinkers" (i.e. low-risk), oral thiamine should be given at a minimum dose of 300 mg/day during detoxification. If, however, the patient is at high risk of developing WE, 250 mg thiamine (or one pair of Pabrinex ampoules) intramuscularly (im) or

> **Box 10.6** Summary of pharmacological approaches for alcohol-related problems
>
> **Withdrawal regimes**
> - Benzodiazepines are the treatment of choice (A).
> - Carbamazepine can be chosen as an alternative to benzodiazepines (A).
> - Chlormethiazole is reserved for inpatient settings (A).
>
> **Seizures**
> - Benzodiazepines are recommended for withdrawal previously complicated by seizures (A).
> - Carbamazepine can be chosen as an alternative (A).
> - To prevent a second seizure, lorazepam can be used (A).
>
> **Delirium**
> - Benzodiazepines are recommended for the prevention (A) and treatment (B) of delirium.
>
> **Others**
> - Evidence does not support the use of other medications, e.g. α_2 agonists, magnesium or antipsychotics.

intravenously (iv) once daily for 3 to 5 days is suggested. For suspected or actual WE, the recommendation is more than 500 mg (two pairs of ampoules) im or iv three times a day for 3 days, followed by 250 mg once daily for 3 to 5 days, depending on the response (i.e. for as long as there is no improvement). Although the risk of anaphylaxis for Parentrovite (the predecessor of Pabrinex) was very small, intravenous preparations should be given in facilities where anaphylactic shock can be treated.

Korsakoff's syndrome

The review concluded that it was not possible to make specific recommendations, despite the fact that a few case reports or small trials have shown improvement with fluvoxamine and donepezil.

Preventing relapse

Acamprosate

A series of meta-analyses and systematic reviews have all found acamprosate to be twice as good as a placebo response (i.e. Category Ia), and the number of treatments needed to prevent one relapse was 11 (Berglund *et al.*, 2003; Slattery *et al.*, 2003). Rates of abstinence ranged from about 25% to 50% at 3, 6 and 12 months. However, psychosocial interventions were part of all "acamprosate" interventions, which raises the question of whether patients who are prescribed it need to participate in psychosocial interventions as well. It appears that the "routine" alcohol-dependent patient (rather than one with complications of psychiatric, social or organic disorder) is more likely to benefit. Sex, age of onset and severity of dependence are not predictive. The addition of disulfiram improved outcome.

Naltrexone

There is Category Ia evidence to support the use of naltrexone (compared with placebo), but not over acamprosate or disulfiram. It is not licensed in the United Kingdom (but is in the United States). Better outcomes are attained if patients are compliant, have high levels of craving or have poor cognitive ability.

There is Category Ia evidence to suggest that there is no difference in outcome between naltrexone and acamprosate and Category Ib evidence indicating that acamprosate and naltrexone combined are superior to placebo but that this combination is only better than acamprosate alone, not better than naltrexone alone.

Disulfiram

There is Category Ia evidence that supervision of patients is key to its efficacy, for which there is evidence at Category Ib level.

Other pharmacological agents

There is a plethora of Category Ib evidence. In general, the statement recommended that acamprosate and naltrexone be considered as treatment options (A) and that disulfiram be considered in those for whom there are no contraindications and in whom

intake is supervised (B). However, Selective Serotonin Reuptake Inhibitors (SSRIs) should be avoided (or used with caution) in Type 2 alcoholism.

Comorbidities: alcohol with nicotine dependence, depression, anxiety, bipolar disorder and schizophrenia

Alcohol and nicotine dependence

Behavioural programmes and nicotine replacement therapy (NRT) may be effective to increase smoking abstinence rates in patients in alcohol treatment programmes, and all patients should be supported in their attempts to stop smoking.

Alcohol and other psychiatric disorders

As discussed earlier, the relationships between alcoholism and other psychiatric disorders are sometimes complex, and it is not always easy to achieve abstinence from alcohol to make an adequate assessment of the nature of the relationship. Ideally, detoxification should be the first step, with assessment after 3 to 4 weeks of abstinence. Assessment of suicidal risk is as important, especially if medication is going to be prescribed. Then, due to relatively little evidence on what works well, a practical clinical approach is recommended, so safety is the main consideration. Findings overall indicate that antidepressant medication is beneficial for depressive symptoms but has little impact on drinking behaviour (Nunes & Levin, 2004). Thus if patients have clear evidence of depression, use of antidepressants is indicated, but with due caution. Tricyclic antidepressants are not recommended because of risk of cardiotoxicity and overdose.

In those alcohol-dependent patients with anxiety, complete withdrawal is advised. Buspirone is *not* recommended, but SSRIs are. In addition, assessment by a specialist addiction service is recommended before embarking on a benzodiazepine regime.

There is little evidence regarding the use of medication in alcohol and bipolar disorders or alcohol and schizophrenia. Data on the value of atypical antipsychotics are preliminary (Jeffrey *et al.*, 2002).

General policy approaches

Governments around the world have attempted to deal with alcohol-related problems. Babor rated the UK Strategy according to a set of guidelines he and others had developed (Babor *et al.*, 2003). Almost 90% of the recommendations were "untested" or "ineffective" policy options. Five areas were well supported by research (e.g. early identification of problem drinkers, server training). In some of the areas supported by the Strategy, there was evidence that these would not be effective (e.g. product labels, responsible drinking messages, designated driver programmes). Three areas had insufficient research evidence (e.g. good policing, information dissemination).

On an international level, Anderson (2004) noted the evidence suggesting that three types of policy are effective:

1. Population-based, including taxation, advertising, regulation of density of outlets, hours and days of sale, drinking locations and minimum drinking age
2. Problem-directed policies (e.g. drunk driving)
3. Interventions aimed at individual drinkers (e.g. primary care–based brief interventions)

A recent WHO report further underlines the fact that taxes are the most cost-effective option in terms of preventing ill health or premature death. However, brief interventions prevent more ill health and death, although at a greater cost. It is acknowledged that in many parts of the world, some effective elements have been adopted in alcohol policies, but others have not, notably alcohol taxation and advertising. The potential for collective action across national boundaries is emphasised (WHO, 2004).

Conclusions

We are beginning to elucidate and pinpoint some specific direct connections with organic changes in the nervous system in chronic alcohol misusers. This information is emerging from genetics, imaging, neurotransmitter studies and neuropsychological approaches. The focus on the neurosciences has not made highly sophisticated understanding of what drives and maintains drinking behaviour redundant. These approaches have led to valuable treatment interventions for the less dependent drinker being delivered across a wide range of health and social care services, in tandem with pharmacological treatments when appropriate.

REFERENCES

Anderson, P. (2004). Editorial: state of the world's alcohol policy. *Addiction* **99**:1367–9.

Anderson, R. A., Jr., Willis, B. R., Oswald, C., *et al.* (1983). Ethanol induced male infertility: impairment of spermatozoa. *J Pharmacol Exp Ther* **225**:479–86.

American Psychiatric Association (1994). *Diagnostic and Statistical Manual of Mental Disorders*, 4th edn. (DSM-IV). Washington, DC: American Psychiatric Association.

Assanangkornchai, S., Noi pha, K., Saunders, J. B., *et al.* (2003). Aldehyde dehydrogenase 2 genotypes, alcohol flushing symptoms and drinking patterns in Thai men. *Psychiatry Res* **118**:9–17.

Babor, T., Caetano, R., Casswell, S., *et al.* (2003). *Alcohol: No Ordinary Commodity*. Oxford: Oxford University Press.

Ball, D. (2004). Genetic approaches to alcohol dependence. *Br J Psychiatry* **185**:449–51.

Baptista, A., Bianchi, L., Groote, J. D., *et al.* (1981). Alcoholic liver disease: morphological manifestations. Review by an international group. *Lancet* **1**:707–11.

Barnow, S., Schuckit, M. A., Lucht, M., *et al.* (2002). The importance of a positive family history of alcoholism, parental rejection and emotional warmth, behavioral problems and peer substance use for alcohol problems in teenagers: a path analysis. *J Stud Alcohol* **63**:305–15.

Becker, U. (1993). The influence of ethanol and liver disease on sex hormones and hepatic oestrogen receptors in women. *Dan Med Bull* **40**:447–59.

Becker, U., Deis, A., Sorensen, T. I., *et al.* (1996). Prediction of risk of liver disease by alcohol intake, sex, and age: a prospective population study. *Hepatology* **23**:1025–9.

Berglund, M., Thelander, S., & Jonsson, E. (2003). *Treating Alcohol and Drug Abuse: An Evidence Based Review.* Weinheim, Germany: Wiley-VCH Verlag.

Beyers, J. M., Toumbourou, J. W., Catalano, R. F., *et al.* (2004). A cross-national comparison of risk and protective factors for adolescent substance use: the United States and Australia. *J Adolesc Health* **35**:3–16.

Bierut, L. J., Saccone, N. L., Rice, J. P., *et al.* (2002). Defining alcohol-related phenotypes in humans. The Collaborative Study on the Genetics of Alcoholism. *Alcohol Res Health* **26**:208–13.

Blum, K., Noble, E. P., Sheridan, P. J., *et al.* (1990). Allelic association of human dopamine D2 receptor gene in alcoholism. *JAMA* **263**:2055–60.

Bohman, M. (1978). Some genetic aspects of alcoholism and criminality. A population of adoptees. *Arch Gen Psychiatry* **35**:269–76.

Brady, K. T., & Sonne, S. C. (1995). The relationship between substance abuse and bipolar disorder. *J Clin Psychiatry* **56**:19–24.

Brooke, D., Edwards, G., Taylor, C., *et al.* (1991). Addiction as an occupational hazard: 144 doctors with drug and alcohol problems. *Br J Addict* **86**:1011–16.

Cadoret, R., Troughton, E., Woodworth, G., *et al.* (1994). Evidence of heterogeneity of genetic effect in Iowa adoption studies. *Ann N Y Acad Sci* **708**:59–71.

Campo, S., Brossard, D., Frazer, M. S., *et al.* (2003). Are social norms campaigns really magic bullets? Assessing the effects of students' misperceptions on drinking behavior. *Health Commun* **15**:481–97.

Carrigan, M. H., & Randall, C. L. (2003). Self-medication in social phobia: a review of the alcohol literature. *Addict Behav* **28**:269–84.

Carroll, J. F. X. (1984). The substance abuse problem checklist: a new clinical aid for drug and/or alcohol dependency treatment. *J Subst Abuse Treat* **1**:31–6.

Catalano, R. F., & Hawkins, J. D. (1996). The Social Development Model. *Delinquency and Crime.* Cambridge: Cambridge University Press: pp. 149–97.

Charness, M. E. (1993). Brain lesions in alcoholics. *Alcohol Clin Exp Res* **17**:2–11.

Chick, J. (1989). Delirium tremens. *BMJ* **298**:3–4.

Clifford, C. A., Hopper, J. L., Fulker, D. W., *et al.* (1984). A genetic and environmental analysis of a twin family study of alcohol use, anxiety, and depression. *Genet Epidemiol* **1**:63–79.

Cloninger, C. R., Bohman, M., Sigvardsson, S., *et al.* (1981). Inheritance of alcohol abuse. Cross-fostering analysis of adopted men. *Arch Gen Psychiatry* **38**:861–8.

Conway, K. P., Swendsen, J. D., Merikangas, K. R., *et al.* (2003). Alcohol expectancies, alcohol consumption, and problem drinking: the moderating role of family history. *Addict Behav* **28**:823–36.

Cook, C. C., Hallwood, P. M., Thomson, A. D., *et al.* (1998). B Vitamin deficiency and neuropsychiatric syndromes in alcohol misuse. *Alcohol Alcohol* **33**:317–36.

Cook, C. H., & Gurling, H. H. D. (1990). The genetic aspects of alcoholism and substance abuse: a review. In G. Edwards & M. Lader, eds. *The Nature of Drug Dependence.* Oxford: Oxford Medical Publications.

Cotton, N. S. (1979). The familial incidence of alcoholism: a review. *J Stud Alcohol* **40**:89–116.

Crawford, V., Crome, I. B. & Clancy, C. (2003). Co-existing problems of mental health and substance misuse (dual diagnosis): a literature review. *Drugs Educ Prevent Policy* **10**:S1–S74.

Crisp, A. H., Gelder, M. G., Rix, S., *et al.* (2000). Stigmatisation of people with mental illnesses. *Br J Psychiatry* **177**:4–7.

Crome, I. B. (1995). *The experiences of withdrawal and craving in alcohol and opiate dependence* [MD thesis]. Birmingham: University of Birmingham.

Crome, I. B., Ghodse, H., Gilvarry, E., *et al.*, eds. (2004). *Young People and Substance Misuse.* London: Gaskell.

Crome, I. B., & Shaikh, N. (2004). Undergraduate medical education in substance misuse in Britain III: can medical students drive change? *Drugs Educ Prevent Policy* **11**:483–503.

Crome, I. B. (1999). Substance misuse and psychiatric comorbidity: towards improved service provision. *Drugs Educ Prevent Policy* **6**:154–71.

Crome, I. (2004). The process of assessment. In I. B. Crome, A. H. Ghodse, E. Gilvarry, *et al.*, eds. *Young People and Substance Misuse.* London: Gaskell, pp. 129–39.

Currie, S. R., Clark, S., Hodgins, D. C., *et al.* (2004). Randomised controlled trial of brief cognitive behavioural interventions for insomnia in recovering alcoholics. *Addiction* **99**:1121–32.

Davidson, R. J., & Raistrick, D. (1986). The validity of the Short Alcohol Dependence Data (SADD) questionnaire. *Br J Addict* **81**:217–22.

Dee, T. S. (2001). Alcohol abuse and economic conditions: evidence from repeated cross-sections of individual-level data. *Health Econ* **10**:257–70.

Drummond, D. C. (1990). The relationship between alcohol dependence and alcohol related problems in a clinical population. *Br J Addict* **85**:357–66.

Drummond, D. C. (2000). What does cue-reactivity have to offer clinical research? *Addiction* **95**(Suppl 2):S129–44.

Dufour, D. R., Lott, J. A., Nolte, F. S., *et al.* (2000). Diagnosis and monitoring of hepatic injury. I. Performance characteristics of laboratory tests. *Clin Chem* **46**:2027–49.

Edwards, G., & Gross, M. M. (1976). The alcohol dependence: a provisional description of a clinical syndrome. *BMJ* **1**:1058–61.

Edwards, G., Marshall, E. J., & Cook, C. C. H. (2003). *The Treatment of Drinking Problems: A Guide for the Helping Professions*, 4th edn. Cambridge: Cambridge University Press, chapter 4.

Eustace, L. W., Kang, D. H., Coombs, D., *et al.* (2003). Fetal alcohol syndrome: a growing concern for health care professionals. *J Obstet Gynecol Neonatal Nurs* **32**:215–21.

Ewing, J. A. (1984). Detecting alcoholism: the CAGE questionnaire. *JAMA* **252**:1905–97.

Feinman, J. A., & Dunner, D. L. (1996). The effect of alcohol and substance abuse on the course of bipolar affective disorder. *J Affect Disord* **37**:43–9.

Finlayson, N., Hayes, P., Simpson, K., *et al.* (2000). Diseases of the liver and biliary system. In C. Haslett, E. R. Chilvers, J. A. A. Hunter, & N. A. Boon, eds. *Davidson's Principles and Practice of Medicine*. London: Churchill Livingstone.

Gabriel, S., Grossmann, A., Hoppner, J., *et al.* (1999). Marchiafava-Bignami syndrome. Extrapontine myelinolysis in chronic alcoholism. *Nervenarzt* **70**:349–56.

Gaziano, J. M., Gaziano, T. A., Glynn, R. J., *et al.* (2000). Light-to-moderate alcohol consumption and mortality in the Physicians' Health Study enrollment cohort. *J Am Coll Cardiol* **35**:96–105.

Goldberg, J. F., Garno, J. L., Leon, A. C., *et al.* (1999). A history of substance abuse complicates remission from acute mania in bipolar disorder. *J Clin Psychiatry*, **58**:18–21.

Goodwin, D. W., Schulsinger, F., Hermansen, L., *et al.* (1973). Alcohol problems in adoptees raised apart from alcoholic biological parents. *Arch Gen Psychiatry* **28**:238–43.

Goodwin, D. W., Schulsinger, F., Moller, N., *et al.* (1974). Drinking problems in adopted and nonadopted sons of alcoholics. *Arch Gen Psychiatry* **31**:164–9.

Gottheil, E., Murphy, B. F., Skoloda, T. E., *et al.* (1972). Fixed interval drinking decisions. *Q J Stud Alcohol* **33**:325–40.

Gurling, H. M. D., Clifford, C. A., Murray, R. M., *et al.* (1981). Investigations into the genetics of alcohol dependence, and into its effects on brain function. In L. Gedda, P. Parisi, & W. E. Nance, eds. *Twin Research 3: Epidemiological and Clinical Studies*. New York: Alan Liss.

Harper, C., Dixon, G., Sheedy, D., *et al.* (2003). Neuropathological alterations in alcoholic brains. Studies arising from the New South Wales Tissue Resource Centre. *Prog Neuropsychopharmacol Biol Psychiatry* **27**:951 61.

Harper, C. G., Giles, M., Finlay-Jones, R., *et al.* (1986). Clinical signs in the Wernicke-Korsakoff complex: a retrospective analysis of 131 cases diagnosed at necropsy. *J Neurol Neurosurg Psychiatry* **49**:341–5.

Hasin, D. S., Grant, B. F., Harford, T. C., *et al.* (1988). The drug dependence syndrome and related disabilities. *Br J Addict* **83**:45–55.

Hawkins, J. D., Catalano, R. F., Miller, J. Y., *et al.* (1992). Risk and protective factors for alcohol and other drug problems in adolescence and early adulthood: implications for substance abuse prevention. *Psychol Bull* **112**:64–105.

Head, J., Stansfeld, S. A., Seigrist, J., *et al.* (2004). The psychosocial work environment and alcohol dependence: a prospective study. *Occup Environ Med* **61**:219–24.

Heather, N., Peters, T. J., & Stockwell, T., eds. (2001). *The International Handbook of Alcohol Dependence and Problems*. Chichester: Wiley.

Heather, N., & Robertson, I. (1997). *Problem Drinking – The New Approach*, 3rd edn. Oxford: Oxford University Press.

Hibbell, B., Anderson, B., Bjarnason, T., *et al.* (1999). *Alcohol and Other Drug Use Among Students in 30 European Countries* (the 1999 ESPAD Report). Stockholm: Council for Information on Alcohol and Other Drugs, Council for Europe, Pompidou Group.

Higgins, E., & du Vivier, A. (1999). Alcohol intake and other skin disorders. *Clin Dermatol* **17**:437–41.

Higgins, E. M., & du Vivier, A. W. (1992). Alcohol and the skin. *Alcohol Alcohol* **27**:595–602.

Hill, S. Y., & Yuan, H. (1999). Familial density of alcoholism and onset of adolescent drinking. *J Stud Alcohol* **60**:7–17.

Hirschi, T. (1969). *Causes of Delinquency*. Berkeley: University of California Press.

Holmes, S. J., & Robins, L. N. (1987). The influence of childhood disciplinary experience on the development of alcoholism and depression. *J Child Psychol Psychiatry* **28**:399–415.

Hulse, G. K., & Tait, R. J. (2002). Six month outcomes associated with a brief alcohol intervention for adult inpatients with psychiatric disorders. *Drug Alcohol Rev* **21**:105–12.

Jeffrey, D. P., Ley, J., McLaren, S., *et al.* (2002). Psychosocial treatment programmes for people with both severe mental illness and substance misuse (Cochrane review). *The Cochrane Library*, **2**.

Jernigan, D. H., Monteiro, M., Room, R., *et al.* (2000). Towards a global alcohol policy: alcohol, public health and the role of WHO. *Bull World Health Organ* **78**:491–9.

Joseph, J. (2002). Twin studies in psychiatry and psychology: science or pseudoscience? *Psychiatr Q* **73**:71–82.

Kaij, L. (1960). *Alcoholism in Twins.* Stockholm: Almqvist & Wiksell.

Kandel, D. B. (1985). On processes of peer influences in adolescent drug use: a developmental perspective. *Adv Alcohol Subst Abuse* **4**:139–63.

Kendler, K. S., Heath, A. C., Neale, M. C., *et al.* (1992). A population-based twin study of alcoholism in women. *JAMA* **268**:1877–82.

Khan, S., Murray, R. P., Barnes, G. E., *et al.* (2002). A structural equation model of the effect of poverty and unemployment on alcohol abuse. *Addict Behav* **27**:405–23.

Khantzian, E. J. (1990). Self-regulation and self-medication factors in alcoholism and the addictions. Similarities and differences. *Recent Dev Alcohol* **8**:255–71.

Khantzian, E. J. (1997). The self-medication hypothesis of substance use disorders: a reconsideration and recent applications. *Harv Rev Psychiatry* **4**:231–44.

Koskenvuo, M., Langinvainio, H., Kaprio, J., *et al.* (1984). Health related psychosocial correlates of neuroticism: a study of adult male twins in Finland. *Acta Genet Med Gemellol (Roma)* **33**:307–20.

Kosten, T. R., Rounsaville, B. J., Babor, T. F., *et al.* (1987). Substance abuse disorders in the DSM III R: evidence of the dependence syndrome across different psychoactive substances. *B J Psychiatry* **151**, 834–43.

Kucheria, K., Saxena, R., Mohan, D., *et al.* (1985). Semen analysis in alcohol dependence syndrome. *Andrologia* **17**:558–63.

Lingford-Hughes, A. R., Welch, S., & Nutt, D. J. (2004). Evidence based guidelines for the pharmacological management of substance misuse, addiction and comorbidity: recommendations from the British Association for Psychopharmacology. *J Psychopharmacol* **18**:293–335.

Lishman, W. (1987). *Organic Psychiatry: The Psychological Consequences of Cerebral Disorder.* Oxford: Blackwell Scientific.

Lishman, W. A. (1990). Alcohol and the brain. *Br J Psychiatry* **156**:635–44.

Lowman, C., Hunt, W. A., Litten, R. Z., *et al.* (2000). Research perspectives on alcohol craving: an overview. *Addiction* **95**(Suppl 2): S45–54.

MacAndrew, C., & Edgerton, R. (1969). *Drunken comportment: A Social Explanation.* Chicago: Aldine.

Marinelli, D., Gaspari, L., Pedotti, P., *et al.* (2004). Mini-review of studies on the effect of smoking and drinking habits on semen parameters. *Int J Hyg Environ Health* **207**:185–92.

McLellan, A. T., Luborsky, L., Woody, G. E., *et al.* (1980). An improved diagnostic evaluation instrument for substance abuse patients: the Addiction Severity Index. *J Nerv Ment Dis* **168**:26–33.

Mello, N. K., & Mendelson, J. H. (1965). Operant analysis of drinking patterns of chronic alcoholics. *Nature* **206**:43–6.

Miller, W. R., Brown, J. M., Simpson, T. L., *et al.* (1995). What works? a methodological analysis of the alcohol treatment outcome literature. In R. K. Hester & W. R. Miller, eds. *Handbook of Alcoholism Treatment Approaches: Effective Alternatives.* Boston, Massachusetts: Allyn & Bacon, pp. 12–44.

Miller, W. R., & Wilbourne, P. L. (2002). Mesa Grande: a methodological analysis of clinical trials of treatments for alcohol use disorders. *Addiction* **97**:265–77.

Moyer, A., Finney, J. W., Swearingen, C. E., *et al.* (2002). Brief interventions for alcohol problems: a meta-analytic review of controlled investigations in treatment-seeking and non-treatment-seeking populations. *Addiction* **97**:279–92.

Newlin, D. B., Miles, D. R., van den Bree, M. B., *et al.* (2000). Environmental transmission of DSM-IV substance use disorders in adoptive and step families. *Alcohol Clin Exp Res* **24**:1785–94.

Noble, E. P. (1996). Alcoholism and the dopaminergic system: a review. *Addict Biol* **1**:333–48.

Nunes, E., & Levin, F. (2004). Treatment of depression in patients with alcohol or other drug dependence: a meta-analysis. *JAMA* **291**:1887–96.

Nurnberger, J. I., Jr., Wiegand, R., Bucholz, K., *et al.* (2004). A family study of alcohol dependence: coaggregation of multiple disorders in relatives of alcohol-dependent probands. *Arch Gen Psychiatry* 61:1246–56.

Ogden, E. J., & Moskowitz, H. (2004). Effects of alcohol and other drugs on driver performance. *Traffic Inj Prev* 5:185–98.

Osier, M. V., Pakstis, A. J., Soodyall, J., *et al.* (2002). A global perspective on genetic variation at the ADH genes reveals unusual patterns of linkage disequilibrium and diversity. *Am J Hum Genet* 71:84–99.

Paredes, A., Hood, W. R., Seymour, H., *et al.* (1973). Loss of control in alcoholism: an investigation of the hypothesis, with experimental findings. *Q J Stud Alcohol* 34:1146–61.

Parish, L. C., & Fine, E. (1985). Alcoholism and skin disease. *Int J Dermatol* 24:300–1.

Paschall, M. J., Flewelling, R. L., Russell, T., *et al.* (2004). Why is work intensity associated with heavy alcohol use among adolescents? *J Adolesc Health* 34:79–87.

Pickens, R. W., Svikis, D. S., McGue, M., *et al.* (1991). Heterogeneity in the inheritance of alcoholism. A study of male and female twins. *Arch Gen Psychiatry* 48:19–28.

Plant, M. A. (1979). Occupations, drinking patterns and alcohol-related problems: conclusions from a follow-up study. *Br J Addict Alcohol Other Drugs* 74:267–73.

Poschl, G., & Seitz, H. K. (2004). Alcohol and cancer. *Alcohol Alcohol* 39:155–65.

Poschl, G., Stickel, F., Wang, X. D., *et al.* (2004). Alcohol and cancer: genetic and nutritional aspects. *Proc Nutr Soc* 63:65–71.

Preedy, V. R., Ohlendieck, K., Adachi, J., *et al.* (2003). The importance of alcohol-induced muscle disease. *J Muscle Res Cell Motil* 24:55–63.

Prescott, C. (2003). Sex differences in the genetic risk for alcoholism [on-line]. National Institute on Alcohol Abuse and Alcoholism. Available at http://pubs.niaaa.nih.gov/publications/arh26-4/264-273.htm.

The Prime Minister's Strategy Unit (2003). *Alcohol Project: Interim Analytical Report.* London: Cabinet Office.

Prochaska, J. O., & DiClemente, C. C. (1984). *The Transtheoretical Approach: Crossing the Traditional Boundaries of Therapy.* Homewood: Dow Jones/Irwin.

Raistrick, D. (2001). Alcohol withdrawal and detoxification. In N. Heather, T. J. Peters and T. Stockwell, eds. *International Handbook of Alcohol Dependence and Problems.* Chichester: Wiley.

Raistrick, D., Bradshaw, J., Tober, G., *et al.* (1994). Development of the Leeds Dependence Questionnaire (LDQ):

a questionnaire to measure alcohol and opiate dependence in the context of a treatment evaluation package. *Addiction* 89:563–572.

Raistrick, D., Dunbar, G., & Robinson, D. (1983). Development of a questionnaire to measure alcohol dependence. *Br J Addict* 78:98–95.

Rambaldi, A., & Gluud, C. (2002). Propylthiouracil for alcoholic liver disease. *Cochrane Database Syst Rev.* CD002800.

Raw, M., McNeill, A., & West, R. (1998). Smoking cessation guidelines for health professionals: a guide to effective smoking cessation interventions for the health care system. *Thorax* 53(Suppl. 5):S1–S37.

Regier, D. A., Farmer, M. E., Rae, D. S., *et al.* (1990). Comorbidity of mental disorders with alcohol and other drug abuse. Results from the Epidemiologic Catchment Area (ECA) Study. *JAMA* 264:2511–18.

Ries, R. K., Russo, J., Wingerson, D., *et al.* (2000). Shorter hospital stays and more rapid improvement among patients with schizophrenia and substance use disorder. *Psychiatr Serv* 51:210–15.

Romberger, D. J., & Grant, K. (2004). Alcohol consumption and smoking status: the role of smoking cessation. *Biomed Pharmacother* 50:77–83.

Room, R. (2001). Intoxication and bad behaviour: understanding cultural differences in the link. *Soc Sci Med* 53:189–98.

Rounsaville, B. J., Bryant, K., Babor, T., *et al.* (1993). Cross-system agreement for substance use disorders: DSM-III-R, DSM-IV, and ICD-10. *Addiction* 88:337–48.

Ruhm, C. J., & Black, W. E. (2002). Does drinking really decrease in bad times? *J Health Econ* 21:659–78.

Rush, B. (1790). *An Inquiry into the Effects of Ardent Spirits on the Human Body and Mind, with an Account of the Means for Preventing and of the Remedies for Curing Them* (8th edn., 1814). Brookfields: E. Merriam. Reprinted in *Q J Stud Alcohol* 4:325–41.

Saitz, R., Harlon, N. J., Larson, M. J., *et al.* (2005). Primary medical care and reductions in addiction severity: a prospective cohort study. *Addiction* 100:70–8.

Saunders, J. B., Aasland, O. G., Babor, T. F., *et al.* (1993). Development of the Alcohol Use Disorders Identification Test (AUDIT): WHO collaborative project on early detection of persons with harmful alcohol consumption II. *Addiction*, 88:791–804.

Schuckit, M. A., & Smith, T. L. (1997). Assessing the risk for alcoholism among sons of alcoholics. *J Stud Alcohol* 58:141–5.

Schuckit, M. A., & Smith, T. L. (2001). Correlates of unpredicted outcomes in sons of alcoholics and controls. *J Stud Alcohol* **62**:477–85.

Selzer, M. L. (1971). The Michigan Alcoholism Screening Test: the quest for a new diagnostic instrument. *Am J Psychiatry* **127**:1653–8.

Sesso, H. D. (2001). Alcohol and cardiovascular health: recent findings. *Am J Cardiovasc Drugs* **1**:167–72.

Shand, F., Gates, J., Fawcett, J., & Mattick, R. (2003). *The Treatment of Alcohol Problems: A Review of the Evidence.* Australia: National Drug and Alcohol Research Centre, Department of Health and Ageing.

Shibuya, A., & Yoshida, A. (1988). Frequency of the atypical aldehyde dehydrogenase-2 gene (ALDH2(2)) in Japanese and Caucasians. *Am J Hum Genet* **43**:741–3.

Sigvardsson, S., Bohman, M., *et al.* (1996). Replication of the Stockholm Adoption Study of alcoholism. Confirmatory cross-fostering analysis. *Arch Gen Psychiatry* **53**:681–7.

Skinner, H. A., & Allen, B. A. (1983). Differential assessment of alcoholism: evaluation of the alcohol use inventory. *J Stud Alcohol* **44**:852–62.

Skinner, H. A., & Allen, B. A. (1982). Alcohol dependence syndrome: measurement and validation. *J Abnorm Psychol* **91**:199–209.

Skinner, H. A., & Horn, J. L. (1984). *Alcohol Dependence Scale: User's Guide.* Toronto: Addiction Research Foundation.

Slap, G., Goodman, E., *et al.* (2001). Adoption as a risk factor for attempted suicide during adolescence. *Pediatrics* **108**:E30.

Slattery, J., Chick, J., Cochrane, M., *et al.* (2003). *Prevention of relapse in alcohol dependence* (Health Technology Assessment Report 3). Glasgow: Health Technology Board for Scotland.

Stockwell, T. R., Hodgson, R. J., Rankin, H. J., *et al.* (1979). The development of a questionnaire to measure severity of alcohol dependence. *Br J Addiction* **74**:79–87.

Stockwell, T., Murphy, D., & Hodgson, R. (1983). The Severity of Alcohol Dependence Questionnaire: its use, reliability and validity. *Br J Addiction* **78**:145–55.

Sullivan, J. T., & K. Sykora, *et al.* (1989). Assessment of alcohol withdrawal: the revised clinical institute withdrawal assessment for alcohol scale (CIWA-Ar). *Br J Addict* **84**:1353–7.

Svensson, R. (2003). Gender differences in adolescent drug use: the impact of parental monitoring and peer deviance. *Youth Soc* **34**:300–29.

Thom, B., & Tellez, C. (1986). A difficult business: detecting and managing alcohol problems in general practice. *Br J Addiction* **81**:405–18.

Thomson, A. D., C. C. Cook, *et al.* (2002). The Royal College of Physicians report on alcohol: guidelines for managing Wernicke's encephalopathy in the accident and Emergency Department. *Alcohol Alcohol* **37**:513–21.

Tome, S., & Lucey, M. R. (2004). Review article: current management of alcoholic liver disease. *Aliment Pharmacol Ther* **19**:707–14.

Trotter, T. (1804). *An Essay, Medical, Philosophical and Chemical, on Drunkenness, and Its Effects on the Human Body.* London: T. N. Longman & G. Rees. Facsimile reproduction 1988 with an introduction by Roy Porter. London: Routledge.

Turner, R. T. (2000). Skeletal response to alcohol. *Alcohol Clin Exp Res* **24**:1693–1701.

Turner, R. T., & Sibonga, J. D. (2001). Effects of alcohol use and estrogen on bone. *Alcohol Res Health* **25**:276–81.

Vaillant, G. E. (1983). *The Natural History of Alcoholism.* Cambridge, Massachusetts: Harvard University Press.

Velleman, R., & Orford, J. (1993). The adult adjustment of offspring of parents with drinking problems. *Br J Psychiatry* **162**:503–16.

Viola, A., Nicoli, F., *et al.* (2001). Applications of magnetic resonance spectrometry (MRS) in the study of metabolic disturbances affecting the brain in alcoholism. *Pathol Biol (Paris)* **49**:718–25.

Walters, G. D. (2002). The heritability of alcohol abuse and dependence: a meta-analysis of behavior genetic research. *Am J Drug Alcohol Abuse* **28**:557–84.

Whitfield, J. B., Zhu, G., *et al.* (2004). The genetics of alcohol intake and of alcohol dependence. *Alcohol Clin Exp Res* **28**:1153–60.

Wilk, A. I., Jensen, N. M. & Havighurst, T. C. (1997). Meta-analysis of randomized controlled trials addressing brief interventions in heavy alcohol drinkers. *J Gen Int Med* **12**:274–83.

Windle, M. (1977). Effect of parental drinking on adolescents. *Research in Brief. Buffalo,* New York: Research Institute on Addictions.

World Health Organisation (2004). *Global Status Report on Alcohol Policy*. Geneva: World Health Organisation.

World Health Organisation (1992). *ICD–10 Classification of Mental and Behavioural Disorders*. Geneva: World Health Organisation.

World Health Organisation (1952). *Expert Committee on Mental Health, Alcoholism Subcommittee, Second Report* (WHO Technical Report Series No. 48). Geneva: World Health Organisation.

Yoshida, A., Huang, I. Y., Ikawa, M., *et al.* (1984). Molecular abnormality of an inactive aldehyde dehydrogenase variant commonly found in Orientals. *Proc Natl Acad Sci U S A* **81**:258–61.

Zimberg, S. (1993). Introduction and general concepts of dual diagnosis. In J. Solomon, S. Zimberg & E. Shollar, eds. *Dual Diagnosis – Evaluation, Treatment, Training and Program Development*. New York: Plenum.

11

Drug use and drug dependence

Wayne Hall and Michael Farrell

Drug use disorders (which include harmful use and dependence on alcohol or other drugs) typically involve impaired control over the use of drugs. Obtaining, using and recovering from the effects of the drug consumes a disproportionate amount of the users' time, and they continue to take drugs in the face of problems that they know to be caused by them. They typically become tolerant to the effects of drugs, requiring larger doses to achieve the desired psychological effect, and abrupt cessation of use often produces a withdrawal syndrome. Many experience other psychological and physical health problems, and their alcohol or drug use often adversely affects the lives of their spouses, children, other family members, friends and workmates.

The focus of much research and treatment intervention has been on dependent patterns of drug use. The original description of alcohol dependence (Edwards & Gross, 1976) has since been extended to nicotine, benzodiazepines and other sedatives, opioids, stimulants and a range of other psychoactive drugs. Operational and diagnostic guidelines for the diagnosis of dependence have been delineated in *International Classification of Diseases* (ICD-10) and the *Diagnostic and Statistical Manual of Mental Disorders* (4th edition, text revision DSM-IV-R). Harmful use is defined as a pattern of psychoactive drug use that causes damage to health, either mental or physical, that can occur in the absence of actual dependence.

Harm reduction is a term that has been used as equivalent to *harm minimisation*. These are essentially practical strategies that can be mobilised to reduce some of the adverse consequences of drug use, such as the provision of clean injecting equipment to reduce the risk of spread of HIV among injecting-drug users or the prescription of a substitute oral opioid or stimulant drug to dependent users.

Some of the complexities of drug policy are related to the illegality of the substances and the complex way in which the legal consequences are intertwined with patterns of use. As an approach to this chapter, we explore the issues as far as appropriate health interventions are concerned, many of which would be delivered in a similar manner irrespective of the legal status of the substance.

Patterns of drug use are now so ubiquitous in modern society that it behoves modern mental health professionals to have as part of their core clinical skills a capacity to incorporate drug screening and assessment into a generic mental health assessment. Drug problems are extremely common in general mental health services, and mental health problems are common in those with drug dependence so that the skills of professionals who work in each of these services need to be shared.

This chapter describes the major forms of drug use and dependence in developed countries, that is, cannabis, amphetamines, cocaine and heroin. In each case, we outline patterns of use, problems

Essential Psychiatry, ed. Robin M. Murray, Kenneth S. Kendler, Peter McGuffin, Simon Wessely, David J. Castle. Published by Cambridge University Press. © Cambridge University Press 2008.

experienced by users and interventions to assist dependent users.

Cannabis

Cannabis is the most widely used illicit drug globally, with around 150 million users, or 3.7% of the world's population aged 15 years and older (United Nations Office for Drug Control and Crime Prevention [UNODCCP], 2003). Europe generally has lower rates of use than Australia, Canada and the United States, with the highest rates in the United Kingdom, Denmark and France (European Monitoring Centre for Drugs and Drug Addiction [EMCDDA], 2002; Hall & Pacula, 2003).

The "natural history" of cannabis use in the United States typically begins in the mid to late teens and reaches its peak in the early 20s before declining in the mid to late 20s. Only a minority of young adults continue to use cannabis into their 30s (Bachman et al., 1997, Chen & Kandel, 1995). Getting married and having children substantially reduces rates of cannabis use (Bachman et al., 1997).

Acute effects

The most common unpleasant effects of cannabis use are anxiety and panic reactions that most often occur in users who are unfamiliar with the drug's effects. Psychotic symptoms such as delusions and hallucinations may occur with high doses. There are no cases of fatal cannabis poisoning in the medical literature, and the fatal dose in humans is likely to exceed what recreational users are able to ingest (Hall & Pacula, 2003).

Cannabis intoxication impairs a wide range of cognitive and behavioural functions that are involved in tasks such as driving an automobile or operating machinery (Beardsley & Kelly, 1999; Jaffe, 1985). Cannabinoids are found in the blood of substantial proportions of persons killed in motor vehicle accidents (Bates & Blakely, 1999; Chesher, 1995; Walsh & Mann, 1999), but these findings have

been difficult to evaluate because they have not distinguished between past and recent cannabis use (Ramaekers et al., 2004). More recent research using better indicators of recent cannabis use has found a dose-response relationship between cannabis and risk of motor vehicle crashes (Ramaekers et al., 2004). Cannabis used in combination with alcohol substantially increases risk of accidents (Bates & Blakely, 1999; Ramaekers et al., 2004).

The health effects of chronic cannabis use

Cannabis smoke is a potential cause of cancer because it contains many of the same carcinogenic substances as cigarette smoke (Marselos & Karamanakos, 1999). Cancers have been reported in the aerodigestive tracts of young adults who were daily cannabis smokers (Hall & MacPhee, 2002) and a case-control study found an association between cannabis smoking and head and neck cancer (Zhang et al., 1999). However, a prospective cohort study of 64000 adults did not find any increase in rates of head and neck or respiratory cancers among habitual cannabis users (Sidney et al., 1997). Further studies are needed to clarify these issues.

Regular cannabis smoking impairs the functioning of the large airways and causes chronic bronchitis (Tashkin, 1999; Taylor et al., 2002). Given that tobacco and cannabis smoke contain similar carcinogenic substances, it is likely that chronic cannabis smoking increases the risks of respiratory cancer (Tashkin, 1999).

Psychological effects of chronic cannabis use

A cannabis dependence syndrome occurs in heavy chronic users of cannabis (American Psychiatric Association, 1994). Regular cannabis users develop tolerance to THC, some experience withdrawal symptoms on cessation of use (Kouri & Pope, 2000) and some report problems controlling their cannabis use (Hall & Pacula, 2003). The risk of dependence is about 1 in 10 among those who ever use the drug, between 1 in 5 and 1 in 3 among those who use cannabis more than a few times and around 1 in 2 among daily users (Hall & Pacula, 2003).

Long-term daily cannabis use does not severely impair cognitive function, but it may exert subtle effects on memory, attention and the integration of complex information (Solowij, 1998; Solowij *et al.*, 2002). It remains uncertain whether these effects are due to the cumulative effect of regular cannabis use on cannabinoid receptors in the brain or they are the residual effects of THC that will disappear after an extended period of abstinence (Hall & Pacula, 2003).

There is now good evidence that chronic cannabis use may precipitate psychosis in vulnerable individuals (e.g. Arseneault *et al.*, 2002; van Os *et al.*, 2002; Zammit *et al.*, 2002). It is less likely that cannabis use can cause schizophrenia de novo because the incidence of schizophrenia has either remained stable or declined while cannabis use has increased among young adults (Degenhardt *et al.*, 2003).

The effects of adolescent cannabis use

The gateway hypothesis

Among adolescents in developed societies alcohol and tobacco have typically been used before cannabis, which in turn, has been used before hallucinogens, amphetamine, heroin and cocaine (Kandel, 2002). Generally, the earlier the age of first use, and the greater the involvement with any drug in the sequence, the more likely a young person is to use the next drug in the sequence (Kandel, 2002). The role played by cannabis in this sequence remains controversial (Hall and Lynskey, in press; Hall & Pacula, 2003).

The simplest hypothesis is that cannabis use has a pharmacological effect that increases the risk of using later drugs in the sequence. Equally plausible hypotheses are that it is due to a combination of (1) early recruitment into cannabis use of nonconforming and deviant adolescents who are likely to use alcohol, tobacco and illicit drugs; (2) a shared genetic vulnerability to dependence on alcohol, tobacco and cannabis; and (3) socialisation

of cannabis users within an illicit drug using subculture which increases the opportunity, and encouragement to use other illicit drugs (Hall & Pacula, 2003).

Adolescent psychosocial outcomes

Cannabis use is associated with early leaving of high school, early family formation, poor mental health and involvement in drug-related crime. In the case of each of these outcomes, the strong associations in cross-sectional data are more modest when account is taken of the fact that cannabis users show characteristics before they use cannabis which predict these outcomes, for example, have lower academic aspirations and poorer school performance than peers who do not use (Lynskey & Hall, 2000; McLeod *et al.*, 2004). Nonetheless, the evidence increasingly suggests that regular cannabis use adds to the risk of these outcomes in adolescents already at risk (Hall & Pacula, 2003).

Interventions for cannabis dependence

Although many dependent cannabis users may succeed in quitting without professional help, there are some who are unable to stop on their own and will need assistance. There has not been a great deal of research on pharmacological treatments for cannabis dependence although a recent study trialled divalproex sodium with promising results (Levin *et al.*, 2004). There has been limited research on the effectiveness of different types of psychosocial treatments for dependent cannabis use (Budney *et al.*, 2000; Copeland *et al.*, 2001; Stephens *et al.*, 1994). These have involved short-term cognitive-behavioural treatments modelled on similar treatments for alcohol dependence, usually given in three to six sessions on an outpatient basis.

In all of these studies rates of abstinence at the end of treatment have been modest (20%–40%) and subsequent high rates of relapse mean that rates of abstinence after 12 months have been modest (Budney & Moore, 2002). Nonetheless, treatment does substantially reduce cannabis use and problems. These outcomes are not very different from those observed in the treatment for alcohol and other forms of drug dependence (Budney & Moore, 2002). Much more research is needed before sensible advice can be given about the best ways to achieve abstinence from cannabis.

Cocaine

After cannabis, cocaine is one of the most widely used illicit drugs in developed and developing societies. Globally, 14 million people were estimated to have used cocaine in 2003, with treatment demand second only to heroin (UNODCCP, 2003). The highest rates of reported cocaine use are in the United States. Rates of cocaine use in the United States increased from the mid-1970s until 1985 when 5.7 million Americans aged 12 years and older reported using cocaine in the previous month. Rates of cocaine use have declined steadily since 1985. In 2000, 11.2% of Americans over age 12 reported that they had used cocaine at some time in their lives, and 0.4% (800,000 people) reported weekly cocaine use (Substance Abuse and Mental Health Services Administration [SAMHSA], 2001).

The reported prevalence of cocaine use in other developed societies is much lower than that in the United States. In Europe, for example, rates of lifetime cocaine use range from 0.5% to 5% (EMCDDA, 2003) compared with 12.3% among American adults in 2001 (SAMHSA, 2001).

The adverse health effects of cocaine

Most cocaine use is infrequent, but regular cocaine use (monthly or more frequently) can be a major public health problem. Regular cocaine users who inject cocaine or smoke crack cocaine are especially likely to develop dependence and to experience problems related to their cocaine use (Platt, 1997). In the United States, it has been estimated that one in six of those who ever use cocaine become dependent on the drug (Anthony et al., 1994). High rates of cocaine dependence are found among persons treated for alcohol and drug problems and among arrestees in the United States (Anglin & Perrochet, 1998).

In large doses, cocaine may be harmful in both cocaine-naïve and tolerant individuals (Platt, 1997; Vasica & Tennant, 2002). The vasoconstrictor effects of cocaine taken in large doses places great strain on a number of the body's physiological systems (McCann & Ricaurte, 2000). Effects on the cardiovascular system can result in a range of difficulties from chest pain through to fatal cardiac arrest (Lange & Hillis, 2001). Neurological problems include cerebral vascular accidents such as strokes or seizures.

Adverse health effects from cocaine are potentially fatal and can occur among healthy users irrespective of cocaine dose and frequency of use (Lange & Hillis, 2001; Vasica & Tennant, 2002). Although the likelihood of health problems may increase with dose and frequency of use, there is wide interindividual variation in reactions to cocaine and therefore no specific combination of conditions under which adverse health effects occur can be predicted. There is no antidote to cocaine overdose as there is for an overdose of heroin (Platt, 1997).

The impact of cocaine on mental health is also complex. Although cocaine can produce feelings of pleasure, it may also result in negative psychological symptoms such as anxiety, depression, paranoia, hallucinations and agitation (American Psychiatric Association, 1994). Regular cocaine users experience high rates of psychiatric disorders. In the United States, regular cocaine users report high rates of anxiety and affective disorders (Gawin & Ellinwood, 1988; Platt, 1997). The repeated use of large doses of cocaine can also produce a paranoid psychosis (Majewska, 1996; Manschreck et al., 1988; Platt, 1997; Satel & Edell, 1991). Persons who are acutely intoxicated by cocaine can become violent, especially those who develop a paranoid psychosis (Platt, 1997).

Animal studies suggest that cocaine use may be neurotoxic in large doses, that is, it can produce permanent changes in the brain and neurotransmitter systems (Majewska, 1996; Platt, 1997). It is unclear whether it is also neurotoxic in humans. Previous studies have documented a variety of neuropsychological effects of cocaine use including deficits in memory and problem solving (Beatty *et al.*, 1995; Hoff *et al.*, 1996; O'Malley *et al.*, 1992). More recently, a twin study indicated that cocaine may lead to impaired attention and motor skills up to 1 year after the conclusion of heavy use (Toomey *et al.*, 2003).

The method in which cocaine is administered can result in adverse health effects (Platt, 1997). "Snorting" cocaine can lead to rhinitis, damage to the nasal septum and loss of sense of smell. Smoking cocaine can lead to respiratory problems, and injecting cocaine leads to the risk of infections and contracting blood-borne viruses associated with all injecting drug use.

Users who inject cocaine, either on its own or in combination with heroin ("speedballs"), inject much more frequently than other injecting drug users and, as a consequence, engage in more needle sharing and more sexual risk taking and have higher rates of HIV infection (Chaisson *et al.*, 1989; Schoenbaum *et al.*, 1989; van Beek *et al.*, 2001). Associations between cocaine use and HIV risk taking has been reported in Europe (Torrens *et al.*, 1991), Australia (Darke *et al.*, 1992) and the United States (Chaisson *et al.*, 1989). Injecting cocaine users report more problems related to injecting drug use such as vascular problems, abscesses and infections, than other injecting drug users (Darke *et al.*, 1992).

The link between cocaine use and HIV risk is not restricted to those who inject cocaine. Crack smoking has been linked to higher levels of needle risk, sexual risk taking and HIV infection (Chaisson *et al.*, 1989; Chirgwin *et al.*, 1991; Des Jarlais *et al.*, 1992; Grella *et al.*, 1995). Two mechanisms probably underlie the relationship between cocaine use and HIV infection. First, the short half-life of cocaine promotes a much higher frequency of injecting than that seen in heroin injectors. Second, cocaine itself disinhibits and stimulates users, encouraging them to take greater risks with sexual activity and needle use (Darke *et al.*, 2000).

Cocaine is associated with a heightened risk of intentional injuries and injuries in general. A recent review reported that 28.7% of people with intentional injuries and 4.5% of injured drivers tested positive for cocaine (Macdonald *et al.*, 2003). Users are also at risk of death from an accidental overdose of cocaine. A recent study of accidental deaths from drug overdose in New York between 1990 and 1998 found that 70% of deaths were caused by cocaine, often in combination with opiates (Coffin *et al.*, 2003). The causes of cocaine-related deaths are usually related to cardiovascular complications (Vasica & Tennant, 2002) but may also be due to brain haemorrhage, stroke and kidney failure (Brands *et al.*, 1998). Injection of cocaine is most likely to cause risk of overdose, followed by smoking, with intranasal use involving the lowest risk (Pottieger *et al.*, 1992).

Interventions for cocaine dependence

Pharmacological interventions

There are no effective pharmacological treatments for cocaine dependence (Kreek, 1997; McCance, 1997; Mendelson & Mellon, 1996; Nunes, 1997; Silva de Lima *et al.*, 2002; van den Brink & van Ree, 2003). Development and evaluation of pharmacological therapies for cocaine dependence is complicated by the multiple interactive processes that may have contributed, for example, coexisting substance abuse or mental health issues (Mendelson & Mellon, 1996). Many of the approaches to the treatment of cocaine dependence have also been used in treating patients with alcoholism and other substance abuse disorders.

Psychotherapy and cognitive-behavioural therapy

The lack of evidence for pharmacological therapy means that treatment for cocaine dependence currently relies on cognitive-behavioural techniques combined with contingency management strategies. Unfortunately, psychosocial treatments for cocaine dependence are also of limited effectiveness. Treatments such as therapeutic communities, cognitive-behavioural treatments, contingency management and 12-step-based self-help approaches benefit cocaine-dependent persons in reducing rates of cocaine use and improving their health and well-being, but rates of relapse to cocaine use after treatment remain high (Platt, 1997).

A multicenter investigation examining the efficacy of four psychosocial treatments for cocaine-dependent patients concluded that individual drug counselling in combination with group drug counselling showed the most promise for effective treatment of cocaine dependence over two forms of traditional psychotherapy (Crits-Christoph et al., 1999). Community reinforcement involving an intensive biopsychosocial multifaceted approach to lifestyle change has shown positive effects over 4 to 6 weeks and has the advantage of tailoring to individual goals (Roozen et al., 2004).

The few studies of the long-term effects of treatment have not shown particularly encouraging results. A 1-year follow-up of the US Drug Abuse Treatment Outcome Studies reported that reductions in the use of cocaine in the year following treatment were associated with longer duration of treatment, particularly 6 months or more in long-term residential or outpatient treatments (Hubbard et al., 2003). A 5-year national follow-up study of 45 US treatment programs found that only 33% of the sample had highly favourable outcomes (Flynn et al., 2003).

Amphetamines

According to the World Health Organization (WHO), amphetamines and methamphetamines are the most widely abused illicit drugs after cannabis, with an estimated 35 million users worldwide (Rawson et al., 2002). Globally, Europe is the main centre of amphetamine production, particularly the Netherlands, Poland and Belgium, with production increasing in Eastern Europe (UNODCCP, 2003). Half of all Western European countries reported an increase in amphetamine abuse in 2000, but in 2001 only a third did so (UNODCCP, 2003). Lifetime use of amphetamines is reported to be between 0.5% and 6% among European Union countries with the exception of the United Kingdom where the figure is 11%.

The adverse health effects of amphetamine use

Amphetamine users who inject the drug are at high risk of blood-borne infections through needle sharing. Amphetamine users are as likely as opioid users to share injection equipment (Darke et al., 1995a, 1995b; Hall et al., 1993; Hando & Hall, 1994; Kaye & Darke, 2000; Loxley & Marsh, 1991). In addition, the youthfulness of amphetamine users places them at risk of sexual transmission of diseases such as HIV and hepatitis B virus (HBV) although not hepatitis C virus (HCV). Primary amphetamine users have been demonstrated to be a sexually active group, and small proportions engage in paid sex to support drug use (Darke et al., 1995a; Hando & Hall, 1994). Among gay and bisexual men, amphetamines may be used to enhance sexual encounters, and this may lead to unprotected anal intercourse and increased risk of HIV infection (Urbina & Jones, 2004).

High-dose amphetamine use, especially by injection, can result in a schizophreniform paranoid psychosis, associated with loosening of associations, delusions and hallucinations (Gawin & Ellinwood, 1988; Jaffe, 1985). The psychosis could be reproduced by the injection of large doses in addicts (Bell, 1973) and by the repeated administration of large doses to normal volunteers (Angrist et al., 1974).

High proportions of regular amphetamine injectors describe symptoms of anxiety, panic attacks, paranoia and depression (Hall et al., 1996; McKetin & Mattick, 1997, 1998). The emergence of such symptoms is associated with injecting the drugs, greater frequency of use and dependence upon amphetamines (Hall et al., 1996; McKetin & Mattick, 1997, 1998).

In sufficiently high doses, amphetamines can be lethal (Derlet *et al.*, 1989). However, the risk is low compared with the high risks of overdose associated with central nervous system depressants such as heroin. Typically, amphetamine-related deaths are associated with the effects of amphetamines on the cardiovascular system, such as cardiac failure and cerebral vascular accidents (Mattick & Darke, 1995).

There is evidence that amphetamines are neurotoxic (Robinson & Becker, 1986). Evidence from animal studies indicates that heavy amphetamine use results in dopaminergic depletion (Ellison, 1992; Fields *et al.*, 1991). The few studies of the neuropsychological effects of amphetamine abuse report findings similar to those found in cocaine abuse. Deficits in memory and attention have been attributed to amphetamine use (McKetin & Mattick, 1997, 1998). More recently, a twin study indicated that amphetamine abuse might lead to impaired attention and motor skills up to 1 year after the conclusion of heavy use (Toomey *et al.*, 2003).

Interventions for amphetamine dependence

Treatment for methamphetamine abuse has been a relatively recent development and has generally been based on previous treatments for cocaine abuse (Huber *et al.*, 1997). A Cochrane Review concluded that evidence for success in treatment of amphetamine dependence is limited with no pharmacological treatment demonstrated to be effective (Srisurapanont *et al.*, 2003). Although some promising interventions have been identified to assist methamphetamine abusers, no single treatment option has been established as better than any other in a randomised controlled trial (Cretzmeyer *et al.*, 2003).

Heroin and other illicit opioid dependence

In household surveys, 1% to 2% of adults in developed countries (such as Australia, Europe and the United States) report that they have used heroin at some time in their lives (Australian Institute of Health and Welfare [AIHW], 1999; EMCDDA, 2002; Makkai & McAllister, 1998; SAMHSA, 2002). The highest rates of reported use are typically among adults aged 20 to 29 years (AIHW, 1999; SAMHSA, 2002).

A minority of those who report heroin use (around one in four) continue to use the drug often enough and for long enough to become dependent on it (Anthony *et al.*, 1994). Persons who are heroin dependent have impaired control over their use of heroin in that they continue to use it in the face of problems that they know (or believe) to be caused by their use. These problems include being arrested or imprisoned, interpersonal and family problems, infectious diseases and drug overdoses. Many heroin users who seek treatment have typically been daily heroin injectors, although in both Europe (EMCDDA, 2002) and North America (Office of National Drug Control Policy, 2001), heroin users now also smoke or chase the drug (inhale the fumes released when heroin is heated; UNODCCP, 2003).

Household surveys are known to underestimate the prevalence of heroin dependence (Hall *et al.*, 2000), and indirect methods produce better estimates (Hartnoll *et al.*, 1985). These estimates suggest that the population prevalence of heroin dependence in Australia is less than 1% of adults aged 15 to 54 years (Hall *et al.*, 2000). Very similar estimates have been derived in the United Kingdom and the European Union (EMCDDA, 1997, 2002).

Research in the United States indicates that dependent heroin users who seek treatment or come to attention through the legal system may continue to use heroin for decades (Goldstein & Herrera, 1995; Hser *et al.*, 1993). In this population, daily heroin use is punctuated by periods of abstinence, drug treatment or imprisonment. In the year after any episode of drug treatment, the majority of users relapse to heroin use (Gerstein & Harwood, 1990). When periods of voluntary and involuntary abstinence during treatment or imprisonment are included, dependent heroin users use heroin daily for 40% to 60% of their addiction careers (Ball *et al.*, 1983; Maddux & Desmond, 1992). The average duration of addiction careers has been estimated to be

20 years (Ball *et al.*, 1983), meaning that 20 years after initiating heroin use in the mid to late teens, approximately half will still be using heroin with the remainder having become abstinent or having died from drug-related causes (Hall *et al.*, 1999).

Mortality, morbidity and heroin dependence

Long-term heroin users have a substantially increased risk of premature death from drug overdoses, violence, suicide and alcohol-related causes (Darke *et al.*, 1999; Goldstein & Herrera, 1995; Hulse *et al.*, 1999). Cohort studies of the mortality of heroin users treated before the advent of HIV indicated that they were 13 times more likely to die prematurely than their age peers (English *et al.*, 1995; Hulse *et al.*, 1999). Analyses of premature mortality due to illicit drug use in Australia indicated that one of the most frequent causes of death among heroin users is opioid overdose (Hall *et al.*, 1999). In countries with a high prevalence of HIV infection among injecting drug users, deaths from AIDS are a major contributor to premature death among heroin users (EMCDDA, 2002; UNAIDS/WHO, 2002). Fatal opioid overdose deaths have increased in many but not all developed societies over the past several decades (Donoghoe *et al.*, 1998; EMCDDA, 2002).

The risk of fatal opioid overdose is higher among heroin injectors who are male and increases with the duration of heroin dependence. The male excess only partially reflects the higher prevalence of heroin dependence among males (2:1; Hall *et al.*, 1999); it probably reflects in part the greater propensity of males who use illicit opioids to use alcohol and engage in other risk behaviour (Hall *et al.*, 1999). The risk of fatal overdose is also higher among those who use heroin with alcohol and benzodiazepines and among users who return to heroin use after a period of abstinence, be it voluntary or coerced (Darke & Zador, 1996; Tagliaro *et al.*, 1998; Warner-Smith *et al.*, 2001).

In some parts of the United States, Southeast Asia and Eastern Europe, the sharing of contaminated needles, syringes and other injecting equipment accounts for a substantial proportion of HIV infections (EMCDDA, 2002; UNAIDS/WHO, 2002). The prevalence of HCV is even higher among injecting drug users; it is between 50% and 60% in Australia (National Centre in HIV Epidemiology and Clinical Research, 1998) and between 20% and 90% in the European Union (EMCDDA, 2002). Chronic infection has been estimated to occur in 75% of infections, and 3% to 11% of chronic HCV carriers will develop liver cirrhosis within 20 years (Hepatitis C Virus Projections Working Group, 1998).

Heroin-related deaths (whether by overdose, suicide or HIV/AIDS) primarily occur among young adults and so account for a substantial number of life years lost in some developed societies. In Australia in 1996, for example, deaths from illicit drugs (which were almost wholly due to illicit opioids) accounted for 2.2% of life years lost with each death accounting for an average of 22 years of life lost (Mathers *et al.*, 1999). In some parts of Europe, namely, Scotland and Spain, opiate-related deaths account for as many as 25% to 33% of deaths in young adult males (EMCDDA, 2002).

Interventions to reduce heroin-related harms

Blood-borne virus infection

Foremost among interventions to reduce blood-borne virus infection (BBV) arising from illicit injecting opioid use is the provision of clean needles and syringes and other injecting equipment to reduce users' risks of contracting or transmitting BBV. This intervention has been widely supported in developed societies but has been incompletely adopted in developing countries which have problems with illicit injecting drug use (UNAIDS/WHO, 2002). In the case of infection with HBV, vaccination is available for injecting drug users.

Opioid overdose deaths

A number of strategies can potentially reduce opioid overdose deaths (Darke & Hall, 2003; Sporer, 2003). One is to educate injecting drug users about the dangers of polydrug use and injecting alone (McGregor *et al.*, 2001). The risks of fatal opioid overdose are heightened by the concurrent use of other central nervous system depressant drugs, particularly benzodiazepines and alcohol (Darke & Zador, 1996; Warner-Smith *et al.*, 2001). It is therefore important that heroin users are informed about the risks of using heroin with alcohol and other depressant drugs. Heroin users also need to be discouraged from injecting in the streets or alone, thereby denying themselves assistance in the event of an overdose. These strategies have not been rigorously evaluated to date.

A second strategy is to improve bystander responses to opioid overdoses. This includes encouraging drug users who witness overdoses to seek medical assistance and to use simple but effective resuscitation techniques until help arrives. A more controversial option would be to distribute naloxone to opioid injectors. Naloxone is a narcotic antagonist that rapidly reverses the effects of acute narcosis, including respiratory depression, sedation and hypotension. Distributing or selling naloxone over the counter to high-risk heroin users may be one way to reduce the number of opioid overdose deaths (Darke & Hall, 1997; Strang *et al.*, 1996). None of these interventions has yet been formally evaluated.

A third strategy is to reduce the risks of injecting by providing supervised injecting facilities (SIS) in areas of concentrated injecting opioid use (Dolan *et al.*, 2000; Kimber *et al.*, 2003; Mattick, Breen, *et al.*, 2003). SISs have been proposed as a public health measure that will reduce the high rates of drug overdose deaths and morbidity from BBV infections among injectors who inject in public places (Dolan *et al.*, 2000). SISs may also enhance public amenity by reducing the visibility of injecting drug use and provide a point of contact with services for injecting drug users who are not in treatment. SISs have been trialled in Europe, but their impact on overdose deaths has not been rigorously evaluated. An SIS was recently evaluated in Australia, but the ability of the evaluation to detect any impact on fatal or nonfatal overdose or BBV infection was limited

by the concurrent onset of a marked heroin shortage that produced a 40% (Degenhardt *et al.*, 2004) decline in overdose deaths and by the limited operating hours and eligibility criteria for the clientele of the SIS (Medically Supervised Injection Center Evaluation Committee, 2003).

A fourth strategy is to increase entry to methadone maintenance and other forms of treatment among older high-risk opioid dependent persons. The risk of overdose death is substantially reduced in individuals who are enrolled in methadone maintenance treatment (Caplehorn *et al.*, 1994; Gearing & Schweitzer, 1974).

Treatment interventions for dependent opioid users

Detoxification and withdrawal

Detoxification is supervised withdrawal from a drug of dependence with the aim of minimising the severity of withdrawal symptoms. It is *not* a treatment for heroin dependence but is one of the interventions most often sought by dependent heroin users (Marsh *et al.*, 1990). It provides heroin users with a respite from opioid use and an occasion to reconsider their drug use, and it may be a prelude to abstinence-based treatment; however, it has minimal if any enduring impact on heroin dependence when provided as a stand-alone intervention (Mattick & Hall, 1996).

Naltrexone is an opiate receptor antagonist, that is, a drug that blocks the analgesic and euphoric effects of heroin and other opiates (such as methadone) by binding to opiate receptors, without producing opiate effects (Dole & Nyswander, 1967). It can be used to shorten the withdrawal process by accelerating its completion. Ultra-rapid opioid detoxification (UROD) involves accelerating withdrawal by giving opiate-dependent people large doses of naltrexone under general anaesthetic to avoid the unpleasant symptoms of naltrexone-induced withdrawal (Hall & Mattick, 2000). As with more traditional ways of achieving abstinence, there is no evidence that accelerated withdrawal *in itself* reduces the high rate of relapse to heroin use in the absence of further treatment (Hall & Mattick, 2000).

Abstinence-oriented approaches to treatment

Abstinence-oriented treatments aim to achieve enduring abstinence from all opioid drugs. They usually involve supervised withdrawal from opiates followed by the provision of some type of intervention to reduce the high rate of relapse to opioids that occurs after simple withdrawal (Mattick & Hall, 1996). The interventions provided may include social and psychological support only, or such support supplemented by pharmacological methods.

Such approaches include residential treatment in therapeutic communities (TCs) and outpatient drug counselling (DC). Both approaches may be assisted by encouraging patients to become involved in self-help (SH) groups, such as Narcotics Anonymous. All of these treatment approaches share a commitment to achieving abstinence from all opioid and other illicit drugs; they do not substitute other opioid drugs for heroin. Instead, they use group and psychological interventions to assist dependent heroin users to remain abstinent. TCs and DC are usually provided through specialist addiction or mental health services. The former are residential and the latter are usually provided on an outpatient basis.

There have been no randomised-controlled trials for TCs or outpatient DC. Most of the evidence on the effectiveness of TC and DC programs comes from observational studies such as the Drug Abuse Reporting Program (Simpson & Sells, 1982), the Treatment Outcome Prospective Study in the United States (Hubbard et al., 1989) and the National Treatment Outcome Study in the United Kingdom (Gossop et al., 1997, 1998).

TCs and DC are more demanding of drug users and are less successful than MMT in attracting and retaining dependent heroin users in treatment. They nonetheless substantially reduce heroin use and crime in those who remain in treatment for at least 3 months (Gerstein & Harwood, 1990; Gossop et al., 1997, 1998). There is some evidence that TCs

may be more effective if they are used in combination with legal coercion to ensure that heroin users are retained in treatment long enough to benefit from it (Gerstein & Harwood, 1990).

Self-help groups

These groups are run by recovering drug users using the 12-step philosophy of Alcoholics Anonymous (AA). They include Narcotics Anonymous, Cocaine Anonymous and Marijuana Anonymous. Some individuals use these groups as their sole form of support for abstinence, whereas for others they provide an adjunctive support for abstinence in addition to professional assistance. Self-help groups particularly complement TCs, which are often based on the same principles of abstinence-oriented treatment. Such groups are usually not open to people who are involved in opioid substitution treatment.

The most extensive research on self-help has been in the treatment of alcohol dependence where participation in AA has been found to be associated with higher rates of abstinence from alcohol (e.g. Tonigan et al., 1996, 2003). The major threat to the validity of this conclusion has been the effects of self-selection. Because participants are not randomly assigned to participation in AA groups, the good outcome of those who attend AA meetings may reflect self-selection of more motivated participants into self-help groups. If this were true, then AA attendance would be an indicator of greater commitment to abstinence as a goal rather than a contributory cause of sustained abstinence. More recent studies have attempted to control for this possibility using sophisticated statistical methods to correct for self-selection bias. The results of these analyses have been mixed, with some showing persistence of an effect of self-help after correction (e.g. Tonigan et al., 2001), whereas others have not (Fortney et al., 1998).

Opioid maintenance treatment

Oral opioid maintenance treatment substitutes a long-acting, orally administered opioid drug for the shorter-acting heroin. It aims to stabilise dependent heroin users so that they become more accessible and amenable to rehabilitation. They are among the most popular forms of treatment with heroin users (Marsh *et al.*, 1990; Ward *et al.*, 1998). Oral methadone maintenance treatment (MMT) is the most common form of drug substitution worldwide; it is taken once daily (Ward *et al.*, 1998). When given in high or "blockade" doses, methadone blocks the euphoric effects of injected heroin, providing an opportunity for the individual to improve his or her social functioning by taking advantage of the psychotherapeutic and rehabilitative services that are an integral part of many treatment programs. Other oral opioids are now available for maintenance purposes in some countries. These include the partial agonist buprenorphine and the longer acting form of methadone LAAM (Ward *et al.*, 1998).

A small number of randomised-controlled trials have evaluated the effectiveness of MMT compared with placebo or no treatment. All produced positive results, despite small sample sizes that worked against finding an effect (Hall *et al.*, 1998; Mattick, Kimber, *et al.*, 2003). Larger observational studies have also found that patients in MMT decreased their heroin use and criminal activity while they remained in treatment (Gerstein & Harwood, 1990; Hall *et al.*, 1998; Simpson & Sells, 1990). MMT also substantially reduces the transmission of HIV via needle sharing (Ward *et al.*, 1992). MMT is the best-supported form of opioid maintenance treatment in terms of retention in treatment and its impact on illicit opioid use (Farre *et al.*, 2002; Marsch, 1998; Mattick, Breen, *et al.*, 2003; Ward *et al.*, 1998).

Buprenorphine is a mixed agonist-antagonist that has partial agonist effects similar to those of morphine, while blocking the effects of pure agonists such as heroin. When given in high doses, its effects can last for up to 3 days, and its antagonist effects substantially reduce the risk of overdose and abuse (Oliveto & Kosten, 1997; Ward *et al.*, 1998). Because of its long half-life, buprenorphine may be given every second or third day. Meta-analyses of controlled trials of buprenorphine have found it to be effective in the treatment of heroin dependence (Mattick, Kimber, *et al.*, 2003).

Injectable heroin maintenance (HMT) has been proposed as a way to attract into drug treatment heroin users who are not interested in or have failed to respond to oral forms of opioid maintenance. Its principal attraction is that it provides heroin-dependent people with their preferred drug, heroin, by their preferred route of administration, injection (Bammer, 1995). The option of prescribing injectable heroin has been part of the British system since 1926, although it has only rarely been used (Stimson & Metrebian, 2003; Strang & Gossop, 1994). It has recently been trialled in the Netherlands (Central Committee on the Treatment of Heroin Addicts [CCBH], 2002) and Switzerland (Perneger *et al.*, 1998; Rihs-Middel, 1997; Uchtenhagen *et al.*, 1997, 1998).

Perneger *et al.* (1998), for example, reported on a randomised clinical trial of HMT in persons who had failed at existing treatment. Heroin was self-administered on-site and accompanied by comprehensive health and social services. The study showed that it was feasible to stabilise and safely maintain heroin addicts on injectable heroin for 6 months and, in the process, to produce substantial improvements in the health and social well-being of participants. The Swiss heroin trials also demonstrated that it is feasible to maintain opioid-dependent persons on injectable heroin for up to 2 years (Bammer *et al.*, 2003). The prescription of injectable heroin benefited the trial participants, but there was no comparison condition with which to compare its effects (Rehm *et al.*, 2001; Uchtenhagen *et al.*, 1998). A recent Dutch RCT (CCBH, 2002) broadly confirmed the findings of Perneger *et al.*'s study.

Legally coerced treatment

The most common intervention received by persons who are dependent on illicit opioids in most developed societies such as Australia, United Kingdom, United States and Europe is imprisonment for drug-related or property offences (EMCDDA,

2003; Gerstein & Harwood, 1990). Imprisonment is not intended to be a health intervention, but its effectiveness as an intervention can be evaluated in terms of its impact on heroin use. It is not a very effective way to reduce opioid dependence when judged by the high recidivism reported in longitudinal studies of dependent heroin users (e.g. Hser *et al.*, 1993; Manski *et al.*, 2001).

The lack of an impact of imprisonment per se on opioid dependence has led to experimentation with legally coerced treatment – that is, treatment for opioid dependence which is entered under legal coercion by persons who have been charged with or convicted of an offence to which their drug dependence has contributed (Hall, 1997). It is most often provided as an alternative to imprisonment, and usually under the threat of imprisonment if the person fails to comply with treatment (Hall, 1997; Manski *et al.*, 2001; Spooner *et al.*, 2001). One of the major justifications for treatment under coercion is that it is an effective way to treat offenders' drug dependence that will reduce the likelihood of their reoffending (Gerstein & Harwood, 1990).

A consensus view on treatment under coercion prepared for WHO (Porter *et al.*, 1986) concluded that compulsory treatment was legally and ethically justified only if (1) the rights of the individuals were protected by due process and (2) if effective and humane treatment was provided. In the absence of due process, coerced treatment could become de facto imprisonment without judicial oversight. In the absence of humane and effective treatment, coerced drug treatment could become a cost-cutting exercise to reduce prison overcrowding.

Some proponents of coerced treatment argue that offenders should be allowed two constrained choices (Fox, 1992). The first such choice would be whether they participate in drug treatment at all. If they decline to do so, then they would be dealt with by the criminal justice system in the same way as anyone charged with their offence. The second constrained choice for those who agreed to participate in drug treatment would be a choice of type of treatment. There is some empirical support for these

recommendations in that there is better evidence for the effectiveness of coerced treatment that requires some *voluntary interest* by the offender (Gerstein & Harwood, 1990; Hall, 1997).

Research into the effectiveness of legally coerced treatment for opioid dependence has been largely limited to observational studies of heroin-dependent offenders entering treatment under various forms of legal coercion (Hall, 1997; Wild *et al.*, 2002). Evidence of the effectiveness of treatment under coercion has been provided by Anglin and colleagues' studies of the California Civil Addict Program (CAP; Anglin, 1988). These quasi-experimental studies compared heroin-dependent offenders who entered CAP between 1962 and 1964 with that of a group of similar offenders who were processed by the criminal justice system during the same period. It found that compulsory hospital treatment followed by close supervision in the community produced substantial reductions in heroin use and crime among CAP participants. The reductions also occurred sooner among CAP participants than among those who were imprisoned (Anglin, 1988).

The effectiveness of less coercive forms of treatment as alternatives to imprisonment has been supported by analyses of the effect of "legal pressure" (i.e. treatment while on probation or parole) on the outcome of community-based drug treatment for heroin-dependent offenders (Hubbard *et al.*, 1988, 1989). The Drug Abuse Reporting Program (DARP; Simpson *et al.*, 1986) and the Treatment Outcome Program Studies (TOPS) (Hubbard *et al.*, 1989) both showed that drug-dependent individuals who entered community-based therapeutic communities and drug-free outpatient counselling under "legal pressure" did as well as those individuals who did not (Hubbard *et al.*, 1988; Simpson & Friend, 1988).

There is also evidence for the effectiveness of legally coerced MMT. The strongest evidence comes from the results of one of the few studies in which illicit drug offenders were randomly assigned to parole with and without community-based methadone maintenance treatment (Dole *et al.,* 1969). This showed a much greater reduction in heroin use and substantially lower rates of incarceration among those enrolled in methadone maintenance treatment in the year after release from prison. These are supported by observational studies of MMT under coercion in California (Anglin *et al.,* 1989; Brecht *et al.,* 1993). These studies found no major differences in response to treatment between those who enrolled under legal coercion and those who did not. Similar results have been obtained from analyses of the effects of legal coercion on methadone treatment in the TOPS study (Hubbard *et al.,* 1988) and in New York methadone programs (Joseph, 1988).

Service organisation and delivery

Given the prevalence of drug-dependence problems in modern society and the often marginalised status of drug users, services need to be organised in a manner that maximises access to interventions. These problems are some of the most common disorders in the community, but those afflicted by them are among the least likely to be in contact with treatment services.

Community-based services through generic practitioners and specialist practitioners and services need to be organised to maximise access. Many countries organise some form of community-based multidisciplinary services that are generally staffed by a mixture of health and social care professionals. They increasingly have input from staff in criminal justice agencies. These services aim to provide a mix of psychosocial and pharmacological interventions in a manner that maximises the benefits of a combined approach.

The rising prevalence of drug problems has put additional pressures on mental health services and prompted the development of a range of strategies to intervene with people affected by these problems. In North America, there has been considerable interest in the development of specialist "dual diagnosis" services, but in other countries, such as the United Kingdom, the main thrust has been to develop liaison teams to link Community Mental Health and Drug Services in ways that enhance the core skills of both services. At present there are no good data on which approach is more effective for what patients.

In addition, services are needed for marginalised groups, such as drug-dependent prisoners and the homeless, among whom alcohol and drug problems constitute a major burden. Models for addressing such needy populations vary considerably but usually mirror the structures of community based multidisciplinary teams.

Conclusions

The twenty-first century is likely to see drug problems persist as a core part of the mental health and social problems. Moreover, it is likely that new drugs will emerge that produce new problems and require their special responses. Changes in drug-use patterns will present an ongoing challenge to clinical services and to the overall organisation and pattern of service delivery. Its difficult to know which forms of technological change will offer new and exciting treatment opportunities (Hall, 2004), but whatever new interventions are developed will need to be delivered within a supportive psychosocial framework the need for which is unlikely to change significantly over the coming decades.

REFERENCES

American Psychiatric Association. (1994). *Diagnostic and Statistical Manual of Mental Disorders,* 4th edn. (DSM-IV). Washington, DC: American Psychiatric Association.

Anglin, M. D. (1988). The Efficacy of Civil Commitment in Treating Narcotic Drug Addiction. In C. G. Leukefeld and F. M. Tims, eds. *Compulsory Treatment of Drug Abuse: Research and Clinical Practice.* Rockville, Maryland: National Institute on Drug Abuse.

Anglin, M. D., Brecht, M. L., & Maddahain, E. (1989). Pretreatment characteristics and treatment performance of legally coerced versus voluntary methadone maintenance admissions. *Criminology* **27**:537–57.

Anglin, M. D., & Perrochet, B. (1998). Drug use and crime: a historical review of research conducted by the UCLA Drug Abuse Research Center. *Subst Use Misuse* 33:1871–914.

Angrist, B., Sathananthan, G., Wilk, S., & Gershon, S. (1974). Amphetamine psychosis: behavioural and biochemical aspects. *J Psychiatr Res* 11:13–23.

Anthony, J. C., Warner, L., & Kessler R. (1994). Comparative epidemiology of dependence on tobacco, alcohol, controlled substances and inhalants: basic findings from the National Comorbidity Survey. *Exp Clin Psychopharmacol* 2:244–68.

Arseneault, L., Cannon, M., Poulton, R., *et al.* (2002). Cannabis use in adolescence and risk for adult psychosis: longitudinal prospective study. *BMJ* 325:1212–13.

Australian Institute of Health and Welfare (AIHW) (1999). 1998 National Drug Strategy Household Survey: First Results (Drug Statistics Series No.1). Canberra: AIHW.

Bachman, J. G., Wadsworth, K. N., O'Malley, P. M., *et al.* (1997). *Smoking, Drinking, and Drug Use in Young Adulthood: The Impacts of New Freedoms and New Responsibilities.* Mahwah, New Jersey: Lawrence Erlbaum.

Ball, J. C., Shaffer, J. W., & Nurco, D. N. (1983). The day-to-day criminality of heroin addicts in Baltimore – a study in the continuity of offence rates. *Drug Alcohol Depend* 12:119–42.

Bammer, G. (1995). Report and recommendations of stage 2 feasibility research into the controlled availability of opioids. Technical Report (Opioids Working Papers, Stage 2). Canberra: National Centre for Epidemiology and Population Health, Australian National University and the Australian Institute of Criminology.

Bammer, G., Van Den Brink, W., Gschwend, V., *et al.* (2003). What can the Swiss and Dutch trials tell us about the potential risks associated with heroin prescribing? *Drug Alcohol Rev* 22:363–71.

Bates, M. N., & Blakely, T. A. (1999). Role of cannabis in motor vehicle crashes. *Epidemiol Rev* 21:222–32.

Beardsley, P., & Kelly, T. (1999). Acute effects of cannabis on human behavior and central nervous system functions. In H. Kalant, W. Corrigall, W. D. Hall, & R. Smart, eds. *The Health Effects of Cannabis.* Toronto: Centre for Addiction and Mental Health, pp. 127–265.

Beatty, W. W., Katzung, V. M., Moreland, V. J., & Nixon, S. J. (1995). Neuropsychological performance of recently abstinent alcoholics and cocaine abusers. *Drug Alcohol Depend* 37:247–53.

Bell, D. S. (1973). The experimental reproduction of amphetamine psychosis. *Arch Gen Psychiatry* 29:35–40.

Brands, B., Sproule, B., & Marshman, J. (1998). *Drugs and Drug Abuse,* 3rd edn. Ontario: Addiction Research Foundation.

Brecht, M. L., Anglin, M. D., & Wang, J. C. (1993). Treatment effectiveness for legally coerced versus voluntary methadone maintenance clients. *Am J Drug Alcohol Abuse* 19:89–106.

Budney, A. J., Higgins, S. T., Radonovich, K. J., & Novy, P. L. (2000). Adding voucher-based incentives to coping skills and motivational enhancement improves outcomes during treatment for marijuana dependence. *J Consult Clin Psychol* 68:1051–61.

Budney, A. J., & Moore, B. A. (2002). Development and consequences of cannabis dependence. *J Clin Pharmacol* 42:28S–33S.

Caplehorn, J. R., Dalton, S., Cluff, M. C., & Petrenas, A. M. (1994). Retention in methadone maintenance and heroin addicts' risk of death. *Addiction* 89:203–7.

Central Committee on the Treatment of Heroin Addicts (CCBH). (2002). Medical co-prescription of heroin: two randomized controlled trials. Utrecht: CCBH.

Chaisson, R. E., Bacchetti, P., Osmond, D., *et al.* (1989). Cocaine use and HIV infection in intravenous drug users in San Francisco. *JAMA* 261: 561–5.

Chen, K., & Kandel, D. B. (1995). The natural history of drug use from adolescence to the mid-thirties in a general population sample. *Am J Public Health* 85:41–7.

Chesher, G. (1995). Cannabis and road safety: an outline of research studies to examine the effects of cannabis on driving skills and actual driving performance. In Parliament of Victoria Road Safety Committee, ed. *The Effects of Drugs (Other than Alcohol) on Road Safety.* Melbourne: Road Safety Committee.

Chirgwin, K., DeHovitz, J. A., Dillon, S., & McCormack, W. M. (1991). HIV infection, genital ulcer disease, and crack cocaine use among patients attending a clinic for sexually transmitted diseases. *Am J Public Health* 81:1576–9.

Clark, N., Lintzeris, N., Gijsbers, A., Whelan, G., *et al.* (2003). LAAM maintenance vs methadone maintenance for heroin dependence [Cochrane Review]. *The Cochrane Library,* 3. Chichester: Wiley.

Coffin, P. O., Galea, S., Ahern, J., *et al.* (2003). Opiate, cocaine and alcohol combinations in accidental drug overdose deaths in New York City, 1990–1998. *Addiction* 98:739–47.

Copeland, J., Swift, W., Roffman, R., & Stephens, R. (2001). A randomized controlled trial of brief cognitive-behavioral interventions for cannabis use disorder. *J Subst Abuse Treat* **21**:55–64.

Cretzmeyer, M., Sarrazin, M. V., Huber, D. L., *et al.* (2003). Treatment of methamphetamine abuse: research findings and clinical directions. *J Subst Abuse Treat* **24**: 267–77.

Crits-Christoph, P., Siqueland, L., Blaine, J., *et al.* (1999). Psychosocial treatments for cocaine dependence: National Institute on Drug Abuse Collaborative Cocaine Treatment Study. *Arch Gen Psychiatry* **56**:493–502.

Darke, S., Baker, A., Dixon, J., *et al.* (1992). Drug use and HIV risk-taking behaviour among clients in methadone maintenance treatment. *Drug Alcohol Depend* **29**:263–8.

Darke, S., & Hall, W. D. (1997). The distribution of naloxone to heroin users. *Addiction* **92**:1195–9.

Darke, S., & Hall, W. D. (2003). Heroin overdose: research and evidence-based intervention. *J Urban Health* **80**:189–200.

Darke, S., Kaye, S., & Ross, J. (1999). Transitions between the injection of heroin and amphetamines. *Addiction* **94**:1803–11.

Darke, S., Ross, J., & Cohen, J., *et al.* (1995). Injecting and sexual risk-taking behaviour among regular amphetamine users. *AIDS Care* **7**:17–24.

Darke, S., Ross, J., & Hall, W. D. (1995). Benzodiazepine use among injecting heroin users. *Med J Aust* **162**: 645–47.

Darke, S., Ross, J., Hando, J., *et al.* (2000). Illicit drug use in Australia: epidemiology, use patterns and associated harm. *Nat Drug Strat Mongr* 43. Canberra: Department of Health and Aged Care.

Darke, S., & Zador, D. (1996). Fatal heroin "overdose": a review. *Addiction* **91**:1765–72.

Degenhardt, L., Hall, W. D., & Lynskey, M. (2003). Testing hypotheses about the relationship between cannabis use and psychosis. *Drug Alcohol Depend* **71**:37–48.

Degenhardt, L., Hall, W. D., Warner-Smith, M., & Lynskey, M. (2004). Illicit drug use. In M. Ezzati, A. Lopez, & C. Murray, eds. *Comparative Risk Assessment*. Geneva: World Health Organization.

Derlet, R. W., Rice, P., Horowitz, B. Z., & Lord, R. V. (1989). Amphetamine toxicity: experience with 127cases. *J Emerg Med* **7**:157–61.

Des Jarlais, D. C., Wenston, J., Friedman, S. R., *et al.* (1992). Crack cocaine use in a cohort of methadone maintenance patients. *J Subst Abuse Treat* **9**:319–25.

Dolan, K., Kimber, J., Fry, C., *et al.* (2000). Drug consumption facilities in Europe and the establishment of supervised injecting centres in Australia. *Drug Alcohol Rev* **19**:337–46.

Dole, V. P., & Nyswander, M. E. (1967). Heroin addiction – a metabolic disease. *Arch Int Med* **120**:19–24.

Dole, V. P., Robinson, J. W., Oracca, J., *et al.* (1969). Methadone treatment of randomly selected addicts. *N Engl J Med* **280**:1372–5.

Donoghoe, M., Hall, W. D., Ball, A., & Lopez, A. (1998). *Opioid Overdose: Trends, Risk Factors, Interventions and Priorities for Action.* Geneva: World Health Organisation.

Edwards, G., & Gross, M. (1976). Alcohol dependence: provisional description of a clinical syndrome. *Br Med J* **6017**:1058–61.

Ellison, G. (1992). Continuous amphetamine and cocaine have similar neurotoxic effects in lateral habenular and fasciculus retroflexus. *Brain Res* **598**:353–6.

English, D., Holman, C., Milne, E., *et al.* (1995). The quantification of drug caused morbidity and mortality in Australia, (1995). Canberra: Commonwealth Department of Human Services and Health.

European Monitoring Centre for Drugs and Drug Addiction (EMCDDA) (2003). *Annual Report 2003: The State of the Drugs Problem in the European Union and Norway.* Luxembourg: EMCDDA.

European Monitoring Centre for Drugs and Drug Addiction (EMCDDA) (2002). Annual Report on the State of the Drugs Problem in the European Union, 2001. Lisbon: EMCDDA.

European Monitoring Centre for Drugs and Drug Addiction (EMCDDA) (1997). *Estimating the Prevalence of Problem Drug Use in Europe.* EMCDDA Scientific Monograph Series 1. Luxembourg: EMCDDA.

Farre, M., Mas, A., Torrens, M., *et al.* (2002). Retention rate and illicit opioid use during methadone maintenance interventions: a meta-analysis. *Drug Alcohol Depend* **65**:283–90.

Fields, J. Z., Wichlinski, L., Drucker, G. E., *et al.* (1991). Long-lasting dopamine receptor up-regulation in amphetamine-treated rats following amphetamine neurotoxicity. *Pharmacol Biochem Behav* **40**:881–6.

Flynn, P. M., Joe, G. W., Broome, K. M., *et al.* (2003). Looking back on cocaine dependence: reasons for recovery. *Am J Addict* **12**:398–411.

Fortney, J., Booth, B., Zhang, M., *et al.* (1998). Controlling for selection bias in the evaluation of Alcoholics Anonymous as aftercare treatment. *J Stud Alcohol* **59**:690–7.

Fox, R. (1992). The compulsion of voluntary treatment in sentencing. *Criminal Law J* **16**:37–54.

Gawin, F. H., & Ellinwood, E. H., Jr. (1988). Cocaine and other stimulants. actions, abuse, and treatment. *N Engl J Med* **318**:1173–82.

Gearing, F. R., & Schweitzer, M. D. (1974). An epidemiologic evaluation of long-term methadone maintenance treatment for heroin addiction. *Am J Epidemiol* **100**: 101–12.

Gerstein, D., & Harwood, H. (1990). *Treating Drug Problems Volume 1: A Study of Effectiveness and Financing of Public and Private Drug Treatment Systems.* Washington, DC: National Academy Press.

Goldstein, A., & Herrera, J. (1995). Heroin addicts and methadone treatment in Albuquerque: a 22-year follow-up. *Drug Alcohol Depend* **40**:139–50.

Gossop, M., Marsden, J., Stewart, D., *et al.* (1997). The National Treatment Outcome Research Study in the United Kingdom: six month follow-up outcomes. *Psychol Addict Behav* **11**:324–37.

Gossop, M., Marsden, J., & Stewart, D. (1998). NTORS at one year: changes in substance use, health and criminal behaviour one year after intake. London: Department of Health.

Grella, C. E., Anglin, M. D., & Wugalter, S. E. (1995). Cocaine and crack use and HIV risk behaviors among high-risk methadone maintenance clients. *Drug Alcohol Depend* **37**:15–21.

Hall, W. D. (1997). The role of legal coercion in the treatment of offenders with alcohol and heroin problems. *Aust N Z J Criminol* **30**:103–20.

Hall, W. D. (2004). Neuroscience research on the addictions: a prospectus for future ethical and policy analysis. *Addict Behav* **29**:1481–95.

Hall, W. D., Bell, J., & Carless, J. (1993). Crime and drug use among applicants for methadone maintenance. *Drug Alcohol Depend* **31**:123–9.

Hall, W. D., Hando, J., Darke, S., & Ross, J. (1996). Psychological morbidity and route of administration among amphetamine users in Sydney, Australia. *Addiction* **91**:81–7.

Hall, W. D., & Lynskey, M. (in press). Testing hypotheses about the relationship between cannabis use and the use of other illicit drugs. *Drug Alcohol Rev.*

Hall, W. D., Lynskey, M., & Degenhardt, L. (1999). *Heroin Use in Australia: Its Impact on Public Health and Public Order.* NDARC Monograph 42. Sydney: National Drug and Alcohol Research Centre.

Hall, W. D., & MacPhee, D. (2002). Cannabis use and cancer. *Addiction* **97**:243–7.

Hall, W. D., & Mattick, R. P. (2000). Is ultra-rapid opioid detoxification a viable option in the treatment of opioid dependence? *CNS Drugs* **14**:251–5.

Hall, W. D., & Pacula, R. L. (2003). *Cannabis Use and Dependence: Public Health and Public Policy.* Melbourne: Cambridge University Press.

Hall, W. D., Ross, J. E., Lynskey, M. T., *et al.* (2000). How many dependent heroin users are there in Australia? *Med J Aust* **173**:528–31.

Hall, W. D., Ward, J., & Mattick, R. (1998). The effectiveness of methadone maintenance treatment 1: heroin use and crime. In J. Ward, R. Mattick and W. Hall, eds. *Methadone Maintenance Treatment and Other Opioid Replacement Therapies.* Amsterdam: Harwood Academic.

Hando, J., & Hall, W. D. (1994). HIV risk-taking behaviour among amphetamine users in Sydney, Australia. *Addiction* **89**:79–85.

Hartnoll, R., Mitcheson, M., Lewis, R., & Bryer, S. (1985). Estimating the prevalence of opiod dependence. *Lancet* **1**:203–5.

Hepatitis C Virus Projections Working Group (1998). *Estimates and Projections of the Hepatitis C Virus Epidemic in Australia.* Sydney: National Centre in HIV Epidemiology and Clinical Research.

Hoff, A. L., Riordan, H., Morris, L., *et al.* (1996). Effects of crack cocaine on neurocognitive function. *Psychiatry Res* **60**:167–76.

Haer, Y. I., Anglin, D., & Powers, K. (1993). A 24-year follow-up of California narcotics addicts. *Arch Gen Psychiatry* **50**:577–84.

Hubbard, R., Marsden, M., Rachal, J. V., *et al.* (1989). *Drug Abuse Treatment: A National Study of Effectiveness.* Chapel Hill: University of North Carolina Press.

Hubbard, R. L., Collins, J. J., Rachal, J. V., & Cavanaugh, E. R. (1988). The criminal justice client in drug abuse treatment. In C. G. Leukefeld and F. M. Tims, eds. *Compulsory Treatment of Drug Abuse: Research and Clinical Practice.* Rockville, Maryland: National Institute on Drug Abuse.

Hubbard, R. L., Craddock, S. G., & Anderson, J. (2003). Overview of 5-year followup outcomes in the drug abuse treatment outcome studies (DATOS). *J Subst Abuse Treat* **25**:125–34.

Huber, A., Ling, W., Shoptaw, S., *et al.* (1997). Integrating treatments for methamphetamine abuse: a psychosocial perspective. *J Addict Dis* **16**:41–50.

Hulse, G. K., English, D. R., Milne, E., & Holman, C. D. (1999). The quantification of mortality resulting from the regular use of illicit opiates. *Addiction* **94**:221–9.

Jaffe, J. (1985). Drug addiction and drug abuse. In A. Gilman, L. Goodman & F. Murad, eds. *The Pharmacological Basis of Therapeutics*. New York: Macmillan, pp. 532–81.

Joseph, H. (1988). The criminal justice system and opiate addiction: a historical perspective. In C. G. Leukefeld & F. M. Tims, eds. *Compulsory Treatment of Drug Abuse: Research and Clinical Practice*. Rockville, Maryland: National Institute on Drug Abuse.

Kandel, D. B., ed. (2002). *Stages and Pathways of Drug Involvement: Examining the Gateway Hypothesis*. New York: Cambridge University Press.

Kaye, S., & Darke, S. (2000). A comparison of the harms associated with the injection of heroin and amphetamines. *Drug Alcohol Depend* **58**:189–95.

Kimber, J., Dolan, K., van Beek, I., *et al.* (2003). Drug consumption facilities: an update since 2000. *Drug Alcohol Re* **22**:227–33.

Kouri, E. M., & Pope, H. G. (2000). Abstinence symptoms during withdrawal from chronic marijuana use. *Exp Clin Psychopharmacol* **8**:483–92.

Kreek, M. J. (1997). Opiate and cocaine addictions: challenge for pharmacotherapies. *Pharmacol Biochem Behav* **57**:551–69.

Lange, R. A., & Hillis, L. D. (2001). Cardiovascular complications of cocaine use. *N Engl J Med* **345**:351–8.

Levin, F. R., McDowell, D., Evans, S. M., *et al.* (2004). Pharmacotherapy for marijuana dependence: a double-blind, placebo-controlled pilot study of divalproex sodium. *Am J Addict* **13**:21–32.

Loxley, W., & Marsh, A. (1991). *Nodding and Speeding: Age and Injecting Drug Use in Perth. National Centre for Research into the Prevention of Drug Abuse*. Perth: Curtin University of Technology.

Lynskey, M., & Hall, W. D. (2000). The effects of adolescent cannabis use on educational attainment: a review. *Addiction* **96**:433–43.

Macdonald, S., Anglin-Bodrug, K., Mann, R. E., *et al.* (2003). Injury risk associated with cannabis and cocaine use. *Drug Alcohol Depend* **72**:99–115.

Maddux, J. F., & Desmond, D. P. (1992). Methadone maintenance and recovery from opioid dependence. *Am J Drug Alcohol Abuse* **18**:63–74.

Majewska, M. D., ed. (1996). *Neurotoxicity and Neuropathology Associated with Cocaine Abuse*. NIDA Research Monograph, Vol. 163. Rockville, Maryland: US Department of Health and Human Services.

Makkai, T., & McAllister, I. (1998). *Patterns of Drug Use in Australia, 1985–95*. Canberra: Australian Government Publishing Service.

Manschreck, T. C., Laughery, J. A., Weisstein, C. C., *et al.* (1988). Characteristics of freebase cocaine psychosis. *Yale J Biol Med* **61**:115–22.

Manski, C. F., Pepper, J. V., & Petrie, C. V., eds. (2001). *Informing America's Policy on Illegal Drugs: What We Don't Know Keeps Hurting Us*. Washington, DC: National Academy Press.

Marsch, L. A. (1998). The efficacy of methadone maintenance interventions in reducing illicit opiate use, HIV risk behavior and criminality: a meta-analysis. *Addiction* **93**:515–32.

Marselos, M., & Karamanakos, P. (1999). Mutagenicity, developmental toxicity and carcinogeneity of cannabis. *Addict Biol* **4**:5–12.

Marsh, K., Joe, G., Simpson, D., & Lehman, W. (1990). Treatment history. In D. Simpson and S. Sells, eds. *Opioid Addiction and Treatment: A 12 Year Follow-Up*. Malabar, Florida: Krieger.

Mathers, C., Vos, T., & Stephenson, C. (1999). *The Burden of Disease and Injury in Australia*. Canberra: Australian Institute of Health and Welfare.

Mattick, R. P., Breen, C., Kimber, J., & Davoli, M. (2003). Methadone maintenance therapy versus no opioid replacement therapy for opioid dependence [Cochrane Review]. *Cochrane Library*, **3**. Chichester: Wiley.

Mattick, R. P., & Darke, S. (1995). Drug replacement treatments: is amphetamine substitution a horse of a different colour? *Drug Alcohol Rev* **14**:389–94.

Mattick, R. P., & Hall, W. D. (1996). Are detoxification programmes effective? *Lancet* **347**:97–100.

Mattick, R. P., Kimber, J., Breen, C., & Davoli, M. (2003). Buprenorphine maintenance versus placebo or methadone maintenance for opioid dependence [Cochrane Review]. *Cochrane Library*, **3**. Chichester: Wiley.

McCance, E. F. (1997). *Overview of Potential Treatment Medications for Cocaine Dependence*. NIDA Research Monograph. Rockville, Maryland: US Department of Health and Human Services, pp. 36–72.

McCann, U. D., & Ricaurte, G. A. (2000). Drug abuse and dependence: hazards and consequences of heroin, cocaine and amphetamines. *Curr Opin Psychiatry* **13**:321–5.

McGregor, C., Ali, R., Christie, P., & Darke, S. (2001). Overdose among heroin users: evaluation of an intervention in South Australia. *Addict Res* **9**:481–501.

McKetin, R., & Mattick, R. P. (1997). Attention and memory in illicit amphetamine users. *Drug Alcohol Depend* **48**:235–42.

McKetin, R., & Mattick, R. P. (1998). Attention and memory in illicit amphetamine users: comparison with non-drug-using controls. *Drug Alcohol Depend* **50**: 181–4.

McLeod, J., Oakes, R., Copello, A., *et al.* (2004). Psychological and social sequelae of cannabis and other drug use by young people: a systematic review of longitudinal, general population studies. *Lancet* **363**:1579–88.

Medically Supervised Injecting Centre Evaluation Committee (2003). Final Report on the Evaluation of the Sydney Medically Supervised Injecting Centre. MSIC Evaluation Committee Authors: J. Kaldor, H. Lapsley, R. P. Mattick, D. Weatherburn, A. Wilson, Sydney.

Mendelson, J. H., & Mellon, N. K. (1996). Management of cocaine abuse and dependence. *N Engl J Med* **334**:965–72.

National Centre in HIV Epidemiology and Clinical Research (1998). HIV/AIDS and related diseases in Australia: annual surveillance report 1998. Sydney: National Centre in HIV Epidemiology and Clinical Research.

Nunes, E. V. (1997). *Methodologic Recommendations for Cocaine Abuse Clinical Trials: A Clinician-Researcher's Perspective*. In NIDA Research Monograph. Rockville, Maryland: US Department of Health and Human Services, pp. 73–95.

Office of National Drug Control Policy (ONDCP) (2001). Pulse check: trends in drug abuse, November 2001. Washington, DC: Executive Office of the President.

Oliveto, A., & Kosten, T. (1997). Buprenorphine. In S. Stine & T. Kosten, eds. *New Treatments for Opioid Dependence*. New York: Guilford Press.

O'Malley, S., Adamse, M., Heaton, R. K., & Gawin, F. H. (1992). Neuropsychological impairment in chronic cocaine abusers. *Am J Drug Alcohol Abuse* **18**:131–44.

Perneger, T. V., Giner, F., del Rio, M., & Mino, A. (1998). Randomised trial of heroin maintenance programme for addicts who fail in conventional drug treatments. *BMJ* **317**:13–18.

Platt, J. J. (1997). *Cocaine Addiction: Theory, Research and Treatment*. Cambridge, Massachusetts: Harvard University Press.

Porter, L., Arif, A., & Curran, W. (1986). *The Law and the Treatment of Drug and Alcohol Dependent Persons – A Comparative Study of Existing Legislation*. Geneva: World Health Organization.

Pottieger, A. E., Tressell, P. A., Inciardi, J. A., & Rosales, T. A. (1992). Cocaine use patterns and overdose. *J Psychoactive Drugs* **24**:399–410.

Ramaekers, J. G., Berghaus, G., van Laar, M., & Drummer, O. H. (2004). Dose related risk of motor vehicle crashes after cannabis use. *Drug Alcohol Depend* **73**: 109–19.

Rawson, R., Anglin, M., & Ling, W. (2002). Will the methamphetamine problem go away? *J Addict Dis* **21**:5–19.

Rehm, J., Gschwend, P., Steffen, T., *et al.* (2001). Feasibility, safety, and efficacy of injectable heroin prescription for refractory opioid addicts: a follow-up study. *Lancet* **358**:1417–1423.

Rihs-Middel, M. (1997). The prescription of narcotics under medical supervision and research relating to drugs at the federal Office of Public Health. In M. Rihs-Middel, ed. *The Medical Prescription of Narcotics; Scientific Foundations and Practical Experiences*. Seattle, Washington: Hogrefe & Huber.

Robinson, T. E., & Becker, J. B. (1986). Enduring changes in brain and behavior produced by chronic amphetamine administration: a review and evaluation of animal models of amphetamine psychosis *Brain Res* **396**: 157–98.

Roozen, H. G., Boulogne, J. J., van Tulder, M. W. *et al.* (2004). A systematic review of the effectiveness of the community reinforcement approach in alcohol, cocaine and opioid addiction *Drug Alcohol Depend* **74**:1–13.

Satel, S. L., & Edell, W. S. (1991). Cocaine-induced paranoia and psychosis proneness. *Am J Psychiatry* **148**:1708–11

Schoenbaum, E. E., Hartel, D., Selwyn, P. A., *et al.* (1989). Risk factors for human immunodeficiency virus infection in intravenous drug users. *N Engl J Med* **321**:874–9.

Sidney, S., Beck, J. E., Tekawa, I. S., *et al.* (1997). Marijuana use and mortality. *Am J Public Health* **87**:585–590.

Silva de Lima, M., Garcia de Oliveira Soares, B., Alves Pereira Reisser, A., & Farrell, M. (2002). Pharmacological treatment of cocaine dependence: a systematic review. *Addiction* **97**:931–49.

Simpson, D., & Sells, S. (1982). Effectiveness of treatment for drug abuse: an overview of the DARP research program. *Adv Alcohol Subst Abuse* **2**:7–29.

Simpson, D., & Sells, S., eds. (1990). *Opioid Addiction and Treatment: A 12-Year Follow-Up*. Malabar, Florida; Krieger.

Simpson, D. S., & Friend, H. J. (1988). Legal status and long-term outcomes for addicts in the DARP followup project. In C. G. Leukefeld and F. M. Tims, eds. *Compulsory Treatment of Drug Abuse: Research and Clinical*

Practice. Rockville, Maryland: National Institute on Drug Abuse.

Simpson, D. S., Joe, G. W., Lehman, W. E. K., & Sells, S. B. (1986). Addiction careers: etiology, treatment and 12-year followup outcomes. *J Drug Issues* **16**:107–21.

Solowij, N. (1998). *Cannabis and Cognitive Functioning*. Cambridge: Cambridge University Press.

Solowij, N., Stephens, R. S., Roffman, R. A., *et al.* (2002). Cognitive functioning of long-term heavy cannabis users seeking treatment. *JAMA* **287**:1123–31.

Spooner, C., Hall, W. D., & Mattick, R. P. (2001). An overview of diversion strategies for Australian drug-related offenders. *Drug Alcohol Rev* **20**:281–94.

Sporer, K. A. (2003). Strategies for preventing heroin overdose. *BMJ* **326**:442–4.

Srisurapanont, M., Jarusuraisin, N., & Kittirattanapaiboon, P. (2003). Treatment for amphetamine dependence and abuse [Cochrane Review]. In *The Cochrane Library*, **2**. Chichester: Wiley.

Stephens, R. S., Roffman, R. A., & Simpson, E. E. (1994). Treating adult marijuana dependence – a test of the relapse prevention model. *J Consult Clin Psychol* **62**:92–9.

Stimson, G., & Metrebian, N. (2003). *Prescribing Heroin: What Is the Evidence?* York: Joseph Rowntree Foundation.

Strang, J., Darke, S., Hall, W. D., *et al.* (1996). Heroin overdose: the case for take-home naloxone – home based supplies of naloxone would save lives. *BMJ* **312**:1435–6.

Strang, J., & M. Gossop, eds. (1994). Heroin Addiction and Drug Policy: The British System. Oxford University Press, New York.

Substance Abuse and Mental Health Services Administration (SAMHSA) (2001). Summary of Findings from the 2000 National Household Survey on Drug Abuse. Rockville, Maryland: Office of Applied Statistics, Substance Abuse and Mental Health Services Administration.

Substance Abuse and Mental Health Services Administration (SAMHSA) (2002). *Results from the 2001 Household Survey on Drug Abuse: Volume 1. Summary of National Findings*. Rockville, Maryland: Office of Applied Statistics, Substance Abuse and Mental Health Services Administration.

Tagliaro, F., De Battisti, Z., Smith, F. P., & Marigo, M. (1998). Death from heroin overdose: findings from hair analysis. *Lancet* **351**:1923–5.

Tashkin, D. P. (1999). Effects of cannabis on the respiratory system. In H. Kalant, W. Corrigall, W. D. Hall, & R. Smart, eds. *The Health Effects of Cannabis*. Toronto: Centre for Addiction and Mental Health, pp. 311–45.

Taylor, D. R., Fergusson, D. M., Milne, B. J., *et al.* (2002). A longitudinal study of the effects of tobacco and cannabis exposure on lung function in young adults. *Addiction* **97**:1055–1061.

Tonigan, J., Toscova, R., & Miller, W. (1996). Meta-analysis of the literature on Alcoholics Anonymous: sample and study characteristics moderate findings. *J Stud Alcohol* **57**:65–72.

Tonigan, J. S., Connors, G. J., & Miller, W. R. (2003). Participation and involvement in Alcoholics Anonymous. In T. F. Babor and F. K. Del Boca, eds. *Treatment Matching in Alcoholism*. Cambridge: Cambridge University Press, pp. 184–204.

Tonigan, J. S., Miller, W. R., & Connors, G. J. (2001). Prior Alcoholics Anonymous involvement and treatment outcome: matching findings and causal chain analyses. In R. H. Longabaugh and P. W. Wirtz, eds. *Project Match Hypotheses: Results and Causal Chain Analyses*. Bethesda, Maryland: National Institute on Alcohol Abuse and Alcoholism, pp. 276–84.

Toomey, R., Lyons, M. J., Eisen, S. A., *et al.* (2003). A twin study of the neuropsychological consequences of stimulant abuse. *Arch Gen Psychiatry* **60**:303–10.

Torrens, M., San, L., Peri, J. M., & Olle, J. M. (1991). Cocaine abuse among heroin addicts in Spain. *Drug Alcohol Depend* **27**: 29–34.

Uchtenhagen, A., Dobler-Miklos, A., & Gutzwiller, F. (1997). Medically controlled prescription of narcotics: fundamentals, research plan, first experiences. In M. Rihs-Middel, ed. *The Medical Prescription of Narcotics; Scientific Foundations and Practical Experiences*. Seattle, Washington: Hogrefe & Huber.

Uchtenhagen, A., Gatzwiller, F., & Dobler-Mikola, A. (1998). *Medical Prescription of Narcotics Research Programme: Final Report of the Principal Investigators*. Zurich: Institut fur Sozial-und Praventivmedizin der Universitat Zurich.

UNAIDS/WHO. (2002). *AIDS Epidemic Update December 2002*. Geneva: Joint United Nations Programme on HIV/AIDS.

United Nations Office for Drug Control and Crime Prevention (UNODCCP). (2003). *Global Illicit Drug Trends 2003*. New York: United Nations Office for Drug Control and Crime Prevention.

Urbina, A., & Jones, K. (2004). Crystal methamphetamine, its analogues, and hiv infection: medical and psychiatric aspects of a new epidemic. *Clin Infect Dis* **38**:890–4.

van Beek, I., Dwyer, R., & Malcolm, A. (2001). Cocaine injecting: the sharp end of drug-related harm! *Drug Alcohol Rev* **20**:333–42.

Van Den Brink, W., & van Ree, J. M. (2003). Pharmacological treatments for heroin and cocaine addiction. *Eur Neuropsychopharmacol* **13**:476–87.

van Os, J., Bak, M., Hanssen, M., *et al.* (2002). Cannabis use and psychosis: a longitudinal population-based study. *Am J Epidemiol* **156**:319–27.

Vasica, G., & Tennant, C. C. (2002). Cocaine use and cardiovascular complications. *Med J Aust* **177**:260–2.

Walsh, G. W., & Mann, R. E. (1999). On the high road: driving under the influence of cannabis in Ontario. *Can J Public Health–Rev Can Sante Publique* **90**:260–3.

Ward, J., Darke, S., Hall, W. D., & Mattick, R. (1992). Methadone-maintenance and the human-immunodeficiency-virus – current issues in treatment and research. *Br J Addict* **87**:447–53.

Ward, J., Hall, W. D., & Mattick, R. P. (1998). *Methadone Maintenance Treatment and Other Opioid Replacement Therapies.* Amsterdam: Harwood Academic.

Warner-Smith, M., Darke, S., Lynskey, M., & Hall, W. D. (2001). Heroin overdose: causes and consequences. *Addiction* **96**:1113–25.

Wild, T. C., Roberts, A. B., & Cooper, E. L. (2002). Compulsory substance abuse treatment: an overview of recent findings and issues. *Eur Addic Res* **8**:84–93.

Zammit, S., Allebeck, S., Andreasson, I., *et al.* (2002). Self reported cannabis use as a risk factor for schizophrenia in Swedish conscripts of 1969: historical cohort study. *Br Med J* **325**:1199–1201.

Zhang, Z. F., Morgenstern, H., Spitz, M. R., *et al.* (1999). Marijuana use and increased risk of squamous cell carcinoma of the head and neck. *Cancer Epidemiol Biomark Prevent* **8**:1071–8.

12

Affective disorders

Peter McGuffin

Depressive *symptoms* are frequent in psychiatric practice and are among the most common complaints in primary care. They are also common in patients presenting to other hospital specialties, and community surveys suggest that depressive *syndromes* are highly prevalent, with many cases never coming to the attention of doctors or other healthcare professionals. The risk of depression over a lifetime has been estimated at 7 of 10 women and 4 of 10 men; in many cases, these would be considered "minor" (but still possibly clinically significant) depressive episodes (Bebbington *et al.,* 1989). Not surprisingly, the differentiation between "normal" depressive symptoms and milder forms of depressive disorder is often difficult and blurred. Only the more severe forms of depressive disorder give an appearance of a qualitative difference from normality.

By contrast, manic states, disorders that are much less frequent than depression, appear to be more distinct from normal experience. However, even here it is possible to envisage a continuum between "normal" high spirits and frank elation. Given the blurred boundaries, it is understandable that the classification of affective disorders is problematic. Furthermore, although the concept of affective illness is often thought to be an ancient one, given that descriptions of manic and melancholic states date back to classical Greece, this is probably a mistaken view. Berrios (1992) has pointed out that what is now called depression does not correspond closely with early notions of melancholia, and current thinking about what constitutes mania or depression dates back only as far as the late nineteenth century. Like most other psychiatric disorders, affective illness is entirely defined in terms of its signs and symptoms. As yet there is no known pathophysiology and no reliable objective tests. Consequently we must accept that the modern definitions remain provisional and that they, too, will be subject to evolution and change.

Many of the component features of affective disorder are described in Chapter 1, but here we consider how the symptoms and signs cluster together and examine the psychopathology of affective states. There are two main types of episode, depressive and manic. Classification is considered in more detail later in the chapter, but for now it is sufficient to note that those who have had one or more episodes of depression are classed as having unipolar disorder, whereas those who suffer both manic and depressive episodes or, less commonly, manic episodes alone are classed as having bipolar disorder.

Psychopathology

Depressive states

Depression as a symptom in clinical practice is exceeded in frequency only by pain, and techniques

Essential Psychiatry, ed. Robin M. Murray, Kenneth S. Kendler, Peter McGuffin, Simon Wessely, David J. Castle. Published by Cambridge University Press. © Cambridge University Press 2008.

for inquiring about both are rather similar. Thus it is important to know how long the depressed mood has been present, or whether it is there all the time; whether anything relieves or exacerbates it; and whether it shows any spontaneous variation in severity. One can gauge severity by asking patients whether their depressed mood is the worst is has ever been and what it makes them want to do (e.g. "hide myself away", or have thoughts of self-harm or suicide). Severe depression is usually persistent, unresponsive to external events that might normally be expected to bring cheer and shows a diurnal variation, with exacerbations in the morning and a perceptible lessening as the day goes on.

The relative frequencies of the symptoms associated with depressive disorder in a large study carried out in Birmingham, Cardiff and London (United Kingdom) are shown in Table 12.1 (Korszun et al., 2004). Among such symptoms, anhedonia, the inability to experience pleasure, is usually prominent. The patient has a diminished enjoyment of both work and leisure pursuits and typically has diminished libido and a decreased appetite for food. Loss of weight may follow, and disturbed sleep with early morning waking is characteristic. Other patterns of sleep disturbance might also occur, with difficulty falling asleep (initial insomnia) or recurrent waking during the night (middle insomnia).

Lack of energy is a common symptom, together with lack of interest, poor concentration and difficulty sustaining attention. Patients with such symptoms often complain of difficulty in reading a newspaper article or following a television programme and sometimes complain of poor memory. Under these circumstances, testing usually reveals that recall of information is intact but registration of new material is inefficient and speed of thinking is reduced. On examination, slowness of movement may also be evident, described as psychomotor retardation. In severe cases, lack of interest may show in lack of self care and an unkempt appearance. Typically, the patient has a sad and miserable facial expression, but this is not always so even in some quite severe cases in which the patient may

Table 12.1 Frequency of symptoms in a depression case control study

Symptom	Frequency %
Depressed mood	98.97
Loss of reactivity	99.38
Anhedonia	99.59
Loss of interest	95.05
Loss of energy or drive	95.26
Hopelessness	93.40
Loss of self-esteem	88.04
Subjectively inefficient thinking	90.31
Fatigability and exhaustion	59.79
Suicidality	64.95
Subjective feeling of retardation	61.44
Irritability	53.61
General rating of anxiety	55.26
Loss of appetite	68.45
Pathological guilt	65.57
Subjectively described restlessness	42.89
Morning depression	45.98
Early waking	52.37
Loss of libido	42.89
Preoccupation with death or catastrophe	36.49
Free floating anxiety	49.69
Hypersomnia	27.84
Guilty ideas of reference	29.48
Anxious foreboding with autonomic symptoms	31.55
Gain of weight	18.56
Gain of appetite	9.90
Delusions of guilt or worthlessness	1.44
Hypochondriacal delusions	1.24
Auditory hallucinations	2.89
Delusions of catastrophe	0.82

$N = 485$. From Korszun et al., 2003

strive to appear normal and put on a brave face (so-called "smiling depression"). In addition to assessing the subjective depth of the patient's low or dysphoric mood, one should always make an objective judgement on the basis of appearance. Tearfulness at interview must be interpreted against the context of recent life happenings, the patient's cultural and social background and gender. Sometimes in depressed patients, the most visible emotions may be irritability or hostility rather than frank despair.

The content of thought usually includes poor self-regard, which may amount to feelings of worthlessness or guilt. The patient may also spontaneously make self-depreciative comments ("I'm no good, I don't deserve help"). Whether spontaneously mentioned or not, it is mandatory in depressed patient to enquire carefully about suicidal thoughts. Far from putting ideas into the patient's head, enquiring about suicidal thoughts is usually a comfort to patients, whose ideas about ending their own life may have signified to them that they were "going crazy". A positive reply to a question such as, "have things seemed so bad that life is not worth going on with?" should lead onto exploring whether a means of suicide has been considered. If so, one should find out what plans have been made to carry out an attempt and whether the patient thinks it is likely that they will act on such plans. In the same context, it is worth asking about whether the patient has any hope for the future. The belief that all is hopeless and there will be no escape from current misery, if accompanied by suicidal ideas, usually indicates a high risk that such ideas will be acted upon. Box 12.1 details factors associated with suicidality in depression.

Abnormal beliefs and perceptions in depression

In a minority of patients, abnormal ideas take on the quality of fixed beliefs that may become of delusional intensity. Usually these can be seen as arising understandably out of a severe depressed mood (Jaspers, 1963). Hence there are described as mood congruent. These include delusions of worthlessness, which can be seen as an extreme form of self-depreciative ideas. Delusions of guilt or blame may result in persistent worrying over real or imagined misdemeanours. In some cases, delusions of guilt may become more bizarre, such as the man who believed he had become "the worst devil created by Satan" or another who believed that he was responsible for the deaths of British soldiers killed in the 1991 Gulf War.

> **Box 12.1** Features predictive of suicide
>
> Persistent or pervasive thoughts of suicide accompanied by hopelessness
> Well worked out plans for self destruction (including plans to avoid discovery)
> Preparations for death (e.g. making a new will)
> High level of irritability or impulsivity
> Low mood accompanied by alcohol or other substance misuse
> Family history of suicide
> Male
> Middle aged
> Single, divorced or separated

Persecutory beliefs may again be in keeping with the mood state, in which the patient says that he or she deserves to be tormented and punished. Delusions of reference may include patients' belief that they are being marked out and talked about behind their backs because of their wickedness. Delusions of poverty, that the patient is bankrupt or in severe debt, are rarer and seems to occur most often in older patients. Also fairly rare, but striking when they are encountered, are nihilistic delusions in which the patient believes that some part of the anatomy such as their brain or intestines has disappeared or rotted away. An example is the case of a man who believed that all his "giblets" had been flushed away down the toilet pan.

Hallucinations may occur as voices that are mood congruent in their content. For example, they may confirm that the patient is guilty of a crime and deserves persecution or punishment. Hallucinations in depressed patients are not usually either as vivid or as continuous as the typical derogatory voices heard by people with schizophrenia (Hamilton, 1985). Rarely, tactile hallucinations can occur as "a funny sensation" on the skin or in the viscera, which may be interpreted as evidence that internal organs are disappearing. Unpleasant tastes or smells are occasionally described by severely depressed patients who often believe that they are emitting the smell themselves, and again they may interpret this as confirmation that their flesh or some internal organ is rotting.

Psychomotor disturbance may accompany severe depression, whether or not the patient also has delusions or hallucinations. Retardation is exhibited as marked slowness of both action and speech so that there is a perceptible delay, or latency, in the patient's response to questions. In the most extreme cases, retardation can progress to mutism and depressive stupor in which the patient appears awake but lies motionless and muted, usually refusing to eat or drink and sometimes being incontinent. A different type of psychomotor disturbance is agitation, when the patient carries out a series of repetitive movements usually with a facial appearance of obvious anguish and despair. The movements typically include wringing of hands, rocking back and forth and pacing up and down but also include repetitive self-punitive movements such as banging the head against a wall, scratching flesh or pulling hair.

Other patterns of depression

Most variability in depressive disorders can simply be considered as being on a continuum from mild to severe. However, toward the mild to moderate end of the spectrum, there may be additional symptoms not typically associated with severe depression. Most commonly these include symptoms of anxiety which frequently overlap with and are difficult to disentangle from depressive features. Some patients with mild or moderate depression also show "reversed functional shift". That is, instead of the classic "endogenous" pattern of biological symptoms consisting of early morning waking, decreased appetite and weight loss, the patient shows somnolence, including a tendency to sleep through the day and an increase in appetite and weight gain. Other patients may show the psychological symptoms of depression with few or none of the somatic features. Such patients have in the past been referred to as showing a reactive or neurotic pattern of depression which was seen to be more related to adversity and misfortune than was depression with endogenous

> **Box 12.2** "Atypical" depression
>
> Mood worse in the evenings
> Increased appetite
> Weight gain
> Increased need for sleep

features. As discussed later in the section on aetiology, modern objective evidence does not support such a tidy dichotomy. See Box 12.2 for a list of atypical depressive symptoms.

Some sufferers from recurrent depression experience symptoms only during autumn or winter. The classic pattern for *seasonal affective disorder* (SAD) is to remit during spring and summer, to recur in consecutive autumns and winters and to be associated with an increase in appetite, weight and the need to sleep. Carbohydrate craving is a common feature. Whether SAD is an entity distinct from other forms of depression is controversial (Sohn & Lam, 2005), but the current classifications such as *Diagnostic and Statistical Manual of Mental Disorders* (4th edn., DSM-IV; American Psychiatric Association, 1994) categorise it as a subform of depressive disorder "with a seasonal pattern". In practice, late autumn and winter exacerbation of depressed mood is fairly common even in those whose episodes are not wholly confined to these seasons and also occurs in some patients who have bipolar disorder.

Mania

Typical manic patients look and feel elated, but their exuberance and cheerfulness may turn to irritability as the episode wears on and others attempt to control and constrain their manic behaviour. Indeed, one fairly common finding in patients who have multiple episodes of mania is that irritability tends to become a more prominent component (Winokur *et al.*, 1969). The patient's subjective description of elation is frequently described as feeling "high". In most cases, particularly in the first episode, the patient may not admit that anything is amiss, but in time many patients acquire sufficient insight to recognise (or can be taught to detect) when they are going "over the top", becoming "too cheerful to be normal".

It is of course not the mood changes as such that make manic states dangerous and disabling, but rather it is the accompanying symptoms and behaviours that arise out of the expansive and heightened sense of well-being. In a manic state, the patient typically feels full of energy, which manifests in overactivity and sometimes in reckless behaviour. There is a decreased need for sleep and an increased appetite for sex. Typically there is also an increased appetite for food, but the patient may not indulge this because they are "too busy to eat".

Recklessness and lack of judgement frequently lead to lavish spending sprees, such as the university student who managed to exceed her credit card limit several times within a week, or the man who thought that the portable radios in his local electrical store were such a good bargain that he bought 40.

Social disinhibition is a common feature, which may show as an overfamiliarity with strangers or people in authority. Sometimes this may be fairly benign, for example, walking into a room of strangers and insisting on shaking hands with everyone. However, it can result in behaviours of an embarrassing or sexual nature. For example, a newly admitted woman in her late 50s announced in the ward round, "I love sex" and then ran over to the consultant psychiatrist and attempted to fondle him intimately.

Speech in mania is typically rapid and increased in quantity. The patient's flow is difficult to interrupt and may be quite unstoppable. In normal conversation, even the most habitually garrulous of individuals respond to nonverbal cues and attend to hints that others wish to enter into the conversation. Manic patients with pressure of speech lose all sense of such conversational niceties. A usual accompaniment is flight of ideas, in which thoughts move rapidly from one topic to another with tenuous but understandable connections. These may

be based on rhymes or "clang associations" or other irrelevant aspects of content. For example, asked to explain the proverb "a stitch in time saves nine", a young woman replied, "it's when you've got a cut and need a stitch. A stitch in time saves nine. Nine lives. Nine lives like a cat. I've got a little black cat actually".

Not all patients show typical pressure of speech and flight of ideas, but most during a manic episode will, if asked, report that their thoughts are going rapidly or "crowding in" to their head. Lesser degrees of speech disorder, in which speech is verbose, rapid and difficult to follow, although not showing full-blown flight of ideas, is sometimes described as prolixity.

Nearly all patients suffering from the mania have an increased feeling of self-worth and importance. Their thought content consists of ambitious plans to which they see no obstacle and a self-assessment that exceeds realistic expectations. Although most patients are at least partially amenable to firm, gentle persuasion not to act on their beliefs, direct confrontation, as previously mentioned, may provoke an irritable or even violent outburst.

Abnormal beliefs and perceptions in mania

Grandiose delusions are the most common and take the form of a delusion of identity, such as being a wealthy or famous person or a divine being, or a delusion of special powers or abilities. Persecutory beliefs and delusions of reference may also occur and tend to be congruent with the overall mood of grandiosity and expansiveness. In general, delusions in manic states are less persistent than those in schizophrenia, but sometimes mood-incongruent delusions such as delusions of passivity may occur. How such patients should be classified is controversial, but most authorities (e.g. American Psychiatric Association, 1994; Goodwin & Jamison, 1990) now allow that passivity and other Schneiderian first-rank symptoms of schizophrenia (see Chapter 13) can also occur in manic states.

Many patients report that their perceptions are generally more vivid during manic episodes, but in addition other abnormal perceptions, particularly auditory hallucinations, may occur in some cases (Goodwin & Jamison, 1990). These usually take the form of voices in which the content is in keeping with the patient's prevailing persecutory or grandiose beliefs. Typically auditory hallucinations in mania are less persistent and less continuous than those in schizophrenia (Hamilton, 1985).

Mixed states

The co-occurrence of depressive and manic states is not uncommon. Winokur *et al.* (1969) reported that 68% of manic episodes were associated with some degree of depressed mood, and Goodwin and Jamison (1990), in reviewing several clinical studies of mania, calculated that depression occurred in 72% of episodes. Mixed states are usually seen in the patient who is in the process of appearing to recover from a manic state and who is about to develop a downward swing in depression or alternately in patients presenting in a depressive state and about to swing into mania. Less commonly, however, both depressive and manic symptoms are persistent in the same patient at the same time and remain evident for days or even weeks. The overall picture can be puzzling to both the clinician and the patient his or herself. Irritability with overactivity is a much more usual picture than frank elation, but the mood is volatile and can quickly turn to tearful despair. Persistent delusions are unusual, but there may be a strange mixture of persecutory ideation, guilt and a vague grandiosity. Mixed affective states, therefore, can present formidable diagnostic difficulties, particularly if the patient is being seen for the first time and when the clinician does not have the benefit of a previous history of mania or depression. Mixed states occurred in 16% of manic depressive patients in one of the most carefully documented series (Winokur *et al.*, 1969), but other studies, possibly using the term more loosely, describe mixed states as occurring in up to two thirds of patients (Goodwin & Jamison 1990).

Classification

The history of the classification of affective disorders is one of controversy and confusion (Farmer & McGuffin, 1989; Kendell, 1976) that is only partially resolved in the current editions of the *International Classification Diseases* (10th revision; ICD-10; World Health Organisation, 1992) or the DSM-IV (American Psychiatric Association, 1994). As noted earlier, affective disorders are syndromes consisting of groups of signs and symptoms that cannot yet be considered as having a well-understood aetiology and pathogenesis. Therefore, current classifications have to be thought of as a set of working hypotheses or convention. They are designed to assist communication between clinicians, facilitate description and help predict outcome and response to treatment. They are nevertheless only conventions and should not be thought of as immutable. Indeed, although there has been considerable convergence in the most recent editions of DSM and ICD, there are still some differences in the way that affective disorders are divided, the terms that are used to describe the disorders and in the constituent items making up the criteria.

The classification of affective disorders in ICD-10 and DSM-IV is summarised and compared in Table 12.2. One of the contrasts is that ICD-10 exists in different versions, principally a descriptive version for clinical use and a fully operational set of criteria of the use in research. DSM-IV has only one version and gives operational criteria for all categories of disorder (see Chapter 2).

Both classification systems contain main symptoms of mania in depression that are broadly similar. Indeed the definitions of mania are virtually identical, consisting of elevated, expansive or irritable mood together with three symptoms (four if the mood is only irritable) probabilistic, including increased self-esteem or grandiosity, decreased need to sleep, pressure of talk, flight of ideas,

Table 12.2 Comparison of ICD-10 and DSM-IV classification of affective disorders

	ICD-10	DSM-IV

Main syndromes	Manic/hypomanic episode
	Depressive episode
	  Mild
	  Moderate
	  Severe
		Manic/hypomanic episode'
		Major depressive episode
		Mixed episode

Subcategories	With/without psychotic symptoms (only in mania or *severe* depression) Mood congruent/mood incongruent psychotic symptoms (only in mania)	With/without psychotic features Mood congruent/mood incongruent psychotic features With/without catatonic features With/without postpartum onset With/without atypical features
Description of course	Single episode or recurrent	Single episode or recurrent, and if recurrent, there are specifiers for recovery between episodes Rapid cycling and seasonal pattern

DSM-IV = *Diagnostic and Statistical Manual of Mental Disorders,* 4th edn.; ICD-10; *International Classification of Diseases,* 10th revision.

distractibility and increased activity and reckless behaviour (such as sexual indiscretion or spending sprees). To fulfil the criteria for mania, the mood disorder has to be present for a week, or the patient requires hospitalisation, but for hypomania a duration of only four days is required.

The classification schemes differ in their approach to depression. Whereas DSM-IV contains a single category of major depression, ICD-10 subdivide depressive episodes into mild, moderate and severe types. The terms used to describe depressive symptoms and the classifications differ slightly, but overall the list of symptoms in depressive disorders is virtually identical, with only one symptom ("loss of confidence or self-esteem") being present in ICD-10 but not in DSM-IV. Both ICD-10 and DSM contain exclusion criteria for a depressive episode specifying that manic symptoms should not be present and the disorder should not result from a psychoactive drug or from a general medical condition. In addition, DSM but not ICD-10 specifies that the symptoms should cause "clinically significant distress or impairment" and that they should not be "better accounted for by bereavement".

Both ICD-10 and DSM classify a disorder with chronic lower-level depressive symptoms that do not fulfil the criteria for depressive disorder as *dysthymia*. The term is less used in the United Kingdom and the rest of Europe than North America. This could be because dysthymia is assigned the same code number (300.4) as depressive neurosis was in the earlier international classification ICD-9. In fact, the bulk of European patients previously diagnosed as having depressive neurosis would fulfil DSM-IV criteria for major depression. The separation of depressive disorders into neurotic and endogenous types is no longer permissible under either "official" classification scheme, but whether these terms will be forever abolished remains to be seen. A majority of experienced clinicians would probably still regard the presence of endogenous features as useful when deciding to prescribe drug treatments or electroconvulsive therapy (see Chapter 27), but there is also increasing acceptance that depressive disorders can be viewed on a dimension of severity, as in the ICD-10 categories of mild moderate and severe depression and that there is no clear-cut line of demarcation between overt

Table 12.3 Symptoms of depressive disorder in ICD-10 and DSM-IV

1. Depressed mood for 2 weeks
2. Loss of interest
3. Fatigue or decreased energy
4. Loss of confidence or self-esteem
5. Self-reproach or guilt
6. Recurrent thoughts of death, suicide or suicidal behaviour
7. Diminished concentration or indecisiveness
8. Agitation and retardation
9. Sleep disturbance (insomnia or hypersomnia)
10. Appetite and weight change (increase or decrease)

DSM-IV = *Diagnostic and Statistical Manual of Mental Disorders*, 4th edn ; ICD-10 *International Classification of Diseases*, 10th revision.
DSM-IV: major depression: five symptoms including 1 or 2 (4 is not listed).
ICD-10: Severe depression: at least eight symptoms including 1 and 2 or 3.
Moderate depression: at least six symptoms including two of 1, 2 or 3.
Mild depression: at least four symptoms including two of 1 and 2 or 3.

depressive disorder and "normal" symptoms of low mood. This has important implications for epidemiological studies and may explain why recent studies give quite wide disparities in prevalence estimates.

Other classes, categories and dimensions of depression

Both ICD-10 and DSM-IV classification allow that subcategories of depression may occur depending, for example, on whether psychotic symptoms are present (Table 12.3). The notion of an endogenous subcategory also lives on in the ICD-10 category of severe depression with somatic symptoms (e.g. prominent sleep or appetite disturbance) and in DSM-IV melancholia. A less explicit feature of both systems in the distinction between primary and secondary depression but both ICD-10 and DSM-IV criteria imply that depressive disorder is a diagnosis applicable only when the syndrome is not a result of some other (nonaffective) condition. The modern concept of primary versus secondary affective disorders is largely based on the views of the Washington University, St Louis School (Robins & Guze, 1972), who proposed that depression following alcohol or drug abuse, medical illness, personality disorder, schizophrenia, organic brain disease and a variety of other psychiatric disorders should be classified as "secondary". Only depressive disorders in which mood disorder occurs first should be classified "primary". Although this dichotomy has been widely used, particularly in North America, it has not been successfully validated by biological or treatment criteria (Grove *et al.*, 1987).

Other attempts to delineate homogenous subgroups of depression have used multivariate statistical methods (Farmer & McGuffin, 1989). None of the proposed subcategories have won general acceptance, but interestingly a study of more than 400 community-living people who reported depressive symptoms found that the most common clusters of symptoms was nearly identical to the DSM-III category of major depression (Blazer *et al.*, 1988). Other minor clusters derived by multivariate classification included a mixed anxiety-depression syndrome and a depressive syndrome associated with premenstrual symptoms in young women. Another approach has been to use latent class analysis (e.g. Sullivan & Kendler, 1998), but the main criticism of such studies is that there is usually no attempt to explore the stability or validity of categories or dimensions. A recent exception was the study of Korzsun *et al.* (2004) in which the investigators derived four dimensions using factor analysis on a large series of affected sibling pairs and were able to demonstrate support using confirmatory factor analysis on an independent sample. The dimensions consisted of (1) "core" depressive symptoms plus psychomotor retardation; (2) anxiety; (3) agitation, guilt and suicidality; and (4) appetite gain with hypersomnia. Only the last of these failed to show significant correlation in siblings.

Epidemiology

Research into the epidemiology of depression has the same difficulty as studies of other common conditions such as obesity and hypertension – that is, where does the threshold between normality and disorder lie? However, there is an additional problem, that although it may be relatively straightforward to ensure that weighing machines or sphygmomanometers are calibrated in the same way, it may not be true that different psychiatric researchers elicit and describe signs and symptoms in a standard fashion. The general solution to this problem has been to use not only explicit diagnostic criteria but also standardised interviews for research (see Chapter 2).

Several standardised interviews have been devised but in general the choice is between semistructured interviews such as the schedules for clinical assessment in neuropsychiatry (SCAN; Wing et al., 1990), or more highly structured instruments such as the diagnostic interview schedule (DIS) and the composite international diagnostic interview (CIDI; Robins et al., 1988). The SCAN was originally designed for use by experienced clinicians, whereas the DIS and CIDI were designed to be easily used by trained lay interviewers. One study has shown that the forerunner of the SCAN (the Present State Examination) and CIDI produce similar results at the level of diagnostic classification (Farmer et al., 1987). However, this was a hospital-based study on a comparatively small number subjects, and the results of some community-based studies have been less reassuring. For example, Brugha and colleagues (1999) compared a fully structured interview administered by lay interviewers with SCAN and found that the lay interviewers overestimated the prevalence of cases.

Further methodological problems arise if, as is the case in genetic epidemiology, the task is to estimate lifetime prevalence rather than prevalence over a limited recent time period. Here one of the difficulties may be failure of subjects to remember symptoms. Rice and colleagues (1992) examined the stability of diagnosis in families ascertained through a depressed proband. Relatives were interviewed at two time points 6 years apart, and the authors explored the factors predicting which of those who received a lifetime diagnosis of major depression at their first interview continued to fulfil diagnostic criteria at their second interview. These consisted of only 74% of those diagnosed with lifetime-ever depression at the initial interview. However, this figure rose to 96% when the definition of a case was more stringent, requiring eight or more symptoms plus receipt of treatment. Interestingly, Kendler et al. (1993) found an even larger degree of diagnostic instability, or unreliability, in their community-based study of female twins. The agreement on a lifetime diagnosis of depression based on interview and a self-completed questionnaire was modest (kappa coefficient 0.34). The authors derived an "index of caseness" based on the number of depressive symptoms, treatment seeking, number of episodes and degree of impairment. They found that there was better reliability the higher the index of caseness.

This problem of diagnostic instability could partly explain why lifetime prevalence estimates appear to vary so widely. For example, in an analysis of international data the rates ranged from 1.5% in Taiwan to 19% in Lebanon (Weissman et al., 1996). The same report found a 1-year prevalence that ranged from 0.8% in Taiwan to 5.8% in New Zealand. The US national comorbidity study found an even larger 12-month prevalence of 7% (Kessler et al., 2003), and a multisite European study found an average prevalence of 8.5% (Ayuso-Mateos et al., 2001).

Gender

There is a consistent finding across the Western studies that depression is approximately twice as common in women as in men (Ayuso-Mateos et al., 2001; Weissman et al., 1996). This holds whether the period considered is 1 month or an entire lifetime. For example, Bebbington and colleagues (1989) found a 1-month prevalence of 9.2% in women and 4.9% in men in the United Kingdom, and in the US ECA study, Weissman and colleagues (1988) found a lifetime prevalence of 7% in women and 2.6% in men.

Although this pattern is consistent for Western cultures, it is not always the case elsewhere. For example, Orley and Wing (1979) found lower male-female differences in the rates of depression in Uganda, and in Taiwan Hwu *et al.* (1989) found that the male-female ratio for a lifetime prevalence of major depression exceeded two in small towns and rural areas but was only 1.4 among urban dwellers. These findings suggest that social and cultural factors must contribute to the differing rates of depression in men and women. Jenkins (1985) tried to address this problem directly by studying a sample of British civil servants and carefully matching the sexes for a range of social variables. Taking a very broad perspective on psychiatric morbidity, which covered approximately a third of the sample, there was no overall difference between men and women, but women showed slightly more depressive symptoms including low mood. Although these findings suggest that there is little difference between the sexes when social factors are controlled for, the subjects were all comparatively young (20–35 years), and the women were nearly all childless. The breadth of definition of depression alone does not seem to be a factor in reducing sex differences. For example, as noted earlier, Bebbington *et al.* (1989) estimated that the lifetime risk of minor depression to age 65 is 46% for men and 72% for women.

Social class

Although most studies in the United Kingdom focussing on women have found an association between depression and lower social class (e.g. Brown & Harris 1978; Surtees *et al.* 1986), no association between social class and major depression was found in the United States in the ECA study. It has also often been suggested that depression is associated more with urban than with rural dwelling, and this was quite striking in a recent European study at the UK and Irish sites (Ayuso-Mateos *et al.*, 2001), although the data from elsewhere are inconsistent. For example, the ECA study was conducted in five sites in the United States. In one of these (Durham, North Carolina), depression was about twice as common in urban as in rural areas, whereas in St Louis, depression was actually more prevalent in the rural sample (Weissman *et al.*, 1988).

Ethnic factors

Within countries such as the United States, quite marked ethnic differences have been reported, but this again is at least partially confounded by socioeconomic issues. For example, Dunlop *et al.* (2003) found significantly higher rates of depression among Hispanic and African Americans than among whites in a cohort of 55 to 65 year olds. However, after adjusting for economic differences and physical healthcare needs, Hispanics and whites showed similar rates of depression, and African Americans actually showed a slightly lower rate. One of the few studies ever conducted on black Africans in rural Africa found very high rates of depression compared with urban United Kingdom (Orley & Wing, 1979), and, as noted earlier, among the lowest frequencies of depression are those from studies in Taiwan (Hwu *et al.*, 1989). Unfortunately, unlike within-national ethnic differences, there are insufficient data to decide whether between-national differences are explicable by social confounders.

Cohort effects

Several studies have suggested an increase in incidence of depression among younger cohorts (Bebbington *et al.*, 1989; Joyce *et al.*, 1990; Klerman & Weissman, 1989); in addition, there appears to be an increased lifetime prevalence of depression among younger groups. This is paradoxical, given that older subjects have lived through more of the period of risk for becoming depressed. A long-term follow-up in Sweden (Hagnell, 1986) suggests that this finding is not entirely due to older people simply forgetting past episodes of depression. There was a very marked increase in the rates of depression reported by young adults in the period 1957–1972 compared with 1947–1957. The differences were particularly striking for men, in whom there appeared to be a 10-fold difference. Although this might reflect a true increase in depressive disorders in recent years, other explanations need to be considered. In particular, there may now be a greater willingness of younger cohorts to volunteer emotional symptoms, but it is also possible that in the Swedish study, in which operational criteria were not used, the breadth of diagnosis of depression simply increased. Against this, one of the most recent longitudinal analyses in women indicated a decline in depression with age in more recent cohorts but increases in earlier ones, suggesting that increases in depression in younger women in successive cohorts may be offset by decreases in middle age (Kasen *et al.*, 2003).

Bipolar disorder

Lifetime prevalence estimates of bipolar disorder are much lower and, in general, more consistent than for unipolar depression, ranging from 0.3% in the United Kingdom (Cardno *et al.*, 1999) and Taiwan (Weissman *et al.*, 1996) to 1.5% in New Zealand (Weissman *et al.*, 1996). The lifetime prevalence of bipolar disorder in the United States as estimated by the ECA study was in the range of 0.7% to 1.6% (Smith & Weissman, 1991). One-month prevalences of mania in studies using the PSE range from 0.08% (Vazquez-Barquero *et al.*, 1986) to 0.8% (Bebbington *et al.*, 1981). The greater consistency in bipolar than unipolar prevalence estimates may well reflect a lesser "boundary problem"; mania is more distinct from "normal" mood changes than is depression. However, some authors (e.g. Angst *et al.*, 2003) have argued that current concepts of bipolarity are too narrow and that the inclusion of "subthreshold" forms of mania results in a lifetime risk in Switzerland of close to 11%.

Unlike unipolar disorder, there is no evidence of sex differences in the rates of bipolar I disorder, although women are over-represented in bipolar II disorder (Weissman *et al.*, 1996). The age of onset tends to be earlier than unipolar disorder, with a mean age of first onset of 21 years for bipolar disorder in the ECA study compared with 27 years for unipolar disorder. Hospital first admission rates and

---

Box 12.3 Comparison between unipolar and bipolar disorder

Unipolar disorder	Bipolar disorder
Episodes of depression	Episodes of depression and mania (or hypomania in bipolar II disorder) or episodes of mania alone
Twice as common in women	Equally common in women and men (but excess of women in bipolar II)
Increased risk of depression in relatives	Increased risk of both depression and mania in relatives

---

first contact in the United Kingdom vary between ethnic groups with particularly high admission rates for mania among African-Caribbeans (Van Os *et al.*, 1994).

Studies, particularly in the United States (Faris & Dunham, 1939; Weissman & Myers, 1978), suggest an association of bipolar disorder with social class. This is in the opposite direction to that sometimes suggested for unipolar disorder, in that patients with bipolar disorder tend to have *higher* socioeconomic status than the population at large. The reasons for this association are unknown, but the most popular speculation is that susceptibility to mania is associated with energy, drive and creativity rather than there being any stressors peculiar to those of higher social class that predispose to mania (Goodwin & Jamison, 1990).

Box 12.3 compares unipolar and bipolar forms of depression.

Aetiology

The causation of affective disorders is complicated but in general terms can be considered to reflect an interplay between constitutional or biological factors (which are at least in part genetic) and reaction to environmental insults, which include both physical and psychosocial factors. Evidence on the causes of affective disorders comes from a wide variety of sources.

Animal studies

As in other psychiatric disorders, researchers interested in the biological substrate of mood change are hampered by the lack of an animal model that will do justice to the complexity of human behaviour. There is no really convincing animal model of mania. Nevertheless several ingenious models of depression have been devised that have turned out to be useful in informing cognitive-behavioural theories of depression and in providing ways to test the effectiveness of antidepressant drugs.

Probably the best-known animal model of depression is the "learned helplessness" paradigm put forward by Seligman (1975). In his original experiments, carried out on dogs, Seligman exposed the animals to recurrent aversive stimuli in the form of electric shocks from which they were unable to escape. Subsequently, the same animals were placed in a situation in which they were again given electric shocks but from which escape was possible. Unlike normal animals, which quickly learn to avoid the aversive stimuli, the dogs previously exposed to uncontrollable stress showed a marked impairment in learning to escape shocks. It was proposed that these dogs had learned to surrender to the inevitability of painful stimuli in a way that is analogous to the painful, hopeless despair of depressed humans. The paradigm has been criticised on the basis that in humans, how the environment is perceived and conceptualised may be as important as the events that actually occur. Learned helplessness theory has subsequently been modified to take into account "attributional style" (Abramson et al., 1978).

More recent animal work has mainly focused on rats. It has also been shown that there is a genetic component to learning a helpless response to uncontrollable electric foot-shock in that such behaviour can be selected for in breeding studies. Indeed, a rat line has been produced that shows

"congenital helplessness" – helpless behaviour without exposure to shock (Henn, 1996; Henn & Vollmayr, 2005). Other researchers have favoured less traumatic ways of producing a depressed-like state, such as exposing the laboratory animals to chronic, mild and unpredictable stress (Willner et al., 1991). Components include change of cage mates, periods of food or water deprivation, tilting the cage and illumination at night or intermittent exposure to a predator (Henn & Vollmayr, 2005). Rats treated in this way, unlike normal animals, fail to increase their intake when a sweetener such as saccharin or sucrose is added to their drinking water. This has been put forward as an analogue of anhedonia (i.e. loss of interest or pleasure, one of the core features of depression as defined in ICD-10 and DSM-IV).

Other proposed animal models are based on studies of separation. This includes both separation of young animals from their mothers and mature animals from their peers. Both approaches produce a "protest despair" reaction that may be more analogous to grief reactions in humans than depression as such. Nevertheless, the behaviour is preventable by treatment with imipramine (Suomi et al., 1978). Separation models have been used mainly in primates such as rhesus macaque monkeys, and, again, there appear to be genetic effects on the extent to which separated monkeys show behavioural or endocrine responses (Barr et al., 2003).

Genetics

It is a consistent finding that affective disorders tend to aggregate in families. Table 12.4 summarises the results of studies of the first degree relatives of index cases (or probands) suffering from unipolar or bipolar disorder. The rates are given as lifetime risks (i.e. the figures are age-corrected to take into account the probable proportion of relatives unaffected at the time of the studies but who will later become affected). Although in absolute terms, the range of lifetime risks in first-degree relatives is large, and this may reflect differences in diagnostic criteria, the

Table 12.4 Affective illness in the first-degree relatives of unipolar (UP) and bipolar (BP) probands

| | | | Relatives | |
| | | | Morbid risk,[a] range (%) | |
Proband type	No. of studies	Age-corrected[b] n at risk	BP	UP
BP	12	3,710	7.8 (1.5–17.9)	—
		3,648	—	11.4 (0.5–22.4)
UP	7	2,319	0.6 (0.3–2.1)	9.1 (5.9–18.4)

Data from studies reviewed by McGuffin & Katz (1986).

[a] Weighted means.

[b] Corrected denominator ("Bezugsziffer") to allow for relatives who have not lived through the period of risk.

overall pattern suggests that affective disorders are more common in the relatives of affected probands than in the population at large. There are two other, more specific findings to note. The first is that the overall risk of affective disorders is higher in the relatives of bipolar probands; the second is that relatives of bipolar probands have an increased risk of both unipolar and bipolar disorder, whereas in the relatives of probands with unipolar disorder there is only an excess of unipolar cases.

As in other disorders, two types of "experiments of nature", twin studies and adoption studies, have enabled researchers to decide whether the familiality of affective disorders is explicable purely in terms of shared genes, shared family environment or a combination of the two. Twin studies have consistently shown higher concordance for mood disorders in monozygotic than dizygotic pairs. Sullivan and colleagues (2000) performed a meta-analysis of published twins studies of depression and concluded that the mean heritability (the proportion of variance in liability to the disorder) was 37%. However, in doing so they lumped together four population-based and one hospital-based study. On its own, the hospital-based twin study actually suggested a heritability of more than 70% (McGuffin *et al.,* 1996). Although this might suggest that more severe depression requiring specialist referral is more heritable than depression detected in community samples, there is another

possible explanation. This has to do with the unreliability of the diagnosis of depression in surveys using lay interviewers, which has already been discussed in relation to epidemiological studies. The one community-based twin study that took unreliability of diagnosis into account in the statistical analysis and used assessment at two time points also found a heritability of about 70% (Kendler *et al.,* 1993).

There have been many twin studies suggesting an important role of genes in bipolar disorder (reviewed by Jones *et al.,* 2004), however most of these have been small. The two largest studies based on hospital-based twin registers in Denmark and the United Kingdom are summarised in Table 12.5. Both studies suggest a heritability for unipolar depression of around 70% and a heritability of 80% for bipolar disorder but also suggest that there is a genetic overlap between the two conditions. McGuffin *et al.* (2003) explored this further and concluded that although such an overlap is substantial, most of the genetic liability to bipolar disorder is specific to the manic syndrome.

An adoption study in Sweden, based mainly on health insurance records (Von Knorring *et al.,* 1983), surprisingly found little evidence of either a genetic or family environmental component in affective illness. However, when a Danish study compared hospital records of the biological relatives of adoptees with affective illness with adopted relatives and

Table 12.5 Probandwise concordance for unipolar (UP) and bipolar (BP) affective disorder in twins

Study		Proband	n	Co-twin		
				UP %	BP %	Affective disorder %
Bertelson *et al.* (1977)	MZ	UP	35	43	9	64
		BP	34	18	62	79
	DZ	UP	17	18	6	24
		BP	37	11	8	19
McGuffin *et al.* (2003)	MZ	UP	68	44	2	46
		BP	30	27	40	67
	DZ	UP	109	20	0	20
		BP	37	14	5	19

relatives of matched control adoptees (Wender *et al.*, 1986), an 8-fold increase in unipolar depression in the biological relatives of adoptees with affective illness was found, as well as a 15-fold increase in the rate of suicide. In another study that examined the parents of adoptees suffering from bipolar disorder, 28% of the biological parents had an affective illness compared with 12% of adopting parents (Mendlewicz & Rainer, 1977). A majority of the affected biological parents of bipolar probands had unipolar rather than bipolar disorder, which is, however, compatible with the most recent twin analyses (McGuffin *et al.*, 2003).

The data discussed thus far suggest that affective disorders are polygenic. That is, they result from the combined effects of several, perhaps many genes each of which on their own have small effects. Single gene forms, if they exist at all, must be extremely rare, and the existing data are mathematically incompatible with either a single gene model or models proposing multiple single gene forms with incomplete penetrance (Craddock *et al.*, 1995). Furthermore, a recent twin analysis challenged the conventional wisdom that bipolar disorder and schizophrenia are genetically distinct, instead suggesting that although specific genes contribute to the liability to each classic syndrome, there are also some genes that contribute to the liability to both disorders (Cardno *et al.*, 2002).

Molecular genetics

Broadly there are the two ways that geneticists seek to find the genes involved in affective disorder (see Chapter 5). These are linkage and association studies. In *linkage studies* researchers now typically use several hundred genetic markers as evenly spaced as possible throughout the genome to try to establish the location of genes involved in susceptibility by identifying markers that are shared at a greater than chance level by multiple affected members within families or in pairs of affected siblings. The location is then narrowed down, and candidate genes within the region are examined. In *association studies* the most common approach is to compare variations within functional candidate genes (that is, genes that encode proteins thought to be involved in the disorder) in cases versus well control subjects. Very recently it has become feasible to search the entire genome using an association approach, although this requires somewhere in the region of half a million markers.

To date gene finding studies have been more consistent in bipolar than unipolar disorder, but interesting findings are beginning to emerge in both conditions. Badner and Gershon (2002) carried out a meta-analysis of linkage studies in both schizophrenia and bipolar disorder and showed that there is significant evidence of linkage for bipolar disorder on chromosomes 13 and 22 in regions that overlap with regions implicated in schizophrenia. A subsequent search through the chromosome 13 linkage region of schizophrenia identified a novel gene, *G72* (also known as D amino acid oxidase activator, *DAOA*) that appears to be associated with susceptibility to the disorder (Chumakov *et al.*, 2002). Other studies have now also implicated *G72* in bipolar disorder (Chen *et al.*, 2004; Hattori *et al.*, 2003; Schumacher *et al.*, 2004). We can conclude that molecular genetic studies are beginning to confirm the suggestion from the twin analysis mentioned earlier (Cardno *et al.*, 2001) that some of the genes that contribute to bipolar disorder also contribute to the liability to schizophrenia. A genomewide association study of 2000 cases of bipolar disorder and 3000 control subjects has confirmed that there are no genes of large effect but has identified a number of novel loci that are likely to be involved in susceptibility (Wellcome Trust Case Control Consortium, 2007).

Studies in unipolar disorder have been reviewed by Levinson (2006), who notes that two whole genome scans suggest linkage on chromosomes 12 and 15. Subsequently another whole genome scan has been conducted lending support for findings in both these regions (McGuffin *et al.*, 2005). Among the interesting candidate genes in unipolar depression is a brain derived neurotrophic factor (BDNF). BDNF shows decreased expression in hippocampus after stress or corticosteroid treatment and enhanced expression in the hippocampus and the cerebral cortex of rats treated with antidepressants. A functional variant in the gene was originally associated with bipolar disorder, but a large case-control study has cast doubt on this finding (Green *et al.*, 2006). However, other variants within this gene now appear to be significantly associated with unipolar depression (Schumacher *et al.*, 2005). An even more intriguing story surrounds the serotonin transporter gene, which has a variant in its promoter region that results in either higher or lower activity. There is evidence of an interaction with stressors such as early adversity or recent life events resulting in depressive symptoms (Caspi *et al.*, 2003), a finding that has been subsequently replicated in other (but not all)

studies (Eley *et al.*, 2004; see review by Zammit & Owen, 2006).

Neurochemistry

Because, in life, the brain is the most inaccessible of organs, progress in understanding the precise neurochemistry of mood changes has been difficult. Pharmacological studies provided the original basis for the catecholamine hypothesis of depression, which stated quite simply that low mood is associated with low synaptic concentrations of noradrenaline (NA) (Schildkraut, 1965). This was based on the idea that the catecholamine-depleting drug reserpine apparently caused depressive symptoms, whereas a variety of antidepressant drugs of the tricyclic group increase availability of NA by inhibiting presynaptic reuptake. However, it became clear that some such drugs also inhibit reuptake of serotonin or 5-hydroxy-tryptamine (5-HT) and that the precursor of 5-HT, L-tryptophan, has an antidepressant effect (Coppen, 1967). These observations led to the indoleamine hypothesis, that low synaptic concentrations of 5-HT bring about depression.

Although it has subsequently been found that a majority of effective antidepressant drugs have marked effects on indoleamine or catecholamine transmissions (or both) (Charney & Nelson, 1981), there is discrepancy between the time taken for synaptic concentrations of NA and 5-HT to increase (almost immediate) and the delay seen in clinical practice before antidepressant effects become apparent (2–3 weeks). A further problem is that studies of 5-HT or NA or their metabolites in blood, urine or cerebrospinal fluid of depressed patients have in the main failed to show any decrease (Charney & Nelson, 1981). Subsequently it has been proposed that the therapeutic effects of antidepressants depend on alterations in neuroreceptor density and sensitivity, and there is considerable evidence for this from animal studies using both ligand binding methods to assess receptor number and affinity directly or by techniques looking at neuroreceptor gene expression as reflected in specific mRNA levels (Buckland *et al.*, 1992).

The situation is further complicated by findings that some tricyclic drugs such as nortriptyline and desipramine and the newer compound reboxetine are relatively selective for NA reuptake, whereas compounds such as fluoxetine, citalopram and paroxetine are selective serotonin reuptake inhibitors (SSRIs). Both selective NA and 5-HT reuptake inhibition are effective in ameliorating the symptoms of depression, and although it may be postulated that different groups of patients are differentially responsive to different types of neurotransmitter reuptake inhibition, there is no good evidence to support this. Perhaps the most promising pointer to individual differences comes from studies of monoamine depletion. It is possible to deplete research subjects of tryptophan, the precursor of 5-HT, by giving them by drink or capsule form a mixture of amino acids without tryptophan. Induction of transient depressive symptoms occurs in some subjects – perhaps not surprisingly, most commonly those with a past history of depression (Neumeister et al., 2004). However, there is also some evidence of genetic differences in that subjects carrying the low activity form of the serotonin transporter polymorphism mentioned earlier (see section on genetics) are also more likely to show symptoms of low mood following tryptophan depletion (Neumeister, 2003). It has been suggested that the proportion of subjects who show mood changes following tryptophan depletion parallels that of those who show a "discontinuation" syndrome when they stop taking serotonin reuptake inhibitors, and therefore these result from common mechanisms (Delgado, 2006). There are to date no genetic data on this question.

A more general hypothesis that unifies at the expense of being somewhat vague is that there is an overall dysregulation of neurotransmission in depression (Siever & Davis, 1985). This is likely to affect more than one neurotransmitter system, which antidepressants may favourably alter by a variety of mechanisms, including alterations in receptor sensitivity. Receptor studies have concentrated on binding of various ligands to lymphocytes (or virally transformed lymphoblasts) and platelets.

One of the more provocative early findings was from the study of Wright et al. (1984) in which bipolar patients and their ill relatives showed decreased numbers of beta-adrenoreceptors on lymphoblasts. Although this could not be replicated in subsequent studies (Berrettini et al., 1987; Kay et al., 1993), downregulation of beta-adrenoreceptors with an agonist, isoprenaline, was less efficient in cells from bipolar patients than control lymphoblasts (Kay et al., 1993). Furthermore, incubation of the bipolar patients' lymphoblasts with lithium selectively enhanced their downregulation by isoprenaline. Evidence of decreased binding to alpha-2 adrenoreceptors in platelets has come from a study (Piletz et al., 1991) that suggested a difference between patients and control subjects which was abolished by antidepressant treatment. It is not clear whether this phenomenon is related to the blunted response to stimulation of alpha-2 receptors in depressed patients, shown by neuroendocrine tests (discussed later). Serotonergic function has also been studied by receptor binding assays on platelets, with some results suggesting decreased binding in patients with depression compared to manic patients (Ellis et al., 1991). This would fit with a general hypothesis of decreased serotonergic transmission in depression or more specifically, with the findings of a blunted prolactin response in depressed subjects following challenge with a serotonin releasing agent D-fenfluramine (O'Keane & Dinan, 1991).

Postmortem studies of the brain of depressed subjects who have died by suicide have produced somewhat conflicting results relating to beta-adrenoreceptor binding. Two groups have reported increased numbers of binding sites in the frontal cortex (Blegon & Israeli, 1988; Mann et al., 1986), whereas a third (De Paermentier et al., 1990) found decreased binding in most cortical areas with particular decreases in the frontal cortex of victims of violent suicide. Postmortem studies of serotonin binding are also difficult to interpret overall. Lawrence et al. (1990) reported no difference in serotonin uptake sites between suicide victims or control subjects, but findings elsewhere have suggested either increased or decreased numbers of binding sites, with the majority indicating an increase in serotonin receptors in frontal cortex (Ball & Whybrow, 1993).

Few investigators have focused attention specifically on the role of dopamine (DA) in depression, and this is because drugs such as amphetamines and, even more potently, cocaine, which bring about the release of DA into synapses, do not appear to have a useful or consistent antidepressant effect. However, amphetamines have been implicated in the development of manic-type states, as have other dopamine agonists, including bromocriptine and L-dopa. The exact role of dopamine in the initiation of manic states is unclear, but there is little doubt that a common mode of action of nearly all currently used drugs (with the exception of lithium) that are effective in alleviating manic symptoms is that they exert a postsynaptic blockade of dopamine receptors.

The suggestion that dopamine underactivity may play a role in depression is best supported by the observation that dopamine release appears to be a common feature in all highly rewarding or pleasurable activities. Thus dopamine levels in the brain can be shown to be increased during sexual arousal and in association with administration of a wide variety of drugs used for "kicks", such as alcohol, cocaine or opioids (Uhl *et al.*, 1993). Therefore it maybe that loss of interest and diminished capacity to experience pleasure, which forms a core feature of current concepts of depression, is related to an impairment in dopaminergic transmission.

Neuroendocrinology

Two early clinical observations have played an important role in stimulating research on the relationship between hormonal disturbance and affective disorders. The first was the existence of an obvious relationship between myxoedema and depressed mood. Patients with hypothyroidism, particularly in the early stages when physical signs are not prominent, can present with persistent mood changes that are easily mistaken for primary depression. Mood changes are a prominent feature

of Cushing's syndrome, again usually presenting with a depressive picture. Subjectively mood change is also a common experience in patients taking corticosteroids in high doses. Some subjects experience depressive symptoms, but others report a heightened sense of well-being that may amount to mild elation. Most work has therefore centred on the hypothalamic-pituitary-adrenocortical (HPA) and the hypothalamic-pituitary-thyroid (HPT) systems, but other endocrine abnormalities have also been explored.

The hypothalamic-pituitary-adrenocortic system

The finding that depression occurs in patients with adrenal tumours but is not found in association with Nelson's syndrome in which there is elevated corticotropin (ACTH) and low corticosteroid levels suggests that cortisol rather than ACTH levels are causally linked with depression (Kelly *et al.*, 1980). However, since at least a quarter of a century ago, raised cortisol levels in depressed patients have been known to occur and were first interpreted as a nonspecific reaction to stress. Better understanding of the physiology of the HPA system led to the development of more complex theories concerning increased HPA activity in depressive disorders. The essentials of the control of HPA activity are as follows: external stress that may be psychosocial or physical (e.g. infection) results in impulses conveyed through relevant brain areas to the hypothalamus, where corticotrophin releasing hormone (CRH) is produced. This permits the release of ACTH in the pituitary, which in turn stimulates secretion of mineralocorticoid and glucocorticoid steroids by the adrenal cortex. There is then a negative feedback mechanism to the hypothalamus, inhibiting further secretion of CRH together with additional negative feedbacks to higher centres and the pituitary directly.

Elevated levels of CRH in cerebrospinal fluid has been demonstrated in depressed patients (Nemeroff *et al.*, 1984). CRH receptors have also been shown to be downregulated in the brains of those dying of suicide, which would be in keeping with the theory that there is overproduction of CRH in depression (Nemeroff *et al.*, 1988). Further evidence of HPA overactivity comes from studies using human CRH, which when given intravenously to depressed subjects results in a blunted ACTH response compared with control subjects. By contrast, cortisol response to CRH in depressed patients appears not to differ from control subjects. This has been interpreted as indicating a hypersensitive adrenocortex in depressed subjects, resulting from persistent exposure to high levels of ACTH (Holsboer *et al.*, 1987).

Much research has focused on the dexamethasone suppression test (DST) in depression, particularly in subjects with an endogenous pattern of symptoms (Carroll *et al.*, 1981), and there was initial optimism that the DST might have a useful diagnostic role. The test depends on the fact that normal subjects show suppressed plasma cortisol levels throughout the following day after a dose of 1 to 2 mg of dexamethasone. A high proportion of severely depressed subjects showed an "escape" from this suppression effect and continued to produce cortisol at normal or even slightly elevated levels. Although this phenomenon would then be in keeping with the hypothesis of HPA overactivity in depression, the DST shows only modest sensitivity (i.e. it "misses" 20%–30% of depressives) and incomplete specificity (i.e. the test is positive in as many as 10% of normal control subjects and an even higher proportion of nondepressed psychiatric patients). Furthermore, in subjects with recurrent depression, an abnormal DST may occur in some but not in other episodes (Coryell *et al.*, 1990). A more recent development has been the introduction of the combined dexamethasone/corticotropin releasing hormone test (dex/CRH test; Ising *et al.*, 2005). The neuroendocrine response to dex/CRH is elevated during major depressive episodes and tends to normalise after treatment. It is also said to be a useful marker of response to treatment with antidepressants. Interestingly, there is some evidence that bipolar patients also show an elevated cortisol response to dex/CRH, but this does not normalise in remitted patients, suggesting that this test may provide a potential trait marker for bipolar disorder (Watson *et al.*, 2004).

In summary, HPA overactivity undoubtedly occurs in depressive disorders. However, it is neither a constant feature nor one that is highly specific. The issue of whether HPA overactivity plays a causal role or whether it is a secondary manifestation of other neurochemical or other endocrine abnormalities remains unresolved, but it has been argued that HPA changes are more likely to cause alterations in central monoamines than the other way round. This hypothesis derives from the well established relationship between HPA overactivity and chronic stress (Dinan, 1994). It suggests that changes in monoamines are secondary and are perhaps mediated in depression susceptible individuals by high levels of glucocorticoid receptors on central neurons.

The hypothalamic-pituitary-thyroid system

Here the control mechanisms are analogous to those in the HPA system. Thyrotrophin-releasing hormone (TRH), produced in the hypothalamus, permits secretion of thyroid-stimulating hormone (TSH) by the pituitary, which in turn stimulates release of thyroxin (T_4) and triiodothyronine (T_3) by the thyroid gland. Again there are inhibitory feedback mechanisms to the hypothalamus as well as directly to the pituitary.

Small reductions in plasma concentrations of T_3 have been reported in depressed subjects (Rupprecht *et al.*, 1989). Similar modest changes have also been reported in fasting control subjects and in anorexia nervosa patients, so that slight reduction in T_3 may simply reflect loss of weight in depressed patients.

Although there is no convincing evidence of lowered basal TSH in depression, many studies have shown a reduced TSH response to TRH, and there is also evidence of increased TRH production in depression (Checkley, 1992).

Antithyroid antibodies show raised titres in depressed patients compared with control subjects

> **Box 12.4** Hypothalamic-pituitary-adrenocortical axis changes in depression
>
> Raised cortisol (measured in blood or saliva)
> Abnormal dexamethasone suppression test in up to 80%
> Abnormal dexamethasone-corticotrophin releasing hormone (CRH) response
> Raised CRH in cerebrospinal fluid
> Down regulated CRH receptors

(Haggerty *et al.*, 1987). Furthermore, increased levels of thyroid antibodies are associated with depressive symptoms in the postpartum period, even though there is no significant association between such symptoms and thyroid hormone or TSH levels (Harris *et al.*, 1992).

In summary, a number of mainly rather subtle changes in the HPT system have been reported in affective disorders, but it is not known to what extent any of these have a pathogenic role. The fairly consistent evidence of raised thyroid antibodies in association with depressive symptoms, independent of changes in hormonal level, is intriguing and warrants further investigation.

Other systems

Pituitary hormones other than ACTH and TSH have been the subject of less intensive scrutiny in affective disorders. Although there is little convincing evidence of abnormal growth hormone (GH) secretion in depression, there is fairly consistent evidence of reduced GH responses to a variety of agents. Thus, the GH response to the alpha-2 agonist clonidine and the tricyclic compound desipramine has been reported as blunted in depressed patients. Although it is possible that these findings reflect a defect at alpha-2 receptors, a blunted GH response to clonidine or desipramine also occurs in other psychiatric disorders (Checkley, 1992).

The release of prolactin by the pituitary is inhibited by dopamine. Therefore the fact that prolactin

levels have consistently been found to be normal in depressed subjects argues against any generalised abnormality of dopaminergic systems (discussed earlier). There is, however, some evidence of an increased prolactin release when a dopamine antagonist is given to patients with bipolar disorder (Joyce *et al.*, 1987). It is thought that prolactin release depends partially on stimulation of 5-HT1 receptors, and one of the effects of antidepressants such as clomipramine, which affects 5-HT reuptake, is to augment the prolactin response to the 5-HT precursor tryptophan. By contrast, the prolactin response to tryptophan is reduced in depressed subjects (Cowen & Charig, 1987). It has been argued that this, plus evidence of reduced neuroendocrine response to 5-HT-releasing agents (O'Keane & Dinan, 1991) and an absence of blunted response to 5-HT agonists, suggests an abnormality involving decreased 5-HT release rather than decreased receptor sensitivity (Cowen, 1993). One of the circumstantial reasons for focusing on hypothalamic-pituitary activity in affective disorder is that diurnal variations are a constant feature of hormonal secretion and of mood in severe depression.

As mentioned earlier, some patients show a longer cyclical phenomenon, that of seasonal affective disorder (SAD). This is characterised by a tendency towards depression, social withdrawal and increased sleep in winter months (Thompson & Isaacs, 1988). The existence of SAD has in turn led to interest in a possible role of melatonin in depression. This substance, secreted by the pineal gland, is known to have a role in the seasonal sexual activity of some mammals, and bright light lowers melatonin blood levels in a variety of mammals, including humans. Circadian rhythm of melatonin in saliva or plasma, or of the melatonin metabolite 6-sulphatoxymelatonin in urine, is governed by the suprachiasmatic nucleus, the endogenous oscillatory pacemaker. Onset of melatonin secretion under dim light conditions (the dim light melatonin onset, or DLMO) has been used clinically to evaluate problems related to the onset or offset of sleep in those with mood disorders (Pandi-Perumal *et al.*, 2006). There is also good evidence that exposure to bright light is as effective as antidepressants such as flu-oxetine in patients with a seasonal (winter) pattern of affective disorder (Lam *et al.*, 2006). However, definitive evidence that this is directly mediated by an overall suppression of melatonin levels is lacking.

Sleep architecture as a clue to brain physiology

Although there is no evidence of abnormalities in the electroencephalogram (EEG) during waking hours, much attention has been paid to "sleep architecture" abnormalities as reflected in EEG patterns. The most consistent abnormality has been of a reduction in depressed subjects of the time between onset of sleep and first appearance of rapid eye movement (REM) sleep. This so-called reduced REM latency appears to be most strongly associated with an endogenous pattern of depressive symptoms and seems to be most pronounced in elderly subjects (Kupfer *et al.*, 1983). Although REM latency decreases with age even in normal subjects, the decrease appears to be more marked in those with depression, and it may be possible to discriminate between elderly depressed and demented patients in a reliable way, based purely on EEG recordings made during sleep (Reynolds *et al.*, 1988).

An important question, therefore, is the one that arises recurrently in studies of the biology of depression: whether the phenomenon of altered REM latency provides some clue about vulnerability to depression rather than being merely a secondary phenomenon that disappears after recovery from depression. Evidence that decreased REM latency may be a persistent trait comes from studies of patients in remission, some of whom, again particularly those who have had an endogenous pattern of symptoms, show a persistent reduction in REM sleep latency (Modell *et al.*, 2005; Rush *et al.*, 1986). Support for the idea that a decrease in REM latency may be an enduring trait rather than a transient state also comes from family studies, in which it has been reported that the relatives of depressed patients are more likely than control subjects to show reduced REM latency (Giles *et al.*, 1988) as well

as increased REM density, the total amount of REM sleep (Modell *et al.*, 2005).

Brain imaging studies

Brain imaging studies and the principles underlying them are discussed in more detail in Chapter 4. It is worth noting that initially the structural brain abnormalities that could be detected in affective disorders showed an overall pattern of results that was much less consistent than that for schizophrenia. Most authors carrying out computed tomography or magnetic resonance imaging (MRI) brain scans reported no change either in young bipolar patients (Harvey *et al.*, 1994; Johnstone *et al.*, 1989) or in a mixture of patients having bipolar or unipolar disorders (Weinberger *et al.*, 1982). A few reported an increase in the size of lateral cerebral ventricles, most commonly associated with psychotic symptoms (Scott *et al.*, 1983) or mania (Andreasen *et al.*, 1990; Nasrallah *et al.*, 1982). Some reports suggested that cerebral ventricular enlargement is a feature of severe affective disorder in the elderly (Abas *et al.*, 1990; Dolan *et al.*, 1985), but others found no difference from age-matched control subjects (Jacoby & Levy, 1980).

More recent studies have focused on more subtle and localised abnormalities. There is now reasonably consistent evidence of reduced hippocampal volume in patients with recurrent unipolar depression, but this is not found in those at an early stage of the illness (Campbell & MacQueen, 2006). There have also been a number of reports of reduction in amygdala volume in patients with bipolar disorder (e.g. Blumberg *et al.*, 2003).

Functional MRI studies have also shown changes in the amygdala. For example, Fu *et al.* (2004) showed that depressed patients compared with control subjects had increased amygdala activation when shown sad faces. This improved on treatment with antidepressants, as did activation in other associated brain regions, and the authors concluded that functional MRI changes in the anterior cingulate may provide a useful surrogate marker of antidepressant response.

Physical illness

There is a strong relationship between affective change, particularly depression, and the presence of debilitating physical disorders, and hospital in-patients on general wards have consistently been found to have high rates of affective disturbance (see Chapters 21 and 23). The importance of recognising this is twofold. First, knowing that depression is a frequent accompaniment or aftermath of physical disorder is important in managing the condition and, second, the association with depression may give some clue as to the mechanisms involved in the aetiology of depression as a whole.

Among the acute infections, *viral illnesses* seem to be particularly prone to produce mood change as sequelae. Infectious mononucleosis is a classic cause of persistent low mood, usually accompanied by fatigue in young patients, but a similar state is quite common after other acute conditions such as infectious hepatitis. The association between depressive symptoms, chronic fatigue and a wide variety of acute viral illnesses, including common ones such as influenza, has recently become the subject of much research and considerable controversy. The latter centres on the extent to which postviral fatigue or chronic fatigue syndrome can be explained partly or even entirely as a subform of affective disorder. There is undoubtedly a high rate of depressive symptoms among patients presenting with chronic fatigue. However, in recent studies only about one third to one half of patients fulfil criteria for depressive disorder (Farmer *et al.*, 1995).

Less controversial is the association between mood change and brain disorders. Although euphoria is classically described as a feature of late-stage *multiple sclerosis*, associated with marked demyelination in prefrontal areas, depression is a more frequently encountered mood change (David, 2007). Depressive disorders are also more frequently seen among patients with *Parkinson's disease* than in other disorders not involving the central nervous system, producing a similar level of chronic disability (Mindham, 1970).

Among the common neurological disorders, most recent interest has focused on the relationship between depression and *stroke*. It has long been recognised that depression is a common sequel to a stroke, but recent work suggests that poststroke depression is strongly associated with increased mortality (Morris *et al.*, 1993). There is no evidence as yet on whether antidepressant treatment improves long-term survival.

Intriguingly, the site of the lesion in strokes may provide an indication of the brain areas predominantly involved in affective disorders. A study using cerebral blood flow measures found that lesions in the left anterior and right posterior cortex were associated with depression (Yamaguchi *et al.*, 1992). Two other studies provide support for involvement of the left anterior hemisphere in poststroke depression (Astrom *et al.*, 1993; Herrmann *et al.*, 1993).

There has been recent growing interest in the association between mood disorders and common physical disorders, leading to speculation about common aetiological mechanisms (Farmer *et al.*, 2008). In particular, there is accumulating evidence that patients with either bipolar disorder (Taylor & Macqueen, 2006) or unipolar depression (Toalson *et al.*, 2004) have an increased risk of "metabolic syndrome" consisting of insulin resistance, obesity, diabetes and an associated increased risk of coronary heart disease and hypertension. However, there is also some evidence suggesting that patients with depression, even in the absence of known cardiac risk factors, still have a high risk of cardiovascular disease because of endothelial dysfunction, perhaps mediated through increased HPA axis activity and increased exposure to cortisol (Broadley *et al.*, 2006).

Psychosocial adversity

To many the relationship between "stress" and "depression" seems obvious and hardly even a subject that needs research. Certainly most members of the lay public or contributors to the popular media tend to explain depression or suicidal behaviour as a response to untoward events or stressful lifestyle rather than constitutional or biological factors (see, for example, Manchip's [1994] discussion of media coverage of the death by suicide of the rock star Kurt Cobain).

However, there are several reasons why it is more difficult than appears at first sight to show a relationship between adversity and depression. These include the fact that some events may be generated by the patient's own behaviour, and hence in turn influenced by the occurrence of a disorder such as depression, as well as that people generally seek explanations for a state that they find themselves in. Thus a depressed patient in a search for meaning may attribute the onset of his or her disorder to a particular event, whereas the same or similar events may impinge on others with no resultant mood disorder. A further and related problem is how to categorise and measure the severity of an event, given that the impact of the same event on different individuals may differ. There is a reasonable consensus that semistructured interview methods are superior to self-completed questionnaires in assessing life events, and one of the widely used instruments is that devised by Brown and Harris (1978). Their Life Events and Difficulty Schedule (LEDS) is a semistructured interview designed to detect the occurrence of life events over a recent period (usually the previous 6–12 months). After interviewing a subject using the LEDS, the researcher reports the result to a panel of raters who are provided with no information about the patient's mental state. Ratings are made of the degree of threat of the event, whether it is independent, possibly independent or dependent on the subject's own actions, and of a number of other characteristics of the event such as whether it is "self-focused" (i.e. directly focused on the subject) or "other focused". There is now an overwhelming body of evidence both from Brown and Harris's own work and from a number of other studies (e.g. Bebbington *et al.*, 1981, 1988; Brugha & Conroy, 1985; Roy *et al.*, 1985) that there is an excess of events before the onset of the disorder in depressed subjects compared with control subjects.

Studies using the LEDS have reported that it is threatening events that are predominantly associated with depression, but other workers using different terminologies (e.g. Paykel *et al.*, 1969) have found that "exit" events such as death of a loved one or departure by some other means such as divorce are most strongly associated with depression. More recent work using the LEDS has highlighted the role of events involving either loss or humiliation, with humiliation probably being a more common precipitator of depression in men than women (Farmer & McGuffin, 2003).

The fact that independent events are associated with depression supports the view that the event has a causal role in the depression rather than the behaviour of the depressed person causing the event. A causal role is also supported by the temporal relationship between life events and depression, with reported events showing a peak before rather than after the onset of the disorder (see, e.g., Bebbington *et al.*, 1988). There is also evidence that the presence of social support from relatives, friends or a spouse with whom there is a caring, intimate relationship has some buffering or protective effect against a depressive response to adversity (Champion, 1990). Another fairly consistent finding is that life events are more commonly associated with first than with subsequent episodes of depression (Farmer & McGuffin, 2003).

The hypothesis that loss of parents during childhood increases the risk of depression in adult life has received much attention. Much of this derives from psychoanalytic theory and the notion that secure attachment to parents, particularly to the mother, is important in the development of mental health (Bowlby, 1951). Brown *et al.* (1977) proposed that loss of a mother, either by death or separation, before the age of 11 years, was associated with an increased risk of depression in adult life, and Brown and Harris (1978) incorporated maternal loss within their concept of vulnerability. However, a number of studies, including the largest controlled series (Birtchnell, 1972), have failed to find any convincing relationship between adult depression and the loss by death of parents during childhood.

A different form of early adversity that has attracted considerable attention is childhood physical or sexual abuse (Moskavina *et al.,* 2006). Although the available evidence favours a relationship with adult depressive and childhood abuse, this is largely based on retrospective accounts, and there is some evidence of recall bias in that there is a modest correlation between current low mood and self-report of abuse (Moskavina *et al.,* 2006).

Psychosocial adversity in the form of life events or chronic difficulties appears to be as strongly associated with an endogenous pattern of depressive symptoms as with a neurotic or "reactive" pattern (Bebbington *et al.,* 1988). This would argue against the existence of two broad groups of depressive disorders, one largely resulting from psychosocial stresses and the other from constitutional or biological factors. The same researchers also found no evidence that depression following life events was any less familial than depression arising "out of the blue" (McGuffin *et al.,* 1988). However, an unexpected finding was that the first-degree relatives of depressed patients reported high rates of threatening life events whether or not they themselves were depressed. This was partly replicated by a study of the siblings of depressed patients (Farmer *et al.,* 2000), but the familial effect could be entirely explained by events that impinged both on the depressed index case and their brothers or sisters.

In contrast, twin studies on nondepressed or depressed subjects confirm that there is a familial component at least when life events are measured by questionnaires and that this may even receive a modest influence from genetic factors (Kendler *et al.,* 1991; Plomin 1990; Thapar & McGuffin, 1996). In one twin study, the effect was more pronounced with self-reports of events than events reported by the twins' parents, suggesting that self-reports of events may be influenced by heritable traits affecting personality. Evidence from a twin study (Kendler *et al.,* 1993) and, as mentioned earlier, from studies of a *5HTTLPR* polymorphism (Zammit & Owen, 2006) implicates genetic factors in individual difference in response to life events and adult response to childhood abuse (Caspi *et al.,* 2003).

Box 12.5 Social factors in depression

Onsets associated with recent independent (uncontrollable), threatening events; this effect most pronounced in first episodes

Loss (or "exit") and humiliation events are most potent types

Effects of adversity buffered by having a close confidante and/or good social support

Childhood abuse probably associated with adult depression (but there may be problems of retrospective recall)

Evidence of difference in genetic susceptibility to adversity

---

Psychological theories and the role of personality

Psychoanalytic theories

Psychoanalytical speculations about the origins of depression date back to Freud's writings of over a century ago, and his theories were crystallised in a classic paper, "Mourning and Melancholia" (Freud, 1917). Here he compared severe depression to a state of bereavement, noting that one of the key differences is that during normal grief, self-regard is usually unimpaired. Freud was, in fact, circumspect about the role of psychogenic factors in melancholia, acknowledging that the symptoms often "suggest somatic rather than psychogenic affections". He therefore confined his discussion to cases in which the role of psychogenic factors seemed most likely. For Freud these were situations involving loss or rejection, in which the melancholic patient identifies the lost object with his own ego by a process of introjection. He then turns the hostility generated by the loss into self-reproach and guilt.

A more explicit formulation in terms of object relations theory was evolved by Klein (1935), who postulated that passage through a "depressive position" is a necessary stage of normal development occurring in infancy. This occurs when the infant first reacts to separation from the mother and her breast with hostility and then realises that his destructive anger may have the consequence of damaging or even destroying the object of his love.

Winnicott (1958) put forward the idea that a successful passage through the depressive position was necessary for the arrival at a "stage of concern" in which the child first develops the capacity to care for others and to recognise the effect upon them of his own emotion.

Although in common with psychoanalytic theory as a whole, Freudian and post-Freudian explanations of depression do not generate testable hypotheses about the cause of depression, they are sometimes useful in interpreting the meaning of depressive symptoms in individual patients. In particular, the self-deprecation of a profoundly depressed patient expressing ideas of guilt and self-blame becomes more understandable when viewed as the angry and frustrated response to external events being turned inward on the self. Nevertheless, such insights into how patients' symptoms may evolve do not necessarily lead to therapeutic benefits.

Cognitive theories

Dissatisfaction with the explanatory power and therapeutic utility of psychoanalytic theory led Beck (1976) to put forward his cognitive theory of depression (see also Chapter 28). Beck proposed that the depressed individual is characterised by a cognitive triad consisting of a negative view of self, current experiences and the future, and that this influences the organisation of thought in a way that selectively attends to depressive ideas.

Beck considered that the cognitive triad of the depressed patient is maintained even in the face of contradictory evidence because of a style of thought, a "schema" that the depressed individual acquires early in life, partly in response to childhood experience. This may lie dormant or inactive for a long period but is then evoked by adverse circumstances. Once activated, a negative cognitive schema overcomes the individual's capacity for voluntary control over his or her thoughts, and negative ideas and attitudes spring up in an autonomous or automatic way. The individual tends to make inferences in an arbitrary fashion, in a way that is unrelated to actual evidence and to overgeneralise so that one unpleasant event or idea colours other unrelated experiences.

A key question that has received comparatively little attention is whether a depressive "cognitive style" is a trait that predisposes to developing depression or whether it is simply something associated with the state of being depressed. To measure his cognitive triad, Beck devised a dysfunctional attitude scale (DAS), which he and other workers subsequently modified (Power et al., 1994). This version of the scale was administered by Farmer and colleagues (2001) to depressed patients (before and after recovery), their siblings and a set of age-matched psychiatrically healthy control subjects and their siblings. Although there was evidence for a degree of temporal stability and familiality for some DAS subscales, the authors concluded that dysfunctional attitudes were predominantly influenced by current low mood and therefore mainly reflected the state of being depressed rather than a familial vulnerability to depressive disorder.

The notion of a fixed and maladaptive response-set in depression is also a feature of "learned helplessness" theories of depression, which were discussed earlier in the context of animal models. The reformulated theory of learned helplessness (Abramson et al., 1978) takes into account the attributional style of the depressed individual. That is, if people experience an unpleasant event over which they have no control, they will seek to interpret its occurrence. Characteristically, depressed subjects attribute the causes of events to factors external to themselves and tend to regard outcomes as noncontingent, that is, independent of anything they actually do. Such attributions are associated with low self-esteem, in which the depressed individual feels that he or she has no control over the things that happen to him or her and hence develops a state of hopelessness and self-blame.

The influence of personality traits

The extent to which depression is related to enduring and overt personality traits (as opposed to schemas that lie dormant and hidden from view) is controversial. The problem is difficult to resolve, partly because most questionnaires that purport to measure stable personality traits are partly confounded by emotional states. Thus, for example, neuroticism, N, or emotional instability as measured using the Eysenck Personality Questionnaire (EPQ) (Eysenck & Eysenck, 1975) shows an increase in scores in subjects when they are depressed (Kendell & DiScipio, 1968). Thus a study of relatives of depressed patients found the highest N scores in those relatives who were themselves depressed at the time of the study and the lowest levels in those who were neither currently depressed nor had a past history of depression. Relatives who were well at the time of the study, but who had been depressed in the past, had intermediate scores (Katz & McGuffin, 1987). Familial aspects were explored further by Farmer *et al.* (2002). Both neuroticism (N) and extraversion (E) were familial and correlated with mood and life event measures. There were no differences for N or E between the never-depressed siblings of probands with depression and control subjects. Regression analyses showed that the major influence on neuroticism was current mood. The authors concluded that neuroticism is flawed as a measure of trait vulnerability to depression. Interestingly, however, in keeping with previous work, subjects in the study who were currently depressed showed lower levels of extraversion.

The same authors (Farmer *et al.*, 2003) subsequently explored another dimension allied to extraversion, "novelty seeking", as measured by Cloninger's Temperament and Character Inventory (TCI; Cloninger *et al.*, 1993). This dimension again appeared to be inversely related to current depressive symptoms but it also showed some traitlike characteristics, suggesting that high scorers may be resilient to the development of depression. The study also suggested that other measures on Cloninger's scales, harm avoidance, reward dependence and self-directedness have stable, traitlike characteristics that may be related to the familiality of depression.

Course and outcome

Bipolar disorder

In general the age of onset of bipolar disorder is lower than that for unipolar depression and occurs in the 20s or early 30s. In contrast to schizophrenia, there are no sex differences in age of onset (Burke *et al.*, 1990; Winokur 1975), but, like schizophrenia, onset in late middle age or in the elderly is uncommon (see Chapter 13). Angst *et al.* (1973) found that 88% of cases had their onset before age 49.

According to Kraepelin (1921), the majority of manic episodes lasted for several months, but nowadays chronic mania is virtually never seen, and about half of episodes of mania last a month or less (Coryell *et al.*, 1989). The mean duration of episodes in modern studies is around 2 to 3 months (Angst *et al.*, 1973; Coryell *et al.*, 1989; Winokur *et al.*, 1969).

More than half of patients with bipolar disorder begin their illness with an attack of mania rather than depression (Dunner *et al.*, 1976; Winokur *et al.*, 1969). Although Kraepelin (1921) maintained that nearly half of patients presenting with mania would never have a further attack of affective illness, more recent studies suggest less favourable outcomes. For example, in follow-ups at 5 years, Coryell *et al.* (1989) found that only 11% of patients originally presenting with mania had not had a further attack of mania or depression, and in a follow-up of 393 patients lasting between 1 and 12 years, Angst *et al.* (1973) found that less than 1% had only had one episode. A recent review concluded that the majority of patients experience recurrent episodes and some persistence of symptoms between episodes with residual impairment in functioning.

Another of Kraepelin's observations was that the time to relapse decreases over the first two or three episodes. This has been confirmed in other studies (Angst *et al.*, 1973; Dunner *et al.*, 1979). In some patients, the course of the illness also tends to show a clustering effect with bouts of recurrences being interspersed with longer episodes of remission (Winokur, 1975).

Excess mortality in patients with bipolar disorder was a feature of some early studies, and this appears to be due to a variety of physical causes, of which cardiovascular disease was probably the most important. However, such excess of mortality appears to be more pronounced in patient samples identified before 1950 (Tsuang *et al.*, 1980) and is less of a feature of more recent follow-up studies (e.g. Martin *et al.*, 1985). The risk of suicide, however, is high (Black *et al.*, 1987), and although there have been suggestions that the risk of death by suicide is lower than for unipolar disorder, some studies (e.g. Morrison, 1982) suggest that the risk is higher, but others found no difference (Perris & d'Elia 1966; Tsuang, 1978). A recent meta-analysis found that the risk of suicide was substantially reduced in patients on long-term lithium treatment (Cipriani *et al.*, 2005).

Kraepelin's assertion that manic-depressive illness has a better long term outcome than schizophrenia is largely borne out by modern studies. However, the range of outcomes is wide, and long term deterioration is by no means rare. Tsuang *et al.* (1979) found that a quarter of patients continued to have incapacitating symptoms at a 40-year follow up, and McGlashan (1984) found that, 15 years after their initial episode, about a third of patients had more or less persistent and unremitting incapacity.

Unipolar disorder

It is difficult to make hard and fast divisions in describing the course and outcome of unipolar versus bipolar disorder, because even though the majority of patients with unipolar disorder will never have a manic episode, a substantial minority of between 4% and 20% (Akiskal, 1983; Coryell *et al.*, 1989; Lee & Murray, 1988) do eventually present with mania. There is a bigger variation in the age of onset for unipolar than for bipolar disorder, with the mean age of onset being later. In general, episodes of unipolar disorder tend to last longer than bipolar disorder, but most episodes of severe depression do not persist for more than 6 months,

and the average recovery rate after 1 year from a survey of recent studies was 64% (Piccinelli & Wilkinson, 1994). The same review found that just over a quarter of patients had a recurrence of depression within a year of the index episode, and 15% of patients had persistent depression with symptoms sustained throughout the follow-up period. Short-term outcome and social functioning appears to be influenced by personality, with evidence that extraversion is correlated with better outcome (Ranjith *et al.*, 2005).

Medium-term follow-ups suggest that the great majority of patients, more than 80%, have recovered after 2 years (Coryell *et al.*, 1987). However, in those who have failed to recover by this stage, there is thereafter only a very gradual improvement, so that at 5 years the recovery rate reaches 90% (Coryell *et al.*, 1989) with the remaining 10% having persistent and unremitting symptoms. Reported recurrence rates in medium-term follow-up studies have been high, with further episodes of between 2 and 5 years reported in 46% to 74% of cases (Piccinelli & Wilkinson, 1994).

There have been four careful long-term follow-up studies of unipolar depression taking place over periods of greater than 10 years (Angst, 1986; Kiloh *et al.*, 1988; Lee & Murray, 1988; Surtees & Barcley, 1994). One of these studies (Surtees & Barcley, 1994) focused on a selective group of patients whom the authors termed "veteran depressives", who had already had multiple episodes of disorder. The other three studies were probably more representative but focused on the severe end of the spectrum, taking as their index case subjects who had in-patient treatment for their depression. In these studies, the weighted average recovery rate, defined as a sustained recovery throughout the entire follow-up period, was 24% (Piccinelli & Wilkinson, 1994). The recovery rate was lowest in the London (UK) study of Lee and Murray (1988). However, the range of recovery rates was fairly small (18%–30%). Greater disparity was found between the UK and Australian studies when outcome was measured on a scale devised by Lee and Murray. This found that only 15% of the London series had an outcome characterised as "very good" compared with 39% of patients in the Australian series. The study by Surtees and Barcley (1994) in Edinburgh, despite the selective nature of their sample, produced results that were more similar to the Australian findings, with 34% of cases having an outcome classified as "very good".

Taken overall, therefore, the findings of long-term follow-up of hospital depressives go against the "traditional" or Kraepelinian view that depression has a relatively benign prognosis. Indeed, 34% of patients in the Lee and Murray (1988) study were categorised as having a very poor outcome, as were exactly the same proportion of patients in the Edinburgh follow-up (Surtees & Barcley, 1994) using the same operationalised outcome criteria.

Although it is often quoted that the risk of death by suicide in patients who have major depression is around 15% (Guze & Robins, 1970), more recent estimates are far lower (see also Chapter 20). For example, a review that used statistical modelling to take into account limited follow-up periods in published studies found that the lifetime risk of suicide and depression was approximately 6% (Inskip *et al.*, 1998). The apparent reduction in the rate of suicide could result from improved treatment, but there are methodological issues that need to be taken into account. For example, earlier studies mainly focused on more severe, in-patient-treated cases. In addition, Guze and Robins (1970) used proportionate mortality to estimate suicide risks. This approach divides the number of suicides by the number of subjects in the population who died from all causes during the follow-up period. Because the suicides are more common soon after hospitalisation and early in the course of the illness, and because suicide is among the more common causes of death in younger adults, using proportionate mortality probably overestimates the frequency of suicide in those suffering from depressive disorder (Bostwick & Pankratz, 2000).

Conclusions and forward view

We noted at the beginning of this chapter that our current classification of affective disorders has to be regarded as provisional and liable to change. Part of the problem is that depressed mood is such a ubiquitous symptom and that, even when associated symptoms are taken into account, there is no clear demarcation between "normal" low mood and disorder. Indeed, when minor syndromes are included, most women and 40% of men are likely to be "affected" at some point in their lives (Bebbington *et al.*, 1989). It is, therefore, as discussed earlier in the epidemiology section of this chapter, difficult to give accurate estimates of the frequency of mood disorders in the general population without qualifying this not only with what classification scheme was used but also what type of diagnostic methods were applied. These problems have led to the suggestion that categorical diagnoses should be replaced by dimensions, and there is currently much discussion on this in the lead up to the new diagnostic systems that will form the basis of DSM-V and ICD-11. At present it seems most likely that dimensional measures will be added alongside categorical definitions of at least some psychiatric disorders rather than replacing categories entirely (see also Chapter 2).

Meanwhile another issue that will need to be addressed by new classifications is that the traditional boundaries between categories of psychiatric disorder are not distinct at an aetiological level. This is best exemplified by the quantitative genetic studies discussed earlier in the chapter suggesting an overlap between the genes that contribute to anxiety and depression, that contribute to unipolar depression and bipolar disorder and that contribute to bipolar disorder and schizophrenia. The overlap between bipolar disorder and schizophrenia presents perhaps the biggest challenge as molecular genetic studies continue to reveal polymorphisms in genes that appear to be associated with liability to each of these major Kraepelinian categories. However, psychiatry is not alone in this respect, and elsewhere in medicine current studies are revealing genes that play a role in multiple phenotypically different common disorders (Wellcome Trust Case-Control Consortium, 2007). In summary, the tasks that twenty-first-century studies of the affective disorders now face are dealing with the ambiguity of the clinical phenotypes and dealing with a level of complexity of gene-environment interplay that few had anticipated (but which nevertheless is bit by bit just beginning to be understood).

REFERENCES

Abas, M., Sahakian, B., & Levy, R. (1990). Neuropsychological deficits and CT scan changes in elderly depressives. *Psychol Med* 2 : 507–20.

Abramson, L., Seligman, M , & Teasdale, J. (1978). Learned helplessness in humans: critique and reformulation. *J Abnorm Psychol* 87:49–74.

Akiskal, H. S. (1983). Dysthymic disorder: psychopathology of proposed chronic depressive subtypes. *Am J Psychiatry* 140:11–20.

Alloway, R., & Bebbington, P. (1987). The buffer theory of social support – a review of the literature. *Psychol Med* 17:91–108.

American Psychiatric Association (1994). *Diagnostic and Statistical Manual of Mental Disorders,* 4th edn. Washington, DC: American Psychiatric Association.

Andreasen, N., Swayze, V., Flaum, M., *et al.* (1990). Ventricular abnormalities in affective disorder: clinical and demographic correlates. *Am J Psychiatry* 147:893–900.

Angst, J. (1986). The course of affective disorders. *Psychopathology* 19(Suppl 2) 47–52.

Angst, J., Baastrup, P., Grof, P., *et al.* (1973). The course of monopolar depression and bipolar psychoses. *Psychiatria Neurologia Neurochirurgia* 76:489–500.

Angst, J., Gamma, A., Benazzi, F., *et al.* (2003). Toward a re definition of subthreshold bipolarity: epidemiology and proposed criteria for bipolar-II, minor bipolar disorders and hypomania. *J Affect Disord* 73:133–46.

Astrom, M., Adolfsson, R., & Asplund, K. (1993). Major depression in stroke patients. A 3-year longitudinal study. *Stroke* 24:976–82.

Ayuso Mateos, J. L., Vazquez-Barquero, J. L., Dowrick, C., *et al.* (2001). Depressive disorders in Europe: prevalence figures from the ODIN study *Br J Psychiatry* 179:308–316.

Badner, J., & Gershon, E. (2002). Meta-analysis of whole-genome linkage scans of bipolar disorder and schizophrenia. *Molec Psychiatry* 7:405–11.

Ball, W., & Whybrow, P. (1993). Biology of depression and mania. *Curr Opin Psychiatry* 6:27–34.

Barr, C. S., Newman, T. K., Becker, M. L., *et al.* (2003). The utility of the non-human primate; model for studying gene by environment interactions in behavioral research. *Genes, Brain and Behavior* 2:336–40.

Bebbington, P., Hurry, J., & Tennant, C. (1988). Adversity and the symptoms of depression. *Int J Soc Psychiatry* 34:163–71.

Bebbington, P., Hurry, J., Tennant, C., *et al.* (1981). Epidemiology of mental disorders in Camberwell. *Psychol Med* 11:561–79.

Bebbington, P., Katz, R. McGuffin, P., *et al.* (1989). The risk of minor depression before age 65: results from a community survey. *Psychol Med* 19:393–400.

Beck, A. (1976). *Cognitive Therapy and the Emotional Disorders.* New York: International Universities Press.

Berrettini, W., Cappellari, C., Nurnberger, J., & Gershon, E. (1987). Beta-andregernic receptor on lymphoblasts. A study of manic-depressive illness. *Neuropsychobiology* 17:15–18.

Berrios, G. (1992). History of the affective disorders. In E. Paykel, ed. *Handbook of Affective Disorders,* Edinburgh: Churchill Livingstone, pp. 43–56.

Biegon, A., & Israeli, M. (1988). Regionally selective increases in beta-adrenergic receptor density in the brains of suicide victims. *Brain Res* 442:199–203.

Birtchnell, J. (1972). Early parent death and psychiatric diagnosis. *Soc Psychiatry* 7:202–10.

Black, D. W., Winokur, G., & Nasrallah, A. (1987). Suicide in subtypes of major affective disorder. A comparison with general population suicide mortality. *Arch Gen Psychiatry* 44:878–80.

Blazer, D., Swartz, M., Woodbury, M., *et al.* (1988). Depressive symptoms and depressive diagnoses in a community population. Use of a new procedure for analysis of psychiatric classification. *Arch Gen Psychiatry* 45:1078–84.

Blumberg, H. P., Kaufman, J., Martin, A., *et al.* (2003). Amygdala and hippocampal volumes in adolescents and adults with bipolar disorder. *Arch Gen Psychiatry* 60:1201–8.

Bostwick, J., & Pankratz, V. S. (2000). Affective disorders and suicide risk: a reexamination. *Am J Psychiatry* 157:1925–32.

Bowlby, J. (1951). *Maternal Care and Mental Health.* Geneva: World Health Organisation.

Broadley, A. J., Korszun, A., Abdelaal, E., *et al.* (2006). Metyrapone improves endothelial dysfunction in patients with treated depression. *J Am Coll Cardiol* 48:170–5.

Brown, G., Davidson, S., Harris, T., *et al.* (1977). Psychiatric disorder in London and North Uist. *Soc Sci Med* 11:367–77.

Brown, G., & Harris, T. (1978). *Social Origins of Depression. A Study of Psychiatric Disorder in Women.* London: Tavistock.

Brugha, T., Bebbington, P., Jenkins, R., *et al.* (1999). Cross validation of a general population survey diagnostic interview: a comparison of CIS-R with SCAN ICD-10 diagnostic categories. *Psychol Med* **29**:1029–42.

Brugha, T., & Conroy, R. (1985). Categories of depression: reported life events in a controlled design. *Br J Psychiatry* **147**:641–6.

Buckland, R., O'Donovan, M., & McGuffin, P. (1992). Changes in dopamine D1, D2 and D3 receptors mRNA levels in rat brain following antipsychotic treatment. *Psychopharmacology* **106**:479–83.

Burke, K. C., Burke, J. D., Jr., Regier, D. A., & Rae, D. S. (1990). Age at onset of selected mental disorders in five community populations. *Arch Gen Psychiatry* **47**:511–18.

Campbell, S., & MacQueen, G. (2006). An update on regional brain volume differences associated with mood disorders. *Curr Opin Psychiatry* **19**:25–33.

Cardno, A. G., Coid, B., MacDonald, A. M., *et al.* (1999). Heritability estimates for psychotic disorders: the Maudsley Twin Psychosis series. *Arch Gen Psychiatry* **56**:162–8.

Cardno, A. G., Rijsdijk, F. V., Sham, P. C., *et al.* (2002). A twin study of genetic relationships between psychotic symptoms. *Am J Psychiatry* **159**:539–45.

Cardno, A. G., Sham, P. C., Murray, R. M., & McGuffin, P. (2001). Twin study of symptom dimensions in psychoses. *Br J Psychiatry* **179**:39–45.

Carroll, B., Feinberg, M., Smouse, P., *et al.* (1981). The Carroll Rating Scale for depression. Development, reliability and validation. *Br J Psychiatry* **138**:194–200.

Caspi, A., Sugden, K., Moffitt, T. E., *et al.* (2003). Influence of life stress on depression: moderation by a polymorphism in the 5-HTT gene. *Science* **301**:386–9.

Champion, L. (1990). The relationship between social vulnerability and the occurrence of severely threatening life events. *Psychol Med* **20**:157–61.

Charney, D., & Nelson, J. (1981). Delusional and nondelusional unipolar depression: further evidence for distinct subtypes. *Am J Psychiatry* **138**:328–33.

Checkley, S. (1992). Neuroendocrine mechanisms and the precipitation of depression by life events. *Br J Psychiatry* **160**:7–17.

Chen, Y. S., Akula, N., Detera-Wadleigh, S. D., *et al.* (2004). Findings in an independent sample support an association between bipolar affective disorder and the G72/G30 locus on chromosome 13q33. *Molec Psychiatry* **9**:87–92; image 5.

Chumakov, I., Blumenfeld, M., Guerassimenko, O., *et al.* (2002). Genetic and physiological data implicating the new human gene G72 and the gene for D-amino acid oxidase in schizophrenia. *Proc Nat Acad Sci U S A* **99**:13675–80.

Cipriani, A., Pretty, H., Hawton, K., & Geddes, J. R. (2005). Lithium in the prevention of suicidal behavior and all-cause mortality in patients with mood disorders: a systematic review of randomized trials. *Am J Psychiatry* **162**:1805–19.

Cloninger, C. R., Scrakic, D. M., & Przybeck, T. R. (1993). A psychobiological model of temperament and character. *Arch Gen Psychiatry* **50**:975–90.

Coppen, A. (1967). The biochemistry of affective disorders. *Br J Psychiatry* **113**:1237–64.

Coryell, W., Endicott, J., & Keller, M. (1987). The importance of psychotic features to major depression: course and outcome during a 2-year follow-up. *Acta Psychiatrica Scand* **75**:78–85.

Coryell, W., Keller, M., Endicott, J., *et al.* (1989). Bipolar II illness: course and outcome over a five-year period. *Psychol Med* **19**:129–41.

Coryell, W., Keller, M., Lavori, P., & J, E. (1990). Affective syndromes, psychotic features and prognosis. I. Depression. *Arch Gen Psychiatry* **47**:651–7.

Cowen, P. (1993). Serotonin receptor subtypes in depression: evidence from studies in neuroendocrine regulation. *Clin Neuropharmacol* **16**:S6–S18.

Cowen, P., & Charig, E. (1987). Neuroendocrine responses to intravenous tryptophan in major depression. *Arch Gen Psychiatry* **44**:958–66.

Craddock, N., Khodel, V., Van Eerdewegh, P., & Reich, T. (1995). Mathematical limits of multilocus models: the genetic transmission of bipolar disorder. *Am J Hum Genet* **57**:690–702.

David, A. (2007). *Lishman's Organic Psychiatry: A Textbook of Neuropsychiatry.* Oxford: Blackwell.

De Paermentier, F., Cheetham, S. C., Crompton, M. R., *et al.* (1990). Brain beta-adrenoceptor binding sites in anti-depressant-free depressed suicide victims. *Brain Res* **525**:71–7.

Delgado, P. L. (2006). Monoamine depletion studies: implications for antidepressant discontinuation syndrome. *J Clin Psychiatry* **67**(Suppl 4):22–6.

Dinan, T. (1994). Glucocorticoids and the genesis of depressive illness. A psychobiological model. *Br J Psychiatry* **164**:365–71.

Dolan, R., Calloway, S., & Mann, A. (1985). Cerebral ventricular size in depressed subjects. *Psychol Med* 15:873–8.

Dunlop, D. D., Song, J., Lyons, J. S., *et al.* (2003). Racial/ethnic differences in rates of depression among preretirement adults. *Am J Public Health* 93:1945–52.

Dunner, D. L., Fleiss, J. L., & Fieve, R. R. (1976). The course of development of mania in patients with recurrent depression. *Am J Psychiatry* 133:905–8.

Dunner, D. L., Murphy, D., Stallone, F., & Fieve, R. R. (1979). Episode frequency prior to lithium treatment in bipolar manic-depressive patients. *Compr Psychiatry* 20:511–15.

Eley, T., Sugden, K., Corsico, A., *et al.* (2004). Gene-environment interaction analysis of serotonin system markers with adolescent depression. *Molec Psychiatry* 9:908–15.

Ellis, P., Mellsop, G., Beeston, R., & Cooke, R. (1991). Platelet tritiated imipramine binding in patients suffering from mania. *J Affect Disord* 22:105–10.

Eysenck, H., & Eysenck, S. (1975). *Manual of the Eysenck Personality Inventory.* London: Hodder & Stoughton.

Faris, R., & Dunham, H. (1939). *Mental Disorders in Urban Areas. An Ecological Study of Schizophrenia and Other Psychoses.* Chicago: University of Chicago Press.

Farmer, A., Harris, T., Redman, K., *et al.* (2000). The Cardiff Depression Study – a sib pair study of life events and familiality in major depression. *Br J Psychiatry* 176:150–5.

Farmer, A., Harris, T., Redman, K., *et al.* (2001). The Cardiff Depression Study: a sib-pair study of dysfunctional attitudes in depressed probands and healthy control subjects. *Psychol Med* 31:627–33.

Farmer, A., Korszun, A., Owen, M. J., *et al.* (2008). Medical disorders in people with recurrent depression. *Br J Psychiatry* 192: 351–5.

Farmer, A., Mahmood, A., Redman, K., *et al.* (2003). A sib-pair study of the Temperament and Character Inventory scales in major depression. *Arch Gen Psychiatry* 60:490–6.

Farmer, A., & McGuffin, P. (2003). Humiliation, loss and other types of life events and difficulties: a comparison of depressed subjects, healthy controls and siblings. *Psychol Med* 33:1169–75.

Farmer, A., Redman, K., Harris, T., *et al.* (2002). Neuroticism, extraversion, life events and depression. *The Cardiff Depression Study.* *Br J Psychiatry* 181:118–22.

Farmer, A. E., Katz, R., McGuffin, P., & Bebbington, P. (1987). A comparison between the Present State Examination and the Composite International Diagnostic Interview. *Arch Gen Psychiatry* 44:1064–8.

Farmer, A. E., & McGuffin, P. (1989). The classification of the depressions: contemporary confusion revisited. *Br J Psychiatry* 155:437–43.

Farmer, A. E., Jones, I., Hillier, J., *et al.* (1995). Neuraesthenia revisited: ICD-10 and DSM-III-R psychiatric syndromes in chronic fatigue patients and comparison subjects. *Br J Psychiatry* 167:503–6.

Freud, S. (1917). *Mourning and Melancholia.* Standard Edition, Vol. 14. London: Hogarth Press.

Fu, C. H., Williams, S. C., Cleare, A. J., *et al.* (2004). Attenuation of the neural response to sad faces in major depression by antidepressant treatment: a prospective, event-related functional magnetic resonance imaging study. *Arch Gen Psychiatry* 61:877–89.

Giles, D., Biggs, M., Rush, A., & Roffwarg, H. (1988). Risk factors in families of unipolar depression. I. Psychiatric illness and reduced REM latency. *J Affect Disord* 14:51–9.

Goodwin, F. K., & Jamison, K. R. (1990). *Manic-Depressive Illness.* New York: Oxford University Press.

Green, E. K., Raybould, R., Macgregor, S., *et al.* (2006). Genetic variation of brain-derived neurotrophic factor (BDNF) in bipolar disorder: case-control study of over 3000 individuals from the UK. *Br J Psychiatry* 188:21–5.

Grove, W., Andreasen, N., Clayton, P., *et al.* (1987). Primary and secondary affective disorders: baseline characteristics of unipolar patients. *J Affect Disord* 13:249–57

Guze, S. B., & Robins, E. (1970). Suicide and primary affective disorders. *Br J Psychiatry* 117:437–8.

Haggerty, J. J., Simon, J., Evans, D., & Nemeroff, C. (1987). Relationship of serum TSH concentration and antithyroid antibodies to diagnosis and DST response in psychiatric inpatients. *Am J Psychiatry* 144:1492–3.

Hagnell, O. (1986). The 25-year follow-up of the Lundby study: incidence and risk of alcoholism, depression and disorders of the senium. In J. Barret & R. Rose, eds. *Mental Disorders in the Community: Findings from Psychiatric Epidemiology.* New York: Guildford Press.

Hamilton, M. (1985). *Fish's Clinical Psychopathology.* Bristol: John Wright & Sons.

Harris, B., Othman, S., Davis, J., *et al.* (1992). Association between postpartum thyroid dysfunction and thyroid antibodies and depression. *BMJ* 305:152–6.

Harvey, I., Persaud, R., Ron, M., *et al.* (1994). Volumetric MRI measures in bipolars compared with schizophrenics and healthy controls. *Psychol Med* 24:689–99.

Hattori, E., Liu, C., Badner, J. A., *et al.* (2003). Polymorphisms at the G72/G30 gene locus, on 13q33 are associated with bipolar disorder in two independent pedigree series. *Am J Hum Genet* 72:1131–40.

Henn, F. (1996). The psychobiology of depression: data for animal models. In H. Hafner & E. Wolpert, eds. *New Research in Psychiatry*. Seattle, Washington: Hogrede & Huber, pp. 1–10.

Henn, F. A., & Vollmayr, B. (2005). Stress models of depression: forming genetically vulnerable strains. *Neurosci Biobehav Rev* 29:799–804.

Hermann, M., Bartels, C., & Wallesch, C. (1993). Depression in acute and chronic aphasia: symptoms, pathoanatomical-clinical correlations and functional implications. *J Neurol Neurosurg Psychiatry* 56:672–8.

Holsboer, F., Gerken, A., Stalla, G., & Muller, O. (1987). Blunted aldosterone and ACTH release after human CRH administration in depressed patients. *Am J Psychiatry* 144:229–31.

Hwu, H.-G., Yeh, E.-K., & Change, L.-Y. (1989). Prevalence of psychiatric disorders in Taiwan defined by the Chinese Diagnostic Interview Schedule. *Acta Psychiatrica Scand* 79:136–47.

Inskip, H. M., Harris, E. C., & Barraclough, B. (1998). Lifetime risk of suicide for affective disorder, alcoholism and schizophrenia. *Br J Psychiatry* 172:35–7.

Ising, M., Kunzel, H. E., Binder, E. B., *et al.* (2005). The combined dexamethasone/CRH test as a potential surrogate marker in depression. *Prog Neuro-Psychopharmacol Biol Psychiatry* 29:1085–93

Jacoby, R., & Levy, R. (1980). Computed tomography in the elderly: 3. Affective disorder. *Br J Psychiatry* 136:270–5.

Jaspers, K. (1963). *General Psychopathology* (translated from 7th edn. by J. Hoenig & M. W. Hamilton). Manchester: Manchester University Press.

Jenkins, R. (1985). Sex differences in minor psychiatric morbidity. *Psychol Med* 15:1–53.

Johnstone, E., Owens, D., Crow, T., *et al.* (1989). Temporal lobe structure as determined by nuclear magnetic resonance in schizophrenia and bipolar affective disorder. *J Neurol Neurosurg Psychiatry* 52:736–41.

Jones, I., Kent, L., & Craddock, N. (2004). Genetics of affective disorders. In P. McGuffin, M. Owen & I. Gottesman, eds. *Psychiatric Genetics and Genomics*. Oxford: Oxford University Press, pp. 211–46.

Joyce, P., Donal, R., Livesey, J., & Abbott, R. (1987). The prolactin response to metaclopramide is increased in depression and in euthymic rapid cycling bipolar patients. *Biol Psychiatry* 22:508–12.

Joyce, P., Oakley-Browne, M., Wells, J., *et al.* (1990). Birth cohort trends in major depression: increasing rates and earlier onset in New Zealand. *J Affect Disord* 18: 83–9.

Kasen, S., Cohen, P., Chen, H., & Castille, D. (2003). Depression in adult women: age changes and cohort effects. *Am J Public Health* 93:2061–6.

Katz, R., & McGuffin, P. (1987). Neuroticism in familial depression. *Psychol Med* 17:155–61.

Kay, G., Sargeant, M., McGuffin, P., *et al.* (1993). The lymphoblast B-adrenergic receptor in bipolar depressed patients. I. Characterization and down-regulation. *J Affect Disord* 27:163–72.

Kelly, W., Checkley, S., & Bender, D. (1980). Cushing's syndrome, tryptophan and depression. *Br J Psychiatry* 136:125–32.

Kendell, R. E. (1976). The classification of depressions: a review of contemporary confusion. *Br J Psychiatry* 129:15–28.

Kendell, R. E., & DiScipio, W. J. (1968). Eysenck personality inventory scores of patients with depressive illnesses. *Br J Psychiatry* 114:767–70.

Kendler, J. S., Neale, M., Kessler, R., *et al.* (1993). The lifetime history of major depression in women: reliability of diagnosis and heritability. *Arch Gen Psychiatry* 50:863–70.

Kendler, K., Kessler, R., Heath, A., *et al.* (1991). Coping: a genetic epidemiological investigation. *Psychol Med* 21:337–46.

Kessler, R., Berglund, P., Demler, O., *et al.* (2003). The epidemiology of major depressive disorder: results from the National Comorbidity Survey Replication (NCS-R). *JAMA* 289:3095–3105.

Kiloh, L. G., Andrews, G., & Neilson, M. (1988). The long-term outcome of depressive illness. *Br J Psychiatry* 153:752–7.

Klein, M. (1935). A contribution to the psychogenesis of manic-depressive states. *Int J Psychoanal 16*. In Vol. 1. London: Hogarth Press, 1975, pp. 262–89; and Virago Press, 1997.

Klerman, G., & Weissman, M. (1989). Increasing rates of depression. *JAMA* 261:2229–35.

Korszun, A., Moskvina, V., Brewster, S., *et al.* (2004). Familiality of symptom dimensions in depression. *Arch Gen Psychiatry* 61:468–74.

Kraepelin, E. (1921). *Manic Depressive Insanity and Paranoia*. Edited by G. M. Robertson, translated by R. M. Barclay. Edinburgh: Livingstone.

Kupfer, D., Spker, D., Rossi, A., *et al.* (1983). Recent diagnostic and treatment advances in REM sleep and depression. In P. Clayton & J. Barrett, eds. *Treatment of Depression: Old Controversies and New Approaches*. New York: Raven Press, pp. 31–52.

Lam, R. W., Levitt, A. J., Levitan, R. D., *et al.* (2006). The Can-SAD study: a randomized controlled trial of the effectiveness of light therapy and fluoxetine in patients with winter seasonal affective disorder. *Am J Psychiatry* **163**:805–12.

Lawrence, K. M., De Paermentier, F., Cheetham, S. C., *et al.* (1990). Brain 5-HT uptake sites, labelled with [3]paroxetine, in antidepressant-free depressed suicides. *Brain Res* **526**:17–22.

Lee, A. S., & Murray, R. M. (1988). The long-term outcome of Maudsley depressives. *Br J Psychiatry* **153**:741–51.

Levinson, D. F. (2006). The genetics of depression: a review. *Biol Psychiatry* **60**:84–92.

Manchip, S. (1994). That stupid club. *BMJ* **308**:1447–8.

Mann, J., Stanley, M., McBridge, P., & McEwen, B. (1986). Increased serotonin2 and beta-adrenergic receptor binding in the frontal cortices of suicide victims. *Arch Gen Psychiatry* **43**:954–9.

Martin, R. L., Cloninger, C. R., Guze, S. B., & Clayton, P. J. (1985). Mortality in a follow-up of 500 psychiatric outpatients. II. Cause-specific mortality. *Arch Gen Psychiatry* **42**:58–66.

McGlashan, T. H. (1984). The Chestnut Lodge follow-up study. II. Long-term outcome of schizophrenia and the affective disorders. *Arch Gen Psychiatry* **41**:586–601.

McGuffin, P., Katz, R., Aldrich, J., & Bebbington, P. (1988). The Camberwell Collaborative Depression Study. II. Investigation of family members. *Br J Psychiatry* **152**:766–74.

McGuffin, P., Katz, R., Rutherford, J., & Watkins, S. (1996). A hospital based twin register of the Heritability of DSM-IV Unipolar Depression. *Arch Gen Psychiatry* **53**:129–36.

McGuffin, P., Knight, J., Breen, G., *et al.* (2005). Whole genome linkage scan of recurrent depressive disorder from the Depression Network (DeNt) Study. *Hum Molec Genet* **14**:3337–45.

McGuffin, P., Rijsdijk, F., Andrew, M., *et al.* (2003). The heritability of bipolar affective disorder and the genetic relationship to unipolar depression. *Arch Gen Psychiatry* **60**:497–502.

Mendlewicz, J., & Rainer, J. D. (1977). Adoption study supporting genetic transmission in manic-depressive illness. *Nature* **268**:327–9.

Mindham, R. (1970). Psychiatric symptoms in parkinsonism. *J Neurol Neurosurg Psychiatry* **33**:188–91.

Modell, S., Ising, M., Holsboer, F., & Lauer, C. J. (2005). The Munich vulnerability study on affective disorders: premorbid polysomnographic profile of affected high-risk probands. *Biol Psychiatry* **58**:694–9.

Morris, P., Robinson, P., Andrzejewski, P., *et al.* (1993). Association of depression with 10-year post stroke mortality. *Am J Psychiatry* **150**:124–9.

Morrison, J. R. (1982). Suicide in a psychiatric practice population. *J Clin Psychiatry* **43**:348–52.

Moskvina, V., Farmer, A., Swainson, V., *et al.* (2006). Interrelationship of childhood trauma, neuroticism, and depressive phenotype. *Depress Anxiety* **23**:1–6.

Nasrallah, H., McCalley-Whitters, M., & Jacoby, C. (1982). Cerebral ventricular enlargement in young manic males: a controlled study. *J Affect Disord* **4**:15–19.

Nemeroff, C., Owens, M., Bissette, G., *et al.* (1988). Reduced corticotrophin releasing factor binding sites in the frontal cortex of suicide victims. *Arch Gen Psychiatry* **45**:577–9.

Nemeroff, C., Widerlov, E., Bissette, G., *et al.* (1984). Elevated concentrations of corticotrophin-releasing factor-like immunoreactivity in depressed patients. *Science* **226**:1342–4.

Neumeister, A. (2003). Tryptophan depletion, serotonin, and depression: where do we stand? *Psychopharmacol Bull* **37**:99–115.

Neumeister, A., Nugent, A. C., Waldeck, T., *et al.* (2004). Neural and behavioral responses to tryptophan depletion in unmedicated patients with remitted major depressive disorder and controls. *Arch Gen Psychiatry* **61**:765–73.

O'Keane, V., & Dinan, T. (1991). Prolactin and cortisol responses to d-fenfluramine in major depression: evidence for diminished responsivity of central serotonergic function. *Am J Psychiatry* **148**:1009–15.

Orley, J., & Wing, J. (1979). Psychiatric disorders in two African villages. *Arch Gen Psychiatry* **36**:513–20.

Pandi-Perumal, S. R., Smits, M., Spence, W., *et al.* (2007). Dim light melatonin onset (DLMO). A tool for the analysis of circadian phase in human sleep and chronobiological disorders. *Prog Neuropsychopharmacol Biol Psychiatry* **31**:1–11.

Paykel, E., Myers, J., Dienelt, M., *et al.* (1969). Life events and depression: a controlled study. *Arch Gen Psychiatry* **21**:753–60.

Perris, C., & d'Elia, G. (1966). A study of bipolar (manic-depressive) and unipolar recurrent depressive psychoses. X. Mortality, suicide and life-cycles. *Acta Psychiatr Scand Suppl* **194**:172–89.

Piccinelli, M., & Wilkinson, G. (1994). Outcome of depression in psychiatric settings. *Br J Psychiatry* **164**:297–304.

Piletz, J., Serasua, M., Chotani, M., *et al.* (1991). Relationship between membrane fluidity and adrenoreceptor binding in depression. *Psychiatry Res* **31**:1–12.

Plomin, R. (1990). The role of inheritance in behavior. *Science* **248**:183–8.

Power, M. J., Katz, R., McGuffin, P., *et al.* (1994). The dysfunctional attitude scale (DAS). A comparison of forms A and B and proposals for a new sub-scaled version. *J Res Person* **28**:263–76.

Ranjith, G., Farmer, A., McGuffin, P., & Cleare, A. J. (2005). Personality as a determinant of social functioning in depression. *J Affect Disord* **84**:73–6.

Reynolds, C., Kupfer, D., Houck, P., *et al.* (1988). Reliable discrimination of elderly depressed and demented patients by electroencephalographic sleep data. *Arch Gen Psychiatry* **45**:258–64.

Rice, J. P., Rochberg, N., Endicott, J., *et al.* (1992). Stability of psychiatric diagnoses. An application to the affective disorders. *Arch Gen Psychiatry* **49**:824–30.

Robins, E., & Guze, S. (1972). Classification of affective disorders: the primary-secondary, the endogenous-reactive, and the neurotic-psychotic concepts. In T. Williams, M. Katz & J. Shields (Eds). *Recent Advances in the Psychobiology of the Depressive Illnesses.* Washington, DC: US Government Printing Office, pp. 283–93.

Robins, L., Wing, J., Wittche, H., *et al.* (1988). The Composite International Diagnostic Interview. An epidemiological instrument suitable for use in conjunction with different diagnostic systems and in different cultures. *Arch Gen Psychiatry* **45**:1969–77.

Roy, A., Breier, A., & Doran, A. (1985). Life events in depression. Relationship to subtypes. *J Affect Disord* **9**:143–8.

Rupprecht, R., Rupprecht, C., Rupprecht, M., *et al.* (1989). Triiodothyronine, thyroxine and TSH response to dexamethasone in depressed patients and normal controls. *Biol Psychiatry* **25**:22–32.

Rush, A., Erman, M., Giles, D., *et al.* (1986). Polysomnographic findings in recently drug-free and clinically remitted depressed patients. *Arch Gen Psychiatry* **43**:873–84.

Schildkraut, J. (1965). The catecholamine hypothesis of affective disorders: a review of supporting evidence. *Am J Psychiatry* **122**:509–22.

Schumacher, J., Jamra, R. A., Becker, T., *et al.* (2005). Evidence for a relationship between genetic variants at the brain-derived neurotrophic factor (BDNF) locus and major depression. *Biol Psychiatry* **58**:307–14.

Schumacher, J., Jamra, R. A., Freudenberg, J., *et al.* (2004). Examination of G72 and D-amino-acid oxidase as genetic risk factors for schizophrenia and bipolar affective disorder. *Mol Psychiatry* **9**:203–7.

Scott, M., Golden, C., Reudrich, S., & Bishop, R. (1983). Ventricular enlargement in major depression. *Psychiatry Res* **8**:91–3.

Seligman, M. E. P. (1975). *Helplessness. About Depression, Development and Death.* San Francisco: Freeman.

Siever, L., & Davis, K. (1985). Overview: toward a dysregulation hypothesis of depression. *Am J Psychiatry* **142**:1017–31.

Smith, A., & Weissman, M. (1991). Epidemiology. In E. Paykel, ed. *Handbook of Affective Disorders.* Edinburgh: Churchill Livingstone,, pp. 111–30.

Sohn, C. H., & Lam, R. W. (2005). Update on the biology of seasonal affective disorder. *CNS Spectr* **10**:635–46.

Sullivan, P. F., & Kendler, K. S. (1998). Typology of common psychiatric syndromes. An empirical study. *Br J Psychiatry* **173**:312–19.

Sullivan, P. F., Neale, M., & Kendler, K. S. (2000). Genetic epidemiology of major depression: review and meta-analysis. *Am J Psychiatry* **157**:1552–62.

Suomi, S., Seaman, S., & Lewis, J. (1978). Effects of imipramine treatment on separation induced social disorders in rhesus monkeys. *Arch Gen Psychiatry* **35**:321–5.

Surtees, P. G., & Barkley, C. (1994). Future imperfect: the long-term outcome of depression. *Br J Psychiatry* **164**:327–41.

Surtees, P. G., Miller, P., Ingham, J., *et al.* (1986). Life events and onset of affective disorder: a longitudinal general population study. *J Affect Disord* **10**:37–50.

Taylor, V., & Macqueen, G. (2006). Associations between bipolar disorder and metabolic syndrome: a review. *J Clin Psychiatry* **67**:1034–41.

Thapar, A., & McGuffin, P. (1996). Genetic influences on life events in childhood. *Psychol Med* **26**:813–20.

Thompson, C., & Isaacs, G. (1988). Seasonal affective disorder – a British sample. Symptomatology in relation to mode of referral and diagnostic subtype. *J Affect Disord* **14**:1–11.

Toalson, P., Ahmed, S., Hardy, T., & Kabinoff, G. (2004). The metabolic syndrome in patients with severe mental illnesses. *Prim Care Companion J Clin Psychiatry* **6**:152–158.

Tsuang, M. T. (1978). Suicide in schizophrenics, manics, depressives, and surgical controls. A comparison with general population suicide mortality. *Arch Gen Psychiatry* **35**:153–5.

Tsuang, M. T., Woolson, R. F., & Fleming, J. A. (1979). Long-term outcome of major psychoses. I. Schizophrenia and affective disorders compared with psychiatrically symptom-free surgical conditions. *Arch Gen Psychiatry* **36**:1295–1301.

Tsuang, M. T., Woolson, R. F., & Fleming, J. A. (1980). Causes of death in schizophrenia and manic-depression. *Br J Psychiatry* **136**:239–42.

Uhl, G., Blum, K., Noble, E., & Smith, S. (1993). Substance abuse vulnerability and D2 receptor genes. *Trends in Neurosciences* **16**:83–8.

Van Os, J., Castle, D. J., Takei, N., *et al.* (1994). Psychotic illness in ethnic minorities: clarification from the 1991 census. *Psychol Med* **26**:203–8.

Vazquez-Barquero, J., Diez-Manrique, J., Pena, C., *et al.* (1986). Two stage design in a community survey. *Br J Psychiatry* **149**:88–97.

Von Knorring, A., Cloninger, C., Bohman, M., & Sigvardsson, S. (1983). An adoption study of depressive disorders and substance abuse. *Arch Gen Psychiatry* **40**:943–50.

Watson, S., Gallagher, P., Ritchie, J. C., *et al.* (2004). Hypothalamic-pituitary-adrenal axis function in patients with bipolar disorder. *Br J Psychiatry* **184**:496–502.

Weinberger, D., Delisi, L., Perman, G., *et al.* (1982). Computerised tomography in schizophreniform disorder and other acute psychiatric disorders. *Arch Gen Psychiatry* **39**:778–83.

Weissman, M. M., Bland, R. C., Canino, G. J., *et al.* (1996). Cross-national epidemiology of major depression and bipolar disorder. *JAMA* **276**:293–9.

Weissman, M., Leaf, D., Tischler, G., *et al.* (1988). Affective disorders in five United States communities. *Psychol Med* **18**:141–53.

Weissman, M., & Myers, J. (1978). Rates and risks of depressive symptoms in a United States urban community. *Acta Psychiatr Scand* **57**:219–31.

Wellcome Trust Case Control Consortium (2007). Genome-wide association study of 14,000 cases of seven common diseases and 3,000 shared controls. *Nature* **447**: 661–83.

Wender, P. H., Seymour, S. K., Rosenthal, D., *et al.* (1986). Psychiatric disorders in the biological and adoptive families of adopted individuals with affective disorders. *Arch Gen Psychiatry* **43**:923–9.

Willner, P., Sampson, D., Papp, M., *et al.* (1991). Animal models of anhedonia. In P. Soubrie, ed. *Anxiety, Depression and Mania*. Basel: Karger, pp. 71–100.

Wing, J. K., Babor, T., Brugha, T., *et al.* (1990). SCAN. Schedules for clinical assessment in neuropsychiatry. *Arch Gen Psychiatry* **47**:589–93.

Winnicott, D. (1958). *Collected Papers*. New York: Basic Books.

Winokur, G. (1975). The Iowa 500: heterogeneity and course in manic-depressive illness (bipolar). *Compr Psychiatry* **16**:125–31.

Winokur, G., Clayton, P., & Reich, T. (1969). *Manic Depressive Illness*. St Louis: C. V. Mosby.

World Health Organisation (WHO) (1992). *The ICD-10 Classification of Mental and Behavioural Disorders*. Geneva: WHO.

Wright, A. F., Crichton, D. N., & Loudon, J. B., *et al.* (1984). B-adrenoceptor binding defects in cell lines from families with manic-depressive disorder. *Ann Hum Genet* **48**:201–14.

Yamaguchi, S., Kobayashi, S., Koido, H., & Tsunematsu, T. (1992). Longitudinal study of regional cerebral blood flow changes in depression after stroke. *Stroke* **23**:1716–22.

Zammit, S., & Owen, M. J. (2006). Stressful life events, 5-HTT genotype and risk of depression. *Br J Psychiatry* **188**:199–201.

13

Schizophrenia and related disorders

Robin M. Murray and Kimberlie Dean

Schizophrenia is a frightening illness in which intrusive "voices" (*auditory hallucinations*) frequently torment the individual with abusive or derogatory comments, and ideas weave together to form false beliefs (*delusions*). The sufferer may be convinced he is under surveillance or enmeshed in a conspiracy of huge religious or political significance. He may believe that his thoughts are no longer private or that they are controlled by an external, and usually malevolent, will.

The onset of psychosis may be characterised by *delusional mood* consisting of intense puzzlement, with familiar surroundings seeming strange, relationships seeming changed and a feeling that something inexplicable or sinister is going on. Patients may also suffer perceptual abnormalities such as faces changing shape or experience odd smells or tastes (e.g. of blood or poison). In addition to auditory hallucinations, some patients have somatic hallucinations (e.g. of a sexual nature) or, less commonly, visual hallucinations. Delusions are most frequently of a paranoid nature but may also be religious, grandiose or sexual.

Most people recover from their first schizophrenic episode within a few weeks of receiving antipsychotic drugs, but with each succeeding episode, the hallucinations and delusions (termed *positive symptoms*) may become more resistant to treatment. Nayani and David (1995) have shown how the psychotic experiences appear to gradually "colonise" the healthy parts of the mind. In particular, they describe how delusional explanations gradually become more complex and bizarre. In this way, one patient interpreted the ordinary anxiety-related experience of tightness of the throat as "a penis being forced down my throat and suffocating me".

Thought disorder. Patients may show derailment of thought or the so-called knight's-move thinking, and illogical speech may deteriorate to the point that it becomes incoherent. There may be dislocation of words or, occasionally, the creation of new private words (neologisms), sometimes by the condensation of others; for example, a patient whose initials were K.A.O. described his personal philosophy as "Kaosophy". Individuals with schizophrenia may also give private idiosyncratic meanings to words that already exist.

Other features have been described and grouped together as *negative symptoms*. These include the features shown in Box 13.1.

Box 13.1 Negative symptoms of schizophrenia

- social withdrawal
- loss of motivation and initiative
- apathy
- slowness of thought and action
- poverty of thought and speech
- emotional blunting (flattening of affect)

Essential Psychiatry, ed. Robin M. Murray, Kenneth S. Kendler, Peter McGuffin, Simon Wessely, David J. Castle. Published by Cambridge University Press. © Cambridge University Press 2008.

TABLE 13.1 Frequency of symptoms in the International Pilot Study of Schizophrenia

Symptom	Frequency (%)
Lack of insight	97
Ideas of reference	70
Flatness of affect	66
Delusions of persecution	64
Thoughts spoken aloud	50
Auditory hallucinations	74
Suspiciousness	66
Delusional mood	64
Thought alienation	52

Data taken from WHO's International Pilot Study of Schizophrenia.

Negative symptoms tend to accumulate gradually and, when they are severe, such symptoms, which often occur together, are sometimes termed the *schizophrenic defect state* (Carpenter *et al.*, 1988). Although they tend to be most prominent in patients with chronic illness, they can be exacerbated during acute episodes and improve during remission. Negative symptoms are often accompanied by cognitive impairment, especially executive (frontal lobe) and memory (temporal lobe) deficits. Positive symptoms are easier to elicit and to measure reliably than negative symptoms, but the latter are more persistent and appear to be of more serious prognostic importance. The relative importance of positive and negative symptoms are discussed by David and Appleby (1992), and a comprehensive overview of the phenomenology of schizophrenia is provided in Chapter 1.

Patients with schizophrenia frequently have little insight into their condition. Indeed, in the International Pilot Study on Schizophrenia (IPSS) carried out in nine countries, lack of insight was the commonest symptom among 306 typical schizophrenic patients (shown in Table 13.1)

The classical subtypes

Schizophrenia was classically subdivided into hebephrenic, catatonic, paranoid and simple subtypes. However, we now know that the differences between these subtypes are of a pathoplastic nature determined in part by age of onset and that patients can change their predominant symptomatology on successive admissions. *Hebephrenia* was used to describe profoundly disturbed young patients with marked thought disorder, but the term is rarely used now. The term *catatonia* was applied to those with pronounced psychomotor abnormalities – stupor or excitement, posturing including waxy flexibility, stereotypes and negativism. Nowadays, catatonic schizophrenia should be diagnosed with caution and always in the presence of other more typical symptoms, not only because it has become much less common in the Western world but also because catatonic symptoms may also occur in both affective disorder and neurological conditions (see also Chapter 14).

Paranoid schizophrenia refers to those cases in which the patient's mental state is dominated by systematised delusions whether of persecution, grandiosity, fantastic or religious nature. Patients with paranoid schizophrenia are less likely to have pronounced thought disorder or to progress to a defect state, perhaps because they frequently have a later onset. Sometimes the term *paraphrenia* is used to describe those who develop this syndrome very late in life; it is more common in women and in the deaf, whose handicap may render them particularly susceptible to ideas of reference and persecution. *Simple schizophrenia* is rarely diagnosed nowadays, but the diagnosis used to be made in patients in whom there was little in the way of positive symptoms but there was a gradual deterioration in personality with increasing emotional bluntness; occasional brief psychotic episodes were used to substantiate the diagnosis.

The concept of schizophrenia

Development of the concept

In the early nineteenth century, many psychiatrists believed in the existence of a single unitary psychosis, *Einheitpsychose*, which could manifest itself in various forms. Then, in 1851, the French psychiatrist Falret delineated *folie circulaire* or manic depressive psychosis, and shortly thereafter his compatriot Morel applied the term *démence précoce* to a deteriorating psychosis in a patient whose withdrawal, bizarre mannerisms and personal neglect had begun in adolescence. Hecker subsequently employed the term *hebephrenia* for a similar picture, and in 1874 Kahlbaum published a monograph on catatonia, which he described as a cyclical condition characterised by stereotyped movement, mannerisms and occasional outbursts of intense excitement, automatic obedience, negativism and stupor. Kahlbaum considered hebephrenia and catatonia quite distinct from one another and also from paranoia, a term that he reserved for those with primary systematised delusions.

In 1896, Emil Kraepelin (see Kraepelin, 1919) brought hebephrenia, catatonia and paranoia together into the single entity of dementia praecox, the characteristics of which he thought included hallucinations, delusions, a decrease in attention towards the outside world, lack of curiosity, disorder of thought, lack of insight and judgement, emotional blunting, negativism and stereotypes. Kraepelin believed that this was a disease which usually had its onset in early adult life (hence "praecox") and generally, although not invariably, progressed to a pervasive impairment of cognitive and behavioural function (hence "dementia").

The Swiss psychiatrist Eugene Bleuler (1911/1974) did not regard dementia praecox as a disease per se but spoke instead of the group of "schizophrenias", a term he introduced because "the disconnection or splitting of the psychic functions is an outstanding feature". Bleuler distinguished primary symptoms – altered associations (thought disorder), affective blunting, ambivalence and autism (a turning away from the external environment into a private world of fantasy) from secondary symptoms such as delusions and hallucinations, which he considered could occur in other illnesses. Unfortunately, Bleuler's primary symptoms were so difficult to define that they allowed clinicians a great deal of diagnostic latitude.

Table 13.2 Schneider's first-rank symptoms

Auditory hallucinations of specific type
(a) Audible thoughts: voices repeating or anticipating the patient's thoughts out loud
(b) Two or more voices discussing the patient in the third person
(c) Voices commenting on the patient's behaviour

Thought interference of specific type
(a) Thought withdrawal
(b) Thought insertion
(c) Thought broadcasting so that thoughts are conveyed to others

Feelings, impulses or acts experienced as being under external control
Delusional perception (a form of primary delusion): an unshakeable belief arising in an unaccountable manner from some commonplace event

Schneider's criteria

The most influential attempt at a more precise definition of schizophrenia was that of Kurt Schneider (1950), who regarded certain symptoms as being *of first rank* importance in differentiating schizophrenia from other conditions. Schneider considered that whenever any of these were found in the absence of organic disease or drug intoxication, one could make a diagnosis of schizophrenia (Table 13.2).

Wing and his colleagues (1978) described first-rank symptoms, and how to elucidate them, in detail, stating, for example, that "Typically thought insertion is described by the patient in terms of some causal idea, such as a radio set implanted in the brain, or rays directed from another planet, or telepathy". Similarly, delusions of control are often elaborated thus: "the patient says that someone else's words are coming out using his voice or that his handwriting is not his own, or that he is a zombie or robot whose very movement is determined by some alien power". Another first-rank symptom is delusional perception, in which a fully fledged delusion arises from some occurrence that others would regard as quite normal; for example, a nurse passing an innocent remark about the weather conveyed to one patient the certainty that he was going to be murdered.

Schneider's criteria have been much criticised. Indeed, in the IPSS carried out in nine countries, only 58% of 1202 acute patients with a hospital diagnosis of schizophrenia had one or more first-rank symptoms (World Health Organisation [WHO], 1973), whereas these symptoms occurred in some nonschizophrenia patients, especially those suffering from mania.

Criticism of the concept

Since the invention of the concept of dementia praecox/schizophrenia, it has attracted dissent. In the 1960s, "antipsychiatrists" such as Thomas Szasz and R. D. Laing regarded schizophrenia as a medical fiction invented for the needs of society, relatives and psychiatrists rather than sufferers. Sociologists also drew attention to the negative aspects of receiving a diagnosis of schizophrenia and considered that some of the symptoms were a consequence of being labelled as mad. Certainly after an individual is diagnosed with schizophrenia, his relations with family, employers and doctors can be considerably altered for the worse. It is easy to conceive how a social reaction might pressurise an individual into deviancy, but as Wing *et al.* (1974) stated, "it is difficult to imagine how a similar reaction would force him to adopt the central schizophrenic syndrome since this would need special coaching from an expert".

Psychologists also made assaults on the concept of schizophrenia. Rosenhan and colleagues (1973) managed to get themselves admitted to mental hospitals and diagnosed with schizophrenia merely by declaring that they heard voices saying "empty", "hollow" and "thud". This study, which illustrated the dangers of both sloppy diagnostic practice and "labelling", was a useful polemic against the practice of bad psychiatry but cannot be regarded as a serious criticism of the concept of schizophrenia.

More recent attacks have come from Mary Boyle (2002), whose thesis is that schizophrenia did exist a century ago when it was a secondary consequence of viral and other neurological disorders, but although such neurological disorders have largely been eliminated, the concept is now erroneously applied to nonorganic conditions. A further assault has come from Richard Bentall (2004), who regards a diagnosis of schizophrenia with its implications of likely deterioration as harmful to patients and their care. Perhaps most painfully, one of the United Kingdom's main nosologists who spent his life researching the nosology of psychosis concluded, "It is important to loosen the grip which the concept of 'schizophrenia' has on the minds of psychiatrists. Schizophrenia is an idea whose very essence is equivocal, a nosological category without natural boundaries, a barren hypothesis. Such a blurred concept is 'not a valid object of scientific enquiry'" (Brockington, 1992, p. 207).

Some psychiatrists react to such criticisms by totally denying their validity and by reasserting a simplistic medical disease model of schizophrenia. However, this is less than satisfactory because there remains widespread confusion regarding the meaning, boundaries and even value of the term schizophrenia. Some authorities define schizophrenia on the basis of symptomatology and some by characteristic course, whereas some consider it merely a syndrome and others regard it as a disease process not necessarily revealed in overt behaviour. The origin of the confusion is that we have failed to understand fully either the aetiology or pathogenesis of the conditions referred to under the term schizophrenia, and it is likely that our confusion will continue until the aetiology and pathogenesis are firmly established.

Operational definitions

Operational definitions were developed as an attempt to improve the reliability of the diagnosis of schizophrenia, most of them based on the classification systems outlined in Chapter 2. The first was the Present State Examination (PSE/CATEGO) system of Wing *et al.* (1974), in which the criteria are based mainly on Schneider's first-rank symptoms. The PSE/CATEGO system was used to show that although psychiatrists in New York diagnosed schizophrenia more frequently than their counterparts in London, the project psychiatrists employing the PSE diagnosed the disorder in much the same proportions in each city (Cooper *et al.*, 1972). A similar but wider study, the IPSS, was carried out under the auspices of WHO (1973). The IPSS used the PSE to examine 1202 patients in nine countries. The three European and four developing countries had similar criteria for diagnosing schizophrenia, but once again the prevailing concept was broader in the United States and also in Russia.

Since that time, a curious change has occurred. The predominantly European-based international concept of schizophrenia has remained relatively unchanged, becoming operationalised in the 10th revision of the *International Classification of Diseases* (ICD-10; WHO, 1992). However, American psychiatrists produced a series of stricter operational definitions with the paradoxical result that the American concept of schizophrenia became narrower than that in use in Europe (Andreasen & Carpenter, 1993). The more important of these definitions have included the Research Diagnostic Criteria (or RDC; Spitzer *et al.*, 1978) and the third and fourth editions of the *Diagnostic and Statistical Manual of Mental Disorders* (DSM-III, DSM-III-R and DSM-IV; American Psychiatric Association, 1980, 1994). Like the PSE/CATEGO system which has now become the SCAN (Schedule for Clinical Assessment in Neuropsychiatry), these definitions emphasise Schneiderian phenomenology, but unlike it, they also incorporate a longitudinal component; thus the DSM-IV demands the presence of active symptoms for 1 month (like ICD-10) and some signs of disturbance persisting for 6 months (unlike ICD-10). Table 13.3 provides a comparison of the criteria for ICD-10 and the text revision of DSM-IV (DSM-IV-TR) definitions of schizophrenia, which are the systems currently most in use.

Brockington *et al.* (1978), who compared 10 operational definitions of schizophrenia as applied to 119 psychotic patients, found that the number who qualified as schizophrenic on the various criteria ranged from 3 to 45! There were wide variations in the reliability, concordance and predictive powers of different criteria; thus Schneider's first-rank symptoms were only weak predictors of future course, whereas the RDC were relatively successful in identifying the poor prognosis group. The investigators concluded that "inarticulate confusion" has been replaced "by a babel of precise but differing formulation of the same concept".

The borders of schizophrenia

Despite the use of reliable definitions of schizophrenia such as the DSM-IV and ICD-10 criteria, the boundaries of schizophrenia remain indistinct, and it merges on one side with bipolar disorder (manic depression) and on the other with schizotypal and paranoid personality disorder.

Schizoaffective disorder

Controversy has focused on whether patients with both schizophrenia and affective symptoms should be considered within the limits of schizophrenia. Kasanin (1933) coined the term *schizoaffective psychosis* for those patients with a sudden onset and marked emotional turmoil, whereas Langfeldt (1939) distinguished between *process schizophrenia* (roughly equivalent to Kraepelin's dementia praecox) and *schizophreniform* illness with precipitating factors, a strong affective component, often disturbance of consciousness and on the whole a good prognosis. Numerous other terms have been used, but the status of such individuals remains a persistent enigma. Because of the frequency of affective disorder in their families and their remitting course, many regard these patients as having a variant of affective disorder, whereas others consider that there is a continuum of psychosis (Crow, 1990;

TABLE 13.3 Diagnostic criteria for schizophrenia: ICD-10 versus DSM-IV-TR

ICD-10	DSM-IV-TR
1. At least one of A or two of B	1. At least two of A (only one of A required if delusions are bizarre or hallucinations consist of running commentary or discussing voices)
2. Features present for most of the time during an episode of illness lasting at least 1 month	2. Continuous signs of disturbance for at least 6 months with at least 1 month of acute phase symptoms (A)
3. Exclusions: the disorder must not be attributable to mood disorder, organic brain disorder or substance use disorder	3. Exclusions: the disorder must not be attributable to schizoaffective or mood disorder with psychotic features, the direct effects of a substance or a general medical condition
	4. Social/occupational dysfunction (below the level of expected functioning)
A	A
• Thought echo, thought insertion or withdrawal, or thought broadcasting	• Delusions
• Delusions of control, influence or passivity; delusional peception	• Hallucinations
• Hallucinatory voices giving a running commentary or discussing the patient or coming from some part of the body	• Disorganised speech
	• Grossly disorganised or catatonic behaviour
• Persistent delusions that are culturally inappropriate and completely impossible	• Negative symptoms
B	
• Persistent hallucinations in any modality	
• Neologisms, breaks or interpolations in the train of thought resulting in incoherent or irrelevant speech	
• Catatonic behaviour	
• Negative symptoms (apathy, paucity of speech, blunting or incongruity of affect)	
• Persistent hallucinations in any modality	

DSM-IV = *Diagnostic and Statistical Manual of Mental Disorders*, 4th edn.; ICD-10; *International Classification of Diseases*, 10th revision.

Murray *et al.*, 2004; Pope & Lipinski, 1978; Procci, 1976).

Psychosis as a dimension

The issue of whether schizophrenic symptoms are qualitatively different from normal human behaviour has not been resolved. Claridge (1972) regarded the schizophrenic predisposition as a continuously variable personality dimension. More recently, it has become clear that a proportion of the general adult population experience brief or isolated psychotic phenomena without coming into contact with psychiatric services. Most European authorities now consider that liability to psychosis exists as a continuous trait in populations and that individuals categorised as schizophrenic lie at the extreme end of this continuum. Hypertension provides a useful analogy. Blood pressure in the whole population approximates a normal distribution, but once the diastolic blood pressure exceeds 85 mm of mercury, then adverse consequences ensue. Therefore, a cut-off is imposed so that the individual is regarded as hypertensive and in need of treatment. In a similar way, schizophrenia can be seen as that part of the distribution of psychotic symptoms which is beyond a threshold indicating the need for treatment. The well relatives of those with schizophrenia lie proximal to those with schizophrenia on this dimension. They often show paranoid or schizoid or schizotypal characteristics, and their performance on cognitive tests is intermediate between that of patients and normal subjects. Thus, schizophrenia merges into schizotypal and paranoid personality; together with schizophrenia, these conditions are sometimes termed the *schizophrenia spectrum*. Tsuang *et al.* (2001) included the personality and cognitive difficulties shown by relatives under the rubric *schizotaxia*.

The current position

The current classification of the psychoses is extremely unsatisfactory, but as yet there is no viable alternative to the use of the term schizophrenia. In the absence of evidence to the contrary, schizophrenia is best considered as a syndrome that may cover several conditions. A relatively restrictive concept should be applied conservatively both in the interests of diagnostic homogeneity and because of the adverse consequences of labelling doubtful cases as schizophrenic. Schneider's first-rank symptoms are included in most contemporary definitions, but schizophrenia should not be diagnosed solely on their basis if other evidence points to an affective disorder. Furthermore, the transient presence of first-rank symptoms does not necessarily imply a poor prognosis (Brockington *et al.*, 1978). Thus the length of the symptoms and the degree of incapacity should also be taken into account in the diagnostic formulation, as should the presence of negative symptoms. The ICD-10 criteria represent a reasonable compromise, but, given the range of currently available operational definitions and uncertainty about validity, some investigators advocate a "polydiagnostic" approach in research; in the so-called OPCRIT (operational criteria) system, clinical data are collected in sufficient detail for several definitions to be applied (Craddock *et al.*, 1996).

Differential diagnosis

A diagnosis should not be made simply on the basis of positive findings of schizophrenia, but must include an absence of features more characteristic of other syndromes. The conditions to be excluded include the following.

Illicit drugs and psychosis

Psychostimulant drugs such as amphetamine (and methamphetamine) and cocaine can produce a psychosis mimicking schizophrenia (Curran *et al.*, 2004). Indeed, the symptoms of amphetamine psychosis can be identical with those of paranoid schizophrenia (Connell, 1958). Amphetamine psychosis is most frequently observed in individuals who have consumed large quantities of the drug over prolonged periods and usually resolves within a few days of ceasing the abuse. Chen *et al.* (2003, 2005) showed that methamphetamine users who develop psychosis differ from those who do not primarily in two ways: (1) greater risk of schizophrenia in relatives and (2) more schizotypal childhood personality. Furthermore these same two factors were the best predictors of how long the psychosis would last. The authors concluded that there is a distribution of liability to psychosis through the general population: that those with little or no liability are unlikely to develop psychosis, whereas those with a higher liability are more likely to develop psychosis and those with highest may develop a persistent psychosis.

Psychoses can also be induced by hallucinogens such as LSD, "ecstasy" and phenylcyclidine (PCP or "angel dust"). LSD tends to cause visual rather than auditory hallucinations, whereas PCP, unlike other hallucinogens, can mimic negative as well as positive symptoms. Debate continues over whether individuals who develop drug-related psychoses are constitutionally predisposed, and there is some evidence that patients who develop apparently genuine schizophrenia following drug abuse breakdown at an earlier stage than those who have not taken drugs. Tsuang *et al.* (1982) contrasted patients with drug-associated psychosis whose illnesses lasted more and less than six months, respectively. Those with the longer-lasting psychoses had more "schizophrenic" symptoms, poorer premorbid personalities and greater familial risks of psychosis. Clearly this group had more affinity to schizophrenia proper.

In recent years, it has also been shown that acute intoxication with cannabis can precipitate psychosis, sometimes termed *cannabis psychosis.* Persistent heavy cannabis use is also associated with schizophrenia, but in this case, the symptoms seem to be identical with schizophrenia. Therefore the condition is better regarded as a variety of schizophrenia rather than a specific psychosis (Henquet *et al.,* 2005)

Organic conditions

Distinction can usually be made from psychosis associated with gross cerebral pathology, infection or metabolic disorder because of the presence of clouding of consciousness, physical signs or laboratory abnormalities in such conditions (Lishman, 1997), but any individual presenting schizophrenic symptoms for the first time should receive a careful workup, including electroencephalogram and magnetic resonance imaging (MRI). In a small proportion (approximately 4%–6%) definite organic pathology is found (Johnstone, 1994). The best established relationship is with temporal lobe epilepsy, which Slater *et al.* (1963) established may cause "symptomatic schizophrenia". Most puerperal psychoses are not schizophrenic, but a minority are or later clearly become so (see Chapter 19).

Paranoid states

The exact classification of the paranoid states has long been a matter of controversy (Kendler,

1980). Some authorities regard the differences between paranoid personality, paranoia and paranoid schizophrenia as merely a matter of degree. Individuals with *paranoid personality* are generally rigid and inflexible, suspicious and morbidly sensitive. They may be of rather dominant nature and their friendships of short duration. The so-called overvalued idea or *idée fixe* may be prominent. *Paranoia* (or delusional disorder) is a relatively rare condition characterised by an intricate, complex and elaborate delusional system without hallucinations. The delusions are systematised, firmly knit and more or less isolated so that the rest of the personality remains relatively intact. Paranoia is rare before 30 years of age. Many with paranoia are single, and they are rarely bothered by others provided they are not dangerous to themselves or others. Occasionally, however, an individual with paranoia may consider that he or she has unique abilities and may seek political expression of his or her views. Recently, interest in "querulous paranoia" has been revived, precipitated by the increase in provision of official avenues for complaints of various kinds (Mullen & Lester, 2006).

In *erotomania* (also known as Clerambault's syndrome; Enoch & Ball, 2001), an individual, usually female, presents ideas that she is loved by another person who does not make a direct avowal but indicates his love in many indirect ways. The person cast in the role of lover is often of higher status and is pestered by unwelcome letters or visits.

Morbid jealousy (Othello syndrome) is characterised by delusions of infidelity and a search for evidence of adultery. Spouses may be followed or their underwear repeatedly examined for seminal stains. Improbable accusations may be succeeded by violence and occasional homicide of the wife or her supposed lover. Morbid jealousy may occur in paranoid states, schizophrenia, alcoholism or depressive psychosis.

In *folie à deux* a delusion is transmitted from one person to another so that the second comes to share the psychopathology of the first. Usually the two persons are living together, perhaps as husband and wife or mother and daughter. The person to whom the delusions are transmitted is often passive and dependent and usually recovers within a few months if the two are separated. *Folie a deux* and the other eponymous conditions have been well reviewed by Enoch and Ball (2001).

Other psychotic conditions

The boundaries between schizophrenia and affective disorder can be vague. One should be particularly aware of the intensifications of affect that may be an early symptom of schizophrenia and of the occurrence of first-rank symptoms and of over-inclusive thinking in mania. Even when the greatest care is taken, patients diagnosed on their initial hospitalization with schizophrenia will sometimes need to be reclassified as having affective disorder and vice versa. It may at times be difficult to differentiate between obsessive-compulsive disorder and schizophrenia, but a careful history should demonstrate that that the nature of the phenomena are different (see Chapter 8).

Epidemiology

Schizophrenia typically presents in late adolescence or in early adult life; prepubertal children rarely manifest Schneiderian symptoms (Pilowsky & Murray, 1991). Males tend to have an earlier onset than females – the mean age of first admission in the United Kingdom is about 22 years for men and 27 years for women (Castle & Murray, 1991; Kirkbride *et al.,* 2006). Females with schizophrenia also tend to have a milder illness with fewer negative symptoms and a better outcome than males, and as a result they are less likely to meet the strictest diagnostic criteria. A recent systematic review reveals that the incidence of schizophrenia is actually higher among males (mean rate ratio 1.4; McGrath *et al.,* 2004).

Geographic and temporal variations

Most authorities quote a lifetime risk of schizophrenia of between 0.5% and 1%, the former being the average risk of narrowly defined schizophrenia (e.g. DSM-IV) and the latter that of broader definitions (e.g. ICD-10). However, some went further and claimed that the incidence does not vary by time or place, even though such an occurrence would have made schizophrenia unique among diseases! This curious belief stemmed from a WHO study (Jablensky *et al.,* 1992) which is frequently quoted as showing that there was no significant variation between countries in the incidence of nuclear schizophrenia as defined by the PSE/CATEGO system. However, it is more correct to say that the study had insufficient power to detect significant differences. Furthermore, when a "broad" concept of schizophrenia was examined, the incidence varied fourfold. Subsequently many studies have shown variation in incidence. In particular, a systematic review by McGrath *et al.* (2004) concluded that the incidence of schizophrenia shows prominent worldwide variation (up to fivefold).

Urbanicity

It has been known for many years that the prevalence of schizophrenia is greater in cities. In the 1930s, Faris and Dunham (1939) reported higher admission rates for schizophrenia in the central areas of lowest socioeconomic status in Chicago than in the more affluent suburbs. This pattern was soon confirmed in other large cities in the United States and Europe. Two main explanations have been proposed. Until recently, the first "drift hypothesis" was predominant. This claimed that schizophrenics and pre-schizophrenics are downwardly mobile, either because of their social and occupational incompetence or because they actively seek out anonymity and isolation in the decaying areas of large cities. However, there has been a revival of interest in the second theory, social causation through factors such as poverty, poor nutrition and healthcare or inadequate education. Studies from Sweden (Lewis *et al.,* 1992) and Denmark (Pedersen & Mortensen, 2001) suggest that the incidence of schizophrenia is indeed greater among those born or brought up in urban areas, and that the larger the town and the longer the individual has lived in the city, the greater the risk. The AESOP (Aetiology and Ethnicity of Schizophrenia and Other Psychoses) study in three English cities demonstrated that the incidence in South London was double that in Nottingham and Bristol and that even within one city, there were wide variations in the rates (Fearon *et al.*, 2006); the highest rates were found in the areas with least social cohesion (Kirkbride *et al.*, 2006).

Does the incidence of schizophrenia also vary by time? The "recency" hypothesis was initiated by Hare (1983), who noted that admissions to hospital for insanity greatly increased throughout the nineteenth century in the United Kingdom and the United States. Hare postulated that this reflected an increase in the incidence of schizophrenia, only to be countered by Scull (1984), who claimed that the asylums were built simply because the newly industrialised society was less able to cope with the mentally ill than the largely agricultural society it replaced. Whatever the reason, it does seem that the rise in the incidence was a consequence of the rise of cities, an interpretation consistent with the risk-increasing effects of urbanization noted earlier.

Migration

A well-replicated finding is that certain migrant groups have a higher than expected incidence of schizophrenia. As long ago as 1932, Odegaard (1932) found that schizophrenia occurred more commonly among Norwegians who emigrated to America than those who were left behind. A metanalysis (Cantor-Graae & Selten, 2005) has confirmed that risk is generally elevated among migrants, although the extent of this depends on the migrant group. The best documented example is that of African-Caribbean people who migrated to the United Kingdom among whom high rates of schizophrenia have been frequently reported. Initially it was thought that these findings might be consequent on underestimation of the number of immigrants in the population, but studies using operational criteria for schizophrenia and population registers have replicated the earlier findings. Thus a London study showed that the first

contact rates of RDC and DSM-III-R schizophrenia over a 20-year period were between 4 and 8 times greater among African-Caribbean than white individuals (Wessely *et al.*, 1991). The results of the more recent AESOP study in three English cities indicated a ninefold increase in incidence among African-Caribbeans, mostly living in London (Fearon *et al.*, 2006): see Figure 13.1. The reasons for such elevated rates among particular ethnic minority groups are not well understood, but social and psychological factors appear to be of greater importance than biological risks.

Boydell *et al.* (2006) further demonstrated that the operationally defined incidence of schizophrenia in South London had doubled between 1964 and 1999 and pointed to migration and drug abuse as possible contributing factors. Migrants were especially vulnerable if relatively isolated in localities where their own ethnic group were in a small minority (Boydell *et al.*, 2001).

Developed versus developing countries

A number of studies have claimed that schizophrenia in less-developed countries tends to have a more acute onset and a more benign outcome than in more industrialised countries (Susser & Wanderling, 1994); the reason for this is unknown. It may be due to better family support or to easier integration into the rather simpler work environment in less-developed countries. However, another possibility is that acute remitting psychoses constitute a higher proportion of schizophrenia in the less-developed world.

Genetics

The classic evidence for a genetic predisposition to schizophrenia has come from three main sources.

Studies of relatives

The lifetime expectancy for schizophrenia, broadly diagnosed, in the general population is less than 1%, but much higher figures have been found in

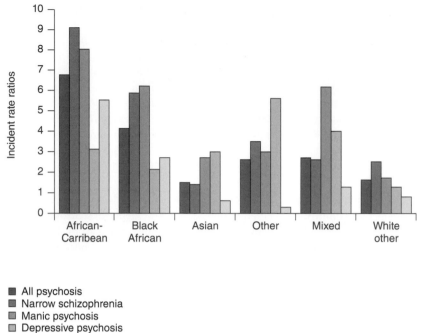

Figure 13.1 Age-adjusted incident rate ratios in ethnic minority groups (AESOP study)

relatives of people with schizophrenia (Gottesman, 1991). One of the most convincing studies is that of Kendler *et al.* (1993), who carried out a case-controlled epidemiological study in rural Ireland based on all patients with schizophrenia on the Roscommon County Case Register. The lifetime risk of schizophrenia in the first-degree relatives of those with schizophrenia was 6.5% compared with 0.5% in the relatives of the control subjects. The closer the genetic relationship the higher the risk, rising as high as 46% among children, both of whose parents have had schizophrenia.

Studies of twins

The increased frequency of schizophrenia in the families of patients is compatible with transmission of the disorder either through genes or the family environment. Because monozygotic (MZ) twins have exactly the same genes whereas dizygotic (DZ) twins share, on average, only half their genes, if pairs of MZ twins share the same psychopathology more often than DZ twins, this can be taken as evidence of a genetic contribution to the disorder. Studies have consistently shown higher concordance rates (i.e. both twins schizophrenic) for MZ than DZ twins. Gottesman *et al.* (1991) pooled the available figures to give a concordance rate of 47% for 261 MZ co-twins and 14% for 329 DZ co-twins.

These twin studies preceded the introduction of operational definitions of schizophrenia. When studies with such definitions were carried out, the rates for both monozygotic and dizygotic twins were both lower, but the disparity between the two remained. Thus in the latest and largest study, which examined 108 consecutive pairs of twins seen at the Maudsley Hospital in London, Cardno *et al.* (1999) reported probandwise concordance rates for DSM-III-R schizophrenia of 42.6% in MZ twins and 0% in DZ twins. As can be seen in Table 13.4, concordance rates for schizophrenia using other operational definitions were not dissimilar.

Table 13.4 Probandwise concordance rates in the Maudsley twins for three operational definitions of schizophrenia (Cardno *et al.*, 1999)

Diagnoses	Probandwise Concordance Rate, No. (%) [95% CI*]†	
	Monozygotic	Dizygotic
Research Diagnostic Critera lifetime-ever		
Schizophrenia	20/49 (40.8) [26.9 to 54.7]	3/57 (5.3) [0.0 to 11.2]
Schizoaffective disorders, all	9/23 (39.1) [18.7 to 59.5]	1/22 (4.5) [0.0 to 13.4]
Manic	4/13 (30.8) [4.7 to 56.9]	0/10 (0.0)
Depressed	5/12 (41.7) [12.6 to 70.8]	0/13 (0.0)
Affective psychoses, all	15/40 (37.5) [22.3 to 52.7]	5/43 (11.6) [1.9 to 21.3]
Mania	8/22 (36.4) [15.8 to 57.0]	2/27 (7.4) [0.0 to 17.5]
Mania and hypomania	11/25 (44.0) [24.1 to 63.9]	3/33 (9.1) [0.0 to 19.1]
Depressive psychosis	2/20 (10.0) [0.0 to 23.5]	1/20 (5.0) [0.0 to 14.8]
Unspecified functional psychosis	5/33 (15.2) [2.8 to 27.6]	1/32 (3.1) [0.0 to 9.2]
OPCRIT‡ main lifetime		
DSM-III-R schizophrenia	20/47 (42.6) [28.3 to 56.9]	0/50 (0.0)
ICD-10§ schizophrenia	21/50 (42.0) [28.2 to 55.8]	1/58 (1.7) [0.0 to 5.1]

*CI indicates confidence interval.

†Some twins qualified for more than 1 Research Diagnostic Criteria diagnosis on a lifetime-ever basis. One monozygotic and 1 dizygotic proband did not fulfill criteria for any Research Diagnostic Criteria psychotic diagnosis.

‡OPCRIT is a computer diagnostic program created by one of US (RM.).

§ICD-10 indicates *International Statistical Classification of Diseases*, 10th Revision.

Adoption studies

Adoption studies can also be used to disentangle genetic and environmental effects. Heston and Denney (1968) followed up 47 adopted-away offspring of chronic schizophrenic mothers and a well-matched control group of 50 adoptees born to mothers without psychiatric disorder; all the children had been separated from their mothers by age 2 weeks. There were five with schizophrenia among the offspring of mothers with schizophrenia, and none in the control group.

The Danish-American study of Rosenthal *et al.* (1971) examined the frequency of schizophrenia among the adopted-away offspring of parents who were known to have schizophrenia and among a control group of adoptees whose biological parents were free of psychiatric illness. Subjects were blindly rated as to whether they had acute or chronic schizophrenia, borderline schizophrenia or personality disorder, and all these diagnoses were included under the rubric *schizophrenia spectrum disorder*. Of the index cases, 32% received the latter label compared with 18% of control adoptees. As part of the same collaboration, Kety *et al.* (1975) blindly rated assessments of the biological and adoptive relatives of 33 adoptees with schizophrenia. There was a significant concentration of definite schizophrenia in the former but not in the latter group.

A large adoption study has also been carried out in Finland by Tienari *et al.* (2004). Offspring of mothers with schizophrenia had much higher risk of developing psychosis than did the offspring of control mothers. This study also found evidence of an interaction between genes and early social environment in that the risk of psychosis was greatest in those

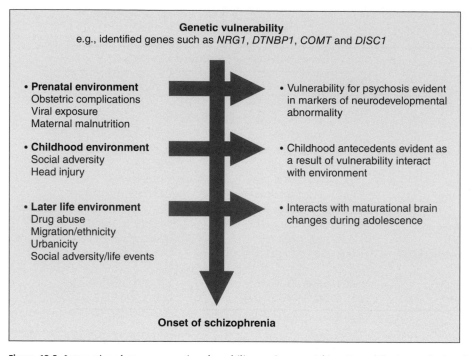

Figure 13.2 Interactions between genetic vulnerability, environmental insuits and the increasingly vulnerable individual

offspring of mothers with schizophrenia adopted into poorly functioning families.

Genetic models

Almost all authorities regard the genetic contribution as the most important of the known aetiological factors, with estimates of the heritability of liability ranging up to 85%. What is transmitted in families includes a predisposition to such features as minor cognitive deficits, poor psychosocial functioning, suspiciousness and oddness as well as to psychotic illness, schizotypal personality and paranoid personality disorder (Kendler *et al.*, 1993).

The evidence is incompatible with the idea that there is a single major gene for schizophrenia. The predominant model is the polygenic multifactorial model which states that many genes each of small effect combine with a variety of environmental factors and that schizophrenia results once a critical threshold of liability is passed. Such models do not exclude the possibility of one or two major genes operating against a polygenic background. The fact that an individual can have the same genes as their co-twin with schizophrenia but have a better than even chance of remaining nonpsychotic indicates that it is not schizophrenia per se which is inherited but rather a susceptibility to it.

Mata *et al.* (2003) showed that schizotypal personality scores in nonpsychotic relatives were significantly correlated with the presence of delusions and hallucinations in the probands; indeed they were also correlated with premorbid schizotypal traits in the childhood of the probands. Thus it seems that certain families transmit schizotypal traits which manifest themselves in childhood; some family members remain schizotypal throughout life, but in others this deviant personality type is compounded by other (genetic or environmental) factors so that the individual passes a threshold for the expression of delusions and hallucinations.

Molecular genetics

For almost 20 years, researchers have been using molecular techniques to seek the genes that predispose to schizophrenia. In linkage studies, large families with several members affected with schizophrenia are studied to try and find a genetic marker that co-segregates with the disease. Linkage studies suggest that no gene can exist which increases the risk of schizophrenia by more than a factor of three and that there may be a number of susceptibility genes. Recent findings suggest that some of these may lie within "hot spots" on chromosomes 22, 6 or 13 (reviewed by Harrison & Owen, 2003). The reader is referred to Chapter 5 for a more detailed discussion of molecular genetic techniques.

The second approach, that of association studies, takes a gene that is suspected of involvement in the pathogenesis of the disorder (e.g. a gene involved in dopamine metabolism) or a nonfunctional marker and then compares the frequency of its various alleles in a series of individuals with schizophrenia as opposed to a control group.

In 2002, the deCODE genetics group in Iceland identified 8p21–22 as the likely location of a susceptibility gene and then fine-mapped the region. An association between a 7-marker haplotype in neuregulin 1 (NRG1) and schizophrenia was found. The findings were replicated in Scotland and Wales and from as far away as South Africa and China. There have been negative studies, but the weight of evidence supports association between NRG1 and schizophrenia. Also in 2002, an American-Irish group identified another susceptibility gene, Dysbindin (DTNBP1), on 6p22.3. As with neuregulin1, the at-risk haplotype varies between populations, and the specific allelic variant (or variants) conferring risk remains unknown.

Other putative genes are now emerging, some from clues provided by chromosomal abnormalities found in some people with schizophrenia. These latter are too rare to account for more than a small fraction of schizophrenia cases, but genes in the vicinity become prime positional candidates. Thus up to 25% of sufferers from the velo-cardio-facial syndrome (DiGeorge syndrome), which results from a deletion on 22q11, develop psychosis. Genes in the deleted region have therefore attracted much interest, particularly catechol-O-methyltransferase (COMT), which is an appealing candidate because of its role in dopamine metabolism.

Investigation of a large Scottish family in which a rare balanced translocation of chromosomes 1 and 11 segregated with psychiatric illness led to the identification of a gene at the breakpoint at 1q42, which was termed *Disrupted in Schizophrenia 1* (DISC1). Other groups have subsequently reported positive linkage for DISC1, which may be involved in neuronal migration during development, neurite outgrowth or cytokinesis. The list of possible susceptibility genes continues to grow, but other candidates are not yet well replicated.

Biological abnormalities in the relatives of those with schizophrenia

Relatives have been examined for some of the biological abnormalities which are found in their schizophrenic kin. The nonpsychotic relatives exhibit MRI abnormalities and neurophysiological abnormalities such as an excess of delayed P300 event-related potentials; their prevalence is not as high as in the patients themselves but higher than in normal controls (Blackwood *et al.*, 1991; Bramon *et al.*, 2005). The relatives of patients with schizophrenia have also been reported to be more likely than control subjects to have abnormal eye movements (Holzman *et al.*, 1988) and poor performance on cognitive tests measuring executive and memory functions (Toulopoulou *et al.*, 2003). These findings suggest that what is being transmitted is not genes for schizophrenia per se but rather genes for a variety of characteristics which increase the risk of schizophrenia. Individuals can inherit these characteristics without being psychotic; perhaps schizophrenia only ensues when an individual inherits a number of such endophenotypic

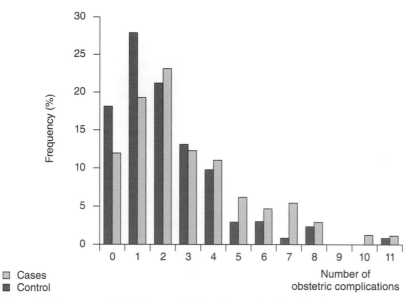

Figure 13.3 Exposure to obstetric complications in people with schizophrenia.

abnormalities and passes a critical threshold of risk.

Early environmental hazards

Schizophrenia is not just a genetic disorder. Thus, environmental risk factors operating throughout the life course have also been identified (see Figure 13.2). Indeed, the discovery of risk factors acting in early life (before and shortly after birth) has been central to the neurodevelopmental hypothesis of schizophrenia (Murray & Lewis, 1987). This hypothesis proposes that environmental risk factors interact with genetic factors during this crucial phase in the formation of the nervous system causing subtle abnormalities that leave the individual vulnerable to psychosis later in life.

Obstetric complications

Many studies have examined the frequency of pregnancy and birth complications (collectively termed *obstetric complications*) in those with

schizophrenia. Cannon and colleagues (2002) conducted a meta-analysis of the population-based studies examining the relationship between obstetric complications and later development of psychosis. They found significant associations with schizophrenia for 10 individual complications, which they grouped into three categories:

1. complications of pregnancy (bleeding, pre-eclampsia, diabetes, rhesus compatibility),
2. abnormal foetal growth and development (low birth weight, congenital malformations, small head circumference), and
3. complications of delivery (asphyxia, uterine atony, emergency C section).

The effect sizes found for these associations were relatively small (odds ratio <2), and it is likely that obstetric complications contribute to the causation of schizophrenia only in combination with other risk factors, particularly susceptibility genes. Patients with schizophrenia are especially likely to have experienced multiple obstetric complications (see Figure 13.3).

Schizophrenic individuals exposed to obstetric hazards are particularly likely to show decreased

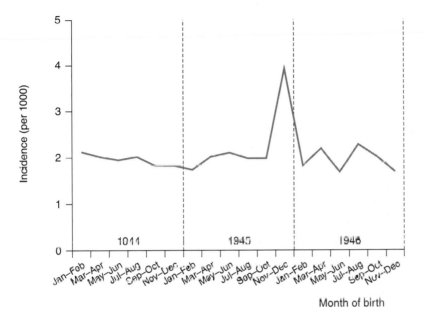

Figure 13.4 Prenatal environmental exposure (famine) and incidence of schizophrenia

volume of the hippocampus (Stefanis *et al.*, 1999). Animal studies have modelled such insults. For example, lesioning the ventral hippocampus in the neonatal rat results in decreased dendritic spine density in the prefrontal cortex and accumbens nuclei; the animals show exaggerated response to amphetamine after reaching maturity.

Prenatal viral infection

One of the most consistently replicated epidemiological features of schizophrenia is the small but significant excess of winter-spring births found in the Northern Hemisphere (approximately 7%–10%) and the reverse in the Southern Hemisphere. Various theories have been put forward to explain this stubborn association, the most widely accepted postulating a teratogenic agent such as infection, diet or temperature which impairs foetal brain development.

One possible explanation is winter infection in mothers, and a number of studies have reported that foetuses exposed to prenatal maternal infections have an increased risk of later development of

psychosis. Prenatal exposure to influenza has been the focus of much research. In particular, several studies have suggested that foetuses exposed during the second trimester to the 1957 A2 influenza pandemic have an increased risk of schizophrenia (Mednick *et al.*, 1988; O'Callaghan *et al.*, 1991). This link with second trimester influenza exposure holds true when the relationship between influenza epidemics and schizophrenic births is assessed over several decades (Sham *et al.*, 1992). However, the association has not always been replicated (McGrath *et al.*, 1994). Association with other viruses has been reported, and most recently there have been claims that the mothers of those with schizophrenia have shown increased titres of antibodies to various infections such as rubella, herpes simple and toxoplasmosis. Animal models have been developed, but the jury remains out on this.

In utero exposure to noninfectious environmental agents, such as maternal malnutrition (see Figure 13.4) (Susser *et al.*, 1998), maternal diabetes (Cannon *et al.*, 2002), smoking (Sacker *et al.*, 1995) and rhesus incompatibility (Hollister *et al.*, 1996),

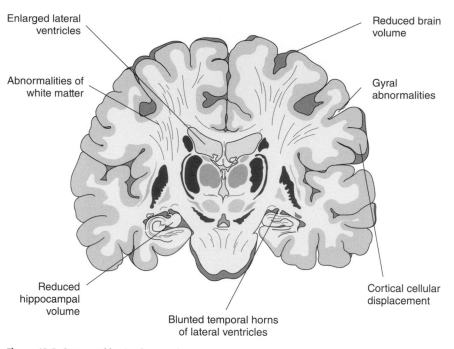

Enlarged lateral
ventricles

Reduced brain
volume

Abnormalities of
white matter

Gyral
abnormalities

Reduced
hippocampal
volume

Cortical cellular
displacement

Blunted temporal horns
of lateral ventricles

Figure 13.5 Structural brain abnormalities in schizophrenia

have also been considered. Maternal body mass index (BMI), childhood BMI and antenatal exposure to famine have all been found to be associated with an increased risk of schizophrenia (Hoek *et al.,* 1998; Jones *et al.,* 1998; Schaefer *et al.,* 2000; Wahlbeck, *et al.,* 2001).

Brain structure and function

MRI studies have consistently demonstrated that people with schizophrenia have increased lateral ventricular volume and also show a slight decrease in cortical volume (2%) with greater decrements (about 5%) in the hippocampus, amygdala and thalamus (Figure 13.5) (Wright *et al.,* 2000). Post-mortem studies largely confirm these volumetric findings. The brain abnormalities are present at the onset of illness, but exactly when do they arise? As noted earlier, it is likely that some are the consequence of damage incurred in prenatal or perinatal life (Cannon *et al.,* 2002); the

absence of cell loss or other signs of neurodegeneration has also supported this developmental view.

However, some may arise later. Velakoulis *et al.* (2006) compared the volumes of the hippocampus and amygdala in (1) patients with chronic schizophrenia, (2) patients with first-episode psychosis, and (3) young people in the so-called prodrome at high risk of developing psychosis. Those with chronic schizophrenia displayed bilateral hippocampal volume reduction, whereas first-episode schizophrenia patients showed only left-sided hippocampal volume reduction; and those at risk for psychosis had normal hippocampal and amygdala volumes. The authors interpreted their findings as suggesting that structural changes in the amygdala-hippocampal complex appear after the onset of psychosis. However, it is also possible that their findings could be a sampling artefact, that is, most of those at risk will recover and therefore will never go on to appear in samples of first onset, or especially chronic, patients.

The same group (Pantelis *et al.*, 2003) demonstrated that subjects at risk for development of psychosis had grey matter abnormalities before development of psychosis but found additional reductions in grey matter when some of the subjects were rescanned following development of a psychotic illness. Job et al. (2005) also examined grey matter changes over time in young adults at high risk of schizophrenia. Those high risk individuals who later developed schizophrenia showed particular reductions in grey matter in the period immediately prior to development of psychosis. Such studies raise the possibility that identification of brain changes might enable us to predict which at risk individuals will go on to develop schizophrenia in the future.

Thus it appears that some brain abnormalities predate the onset of psychosis, whereas others are associated with the onset itself. There is also some evidence of worsening of the abnormalities during the course of the illness. However, it is not yet known whether the latter represents ongoing developmental changes occurring in late adolescence and early adult life, whether they may reflect degenerative change, or even occur secondary to treatment with antipsychotic medication. Cahn *et al.* (2006) demonstrated that global grey matter volumes decreased over time (the first year of illness) in patients with first-episode schizophrenia and that these decreases correlated significantly with outcome. However, the volume decreases were also independently associated with higher cumulative antipsychotic dose. Evidence has been produced that even after short-term treatment, typical and atypical antipsychotics appear to affect brain structure differently. In a longitudinal study investigating antipsychotic effects on brain morphology over a 2-year period, first-episode patients treated with the typical antipsychotic haloperidol experienced reductions in grey matter volume, whereas those on the atypical medication olanzapine did not (Lieberman, Tollefson *et al.*, 2005). Dazzan *et al.* (2005) used voxel-based methods in first episode patients to show that typical antipsychotics were associated with basal ganglia enlargement and reduced volume in cortical areas, whereas atypicals were associated with thalamic enlargement. One possibility is that these differential changes are a consequence of prolonged high D2 dopamine blockade associated with use of typical antipsychotics.

A succession of studies has reported abnormalities at the histological level; these range from disarray of pyramidal cells in the hippocampus through displaced pre-alpha cells in the parahippocampal gyrus to neurones lying deeper than normal in the frontal and temporal cortex. These cytoarchitectural abnormalities are of such a kind that they suggest dysgenesis rather than degeneration (Akbarian, Bunney, *et al.*, 1993; Akbarian, Vinuela, *et al.*, 1993).

This notion of dysgenesis is also supported by evidence that minor physical abnormalities (MPAs) of, for example, eyes, ears and mouth occur in excess in schizophrenia; these anomalies serve as "fossilised" evidence of a deviant foetal development (McGrath *et al.*, 1995). Abnormalities of dermatoglyphics (finger and palm prints) are another pointer to deviant early development (Bramon, Walshe, *et al.*, 2005).

This evidence, plus the literature on obstetric complications and prenatal influenza reviewed earlier, has given rise to the neurodevelopmental hypothesis (Murray, 1994; Murray & Lewis, 1987; Weinberger, 1987), which states that a substantial proportion of schizophrenic patients have experienced a disturbance of the orderly development of the brain, decades before the symptomatic phase of the illness begins.

What is the cause of these abnormalities? Brain growth is largely under genetic control, and Reveley *et al.* (1982, 1984), using computed tomography (CT), found a high heritability for ventricular size in normal twins. However, twins with schizophrenia had larger ventricles than their MZ nonschizophrenic co-twins. Suddath *et al.* (1990), using MRI, confirmed this. One interpretation is that a genetic factor contributes to ventricular enlargement in both twins and that environmental damage may further increase ventricular size in the twin who goes on to develop schizophrenia.

Functional MRI (fMRI) has begun to elucidate some of the abnormal physiology underlying symptoms. Thus auditory hallucinations are associated with activation of Broca's area in prefrontal cortex where "inner speech" is produced, and certain temporal and subcortical areas, which normally process external speech. It is as if the auditory processing system does not recognise the individual's own "inner speech" as self-generated and instead processes it as if it were externally derived. Similarly, fMRI studies have demonstrated that negative symptoms and planning difficulties are associated with an inability to activate prefrontal areas efficiently in response to cognitive challenge.

Crow (1980) divided psychotic symptoms into the positive and the negative. Subsequently, Liddle (1987) carried out a factor analysis that subdivided the positive symptoms and has been replicated several times; Liddle's three factors are (1) psychomotor poverty, which essentially is another name for the negative symptom cluster; (2) disorganisation, which many liken to hebephrenia; and (3) reality distortion, that is, delusions and hallucinations. Liddle later used positron emission tomography (PET) to show that psychomotor poverty was associated with decreased left frontal activity, disorganisation with increased cingulate activity on the right and delusions and hallucinations with increased activity in the left hippocampal region.

Dopamine as "the wind of psychotic fire"

Arvid Carlsson, who won the Nobel Prize for his work on neurotransmitters, suggested in the 1960s that excess brain dopamine underlies schizophrenic symptoms (Carlsson & Lindqvist, 1963). This idea was partly based on the evidence that amphetamine abuse (which results in increased synaptic dopamine) can produce ideas of reference, delusions of persecution and auditory hallucinations (Connell, 1958). When large oral doses of amphetamines are given to normal subjects, psychosis invariably results within a few days (Griffith *et al.*, 1972); indeed intravenous amphetamine can produce the psychosis within

a matter of hours. Furthermore, small doses of amphetamine exacerbate schizophrenic symptoms, and patients with schizophrenia are reportedly unable to differentiate an amphetamine psychosis from their usual symptoms.

The second strand of the dopamine hypothesis rests on the well-known tendency of the typical antipsychotic drugs to cause extrapyramidal symptoms. With the discovery that dopamine was deficient in Parkinson's disease, it appeared likely that these parkinsonian-like effects of antipsychotics were due to production of a functional dopamine deficiency. It was then suggested that the antipsychotic effects were also due to the drugs blockading dopamine receptors. Johnstone *et al.* (1978) demonstrated this clinically by comparing the therapeutic efficacy of different isomers of fluphenthixol. Only one has dopamine-blocking activity and so only it should be antipsychotic; this proved to be the case. With the exception of clozapine, the potency of antipsychotics correlates closely with their dopamine D2 blocking potential.

If blocking dopamine receptors relieves schizophrenic symptoms, and drugs such as amphetamine that flood the receptors with dopamine can cause psychosis, then could overactivity of central dopaminergic neurones underlie the symptomatology of schizophrenia? The first direct evidence came in 1996 when Laruelle *et al.* (1996) demonstrated that acutely psychotic patients release excessive striatal dopamine in response to an amphetamine challenge; furthermore, the degree of dopamine release correlates positively with the severity of positive symptoms and with subsequent response to dopamine blockers. Yet why should an excess of striatal dopamine make someone think that his neighbours are out to poison him or that the CIA has planted a chip in his brain? In 2003, the Canadian researcher Shitij Kapur proposed an attractive theory which linked dopamine dysregulation to clinical symptoms. He pointed out that in the normal individual, the role of mesolimbic dopamine is to provide an external stimulus, or an internal thought, with significance or "salience", that is, to convert its mental representation from a neutral piece of information into one which "grabs the attention" of the individual (Kapur, 2003). Because acute psychosis is associated with increased release of dopamine, increased attention and salience is given inappropriately to what would otherwise have been regarded as insignificant events and perceptions. In this way, an unexpected sound, the comments of a TV newsreader or eye contact with a stranger are transformed from trivial everyday occurrences into highly salient events of great personal meaning to the psychotic individual. Delusions can be understood as an attempt to explain these experiences and resolve the resultant perplexity, confusion and dysphoria.

Carlsson's original theory implied a general hyperdopaminergic state, but the modern view is that excess mesolimbic dopamine is indeed responsible for the positive symptoms, whereas negative symptoms and executive deficits are the result of deficient dopamine in the frontal cortex. It is not clear whether the frontal or mesolimbic abnormalities come first. Many believe that the impaired (and dopamine-deficient) prefrontal cortex fails to "brake" the limbic system, and the resultant increased mesolimbic dopamine causes the increased salience and overreaction to stimuli, which ultimately leads to paranoia and psychosis. However, recently, Kellendonk et al. (2006) used a transgenic mouse model to show that prefrontal cortical function can be impaired in mice by increased dopamine expression in the striatum. Thus mice genetically modified to have increased expression of striatal D2 receptors also developed selective cognitive impairments in working memory and behavioural flexibility. These findings offer a possible molecular explanation of the cognitive deficit in schizophrenia and may explain the inability of antipsychotics to reverse cognitive deficits.

Although it is clear that dopamine dysregulation operates as the final common pathway, the neurochemical origins of schizophrenia do not necessarily lie here. One possibility is that there is an underlying glutamatergic abnormality. This glutamate hypothesis derives from evidence that PCP,

a glutamate agonist, induces a psychotic state closely akin to schizophrenia. Glutamic acid is an important excitatory neurotransmitter that can be toxic to neurones in excess; perhaps excitatory overstimulation may cause neuronal degeneration and secondary dopaminergic overactivity. One possibility is that this neurotoxicity may be produced by hypoxia or other insult to the developing brain; glutamate's activity is exerted via several receptor sites, among the most important of which are N-methyl-D-aspartate and kainate receptors.

Another theory implicates the inhibitory transmitter GABA (gamma-aminobutyric acid). Thus Busatto et al. (1997) have used single-photon PET to show reduced GABA receptors in the left temporal lobe and suggested that reduced inhibitory GABAergic tone contributes to temporal lobe malfunction and to positive symptoms.

The antecedents of schizophrenia

Children destined to develop schizophrenia often have subtle developmental delays and deficits in motor and cognitive function, tend to be solitary and show an excess of social anxiety. These childhood delays and deficits have been taken as indicating that schizophrenia is in part a neurodevelopmental disorder. Researchers have studied individuals at high risk of the condition such as the children of parents with schizophrenia. For example, Mednick et al. (1987) chose 200 pre-adolescent and teenage offspring of mothers with schizophrenia and matched them with 100 low-risk children. Those high-risk children who developed psychiatric problems were distinguished particularly by a history of obstetric complications and on the original testing had shown more deviant autonomic responsivity. Parnas et al. (1982) confirmed that it is particularly those high-risk offspring who have suffered obstetric complications who develop schizophrenia. Other characteristics claimed as occurring more frequently in high-risk children include deficits in attention, poor motor co-ordination, soft neurological signs and disturbance of interpersonal relationships. Fish (1992) suggested that these were all manifestations of an underlying "pandysmaturation".

However, only a minority of those with schizophrenia have parents with schizophrenia, and therefore there is uncertainty over how far one can generalise from "high-risk" studies. Other approaches have therefore been used to elucidate the antecedents of schizophrenia. A particularly original approach was employed by Walker and Lewine (1990), who obtained videotapes of children who subsequently manifested schizophrenia and blindly compared the videos with those of their growing siblings. The pre-schizophrenic children were more likely to show behavioural and motor abnormalities such as clumsiness or odd movements.

Another approach involved following up unselected samples of children into adult life. Jones *et al.* (1994) examined the life histories of 4,746 children who had been born in one week in 1946 in the United Kingdom, and contacted 19 times by the age of 43 years. The 30 children who went on to develop schizophrenia had slightly delayed motor milestones; at age 4, they were more likely to play alone than the other children, and by age 7, they already performed more poorly on cognitive tests; they were especially likely to have had language difficulties. Similar findings were reported from the Dunedin birth cohort study (Cannon, Caspi *et al.*, 2002) which also showed that having minor psychotic symptoms by age 11 years predicted the development of schizophrenia-like psychosis by age 26 years (Poulton *et al.*, 2000).

Thus it is clear that a proportion of those who go on to develop schizophrenia show deficits in motor, cognitive and social performance long before they present with psychotic symptoms. What is not clear is (1) whether there exists a distinct subgroup only that is typified by childhood abnormality and (2) whether the childhood deficits are an early manifestation of a neurodevelopmental lesion or whether they are independent risk factors for later schizophrenia.

Social factors

Schizophrenia lies at the interface between brain functioning and the social environment, and any plausible aetiological model of schizophrenia needs to incorporate the evidence that social factors modulate risk. It has long been known that patients commonly have their first psychotic episode at times of great stress, and those whose relatives show hostility towards them (high expressed emotion) have the worst outcome. Now we also know that being born or brought up in a city increases risk, as does migration from one country to another. The most striking example of the latter is the consistent evidence that Africans and African-Caribbeans living in England show an incidence of schizophrenia at least 6 times that of the native white population. Social isolation and lack of social support may play a role, and, of course animal studies have shown that the mesolimbic dopamine system can be manipulated by social means (reviewed by Di Forti *et al.*, 2007).

Current stress can precipitate psychotic episodes. Brown and Birley (1968) studied those with acute-onset schizophrenia and charted the occurrence of life events for the preceding 3 months; the patients experienced a significantly higher frequency of such events during the 3-week period prior to the onset of their symptoms than did a matched group of nonschizophrenic control subjects. This was true even of independent events that could not have been caused by the patient becoming ill. Brown *et al.* (1972) suggested that life events serve to trigger the florid onset and reappearance of symptoms "in those who are predisposed and are experiencing tense and difficult situations". Numerous other studies (e.g. Bebbington *et al.*, 1993) have confirmed a role for adverse life events, but most authorities regard social adversity as operating on already predisposed individuals to trigger onset or relapse, not as causal factors in their own right.

Considerable effort has been devoted to studying family life after the onset of psychosis: Brown *et al.* (1972) demonstrated that those with schizophrenia are highly responsive to the quality of the emotional relationship between them and the relative with whom they live. These workers could predict relapse by using an index of the emotions shown by the relative that expressed the amount of critical comment, hostility and emotional overinvolvement of that relative; during the 9 months after discharge from hospital, 58% of patients from houses with high "expressed emotion" (high EE) relapsed compared with only 16% from low EE homes. Vaughn and Leff (1976) almost exactly replicated these results. However, there is no evidence that high EE is of importance in contributing to onset of schizophrenia.

Abuse and victimisation

Many investigators have examined the question of whether the behaviour of mothers of those with schizophrenia may have a causal role, but most well-conducted enquiries (Hirsch & Leff, 1975) concluded that the characterisation of the mothers of schizophrenic patients as "schizophrenogenic" cannot be sustained. The question of whether physical or sexual abuse in childhood can increase risk is very controversial. Read *et al.* (1999) argued that evidence supports a diathesis-stress model of psychosis and highlights the similarities between biological sequelae of childhood abuse and those associated with schizophrenia. Others have focused on the psychological impact of childhood trauma which may predispose to later psychotic symptoms via changes in cognitive and affective functioning (Garety *et al.*, 2001). Child abuse is certainly not aetiologically specific for psychosis (Mullen *et al.*, 1993) but within psychosis what evidence there is points towards a particular relationship with positive psychotic symptoms (Read & Argyle, 1999). Of course, such symptoms are not necessarily part of schizophrenia, and indeed, the association has also been found in a general population sample (Janssen *et al.*, 2004). A recent critical review of the evidence for a causal link between child abuse and psychosis concludes that more research is needed

because findings have been inconsistent and previous studies methodologically limited (Morgan & Fisher, 2007).

Following the onset of a psychotic illness, however, evidence for an increased risk of suffering violent victimisation is strong (Hiday *et al.*, 1999; Silver *et al.*, 2005), although an understanding of the nature of the risk and the factors underlying it is limited. Linking early-life and post-illness-onset abuse, in one study childhood abuse was shown to increase risk of later victimisation among those with severe mental illness (Goodman *et al.*, 2001).

Psychology

The tradition of psychological research in schizophrenia stretches back to Kraepelin, who received his scientific training in Wundt's psychological laboratory. One classic line of research considered that in schizophrenia the ability to form normal abstract concepts is lost, and instead concrete ones are formed. Certainly many with chronic schizophrenia appear to think in very concrete terms, as can be demonstrated by asking them to interpret a proverb. Another classic view suggested that those with schizophrenia have difficulty in maintaining the boundaries of concepts so that each concept spreads into others and thus becomes overinclusive.

Neuropsychologists have attempted to explain such findings in terms of the cognitive deficits found in patients with known damage to specific brain regions (Chua & Murray, 1995; David & Cutting, 1994). Thus studies have employed tests known to detect frontal lobe damage. For example, those with schizophrenia perform poorly on the Tower of London Test, which is a measure of planning ability, and on the Wisconsin Card Sort Test, which measures ability to alter cognitive set; they show deficits in such executive and conceptual functions as well as in initiating and monitoring their own actions.

Individuals with schizophrenia also perform poorly on tests of verbal fluency, which is normally associated with activation of the left frontal cortex. This accords with the view, first put forward by Kleist in 1930, that many of the speech abnormalities shown by those with schizophrenia are common to patients with left frontal damage. In a similar way, researchers have examined tests of temporal lobe functions such as memory, although here there is less consensus.

In general the neuropsychological approach has been more successful in relating cognitive deficits to negative rather than positive symptoms. Furthermore, critics say it is not surprising that individuals with schizophrenia perform badly on neuropsychological batteries because they perform badly on almost all forms of testing.

The alternative, experimental approach focuses on abnormalities of attention and perception, which are common in acute schizophrenia. McGhie and Chapman's patients (1961) described how once-familiar objects become different and people may appear distorted in a terrifying manner; they also experienced being bombarded by stimuli, and these authors quote a patient as saying "the sounds are coming through to me but I feel my mind cannot cope with everything. It's difficult to concentrate on any one sound. It's like trying to do two or three different things at one time" (p. 104). McGhie and Chapman (1961) interpreted their findings in terms of Broadbent's "filter theory" of input limitation, which suggests that some with schizophrenia have a deficit in the filter mechanism that should limit sensory input to a level that the brain can deal with.

Gray *et al.* (1991), who were much influenced by Broadbent's filter theory, suggest that those with schizophrenia have a "weakening of the influence of stored irregularities" on their present actions. Such a theory predicts that patients will therefore do better than normal subjects on tasks in which previous experience interferes with performance. One such task is "latent inhibition" in which, as predicted, those with acute schizophrenia perform better than normal controls. Gray and his colleagues believe that a failure of latent inhibition underlies many positive symptoms of schizophrenia.

Some of the most attractive explanatory models of schizophrenic symptoms have come from Frith (1992), who suggested that for normal social interaction it is necessary to have a "theory of mind", that is, some understanding of another person's point of view. He postulated that the schizophrenic patient is unable to discern the mental state of others accurately, and this inability to "read the mind" of others leads to misjudgements and ultimately to paranoia.

Frith explains other symptoms in terms of a failure of internal monitoring. For example, we all use internal speech as we "talk to ourselves" or think. He suggests that schizophrenia patients fail to recognise their inner speech as their own and instead misinterpret it as coming from some external source and therefore label it as "voices". Empirical support for this comes from McGuire *et al.* (1993), who found that when patients were experiencing auditory hallucinations, they showed activation of Broca's area on single-photon PET imaging. McGuire and colleagues (1995) went on to show that although both normal and schizophrenia patients activate Broca's area during inner speech, the normal subjects but not the schizophrenic subjects contemporaneously use certain temporal lobe areas to determine that the speech is internal and not external.

Work implicating the temporal lobes in hallucinations and delusions goes back to Slater *et al.* (1963) who showed that patients with temporal lobe epilepsy had an increased risk of positive "schizophreniform" symptoms. Barta *et al.* (1990) found that reduction of the volume of left anterior superior temporal gyrus (auditory association cortex) correlated with the severity of auditory hallucinations, and Shenton *et al.* (1992) found that left superior temporal gyrus volume reduction was associated with thought disorder. These findings remain to be confirmed.

Outcome

In a classic study, Manfred Bleuler (1974), who followed up a cohort of 208 patients over a 22-year period, made the important observation that on average those with schizophrenia show little further deterioration after 5 years but rather tend to improve. He pointed out that schizophrenia cannot be considered a progressive disease because 20 years after the event, the proportion of recovered patients remains the same as 5 years after the onset. At 5 years, about one-quarter of the schizophrenic patients who were alive were in hospital; thereafter, although individual patients were admitted or discharged, the percentage in hospital remained roughly similar.

There have been many studies of the factors that influence outcome in schizophrenia. There is unanimity that the outlook is bad if the illness leads to hospitalization before age 15 years. This may be not only because earlier breakdown is indicative of more severe illness, but also because the younger patient has not had sufficient time to build up social and occupational skills to aid his rehabilitation. Women have a better prognosis than men (van Os et al., 1996), and marriage appears to have a protective role against future relapse (Vaughan & Leff, 1976).

There is a high correlation between poor premorbid personality and bad outcome and also, as Munro et al. (2002) have suggested, between the latter and low IQ and other difficulties in childhood. A history of good adjustment in social, sexual and occupational functioning indicates a more favourable prognosis, as do catatonic features, and a family history of affective disorder. The more acute the onset of psychosis and the more obvious the precipitants, the greater the chances of recovery, although not surprisingly, chronicity tends to predict chronicity. Lack of insight, emotional withdrawal, and blunting of affect are bad signs.

In a prospective follow-up study, Van Os et al. (1995), examined and then followed up a large series of recent-onset psychotic patients for 4 years. Poor outcome was predicted by CT findings suggestive of cortical atrophy, whereas those patients who had suffered adverse life events had significantly better outcome.

One should only make firm predictions when all the prognostic indicators point in the same direction as even the most disabled patients may improve. Indeed, Harding et al. (1987) recontacted a series of patients with schizophrenia after several decades and showed that even among those who retrospectively met the DSM-III criteria for schizophrenia, and had appeared very ill, a surprising proportion were largely recovered and were living independently.

Although there is known to be a high correlation between poor premorbid personality or functioning and bad outcome, there is current debate about the importance of the "duration of untreated psychosis". On one side it is argued that a long duration of untreated psychosis is literally "neurotoxic", and thus early intervention can improve outcome. Opponents of this concept argue that duration of untreated psychosis is merely a marker of other factors which themselves predict poor outcome, namely, an insidious mode of onset and poor premorbid status.

It must be remembered that those diagnosed with schizophrenia are at elevated risk of premature death due to suicide, particularly during the early phase of illness (Palmer et al., 2005). In addition, risk of morbidity and mortality due to poor physical health is increased among those with severe mental disorders such as schizophrenia (Mortensen, 2003).

Management

This section reviews the essential principles of management for psychosis. First, antipsychotic drugs should be used to induce an initial remission, and in many cases to maintain that remission over a prolonged period. Second, psychological approaches should be considered both in the acute and maintenance phases of treatment. Third, a variety of social measures should be used to provide a social and work environment to suit the patient's particular needs.

Before outlining in detail the principles of management for psychosis, the possibility of prevention and investigation following initial presentation should be considered. At present, the only attempt at prevention is by treating those "prodromal" individuals who are on the brink of developing psychosis. Currently much effort is going into identifying those defined as having the "at-risk mental state", up to 40% of whom develop frank psychosis within 1 or 2 years. Whether to treat them is a matter of heated debate. Some believe that with a combination of psychological treatments and low-dose antipsychotics, we could prevent a significant proportion from developing the illness. Others point out that even if this were true, it would be at the cost of giving antipsychotic drugs to a majority of individuals who would never develop psychosis.

Anyone presenting for the first time with symptoms of schizophrenia deserves thorough investigation. First, given the serious personal implications of receiving a diagnosis of schizophrenia, it is vital to exclude conditions that may be mistaken for it. Second, a detailed exploration of the patient's psychological, social and physical status must be undertaken to elucidate possible aetiological or exacerbating factors. Third, only after a comprehensive assessment of a patient's strengths and particular disabilities can individually tailored treatment be instigated.

Antipsychotic drugs

The discovery of chlorpromazine in the early 1950s enabled people with schizophrenia to be treated as outpatients for the first time and led ultimately to the closure of the old mental hospitals in most Western countries. Subsequently a range of other antipsychotic drugs were developed. Antipsychotic drugs have now been studied in literally hundreds of double-blind trials, almost all of which indicate that they arc superior to placebo in the treatment of both acute and chronic schizophrenia. They remain the mainstay of the treatment of schizophrenia and are overviewed in detail in Chapter 26, to which the reader is referred.

Psychosocial interventions

Treatment of psychosis is rarely successful using pharmacological agents alone. Lack of response,

development of side effects and poor adherence are clearly among the main factors responsible for the inadequacy of reliance on antipsychotic medication. The importance of considering the social environment and the opportunity for benefit from psychological interventions cannot be underestimated. The current UK National Institute for Clinical Excellence (NICE) Guidelines for schizophrenia recommend the following psychosocial interventions because their supportive evidence base is strong (NICE, 2006):

- Cognitive-behavioural therapy
- Family intervention
- Vocational rehabilitation

Psychological treatments

Psychological treatments in general, and cognitive-behavioural therapy (CBT) in particular, have become an increasingly vital component of treatment for schizophrenia. This increasing emphasis on psychological therapies has also highlighted the importance of engagement and the establishment of a "therapeutic alliance", which has proved central to treatment success whatever the mode offered.

Cognitive-behavioural therapy

Initially CBT was used to address the distress associated with psychotic symptoms, but more recently encouraging results have come from studies aimed at a variety of other components of illness. It is specifically recommended by the National Health Service NICE (2006). The authors of the guidelines concluded that there is good evidence for reduction in symptoms over a year with greater benefits associated with longer periods of treatment (6 months).

The model for CBT in schizophrenia relies on the notion that the patient's thoughts and feelings about symptoms of psychosis are important. It emphasises the importance of maintaining a therapeutic relationship and an understanding of illness which is based on the stress-vulnerability relationship. Box 13.2 provides a summary of emerging evidence of the benefits of CBT in the treatment of schizophrenia (Turkington *et al.*, 2004).

Box 13.2 Evidence regarding cognitive-behavioural therapy (CBT) in schizophrenia

- Positive symptoms are reduced when CBT is given as an adjunct to antipsychotic medication amongst those with chronic illness.
- Gains are maintained over time and following the end of active treatment.
- Cost-effectiveness has been demonstrated.
- Other symptom dimensions (depression, negative symptoms) may be improved.
- Improvements in adherence and insight may be seen.
- Relapse rates have been shown to be reduced.
- CBT may be effective in reducing symptoms among those resistant to antipsychotic medication.

There is less support for the effectiveness of CBT for patients in the prodromal phase, those with first-onset psychosis and among those with co-morbid disorders, children and the elderly. Even where evidence of effectiveness is stronger, treatment studies have differed from each other in a number of important respects, which limits comparison. Factors such as the nature of the sample studied, the type of comparator treatment used, the length of treatment and the length of follow-up evaluation have not been consistent across studies. There is, however, sufficient evidence to justify attempts to incorporate CBT into treatment regimes for schizophrenia and to encourage further study, particularly among subgroups of patients with specific needs and challenges.

Cognitive remediation

Cognitive remediation is an intervention designed to address the well-known cognitive deficits associated with schizophrenia (Wykes & Reeder, 2005). Although well established in the treatment of patients with neurological disorders, it has only recently been applied to those with psychosis. Success in terms of improvement on repeated cognitive testing has been reported, but concerns have been raised about the generalisation of improvement in day-to-day functioning. NICE has concluded that there is currently insufficient evidence

to recommend use of cognitive remediation either to improve cognitive performance or other aspects of outcome in schizophrenia (NICE, 2006). Whether future therapeutic developments should focus on general functioning rather than specific deficits is a source of ongoing debate.

Social environment

The social environment has a major impact on outcome in schizophrenia. The first priority in considering psychosocial intervention is to identify and if possible reduce the impact of any source of social stress. It is a curious fact that we expect patients with schizophrenia to cope with social conditions which the rest of us less vulnerable individuals would find intolerable. Not surprisingly, ongoing poverty, social isolation, poor accommodation and difficulties in family relationships are a recipe for disaster.

It is important to strike a balance between under- and overstimulation; an understimulating environment can lead to an exacerbation of negative symptoms, whereas over-stimulation can precipitate the return of positive symptoms. In a classic study, Wing and Brown (1970) studied individuals with chronic schizophrenia residing in hospitals and found that the hospital with the most barren understimulating wards contained patients who were the most withdrawn, silent and affectively blunted. Paradoxically, too vigorous an attempt at rehabilitation led to excessive stimulation and the re-emergence of dormant delusions and hallucinations.

Family therapy

Since the 1960s, there has been a particular interest in the impact of family relationships on outcome for individuals with psychosis. Vaughan and Leff (1976) demonstrated that patients from homes with high expressed emotion constituted a group at higher risk of relapse. This finding was confirmed on the basis of a review of 25 studies from a variety of geographic locations (Bebbington & Kuipers, 1994). On the basis of the notion that modifying family environments might reduce risk of poor outcome,

---

Box 13.3 Elements of family interventions for schizophrenia

- Counselling
- Psychoeducation
- Problem solving
- Self-help groups
- Behavioural therapy
- Crisis-oriented therapy
- Survival skills training

---

interventions for families were developed and positive results reported (Leff *et al.,* 1982). In a meta-analysis of results from a range of family therapies, significant preventative effects on rate of relapse and rehospitalisation were found in addition to benefits on medication compliance (Pilling, Bebbington *et al.,* 2002). The nature of family interventions included in this meta-analysis are shown in Box 13.3.

There is an increasing awareness of the role of family members and others acting as carers in the management of patients with schizophrenia and of the impact of this role on the carers themselves. Carers are found to be more distressed by depressed behaviours or negative symptoms exhibited by relatives with schizophrenia rather than the type of disturbed behaviour associated with acute psychosis (Tucker *et al.,* 1998). In addition to the help given by Mental Health Services, voluntary organisations such as Rethink can also provide valuable understanding, advice and support to both carers and ill relatives.

Vocational and occupational rehabilitation

One of the major aims of rehabilitation should be to return the individual to meaningful occupational activity. Working gives structure to lives, provides social contact, improves self-esteem and can distract the sufferer from the distress of symptoms. Unemployment rates are, however, very high among those with schizophrenia even when compared with others suffering comparable levels of disability. In the recent Clinical Antipsychotic Trials of Intervention Effectiveness (CATIE) study, the following factors were identified as barriers to employment: active symptomatology, neurocognitive impairment and the availability of rehabilitative services (Rosenheck *et al.,* 2006). Prevocational preparation, such as in sheltered workshops, and supported competitive employment schemes are the two main approaches taken to vocational rehabilitation, with evidence of superiority for the latter coming from studies based in the United States (NICE, 2006). There is little evidence to support such schemes in other countries, including the United Kingdom, and clearly much more research is needed.

Stigma and discrimination are often an unfortunate additional burden for those with mental illnesses, particularly schizophrenia, and present another barrier to employment. Public education campaigns to address this problem have been launched by various organisations including the UK Royal College of Psychiatrists ("Changing Minds"). Emerging evidence suggests that educational interventions offered to particular groups in society may be effective in reducing the negative attitudes towards those with mental illness (Pinfold *et al.,* 2003).

Social skills training

Social skills training is a well-established intervention with roots in behavioural and social learning traditions. Impairments in social functioning are well known to occur in schizophrenia and can have a significant impact on outcome. Despite previous reports of positive results for social skills training programmes, doubt has been cast on the evidence base for this intervention (Pilling, Bebbington *et al.,* 2002).

Service-level interventions

Care in the community

See also Chapter 22 for more information on this topic. Inherent in the idea of community care is the belief that most patients with schizophrenia can lead happier and more productive lives in the community than in a hospital ward or nursing home. This approach has been shown to have many advantages – patients prefer it, families are less disrupted and patients can continue to benefit from the support networks available to them in the community. Successful community care demands extensive community facilities, adequate resources and efficient systems of communication and follow-up. Unfortunately the development and funding of community care following deinstitutionalisation has often been inadequate. A series of reports in Britain have been critical of the way in which government policies have resulted in large numbers of patients with chronic psychosis failing to receive adequate support in the community, with disturbing and occasionally violent consequences.

Case or care management systems have been developed in Europe and North America with the intention that the needs of those with mental illnesses living in the community are met and that the various services and agencies involved in care are coordinated. Such management systems are the core of multidisciplinary community mental health teams which have become the mainstay of community care in most developed countries. Despite the widespread existence of community mental health teams (CMHTs), there is little evidence to support their use. Concerns have certainly been raised about the ability of CMHTs to coordinate care adequately and clearly more research is needed.

The past decade has seen enormous changes in the way in which community services for those with schizophrenia and other severe mental illnesses are organised. There has been an increasing trend towards development of highly specialist services (see Box 13.4 for summary) in preference to more generalist CMHTs. Many have argued that the development of such specialist services is not based on good evidence of their advantage over existing models, particularly in local settings.

Box 13.4 Summary of specialist community treatment services

Treatment Service	Principles of treatment
Early onset	Rapid assessment and management of patients with first onset psychosis or, in some cases, prodromal symptoms
Dual diagnosis	Management of patients with both a psychotic illness and a comorbid substance misuse problem
Assertive outreach	Community-based management of patients with severe mental illness and poor engagement with services
Home treatment	An alternative to admission to hospital – at least daily home contact with patients during a relapse or acute onset of illness
Forensic community	Assessment and case management of patients with severe mental illness and significant risk of violence; an assertive approach is generally taken

---

Early onset or prodromal services

There is now a strong emphasis on early identification and treatment of those presenting with a first episode of psychosis. The rationale behind this is the belief that acting early will prevent poor outcome (secondary prevention). Taking this concept further, many have advocated for the development of prodromal services with the aim of identifying and managing risk of conversion to psychosis among those with prodromal symptoms, although this remains controversial. The aim of prodromal services is to reduce the duration of untreated psychosis on the basis that the longer it persists the worse the outcome (Harris *et al.*, 2005).

The Early Psychosis Prevention and Intervention Centre (EPPIC) in Australia is a well-known

---

Box 13.5 US Consensus recommendations regarding dual-diagnosis services

- Screening and assessment to establish substance misuse diagnoses and levels of motivation to change
- Assessment and management of the physical consequences of substance misuse
- Development of individually tailored treatment plans with regular review
- Consideration of psychosocial approaches to treatment including motivational enhancement therapy, relapse prevention and 12-step facilitation in an integrated treatment service
- Medication management of psychotic symptoms with consideration of using atypicals as the first line choice, avoiding sedative medications, minimising risk of overdose and adding addiction treatment where appropriate
- Developing structures for the implementation of services which take into account the funding and regulatory barriers which commonly exist and the need for ongoing research and training of staff

---

Box 13.6 Elements of assertive community treatment

- Multidisciplinary team working with members sharing responsibility for clients (in contrast to case management)
- Focus on care for those with severe mental illnesses with an "assertive" approach taken to those reluctant to engage with services
- An attempt to provide for all the psychiatric and social needs of a patient rather than refer to other agencies
- Emphasis on treatment adherence and provision of care in the home environment wherever possible

---

example of "multielement" service provision for first-episode psychosis (McGorry *et al.*, 1996). The service incorporates inpatient facilities, outpatient case-management, individual/group/family therapy, pharmacological management with an emphasis on low-dose atypical antipsychotics and provision of specialised treatments. Research has been an integral component of many of the early-onset services established, and thus a considerable evidence base is now emerging although few studies have involved a rigorous randomised controlled design. In a recent review, limited support was found for at least short-term benefits for early-onset service interventions, and a recommendation was made for more rigorous assessment and incorporation of study designs which might identify the "key ingredients" of such services (Penn *et al.*, 2005).

Dual-diagnosis interventions

The prevalence of comorbid substance misuse disorders among those with schizophrenia is high. Historically little account was taken of the needs of

patients with psychosis for substance misuse treatments, but more recently there has been a growing awareness that outcomes are poorer for those with untreated substance misuse disorders. Those with severe mental illness have generally been excluded from treatment trials for addiction interventions, and services have developed in parallel with limited cross-training, research or clinical development. Increasingly evidence is emerging to support addiction interventions and integrated services for those with dual diagnosis. In the United States, national consensus recommendations have been made for services as outlined in Box 13.5 (Ziedonis *et al.*, 2005).

Assertive and intensive community treatment services

Poor service engagement and poor treatment adherence is known to be both common and to have a negative impact on outcome for those with schizophrenia. Concerns about the ability of community mental health teams to meet the needs of those with such problems has led to the development of services with a more assertive and/or intensive model of treatment provision. Assertive outreach or assertive community treatment is a well-established model of care based on the principles shown in Box 13.6 (Marshall & Lockwood, 2002).

Studies of assertive care, based mainly in the United States, do demonstrate evidence of benefit in terms of clinical status, social functioning and service contact aims, particularly for those with a low baseline of functioning and poor access to services. The evidence for their superiority over "standard" care in Europe is not, however, well established. In the United Kingdom, a randomised trial of intensive (reduced case loads for key workers) versus standard community care found little benefit for the former (Burns *et al.*, 1999), and certainly the NICE Guidelines for Schizophrenia conclude that although intensive case management results in greater service contact, there is insufficient evidence that this results in any enhanced clinical benefit (NICE, 2006).

Other service innovations

Home treatment, crisis intervention and specialist forensic services have also evolved over recent years. Good results have been reported for the former two in managing acute presentations of psychosis among those with schizophrenia living in the community. Home treatment during such a crisis has been shown to reduce the need for hospitalisation and to be a more acceptable option for patients (NICE, 2006). There has been a growing awareness of the risk to others posed by a small proportion of those with psychosis. Specialist forensic services have been developed to address the dual, and sometimes conflicting, aims of treating severe mental illness and reducing risk of harm to others. More recently specialist forensic clinicians, either in parallel or integrated teams, have begun managing patients in the community in addition to well-established secure units. The evidence base for forensic services in general and community services in particular is not, however, well developed. Such services are, nevertheless, expanding in many Western countries, particularly in response to the awareness that large numbers of patients are receiving none or inadequate care within the criminal justice system. Whether this trend is a direct consequence of the deinstitutionalisation of psychiatric care is a source of ongoing debate.

Conclusions

Schizophrenia remains in many ways an enigma. Although the understanding of the genetic, environmental and neurobiological causative elements has been enhanced with modern research designs and neuroimaging techniques, we are still far from consensus about such fundamental issues as what defines the boundaries of this "disorder". Also, schizophrenia remains a prevalent and highly disabling problem, for which our treatments, albeit improved, are still inadequate. The decades ahead will hopefully bring further advances in the unravelling of the mysteries of psychiatry's "sacred symbol".

REFERENCES

Akbarian, S., Bunney, W. E., Jr., Potkin, S. G., *et al.* (1993). Altered distribution of nicotinamide adenine dinucleotide phosphate-diaphorase cells in frontal lobe of schizophrenics implies disturbances of cortical development. *Arch Gen Psychiatry* **50**:169–77.

Akbarian, S., Vinuela, A., Kim, J. J., *et al.* (1993). Distorted distribution of nicotinamide-adenine dinucleotide phosphate-diaphorase neurons in temporal lobe of schizophrenics implies anomalous cortical development. *Arch Gen Psychiatry* **50**:178–87.

Andreasen, N. C. & Carpenter, W. T., Jr. (1993). Diagnosis and classification of schizophrenia. *Schizophr Bull* **19**:199–214.

Barta, P. E., Pearlson, G. D., Powers, R. E., *et al.* (1990). Auditory hallucinations and smaller superior temporal gyral volume in schizophrenia. *Am J Psychiatry* **147**:1457–62.

Bebbington, P., & Kuipers, L. (1994). The predictive utility of expressed emotion in schizophrenia: an aggregate analysis. *Psychol Med* **24**:707–18.

Bebbington, P., Wilkins, S., Jones, P., *et al.* (1993). Life events and psychosis. Initial results from the Camberwell Collaborative Psychosis Study. *Br J Psychiatry* **162**:72–9.

Bentall, R. (2004). *Madness Explained.* Penguin Books

Blackwood, D. H., St Clair, D. M., Muir, W. J., *et al.* (1991). Auditory P300 and eye tracking dysfunction in schizophrenic pedigrees. *Arch Gen Psychiatry* **48**:899–909.

Bleuler, M. (1974). The long-term outcome of the schizophrenic psychoses. *Psychol Med* **4**:244–54.

Boydell, J., van Os, J., Caspi, A., *et al.* (2006). Trends in cannabis use prior to first presentation with schizophrenia, in South-East London between 1965 and 1999. *Psychol Med* **36**:1441–6.

Boydell, J., van Os, J., McKenzie, K., *et al.* (2001). Incidence of schizophrenia in ethnic minorities in London: ecological study into interactions with environment. *BMJ* **323**:1336–8.

Boyle, M. (2002). *Schizophrenia: A Scientific Delusion?* Hove: Routledge.

Bramon, E., McDonald, C., Croft, R. J., *et al.* (2005). Is the P300 wave an endophenotype for schizophrenia? A meta-analysis and a family study. *Neuroimage*, **27**: 960–8.

Bramon, E., Walshe, M., McDonald, C., *et al.* (2005). Dermatoglyphics and schizophrenia: a meta-analysis and investigation of the impact of obstetric complications upon a-b ridge count. *Schizophr Res* **75**:399–404.

Brockington, I. F. (1992). Schizophrenia: yesterday's concept. *Eur Psychiatry* **7**:203–7.

Brockington, I. F., Kendell, R. E., & Leff, J. P. (1978). Definitions of schizophrenia: concordance and prediction of outcome. *Psychol Med* **8**:387–98.

Brown, G. W., Birley, J. L., & Wing, J. K. (1972). Influence of family life on the course of schizophrenic disorders: a replication. *Br J Psychiatry* **121**:241–58.

Brown, G. W., & Birley, J. L. T. (1968). Crises and life changes and the onset of schizophrenia. *J Health Soc Behav* **9**:203–14.

Burns, T., Creed, F., Fahy, T., *et al.* (1999). Intensive versus standard case management for severe psychotic illness: a randomised trial. UK 700 Group. *Lancet* **353**: 2185–9.

Busatto, G. F., Pilowsky, L. S., Costa, D. C., *et al.* (1997). Correlation between reduced in vivo benzodiazepine receptor binding and severity of psychotic symptoms in schizophrenia. *Am J Psychiatry* **154**:56–63.

Cahn, W., van Haren, N. F., Hulshoff Pol, H. E., *et al.* (2006). Brain volume changes in the first year of illness and 5-year outcome of schizophrenia. *Br J Psychiatry* **189**:381–2.

Cannon, M., Caspi, A., Moffitt, T. E., *et al.* (2002). Evidence for early-childhood, pan-developmental impairment specific to schizophreniform disorder: results from a longitudinal birth cohort. *Arch Gen Psychiatry* **59**:449–56.

Cannon, M., Jones, P. B., & Murray, R. M. (2002). Obstetric complications and schizophrenia: historical and meta-analytic review. *Am J Psychiatry* **159**:1080–92.

Cannon, T. D., van Erp, T. G., Rosso, I. M., *et al.* (2002). Fetal hypoxia and structural brain abnormalities in schizophrenic patients, their siblings, and controls. *Arch Gen Psychiatry* **59**:35–41.

Cantor-Graae, E., & Selten, J. P. (2005). Schizophrenia and migration: a meta-analysis and review. *Am J Psychiatry* **162**:12–24.

Cardno, A. G., Marshall, E. J., Coid, B., *et al.* (1999). Heritability estimates for psychotic disorders: the Maudsley twin psychosis series. *Arch Gen Psychiatry* **56**:162–8.

Carlsson, A., & Lindqvist, M. (1963). Effect of chlorpromazine or haloperidol on formation of 3methoxytyramine and normetanephrine in mouse brain. *Acta Pharmacol Toxicol (Copenh)* **20**:140–4.

Carpenter, W. T., Jr., Heinrichs, D. W., & Wagman, A. M. (1988). Deficit and nondeficit forms of schizophrenia: the concept. *Am J Psychiatry* **145**:578–83.

Castle, D. J., & Murray, R. M. (1991). The neurodevelopmental basis of sex differences in schizophrenia. *Psychol Med* **21**:565–75.

Chen, C. K., Lin, S. K., Sham, P. C., *et al.* (2005). Morbid risk for psychiatric disorder among the relatives of methamphetamine users with and without psychosis. *Am J Med Genet B Neuropsychiatr Genet* **136**:87–91.

Chen, C. K., Lin, S. K., Sham, P. C., *et al.* (2003). Pre-morbid characteristics and co-morbidity of methamphetamine users with and without psychosis. *Psychol Med* **33**:1407–14.

Chua, S., & Murray, R. M. (1995). The neurodevelopmental theory of schizophrenia: evidence concerning structure and neuropsychology. *Acta Neuropsychiat.*, **7**:568–70.

Claridge, G. (1972). The schizophrenias as nervous types. *Br J Psychiatry* **121**:1–17.

Connell, P. H. (1958). *Amphetamine Psychosis.* London: Oxford University Press.

Cooper, J. E., Kendell, R. E., Gurland, B. J., *et al.* (1972). *Psychiatric Diagnosis in New York and London.* Oxford: Oxford University Press.

Craddock, M., Asherson, P., Owen, M. J., *et al.* (1996). Concurrent validity of the OPCRIT diagnostic system. Comparison of OPCRIT diagnoses with consensus best-estimate lifetime diagnoses. *Br J Psychiatry* **169**:58–63.

Crow, T. J. (1980). Positive and negative schizophrenic symptoms and the role of dopamine. *Br J Psychiatry* **137**:383–6.

Crow, T. J. (1990). The continuum of psychosis and its genetic origins. The sixty-fifth Maudsley lecture. *Br J Psychiatry* **156**:788–97.

Curran, C., Byrappa, N., & McBride, A. (2004). Stimulant psychosis: systematic review. *Br J Psychiatry* **185**:196–204.

David, A. S., & Appleby, L. (1992). Diagnostic criteria in schizophrenia: accentuate the positive. *Schizophr Bull*, **18**:551–7.

David, A. S., & Cutting, J. C. (1994). *The Neuropsychology of Schizophrenia*. East Sussex: Lawrence Erlbaum.

Davis, J. M., Chen, N., & Glick, I. D. (2003). A meta-analysis of the efficacy of second-generation antipsychotics. *Arch Gen Psychiatry* **60**:553–64.

Dazzan, P., Morgan, K. D., Orr, K., *et al.* (2005). Different effects of typical and atypical antipsychotics on grey matter in first episode psychosis: the AESOP study. *Neuropsychopharmacology*, **30**:765–74.

Di Forti, M., Lappin, J. M., & Murray, R. M. (2007). Risk factors for schizophrenia — all roads lead to dopamine. *European Neuropsychopharmacology*, **17**(Suppl 2):S101–S107.

Enoch, M., & Ball, H. (2001). *Uncommon Psychiatric Syndromes*, 4th edn. London: Hodder & Stoughton.

Faris, R. E., & Dunham, W. (1939). *Mental Disorders in Urban Areas: An Ecological Study of Schizophrenia and Other Psychoses*. Chicago: University of Chicago Press.

Fearon, P., Kirkbride, J. B., Morgan, C., *et al.* (2006). Incidence of schizophrenia and other psychoses in ethnic minority groups: results from the MRC AESOP Study. *Psychol Med* **36**:1541–50.

Fish, B., Marcus, J., Hans, S., Auerbach, J., & Perdue, S. (1992). Infants at risk for schizophrenia: sequelae of a genetic neurointegrative defect. *Arch Gen Psychiatry* **49**:221–35.

Frith, C. (1992). *The Cognitive Neuropsychology of Schizophrenia*. Hove: Lawrence Erlbaum.

Garety, P. A., Kuipers, E., Fowler, D., *et al.* (2001). A cognitive model of the positive symptoms of psychosis. *Psychol Med* **31**:189–95.

Goodman, L. A., Salyers, M. P., Mueser, K. T., *et al.* (2001). Recent victimization in women and men with severe mental illness: prevalence and correlates. *J Trauma Stress* **14**:615–32.

Gottesman, I. I. (1991). *Schizophrenia Genesis: The Origins of Madness*. New York: Freeman.

Gray, J. A., Feldon, J., Rawlins, J. N. P., *et al.* (1991). The neuropsychology of schizophrenia. *Behav Brain Sci* **14**:1–20.

Griffith, J. D., Cavanaugh, J., Held, J., *et al.* (1972). Dextroamphetamine. Evaluation of psychomimetic properties in man. *Arch Gen Psychiatry* **26**:97–100.

Gupta, S., Sonnenberg, S. J., & Frank, B. (1998). Olanzapine augmentation of clozapine. *Ann Clin Psychiatry* **10**:113–15.

Harding, C. M., Brooks, G. W., Ashikaga, T., *et al.* (1987). The Vermont longitudinal study of persons with severe mental illness, II: long-term outcome of subjects who retrospectively met DSM-III criteria for schizophrenia. *Am J Psychiatry* **144**:727–35.

Hare, E. (1983). Was insanity on the increase? The fifty-sixth Maudsley Lecture. *Br J Psychiatry* **142**:439–55.

Harris, M. G., Henry, L. P., Harrigan, S. M., *et al.* (2005). The relationship between duration of untreated psychosis and outcome: an eight-year prospective study. *Schizophr Res* **79**:85–93.

Harrison, P. J., & Owen, M. J. (2003). Genes for schizophrenia? Recent findings and their pathophysiological implications. *Lancet* **361**:417–19

Henquet, C., Murray, R., Linszen, D., *et al.* (2005). The environment and schizophrenia: the role of cannabis use. *Schizophr Bull* **31**:608–12.

Heston, L. L., & Denney, D. (1968). Interactions between early life experience and biological factors in schizophrenia. In D. Rosenthal & S. Kety, eds. *The Transmission of Schizophrenia*. Oxford, UK: Pergamon Press, pp. 363–70.

Hiday, V. A., Swartz, M. S., Swanson, J. W., *et al.* (1999). Criminal victimization of persons with severe mental illness. *Psychiatr Serv* **50**:62–8.

Hirsch, S. R., & Leff, J. (1975). *Abnormalities in the Parents of Schizophrenics*. Oxford: Oxford University Press.

Hoek, H. W., Brown, A. S., & Susser, E. (1998). The Dutch famine and schizophrenia spectrum disorders. *Soc Psychiatry Psychiatr Epidemiol* **33**:373–9.

Hollister, J. M., Laing, P., & Mednick, S. A. (1996). Rhesus incompatibility as a risk factor for schizophrenia in male adults. *Arch Gen Psychiatry* **53**:19–24.

Holzman, P. S., Kringlen, E., Matthysse, S., *et al.* (1988). A single dominant gene can account for eye tracking dysfunctions and schizophrenia in offspring of discordant twins. *Arch Gen Psychiatry* **45**:641–7.

Jablensky, A., Sartorius, N., Ernberg, G., *et al.* (1992). Schizophrenia: manifestations, incidence and course in different cultures. A World Health Organisation ten country study. In *Psychological Medicine Monograph Supplement 20*. Cambridge: Cambridge University Press.

Janssen, I., Krabbendam, L., Bak, M., *et al.* (2004). Childhood abuse as a risk factor for psychotic experiences. *Acta Psychiatr Scand* **109**:38–45.

Job, D. E., Whalley, H. C., Johnstone, E. C., *et al.* (2005). Grey matter changes over time in high risk subjects developing schizophrenia. *Neuroimage* **25**:1023–30.

Johnstone, E. C. (1994). Brain imaging, psychopathology and neurology. In H. Hafner & W. F. Gattaz, eds. *Search for the Causes of Schizophrenia*. Berlin: Springer-Verlag, pp. 129–40.

Johnstone, E. C., Crow, T. J., Frith, C. D., *et al.* (1978). Mechanism of the antipsychotic effect in the treatment of acute schizophrenia. *Lancet* **1**:848–51.

Jones, P., Rodgers, B., Murray, R., *et al.* (1994). Child development risk factors for adult schizophrenia in the British 1946 birth cohort. *Lancet* **344**:1398–1402.

Jones, P. B., Rantakallio, P., Hartikainen, A. L., *et al.* (1998). Schizophrenia as a long-term outcome of pregnancy, delivery, and perinatal complications: a 28-year follow-up of the 1966 north Finland general population birth cohort. *Am J Psychiatry* **155**:355–64.

Kapur, S. (2003). Psychosis as a state of aberrant salience: a framework linking biology, phenomenology, and pharmacology in schizophrenia. *Am J Psychiatry* **160**: 13–23.

Kasanin, J. (1933). The acute schizoaffective psychoses. *Am J Psychiatry* **13**:97–123.

Kellendonk, C., Simpson, E. H., Polan, H. J., *et al.* (2006). Transient and selective overexpression of dopamine D2 receptors in the striatum causes persistent abnormalities in prefrontal cortex functioning. *Neuron* **49**: 603–15.

Kendler, K. S. (1980). The nosologic validity of paranoia (simple delusional disorder). A review. *Arch Gen Psychiatry* **37**:699–706.

Kendler, K. S., McGuire, M., Gruenberg, A. M., *et al.* (1993). The Roscommon Family Study. I. Methods, diagnosis of probands, and risk of schizophrenia in relatives. *Arch Gen Psychiatry* **50**:527–40.

Kety, S. S., Rosenthal, D., Wender, P. H., *et al.* (1975). Mental illness in the biological and adoptive families of adopted individuals who have become schizophrenic: a preliminary report based on psychiatric interviews. *Proc Annu Meet Am Psychopathol Assoc* 147–65.

Kirkbride, J. B., Fearon, P., Morgan, C., *et al.* (2007). Neighbourhood variation in the incidence of psychotic disorders in Southeast London. *Soc Psychiatry Psychiatr Epidemiol* **42**:438–45.

Kirkbride, J. B., Fearon, P., Morgan, C. (2006). Heterogeneity in incidence rates of schizophrenia and other psychotic syndromes: findings from the 3-center AeSOP study. *Arch Gen Psychiatry* **63**:250–8.

Kleist, K. (1930). Alogical thought disorder [Translated 1987]. In J. Cutting & M. Shepherd, eds. *The Clinical Roots of the Schizophrenic Concept*. Cambridge, UK: Cambridge University Press, pp. 75–9.

Kraepelin, E. (1919). *Dementia Praecox and Paraphrenia*. Translated by R. M. Barclay. Edinburgh: Livingstone.

Langfeldt, G. (1939). *The Schizophreniform States*. Oxford: Oxford University Press.

Laruelle, M., Abi-Dargham, A., van Dyck, C. H., *et al.* (1996). Single photon emission computerized tomography imaging of amphetamine-induced dopamine release in drug-free schizophrenic subjects. *Proc Natl Acad Sci U S A* **93**:9235–40.

Leff, J., Kuipers, L., Berkowitz, R., *et al.* (1982). A controlled trial of social intervention in the families of schizophrenic patients. *Br J Psychiatry* **141**:121–34.

Lewis, G., David, A., Andreasson, S., *et al.* (1992). Schizophrenia and city life. *Lancet* **340**:137–40.

Liddle, P. F. (1987). The symptoms of chronic schizophrenia. A re-examination of the positive-negative dichotomy. *Br J Psychiatry* **151**:145–51.

Lieberman, J. A., Stroup, T. S., McEvoy, J. P., *et al.* (2005). Effectiveness of antipsychotic drugs in patients with chronic schizophrenia. *N Engl J Med* **353**: 1209–23.

Lieberman, J. A., Tollefson, G. D., Charles, C., *et al.* (2005). Antipsychotic drug effects on brain morphology in first-episode psychosis. *Arch Gen Psychiatry* **62**: 361–70.

Lishman, W. A. (1997). *Organic Psychiatry: The Psychological Consequences of Cerebral Disorder*, 3rd edn. Blackwell Science.

Marshall, M., & Lockwood, A. (2002). Assertive community treatment for people with severe mental disorders [Cochrane Review]. Oxford: Update Software, Cochrane Library.

Mata, I., Gilvarry, C. M., Jones, P. B., *et al.* (2003). Schizotypal personality traits in nonpsychotic relatives are associated with positive symptoms in psychotic probands. *Schizophr Bull* **29**:273–83.

McGhie, A., & Chapman, J. (1961). Disorders of attention and perception in early schizophrenia. *Br J Med Psychol* **34**:103–16.

McGorry, P. D., Edwards, J., Mihalopoulos, C., *et al.* (1996). EPPIC: an evolving system of early detection and optimal management. *Schizophr Bull* **22**:305–26.

McGrath, J., Saha, S., Welham, J., *et al.* (2004). A systematic review of the incidence of schizophrenia: the distribution of rates and the influence of sex, urbanicity, migrant status and methodology. *BMC Med* **2**:13.

McGrath, J. J., Pemberton, M. R., Welham, J. L., *et al.* (1994). Schizophrenia and the influenza epidemics of 1954: 1957 and 1959: a southern hemisphere study. *Schizophr Res* **14**:1–8.

McGrath, J. J., van Os, J., Hoyos, C., *et al.* (1995). Minor physical anomalies in psychoses: associations with clinical and putative aetiological variables. *Schizophr Res* **18**:9–20.

McGuffin, P., Farmer, A. E., Gottesman, II, *et al.* (1984). Twin concordance for operationally defined schizophrenia. Confirmation of familiality and heritability. *Arch Gen Psychiatry* **41**:541–5.

McGuire, P. K., Shah, G. M., & Murray, R. M. (1993). Increased blood flow in Broca's area during auditory hallucinations in schizophrenia. *Lancet* **342**:703–6.

McGuire, P. K., Silbersweig, D. A., Wright, I., *et al.* (1995). Abnormal monitoring of inner speech: a physiological basis for auditory hallucinations. *Lancet* **346**: 596–600.

Mednick, S. A., Machon, R. A., Huttunen, M. O., *et al.* (1988). Adult schizophrenia following prenatal exposure to an influenza epidemic. *Arch Gen Psychiatry* **45**:189–92.

Mednick, S. A., Parnas, J., & Schulsinger, F. (1987). The Copenhagen High-Risk Project, 1962–86. *Schizophr Bull* **13**:485–95.

Meltzer, H. Y., & Cola, P. A. (1994). The pharmacoeconomics of clozapine: a review. *J Clin Psychiatry* **55**(Suppl B):161–5.

Morgan, C., & Fisher, H. (2007). Environment and schizophrenia: environmental factors in schizophrenia: childhood trauma – a critical review. *Schizophr Bull* **33**:3–10.

Mortensen, P. B. (2003). Mortality and physical illness in schizophrenia. In R. M. Murray, P. B. Jones, E. Susser, *et al.*, eds. *The Epidemiology of Schizophrenia*. Cambridge: Cambridge University Press, pp. 275–87.

Mullen, P. E., & Lester, G. (2006). Vexatious litigants and unusually persistent complainants and petitioners: from querulous paranoia to querulous behaviour. *Behav Sci Law* **24**:333–49.

Mullen, P. E., Martin, J. L., Anderson, J. C., *et al.* (1993). Childhood sexual abuse and mental health in adult life. *Br J Psychiatry* **163**:721–32.

Munro, J. C., Russell, A. J., Murray, R. M., *et al.* (2002). IQ in childhood psychiatric attendees predicts outcome of later schizophrenia at 21 year follow-up. *Acta Psychiatr Scand* **106**:139–42.

Murray, R. M. (1994). Neurodevelopmental schizophrenia: the rediscovery of dementia praecox. *Br J Psychiatry Suppl* November (**25**):6–12.

Murray, R. M., & Lewis, S. W (1987). Is schizophrenia a neurodevelopmental disorder? *Br Med J (Clin Res Ed)* **295**:681–2.

Murray, R. M., Sham, P., Van Os, J., *et al.* (2004). A developmental model for similarities and dissimilarities between schizophrenia and bipolar disorder. *Schizophr Res* **71**:405–16.

Nayani, T. H., & David, A. S. (1995). The auditory hallucination: a phenomenological survey. *Psychol Med* **26**:177–89.

National Institute for Clinical Excellence. (2006). *Schizophrenia: Full National Clinical Guideline on Core Interventions in Primary and Secondary Care*. London: Gaskell and the British Psychological Society.

O'Callaghan, E., Sham, P., Takei, N., *et al.* (1991). Schizophrenia after prenatal exposure to 1957 A2 influenza epidemic. *Lancet* **337**:1248–50.

Odegaard, O. (1932). Emigration and insanity: a study of mental disease among Norwegian-born population in Minnesota. *Acta Psychiatr Neurol Scand Suppl* **4**:1–206.

Palmer, B. A., Pankratz, V. S., & Bostwick, J. M. (2005). The lifetime risk of suicide in schizophrenia: a reexamination. *Arch Gen Psychiatry* **62**:247–53.

Pantelis, C., Velakoulis, D., McGorry, P. D., *et al.* (2003). Neuroanatomical abnormalities before and after onset of psychosis: a cross-sectional and longitudinal MRI comparison. *Lancet* **361**:281–8.

Parnas, J., Schulsinger, F., Teasdale, T. W., *et al.* (1982). Perinatal complications and clinical outcome within the schizophrenia spectrum. *Br J Psychiatry* **140**:416–20.

Pedersen, C. B., & Mortensen, P. B. (2001). Evidence of a dose-response relationship between urbanicity during upbringing and schizophrenia risk. *Arch Gen Psychiatry* **58**:1039–46.

Penn, D. L., Waldheter, E. J., Perkins, D. O., *et al.* (2005). Psychosocial treatment for first-episode psychosis: a research update. *Am J Psychiatry* **162**:2220–32.

Pilling, S., Bebbington, P., Kuipers, E., *et al.* (2002). Psychological treatments in schizophrenia: II. Meta-analyses of randomized controlled trials of social skills training and cognitive remediation. *Psychol Med* 32:783–91.

Pilling, S., Bebbington, P., Kuipers, E., *et al.* (2002). Psychological treatments in schizophrenia: I. Meta-analysis of family intervention and cognitive behaviour therapy. *Psychol Med* 32:763–82.

Pilowsky, L., & Murray, R. M. (1991). Why don't preschizophrenic children have delusions and hallucinations? *Behav Brain Sci* 41–2.

Pinfold, V., Toulmin, H., Thornicroft, G., *et al.* (2003). Reducing psychiatric stigma and discrimination: evaluation of educational interventions in UK secondary schools. *Br J Psychiatry* 182:342–6.

Pope, H. G., Jr., & Lipinski, J. F., Jr. (1978). Diagnosis in schizophrenia and manic-depressive illness: a reassessment of the specificity of "schizophrenic" symptoms in the light of current research. *Arch Gen Psychiatry* 35:811–28.

Poulton, R., Caspi, A., Moffitt, T. E., *et al.* (2000). Children's self-reported psychotic symptoms and adult schizophreniform disorder: a 15-year longitudinal study. *Arch Gen Psychiatry* 57:1053–8.

Procci, W. R. (1976). Schizo-affective psychosis: fact or fiction? A survey of the literature. *Arch Gen Psychiatry* 33:1167–78.

Read, J., & Argyle, N. (1999). Hallucinations, delusions, and thought disorder among adult psychiatric inpatients with a history of child abuse. *Psychiatr Serv* 50: 1467–72.

Reveley, A. M., Reveley, M. A., Chitkara, B., *et al.* (1984). The genetic basis of cerebral ventricular volume. *Psychiatry Res* 13:261–6.

Reveley, A. M., Reveley, M. A., Clifford, C. A., *et al.* (1982). Cerebral ventricular size in twins discordant for schizophrenia. *Lancet* 1:540–1.

Ritchie, J. H., Dick, D., & Lingham, R. (1994). The Report of the Enquiry into the Care and Treatment of Christopher Clunis. London: HMSO.

Rosenhan, D. L. (1973). On being sane in insane places. *Science* 179:250–8.

Rosenheck, R., Leslie, D., Keefe, R., *et al.* (2006). Barriers to employment for people with schizophrenia. *Am J Psychiatry* 163:411–7.

Rosenthal, D., Wender, P. H., Kety, S. S., *et al.* (1971). The adopted-away offspring of schizophrenics. *Am J Psychiatry* 128:307–11.

Sacker, A., Done, D. J., Crow, T. J., *et al.* (1995). Antecedents of schizophrenia and affective illness. Obstetric complications. *Br J Psychiatry* 166:734–41.

Schaefer, C. A., Brown, A. S., Wyatt, R. J., *et al.* (2000). Maternal prepregnant body mass and risk of schizophrenia in adult offspring. *Schizophr Bull* 26:275–86.

Schneider, K. (1950). *Psychopathic Personalities* (translated by M. Hamilton).

Scull, A. (1984). Was insanity increasing? A response to Edward Hare. *Br J Psychiatry* 144:432–436.

Sham, P. C., O'Callaghan, E., Takei, N., *et al.* (1992). Schizophrenia following pre-natal exposure to influenza epidemics between 1939 and 1960. *Br J Psychiatry* 160:461–6.

Shenton, M. E., Kikinis, R., Jolesz, F. A., *et al.* (1992). Abnormalities of the left temporal lobe and thought disorder in schizophrenia. A quantitative magnetic resonance imaging study. *N Engl J Med* 327:604–12.

Shiloh, R., Zemishlany, Z., Aizenberg, D., *et al.* (1997). Sulpiride augmentation in people with schizophrenia partially responsive to clozapine. A double-blind, placebo-controlled study. *Br J Psychiatry* 171:569–73.

Silver, E., Arseneault, L., Langley, J., *et al.* (2005). Mental disorder and violent victimization in a total birth cohort. *Am J Public Health* 95:2015–21.

Slater, E., Beard, A. W., & Glithero, E. (1963). The schizophrenialike psychoses of epilepsy. *Br J Psychiatry* 109:95–150.

Spitzer, R. L., Endicott, J., & Robins, E. (1978). Research diagnostic criteria: rationale and reliability. *Arch Gen Psychiatry* 35:773–82.

Stefanis, N., Frangou, S., Yakeley, J., *et al.* (1999). Hippocampal volume reduction in schizophrenia: effects of genetic risk and pregnancy and birth complications. *Biol Psychiatry* 46:697–702.

Suddath, R. L., Christison, G. W., Torrey, E. F., *et al.* (1990). Anatomical abnormalities in the brains of monozygotic twins discordant for schizophrenia. *N Engl J Med* 322:789–94.

Susser, E., Hoek, H. W., & Brown, A. (1998). Neurodevelopmental disorders after prenatal famine: The story of the Dutch Famine Study. *Am J Epidemiol,* 147:213–16.

Susser, E., & Wanderling, J. (1994). Epidemiology of nonaffective acute remitting psychosis vs schizophrenia. Sex and sociocultural setting. *Arch Gen Psychiatry* 51:294–301.

Tienari, P., Wynne, L. C., Sorri, A., *et al.* (2004). Genotype-environment interaction in schizophrenia-spectrum disorder. Long-term follow-up study of Finnish adoptees. *Br J Psychiatry* 184:216–22.

Toulopoulou, T., Rabe-Hesketh, S., King, H., *et al.* (2003). Episodic memory in schizophrenic patients and their relatives. *Schizophr Res* **63**:261–71.

Tsuang, M. T., Simpson, J. C., & Kronfol, Z. (1982). Subtypes of drug abuse with psychosis. Demographic characteristics, clinical features, and family history. *Arch Gen Psychiatry* **39**:141–7.

Tsuang, M. T., Stone, W. S., & Faraone, S. V. (2001). Genes, environment and schizophrenia. *Br J Psychiatry Suppl*, **40**:s18–24.

Tucker, C., Barker, A., & Gregoire, A. (1998). Living with schizophrenia: caring for a person with a severe mental illness. *Soc Psychiatry Psychiatr Epidemiol* **33**: 305–9.

Turkington, D., Dudley, R., Warman, D. M., *et al.* (2004). Cognitive-behavioral therapy for schizophrenia: a review. *J Psychiatr Pract* **10**:5–16.

van Os, J., Fahy, T. A., Jones, P., *et al.* (1995). Increased intracerebral cerebrospinal fluid spaces predict unemployment and negative symptoms in psychotic illness. A prospective study. *Br J Psychiatry* **166**:750–8.

van Os, J., Fahy, T. A., Jones, P., *et al.* (1996). Psychopathological syndromes in the functional psychoses: associations with course and outcome. *Psychol Med* **26**:161–76.

Vaughan, C., & Leff, J. (1976). The influence of family and social factors on the course of psychiatric illness. *Br J Psychiatry* 125–37.

Velakoulis, D., Wood, S. J., Wong, M. T., *et al.* (2006). Hippocampal and amygdala volumes according to psychosis stage and diagnosis: a magnetic resonance imaging study of chronic schizophrenia, first-episode psychosis, and ultra-high-risk individuals. *Arch Gen Psychiatry* **63**:139–49.

Wahlbeck, K., Forsen, T., Osmond, C., *et al.* (2001). Association of schizophrenia with low maternal body mass index, small size at birth, and thinness during childhood. *Arch Gen Psychiatry* **58**:48–52.

Walker, E., & Lewine, R. J. (1990). Prediction of adult-onset schizophrenia from childhood home movies of the patients. *Am J Psychiatry* **147**:1052–6.

Weinberger, D. R. (1987). Implications of normal brain development for the pathogenesis of schizophrenia. *Arch Gen Psychiatry* **44**:660–9.

Wessely, S., Castle, D., Der, G., *et al.* (1991). Schizophrenia and Afro-Caribbeans. A case-control study. *Br J Psychiatry* **159**:795–801.

Wing, J. K., & Brown, G. W. (1970). *Institutionalism and Schizophrenia*. Cambridge: Cambridge University Press.

Wing, J. K., Cooper, J. E., & Sartorius, N. (1974). *The Description and Classification of Psychiatric Symptoms: An Instruction Manual for the PSE and CATEGO System*. London: Cambridge University Press.

Wing, J. K. (1978). Clinical concepts of schizophrenia. In: J. K. Wing, ed. *Schizophrenia Towards a New Synthesis*. London: Academic Press.

World Health Organisation (1973). *Report of the International Pilot Study of Schizophrenia*. Geneva: World Health Organisation.

World Health Organisation (1992). *International Classification of Impairments, Disabilities and Handicaps*, 10th revision. Geneva: World Health Organisation.

Wright, I. C., Rabe-Hesketh, S., Woodruff, P. W., *et al.* (2000). Meta-analysis of regional brain volumes in schizophrenia. *Am J Psychiatry* **157**:16–25.

Wykes, T., & Reeder, C. (2005). *Cognitive Remediation Therapy: Theory and Practice*. London: Brunner Routledge.

Ziedonis, D. M., Smelson, D., Rosenthal, R. N., *et al.* (2005). Improving the care of individuals with schizophrenia and substance use disorders: consensus recommendations. *J Psychiatr Pract*, **11**:315–39.

14

Neuropsychiatry

Perminder Sachdev

Neuropsychiatry is an old discipline that can trace its origins to the seventeenth century, much before modern psychiatry was born. After being in hibernation for many years, it has re-emerged in the last three decades, not merely as a borderland between psychiatry and neurology but as a discipline with a distinctive approach and a clinical territory. As a hybrid discipline, however, neuropsychiatry may be regarded as the application of the neurological or neuroscientific paradigm to psychiatric and behavioural syndromes. It brings together the descriptive, nosological and therapeutic strengths of psychiatry; the empirical foundations of neurology; and the assessment skills of neuropsychology to deal with these disorders. Its sister discipline within neurology is behavioural neurology, which covers the same territory but with a neurological bias in training and clinical emphasis (Sachdev, 2005).

The neuropsychiatric approach recognises that all types of behavioural disturbances that occur in psychiatric disorders can also occur in conjunction with neurological disorders. This is implicit in the diagnostic criteria used by most classifications of psychiatric disorders, which consider the presence of a putative organic cause as being exclusionary. Psychiatric classifications, in this regard, are hierarchical, giving pre-eminence to organic brain disease over idiopathic syndromes. Psychiatric diagnoses are syndromal, and the fact that psychiatric and neurological disorders are responsible for similar syndromes does not mean that the pathogenetic mechanisms are the same, even though there is a presumption of significantly shared pathophysiology. This is reason enough for some neuropsychiatric syndromes to be considered as neurological models of psychiatric disorders.

A critique of *organic* and its proposed alternatives

The term *organic* in reference to psychiatric disorders is the topic of much contemporary debate (Sachdev, 1996). Its origins are rooted in the late nineteenth century move to distinguish *functional* (or psychological) disorders from *structural* brain diseases in the spirit of Cartesian dualism. In modern neurobiology, there is an understanding of an interaction of structure and function whereby no disorder of the brain (or mind) can be based solely on disturbance of structure or function alone. In addition to its philosophical baggage, *organic* presents practical problems. According to the 10th revision of the *International Classification of Diseases* (ICD-10; World Health Organisation, 1992), organic mental disorders are "a range of mental disorders grouped together on the basis of their having in common a demonstrable aetiology in cerebral disease, brain injury, or other insult leading to

Essential Psychiatry, ed. Robin M. Murray, Kenneth S. Kendler, Peter McGuffin, Simon Wessely, David J. Castle. Published by Cambridge University Press. © Cambridge University Press 2008.

brain dysfunction". It goes on to say that *organic* is no more and no less than that a syndrome so classified can be attributed to an independently diagnosable cerebral or systemic disease or disorder. The working hypothesis is that the cerebral or systemic dysfunction is directly responsible for the disorder, and not a 'fortuitous association with such a disease or dysfunction, or a psychological reaction to its symptoms'. In practice, however, there are no infallible guidelines to establish a direct association, and the following considerations are generally given. (1) A temporal association between the onset, exacerbation, or remission of the medical condition and the mental disorder. However, there are many exceptions to this. (2) The presence of features that are atypical of the primary mental disorder. (3) Evidence from the literature of a well-established or frequently encountered association between the general medical condition and the phenomenology of a specific mental disorder. The situation is often not ambiguous. We recognise that psychiatric illnesses have multiple aetiological factors (e.g. genetics, coarse brain disease, personality, stress), some of which would be recognised as being "organic" in most cases.

The approach taken by 4th edition of the *Diagnostic and Statistical Manual of Mental Disorders* (DSM-IV) to address the problems associated with *organic* was to retire the term and replace it with *secondary* (or *symptomatic*). It is not being argued that primary psychiatric disorders do not have a basis in brain dysfunction, but that their aetiology is poorly understood and they are therefore *idiopathic*, akin to the primary-secondary dichotomy used in medicine. Although this does not make the process of aetiological determination any easier, it is a philosophically more comfortable position.

The clinical neuropsychiatric assessment

A neuropsychiatric assessment is no more or less than a good psychiatric assessment, comprising a psychiatric and medical history; a detailed mental state examination, including a cognitive examination; a physical examination, especially neurological; a neuropsychological assessment; and laboratory investigations to evaluate general medical disorders and substance abuse, including electrophysiology (electroencephalograms [EEGs], event-related potentials [ERPs]) and neuroimaging (computed tomography [CT], magnetic resonance imaging [MRI], single photon emission computed tomography [SPECT], positron emission tomography [PET]). This assessment differs from a general psychiatric assessment in its emphasis on the medical-neurological factors. In the history, an account from a knowledgeable informant is often very helpful. A history of physical symptoms and behavioural change is important, and changes should be documented chronologically. Changes in appetitive functions such as sleep, eating and sexual interest are important to document. Pointers to brain disease such as seizures, head injury, stroke or transient ischaemic attack (TIA), alcohol and drug use, and evidence of cognitive impairment are all emphasised. Personality change with features such as impulsivity, aggressiveness or disinhibition is another important feature. Perinatal and developmental history is informative, particularly in neuropsychiatric disorders of childhood and young adulthood.

The mental state examination in neuropsychiatry follows the same format as that in general psychiatry except for a more detailed cognitive assessment. A brief cognitive assessment, which should be performed in all cases, is possible at the bedside. For a detailed assessment, a referral to a clinical neuropsychologist is necessary. When making such a referral, the neuropsychologist must be provided with the history and the salient questions the referring physician wishes to be addressed. This is necessary for the examination to be tailored to the patient's needs, abilities and limitations.

The bedside *cognitive state examination (CSE)* must be divided into a number of cognitive domains or systems, each of which must be examined. These are as follows:

1. Alertness and arousal
2. Attention, concentration and working memory

3. Orientation
4. Memory
5. Language
6. Visuospatial and constructive functions
7. Frontal executive functions
8. Other dominant (left) hemisphere functions: calculation, praxis, right-left orientation, finger gnosis, writing
9. Other nondominant (right) hemisphere functions: dressing apraxia, neglect phenomena and agnosias
10. Comportment: insight, judgement, self-awareness and social adaptation.

The assessment of level of consciousness and attentional processes is crucial, because disturbance in these domains can influence performance on other tests. Familiarity with the common bedside tests for each function is important (Hodges, 1994). For most purposes, a screening battery such as Folstein's (1975) Mini-Mental State Examination (MMSE) is a good starting point. It tests orientation, immediate and recent memory, concentration, arithmetic ability, language and praxis. It is easy to administer and takes only 5 to 10 minutes. It has reasonable sensitivity but low specificity and may be used for serial evaluations. The score is out of 30, and 27 or less is indicative of impairment. A score less than 25 is definitely abnormal. The MMSE may be normal in the presence of subtle impairment, and if this is suspected, a detailed evaluation is recommended. It is useful to combine the MMSE with the Clock Drawing Test in which the patient is asked to draw a clock face and then draw in the hands to indicate 10:10. This tests the patient's constructional abilities and, more importantly, planning and organisation ability. To help distinguish these two cognitive functions, the patient is asked to draw the Clock spontaneously, and if the result is not satisfactory, to copy the clock drawn by the examiner in front of patient. The latter assists the patient with frontal executive dysfunction but not one with visuoconstructive problems.

For a detailed discussion of neuropsychological tests and their application, the reader is referred to the classic textbook by Lezak (2004). Tests are rarely pure and are usually influenced by a number of cognitive functions, for example, a simple test such as "serial sevens" may be influenced by impairment of attention, short-term or working memory and calculation ability. A battery of tests is therefore necessary to determine which function is really disturbed. Failure on one test must be followed up with other tests before a dysfunction is established. All cognitive tests are designed to be administered in a particular manner. Significant departure from a standard administration may render the test invalid. Repetition of the same test may lead to an improvement in performance because of what is known as "practice effect". Also, bedside testing has the potential of confounding the formal assessment of a neuropsychologist if that were to follow. Therefore, the clinician should use only the tests that are meaningful for a bedside assessment. Some examples of the tasks used to test certain cognitive domains are provided in Table 14.1.

Memory

Memory is the process by which the brain stores information that has been acquired through learning or experience. It results in a relatively permanent change in the brain, as an "engram" which is subject to further modifications, adaptations and distortions. The process of memorising involves registration, encoding and storage of information. The recall of the stored information is a complex interaction of retrieval cues and the engrams. The traditional subtyping of memory is according to temporal parameters into *ultra-short* (iconic or echoic), *short-term* (working) and *long-term* memory. Baddeley's (1986) concept of *working memory* refers to the process by which information is held on-line for it to be manipulated. In long-term memory, information is stored off-line for minutes to decades. Memory is also subtyped according to content into two broad categories: (1) *Declarative* (or *explicit*) memories are facts that are accessible to conscious recollection. These may be personal (*episodic* memory) or general facts (*semantic* memory). (2) *Procedural* (or *implicit*) memories are stored as skills and automatic operations that cannot be tied to particular times or places and cannot

Table 14.1 Commonly used bedside cognitive tests by level of difficulty

Cognitive domain	Easy	Moderate	Hard
Attention and working memory	Counting 1–20 20–1, Serial 2s	Serial 3s Months forward/backward "World" backwards	Serial 7s Digit span backwards
Episodic memory	Three unrelated object names Name and addres Three shapes	CERAD word list	12–15 word lists (RAULT, CVLT) Logical memory
Language			
– Naming	Common objects and parts BNT items 1–20	*BNT items 21–40	*BNT items 41–60
– Repetition	The table	The book is on the table	No ifs, ands or buts
– Comprehension	Do dogs fly?	Where is the source of light in this room?	Do you prefer a vehicle or a dwelling for transportation?
– Generativity	—	Category lists (animals in 1 min)	FAS list (1 min each)
Parietal lobe function			
– Construction	Greek numbers, interlocking pentagons	Copy a cube House-tree-person	Copy Rey figure
– Praxis	"Cough" "Blow out a match" "Comb your hair" "Salute"	Fold letter and envelope and affix stamp Take stance of boxer	
– Calculations	Simple addition, subtraction	Operations using >3-digit numbers	Word problems (e.g. "what is 15% of 150?")
– R–L orientation	"Show me your. . . left hand, right eye, right hand, left ear, etc.	"Touch my left hand with your right hand" "Touch your left cheek with your right thumb"	. . . with hands crossed over chest
– Finger gnosis	"Show me your. . . right index finger, left little finger. . ."	Ask patient to match fingers tonumber) those on an outline drawn on paper	Identify (name or fingers with eyes closed & examiner touching the finger
– Stereognosis	Key, paper clip, coin, pen	Texture discrimination (cloth, wood, sandpaper)	Skin writing
Fontal lobe function			
– Primitive reflexes	Grasp reflex Palmomental reflex		
– Motor sequencing	Fist-ring test	Palm-fist-cut	Two hands together (fist-palm)
– Response inhibition and preserveration	Go-No go test Trails A Copying repetitive pattern	Trails B	
– Abstraction	Easy similarities and differences	Difficult similarities Easy proverbs	Abstract similarities Difficult proverbs
– Planning and organisation	Clock drawing		

Adapted from Weintraub, 2000. *BNT = Boston Naming Test.

be recalled as facts. Assessment of memory is an important part of any cognitive assessment, and the focus is generally on disturbance in short-term and long-term memory for verbal as well as nonverbal information.

Frontal lobe function

The frontal lobes, which comprise about one-third of the brain, are anatomically and functionally heterogeneous structures. They include the primary motor cortex, premotor cortex, supplementary motor cortex, Broca's area, medial frontal cortex and the prefrontal cortex (dorsolateral and orbitofrontal cortex and frontal eye fields). Disturbance of frontal lobes may lead to, depending on the region affected, motor dysfunction (loss of strength, loss of fine movement, poor programming of movement), voluntary gaze abnormality, expressive dysphasia, executive dysfunction (working memory, planning and organisation, strategy formation), impairment in memory recall, poor temporal memory (recency memory, frequency estimate, self-order recall), loss of divergent thinking, problems in reasoning and abstraction, impaired social and sexual behaviour (disinhibition, risk taking and rule breaking, inflexibility, impaired response inhibition), poor motivation, reduced spontaneity and impaired olfactory discrimination. A comprehensive assessment of frontal lobe function is therefore an elaborate process, but a brief bedside clinical examination is outlined in Box 14.1. It is noteworthy that the frontal lobes are parts of neuronal circuits with subcortical structures, in particular the basal ganglia and thalamus, and disruption of any part of a circuit may produce what we recognise as frontal lobe dysfunction. The description of these parallel corticosubcortical circuits has been of much interest to psychiatry (Cummings, 1993).

Physical examination

Neuropsychiatry has been called "psychiatry with signs", and it is important to examine the patient in detail for neurological and systemic disease

---

Box 14.1 Bedside tasks for examination of frontal lobe function.

1. Observable behaviour: impulse control, delaying gratification, motivation, affective regulation, relationships
2. Motor and expressive language
3. Primitive reflexes: grasp, palmomental, snout, pout, glabellar tap
4. Working memory: digit span backwards, serial 7's
5. Verbal fluency: semantic (e.g. saying as many words – not proper nouns – as possible in 1 minute beginning with the letter F or A or S), category (e.g. naming as many objects in one category as possible in 1 minute, such as animals)
6. Motor sequencing: Luria's hand sequences (e.g. alternating repeatedly between making a fist and a ring with one hand and then the other – fist-ring test, alternating between a fist, palm and cut movement with one had and then the other)
7. Reasoning and conceptualisation: similarities, differences, proverbs
8. Planning and organisation: clock drawing (asking the patient to draw a clock face and put in the hands to indicate 10:10, followed by asking him/her to copy a clock drawn by the examiner).

(DeMyer, 2003). When signs of definite neurological disease are lacking, "soft" or nonlocalising signs (for high-level sensory integration, motor coordination, gait and posture, stereognosis, graphaesethesia, motor inhibition) are often sought (Buchanan & Heinrichs, 1989). Their diagnostic significance is uncertain.

Investigations

Electrodiagnostic techniques have an important role in neuropsychiatric diagnosis. The EEG is a non-specific indicator of brain function and is routinely performed with the patient awake and at rest. Activation procedures that may enhance abnormalities include hyperventilation, photic stimulation, sleep deprivation and drug challenges. The standard electrode placements or "montages" use the 10 to 20 international system. The most important clinical value of EEG is in the evaluation of epilepsy and delirium. It has a role in the differentiation between organic and nonorganic disorders, although cautious interpretation is necessary. It may be of value in some dementias, such as Creutzfeldt-Jakob disease and subacute sclerosing panencephalitis. Although many quantitative methods of analysis of EEG are now available, the most common method remains a visual analysis by an expert encephalographer (Ebersole & Pedley, 2003). Quantitative EEG (QEEG) permits the determination of relative predominance or power of the different frequency bands, which can be condensed into a topographic map. This technique has been applied to differential diagnosis in psychiatry, the diagnosis and prognostication of attention-deficit/hyperactivity disorder and other applications. However, its validity as a diagnostic tool remains to be established.

Event-related potentials (ERPs) are useful for determining the integrity of sensory pathways. Sleep studies using EEG and other measures have many indications (Kryger et al., 2000). A recent development in EEG has been the study of cortical oscillations in the gamma-band (30–100 Hz), suggesting a role of these signals for cognitive functions, including visual perception, attention, learning and memory (Kaiser & Lutzenberger, 2005).

Magneto-encephalography (MEG) measures the small magnetic fields generated by neuronal currents and may be regarded as the magnetic counterpart of the EEG. It has advantages over the latter in spatial localisation of the signal and a broader range in frequency resolution. However, it is an expensive technique, owing to the very low signal-to-noise ratio and the need for shielding of the magnetometer from ambient magnetic noise. Most studies indicate that MEG seems to be more sensitive than EEG for neocortical spike sources, and MEG dipole analysis appears to be the main clinical application. Other clinical applications are in the process of development (Barkley & Baumgartner, 2003).

Neuroimaging

The recent advances in neuroimaging have had a great impact on neuropsychiatry. The techniques can be broadly divided into structural and functional. The reader is also referred to Chapter 4.

Structural imaging

The two major techniques are CT and MRI. Although CT is cheaper and more readily available, MRI offers a number of advantages. It provides excellent anatomical and spatial resolution, uses no ionising radiation, visualises the posterior fossa and pituitary regions without distortion due to bone, is more sensitive to white matter pathology and is versatile in its ability to scan in any plane. It is also possible to combine in the same scanning session structural MRI with a functional analysis of the brain using magnetic resonance spectroscopy (MRS), perfusion imaging, angiography and functional MRI (fMRI). Structural MRI has had a major impact on neuropsychiatric assessment and diagnosis (Symms et al., 2004). As a research tool as well, structural imaging has been extensively adapted by neuropsychiatry, especially since the availability of advanced computerised methods of analysis (Ashburner et al., 2003).

Functional imaging

These techniques are used primarily to provide information on metabolism, blood flow, neurochemistry or activity of the brain. PET, SPECT and fMRI are the main techniques. SPECT and PET rely on the incorporation of a radioactive nuclide into a drug or substance (called a radiopharmaceutical) which is typically injected intravenously into a patient. The subsequent uptake of the substance by the brain and the measurement of regional brain activities over time are analysed to provide information about metabolism, blood flow, receptor binding and so on. SPECT scanning, which uses gamma-emitters and a gamma camera, is cheaper and available in most nuclear medicine departments. Its resolution is less than that of PET, although with the development of multihead neuro-dedicated cameras has significantly closed the gap. Earlier SPECT studies used xenon-133 by the inhalation method, which provides quantitative data on cerebral blood blow (CBF) but with poor spatial resolution. Most SPECT scanning has used hexamethyl propylene amine oxime (Tc^{99m}-HMPAO; Ceretec) which permits the semi-quantitative estimation of regional cerebral blood flow (rCBF). A number of radiolabelled receptor binding agents are available for SPECT imaging, which include ^{123}I-labelled 3-quinuclidinyl-4-iodobenzilate (QNB) for muscarinic acetylcholine receptors, 3-iodo-6-methoxybenzamide (IBZM) for D_2 dopamine receptors, iomazenil for benzodiazepine receptors, iodoketanserin for $5HT_2$ receptors and β-CIT for the dopamine transporter (Saha *et al.*, 1994).

PET scanning is characterised by the use of short-lived radioactive labels that decay in the brain-emitting positrons. A positron travels a short distance before colliding with an electron, resulting in annihilation and the emission of two photons that travel in opposite directions at 180 degrees to each other. The coincident detection of the photons is the basis for the image reconstruction. The natural collimation provided by the coincident annihilation detection is the reason for the better spatial resolution of PET, although PET images remain somewhat blurry and do not reach the resolution of MRI. The labels commonly used are ^{18}F, ^{15}O, ^{13}N and ^{11}C. The fact that these have half-lives of a few minutes makes it necessary that they be produced in a cyclotron in close geographical proximity to the scanner. The most commonly used PET scans in clinical practice are with ^{18}F-fluoro-deoxyglucose (FDG) which reflect glucose uptake by the cells and thereby regional cerebral metabolism. This has clinical application in dementia, such as Alzheimer's disease in which patients have a reduction in metabolism bilaterally in the temporoparietal regions as an early manifestation. ^{15}O-H_2O provides a measure of rCBF and was the major technique for activation studies before the availability of functional MRI. PET has been extensively used in neurotransmitter and receptor studies for which it is more versatile than SPECT.

Other functional techniques such as fMRI and MRS are rapidly becoming popular. fMRI can be used to measure rCBV or rCBF by injecting the individuals with a paramagnetic contrast agent (e.g. gadolinium) and tracking the bolus through the brain, or alternatively labelling the red blood cells by the technique of arterial spin labelling. More commonly, however, fMRI measures the change in magnetisation due to the blood oxygen level–dependent (BOLD) method, which permits minute changes in blood flow in relation to physiological function to be studied. BOLD fMRI has resulted in an explosion of neuroimaging research with many imaginative applications (Matthews & Jezzard, 2004). It takes advantage of the coupling between neuronal activity and haemodynamics, although many aspects of this relationship remain incompletely understood (Heeger & Ress, 2002).

MRS is a technique by which certain chemicals in targeted brain regions can be measured, akin to a chemical biopsy of the brain. In vivo ^{1}H-MRS and ^{31}P-MRS are the most widely used applications of MRS, but other atoms that are also used include ^{13}C, ^{14}N, ^{19}F and ^{23}Na. Although proton MRS is widely available, it remains largely a research tool, even though its applications in cognitive disorders are developing rapidly (Ross & Sachdev, 2004).

Mental disorders due to a general medical condition (secondary or "organic" mental disorders)

This category of disorders is characterised by the presence of mental symptoms that are judged to be the direct physiological consequence of a general medical condition. These disorders were previously categorised as *organic mental disorders*. DSM-IV distinguishes those mental disorders that are due to a general medical condition from those that are substance induced and those that have no specified aetiology. The latter are, as a shorthand, called *primary mental disorders*, and the former two are *secondary mental disorders*. *Primary* or *idiopathic* mental disorders are sometimes inappropriately referred to as *functional disorders,* with the implication that psychological factors take primacy in the aetiology. Because functional disturbance is part of all psychiatric disorders, the term *functional* is best avoided. There are situations in which psychosocial factors produce an exacerbation of a disorder with a primary "organic" aetiology. It is therefore important in any psychiatric disorder to consider the biological, psychological and social factors, even when the primacy of one or the other factor may be apparent. The secondary mental disorders are categorised by DSM-IV, as shown in Table 14.2.

General principles

In clinical practice, *the clinician must have a high index of suspicion for organic factors in aetiology.* Some features that may act as pointers to possible organic contribution to a syndrome are the presence of cognitive dysfunction; presence of a general medical disorder known to be associated with neuropsychiatric syndromes; presence of an atypical psychiatric syndrome (e.g. a late age of onset, or unusual clinical features); or resistance to treatment, which should prompt revisiting the diagnosis.

In making a diagnosis in this category, the following steps are followed:

1. A syndromal diagnosis is made first, that is, does the patient suffer from delirium, psychosis, mood disorder or other problems?
2. Is a general medical condition present, or can a substance be implicated (as ascertained by history, physical examination and laboratory investigations)?
3. Is the mental disturbance related to the medical condition or substance aetiologically through a physiological mechanism? There are no infallible guidelines to establish such an association, but the following considerations are of assistance:
   a. a temporal association between the onset, exacerbation or remission of the medical condition and the mental disorder (there are many exceptions to this),
   b. the presence of features that are atypical of the primary mental disorder, and

Table 14.2 "Secondary" mental disorders

Cognitive disorders

1. Delirium due to a general medical condition or substance
2. Dementia due to a general medical condition or substance
3. Amnestic disorder due to a general medical condition or substance

Noncognitive disorders

4. Psychotic disorder due to a general medical condition or substance
   4a. With delusions
   4b. With hallucinations
5. Mood disorder due to a general medical condition or substance
   5a. With depressive features
   5b. With major depressive-like episode
   5c. With manic features
   5d. With mixed features
6. Catatonic disorder due to a general medical condition
7. Anxiety disorder due to a general medical condition or substance
   7a. With generalised anxiety
   7b. With panic attacks
   7c. With obsessive-compulsive features
   7d. With phobic symptoms
8. Personality disorder due to a general medical condition*
9. Sexual dysfunction due to a general medical condition or substance
10. Sleep disorder due to a general medical condition or substance

*These syndromes are not generally diagnosed as substance induced. All other syndromes can be caused by general medical conditions or substances.

   c. evidence from the literature of a well-established or frequently encountered association between the general medical condition and the phenomenology of a specific mental disorder.
4. Can the disturbance not be accounted for by another mental disorder? Ruling out a primary mental disorder (such as major depression or schizophrenia) may prove to be difficult.

5. Is the disturbance not exclusively during the course of a delirium?

6. Could multiple aetiologies be implicated?

It must be appreciated that not only are multiple causes involved in many neuropsychiatric syndromes, the same aetiology may be responsible for a variety of syndromes. As an example, corticosteroids may in different patients be associated with depression, euphoria or frank mania; delirium; anxiety; psychosis; or even a picture of dementia. The same can be said for other causes, such as alcohol, brain trauma, epilepsy and so on. What determines which syndrome will develop depends on a number of variables, relating both to the host or the agent, to borrow an infectious diseases analogy. Important host-related variables are age and gender, premorbid personality, past psychiatric illness, education, support systems, quality of relationships and previous experience with this agent. Agent-related variables include type and quality of brain impairment, rate of loss of function, brain regions involved and degree of reversibility of the dysfunction.

Noncognitive secondary disorders

Psychotic disorder due to a general medical condition and substance-induced psychotic disorder

The essential features are prominent hallucinations or delusions that are judged to be due to the direct physiological effects of the medical condition or substance. There are, therefore, two subtypes: (1) with hallucinations and (2) with delusions – depending on which feature is predominant, although both are often present in the same individual (Sachdev, in press).

Hallucinations

Hallucinations may occur in any modality, which is determined by aetiological factors. For example, hallucinogenic drugs most commonly cause visual hallucinations, whereas alcohol tends to induce auditory hallucinations. People who are blind due to cataracts may develop visual hallucinations; in those deaf due to otosclerosis, these are more likely to be auditory. In general, auditory hallucinations most typically occur in primary psychoses, whereas those in other modalities are more likely to be "organic". The hallucinations vary from very simple and unformed to highly complex and organised. The person may have varying degrees of insight into the hallucinations and, in some cases, may develop an elaborate secondary delusional system. The majority of people with hallucinations of organic aetiology in general hospitals have a delirium, and an examination of disturbance in consciousness is therefore important. Hallucinations are common in drug abuse settings. Overall, the commonest hallucination due to medical disorders or substances is visual.

Use of hallucinogens and prolonged use of alcohol are the two commonest causes of hallucinosis. The better-known hallucinogens are ergot and related compounds (lysergic acid diethylamide [LSD], morning glory seeds), phenylalkylamines (mescaline, "STP"), MDMA (3,4-methylenedioxymethamphetamine or "ecstasy") and indole alkaloids (psilocybin, dimethyltryptamine [DMT]). They can cause an acute hallucinosis as a result of intoxication. In some patients who chronically abuse hallucinogens, episodic recurrences of portions of prior hallucinogen-induced experiences (flashbacks) occur. This has been given the name *hallucinogen persisting perception disorder* in DSM-IV. A few develop persistent hallucinatory psychoses. Visual hallucinations also occur in certain central nervous system (CNS) disorders (e.g. epilepsy, migraine, brainstem lesions) or eye diseases (optic neuritis, retinal detachment) and may occur in normal individuals in sleep or sensory deprivation, hypnogogic states and hypnosis.

Alcoholic hallucinosis consists of vivid and persistent auditory hallucinations, often malicious, reproachful or threatening in nature, occurring following cessation or reduction of alcohol ingestion. Olfactory, gustatory and kinaesthetic hallucinations

---

Box 14.2 Causes of secondary hallucinations

1. Visual hallucinations
   a. Ocular pathology (cataracts, macular degeneration)
   b. Optic neuritis
   c. Brainstem pathology
   d. Cerebral hemispheric lesions (geniculo-calcarine lesions, epilepsy)
   e. Neurological illnesses (migraine, narcolepsy)
   f. Medical illnesses (delirium)
   g. Toxins (hallucinogens – LSD, DMT, MDMA, mescaline)
   h. Normal (hypnogogic, sensory or sleep deprivation, imaginary companions, autoscopy)
2. Auditory hallucinations
   a. Ear pathology (deafness)
   b. Brainstem pathology
   c. Cerebral pathology (temporal neocortex, epilepsy)
   d. Toxins (alcohol withdrawal)
   e. Normal (hypnogogic, deprivation)

Box 14.3 Causes of secondary delusions

Central nervous system disorders: cerebrovascular disease, Parkinson's disease, multiple sclerosis, partial complex epilepsy, brain neoplasm, Huntington's disease, HIV encephalopathy, etc.
Drugs: stimulants, corticosteroids, dopaminergic drugs (L-dopa, bromocriptine etc.), phencyclidine, cannabis
Endocrine disorders: Cushing's disease, hypo- or hypercalcemia, hyper- or hypothyroidism, hypopituitarism
Connective tissue diseases: systemic lupus erythematosus, temporal arteritis
Other: porphyria, heavy metal toxicity

---

are rare and likely to be associated with partial complex epilepsy and primary psychiatric disorders. The main organic causes of hallucinations are summarised in Box 14.2.

Treatment is dependent on identifying the aetiology. Drug intoxications are usually time limited and will settle without drug treatment in a safe environment. Drugs with anticholinergic effects should be avoided because street drugs are often "cut" with such drugs. Neuroleptics may sometimes be of benefit. Efforts to correct sensory impairments in the elderly may help.

Delusions

Delusions have been described in a number of neurological disorders. They have to occur in clear consciousness and without significant impairment of cognition for this to be categorised as a secondary psychosis. Although the nature of the delusions varies from patient to patient and to some extent depends on aetiology, delusions are most often persecutory in nature. They may be well organised or fleeting and changeable. Almost any symptom may occur as an associated feature.

The aetiology of delusions is diverse. Drugs are the most common – for example, amphetamines, dopaminomimetics (L dopa, bromocriptine, pergolide), corticosteroids, cannabis and phencyclidine. Amphetamine is the prototypical offender, and given in large amounts over a relatively brief period can lead to psychosis in normal volunteers. CNS disorders such as Huntington's disease, cerebrovascular disease, brain tumours, and multiple sclerosis may be associated with delusions. Psychotic disorders are overrepresented in epileptic patients, in particular those with chronic temporal lobe seizures (discussed later). Other causes are summarised in Box 14.3. Two causes, stimulants and cannabis, are discussed in some detail.

Treatment involves identifying and treating the offending agent or the underlying condition. Short-term symptomatic control may be achieved with neuroleptics.

Stimulant psychosis

A large dose of a stimulant drug can produce a brief psychotic reaction, usually lasting a few hours. This is most commonly seen after intravenous use of methamphetamine or dexamphetamine, but this may be due to the lower doses used orally. The picture resembles an acute paranoid illness and may be indistinguishable from schizophreniform disorder, although a dreamlike quality is often present and there may be an emotional reaction of fear.

The reaction is more likely to occur in those with a previous history of psychotic symptoms. There is some evidence of sensitisation to repeated doses of stimulants, although this remains controversial. The evidence for a more prolonged psychosis after amphetamine use comes from a limited number of human studies but is supported by animal models. It usually occurs in individuals who use high doses repeatedly, often with escalation of the dose. The picture is paranoid-hallucinatory, with visual hallucinations predominating over auditory, and is associated with emotional and autonomic arousal. Formal thought disorder is rare. With the cessation of stimulant use, hallucinations subside in 1 to 2 days, but the delusions may persist for a week or more. However, persistence of symptoms beyond a week after complete urinary clearance of the drug should make one question the aetiological role of stimulants.

The treatment of stimulant psychosis involves abstinence from the drug and the use of antipsychotic medication until symptoms subside. If there is history of more than one episode of psychosis or if the psychosis persists beyond a week, low-dose antipsychotic maintenance for 6 months or more may be advisable. Relapse into drug use should be assertively prevented (Curran *et al.,* 2004).

Cannabis and psychosis

Acute psychosis may rarely occur with cannabis exposure, probably in individuals who are previously vulnerable. The psychosis is usually of paranoid-hallucinatory type, but catatonic features such as negativism, posturing and waxy flexibility may emerge. Affective, usually hypomanic symptoms may be present, and formal thought disorder is usually lacking. The psychosis is short lasting, with a rapid response to antipsychotic drugs, but relapse may occur upon re-exposure to cannabis (McGuire *et al.,* 1994). In the rare case in which the psychosis persists for weeks or months, the question arises whether the patient was already psychotic or pre-psychotic. Cannabis is known to produce short-term exacerbation of pre-existing psychotic

symptoms or precipitate a relapse (Hall & Degenhardt, 2000). There have been a few reports for prolonged depersonalisation after a seemingly brief exposure to cannabis, but these patients are not psychotic. The relationship of chronic cannabis use to prolonged schizophreniform psychosis remains controversial. The five longitudinal studies that have examined this issue concluded that cannabis use in adolescence was associated with an increased risk of schizophrenia in adulthood, after accounting for potential confounding factors. There appears to be a dose-response relationship, and the effect is specific, with rates of depression not consistently being associated with cannabis use. According to one review (Arseneault *et al.,* 2004), cannabis use confers a twofold increase in risk of schizophrenia or schizophreniform disorder (pooled odds ratio = 2.34, confidence interval 1.69–2.95).

Mood disorder due to a general medical condition and substance-induced mood disorder

The clinical phenomenology of this syndrome is similar to that of a primary manic or major depressive episode. Organic factors should be considered and investigated in any patient with depression that is of late onset, atypical in presentation, associated with medical illness or resistant to treatment. Mania is less likely to be secondary in aetiology. The full criteria for one of the affective episodes may not be met; therefore the predominant symptom type may be indicated by using one of the following subtypes: *with depressive features, with major depressive-like episode, with manic features, or with mixed features.*

Depression may be difficult to diagnose in patients with neurological disorder. Many neurological disorders without mood changes are associated with symptoms that are characteristic of depressive episodes – diminished pleasure and interest, weight loss, insomnia, agitation, retardation, fatigue, impaired concentration – and may lead to the misdiagnosis of depression. Experiential manifestations of depression are the most dependable indicators of a depressive syndrome. Patients with dementia may, however, be unable to describe the subjective symptoms, and depression must be inferred from the associated symptoms.

Secondary depression is most commonly caused by toxic or metabolic factors. Medications, especially antihypertensives, are a common aetiology. In fact, no antihypertensive that has a central effect is absolutely safe from this risk. Prior history of depression increases the risk substantially. Other drugs causing depression are corticosteroids, hallucinogens, antipsychotics, amphetamine withdrawal and so on. A number of drugs (corticosteroids, L-dopa, tricyclic and other antidepressants) have been implicated in the triggering of manic episodes, especially in patients with an underlying bipolar illness.

Endocrine disorders are another important aetiological factor. Hypothyroidism commonly presents with depressive symptoms. It is also known to be associated with progressive cognitive decline and frank psychosis. A severely hyperthyroid patient may sometimes resemble a manic patient clinically. The elderly hyperthyroid patient may, on the other hand, appear apathetic and withdrawn, thus creating diagnostic confusion. Major psychiatric disturbances are common in Cushing's syndrome, with depression again being the commonest. Mental disturbances are common in patients on long-term corticosteroids or corticotropin (ACTH), the incidence being related to dose. The most common change observed is euphoria, but mania, depression or delirium may all occur. Depression is commonly associated with cerebrovascular disease (as discussed later) and basal ganglia disorders. The causes of secondary depression and mania are summarised in Table 14.3.

Treatment of secondary depression requires correction of the underlying physiologic abnormality or discontinuation of the offending medication. Depressed mood may nevertheless persist after these efforts, and some patients will also need concurrent antidepressant treatment or electroconvulsive therapy (ECT).

For treatment of secondary mania, neuroleptics may be used to suppress acute symptoms until the

Table 14.3 Medical disorders and substances associated with secondary mood disorder

1. Drugs
   a. Antihypertensives, corticosteroids, and a range of other drugs
   b. Withdrawal from stimulants
   c. Alcohol and sedative-hypnotics abuse
2. Neurologic disorders
   a. Stroke, especially with frontal and basal ganglia involvement
   b. Parkinson's disease and parkinsonism plus syndromes
   c. Epilepsy, especially partial complex
   d. Demyelinating disorders
   e. Alzheimer's disease and other dementias
   f. HIV encephalopathy
   g. Paraneoplastic syndrome (limbic encephalitis)
   h. Brain tumour
3. Endocrine disorders
   a. Hypothyroidism and hyperthyroidism
   b. Adrenal disease (Cushing's disease, Addison's disease)
   c. Parathyroid disorders
4. Infectious diseases
   a. Viral illnesses (hepatitis, influenza), in post-infectious phase
   b. Neurosyphilis
   c. AIDS
   d. Mononucleosis
   e. Chronic fatigue syndrome
5. Autoimmune disorders with vasculitis
   a. Systemic lupus erythematosus
   b. Sjogren's syndrome
   c. Anti-cardiolipin antibody syndrome
6. Other
   a. Malignancy (pancreas, chest, lymphoma)
   b. Deficiencies (vitamin B_{12})
   c. Sleep apnoea
   d. Chronic pain
   e. Migraine

aetiological process is effectively treated. In some cases, the manic process is fairly persistent and may respond to lithium carbonate, carbamazepine, clonazepam or valproate. These agents may also be used in a patient with recurrent episodes.

Depression and Parkinson's disease

Depression is common in Parkinson's disease (PD), with about 50% of PD patients suffering depression at some stage of their illness (Cummings, 1992). The clinical features vary considerably and range from mild dysthymia to severe melancholia. Patients commonly present not with depression, worthlessness or suicidal ideation, but with fatigue, loss of initiative and reduced energy levels. Anxiety and panic symptoms are common. Suicidal ideation is frequently present, but suicide attempts are at a low rate. It is important not to confuse the stooped posture, bradykinesia and masked face of PD for depression, and it is important to enquire about affective and cognitive symptoms. Sleep and appetite disturbances and cognitive slowing are present in the more severe cases. Depression or panic attacks may precede the onset of the motor symptoms of PD in about 30% of cases. The prevalence appears to be greater in younger PD patients, especially women (Poewe & Luginger, 1999).

There has been much speculation on the likely mechanisms of parkinsonian depression. Dysphoria is common in the "off" phase of PD which responds to L-dopa, but dopaminergic drugs do not treat depression in the majority of PD cases. In addition to nigral degeneration, there is a loss of serotonergic neurons in the dorsal raphe and noradrenergic cells in the locus coeruleus, both of which may contribute to depression. The increased incidence of hypothyroidism in PD may also contribute to depression. A high index of suspicion is therefore necessary for depression because it is a potentially treatable cause of worsening of function.

The treatment of depression in PD involves the optimisation of dopaminergic treatment as a first step, although it is not certain that L-dopa has an antidepressant effect. The D2 and D3 receptor agonist pramipexole has been reported to have an antidepressant action, and selegiline may be helpful at higher dosages, at which it probably loses its selectivity for monoamine oxidase-B inhibition. The introduction of an antidepressant, either a tricyclic (TCA) or a selective serotonin reuptake inhibitor (SSRI), is recommended, and most clinicians choose an SSRI, although research studies have been reported more often with TCAs. Orthostatic hypotension, sedation and anticholinergic side effects of TCAs limit their usefulness. In the presence of selegiline, SSRI-induced serotonin syndrome is a consideration, although the reported rate is very low. If a mood stabiliser is used, it is best to select an anticonvulsant over lithium because of potential worsening of PD with the latter. In the presence of sexual dysfunction, nefazodone, bupropion or mirtazapine may be considered. In the more severe or drug-resistant case, ECT is often helpful for both the depression and the PD. Finally, it is important not to neglect psychosocial and psychological aspects, and cognitive therapy has a role in this form of depression (Okun & Watts, 2002).

Catatonic disorder due to a general medical condition

In this disorder, catatonia is judged to be due to the direct physiological effects of a general medical condition. Catatonia is a syndrome of specific motor abnormalities manifested by one or more of the following: motoric immobility (posturing, waxy flexibility, stupor), excessive motor activity (catatonic excitement), extreme negativism, mutism, peculiarities of voluntary movement (mannerisms, opposition, gegenhalten, ambitendence), echolalia or echopraxia. It is associated with disturbance of thought and cognition.

A variety of medical conditions may cause catatonia, especially neurological (e.g. neoplasms, head trauma, cerebrovascular disease, encephalitis, epilepsy) and metabolic conditions (e.g. hypercalcaemia, hepatic encephalopathy, homocystinuria, diabetic ketoacidosis). Patterns of prevalence and onset reflect those of the aetiological conditions. In the differential diagnosis, it is important to consider neuroleptic-induced movement disorders, including neuroleptic malignant syndrome, catatonic schizophrenia, and mood disorder with catatonic features. In childhood, catatonia can occur in association with autism, Prader-Willi syndrome and mental retardation. Fink and Taylor (2003) provided a comprehensive account of the aetiology of catatonia. Acute catatonia is usually treatable, regardless of aetiology, although the treatment algorithm will vary. Benzodiazepines and ECT are the main modalities of treatment. Because of the complex relationship of neuroleptic drugs with catatonia, it is important to be cautious about their use in this condition.

The syndrome of malignant catatonia is characterised by fever, muscle rigidity and autonomic instability and can be fatal if not treated promptly. It is indistinguishable from neuroleptic malignant syndrome in its presentation and should not be treated with neuroleptic drugs. ECT is the treatment of choice.

Anxiety disorder due to a general medical condition or substance-induced anxiety disorder

The essential feature is the presence of clinically significant anxiety judged to be directly due to the physiological effects of a general medical condition or substance. Symptoms can include prominent *generalised anxiety symptoms, panic attacks, social phobia or obsessions and compulsions*. The diagnosis is not made if the anxiety occurs only during the course of delirium.

Endocrine disorders or the use of psychoactive substances usually cause generalised anxiety and panic. Examples of such endocrine disorders are hyper and hypothyroidism, phaeochromocytoma, fasting hypoglycaemia and hypercortisolism. It is commonly caused by intoxication from substances such as caffeine, cocaine or amphetamines or from withdrawal from substances that depress the CNS, such as alcohol and sedatives. Brain tumours in the vicinity of the third ventricle, trauma, cerebrovascular disease, migraine, encephalitis, multiple sclerosis, Parkinson's disease, Huntington's disease, Wilson's disease, and epilepsy involving the diencephalon are unusual but established aetiologies. Other aetiological factors may include pulmonary embolus, chronic obstructive pulmonary disease, aspirin tolerance, collagen-vascular disease

---

> **Box 14.4** Medical causes of obsessive-compulsive symptoms
>
> Tourette's disorder
> Sydenham's chorea
> Parkinson's disease during "on" period
> Postencephalitic parkinsonism
> Progressive supranuclear palsy
> Huntington's disease
> Neuroacanthocytosis
> Carbon monoxide poisoning or anoxia (with bilateral caudate or pallidal lesions)
> Manganese intoxication
> Acute dystonic reactions with oculogyric crises

---

and brucellosis. Vitamin B_{12} deficiency, demyelinating disease and heavy metal intoxication are less likely to present with anxiety as the only symptom, but this can occur.

Lesions of the basal ganglia and frontal cortex often cause obsessive-compulsive symptoms. Obsessive compulsive disorder (OCD) has important associations with Tourette's syndrome, Sydenham's chorea, anoxic injury to the basal ganglia, postencephalitic parkinsonism, neuroacanthocytosis and other basal ganglia disorders. The relationship of OCD with Tourette's syndrome is discussed later. A summary of organic causes of obsessive-compulsive symptoms is presented in Box 14.4.

Treatment requires attention to the underlying condition, as well as to the anxiety symptoms. When pharmacological agents are indicated, conventional anxiolytics and β-receptor antagonists are used. Obsessive-compulsive symptoms are treated with behavioural therapy and serotonin reuptake inhibitors.

Personality change due to a general medical condition

This syndrome designates a change in personality style or traits manifested primarily by reduced drive or by an impaired control of behavioural expression of emotions or impulses or both. There must be evidence of a general medical condition antedating the onset of the syndrome and judged to be causally significant for its occurrence. There should be no clouding of consciousness, significant loss of intellectual abilities, predominant mood disturbance or predominant delusions or hallucinations.

Depending on the predominant symptomatology, DSM-IV suggests the following subtypes: *labile type, disinhibited type, aggressive type, apathetic type, paranoid type, other or combined.*

The most common association is with focal lesions of the brain and in endocrine disorders (hypothyroidism, hypo- and hyperadrenocorticism). Head trauma is an important cause. Subarachnoid haemorrhage, especially with anterior communicating artery aneurysm, is another significant cause. Brain tumours may induce the syndrome, although the overall incidence is low. Its occurrence with temporal lobe epilepsy has been extensively debated, and a syndrome known as Geschwind's syndrome (hypergraphia, circumstantiality, interpersonal viscosity, hyperreligiosity and hyposexuality) has been described. Its occurrence as a consequence of chronic drug use is open to question.

The clinical features depend principally on the nature and localisation of the pathological process. A common pattern is characterised by emotional lability and impairment in impulse control and social judgment. The individual may be belligerent or have temper outbursts and sudden bouts of crying with little or no provocation. Euphoria may mimic hypomania, although the patient usually does not report being happy. Socially inappropriate actions, such as sexual indiscretions, may be engaged in with little concern for the consequences. Inappropriate jocularity and facetiousness (*witzelsucht*), a coarse manner and even frank antisociality may occur. Another pattern is characterised by marked indifference and apathy. The individual may have no interest in his or her usual hobbies and appear unconcerned with events occurring in the immediate environment. Both of these patterns may be associated with damage to the frontal lobes

(the former with orbitomedial lesions, and the latter with dorsolateral prefrontal lesions), and for this reason are sometimes referred to as *frontal lobe syndromes*. Another recognised pattern, seen in some individuals with temporal lobe epilepsy, is a marked tendency to humourless verbosity in writing and speech, religiosity and, occasionally, exaggerated aggressiveness. A common pattern also is the development of suspiciousness or paranoid ideation not amounting to delusions.

Associated features include mild disorders of cognitive function often coexist, such as inattention and mild memory impairment. Irritability and suspiciousness are often present.

Course and prognosis depend on the cause. It may be transient, if it is the result of chronic intoxication, for example, or persistent if it is secondary to structural damage to the brain. It may be succeeded by dementia in cases of brain tumour or Huntington's chorea. Some patients require custodial care or, at least, close supervision to meet their basic needs or to prevent adverse consequences of their impulsivity and inappropriateness. Their behaviour may lead to social ostracism or legal difficulties.

Treatment considerations include treating the underlying condition if possible. Psychopharmacological treatment of the symptoms may be indicated in some cases. Drugs tried include TCA or SSRI antidepressants for organic emotionality and SSRIs, lithium, carbamazepine and propranolol for aggressiveness. The efficacy of drugs has not been sufficiently demonstrated. The patient will usually need counselling; a change in job or even premature retirement may be necessary. The family may need support and concrete advice on how to minimise the patient's tendency to undesirable conduct.

Cognitive disorders

The patient presents with a clinically significant disturbance in cognition that is a change from a previous level of functioning, due to either a general medical condition or a substance or to a combination of factors. If the primary aetiology is not identifiable, there is a strong presumptive evidence of its existence. The disturbance may be related to a number of cognitive domains or restricted to a single domain. Disturbance in multiple domains may occur in clear consciousness (dementia) or with disturbance of consciousness (delirium). Abnormalities of single cognitive domain may involve memory (amnestic syndrome), language (dysphasia), praxis (apraxia) and so on.

Dementia

The general aspects of dementia, including the approach to diagnosis and treatment, are discussed in Chapter 15 and elsewhere (see Ritchie & Lovestone, 2002). The commonest cause of dementia in Western societies is Alzheimer's disease (AD), accounting for about 50% of cases, and is discussed elsewhere in this book. Other common subtypes are vascular dementia (VaD), dementia with Lewy bodies (DLB) and front-temporal dementia (FTDX), which are not discussed here (see Qizilbash, 2002). There are many other causes of dementia that need to be considered in the evaluation of any patient with cognitive decline, and only a few of the non-Alzheimer causes of dementia are discussed briefly here. The early "at-risk" stage of dementia has been referred to as *mild cognitive impairment* (MCI), the definition and accurate delineation of which is undergoing much investigation (Nestor *et al.*, 2004). Causes of dementia, as well as relative frequencies, are shown in Box 14.5.

Early-onset dementia

Dementia before age 65 years is common but still poses a significant challenge to a neuropsychiatrist (Sampson *et al.*, 2004). Data on the prevalence of early-onset dementia (EOD) are incomplete, and reliable figures are not available. Rates varying from 30 to 300 per 100,000 have been reported (Harvey, 2001). About one third of early-onset cases are due to AD, with VaD and FTD being about

---

Box 14.5 Causes of dementia (with commonly accepted relative frequencies)

Alzheimer's disease 50%

Vascular dementia 15%

Mixed Alzheimer's/vascular 20%

Lewy body dementia 17%

Frontal dementias (Pick's/non-Pick's) <15%

Subcortical dementias 4%
>   Progressive supranuclear palsy
>   Huntington's disease
>   Parkinson's disease

Alcohol 6%

Normal pressure hydrocephalus 5%

Trauma, anoxia, infections 3%

Prion disease 2%

---

half as prevalent. DLB is rare in this age group. In the very young, Huntington's disease is an important cause. Prion diseases and dementia of multiple sclerosis (4/100,000) are special cases. Dementia in Down's syndrome is usually of early onset, with rates of 3.4% in the 30s to 40% in the 50- to 59-year age group being reported (Harvey, 2001). EODs are often rapidly progressive and have a high mortality rate. Neuropsychiatric symptoms such as mood disturbance, anxiety, psychosis, personality change and agitation are common and important in the treatment.

Familial Alzheimer's disease

A small proportion of early-onset AD has a family history of dementia with an autosomal pattern. In some of these cases, point mutations have been identified. Mutations of the amyloid precursor protein (APP) gene on chromosome 21 have been reported in about 20 families around the world. The age of onset in this group is about 50 to 55 years, and the clinical picture is fairly typical of AD. The most common genetic form of familial AD is due to the presenilin 1 (PS1) gene mutation on chromosome 14, which is often associated with onset before 40 years. Another mutation, affecting the presenilin 2 gene on chromosome 1, is much rarer. A gene that is a risk factor for both familial and sporadic AD is apolipoprotein E4 allele (Nussbaum & Ellis, 2003).

Fronto-temporal dementias

A proportion of patients presenting in their 50s with dementia do not have the typical picture of cognitive impairment seen in Alzheimer's disease but show behavioural and personality changes generally of insidious onset which may strongly suggest the presence of a depressive disorder or frontal lobe lesion. Some of the group will be shown at post-mortem to have Pick bodies (cytoplasmic basophilic inclusions), but many will have quite nonspecific appearances. These patients have been characterised as the fronto-temporal dementias which neuropathologically are Pick's disease, non-Alzheimer non-Pick's frontal dementia, striatonigral degeneration, corticobasal ganglionic degeneration, hereditary dysphasic dementia, motor neuron disease with dementia and progressive subcortical gliosis. About one third of frontotemporal dementia cases have a family history, and in some of these, a tau gene mutation on chromosome 17 has been identified.

The characteristic features of this group are personality deterioration and behavioural change with apathy, reduced initiative and lack of concern, socially inappropriate actions and disinhibition, a poverty of ideation, poor planning and organisational skills, variable verbal fluency and memory impairment but intact visuospatial function. Additionally, hypochondriacal, obsessional and paranoid symptoms along with hyperphagia, restlessness and distractibility will be seen. There may be two broad groupings with one showing slowness, apathy and adynamia and the other restlessness, overactivity, distractibility and disinhibition. Pathology predominantly affecting the dominant hemisphere will show aphasia as the first severe clinical abnormality.

Neurological signs are generally absent in the early stages, but frontal release signs become evident with progression along with a range of signs, including parkinsonism and rigidity, autonomic abnormalities, dyspraxic features and dystonia, tremor, dysarthria and eye movement disorder. In the Neary *et al.* (1990) series, the mean age of onset was 54 years, and there was no excess of females. Of interest was the fact that a family history of dementia was obtained in 46% of first-degree relatives, in contrast to the 13% of cases with Alzheimer's disease. They estimated that the group of frontal dementias as a whole account for between 15% and 20% of all presenile dementias. The diagnosis is supported by neuroimaging, with structural imaging (CT and MRI) showing frontal and temporal lobe atrophy, which may be asymmetric. Structural imaging may, however, be normal in the early stages, and functional imaging with SPECT or PET may be helpful to detect early abnormality.

Some distinct subsyndromes have been described in fronto-temporal dementia. In semantic dementia, patients lose memory of words, whereas their speech remains fluent with normal syntax. Abilities such as episodic memory, nonverbal reasoning and visuospatial function are preserved. It is associated with striking anterolateral temporal lobe atrophy, usually more on the left side. The mirror image of semantic dementia is progressive nonfluent aphasia in which the phonologic and syntactic aspects of speech are progressively affected. This is associated with perisylvian brain atrophy (Mesulam *et al.*, 2003).

Subcortical dementias

The concept of subcortical dementia is not universally accepted but serves to identify a number of dementing disorders lacking the features of cortical deficits such as aphasia, agnosia and apraxia so clearly seen in Alzheimer's disease. The characteristic features are memory disorder, poor attention, slowed speed of information processing, poor verbal fluency, impaired organisational and planning performance and abnormal visuospatial skills. The three principal members of the group are progressive supranuclear palsy (PSP; Steele-Richardson-Olszewski syndrome), Huntington's disease and Parkinson's disease.

Progressive supranuclear palsy

This is a progressive dementing syndrome with fairly characteristic neurological features. Patients usually present with the provisional diagnosis of Parkinson plus syndrome. The picture is distinct and includes axial rigidity with an erect posture and often tell-tale food stains on the front of the patient's shirt or dress rather than the stooped flexed posture of Parkinson's disease; there is an eye movement disorder with reduction in down-gaze initially and then impaired up-gaze, and a frequent history of falls. Pseudobulbar palsy, mask like facies, brisk jaw jerk and palatal and pharyngeal reflexes, dysphagia and dysarthria are also noted. PSP is more common in men, with an onset usually in the 50s to 60s with duration of illness of 5 to 7 years.

Huntington's disease

This is a progressive degenerative disorder with alterations of behaviour, cognitive function and movement. The disease is an autosomal-dominant disorder with the responsible gene IT-15 located on the short arm of chromosome 4 and encoding for the protein huntingtin. Since 1993, it has been possible to identify at-risk subjects by determining the number of CAG trinucleotide repeats, less than 34 having no risk, those with 34 to 40 having an intermediate risk and those with 41 and above clearly being expected to develop the disease. The Huntington's disease gene is considered specific, and the genetic test can be used for diagnosis, to inform a healthy person about future risk and to assess the risk of a foetus.

The average age of onset is 42 years, but there is a wide range on either side of this with the disease sometimes developing before 10 years or after 80 years. Anticipation is found to occur, with successive generations tending to show an increase in the number of trinucleotide repeats, and an earlier age of onset is associated with paternal transmission. Higher numbers of repeats have an association with an earlier age of onset and a shorter course of the disease, which would generally run for a period of 10 to 12 years, but cases are seen in which the history has extended over 20 years.

An association with affective disorder is noted, and this may precede the onset of the disease by several years, often being associated with features of irritability. When established, the disease also has some association with the development of schizophrenia.

Early movement abnormalities include hypometric saccades, interrupted pursuit eye movements, tongue persistence, impaired rapid alternating movements and akathisia. The typical movement disorder is a progressive choreiform and choreoathetoid pattern of irregular involuntary movements affecting the proximal and peripheral limbs, the face and tongue, and swallowing and speech can become significantly affected, raising the risk of aspiration. In the later stages of the disease, movements will often be much reduced, and patients will generally die from the effects of infection, progressive wasting and cardiac failure.

The dementia is subcortical in type, and memory is often relatively well preserved in the earlier stages, with major difficulties lying in the areas of frontal executive function, planning and organisational tasks, motor and cognitive speed and attention. The dementia may on occasions be the presenting feature, but the movement disorder will usually become apparent within a few years. There is good evidence that behavioural and cognitive abnormalities, as well as reduced brain metabolism on PET scanning, especially in the caudate, are abnormal for long periods before diagnosis, which may be up to 10 years.

The pathology is centred on the caudate nuclei and putamen, with severe neuronal loss and gliosis, but also involves the deeper layers of cerebral cortex. There is a selective loss of gamma-aminobutyric acid-A (GABBA)- and enkephalin- containing cells, which may explain the motor symptoms. Atrophy of the caudate nuclei along with cerebral atrophy is shown on imaging as the process becomes widespread.

There is at present no specific treatment for the disease, and symptomatic measures are all that is possible (Gardian & Vecsei, 2004). Several drugs to delay the onset and slow progression have been developed in animal models and are presently undergoing therapeutic trials.

Parkinson's disease

Current opinion suggests that dementia is increased threefold in the population with Parkinson's disease, generally in the elderly with a later age of onset and in those with rapid disease progression. Figures of 9.4% to 10.9% have been reported, with 4-year follow-up suggesting a figure of 19%. The pattern is that of a subcortical dementia with impairment in frontal executive function with planning and organisation; visuospatial functions are impaired along with speed of information processing, verbal fluency and memory tasks. In a proportion of cases, there are associated deficits suggesting cortical involvement with aphasia, agnosia and apraxia, and an association with AD exists. Again, in this population the overlap with DLB and AD becomes important (Lauterbach, 2004).

Alcohol

Alcohol is considered to be a significant factor in the presentation of about 6% of subjects with dementia, although rates of alcohol abuse are much higher in individuals attending memory clinics (Oslin *et al.*, 1998). Some investigators have cast doubt on the presence of a true alcohol-related dementia (ARD), stating that the reported cases suffer from Wernicke-Korsakoff syndrome, Marchiafava-Bignami, pellagrous encephalopathy or acquired hepatocerebral degeneration (Victor, 1994). Associated factors include those of thiamine deficiency, metabolic disorder (a low-grade hepatic encephalopathy), nutritional deficiencies and a history of head injury,

which make attribution difficult. However, alcohol-related cerebral pathology not due to Wernicke's encephalopathy has been reported, which includes general cerebral atrophy with neuronal loss and neuroglial proliferation, thinning of the corpus callosum and changes in the cerebellum (Harper & Kril, 1985).

Reports of alcoholic dementia refer to a general cognitive impairment but an absence of language disturbance, and features of frontal lobe impairment with affective blunting and poor organisational and planning abilities are prominent. A prolonged period (>5 years) of heavy alcohol abuse (≥5 standard drinks per day for men and ≥4 drinks for women) is generally necessary (Oslin *et al.*, 1998). A period of abstinence will lead to a measure of improvement over time, suggesting that at least a portion of this dementia may be reversible. The structural brain abnormalities on CT scanning are also partially reversible with abstinence. The basis of this reversibility is uncertain and may be due to rehydration of the brain or due to increased protein synthesis and dendritic growth following the cessation of alcohol.

Normal pressure hydrocephalus

This disorder may account for up to 5% of subjects presenting with dementia. It is of particular interest because it remains one of the few dementing syndromes that are potentially reversible. Patients usually present in their 60s and 70s with the triad of progressive dementing syndrome, gait disorder and sphincteric disturbance (urinary incontinence). The dementing syndrome may develop over a few months with prominent memory difficulties and a slowing of mental processing, initially suggestive of depression in some cases. More widespread deficits become apparent, and there may ultimately be a catatonic-like picture. In a proportion of patients, one sees episodes of confusion superimposed on the dementing syndrome. The gait disorder is characterised by small zigzag steps and a tendency to repeated falls and difficulty turning. Spasticity and extensor plantar reflexes may be encountered late in the course of the disorder. The underlying pathology may include former subarachnoid haemorrhage, traumatic brain injury and meningitis; in a significant number, no identifiable pathology is found.

Investigation by CT scanning will reveal the ballooning of the anterior horns of the lateral ventricles, often with periventricular lucency. Further diagnostic help may be provided by lumbar puncture in which 20 to 30 mL of CSF is drained, and the patient may show a recognisable improvement in symptomatology. CSF monitoring over 24 hours is another useful procedure to help identify patients suitable for shunting.

Treatment involves the introduction of a ventriculoperitoneal or ventriculoatrial shunt into the right lateral ventricle, with a favourable outcome being evident in a few weeks in about 40% of cases. However, the presence, severity and duration of dementia are associated with poorer outcome after shunting. Systematic long-term outcome studies have not been conducted.

Trauma, anoxia and infection

In this group is included the traumatic brain injury associated with motor vehicle accidents, the group surviving anoxic episodes secondary to cardiac arrest, hypoglycaemic coma, drowning or asphyxiation, and those with the results of acute encephalitis, neurosyphilis or HIV/AIDS. The group accounts for perhaps 3% of the total population with dementia. Chronic traumatic encephalopathy (*dementia pugilistica*) has been described in professional boxers who have had multiple bouts and suffered repeated head blows (Mendez, 1995).

Prion diseases

The transmissible spongiform encephalopathies, now referred to as prion diseases, include both human and animal forms. The field has become particularly significant in recent times with the suggestion of transmissibility across species, humans developing a variant of Creutzfeldt Jakob disease by transmission of an abnormal prion protein (PrP)

from animals with bovine spongiform encephalopathy (BSE) or "mad cow disease". The human forms are Creutzfeldt Jakob disease (CJD), Gerstmann Straussler Sheinker (GSS) disease and Kuru. The animal forms of prion disease include scrapie in sheep and goats, mink encephalopathy and BSE.

Creutzfeldt Jakob disease

In humans most cases are sporadic, but about 15% of cases have a positive family history, and an iatrogenic form has been identified in which transmission of the abnormal protein has been through neurosurgical procedures, dural grafts, human growth hormone extracts and also corneal transplants. Familial CJD has been related to several mutations on the short arm of chromosome 20. The disease is rare with about one case per million generally being quoted, but this may well be a conservative estimate. There is a rapid course with 75% of cases dying within 12 months. Both sexes are equally affected, and the age of onset is generally in the 60s.

The clinical presentation is with a rapidly progressive dementing picture, sometimes appearing almost that of a confusional state, but a prodrome with anergia, anxiety and depressive features may be seen in some cases, leading to death in 4 to 12 months. Psychotic symptoms are seen quite frequently, and the neurological picture is one of ataxia with motor weakness and rigidity, cortical blindness, myoclonic jerks, dysarthria and sometimes seizures. The clinical picture may be put into a number of subvarieties depending on the predominant neurological features. The hallmark neuropathological lesion is spongiform degeneration of neurones and their processes, seen as vacuoles in the neuropil. Immunohistochemistry displays deposition of a protease-resistant prion protein in association with the vacuoles.

Of major concern has been the development in humans of a *variant* of CJD (*variant CJD*) in the animal form of BSE in the United Kingdom. A major outbreak of BSE occurred in 1986, and around 10 years later a number of cases of variant CJD began to be reported with a much younger age of onset of the disease, a prominent presentation with psychiatric symptomatology and a more protracted history.

Delirium

Delirium (from Latin, *delirio*: "I rave") is one of the commonest neuropsychiatric syndromes encountered by physicians and surgeons, and its prompt detection and management is vitally important. Unfortunately, it is frequently undiagnosed or misdiagnosed as dementia or psychosis. Its onset usually heralds physical illness and calls for immediate medical attention. There are many terms used synonymously with delirium (acute confusional disorder, acute brain syndrome, toxic or metabolic encephalopathy, toxic psychosis, etc.), but it is best to restrict this usage to the term *delirium* to represent a transient global cognitive impairment of presumed organic aetiology. The diagnostic criteria based on DSM-IV are shown in Box 14.6.

Prevalence

Prevalence of delirium is estimated to be about 1% in the general population but much higher in hospitalised patients, with rates of 5% to 15% in acute medical and surgical admissions. The rates in hospitalised elderly (>65 years) may be as high as 35%. The incidence in surgical intensive care units has been reported to range from 18% to 30%.

Risk factors

The extremes of age are particularly vulnerable, with children being affected when suffering febrile illness and the elderly being most vulnerable to the effects of intercurrent infections or medication mismanagement. The presence of dementia raises the risk of delirium, with 40% of demented subjects being confused or delirious on admission. A quarter of the confusional states turn out to be

---

Box 14.6 Diagnostic criteria for delirium

Disturbance of consciousness (reduced clarity of awareness of environment) with reduced ability to focus, sustain and/or shift attention

Change in cognition (memory deficit, disorientation, language disturbance) or development of a perceptual disturbance not better accounted for by pre-existing, established or evolving dementia

Disturbance develops over a short period of time (hours to days) and fluctuates during the course of the day

D1. Evidence from history, physical examination and laboratory findings that the disturbance is caused by the direct physiological consequences of a general medical condition

or

D2. 1. Symptoms in A and B developed during substance intoxication

Medication used is aetiologically related to the disturbance

or

D3. Symptoms in A and B developed during or shortly after a withdrawal syndrome

or

D4. The delirium has more than one aetiology

---

associated with dementia. Depression, acute psychological stress, sleep or sensory deprivation and bereavement increase the risk of delirium. The presence of brain damage, drug or alcohol dependence and impairment in hearing or vision will be relevant in many patients.

Clinical features

Delirium is typically of acute onset, developing over several hours to about 3 days depending on the aetiology. The picture varies during the course of the day and features are often most prominent towards the evening. The duration may be just a day or so or may be prolonged for up to 3 or 4 weeks with a gradual resolution depending on the speed of diagnosis and correction of the underlying pathology.

Clouding of consciousness, shown by reduced alertness and awareness, impaired arousal and particular difficulties with attention, manifest as distractibility and an inability to sustain focused attention, are the hallmarks of the disorder. These may at times be difficult to identify in the milder forms, and there is the impression of a slowed or laboured performance with the patient experiencing difficulty in grasping elements of the admission process and interview. There is often a disorder in the sleep-wake cycle with the individual appearing somnolent during the day, only to become increasingly restless and agitated as night-time approaches. Psychomotor activity may range from apathy and inactivity to restlessness with picking at bedclothes and objects and also marked agitation with hyperactivity and sometimes physical aggression. The whole picture may fluctuate during the course of a day.

Cognition is impaired with often fragmentary and erratic performance, poor registration of information and faulty recall and disorientation particularly of time and place. Language function may be impaired for naming, and paraphasias may occur. Thinking will often be markedly disturbed with rambling, circumstantial and repetitious or irrelevant and disorganised content. Formal thought disorder may be seen, and poorly organised, transient paranoid and persecutory delusional beliefs are present in up to 50% of patients.

Perceptual change is common, with misperceptions, illusions and hallucinations, particularly of visual type, reported in up to 60% of cases. Affective responses are varied, and although will appear almost indifferent to their state, many patients communicate considerable anxiety, agitation, fear, anger or depression and, rarely, a sense of elation.

Differential diagnosis

A common clinical concern is whether the patient has a dementia or a dementia complicated by a secondary delirium. A detailed history with additional information from the family members is critical at such times. An acute psychotic disorder, schizophrenia, agitated depression and sometimes a manic disorder can be mistaken for delirium or vice versa, and it may only be the result of careful observation, examination and extensive investigations that will clarify matters (Rummans *et al.*, 1995).

Investigations

All patients will require a set of investigations, tailored somewhat to the particular leads obtained from the history and physical examination. The following would generally be considered: full blood count and blood film, erythrocyte sedimentation rate, liver function tests, drug assays, urine test, blood cultures, electroencephalograph, electrolytes, blood sugar, urinary drug screen, CSF examination, blood gases, CT scans and chest X-rays. Specialised investigations may be necessary.

Aetiology

It is important to treat delirium as an acute emergency, because the longer the delay the greater is the likely morbidity and risk of death. Physicians and nurses must have a high index of suspicion (Dyer *et al.*, 1995). Every effort should be made to identify the underlying pathology, which is possible in 80% to 95% of cases. Although the possibilities are numerous, it is valuable to have a ready list of the more common causes to consider at the bedside. A useful approach is an adaptation of Gallant's mnemonic "DELIRIUM" (Table 14.4).

Management

The general principle is that the primary cause be identified and treated, but it is important to remember that the treatment itself may potentially compound the problem if not carefully considered. The possibility of drug interactions must always be kept in mind.

Table 14.4 Causes of delirium

1. Drugs
   a. Intoxications / withdrawal of alcohol, benzodiazepines, barbiturates, narcotics
   b. Anticholinergic drugs (atropine, benztropine, benzhexol); anticholinergic effects of neuroleptics and tricyclic antidepressants
   c. Antihistamines
   d. Anticonvulsants (phenytoin, carbamazepine, clonazepam, valproate, vigabatrin)
   e. Antiparkinson drugs (amantadine, L dopa, bromocriptine)
   f. Cardiac drugs (β-blockers, digoxin, theophylline, diuretics, hypotensives)
   g. Anti-inflammatory drugs (non-steroidal drugs, steroids)
   h. Sympathomimetics (ephedrine, amphetamines)
   i. Antibiotics
   j. Antineoplastic drugs
   k. Others (e.g., chlorpropamide, cimetidine, ranitidine, lithium, metrizamide)
2. Endocrine
   Diabetes; thyroid, parathyroid or adrenal dysfunction
3. Epilepsy
   Ictal or post-ictal states
4. Lung disease
   Pneumonia, chronic obstructive airways disease, sleep apnoea
5. Infection
   Encephalitis, meningitis, syphilis, human immunodeficiency virus, septicaemia
6. Injury
   Concussion, subdural, extradural haemorrhage, burns, general and cardiac surgery, fracture neck of femur
7. Intracranial
   Tumour, raised intracranial pressure
8. Renal
   Acute and chronic end-stage failure
9. Intestinal
   Carcinoma, obstruction, ileus
10. Unstable circulation
    Arrhythmia's, congestive cardiac failure, myocardial infarction, congestive heart failure, hypertensive encephalopathy, hypoperfusion, blood loss, shock
11. Metabolic
    Hyponatraemia, hypokalaemia, acidosis / alkalosis, hepatic failure, dehydration

Some general measures to support the delirious patient deserve attention, and these include attention to hydration, nutrition, ventilation, temperature control, skin care to prevent decubitus ulcers, physiotherapy and so on. An optimal sensory, social and nursing environment must be provided, and this may include a well-lighted room, dim light at night, a calendar and clock, a radio or television for sensory stimulation, familiar nurses in attendance and visits of close family and friends. Reorientation, the provision of simple information, careful observation and the prevention of accidents and injury are all important.

Management of an agitated, restless or fearful patient can be challenging. If at all possible, restraint should be minimised because it often serves to further agitate the patient. Shackles should not be used, and tying the patient to the bed with a sheet or to a chair is potentially dangerous. If necessary, a proper restraining jacket should be used. When intravenous or central lines, catheters or nasogastric tubes are in place and their forcible removal by the patient could potentially cause injury, the hands may be loosely bandaged or back slabs applied to the arms. Sometimes drug treatment for the management of agitation may be necessary. A high-potency neuroleptic, such as haloperidol, is safe in such situations. Depending on the patient's weight, age and physical condition, the initial dose of haloperidol may vary from 0.5 to 5 mg intramuscularly, to be repeated hourly if the patient continues to be agitated. When the patient is calm, oral medication, usually in divided doses, should be substituted. Other neuroleptics have been used, and the use of benzodiazepines in delirium also has its proponents. Excess sedation has the potential of worsening the delirium, however. After the confusion has cleared, the medication may be continued for 3 to 5 days.

Review

Regular review is an essential part of the overall management of the delirious patient who carries the added risk of intercurrent infection, dehydration or anaemia and other concerns. When the delirium has resolved, considerable reassurance and support may be required to deal with the often fragmented and frightening recollections the patient may have of the period of delirium. It is advisable in the elderly to pay particular attention to a review of the cognitive status to ensure that there is no underlying dementia.

Neuropsychiatric aspects of cerebrovascular disease

Cerebrovascular disease (CVD) follows ischaemic heart disease and cancer as the third leading cause of death over the age of 50 years. Stroke patients often experience a catastrophic decline in physical, sensory or language ability, as well as neuropsychiatric consequences such as cognitive, mood, behavioural and personality changes. The resulting loss of independence and disability often results in grief and anxiety syndromes and significant stress for caregivers.

Major depression is common in stroke patients, and prevalence rates of 10% to 34% after a stroke have been reported, with the depression most likely to occur 6 months to 2 years after the stroke. The features of the condition are largely the same as for a major depressive episode without stroke. However, owing to language problems, vegetative symptoms and problems in emotional expression directly related to the stroke, diagnosis may be difficult. Reliance on subjective report of depression and the cognitive symptoms of depression must be supplemented by a high index of suspicion in patients showing decline in function after an initial recovery from stroke. Post-stroke depression has been attributed to loss of function because of the stroke, associated vascular cognitive impairment, the occurrence of a life-threatening event or the direct involvement of the mood-related brain regions. In this context, there has been controversy on the relationship of depression to infarction in particular brain regions. There is some evidence that patients with cortical strokes closer to the frontal lobes, and particularly left anterior cortical infarcts, may have an increased incidence of depression, although the evidence for this has been disputed (Carson *et al.*, 2000; Narushima *et al.*, 2003). An association of depression with basal ganglia lesions has also been reported (Steffens *et al.*, 2002). Correct diagnosis and treatment are important because the presence of depression worsens the patient's prognosis and prolongs disability. Distinguishing depression from apathy and abulia may be difficult, and post-stroke emotionalism may be mistaken for depression. Because a psychiatrist may not be available on a stroke unit, the routine use of screening instruments such as the Hospital Anxiety and Depression Scale of the General Health Questionnaire have been recommended so that appropriate referral can occur. Treatment is as for major depression in general, with the recognition that the patient may be more sensitive to medication side effects. The use of antidepressant drugs prophylactically has not received much support in trials, but supportive psychotherapy had a significant but small protective effect. One recent trial argued for early treatment with an antidepressant in the first month after the stroke. Although biological causation has been suggested for post-stroke depression, it is important not to disregard the significant psychological and social occupational effects of the stroke on the individual and his or her family that may be relevant in causing or maintaining depression.

Lability of affect or pathological laughing and crying is common in stroke patients. Usually it takes the form of the patient crying inappropriately and precipitously to minimal or no emotional cues. The patient often has insight and finds the symptom embarrassing and distressing. The disorder usually decreases in intensity with time and may be amplified by major depression but should not be mistaken for the latter in the absence of other features of depression. Some patients respond to treatment with a tricyclic antidepressant (usually imipramine or amitriptyline at dosages of 25–57 mg/day) or an SSRI.

An *apathetic syndrome*, involving the loss of interest, motivation and concern, may also occur and can be differentiated from major depression by the patient denying a depressed mood and sleep and appetite remaining intact. The patient may also demonstrate a lack of awareness of one side of his or her body or visual field (hemineglect) or indifference to physical disability (anosognosia). These syndromes are more likely to arise after parietal lobe infarction, particularly of the right hemisphere. Personality changes post-stroke are common and may take the form of apathy, impulsivity, aggression or coarsening of previous personality traits. An inability to perceive or express emotion (aprosodia) can be the consequence of strokes of the frontal and temporoparietal regions of the right hemisphere in the areas that correspond to Broca and Wernicke's language areas of the dominant hemisphere.

Mania occurring for the first time after stroke is rare but may arise after a subcortical stroke in the limbic areas. Bipolar disorder may occur de novo; in these cases there is an increased prevalence of depression before the stroke and a family history of bipolar disorder.

Psychosis occurring after stroke in the absence of cognitive impairment is rare. However, in vascular dementia, delusions (usually persecutory) and hallucinations can occur in up to 50% of individuals. It can be part of the "sun-downing syndrome", in which the patient with dementia tends to become more confused in the evening or as a feature of delirium. Late-onset schizophrenia has been linked to small vessel disease in some instances, although the reports are not completely consistent (Figure 14.1).

The concept of vascular depression

The high prevalence of depression in stroke patients and the report of white matter disease and basal ganglia vascular abnormality in late-onset depression (LOD) has prompted much discussion on a neurological subtype of depression which is secondary to vascular disease. Criteria for this syndrome have been proposed and the concept defended from different perspectives (Alexopoulos *et al.*, 1997; Steffens & Krishnan, 1998). The relationship between vascular disease and depression is complex, however, and a simple aetiological model of vascular disease causing depression may be too simplistic. Studies of the relationship between vascular disease and depression do not often take all confounding factors into consideration, including the mediating role of physical ill health in general (Jorm *et al.*, 2005). Moreover, depression is known to worsen vascular disease, reversing the direction of the relationship. There may also be common pathophysiological factors such as inflammation (Baldwin, 2005). The concept therefore needs further critical appraisal.

Neuropsychiatric aspects of HIV infection and AIDS

The effects of HIV infection on the individual are diverse and reflect the multiple mechanisms of pathophysiology involved with the disease. HIV invades brain tissue soon after infection and the later immunological compromise of AIDS can lead to secondary brain involvement due to infection, neoplastic infiltration or vascular complications. The patient must also adjust to the consequences of a serious physical illness, deal with the responses of relatives and suffer the impact of social stigma. Predisposing personality disorders or psychoactive substance abuse may interact with the expression of neuropsychiatric disorders (see Box 14.7).

The evidence whether mild cognitive impairment is present soon after acute HIV seroconversion is conflicting, but up to 70% of HIV-positive individuals demonstrate neuro-cognitive deficits in the late stages of the disease. HIV-associated dementia (HAD) has a cumulative prevalence of 25% to 60% until the time of death and is an AIDS-defining condition. This is a subcortical dementia involving HIV infection of the deep white matter and basal ganglia, resulting in personality change as well as a slowing

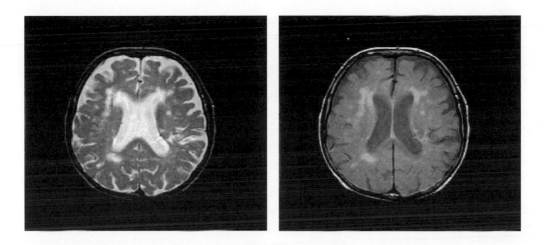

Figure 14.1 T2-weighted and proton density (right) images of an axial brain magnetic resonance imaging scan from an elderly patient with a late-onset schizophrenic disorder. The widespread white matter hyperintensities are possibly ischaemic in aetiology. The patient was hypertensive and diabetic.

Box 14.7 The mechanisms of neuropsychiatric complications of HIV infection

Direct HIV brain infection: encephalitis, meningitis, white matter disease, neuronal cell death
Secondary brain infection: viral, mycotic, protozoan, bacterial
Neoplastic infiltration: e.g. lymphoma
Vascular: embolism and thrombosis secondary to vasculitis and endocarditis
Metabolic effects of systemic disease: hypoxia, "toxaemia"
Iatrogenic: e.g. drug side effects of nucleosides and neurotropics

---

and deterioration in cognitive function and movement. HAD may occasionally be one of the presenting signs of HIV infection. HIV-associated myelopathy is also an AIDS-defining condition. However, HIV-associated minor cognitive or motor disorder is not (Working Group of AAN AIDS Task Force, 1991).

Delirium occurs frequently in AIDS because of the metabolic effects of secondary infections and neoplasms. Fluctuations in consciousness and disorganised or apathetic behaviour, with or without psychosis, indicate probable delirium.

Major depression has a cumulative incidence of 30% throughout the duration of the disease. The differential diagnosis includes the cognitive slowing associated with HAD, malaise associated with systemic illness or adjustment disorder. Suicide rates are 30 to 60 times greater than the general population. Mania is less likely to present de novo in HIV-positive patients. It may present as a consequence of delirium or be a medication side effect. Anxiety is common and often relates to issues concerning the uncertainty of the future and the possibility of infecting others. Some patients can falsely conclude that somatic symptoms associated with anxiety are related to disease progression.

Psychotic episodes (as with mania) may indicate the chance association of a pre-existing psychotic disorder but can be a consequence of delirium, subtle cognitive dysfunction or the focal brain effects of secondary disease. Psychosis resembling a schizophreniform disorder in the absence of clear organic aetiology occurs occasionally and may be due to direct HIV brain infection.

The use of antiretroviral agents decreases the incidence of neuropsychiatric disorders in HIV infection. Low-dose, high-potency neuroleptic medication is appropriate in the management of psychosis, mania and agitated symptoms of delirium, but this population has an increased sensitivity to medication side effects. Antidepressants are effective in major depression, and psychostimulants such as methylphenidate can assist apathetic syndromes.

Psychological treatment is useful for the patient and caregivers in managing anxiety, depression and grief, and support groups offer social and educational assistance.

Neuropsychiatric aspects of traumatic brain injury

Traumatic brain injury has become a modern epidemic, accounting for about one half of all accident-related deaths. After headache, it is the most common cause of neurological presentation, with patients often being young. Neuropsychiatric problems are common in the brain-injured and may be out of proportion to any neurological deficits. They may be in the form of cognitive impairment (dementia, amnestic syndrome, dysphasia or other deficit), affective disorder (depression or mania), personality or behavioural change, anxiety disorder (generalised anxiety disorder, posttraumatic stress disorder, obsessive-compulsive disorder) or, rarely, psychosis. There are many determinants of the psychiatric outcome of brain injury, with the type and extent of injury, the duration of altered consciousness and period of posttraumatic amnesia being influenced by many other host and agent factors. The outcome is often modulated by education, premorbid personality, cultural factors, quality of social network, quality of medical and rehabilitative care and financial incentives for chronicity of problems. The patient's attribution style, coping behaviour and locus of control are all important. Furthermore, the head injury must be considered in the context of the stage of the individual's and the family's life cycle.

A topic of much controversy is the validity of *persistent postconcussional syndrome* (PCS). Approximately 75% of head injuries are mild, and most recover by 3 months. Approximately one third of patients have some symptoms persisting beyond 3 months, and about 10% with mild brain injury develop persistent symptoms beyond 1 year, usually characterised by somatic (headache, dizziness, fatigue, insomnia), cognitive (concentration, memory and executive dysfunction), perceptual (sensitivity to noise and light) and emotional (depression, anxiety, irritability) features. There are few objective features of persisting neurological deficits and neuroimaging is generally normal. Such patients often have a pre-injury history of psychiatric problems and usually have had extensive disruption because of the accident. Other risk factors are female sex, ongoing litigation, low socioeconomic status, prior mild injury and associated somatic injury. In general, there are both physiological and psychological factors in the aetiology of PCS, and the point at which physiogenesis more properly become psychogenesis is hard to establish and may partly be iatrogenic (King, 2003). Early brief psychological intervention appears to have a protective effect.

Psychiatric aspects of epilepsy

Epilepsy is a common disorder, affecting approximately 0.5% of the population. Although in the majority of affected persons epilepsy is compatible with normal mental health, psychiatric disturbance is far from uncommon and greatly outstrips that in the general population. Psychiatric problems are present in about 30% of patients and the figure rises to 50% in those with temporal lobe epilepsy. A survey of epileptics from general practice found that 17% had significant social problems, 8% were incapable of work because of epilepsy and a further 12% were capable of only restricted employment. In a survey of all children from the Isle of Wight study, the overall rate of psychiatric disorder in children with uncomplicated epilepsy was 28.6%, 4 times the control rate, rising to 58.3% in those with brain damage.

The range of psychiatric disorders in epilepsy is wide, with depression, anxiety, psychosis and personality disturbance being overrepresented.

Depression has been linked to the peri-ictal period and the seizure itself, but is most commonly inter-ictal. Suicide rates in epileptics are 3 times those of the general population and are most commonly due to overdoses on anticonvulsants. Even though some anticonvulsants are used as mood stabilisers, certain drugs, such as vigabatrin, topiramate and phenobarbitone, are sometimes associated with depression soon after initiation. Depression in epilepsy is usually treated with SSRIs and serotonin and norepinephrine reuptake inhibitors, but TCAs may be used provided the risk of overdose is kept in mind. There is a small risk of worsening of seizures, somewhat greater with TCAs. There are very few interactions of clinical significance, except that fluvoxamine slows the metabolism of carbamazepine and phenytoin, and carbamazepine, oxcarbazepine and SSRIs all have a tendency to produce hyponatremia. ECT is not contraindicated in epilepsy (Jackson & Turkington, 2005).

Rates of anxiety disorder of 10% to 25% have been reported in epilepsy, usually as generalised anxiety disorder. Some patients with sudden unexpected seizures develop agoraphobic symptoms. Occasionally panic attacks with dissociative symptoms may be confused with complex partial seizures.

The relationship between psychosis and epilepsy and schizophrenia-like psychosis (SLP) has been of particular interest. The psychosis of epilepsy is generally delineated into ictal, post-ictal and inter-ictal. Post-ictal psychoses begin hours or days after a flurry of seizures and are usually brief in duration. Some patients develop brief inter-ictal psychoses that show an alternating pattern between epilepsy and psychosis and may be accompanied by changes in the EEG that have been termed *forced normalisation* (Landolt, 1953). Patients with epilepsy, especially those with temporal lobe epilepsy, have a higher risk of developing chronic SLP, although many aspects of this relationship remain contentious. The majority of investigators support a special but not exclusive relationship with mediobasal temporal lobe epilepsy, with a left temporal bias receiving only limited support. Some suggested risk factors are severe and intractable epilepsy, epilepsy of early onset, secondary generalisation of seizures, certain anticonvulsant drugs and temporal lobectomy. Different neuropathological studies suggest the presence of cortical dysgenesis or diffuse brain damage in such patients (Sachdev, 1998).

Conclusion

The overview presented in this chapter supports the salience of a neuropsychiatric approach for some disorders, as well as a clinical territory for the practicing neuropsychiatrist. Taking this forward will enable the development of a robust specialised field of neuropsychiatry across a number of traditional medical disciplines.

REFERENCES

Alexopoulos, G. S., Meyers, B. S., Young, R. C., *et al.* (1997). "Vascular depression" hypothesis. *Arc Gen Psychiatry* 54:915–22.

Arseneault, L., Cannon, M., Witton, J., *et al.* (2004). Causal association between cannabis and psychosis: examination of the evidence. *Br J Psychiatry* 184:110–17.

Ashburner, J., Csernansky, J. G., Davatzikos, C., *et al.* (2003). Computer-assisted imaging to assess brain structure in healthy and diseased brains. *Lancet Neurol* 2:79–88.

Baddeley, A. D. (1986). *Working Memory*. Oxford: Oxford University Press.

Baldwin, R. C. (2005). Is vascular depression a distinct subtype of depressive disorder? A review of the causal evidence. *Int J Geriatr Psychiatry* 20:1–11.

Barkley, G. L., & Baumgartner, C. (2003). MEG and EEG in Epilepsy. *J Clin Neurophysiol* 20:163–78.

Buchanan, R. W., & Heinrichs, D. W. (1989). The Neurological Evaluation Scale (NES): a structured instrument for the assessment of neurological signs in schizophrenia. *Psychiatry Res* 27:335–350.

Carson, A. J., MacHale, S., Allen, K., *et al.* (2000). Depression after stroke and lesion location: a systematic review. *Lancet* 356:122–6.

Cummings, J. L. (1992). Depression and Parkinson's disease: a review. *Am J Psychiatry* **149**:443–54.

Cummings, J. L. (1993). Frontal-subcortical circuits and human behavior. *Arch Neurol* **50**:873–80.

Curran, C., Byrappa, N., & McBride, A. (2004). Stimulant psychosis: systematic review. *Br J Psychiatry* **185**:196–204.

DeMyer, W. E. (2003). *Technique of the Neurological Examination*. New York: McGraw-Hill Professionals.

Dyer, C. B., Ashton, C. M., & Teasdale, T.A. (1995). Postoperative delirium. A review of 80 primary data-collection studies. *Arch Int Med* **155**:461–5.

Ebersole, J. S., & Pedley, T. A. (2003). *Current Practice of Clinical Electroencephalography*. Philadelphia: Lippincott Williams & Wilkins.

Fink, M., & Taylor, M. A. (2003). *Catatonia*. Cambridge: Cambridge University Press.

Folstein, M. F., Folstein, S. E, & McHugh, P. R. (1975). "Mini-Mental State". A practical method for grading the cognitive state of patients for the clinician. *J Psychiatr Res* **12**:189–98.

Gardian, G., & Vecsei, L. (2004). Huntington's disease: pathomechanism and therapeutic perspectives. *J Neural Transm* **111**:1485–94.

Hall, W., & Degenhardt, L. (2000). Cannabis use and psychosis: a review of clinical and epidemiological evidence. *Aust N Z J Psychiatry* **34**:26–34.

Harper, C., & Kril, J. (1985). Brain atrophy in chronic alcoholic patients: a quantitative pathological study. *J Neurol Neurosurg Psychiatry* **48**:211–17.

Harvey, R. J. (2001). Epidemiology of presenile dementia. In J. R. Hodges, ed. *Early-Onset Dementia: A Multidisciplinary Approach*. Oxford: Oxford University Press, pp. 1–23.

Heeger, D. J., & Ress, D. (2002). What does fMRI tell us about neuronal activity? *Nat Rev Neurosci* **3**, 142–51.

Hodges, J. R. (1994). *Cognitive assessment for clinicians*. Oxford: Oxford University Press.

Jackson, M.J., & Turkington, D. (2005). Depression and anxiety in epilepsy. *J Neurol Neurosurg Psychiatry* **76**:45–7.

Jorm, A. F., Anstey, K. J., Christensen, H., *et al.* (2005). MRI hyperintensities and depressive symptoms in a community sample of 60–64 year olds. *Am J Psychiatry* **162**:699–705.

Kaiser, J., & Lutzenberger, W. (2005). Human gamma-band activity: a window to cognitive processing. *Neuroreport* **16**:207–11.

King, N. S. (2003). Post-concussion syndrome: clarity amid the controversy? *Br J Psychiatry* **183**:276–8.

Kryger, M. H., Roth, T., Dement, W. C., eds. (2000). *Principles and Practice of Sleep Medicine*. Philadelphia: W.B. Saunders.

Landolt, H. (1953). Some clinical electroencephalographical correlations in epileptic psychoses (twilight states). *Electroencephalogr Clin Neurophysiol* **5**: 121.

Lezak, M. D. (2004). *Neuropsychological Assessment*, 4th edn. Oxford: Oxford University Press.

Lauterbach, E. C. (2004). The neuropsychiatry of Parkinson's disease and related disorders. *Psychiatr Clin North Am* **27**:801–25.

Matthews, P. M., & Jezzard, P. (2004). Functional magnetic resonance imaging. *J Neurol Neurosurg Psychiatry* **75**:6–12.

McGuire, P. K., Jones, P., Harvey, I., *et al.* (1994). Cannabis and acute psychosis. *Schizophr Res* **13**: 161–8.

Mendez, M. F. (1995). Neuropsychiatric aspects of boxing. *Int J Psychiatr Med* **23**:249–62.

Mesulam, M. M. (2003). Current concepts: primary progressive aphasia – a language-based dementia. *New Engl J Med* **349**:1535–42.

Narushima, K., Kosier, J. T., & Robinson, R. G. (2003). A reappraisal of poststrokedepression, intra- and inter hemispheric lesion location using meta-analysis. *J Neuropsychiatry Clin Neurosci* **15**:423–30.

Neary, D., Snowden, J. S., Mann, D. M. A., *et al.* (1990). Frontal lobe dementia and motor neuron disease. *J Neurol Neurosurg Psychiatry* **53**:23–32.

Nestor, P. J, Scheltens, P., & Hodges, J. R. (2004). Advances in the early detection of Alzheimer's disease. *Nat Rev Neurosci* **5**(Suppl):S34–S41.

Nussbaum, R. L., & Ellis, C. E.,(2003). Genomic medicine: Alzheimer's disease and Parkinson's disease. *N Engl J Med* **348**:1356–64.

Okun M. N., & Watts, R. L. (2002). Depression associated with Parkinson's disease: clinical features and treatment. *Neurology* **58**(Suppl 1):S63–S70.

Oslin, D., Atkinson, R. M., Smith, D. M., *et al.* (1998). Alcohol related dementia: proposed clinical criteria. *Int J Geriatr Psychiatry* **13**:203–12.

Poewe, W., & Luginger, E. (1999). Depression in Parkinson's disease: impediments to recognition and treatment options. *Neurology* **52**(Suppl 3):S2–S6.

Qizilbash, N. (2002). *Evidence-based dementia practice*. Oxford: Blackwell Science.

Ritchie, K., & Lovestone, S. (2002). The dementias. *Lancet* **360**:1759–66.

Ross, A. J., & Sachdev, P. S. (2004). Magnetic resonance spectroscopy in cognitive research. *Brian Res Rev* **44**:83–102.

Rummans, T. A., Evans, J. M., Krahn, L. E. *et al.* (1995). Delirium in elderly patients: evaluation and management. *Mayo Clin Proc* **70**:989–98.

Sachdev, P. S. (1996). A critique of "organic" and its proposed alternatives. *Aust N Z J Psychiatry* **30**:165–70.

Sachdev, P. (1998). Schizophrenia-like psychosis and epilepsy: the status of the association. *Am J Psychiatry* **155**:325–36.

Sachdev, P. S. (2005). Whither neuropsychiatry? [Editorial]. *J Neuropsychiatry Clin Neurosci* **17**:140–4.

Sachdev, P. S. (ed.). (In press). *Secondary Schizophrenia.* Cambridge. UK: Cambridge University Press.

Sampson, E. L., Warren, J. D., & Rossor, M. N. (2004). Young onset dementia. *Postgrad Med J* **80**:125–39.

Saha, G. B., McIntyre, W. J., & Go, R. T. (1994). Radiopharmaceuticals for brain imaging. *Sem Nucl Med* **24**:324–49.

Steffens, D. C., & Krishnan, K. R. R. (1998). Structural neuroimaging and mood disorders: recent findings, implications for classification, and future directions. *Biol Psychiatry* **43**:705–12.

Steffens, D. C., Krishnan, K. R. R., Crump, C., *et al.* (2002). Cerebrovascular disease and evolution of depressive symptoms in the Cardiovascular Health Study. *Stroke* **33**:1636–44.

Symms, M., Jager, H. R., Schmierer, K., *et al.* (2004). A review of structural magnetic resonance neuroimaging. *J Neurol Neurosurg Psychiatry* **75**:1235–44.

Victor, M. (1994). Alcoholic dementia. *Can J Neurol Sci* **21**:88–99.

Weintraub, S. (2000). Neuropsychological assessment of mental state. In M. M. Mesulam, ed. *Principles of Behavioural and Cognitive Neurology.* New York: Oxford University Press, p. 128.

Working Group of AAN AIDS Task Force (1991). Nomenclature and research case definitions for neurologic manifestations of human immunodeficiency virus type 1 (HIV-1) infection. *Neurology* **41**:778–85.

World Health Organisation (1992). World Health Organisation (1992). *International Classification of Impairments, Disabilities and Handicaps,* 10th revision (ICD-10). Geneva: World Health Organisation.

15

The psychiatry of old age

E. Jane Byrne, Alistair Burns and Sean Lennon

The psychiatry of old age, like the population it serves, has expanded in the last ten years. Demographic change, with an ageing population, has ensured that this will continue to be an area of growth. Fertility and mortality rates are the main determinants of population age structure. The reduction in fertility rates in many Western countries over the latter half of the twentieth century is well established, as is the decline in the mortality of the very old (Murphy, 1990; Preston *et al.,* 1989; Tomassini, 2004). Life expectancy at age 65 years has increased for both men and women – from 13 years and 17 years, respectively, in 1980–1982 to 16 and 19 years, respectively, in 2000–2002 (Government Actuary's Department, 2004). The net result of these changes is an ageing population. Those aged over 85 years have been the fastest growing group over the last 30 years, and these "oldest old" are more likely to have chronic diseases and to suffer social isolation.

Grundy (1992) and Tomassini (2004) have described other important changes affecting the population of old people – the cohort with marked female preponderance (due to World War I) is now largely replaced by a cohort who are more likely to have married and in whom the sex differential is less marked. The older population is now more diverse than ever before in health, income, working patterns and family relationships (Office of National Statistics [ONS]; 2004 Tomassini, 2004).

These "new" cohorts of old people are more likely to have children but less likely to live with them than in former years (ONS, 2004).

In terms of service provision, social deprivation indices (relevant to older people) are related to the prevalence and incidence of mental health problems. At the same time, informal (unpaid) carers for older people are also ageing, with 21% of people in their 50s providing unpaid care for family members, friends or relatives (ONS, 2004).

Old age psychiatric services

The needs of older people with mental health problems are not confined simply to mental health but also physical health and social care needs. It is because of this that the specialist mental health service must be expert at collaboration with other health and social care providers and must have a service model which outreaches to all the settings in which each patient group may be found. In the United Kingdom, the National Service Framework delineates the core elements of a high-quality mental health service for older people (see Box 15.1).

Community care

The community mental health team is the cornerstone of a comprehensive mental health service for older people (Royal College of Psychiatrists College

Essential Psychiatry, ed. Robin M. Murray, Kenneth S. Kendler, Peter McGuffin, Simon Wessely, David J. Castle. Published by Cambridge University Press. © Cambridge University Press 2008.

Report CR110). The role of the team is to assess older people with complex needs and to provide treatment and support to them and their carers.

The community mental health team may not only provide assessment and treatment over an extended period of time but also act to manage crises, possibly reducing the need for hospital admission (Richman *et al.*, 2003). The team can also achieve this outcome by providing support into care homes (Challis, 2002).

These teams operate as a multidisciplinary specialist service. They comprise a range of practitioners, including a consultant psychiatrist, community mental health nurses, clinical psychologists, occupational therapists and social workers. The team should have agreed working referral arrangements with general practitioners (GPs), speech and language therapists, physiotherapists, dieticians, chiropodists/podiatrists, community dental services, pharmacists, district nurses, health visitors and housing workers.

Day hospital care

The old age psychiatry day hospital is described by the National Service Framework for Older People (Department of Health [DoH], 2001) as an "integral part of a comprehensive old age mental health service" which offer intensive assessment and treatment to people with both functional disorders and dementia. They encompass "day care providing a range of stimulating group and one-to-one activities". The day hospital may reduce the admission rate to acute in-patient beds, and it may facilitate early discharge from hospital, as well as reduce carer stress (Gilliard, 1987).

In-patient care

In-patient care for the elderly with mental health problems is best provided separately from younger adult services, both for the efficiency of the service (Draper, 1994) and also to ensure that the different needs of older people can be met in the most suitable environment. Furthermore, the fact that many in-patients have concomitant medical illnesses suggests that co-location with a general hospital is sensible. This gives improved access to appropriate assessments and treatments, allows the planning of joint assessments and provides opportunities for joint training. Finally, there is a higher standard of emergency response for physical illness (Draper & Luscombe, 1998).

Old age in-patient services must be available for both those suffering functional disorders and those with cognitive impairments. In the short-term treatment of those with dementia, improvements are noted particularly in psychopathology (DJernes *et al.*, 1998; Wattis *et al.*, 1994). Favourable outcomes for depressed elderly have also been shown (Baldwin & Jolley, 1986; Wattis *et al.*, 1994). The staff members in these units need a special range of skills to deal with the combination of psychological symptoms, behavioural disturbance and physical illness in this patient group.

Liaison with the general hospital

A comprehensive old age mental health service needs to provide a service both in the community and in the setting of the general hospital, given the high prevalence of mental health disorders among older people within the general hospital setting and the effect of this on outcome. Despite this, liaison old age psychiatry is often a poorly resourced part of the mental health service, and old age psychiatry support to general hospitals is usually provided on an ad hoc consultation model. In such a model a member of the mental health team (usually a psychiatrist) provides assessment and advice but often little more support to the general hospital service. This is inadequate given that older people occupy almost two thirds of general hospital beds.

A more acceptable model of a specialist old age mental health service within the general hospital is the liaison model. Anderson (2004) stated: "Liaison is pro-active, working to raise the profile of mental health, collaborating with general departments and shared care, taking part in joint meetings and developing education and training programmes in mental health. It is available, accessible, can respond quickly and review patients frequently". The model of liaison is multidisciplinary, including psychiatrists, social workers, occupational therapists, psychologists and psychiatric nurses. Such a team is able to provide specific clinical interventions and is also able to provide education and training of general hospital staff members to develop their skills in detection, treatment and management of mental illness among older people. It also improves the ability of the general hospital staff to access services.

The benefits of such a model are seen in high referral rates (Scott *et al.*, 1988) and an improvement in compliance with the treatment recommendations (De Leo *et al.*, 1989). There is some evidence that the clinical outcomes are consequently improved (Strain *et al.*, 1991).

Memory clinics

Memory clinics are increasingly becoming part of local old age mental health services. Their rationale is to provide a specialist service for diagnosis and treatment of people suffering a memory problem. They can play a key role in managing therapy, may participate in research and are a focus for professionals and other caregivers for education. Memory clinics act as a component of a local comprehensive service, and some will become tertiary services for difficult diagnostic and management problems.

The work of a memory clinic, in common with the work of other old age mental health services, is multidisciplinary. Each memory clinic must therefore be appropriately staffed. The doctor's role is not just the diagnosis of the memory disorder but also the assessment of comorbid conditions (Walstra *et al.*, 1997). Nurses are key members of the team, providing skills in identifying dementia and other mental illnesses and being able to provide assessments and treatments in appropriate settings. The psychologist plays a role not only in assessment but also in treatment through psychosocial interventions or specific treatments for memory impairment which are not due to dementia.

The memory clinic functions by carrying out a detailed assessment, collating information and, where possible, making a diagnosis. When a dementing illness is identified, the clinic can help the patient and their carers to understand the consequences of the diagnosis, including providing access to treatment, considering what longer-term support is needed and providing advice on the basis of which the person and his or her family can make plans. This includes giving a prognosis when possible; offering specific advice about planning future care including financial planning, advanced directives (living wills), advice about driving; and, if appropriate, considering the need for genetic counselling.

Dementia

Dementia is a term which describes a chronic and progressive clinical syndrome of the brain expressed in three ways – neuropsychological, neuropsychiatric and activities of daily living. The *neuropsychological* components are amnesia (loss of memory), aphasia (impairment of language), apraxia (the inability to carry out actions despite intact sensory motor function), agnosia (the inability to recognise or associate meaning to sensory perception) and impaired executive function (disturbances in judgement, planning and abstraction).

Neuropsychiatric symptoms describe a range of psychiatric symptoms and behavioural disturbances. Examples of the former are depression, hallucinations, delusions and misidentifications; examples of the latter are agitation, aggression, wandering, sexual disinhibition, sleep disturbance and changes in appetite.

Activities of daily living can be described in terms of those changes which occur early in dementia (instrumental activities of daily living) characterised by an inability to carry out complex tasks, such as driving, using the telephone or handling money, and tasks which become affected in the later stages of dementia (such as dressing, feeding and toileting) – so-called basic activities of daily living.

These three aspects of dementia are common to all forms, with the differentiation between the two main types of dementia being at the level of the onset of progression of deficits rather than the specific presence or absence of one or the other. The reader is referred to Chapter 14 for an overview of dementia across the lifespan; here we concentrate on dementia in the elderly.

Differential diagnosis of dementia

The three main differential diagnoses are depression (pseudodementia), delirium and mild cognitive impairment. Tables 15.1 and 15.2 summarise the main differentiating characteristics of delirium and depression.

Mild cognitive impairment (MCI) refers to the clinical situation in which a person has complaints of memory loss and there is objective evidence of cognitive loss, but no evidence of dementia. The criteria are as follows:

- Complaints of memory loss, preferably corroborated by an informant
- Objective cognitive loss as demonstrated by neuropsychological tests
- Impairments not sufficient to impair professional and social activities
- Normal general cognitive function
- Not satisfying criteria for dementia

People satisfying criteria for MCI have a 12- to 15-fold increased risk of developing Alzheimer's disease at follow-up compared with the normal

Table 15.1 Dementia versus delirium

Dementia	Delirium
Long duration (months, years)	Short duration (days, weeks)
Intervals of normal function rare	Marked variability
Short and long-term memory loss	Short-term memory loss
Deterioration in personality	Preservation of personality
Ideational poverty	Creative ideation
Ill-defined hallucinations	Florid hallucinations
Ill-defined persecution	Prominent persecution
Apathy	Fear and perplexity

population. There do not appear to be any consistent predictive factors of who will go on to develop dementia, but the presence of more severe objective evidence of cognitive loss does indicate a higher chance of developing the disorder. Currently there are no specific treatments for MCI other than treating any comorbid conditions, including depression and following up with repeat neuropsychological tests. Often people in whom there is a family history of dementia are more sensitised to the early symptoms.

Aetiology of the dementia syndrome

The various causes of dementia are summarised in Table 15.3 (see also Box 14.5). Diagnostic criteria for each of the main types of dementia are summarised in Tables 15.4–15.8.

Essentially, the gradual onset of a dementia syndrome without any obvious cause is suggestive of Alzheimer's disease; the presence of sudden periods of change is suggestive of vascular disease; confusional states with parkinsonian features is indicative of dementia with Lewy bodies; personality change with relatively intact memory may indicate a frontal lobe dementia; and a very rapid decline with a characteristic electroencephalogram (EEG) would be consistent with Creutzfeld-Jakob disease. The Hachinski score (Box 15.2) helps

Table 15.2 Pseudodementia and dementia

	Pseudodementia	Dementia (AD)
History	Onset can be dated accurately	Onset vague
	Rapid progression of symptoms	Symptoms slowly progressive
	Symptoms of short duration	Symptoms of long duration
	Previous or family history of depression common	Previous or family history of depression rare
	Family very aware of disabilities early on	Family usually unaware of disability initially
Symptomatology	Patients complain of memory loss	Patients rarely complain of memory loss
	Patients emphasize disability	Patients hide disability
	Symptoms often worse in the morning	Confusion worse in the evening
Examination	Patients convey distress	Labile mood
	Affective change usual	Affective change less common
	'Don't know' answers to questions	Questions tend to be answered incorrectly
	Variability in performance	Performance consistently poor
	Memory gaps usually apparent	Specific memory gaps rare
	Patients make little effort to perform tasks	Patients try hard
	General physical examination and investigations usually normal in both cases	
Investigations		
CT	Usually little evidence of atrophy	Cerebral atrophy and ventricular enlargement
EEG	Usually normal	Pronounced slow activity
SPET	Blood flow patterns usually normal	Parietotemporal and frontal abnormalities often seen
Prognosis	Good	Poor
Treatment	Antidepressants in all cases	Antidepressants if affective disorder severe
	ECT if necessary	ECT not recommended

Box 15.2 The Hachinski ischaemia score

Abrupt onset	Emotional incontinence
Stepwise progression	History of hypertension
Fluctuating course	History of strokes
Nocturnal confusion	Evidence of associated
Relative preservation of	atherosclerosis
personality	
Depression	Focal neurological
	symptoms
Somatic complains	Focal neurological signs

differentiate between vascular dementia and Alzheimer's disease.

Epidemiology

Up to 25 million people worldwide are affected with dementia, a figure which will effectively double by 2020 (Prince, 1997). A number of studies have confirmed that, in any population, the prevalence of Alzheimer's disease doubles with every 5-year increase in an age group (see Table 15.9 and Lobo *et al.*, 2000).

Alzheimer's disease (AD) has been reported as consistently more common than vascular dementia in studies in developed countries. The incidence rises exponentially after age 90, with a tendency to be more common in older women (vascular dementia preferentially affects males).

Risk factors for dementia

Genetic abnormalities have been shown to be risk factors for dementia. For example, early-onset genetic types of AD are associated with abnormalities in the amyloid precursor protein (chromosome 21) and also presenilin 1 (chromosome 14) and presenilin 2 (chromosome 1). Late-onset sporadic AD

Table 15.3 Differential diagnosis of dementia

Alzheimer's disease

Mixed Alzheimer – vascular dementia

Vascular dementia

Frontotemporal lobar degenerations, including
frontotemporal dementia and Pick's disease

Parkinsonian disorders with dementia: dementia with
Lewy bodies, Parkinson's disease

Non-parkinsonian motor disorders with dementia:
Huntington's disease and others

Conventional infectious diseases: AIDS, syphilis, Lyme
disease, chronic meningitis

Prior-related disorders, especially Creutzfeldt-Jakob
disease

Toxic-metabolic disorders

Drugs: alcohol, other recreational drugs, medications

Toxins: heavy metals, organophosphates, other
industrial toxins

Anoxia and hypoglycaemia

Gastrointestinal and hepatic, including hepatic
encephalopathy

Kidney: renal failure and dialysis dementia

Vitamin deficiencies: B_{12}, thiamine, folate, niacin

Endocrinopathies: thyroid, parathyroid, adrenal,
pituitary

Inherited adult onset biochemical disorders, e.g.,
metachromatic leukodystrophy

Kuf's disease

Psychiatric diseases, especially depression

Miscellaneous

Normal pressure hydrocephalus

Posttraumatic and dementia pugilistica

Neoplastic: gliomatosis cerebri, lymphomatosis
cerebri, angioendotheliosis

Epilepsy-related

Sarcoidosis

Mendez & Cummings (2004). Used with permission.

is associated with the presence of apolipoprotein A4 (chromosome 19). Other risk factors include raised cholesterol, raised blood pressure, diabetes and a history of myocardial infarction, as well as the risk factors traditionally associated with dementia in epidemiological studies such as head injury, depression and thyroid disease.

Clinical assessment

History

It is unlikely that patients with dementia will be able to give detailed accounts of their situation and circumstances; thus whenever possible and practical, information about their background should be gleaned from others. Family and carers are the obvious people to ask, together with the person's GP. Much of the diagnosis of dementia is based on the history of the present complaint, and details about when the symptoms started, whether they appeared gradually or suddenly and the rate and degree of progression are important factors. The advent of memory clinics has meant that many more people are presenting themselves for assessment and treatment, but a history should always be backed up with information from an informant.

In addition to asking for symptoms of memory loss and problems with activities of daily living, one needs to ask directly about symptoms which suggest aphasia, apraxia, agnosia and other symptoms such as delusions, hallucinations and paranoid ideas (which may suggest the presence of delirium or dementia with Lewy bodies) and changes in personality and eating preference with poor social awareness (which may indicate frontotemporal dementia). A medical history should be taken with particular relevance to risk factors for cardiovascular or cerebrovascular disease and a history of transient ischaemic attacks. One should also consider the presence of a head injury, so as not to miss a subdural haematoma, or the triad of dementia, gait disturbance and incontinence, which may indicate normal pressure hydrocephalus. A previous history of depression may indicate an affective disorder.

Mental state examination

This follows the same schema as in any other person but with obvious differences in emphasis. Evidence of self-neglect or a smell of stale urine would indicate poor self care and an inappropriate kiss or embrace may signal disinhibition. Paranoid

Table 15.4 Criteria for clinical diagnosis of Alzheimer's disease

I   The criteria for the clinical diagnosis of **probable** Alzheimer's disease include:
- dementia established by clinical examination and documented by the MMSE, Blessed dementia scale or some similar examination and confirmed by neuropsychological tests;
- deficits in two or more areas of cognition;
- progressive worsening memory and other cognitive functions;
- no disturbance of consciousness;
- onset between ages 40 and 90, most often after age 65; and
- absence of systemic disorders or other brain diseases that in and of themselves could account for the progressive deficits in memory and cognition.

II The diagnosis of **probable** Alzheimer's disease is supported by:
- progressive deterioration of specific cognitive functions such as language (aphasia), motor skills (apraxia) and perception (agnosia);
- impaired activities of daily living and altered patterns of behaviour;
- family history of similar disorders, particularly if confirmed neuropathologically; and
- laboratory results of:
  - normal lumbar puncture as evaluated by standard techniques;
  - normal pattern or non-specific changes in EEG, such as increased slow-wave activity; and
  - evidence of cerebral atrophy on CT with progression documented by serial observation.

III Other clinical features consistent with the diagnosis of **probable** Alzheimer's disease, after exlusion of causes of dementia other than Alzheimer's disease include:
- plateaus in the course of progression of the illness;
- associated symptoms of depression, insomnia, incontinence, delusions, illusions, hallucinations, catastrophic verbal, emotional or physical outbursts, sexual disorders and weight loss;
- other neurological abnormalities in some patients, especially with more advanced disease and including motor signs, such as increased muscle tone, myoclonus or gait disorder;
- seizures in advanced disease; and
- CT normal for age.

IV Features that make the diagnosis of **probable** Alzheimer's disease uncertain or unlikely include:
- sudden, apoplectic onset;
- focal neurological findings such as hemiparesis, sensory loss, visual field deficits and incoordination early in the course of the illness; and
- seizures or gait disturbances at the onset or very early in the course of the illness.

V   Clinical diagnosis of **probable** Alzheimer's disease:
- may be made on the basis of the dementia syndrome, in the absence of other neurological, psychiatric or systemic disorder sufficient to cause dementia, and in the presence of variation in the onset, in the presentation, or in the clinical course;
- may be made in the presence of a second systemic or brain disorder sufficient to produce dementia, which is not considered to be the cause of the dementia; and
- should be used in research studies when a single, gradually progressive severe cognitive deficit is identified in the absence of other identifiable cause.

VI Criteria for diagnosis of **definite** Alzheimer's disease are:
- the clinical criteria for probable Alzheimer's disease and histopathological evidence obtained from a biopsy or autopsy.

VII Classification of Alzheimer's disease for research purpose should specify features that may differentiate subtypes of the disorder, such as:
- familial occurrence;
- onset before age 65;
- presence of trisomy-21; and
- coexistence of other relevant conditions, such as Parkinson's disease.

MMSE = Mini-Mental State; CT = computed tomography.

Table 15.5 The criteria for the clinical diagnosis of vascular dementia (VaD)

I The criteria for the clinical diagnosis of VaD include all the following:

- **dementia** defined by cognitive decline from a previously higher level of functioning and manifested by impairment of memory and of two or more cognitive domains (orientation, attention, language, visuospatial functions, executive functions, motor control and praxis), preferably established by clinical examination and documented by neuropsychological testing; deficits should be severe enough to interfere with activities of daily living not due to physical effects of stroke alone. *Exclusion criteria: cases with disturbance of consciousness, delirium, psychosis, severe aphasia or major sensorimotor impairment precluding neuropsychological testing. Also excluded are systemic disorders or other brain diseases (such as AD) that in and of themselves could account for deficits in memory and cognition.*
- **CVD** defined by the presence of focal signs on neurological examination, such as hemiparesis, lower facial weakness, Babinski sign, sensory deficit, hemianopia and dysarthria consistent with stroke (with or without history of stroke), and evidence of relevant CVD by brain imaging (CT or MRI), including multiple large vessel infarcts or a single strategically placed infarct (angular gyrus, thalamus, basal forebrain or PCA or ACA territories), as well as multiple basal ganglia and white matter lacunes or extensive periventricular white matter lesions, or combinations thereof.
- **a relationship between the above 2 disorders** manifested or inferred by the presence of one or more of the following:
  a) onset of dementia within 3 months following a recognized stroke;
  b) abrupt deterioration in cognitive functions; or fluctuating, stepwise progression of cognitive deficits.

II Clinical features consistent with the diagnosis of **probable** vascular dementia include the following:

- early presence of a gait disturbance (small step gait or marche à petits pas, or magnetic apraxic-ataxic or parkinsonian gait);
- history of unsteadiness and frequent, unprovoked falls;
- early urinary frequency, urgency and other urinary symptoms not explained by urological disease;
- pseudobulbar palsy; and
- personality and mood changes, abulia, depression, emotional incontinence or other subcortical deficits, including psychomotor retardation and abnormal executive function.

III Features that make the diagnosis of vascular dementia **uncertain** or **unlikely** include:

- early onset of memory deficit and progressive worsening of memory and other cognitive functions, such as language (transcortical sensory aphasia), motor skills (apraxia) and perception (agnosia), in the absence of corresponding focal lesions on brain imaging;
- absence of focal neurological signs, other than cognitive disturbance; and
- absence of cerebrovascular lesions on brain CT or MRI.

IV Clinical diagnosis of **possible** vascular dementia may be made:

- in the presence of dementia (Section I) with focal neurological signs in patients in whom brain imaging studies to confirm definite CVD are missing; or
- in the absence of clear temporal relationship between dementia and stroke; or
- in patients with subtle onset and variable course (plateau or improvement) of cognitive deficits and evidence of relevant CVD.

V Criteria for diagnosis of **definite** vascular dementia are:

- clinical criteria for **probable** vascular dementia;
- histopathological evidence of CVD obtained from biopsy or autopsy;
- absence of neurofibrillary tangles and neuritic plaques exceeding those expected for age; and
- absence of other clinical or pathological disorder capable of producing dementia.

VI Classification of vascular dementia for research purposes may be made on the basis of clinical, radiological and neuropathological features, for subcategories or defined conditions such as cortical vascular dementia, subcortical vascular dementia and thalamic dementia.

The phrase 'AD with CVD' should be reserved to classify patients fulfilling the clinical criteria for possible AD and who also present clinical or brain imaging evidence of relevant CVD. Traditionally, these patients have been included with VaD in epidemiological studies. The phrase 'mixed dementia', used hitherto, should be avoided.

Table 15.6 Consensus criteria for the clinical diagnosis of probable and possible DLB

The central feature required for a diagnosis of DLB is progressive cognitive decline of sufficient magnitude to interfere with normal social or occupational function. Prominent or persistent memory impairment may not necessarily occur in the early stages but is usually evident with progression. Deficits on tests of attention and of frontal-subcortical skills and visuospatial ability may be especially prominent.

Two of the following core features are essential for a diagnosis of DLB:

- fluctuating cognition with pronounced variations in attention and alertness;
- recurrent visual hallucinations that are typically well formed and detailed;
- spontaneous motor features of parkinsonism.

Features supportive of the diagnosis are:

- repeated falls;
- syncope;
- transient loss of consciousness;
- neuroleptic sensitivity;
- systematized delusions;
- hallucinations and other modalities.

A diagnosis of DLB is less likely in the presence of:

- stroke disease, evident as focal neurological signs or on brain imaging;
- evidence on physical examination and investigation of any physical illness or other brain disorder sufficient to account for the clinical picture.

Table 15.7 Clinical features of frontotemporal dementia

1) Insidious onset and slow progression
2) Early loss of personal and social awareness and insight
3) Early signs of disinhibition
4) Mental rigidity and inflexibility
5) Hyperoraloty, stereotypes and perseverative behaviour
6) Unrestrained exploration of objects and the environment (hypermetormorphosis)
7) Distractability and impulsivity, depression and anxiety
8) Hypochondriasis
9) Emotional unconcern
10) Inertia
11) Disorders of speech
12) Preserved abilities of spatial orientation

Table 15.8 Diagnostic criteria for CJD

Probable CJD
1) Rapidly progressive dementia
2) Periodic sharp waves in the EEG
3) At least 2 of the following 4 findings

- myoclonus
- visual or cerebellar symptoms
- pyramidal and/or extrapyramidal signs
- akinetic mutism

Possible CJD

- Those who fulfil the above clinical criteria but do not have typical EEG
- The presence of 1-3-3 protein in the CSF is a better discriminator between CJD and other dementias than the EEG or MRI scanning.
- Preliminary results suggest that basal ganglia hyperintensity on MRI scans may be a useful diagnostic marker.

ideas may manifest as suspicion and agitation. The patient's consciousness level and any involuntary movements should be assessed.

It is the examination of the cognitive state which deserves special attention. Numerous tests may be of help in detecting cognitive impairment. The Mini-Mental State Examination (Folstein *et al.*, 1975; see also www.nemc.org/psych/mmse.asp) remains a common screening tool for dementia. It is scored out of 30 points and assesses the areas of orientation, registration, recall, language, constructional ability, attention and calculation. It takes between 5 and 10 minutes to administer, and although it has been criticised for not concentrating sufficiently on memory and being heavily affected by education, it remains probably the most readily available test of cognitive function. The Abbreviated Mental Test Score, a 10-item measure, tests memory and orientation and is preferred by some. As a screening test, some like the Clock Drawing Test in which patients are asked to draw a clock face. A number of schema for scoring the result have been proposed (Shulman *et al.*, 1986), but it is probably fair to say that the drawing of a normal clock face effectively excludes a diagnosis of dementia, as long

Table 15.9 Prevalence rates of dementia from EURODEM

	Men	Women
65–69	1.6	1.0
70–74	2.9	3.1
75–79	5.6	6.0
80–83	11.0	12.6
85–89	12.8	20.2
90+	22.1	30.8

After Lobo, Launer, Fratiglioni, *et al.* (2000).

as everything else is equal (i.e. the person has intact motor and sensory function).

The Clinical Dementia Rating Scale (Hughes *et al.*, 1982, updated by Morris, 1993) is probably the most widely used global scale to give an overall severity rating in dementia, ranging from 0 (*none*) to 0.5 (*questionable dementia*) through mild and moderate to severe dementia. Each is rated in six domains: memory, orientation, judgement and problem solving, community affairs, home and hobbies and personal care.

The Neuropsychiatric Inventory (NPI; Cummings *et al.*, 1994) measures 12 behavioural areas (delusions, hallucinations, agitation, depression, anxiety, euphoria, apathy, disinhibition, irritability, aberrant motor behaviour, night-time behaviours and appetite/eating disorders). Each is rated on a 4-point scale of frequency and a 3-point scale of severity. Distress in carers is also measured.

The Bristol Activities of Daily Living Scale (Bucks *et al.*, 1996) contains 20 items rated on a 5-point severity scale looking at basic activities of daily living (e.g. feeding, eating and toiletting) and instrumental activities of daily living (which refer to the performance of more complex tasks such as shopping, travelling, answering the telephone and handling finances).

Investigations

A physical examination should be performed, and blood tests should include full blood count, urea and electrolytes, liver function tests, erythrocyte sedimentation rate, serum protein, glucose, calcium, phosphate, thyroid function tests and vitamin B_{12} and folate. A urine culture should be taken if a urinary tract infection is suspected. A chest X-ray and electrocardiogram should be performed if clinically indicated. Some form of brain imaging should be undertaken: computed tomography (CT) is probably the most widely available, although magnetic resonance imaging (MRI) is sometimes indicated in people with very early disease (see also Chapter 4).

The neurobiology of dementia

Alzheimer's disease

The neuropathology of Alzheimer's disease is the most distinctive of all the dementias. The definitive diagnosis still requires neuropathological confirmation. The most obvious finding on naked-eye examination is generalised atrophy of the cerebral hemispheres but in particular the medial temporal lobes, hippocampus and amygdala. This atrophy consists of narrowing of the gyri and widening of the sulci and increased ventricular size with atrophy of the striatum and a decrease in pigment in the locus coeruleus. The microscopic pathology is characterised by widespread senile (neuritic) plaques and neurofibrillary tangles. Plaques are best seen with silver stains or immunocytochemistry using antibodies to the B amyloid (AB) peptide; the plaques are extra-cellular and consist of a dense core surrounded by less dense material. These neuritic plaques may well be the successor of diffuse plaques which consist of deposits of fibrillary material without any evidence of a central core of amyloid.

Neurofibrillary tangles are abnormal structures inside neurones and are well seen with silver stains or by using immunocytochemical stains of antibodies against their principle component, hyperphosphorylated tau. They are smaller than plaques, and most contain a nucleus, although some tangles are clearly extra-cellular and appear to be the result of neuronal death (a ghost tangle). Other pathological features of Alzheimer's disease include neuronal loss, glial cell reactions, neuropil threads, granulovacuolar degeneration, Hirano bodies and congophilic angiopathy.

The main component of the plaque is a peptide known as AB which is derived from the break-up of the amyloid precursor protein (APP). A number of mutations have been found in the gene coding for APP, and this was the first familial gene to be found in Alzheimer's disease. APP is metabolised by at least three pathways, not all of which result in the creation of AB.

Another group of genetic abnormalities are the presenilin mutations. These are transmembrane proteins and the genes PS1 (linked to chromosome 14) and PS 2 (linked to chromosome 1) have been described. The former appears to be a dominant, early-onset familial chain for Alzheimer's disease. The normal biological roles of APP and presenilin remain unclear.

Apolipoprotein E (ApoE) is linked to chromosome 19 and is a polymorphic gene that exists in three alleles – e2, e3 and e4. E3 is the most common allele followed by e4 and e2. Any individual has any two of these three resulting in either being homozygous (e2/e2, e3/e3, e4/e4) or heterozygous (e2/e3, e2/e4, e3/e4) phenotypes. The presence of either one or two of the e4 alleles has been associated with the development of cardiovascular disease, and a number of studies have documented the greatly increased risk of Alzheimer's disease in people with one or two e4 alleles. ApoE is a lipid transport molecule and is part of liver-synthesised very low-density lipoproteins. There is some evidence to show that e4 may be specifically related to neurofibrillary tangle and amyloid formation.

Despite being overtaken by studies into the molecular genetics of AD, neurochemical abnormalities have been consistently described. Deficits in the cholinergic system seem to be the most prominent, with particular deficiencies in the marker enzymes choline acetyl transferase and acetyl cholinesterase. This led to the cholinergic hypothesis of Alzheimer's disease, and it is this which forms the basis of current drug therapies. It is far from clear why there is selective vulnerability of cholinergic neurones and difficult to reconcile fully the distribution of pathology and cholinergic dysfunction. Less consistent deficits in gamma-aminobutyric acid (GABA), dopamine, noradrenaline and serotonin have also been described.

Vascular dementia

With regard to vascular dementia, the pathology originally was much more straightforward – large cerebral infarctions resulted in the loss of brain tissue, which, either by sheer volume or strategic position, resulted in signs and symptoms of dementia. However, it is increasingly becoming recognised that more progressive accumulation of vascular change can cause damage without evidence of discrete infarction. Large infarctions usually affect the cerebral cortex and underlying white matter, usually in watershed areas (areas at the end of the blood supply territory of different arteries) and are sometimes associated with lacunes. *Microinfarcts* are lesions usually less than 2 mm in diameter.

White matter changes were once considered rare but are now considered central to the understanding of cerebral vascular dementia. The terms Binswager's disease and leukoaraiosis have been used to describe these white matter abnormalities which are universal in people with vascular dementia and also common in Alzheimer's disease. Frontal white matter hyperintensities appear to be associated with depression and those in the periventricular area more with cognitive impairment. There is some evidence that people with vascular dementia may have an increased frequency of the e4 allele and this may partly be related to the core presence of Alzheimer's disease pathology. A specific type of hereditary vascular dementia called CADASIL (cerebral autosomal dominant arteriopathy with subcortical infarcts and leukoencephalopathy) has also been described.

Management of dementia

The clinical management of a person with dementia is considered under three main headings:

- general care and support;
- treatment of cognitive symptoms; and
- management of behavioural and psychological symptoms.

Support and care

Increasingly there has been an appreciation that the traditional medical view of dementia could be broadened with benefit to patients and carers. Maintaining functional ability can be achieved (Lawton & Rubenstein, 2000). Placing the person at the centre of care is a recently evolved concept, spearheaded by the late Tom Kitwood (1997). Much can be done in terms of general support and care to support independence. For example, Beck and colleagues (1997) showed that by teaching nursing assistants strategies to encourage nursing home residents who were cognitively impaired to dress, three quarters became more independent.

Improved communication, social interaction and decreasing negative stigma (all components of person-centred care) can achieve modest improvements in memory, emotions, activities of daily living, communication and, ultimately, quality of life. Memory books can encourage carers to interact more with a person suffering from dementia, and, contrary to popular expectation, people with even advanced dementia can benefit from such interactions. Reality orientation, in which the carer uses visual and verbal cues to help reorientate the individual, can also be effective. Reminiscence therapy (concentrating individually or in groups on things in the past to stimulate memories), however, shows equivocal results, as does validation therapy (a person-centred approach to care aimed at validating rather than correcting a person's memories and perceptions). It can be difficult to tease apart the specific positive effects of such interactions and the benefits of individualised care.

Individual interventions directed towards reducing specific abnormal behaviours are effective and usually based on the ABC construct, that is, a careful analysis of an abnormal behaviour should concentrate on its antecedents (A), the behaviour itself (B) and the consequences (C). For example, say an elderly person with Alzheimer's disease in a nursing home becomes agitated and stands by the door at about 6 PM every night. She gets agitated when staff members try to take her away from the door to sit down to have her tea. On close questioning, it becomes apparent that she believes her husband (who died 25 years earlier) will be coming home from work soon; she is anxious to meet him at the door, worried that she has not been able to prepare his evening meal and worried that he will hit her when he comes home. This understanding could inform to a treatment plan in which the lady helps to lay the tables at around 4:45 PM and feels she is doing something positive which will allay her husband's potential anger when he comes home.

Interventions specifically for carers can reduce distress and enhance knowledge, but with no specific effect on caregiver burden. Such interventions are more successful if patients are involved in them rather than being completely separate. The attributional style of carers is also a marker for the carer/patient relationship. Thus carers with a more positive attributional style suffer less stress than carers with a predominantly negative attitude.

Treatment of cognitive symptoms

A major advance in the treatment of cognitive decline in dementia has been the development of drugs that block the activity of acetylcholinesterase (Box 15.3). The rationale for this approach lies in the understanding that decreased synthesis of

---

Box 15.3 Drugs licensed for Alzheimer's disease (AD) in the United Kingdom

Anticholinesterases (mild to moderate AD)

Tacrine (Cognex)	No longer marketed
Donepezil (Aricept)	5–10 mg
Rivastigmine (Exelon)	6–12 mg
Galantamine (Reminyl)	8–24 mg

Glutaminergic (moderately severe AD)

Memantine (Ebixa)	10–20 mg

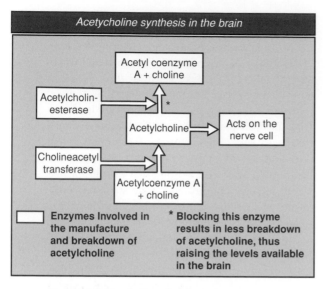

Figure 15.1 The cholinergic approach

acetylcholine and increased breakdown results in a significant diminution of central acetylcholinergic activity in dementia and that this correlates with the degree of cognitive impairment (see Figure 15.1).

Acetylcholinesterase inhibitors are superior to placebo in improving cognitive deficits, global ratings of dementia and activities of daily living in Alzheimer's disease. The duration of effect and long-term safety of the drugs has yet to be fully established. The drugs donepezil, rivastigmine and galantamine should be made available as one component in the management of those people with mild and moderate Alzheimer's disease (MMSE >12), under the following conditions:

- The form of dementia has been confirmed to be Alzheimer's disease.
- Assessment in a specialist clinic, including tests of cognitive, global and behavioural functioning and of activities of daily living has occurred.
- Clinicians exercise judgment about the likelihood of compliance.
- Only specialists (including old age psychiatrists, neurologists and care of the elderly physicians) initiate treatment.
- Carers' views of the patient's condition at baseline and follow-up are sought.

- Further assessments are made, usually 2 to 4 months after reaching maintenance dose of the drug. The drug should be continued only if there has been an improvement or no deterioration in MMSE score and evidence of global improvement on the basis of behavioural and/or functional assessment.
- Patients who continue on the drug should be reviewed every 6 months; the drug should be continued while the MMSE score remains above 12 points and global, functional and behaviour condition remains at a level in which the drug is considered to have a worthwhile effect.

It should be noted that the benefits of these drugs for patients with other forms of dementia (e.g. dementia with Lewy bodies) has not been systematically assessed.

Donepezil, a highly selective reversible inhibitor of acetylcholine, has high oral bioavailability which is unaffected by food, a long plasma half-life of 70 hours permitting once-daily dosing, and almost total plasma protein binding. Pivotal studies show an improvement in both cognition and clinician-rated improvement with a greater effect at the 10-mg compared with the 5-mg dosage. The most common side effects are gastrointestinal and include nausea, vomiting, diarrhoea and anorexia. Some patients develop muscle cramps. Haematological side effects include anaemia, thrombocytopaenia and cardiac side effects include bradyarrhythmia and syncope. Central nervous system side effects include headache, dizziness, insomnia, weakness, drowsiness, fatigue and agitation.

Rivastigmine has an effect both on acetylcholinesterase and butyrylcholinesterase. It has a short half-life (2 hours) and thus needs to be given twice a day and requires slow titration to minimise the cholinergic side effects. Side effects include nausea, vomiting and anorexia.

Galantamine is an anti-cholinesterase agent which also has a modulating effect on nicotinic receptors. It has the expected tolerability problems in keeping with other anti-cholinesterases, the majority being gastrointestinal. It has a half-life between that of donepezil and rivastigmine and needs to be given twice daily at an optimal daily dose between 16 and 24 mg.

Management of behavioural and psychological symptoms

Nonpharmacological treatments can be an effective first-line management strategy for many people with behavioural and psychological symptoms of dementia. When drug treatment is required, antipsychotics are generally the treatment of choice; studies suggest a 60% response rate compared with 40% on placebo. Adverse effects include falls, drowsiness, parkinsonism, akinesia, tardive dyskinesia and cardiac arrhythmias; some may accelerate cognitive decline. A recent warning by the Committee of Safety in Medicines has highlighted an increased incidence of stroke, transient ischemic attacks and other cardiovascular adverse events with the antipsychotics risperidone and olanzapine in the elderly (DoH, 2004). This has promoted the search for alternative agents. There is good evidence that the anticholinesterase drugs may be effective in the management of behavioural and psychological symptoms; rivastigmine has been shown to be effective in dementia with Lewy bodies (McKeith et al., 2000).

A number of non-antipsychotic drugs are also used in the management of patients with dementia. Antidepressants can control agitation and restlessness – not necessarily in patients with obvious depressive features, although obviously they are specifically effective when depression is present. Trazodone seemed to be particularly helpful in controlling screaming. Some anticonvulsants are used to control agitation. A few case reports suggest that lithium improves agitation, but because of its relative toxicity and the need for monitoring, it is not likely to become a treatment of first choice. Buspirone, a gamma-aminobutyric acid antagonist, is said to have some effect on agitated patients. Beta-blockers have traditionally been used to control aggression in younger patients with brain damage. Benzodiazepines should not be forgotten: in cases with a clinical suspicion of Lewy body dementia, a combination of benzodiazepines and chlormethiazole can be effective. Care always needs to be taken with dosing of medications in the elderly, with generally lower dosages required than in younger adults. Table 15.10 provides guidance regarding dosing of psychotropic medications in the elderly.

Recently, interest has been kindled in so-called novel treatments for agitation in dementia with approaches such as aromatherapy and bright light therapy (see Burns et al., 2002). *Aromatherapy* has been used for a number of years for a variety of health problems, the most common agents being lemon balm or lavender. These can be given through skin application or by inhalation. Active agents in aromatherapy oils have been identified (the terpines) which cross the blood-brain barrier easily because of their lipid solubility. *Bright light therapy* has antidepressant and calming effects.

Depression occurs commonly in people with dementia, with a prevalence of 50% to 70% in AD, and even higher rates in vascular dementia and dementia with Lewy bodies. There have not been many studies specifically looking at the effect of drugs for the treatment of depression in dementia, but those which are available show that the treatment is as effective in the presence of cognitive impairment as in its absence. The selective serotonin reuptake inhibitors (SSRIs) seem to be the most appropriate agents, with tricyclic antidepressants (TCAs) being relatively contraindicated in view of their negative cardiovascular and cholinergic side effects. Exercise has also been shown to enhance mood in people with AD (Teri et al., 2003).

Treatment of vascular dementia

There are no specific treatments for vascular dementia. Studies on the anti-dementia drugs, particularly galantamine and memantine, in people with mixed Alzheimer's vascular dementia do suggest some improvement, but the effect is much less marked than for Alzheimer's disease. Interventions to ameliorate the effects of cardiovascular risk factors can have benefit both in the prevention of

Table 15.10 Guidelines regarding starting doses of psychotropic agents in the elderly

Drug and class	Suggesting starting[a] and daily dose (range/maximal; mg/day)
Antipsychotics	
Traditional	
haloperidol	0.25–0.5 (2–4)
thioridazine	12.5–25 (50–100)
thiothixene	0.5–1 (2–4)
Atypical	
clozapine	6.25–12.5 (25–100)
olanzapine	2.5 (5–10)
quetiapine	25 (50–200)
risperidone	0.5 (1–2)
aripiprazole	5 (15)
ziprasidone	unknown
Anxiolytics and sedatives	
Benzodiazepines:	
alprazolam	0.5 (1–2)
lorazepam	0.5 (2–4)
oxazepam	10 (40–60)
Non-benzodiazepines:	
zolpidem	2.5 (5)
buspirone	10 (30–60)
Antidepressants	
trazodone	25–50 (200–300)
Selective serotonin reuptake inhibitors	
citalopram	10 (20)
fluoxetine	10 (20)
sertraline	25–50 (100–200)
Anticonvulsants	
carbamazepine	50–100 (300–500)
divalproex	125–375 (500–1500)
Beta-blockers	
propranolol	20 (50–100)
Others	
selegiline	10
oestradiol/progesterone	0.625/2.5

From Tariot *et al.* (2005). Reproduced with permission.
[a] Suggestions are based on published data as well as anecdotal experience and should be regarded accordingly.

Box 15.4 Testamentary capacity

1. The person should know what the act of making a will means.
2. The person should have a broad understanding of the extent of his or her estate.
3. The person should know who might have a claim on his or her possessions.
4. The person should have no mental disorder affecting points 1, 2 and 3 and not be subject to undue influence.

(Jacoby, 2004)

the emergence of dementia and the treatment of symptoms.

Ethical and legal aspects

Most of the ethical and legal aspects of the care of people with dementia revolve around whether these people have competence (a medical term) or capacity (predominantly a legal term) to make decisions for themselves. Competence is directed towards an individual task; for example, someone may have the ability to agree to a marriage but not to be able to handle complex financial tasks. To be competent, a person should be able to (a) understand information relevant to the required decision; (b) use the information rationally, e.g. make a risk-benefit comparison; (c) appreciate the situation and its consequences; and (d) communicate choices (Jacoby, 2004). A particularly problematic issue is that of competence to make a will, so-called testamentary capacity (Box 15.4).

Various legal mechanisms are available to protect people with dementia and ensure they are adequately cared for. These differ from country to country but can include guardianship and enduring power of attorney.

Delirium

Delirium is discussed in detail in Chapter 14. Here we emphasise those issues pertinent to the elderly. Delirium in old people is common and has high morbidity and mortality, yet it is often unrecognised.

Epidemiology

Folstein *et al.* (1991) found a prevalence of 1.1% in community residents aged 55 years or more and 13.6% of those aged over 80 years. In nursing homes, the prevalence is about 6% (Bienenfeld & Wheeler, 1989; Rovner *et al.*, 1986), whereas in hospital settings, the rates are even higher: 15% to 25% on medical wards (Lindesay *et al.*, 2002), 26% to 61% on surgical wards (Levkoff *et al.*, 1991; Marcantonio *et al.*, 2000) and 13% on psychiatry of old age wards (Kaponen *et al.*, 1989).

Aetiology

Factors that may predispose to delirium include age and pre-existing dementia (Lipowski, 1990; Rolfson, 2002); others such as sensory impairment may act as maintaining factors (Beresin, 1988). Risk factors for the development of delirium in elderly surgical patients include age, previous alcohol or drug abuse and prolonged operations (Whittaker, 1989). Table 15.11 lists the common causes of delirium in the elderly; see also Table 14.4.

Course and outcome

Prospective studies of delirium in old people in hospital have found mean durations of around 3 weeks (Cole & Primeau, 1993; Kaponen & Reikkinen, 1993; Thomas *et al.*, 1988). Delirious patients aged 65 years or more have significantly longer hospital stays than do nondelirious patients (Francis *et al.*, 1990; Thomas *et al.*, 1988).

Mortality rates in all studies are high, ranging from 15% to 30% (Cole & Primeau, 1993; Lipowski, 1992); this is perhaps not surprising in view of the close association of delirium with serious physical illness (Francis *et al.*, 1990).

It is possible that quantitative electroencephalography (QEEG) may prove to be a useful technique

Table 15.11 The commonest causes of acute delirium in old people

Very common	
Heart failure	left ventricular failure
	congestive cardiac failure
Infection	urinary oblique respiratory
Carcinomatosis	
Common	
Cerebrovascular	transient ischaemia
Drugs	anticholinergic (e.g., tricyclic antidepressants, benzhexol); interactions; withdrawal (alcohol, benzodiazepines)
Metabolic	hypoglycaemia; disorders of fluid and electrolyte balance; renal or hepatic failure
Anoxia	respiratory, anaemia, reduced cerebral perfusion

From Lipowski, 1992; Royal College of Physicians, 1981.

in the detection and monitoring of delirium in old people (Leuchter & Jacobsen, 1991).

Management

Comprehensive reviews of the management of delirium can be found in Marcantonio (2002), Burns *et al.* (2003) and in Chapter 14. The two basic principles are to identify and treat the underlying cause and to treat or manage the associated behavioural and psychiatric symptoms (Fairweather, 1991; Lindesay *et al.*, 1990). Identification of delirium may be improved by education and at least one RCT of an intervention designed to prevent delirium by identifying and treating risk factors was successful (Innouye *et al.*, 1999).

Antipsychotic drugs may be indicated in cases of severe agitation or distressing psychiatric symptoms (persecutory delusions), and haloperidol has been advocated as the drug of choice by some (American Psychiatric Association, 1999; Lipowski, 1989; Taylor & Lewis, 1993). Care must be exercised in its use in the elderly, because it has a long half-life (up to 60 hours) and is a powerful inducer of extrapyramidal symptoms; dosages of around 2 mg have been suggested (Fairweather, 1991), but benefit may accrue from dosages as low as 0.5 to 1 mg. Other drugs which have been used in delirium in the elderly include olanzapine and donepezil (Burns *et al.*, 2003).

Manipulation of the environment in which the delirious patient is nursed is often "prescribed", but there is no experimental data on which to base this view (Burns *et al.*, 2003), and there may be downsides such as neglect and disruption to the sleep-wake cycle from 24-hour lighting.

Some people who survive delirium can recall their experiences, often in surprising detail (Andersson, 2002; Crammer, 2002; Levin, 1968; Schofield, 1997). This observation suggests that reassurance might be a helpful technique.

Affective disorders

Depression

Depression is one of the most common problems encountered in old age psychiatry, yet, as with younger patients, there is continuing debate as to its nosology, aetiology, treatment and outcome (see Chapters 12 and 27). The nosological debate focuses on the definitions of major depression (severe depression, depressive illness) and, especially in regard to the latter, the definition of caseness. Some have argued quite persuasively that the expression of depression in old age is inadequately defined by both the *Diagnostic and Statistical Manual of Mental Disorders* (DSM) and the *International Classification of Diseases* (ICD) (Cairne *et al.*, 1994; Gallo & Rabins, 1999) because much of what is called depression consists of affective symptoms which do not reach caseness (as defined by DSM); which are frequently comorbid with other psychiatric disorders, especially anxiety; and which are not included in the nosological definitions. The frequency of the comorbidity of depression in old age with anxiety has led to renewed interest in the concept of generalised neurotic disorder (Larkin *et al.*, 1992).

Epidemiology

Studies of old people have shown that depressive symptoms are much more common than cases of depression. Some of these studies are summarised in Table 15.12. All used structured interviews or depressive symptom rating scales, some of which are linked to diagnostic systems, but only the Epidemiological Catchment Area (ECA) study applied DSM-III (third edition) diagnoses. In a systematic review of community studies of depression in people aged over 55 years, Beekman *et al.* (1999) found that the (weighted average) prevalence was 1.8% for major depression and 9.8% for minor depression; the average prevalence of all depressive syndromes was 13.5%. In the "oldest old", rates of depressive symptoms are higher than in the "young old" (20% compared with 10%; Blazer, 2000). Much higher rates of depressive symptoms are reported in hospital in-patients and in old people living in residential or nursing homes.

Depressive symptoms in old age

There is now good evidence to support the contention that "depression is depression at any age" (Baldwin, 1991). However, depression in old age may be overlooked either because it is seen as an "understandable" consequence of senescence or because it arises in association with physical ill health (Baldwin, 1991; Epstein, 1976; Pitt, 1986). Newmann *et al.* (1996), in a careful appraisal of the experience of depressive symptoms in older women, suggested that "older persons may be at decreased risk for depression in its classical form, although at increase risk for a quieter more unconventional form". This quieter form was given the name of "depletion syndrome of the elderly" (Fogel & Fretwell, 1985) and is characterised by social withdrawal and disengagement rather than by a feeling of despair and emotional distress. Depression without sadness also occurs in older people (Gallo & Rabins, 1999).

Where depression in old age arises with physical illness, it is important to obtain a history of change from the patient and relatives and to look

Table 15.12 Selected community epidemiological studies of depression in old people (≥65 years)

Study	n	Screening instrument/ Diagnostic system	Location	Prevalence of depression
Copeland et al., 1987	1,070	GMS Agecat	Urban UK	11.5% 3%
Morgan et al., 1987	1,042	SAD	Urban UK	10% (65–74 years) 9.5% (75+)
ECA (Johnson et al., 1992; Weissman et al., 1988)	4,701	DIS/ DSM-III	5 communities USA	23% (16% cases)
Lindesay et al., 1989	983	CARE/ Catego	Urban UK	13.5% (including 4.3% severe)
Livingston et al., 1990	932	CARE	Urban UK	15.9%
Fuhrer et al., 1992	4,050	CES-D	Urban & Rural France	13.4%
Copeland et al., 1999 (EURODEP)	13,808	Agecat	8 European countries	12.3%
Ritchie et al., 2004	1,863	DSM-IV	Urban France	3.1%

Agecat = Computer derived diagnostic system linked to GMS; CARE = Comprehensive assessment & referral examination; Catego = A computer diagnostic classification system; CES-D = Centre for epidemiological studies – depression scale; DIS = Diagnostic interview schedule; DSM = *Diagnostic and Statistical Manual of Mental Disorders*; ECA = National Institutes of Mental Health–epidemiological catchment area; GMS = Geriatric mental state schedule; SAD = Symptoms of anxiety and depression scale

for features such as loss of pleasure and depressive thoughts (feelings of guilt, worthlessness). More classical features of depression such as sleep disturbance and fatigue are often less reliable in the context of physical illness (Baldwin, 1991; Cohen-Cole & Stoudemire, 1987)

Aetiology

Although there is some genetic contribution to the aetiology of major affective disorder with onset in old age, this is much weaker than that shown in patients with onset less than 60 years of age. For example, Musetti et al. (1989) found a family history of affective disorder in 45.6% of patients whose illness began before 40 years, 35.5% with onset before 60 years, and 28.6% with onset after 60 years.

The evidence as to whether the ageing process intrinsically predisposes to late-onset affective disorder is equivocal. Epidemiological studies which show that the prevalence of major affective illness declines with age suggest that it does not. Reviews of neurotransmitter changes in depression in relation to ageing have been inconsistent. Depressive symptoms are commoner in older people, and their aetiological relationship with the ageing process – both in biological and psychological terms – is only now beginning to be addressed (discussed later).

Depression is very common in association with some diseases which are more prevalent in old age such as Parkinson's disease (Baldwin & Byrne, 1989) and stroke (House, 1987). The MRC-ALPHA study (Copeland et al., 1999) examined risk factors for depression in a large case-control study in Liverpool. Female gender, physical disability and dissatisfaction with life were associated with depression, whereas age itself was not.

Depression and cerebrovascular disease in late life

CT (MacDonald, 1992) and MRI (Baldwin, 1993) studies have found older depressive patients to have more, albeit mild, cerebral atrophy than age-matched control subjects and a greater incidence of white matter lesions. These findings, inter alia, led to the "vascular depression" hypothesis (Alexopoulos et al., 1997), in which cerebrovascular disease is thought to predispose, precipitate and/or perpetuate depression. Evidence to support this hypothesis has steadily accumulated (see reviews by Byrne & Simpson, 1997; Camus et al., 2004). Particularly cogent is the formulation that the relationship between depression and vascular disease is bi-directional; that is, depression increases the risk of vascular disease and vice versa (Thomas et al., 2008). An example of the perpetuation of depression by cerebrovascular disease is seen in its association with treatment-resistant depression (TRD). TRD in older people is associated with an increased burden of cerebrovascular lesions on MRI scan, and with cognitive impairment (Baldwin & O'Brien, 2002).

Treatment

The treatment of depression in old age has been reviewed by the US Surgeon General (2000), and guidelines have been developed for primary care (Baldwin et al., 2003). The evidence base for the physical treatment of major depression in older people is growing but is still not comprehensive (Chew-Graham et al., 2004).

In terms of medication, choice of antidepressant, relative efficacy and benefits compared to nonpharmacological therapy for acute-phase treatment in the elderly have not yet been fully elucidated. In minor depression, the effects of antidepressants are modest (Roose et al., 2004; Williams et al., 2000). Many patients prefer psychological therapy, which has also shown to be of benefit (Williams et al., 2000).

For moderately severe and severe (nonpsychotic) depression, antidepressants are significantly superior to placebo in controlled trials (Katona & Livingstone, 2002; Wilson et al., 2001). In the "oldest old", those with the most severe depression (>24 on the Hamilton Depression Rating Scale) showed a greater response to citalopram than those with less severe depression. The most severe cases, and those with delusions or other psychotic features, have a better outcome if treated with a combination of antidepressants and antipsychotics or with electroconvulsive therapy (ECT) (Baldwin, 1988).

SSRIs are usually recommended as the first choice for the treatment of moderately severe and severe (nonpsychotic) depression. Their adverse effect profile, compared with that of TCAs, is favourable; they have no significant effects on cardiac rhythm or blood pressure (Katona & Livingston, 2002). Nausea (with or without vomiting) can be troublesome in some patients. Although the SSRIs are generally better tolerated (Birrer & Vemuri, 2004; Katona & Livingston, 2002) in older people, there is still a significant minority who are noncompliant (Birrer & Vemuri, 2004). Further, the efficacy of SSRIs is no better than that of TCAs (Block et al., 1997; Wilson et al., 2001), and in one study it was less (Danish University Antidepressant Group, 1990). Other classes of antidepressants (such as venlafaxine, a serotonin-noradrenaline reuptake inhibitor [SNRI]) have been assessed for acute-phase treatment of depression in older people (Anderson et al., 2000), but data from randomised controlled trials is lacking.

Adverse effects for both SSRIs and TCAs in the elderly can be reduced by a low starting dosage and slow titration (Birrer & Vemuri, 2004). Treatment in the acute phase should be tailored to the individual patient (Baldwin, 1998; Reynolds, 1992; US Surgeon General, 2000).

The duration of treatment for depression in old age is not yet definitively established. Reviewing the available evidence, Flint (1992) concluded that 6 months was not enough and that elderly patients may benefit from a much longer period of treatment. The Old Age Depression Interest

Group (OADIG) study (Jacoby *et al.*, 1993) supported this view: continued treatment with dothiepin for 2 years reduced the risk of relapse by 2.5 times that of the placebo in a group of elderly patients with major depression. A similar reduction in rate of relapse was found by Klysner *et al.* (2002) in a 48-week trial of citalopram in older (>65 years) out-patients. The evidence for the benefit of continuation therapy for the treatment of depression overall (including all age groups) is robust (Geddes *et al.*, 2003). Lithium prophylaxis has been used in the elderly, but adherence can be problematic.

Treatment-resistant depression (TRD) in older depressed patients is variously defined as depression not responding to antidepressants after 4 to 6 weeks or as the failure to respond to two trials of antidepressants, from two classes, in adequate dosage for an adequate period of time (Thase *et al.*, 2002). Augmentation therapy for TRD in older people, for example, using lithium in addition to antidepressants, is at least as effective as it is in younger patients, with about two thirds showing benefit (Finch & Katona, 1989). ECT is both safe and effective in elderly patients (Benbow, 1989; Flint & Ritaf, 1998; Salzman *et al.*, 2002; Tew *et al.*, 1999), and the indications for its use are well established.

Nonpharmacological treatments, including counselling, group therapy, interpersonal psychotherapy (IPT) and cognitive-behavioural therapy (CBT), may also be effective in the treatment of depression in old age (see reviews by US Surgeon General, 2000; Wilkinson *et al.*, 2002). Jarvick *et al.* (1982) found that group psychotherapy (dynamic or cognitive) for elderly depressives was more effective than placebo but less effective than antidepressants. Baldwin (1991) suggested that psychotherapy would be more effective if combined with antidepressants or when used in adequately treated patients, an assertion subsequently validated by Reynolds *et al.* (1999) in a randomised controlled trial of IPT and nortriptyline. A meta-analysis of 17 studies of psychological therapies for depression in older people found that psychological therapy was more effective than no treatment or placebo treatment (Scogin & McElreath, 1994).

Outcome

The results of the initial treatment (<25 weeks) of a depressive episode in old age are good with about 70% improving (Baldwin & Jolley, 1986; Tuma, 2000). However, over the intermediate term (>25 weeks to 1 year), outcome is less favourable (Murphy, 1983), and the longer-term outcome is poor. At 2 years, only around a third are well, a third remain depressed and a fifth are dead (Cole *et al.*, 1999). At 4.5 years, only a quarter of patients are well, a third are dead and 15% have developed dementia (Tuma, 2000). Adverse prognostic factors include the presence of brain "pathology" (such as cerebrovascular disease; Jacoby 1981), a slow or incomplete initial recovery (Godber *et al.*, 1987), adverse life events before onset (Murphy, 1983) and coexistent physical illness (Cole *et al.*, 1999; Tuma, 2000).

Mania

The true prevalence of manic illness in old age has not been fully established but estimates suggest rates of around 0.4% in community samples and 5% in hospitalised elderly patients (Yassa *et al.*, 1988). There is some evidence that an increased inception rate for mania is associated with increasing age (Eagles & Whalley, 1985), although Broadhead and Jacoby (1990) found the mean age of onset of manic episodes in a group of manic patients to be bimodal with a peak at 37 years and another at 73 years. One-year incidence rates for first admission for bipolar disorder in a Finnish study found that 20% were aged over 60 years.

Aetiology

As with depression in old age, genetic factors in mania are probably less important than in younger cohorts (Hays *et al.*, 1998; Stone, 1989). Onset of mania in old age may be linked to cerebral organic disease (Jacoby, 1991). Krauthammer and Klermann (1978) coined the term *secondary mania* to describe such cases. There is still debate as to whether such individuals lack a genetic predisposition. Among elderly manic patients, between 24% and 43% (Broadhead & Jacoby, 1990; Stone, 1989) have demonstrable cerebral pathology; Shulman and Post (1980) reported higher figures for elderly manic men (61%) than women (10%). Neuroimaging studies (reviewed by Steffans & Krishnan, 1998) report an increased tendency to "vascular" lesions in older manic patients, leading to the hypothesis that there is a vascular subtype of mania.

Clinical features

Early studies suggested that mania in late life often has a prominent admixture of depressive features. However, a prospective study (Broadhead & Jacoby, 1990) compared the clinical features of young- and late-onset mania and found no differences between them. The late-onset manias were, however, more likely to have had a depressed phase during their index admission. Also, a substantial minority of those with late-onset mania begin with recurrent depressive disorder (Shulman & Post, 1980; Stone, 1989).

Occasionally manic symptoms in late life may herald the onset of dementia, especially of the frontal lobe type (Gustafson, 1987), but in established Alzheimer's disease this is uncommon.

Treatment

Advice on the treatment of mania in the elderly is based on a paucity of controlled trials; for a review, see Baldwin, 2000. The reader is also referred to Chapter 26.

Lithium
Lithium is a safe and effective treatment for both acute illness and for prophylaxis in elderly manic patients (Foster *et al.*, 1990). Use in the elderly requires careful monitoring of renal and thyroid function and ensuring therapeutic levels are maintained.

Anticonvulsants
Sodium valproate and carbamazepine have both been used, with efficacy, in the treatment of mania

in older people (Shulmann & Hermann, 2001; Young *et al.*, 2004), and lamotrigine (for bipolar depression) and gabapentin (for treatment resistant bipolar disorder) have shown promise in uncontrolled trials in older people (Robillard & Conn, 2002).

Antipsychotics
Antipsychotics may also be effective in the acute phase, either alone or in combination with lithium (Jacoby, 1991). In the elderly, the place of these agents in prophylaxis is still underresearched, and careful monitoring of side effects is required.

Other treatments
ECT has a role in the acute treatment of mania in older people. Transcranial magnetic stimulation (TMS) has been proposed as a safe and effective treatment for mania, but studies in younger adults have been equivocal, and there is a lack of evidence for its use in the elderly.

Outcome

The outcome for an index admission for mania in old age is good, but there are few data regarding longer-term outcome. Shulmann and Post (1980) found that the majority of elderly manic patients suffered from recurrent affective illness.

Very late onset schizophrenia (late paraphrenia)

There is a nosological debate as to how schizophrenia arising in old age should be categorised. The original description by Post (1966) was of "persistent persecutory states", encompassing those elderly patients in whom paranoid symptoms were prominent. The term *late-onset schizophrenia* was used by Manfred Bleuler in 1943 to describe a schizophrenia-like illness arising in old age (without evidence of cognitive impairment or brain disease). Roth (1955) introduced the term *late paraphrenia* as a florid psychosis manifesting for the first time, usually after the age of 60. The International Late Onset Schizophrenia Group (Howard *et al.,* 2000) propose that the evidence (symptomatology, epidemiology, family history) suggests that schizophrenia may arise at any stage in the life cycle from the teenage years to old age; these researchers suggest the terminology *early-onset schizophrenia* (EOS) for those with an age of onset below 39 years, *late-onset schizophrenia* (LOS) for those with an onset between 40 and 59 years and *very late onset schizophrenia-like psychosis* (VLOS) for those with an onset over age 60. This approach is pragmatic, fits the available evidence and has heuristic value; we have therefore adopted this terminology throughout this section.

The nosological status of delusional disorder arising in middle or old age has also been questioned, with some arguing that diagnostic distinction from schizophrenia lacks validity (Hafner *et al.,* 2001; Riechei-Russler *et al.,* 2003).

Epidemiology

The prevalence of VLOS in community samples varies from 0.1% to 0.5% in the population aged over 65 years (Cohen *et al.,* 1990; Howard *et al.,* 2000). The incidence of VLOS is between 17 and 24 per 100,000 per year (Holden, 1987).

Symptoms

VLOS is characterised by female sex, fewer negative symptoms, little formal thought disorder and prominent hallucinations (notably visual). Associations include social isolation, sensory impairment and premorbid paranoid personality traits; family loading for schizophrenia is lower than for early-onset cases (Howard *et al.,* 2000).

Cognitive function

In a community study of cognitive function in schizophrenia (irrespective of age of onset) Kelly and colleagues (2000) found that impaired cognitive function was "pervasive" and most impaired in those aged 60 years or older. In a 6-year follow-up study of institutionalised patients with schizophrenia (*n* = 107) aged between 20 and 80 years, Friedman and colleagues (2001) found that there was a significant age group effect on cognitive decline, with those aged over 50 years at study onset showing the steepest decline. In comparison, AD patients (*n* = 118) showed progressive cognitive decline irrespective of their age at the initiation of follow-up.

Follow-up studies of cognitive function in schizophrenia have usually defined late onset as occurring in middle age (45–50 years). Such studies have shown conflicting results, demonstrating either no difference in rates of cognitive decline between EOS and LOS compared with AD patients or a subgroup of LOS who developed dementia (Brodaty *et al.,* 2003; Palmer *et al.,* 2003). Others found cognitive decline in such patients that did not reach criteria for dementia (Rabins & Lavrisha, 2003).

There is some evidence that late-onset delusional disorder carries a higher risk (than the older population) for subsequent dementia, with nearly one third of such patients becoming demented at 10-year follow-up (Leinonen *et al.,* 2004).

Aetiology

The most robust association in the aetiology of LOS and VLOS is female sex, although the reasons for this are unclear (Howard *et al.,* 2000; Sajatovic *et al.,* 2002; Salokangas *et al.,* 2003). Premorbid paranoid personality has long been associated with the development of VLOS, but often it is difficult to ascertain whether a new illness has supervened or whether the condition is merely an extension of the existing personality with exacerbation of eccentricity, suspiciousness and social isolation. Genetic risk for schizophrenia is intermediate between early-onset cases and the general population (Howard *et al.,* 2000).

The contribution of organic brain lesions has been emphasised by a number of studies which have shown changes on neuroimaging, including enlarged cerebral ventricles, white matter, cerebral infarctions, and cortical atrophy (Burns *et al.,* 1989; Keshavan *et al.,* 1996; Miller *et al.,* 1991; Naguib &

Levy, 1987; Rabins *et al.*, 1987; Sachdev *et al.*, 1999). However, the study by Symonds and colleagues (1997) found no excess of abnormalities on MRI in LOS versus EOS. In very old (>85) nondemented people, basal ganglia calcification was found in more than 60% of those with hallucinations or delusions compared with only 19% of mentally healthy control subjects (Ostling *et al.*, 2003).

Holden (1987) showed that individuals with a diagnosis of late paraphrenia and cerebral organic factors had a poorer prognosis than their nonorganic counterparts.

Management

Antipsychotic medication is the mainstay of management of LOS and VLOS (Howard, 1996). Two randomised controlled trials (comparing risperidone and olanzapine) found significant improvement on standard symptom measures (of schizophrenia and cognition respectively) for both drugs (Jeste *et al.*, 2003).

Treatment response is related to adherence (Howard, 1996), which is enhanced by allocation of a community psychiatric nurse, use of depot antipsychotic medication, or both (see Howard, 1996).

Older people are more likely to experience adverse effects of medications because of the altered pharmacokinetics related to aging. Extrapyramidal symptoms are common and are associated with both typical and atypical antipsychotics. The risk factors for tardive dyskinesia (TD) in older people with schizophrenia include advancing age, the use of typical antipsychotics, female sex and organicity. Orofacial TD was associated with a lower MMSE score in the study by Purandare *et al.* (2003). Because of tolerability issues and altered pharmacokinetics in the elderly, the recommended dosages of antipsychotics for the treatment of LOS and VLOS are between one quarter and one third of the dosages for EOS (Howard, 1996; Zyas & Grossberg, 2002).

Nonpharmacological treatments for psychosis in late life deserve study.

Neurosis

Neurosis in old age has, until the last decade, been a relatively neglected area of enquiry (Lindesay, 1995). Neurotic disorders in old age are often unrecognised (Shah *et al.*, 2001), often chronic (Lindesay, 1995) and are probably associated with both increased mortality and physical illness (Dewey & Chen, 2004; Lindesay, 1995). Conceptual issues remain unresolved. Some advocate viewing neurosis from a unitary perspective in which symptoms change over time (Larkin *et al.*, 1992; Lindesay, 1995; Tyrer, 1985). Obsessive-compulsive disorder is the exception, being less common in old age (Myers *et al.*, 1984) and being relatively constant over time. Others have argued against the unitary theory, and prevalence rates of neurosis in old age are usually reported by symptom type or nosological category (e.g. DSM or ICD); however, Lindesay and Banerjee (1993) have shown that the diagnostic system used greatly influences the observed prevalence rates.

The results of three large epidemiological surveys are shown in Table 15.13. There are great differences in reported rates of all neurotic disorders except panic disorder, which was rarely found in any of the studies. These differences are partly due to the different survey instruments used but may also represent observer differences or sampling effects. The overall prevalence rate for neurosis ranges between 2.5% and 14.2% of the population aged 65 years or older, with community studies showing that between 5% (Kay *et al.*, 1964) and 24% (Bergmann, 1971) of neurosis in older people has its onset in old age. The influence of culture and ethnicity on the prevalence rates remains unresolved (Bhatnagar & Frank 1997; Chong *et al.*, 2001; Saz *et al.*, 1995).

Although neurotic disorders in the young old are more common in females than in males, this sex difference tends to narrow in the very old, largely as a result of the decreasing rates of neurotic disorder in older women (Lindesay, 1998; Nilsson & Persson, 1984). Longitudinal community surveys of depressive neurosis in the United Kingdom (Copeland *et al.*, 1992) and Singapore (Kua, 1993)

Table 15.13 Prevalence of neurotic disorders in older populations

Study	Neurosis	Males	Females	Total
Robins and Regier 1991	Phobic disorder	4.9	7.8	–
	Generalised Anxiety	–	–	2.2
	Panic disorder	0.04	0.08	–
	OCD	0.8	0.9	1.7
Ritchie *et al.*, 2004	Phobic disorder	6.5	13.7	10.7
	Generalised Anxiety	3.0	5.6	4.6
	Panic disorder	0.1	0.5	0.3
	OCD	0.8	0.5	0.5

show high mortality rates (23.2% and 16.1%, respec tively) and changing symptom patterns over the follow-up period. Recovery occurs in only about one in five for neurosis overall (Larkin *et al.*, 1992).

Goldberg and Huxley (1980) showed that anxiety disorders in the elderly do not easily pass through the filters to psychiatric care. It is not clear why this is so, but for anxiety disorders Jarvik and Russell (1979) suggested that the elderly may "freeze" rather than display the classical fight-or-flight anx iety reaction, and thus the true nature of their condition may not be recognised. Larkin *et al.* (1992) suggested that ageism on the part of clinicians may influence attitudes to neurotic disorders in old age, including unwarranted pessimism regarding prognosis and treatablility, reducing the likelihood of psychiatric referral.

Specific neurotic disorders in the elderly

Posttraumatic stress disorder

A recent population study of older people found a 6-month prevalence of posttraumatic stress disorder (PTSD) of 0.9%, with 13.6% of the population showing subsyndromal symptoms (van Zelst *et al.*, 2003). In this study, neuroticism and adverse events in early childhood were risk factors.

PTSD in older people has been most extensively studied in combat veterans (e.g. Schurr, 1991). A conversion of subsyndromal symptoms into full-blown PTSD was noted by Hilton (1997) following the 50th anniversary celebrations of the end of the Second World War in 1994–1995. Whether the chronicity of the disorder in combat veterans is due to lack of either recognition or of treatment remains to be established (Schnurr, 1991).

Somatisation

Psychological distress manifesting as somatic symptoms (somatisation) most often begins in early adult life but may persist into old age. Recent research suggests that somatisation is common in old age, especially among female frequent attenders, and is well recognised by primary care physicians (Wijeratne *et al.*, 2003).

Treatment

Butler (1968) has long advocated a psychotherapeutic approach in older people for the treatment of neurotic disorders and psychological reactions to adverse life events such as loss. Yost *et al.* (1986) outlined adaptations of Beck *et al.*'s (1979) model of cognitive therapy for older people. Morris and Morris (1991) reviewed the studies of behavioural and cognitive therapy in old people with depression and concluded that, when used appropriately, these therapies are beneficial. Although many older people with neurotic disorders are treated with medication (see Chapter 27), an evidence base for their use remains to be established.

Suicide and deliberate self-harm in the elderly

Suicide

Suicide rates increase with age in most studies from the developed world (reviewed by Pritchard, 1992). Although suicide rates in England and Wales have declined overall (including those for the elderly), rates in the oldest old (85+ years) have not fallen

(Shah *et al.*, 2001). The reasons are not yet fully established but may (for the elderly population) include changes in drug prescribing, including the reduction in the prescription of TCAs (Lodhi & Shah, 2004; Shah *et al.*, 2002). Suicide in older people is associated with depression, family conflict, physical illness and loneliness (see Jacoby, 2000). In older people, male suicide rates remain higher than those for females (Shah *et al.*, 2001). Suicidal thoughts are not uncommon in the oldest old with mental health problems and should always be taken seriously.

Older suicides are more likely to suffer from a depressive illness but are less likely to be known to mental health services or to have been treated for depression, compared with younger suicides (Salib & Green, 2003; Waern *et al.*, 2003). Older people may be particularly likely to enter into suicide pacts.

The prevention of suicide in older people is complex and current screening methods are probably inadequate. Thus a high index of suspicion must be exerted in older people who have risk factors such as depression, alcohol abuse, social isolation and chronic painful medical conditions (Jacoby, 2000; O'Connell *et al.*, 2004).

Deliberate self-harm

Deliberate self-harm (DSH) is less common in older than younger people. In one study in Wales, only 5.4% of all cases of DSH seen in a district general hospital over a 12-year period were aged 65 years or older (Pierce, 1987). Of these, the majority were depressed (93%) and female (male:female ratio = 1:1.5). DSH in older people should probably be regarded as a failed suicide attempt because the ratio between attempts (DSH) to completion (suicide) is relatively low (Cattell, 2000) and suicidal intent is high in this group (Marriott *et al.*, 2003; Merrill & Owens, 1990).

Alcohol abuse

Recent community surveys of alcohol abuse in elderly people report prevalence rates of anything up to to 5% of men and 3.2% of women (Iliffe *et al.*,

1991; Liberto *et al.*, 1992). The range of prevalence rates can probably be attributed to the methods of case identification, and the differing socioeconomic status of the populations studied (high socioeconomic status populations tending to have higher prevalence rates).

Clinical picture

It is now established that alcohol abuse in old age comprises two groups. Group I are graduate alcoholics; the majority have features of the alcohol dependence syndrome and have been drinking for many years. They tend to present with physical problems, and the sexes are equally represented. Group II comprise elderly people who began to abuse alcohol in old age; they rarely have symptoms of alcohol dependence syndrome. They present with falls, self-neglect and intermittent confusional states. They are usually female and are often isolated and suffer from chronic ill health (Jolley & Hodgson, 1985; Rosin & Glatt, 1971).

Management

Some elderly alcoholics are in contact with the Alcohol Treatment Services, but they are a small minority (Glatt *et al.*, 1978). There are few data on management of Group II alcoholic abusers. Jolley and Hodgson (1985) suggested that hospital admission might be used to "break the cycle" with a careful assessment of social, psychological and physical problems and appropriate treatment of each as the basis for successful management. They also advocate the use of vitamins and tranquilisers. Perhaps the most important factor is initial recognition of these patients, which is not always easy.

Other psychiatric disorders of old age

Senile self-neglect (Diogenes syndrome)

These patients are characterised by reclusiveness and breakdown of self-care to the extent that they may pose an environmental health hazard. Not infrequently they hoard rubbish and reject help from relatives or statutory services. The condition is not necessarily associated with poverty, with many patients having more than sufficient money.

Men and women are equally affected, and occasional cases of "Diogenes a deux" in married couples have been described (Cole *et al.*, 1992; MacMillan & Shaw 1966). The condition is not common: an annual incidence of 0.5 per 1,000 of the population aged over 60 years was reported by MacMillan and Shaw (1966). Patients form a heterogenous group, both in their symptom profile and their mode of presentation. Post (1982) considered that many are personality disordered, the rest suffer from dementia or paraphrenia. Contact with medical services is rarely initiated by the patients themselves but often by neighbours, although at the time of referral, many are mentally ill or disabled, and mortality is high (Clark *et al.*, 1975; MacMillan & Shaw, 1966). Not infrequently, the environmental hazard is the cause of contact with medical services.

Charles Bonnet syndrome

De Morsier (1938) used this eponym to describe a syndrome of complex visual hallucinosis in mentally normal, but usually visually impaired, old people. Podoll *et al.* (1990) proposed an operational definition which requires the presence of visual hallucinations in clear consciousness and in the absence of cerebral pathology or psychosis; visual impairment is considered a usual but not necessary concomitant. Rates of 1% to 2% of psychiatric elderly out-patients have been reported (Berrios & Brook, 1984; Podoll *et al.*, 1990).

Characteristically the visual hallucinations begin suddenly, last for only brief periods (seconds or minutes) and are more common in the evening or at night. They are vivid, and about a third are simple (patterns). When complex, human forms predominate over inanimate objects. Insight is maintained (Fuchs & Lauter, 1992).

Some authors have attempted to widen the boundaries of the syndrome to include those who subsequently develop cerebral cortical pathology such as cerebrovascular disease, and it has been reported as the presenting feature of Alzheimer's

disease (Crystal *et al.*, 1988) and stroke (Ball, 1991). Even in cases as defined by Podoll *et al.* (1990), mild abnormalities on EEG may be found.

Treatment of visual impairment, when possible (e.g. removal of cataracts) can be successful (Fernandez *et al.* 1997). Visual hallucinations in a 65-year-old women with depression were successfully treated by episodic blindfolding (Naik & Jones, 1993).

Learning disability in the elderly

The aging of the population in developed countries has resulted in increasing numbers of older people with learning disability. The carers of those with learning disability are also aging (Llewllyn *et al.*, 2004).

Older people with learning disability have high rates of both psychiatric and physical disorders (Moss & Patel, 1997). In a population of older people with learning disability aged over 50 years (*n* = 101), 12% had dementia (Moss & Patel, 1997). People with Down syndrome now have a life expectancy of 56 years and are at increased risk of developing dementia. Aged carers of people with learning disability are frequently isolated from the services that are supposed to support their caring role (Llewellyn *et al.*, 2004).

Conclusions

Old age psychiatrists worldwide face a future which is both uncertain and exciting – uncertain because of increasing restraints on resource allocation, exciting because this in itself offers a new challenge for service development. Exciting also because of the growth of the speciality and of research into psychiatric disease of old age. No longer is there any justification for the therapeutic nihilism which so often was associated with the treatment of the mental disorders of old age. Aging populations also bring challenges to specialists and services for learning disability and forensic psychiatry. The specialist in the psychiatry of old age has the means to alleviate distress and bring hope of increasingly effective treatments.

REFERENCES

Alexopoulos, G. S., Meyers, B. S., Young, R. C., *et al.* (1997). "Vascular depression" hypothesis. *Arch Gen Psychiatry* **54**:915–22.

American Psychiatric Association (1999). Practical Guidelines for the treatment of patients with delirium. Washington, DC: American Psychiatric Association.

American Psychiatric Association (2000). *Diagnostic and Statistical Manual of Mental Disorders*, 4th edn., text revision (DSM-IV-R). Washington, DC: American Psychiatric Association.

Ames, D. (1991). Epidemiological studies of depression among the elderly in residential and nursing homes. *Int J Geriatr Psychiatry* **6**:347–54.

Anderson, D. (2004). *Old Age Psychiatrist* **34**:4–5.

Andersson, E. (2002). *Acute Confusion in Orthopaedic Care with the Emphasis on the Patient's View and the Episode of Confusion.* Lund University Medical Dissertations Bulletin No. 10. Department of Nursing, Medical Faculty.

Anderson, I. M., Nutt, D. J. & Deakin, J. F. W. (2000). Evidence-based guidelines for the treatment of depressive disorders with antidepressants: revision of the 1993 British Associationn or Psychopharmacology guidelines. *J Psychopharmacology* **14**: 3–20

Baldwin, R. (1988). Delusional and non-delusional depression in late life: evidence for distinct sub-types. *Br J Psychiatry* **152**:39–44.

Baldwin, R., & Jolley, D. J. (1986). The prognosis of depression in old age. *Br J Psychiatry* **149**:574–83.

Baldwin, R. C. (1991). Depressive illness. In R. Jacoby & C. Oppenheimer, eds. *Psychiatry in the Elderly.* Oxford: Oxford Medical Publications, pp. 676–710.

Baldwin, R. C. (1993). Late life depression and structural brain changes: a review of recent magnetic resonance imaging research. *Int J Geriatr Psychiatry* **8**:115–24.

Baldwin, R. C., & Byrne, E. J. (1989). Psychiatric aspects of Parkinson's disease. *BMJ* **299**:3–4.

Baldwin, R. C. (1998). Re: Geriatric consultation and liaison service. *Int J Geriatr Psychiatry* **13**:820–1.

Baldwin, R. C. (2000). Mood disorders in the elderly. In M. Gelder, J. Lopez-Ibor & N. Andresen, eds. *New Oxford Textbook of Psychiatry.* Oxford: Oxford University Press, pp. 1644–1651.

Baldwin, R.C. & O'Brien, J. (2002). Vascular basis of late-onset depressive disorder. *Br J Psychiatry* **180**: 157–60.

Baldwin, R., Anderson, D., Black, S., *et al.* (2003). Guideline for the management of late-life depression in primary care. *Int J Ger Psychiatry* **18**: 829–38.

Ball, C. J. (1991). The vascular origins of the Charles Bonnet syndrome: four cases and a review of the pathogenic mechanisms. *Int J Geriatr Psychiatry* **6**:673–9S.

Beck, A. T., Rush, A. J., Shaw, B. F., & Emergy, G. (1979). *Cognitive Therapy of Depression.* New York: Guilford Press.

Beck, C., Heacock, P., & Mercer, S., *et al.* (1997). Improving dressing behaviour in cognitively impaired nursing home residents. *Nurs Res* **46**:126–32.

Benbow, S. M. & Marriott, A. (1997). Family therapy with elderly people. *Adv Psychiatr Treatment* **3**:138–45.

Benbow, S. M. (1989). The role of electroconvulsive therapy in the treatment of depressive illness in old age. *Br J Psychiatry* **155**:147–52.

Beresin, E. V. (1988). Delirium in the elderly. *J Geriatr Psychiatry Neurol* **1**:127–43.

Bergmann, K. (1971). The neurosis in old age. In: D. W. K. Kay & A. Walk, eds. *Recent Developments in Psychogeriatrics. Br J Psychiatry*, special publication no. 6, pp. 39–50.

Berrios, G. G., & Brook, P. (1984). Visual hallucinations and sensory delusions in the elderly. *Br J Psychiatry* **144**:662–4.

Bhatnagar, K., & Frank, J. (1997). Psychiatric disorders in elderly from the Indian sub-continent living in Bradford. *Int J Geriatr Psychiatry* **12**:907–12.

Bienenfeld, D., & Wheeler, B. G. (1989). Psychiatric services to nursing homes: a liaison model. *Hosp Commun Psychiatry* **40**:793–4.

Beekman, A. T., Copeland, J. R., Prince, M. J. (1999). Review of community prevalence of depression in late life. *Br J Psychiatry* **174**:307–11.

Blanchard, M. R., Waterreus, A., & Mann, A. H. (1995). The effect of primary care nurse interventions upon older people screened as depressed. *Int J Geriatric Psychiatry* **5**:119–21.

Blazer, D., Hughes, D. C., & George, L. K. (1987). The epidemiology of depression in an elderly community population. *The Gerontologist* **27**:281–7.

Bleuler, M. (1943). Late schizophrenic clinical pictures. *Fortschr Neurol Psychiatr* **15**:259–90.

Broadhead, J., & Jacoby, R. J. (1990). Mania in old age: a first prospective study. *Int J Geriatr Psychiatry* **5**:215–22.

Brodaty, H., Sachdev, P., Koschera, A., *et al.* (2003). Long-term outcome of late-onset schizophrenia: 5-year follow-up study. *Br J Psychiatry* **183**:213–19.

Bruce, M. L., McAvay, G. J., Raue, P. J., *et al.* (2002). Major depression in elderly home health care patients. *Am J Psychiatry* **159**:1367–74.

Bucks, R. S., Ashworth, D. L., Wilcock, G. K., & Siegfried, K. (1996). Assessment of activities of daily living in dementia: development of the Bristol Activities of Daily Living Scale. *Age Ageing* **25**:113–20.

Burns, A., Byrne, E. J., Ballard, C., & Holmes, C. (2002). Sensory stimulation in dementia: an effective option for managing behavioural problems. *BMJ* **325**:1312–13.

Burns, A., Carrick, J., Ames, D., *et al.* (1989). The cerebral cortical appearance in late paraphrenia. *Int J Geriatr Psychiatry* **4**:31–34.

Burns, A., Downs, M., & Kampers, W. (2003). *Current Dementia*. London: Science Press.

Burns, A., Rossor, M., Hecker, J., *et al.* (1999). The effects of donepezil in Alzheimer's disease – results from a multinational trial. *Dement Geriatr Cogn Disord* **10**:237–44.

Burns, A., Spiegel, R., & Qarg, P. (2003). Efficacy of rivastigmine in subjects with moderately severe Alzheimer's disease. *Int J Geriatr Psychiatry* **19**:243–9.

Butler, R. N. (1960). Towards a psychiatry of the life cycle: implications of sociopsychologic studies of the ageing process for the psychotherapeutic situation. In A. Simon & L. J. Epstein, eds. *Ageing in Modern Society. Psychiatric Research Reports*. Washington, DC: American Psychiatric Association, pp. 233–48.

Byrne, E. J., & Simpson, S. (1997). Other dementias. In D. Ames & E. Chiu, eds. *Neuroimaging and the Psychiatry of Late Life*. Cambridge: Cambridge University Press, pp. 145–58.

Caine, E. D., Lyness, J. M., King, D. A., & Connors, L. (1994). Clinical and aetiological heterogeneity of mood disorders in elderly patients. In L. S. Schneider, C. F. Reynolds, B. D. Lobowitz & A. J. Friedhoff, eds. *Diagnosis and Treatment of Depression in Late Life. Results of the NIH Consensus Development Conference*. Washington, DC: American Psychiatric Press, pp. 25–53.

Camus, V., Kraehenbuhl, H., Preisig, M., *et al.* (2004). Geriatric depression and vascular diseases: what are the links? *J Affect Disord* **81**:1–16.

Challis, D., von Abendorff, R., Brown, P., *et al.* (2002). Care management, dementia care and specialist mental health services: an evaluation. *Int J Geriatr Psychiatry* **17**:315–25.

Chew-Graham, C., Baldwin, R., & Burns, A. (2004). Treating depression in later life. *BMJ* **329**:181–2.

Chong, M. Y., Tsang, H. Y., Chen, C. S., *et al.* (2001). Community study of depression in old age in Taiwan: prevalence, life events and socio-demographic correlates. *Br J Psychiatry* **178**:29–35.

Clark, A. N. G., Mankikar, G. D., & Gray, I. (1975). Diogenes syndrome. A clinical study of gross neglect in old age. *Lancet* **1**:366–73.

Cohen, L. J., Test, M. A., & Brown, R. L. (1990). Suicide and schizophrenia: data from a prospective community treatment study. *Am J Psychiatry* **147**:602–7.

Cohen-Cole, S. A., & Stoudemire, A. (1987). Major depression and physical illness. Special considerations in diagnosis and biologic treatment. *Psychiatr Clin North Am* **10**:1–17.

Cole, A. J., Fillett, J. P., & Fairbairn, A. (1992). A case of senile self-neglect in a married couple: "Diogenes a Deux". *Int J Geriatr Psychiatry* **7**:839–41.

Cole, M. G., Bellavance, F., & Mansour, A. (1999). Prognosis of depression in elderly community and primary care populations: a systematic review and meta-analysis. *Am J Psychiatry* **156**:1182–9.

Cole, M. G., & Primeau, F. (1993). Prognosis of delirium in elderly hospital patients. *Can Med Assoc* **149**:41–6.

Copeland, J. R., Chen, R., & Dewey, M. E., *et al.* (1999). Community-based case-control study of depression in older people. Cases and sub-cases from the MRC-ALPHA Study. *Br J Psychiatry* **175**:340–7.

Copeland, J. R. M., Davidons, I. A., Dewey, M. E., *et al.* (1992). Alzheimer's disease, other dementias, depression and pseudodementia: prevalence incidence and three-year outcome in Liverpool. *Br J Psychiatry* **151**:230–9.

Crammer, J. (2002). Subjective experiences of a confusional state. *Br J Psychiatry* **180**:71–75.

Crystal, H. A., Wolfson, L., & Ewing, S. (1988). Visual hallucinations as the first symptoms of Alzheimer's disease. *Am J Psychiatry* **145**:1318.

Cummings, J. L., Mega, M., Gray, K., *et al.* (1994). The Neuropsychiatric Inventory: comprehensive assessment of psychopathology in dementia. *Neurology* **44**:2308–14.

De Leo, D., Beinocchi, A., Cipollona, B., *et al.* (1989). Psychogeriatric consultation within a geriatric hospital: a six-year experience. *Int J Geriatr Psychiatry* **4**:135–41.

De Morsier, G. (1938). Les hallucinations, etude oto-neuro-ophtalmologique. *Rev Otoneurophtalmol* **16**:244–352.

Department of Health. (2001). www.dh.gov.uk/publicationsandstatistics/publications/index.htm.

Department of Health, Public Health Link. (2004). The atypical antipsychotics and stroke. London: Department of Health. Available at http://199.228.212.132/doh/embroadcast.nsf/.

Djernes, J. K., Gulmann, N. C., Abelskov, J. E., *et al.* (1998). Psychopathological and functional outcome in the treatment of elderly in-patients with depressive disorders, dementia, delirium and psychosis. *Int Psychogeriatr* **10**:71–83.

Draper, B. (1994). The elderly admitted to a general hospital psychiatry ward. *Aust N Z J Psychiatry* **28**:288–97.

Draper, B., & Luscombe, G. (1998). Quantification of factors contributing to length of stay in an acute psychogeriatric ward. *Int J Geriatr Psychiatry* 13:1–7.

Eagles, J. M., & Whalley, L. J. (1985). Ageing and affective disorders: the age at first onset of affective disorders in Scotland; 1969–1978. *Br J Psychiatry* 147:180–7.

Epstein, L. J. (1976). Symposium on age differentiation in depressive illness. Depression in the elderly. *J Gerontol* 31:278–82.

Fairweather, D. S. (1991). Delirium. In R. Jacoby & C. Oppenheimer, eds. *Psychiatry in the Elderly*. Oxford: Oxford Medical Publications, pp. 647–75.

Fenandez , A., Lichtein, G., Vieweg, W. V. (1997). The Charles Bonnet Syndrome: a review. *JNMD* 185: 195–200.

Finch, E. J. L., & Katona, C. L. E. (1989). Lithium augmentation in the treatment of refractory depression in old age. *Int J Geriatr Psychiatry* 4:41–6.

Flint, A. J., & Rifat, S. L. (1998). The treatment of psychotic depression in later life: a comparison of pharmacotherapy and ECT. *Int J Geriatr Psychiatry* 13:23–8.

Flint, A. J. (1992). The optimum duration of antidepressant treatment in the elderly. *Int J Geriatr Psychiatry* 7: 617–9.

Fogell, B. S., & Fretwell, M. (1985). Re-classification of depression in the medically ill elderly. *J Am Geriatr Soc* 33:446–8.

Folstein, M. F., Bassett, S. S., Romanowski, A. J., *et al.* (1991). The epidemiology of delirium in the community: the Eastern Baltimore mental Health Survey. *Int Psychogeriatr* 3:169–79.

Folstein, M. F., Folstein, S. E., & McHugh, P. R. (1975). "Mini-Mental State". A practical method of grading the cognitive state of patients for the clinician. *J Psychiatric Res* 12:189–98.

Foster, J. R., Silver, M., & Boksay, I. J. E. (1990). Lithium use in the elderly: Diagnostic and research considerations. *Int J Geriatr Psychiatry* 5:1–8.

Francis, J., Martin, D., & Kapoor, W. N. (1990). A prospective study of delirium in hospitalised elderly. *JAMA* 263:111–15.

Friedman, J. I., Harvey, P. D., Coleman, T., *et al.* (2001). Six-year follow-up study of cognitive and functional status across the lifespan in schizophrenia: a comparison with Alzheimer's disease and normal aging. *Am J Psychiatry* 158:1441–8.

Fuchs, T., & Lauter, H. (1992). Charles Bonnet syndrome and musical hallucinations in the elderly. In C. Katona & R. Levy, eds. *Delusions and Hallucinations in Old Age*. London: Gaskell, pp. 187–98.

Gallo, J. J., Rabins, P. V., & Anthony, J. C. (1999). Sadness in older persons: 13-year follow-up of a community sample in Baltimore, Maryland. *Psychol Med* 29:341–50.

Geddes, J. R., Carney, S. M., Davies, C., *et al.* (2003). Relapse prevention with antidepressant drug treatment in depressive disorders: a systematic review. *Lancet* 361:653–661.

Gilliard, C. J. (1987). Influence of emotional distress among supporters on the outcome of psychogeriatric day care *Br J Psychiatry* 150:219–23.

Glatt, M., Rosin, A., & Jauha, P. (1978). Alcoholism and the elderly. *Age Ageing* 7(Suppl):64–6.

Godber, C., Rosenvinge, H., Wilkinson, D. & Smithies, J. (1987). Depression in old age: prognosis after ECT. *Int J Geriatr Psychiatry* 2:19–24.

Goldberg, D., & Huxley, P. (1980). *Mental Illness in the Community*. London: Tavistock.

Government Actuary's Department. (2004). www.gad.gov.uk/population/index.asp.

Grundy, E. (1992). Sociodemographic change and the elderly population of England and Wales. *Int J Geriatr Psychiatry* 7:75–82.

Gustafson, L., Risberg, J., & Silfverskiold, P. (1981). Cerebral blood flow in dementia and depression. *Lancet* 1: 275.

Hafner, H., Loffler, W., Riecher-Rossler, A., & Hafner-Ranabauer, W. (2001). [Schizophrenia and delusions in middle aged and elderly patients. Epidemiology and etiological hypothesis]. *Nervenarzt* 72:347–357 [in German].

Hays, J. C., Krishnan, K. R., George, L. K., & Blazer, D. G. (1998). Age of first onset of bipolar disorder: demographic, family history, and psychosocial correlates. *Depress Anxiety* 7:76–82.

Hilton, C. (1997). Media triggers of post-traumatic stress disorder 50 years after the Second World War. *Int J Geriatr Psychiatry* 12:862–7.

Holden, N. (1987). Late paraphrenia or the paraphrenias. *Br J Psychiatry* 150:635–9.

House, A. (1987). Mood disorder after stroke: a review of the evidence. *Int J Geriatr Psychiatry* 2:211–21.

Howard, R. (1996). Drug treatment of schizophrenia and delusional disorder in late life. *Int Psychogeriatr* 8:597–608.

Howard, R., Rabins, P. V., Seeman, M. V., & Jeste, D. V. (2000). Late-onset schizophrenia and very-late-onset schizophrenia-like psychosis: an international consensus. The International Late-Onset Schizophrenia Group. *Am J Psychiatry* 157:172–8.

Hughes, C. P., Berg, L., Danzinger, W. L., *et al.* (1982). A new clinical scale for the staging of dementia. *Br J Psychiatry* **140**:556–72 [updated by Morris, 1993].

Iliffe, S., Haine, A., Booroof, A., *et al.* (1991). Alcohol consumption by elderly people: a general practice survey. *Age Ageing* **20**:120–3.

Inouye, S. K., Bogardus, S. T., Charpentier, P. A., *et al.* (1999). A multicomponent intervention to prevent delirium in hospitalized older patients. *N Engl J Med* **340**:669–76.

Jacoby, R. (2004). Ethical and legal aspects of dementia. *Psychiatry* **3**:33–34. Available at http://www.psychiatryjournal.co.uk.

Jacoby, R. J. (1981). Depression in the elderly. *Br J Hosp Med* **25**:40–7.

Jacoby, R. J. (1991). Manic illness. In R. Jacoby & C. Oppenheimer, eds. *Psychiatry in the Elderly*. Oxford: Oxford Medical Publications, pp. 720–6.

Jacoby, R. J. (2000). Suicide and deliberate self harm. In M. Gelder, J. Lopez-Ibor & N. Andreson, eds. *New Oxford Textbook of Psychiatry*. Oxford: Oxford University Press, pp. 1658–61.

Jarvik, L. F., & Russell, D. (1979). Anxiety, ageing and the third emergency reaction. *J Gerontol* **34**:197–200.

Jarvik, L. F.,Mintz, J., Steuer, J., & Gerner, R. (1982). Treating geriatric depression: a 26-week interim analysis. *J Am Geriatr Soc* **30**:713–17.

Jeste, D. V., Barak, Y., Madhusoodanan, S., *et al* (2003). International multisite double-blind trial of the atypical antipsychotics risperidone and olanzapine in 175 elderly patients with chronic schizophrenia. *Am J Geriatr Psychiatry* **11**: 638–647. Erratum in *Am J Geriatr Psychiatry* 2004; **12**:49.

Jolley, D. J., & Hodgson, S. (1985). Alcoholism and the elderly: a tale of women and our times. In B Isaacs, ed. *Recent Advances in Geriatric Medicine*, 3rd edn. Edinburgh: Churchill Livingstone, pp. 113–22.

Kaponen, H. J., & Riekkinen, P. J. (1993). A prospective study of delirium in elderly patients admitted to a psychiatric hospital. *Psychol Med* **23**:103–9.

Katona, C., & Livingston, G. (2002). How well do antidepressants work in older people? A systematic review of number needed to treat. *J Affect Disord* **69**:47–52.

Kay, D. W. K., Beamish, P., & Roth, M. (1964). Old age mental disorders in Newcastle upon Tyne. Part I: a study of prevalence. *Br J Geriatr Psychiatry* **110**:146–58.

Kelly, C., Sharkey, V., Morrison, G., *et al.* (2000). Nithsdale Schizophrenia Surveys. 20. Cognitive function in a catchment-area-based population of patients with schizophrenia. *Br J Psychiatry* **177**:348–53.

Keshavan, M. S., Mulsant, B. H., Sweet, R. A., *et al.* (1996). MRI changes in schizophrenia in late life: a preliminary controlled study. *Psychiatry Res* **60**:117–23.

Kitwood, T. (1997). *Dementia Reconsidered: The Person Comes First*. Buckingham: Open University Press.

Klysner, R., Bent-Hansen, J., Hansen, H. L., *et al.* (2002). Efficacy of citalopram in the prevention of recurrent depression in elderly patients: placebo-controlled study of maintenance therapy. *Br J Psychiatry* **181**:29–35.

Krauthammer, C., & Klerman, G. L. (1978). Secondary mania. *Arch Gen Psychiatry* **35**:1333–9.

Kua, E. H. (1993). Dementia in elderly Malays – preliminary findings of a community survey. *Singapore Med J* **34**:26–8.

Larkin, B. A., Copeland, J. R. M., Dewey, M. E., *et al.* (1992). The natural history of neurotic disorders in an elderly urban population. Findings from the Liverpool study of continuing health in the community. *Br J Psychiatry* **160**:681–6.

Lawton, M., & Rubenstein, L. (2000). *Interventions in Dementia Care: Toward Improving Quality of Life*. London: Springer.

Leinonen, E., Santala, M., Hyotyla, T., *et al.* (2004). Elderly patients with major depressive disorder and delusional disorder are at increased risk of subsequent dementia. *Nord J Psychiatry* **58**:161–4.

Leuchter, A. F., & Jacobsen, S. A. (1991). Quantitative measurement of brain electrical activity in delirium. *Int Psychogeriatr* **3**:231–47.

Levin, M. (1968). Delirium: an experience and some reflections. *Am J Psychiatry* **124**:1120.

Levkoff, S., Clearly, P., Pitzin, B., & Evans, D. S. (1991). Epidemiology of delirium: an overview of research issues and findings. *Int Psychogeritatr* **3**:149–67.

Levkoff, S. E., Evans, D. A., Liptzin, B., *et al.* (1992). Delirium: the occurrence and persistence of among hospitalized elderly patients. *Arch Int Med* **152**:334–40.

Liberto, J. G., Oslin, D. W. & Rushkin, P. E. (1992). Alcoholism in older persons: a review of the literature. *Hosp Comm Psychiatry* **43**: 975–84

Lindesay, J. (1991). Anxiety disorders in the elderly. In R. Jacoby & C. Oppenheimer, eds. *Psychiatry in the Elderly*. Oxford: Oxford Medical Publications, pp. 735–57.

Lindesay, J. (1995). *Neurotic Disorders in the Elderly*. Oxford: Oxford University Press.

Lindesay, J., & Banerjee, S. (1993). Phobic disorders in the elderly: a comparison of three diagnostic systems. *Int J Geriatr Psychiatry* **8**:387–93.

Lindesay, J., MacDonald, A., & Starke, I. (1990). *Delirium in the Elderly*. Oxford: Oxford Medical Publications, pp. 80–97.

Lindesay, J., Rockwood, K., & Rolfson, D. (2002). The epidemiology of delirium. In J. Lindesay, K. Rockwood & A. Macdonald. *Delirium in Old Age*. Oxford: Oxford University Press, pp. 27–50.

Lipowski, Z. J. (1989). Delirium in the elderly patients. *N Engl J Med* **320**:578–92.

Lipowski, Z. J. (1990). *Delirium (Acute Confusional States)*. New York: Oxford University Press.

Lipowski, Z. J. (1992). Delirium and impaired consciousness. In J. G. Evans & T. F. Williams, eds. *Oxford Textbook of Geriatric Medicine*. Oxford: Oxford Medical Publications, pp. 490–6.

Lobo, A., Launer, L., & Fratiglioni, L., *et al.* (2000). Problems of dementia. Major subtypes in Europe. *Neurology* **54**(Suppl 11):S4–S9.

Lodhi, L. M., & Shah, A. (2004). Psychotropic prescriptions and elderly suicide rates. *Med Sci Law* **44**:236–44.

MacDonald, A. (1992). Old age depression and organic brain change. In T. Aries, ed. *Recent Advances in Psychogeriatrics*, 2nd edn. Edinburgh: Churchill Livingstone, pp. 45–58.

MacMillan, D., & Shaw, P. (1966). Senile breakdown in standards of personal and environmental cleanliness. *BMJ* **2**:1032–37.

Marcantonio, E., Ta, T., Duthi, E., & Resnick, N. M. (2002). Delirium severity and psychomotor types: their relationship with outcomes after hip fracture repair. *J Am Geriatr Soc* **50**:850–7.

Marcantonio, E. R., Flacker, J. M., Michaels, M., & Resnick, N. M. (2000). Delirium is independently associated with poor functional recovery after hip fracture. *J Am Geriatr Soc* **48**:618–24.

Marriott, R., Horricks, J., House, A., & Owens, D. (2003). Assessment and management of self-harm in older adults attending accident and emergency: a comparative cross-sectional study. *Int J Geriatr Psychiatry* **18**:645–52.

Mendez, M., & Cummings, J. (2004). *Dementia: A Clinical Approach*, 3rd edn. Butterworth, Heinemann.

Merrill, J., & Owens, J. (1990). Age and attempted suicide. *Acta Psychiatr Scand* **82**:385–8.

Miller, B., Lesser, I., & Boone, K. (1991). Brain lesions in cognitive function in late life psychosis. *Br J Psychiatry* **158**:76–82.

Morris, J. (1993). The CDR: current version and scoring rules. *Neurology* **43**:2412–13.

Morris, R. G., & Morris, L. W. (1991). Cognitive and behavioural approaches with the depressed elderly. *Int J Geriatr Psychiatry* **6**:407–13.

Murphy, E. (1983). The prognosis of depression in old age. *Br J Psychiatry* **142**:111–119.

Murphy, E., Smith E.R., Lindesay J. E. B. (1988) Increased mortality in late life depression. Increased mortality in late-life depression. *Br J Psychiatry* **139**:288–92.

Murphy, M. (1990). Methods of forecasting mortality for population projections. In *Population Projections, Trends, Methods and Uses*. OPCS Occasional Paper 38. London: Office for Population Census and Surveys.

Musetti, L., Perugi, G., Soriani, A., *et al.* (1989). Depression before and after age 65. A re-examination. *Br J Psychiatry* **155**:330–6.

Myers, J. K., Wissman, M. M., Tischler, G. L., *et al.* (1984). Six month prevalence of psychiatric disorders in three communities. *Arch Gen Psychiatry* **41**:959–67.

Naguib, N., & Levy, R. (1987). Late paraphrenia – neuropsychological impairment and structural brain abnormalities on computer tomography. *Br J Geriatr Psychiatry* **2**:83–90.

Naik, P., & Jones, R. (1993). Response of visual hallucinations to blindfolding. *Int J Geriatr Psychiatry* **8**:357–63.

Newmann, J. P., Klein, M. H., Jensen, J. E., & Essex, M. J. (1996). Depressive symptoms experiences among older women: a comparison of alternative measurement approaches. *Psychol & Aging* **11**:112–26.

Nilsson, L. V., & Persson, G. (1984). Prevalence of mental disorders in an urban sample examined at 70, 75 and 79 years of age. *Acta Psychol Scand* **69**:519–27.

Noaghiul, S., & Hibbeln, J. R. (2003). Cross-national comparisons of seafood consumption and rates of bipolar disorders. *Am J Psychiatry* **160**:2222–7.

O'Connell H., Chin A. V., Cunningham, C., & Lawlor, B. A. (2004). Recent developments: suicide in older people. *BMJ* **329**:895–9.

Orrell, M., Baldwin, B., Collins, E., & Katona, C. (1995). A UK national survey of the management of depression by geriatricians and old age psychiatrists *Int J Geriatr Psychiatry* **10**:450–67.

Ostling, S., Andreasson, L. A., & Skoog, I. (2003). Basal ganglia calcification and psychotic symptoms in the very old. *Int J Geriatr Psychiatry* **18**:983–7.

Palmer, B. W., Bondi, M. W., Twamley, E. W., *et al.* (2003). Are late-onset schizophrenia spectrum disorders neurodegenerative conditions? Annual rates of change on two dementia measures. *J Neuropsychiatry Clin Neurosci* **15**:45–52.

Pierce, D. (1987). Deliberate self-harm in the elderly. *Int J Geriatr Psychiatry* **2**:105–10.

Pitt, B. (1991). (NB Pitt 1986 is 'Characteristics of depression in the elderly'). Depression in the general hospital setting. *Br J Geriatr Psychiatry* **6**:363–70.

Podoll, K., Schwan, M., & Noth, J. (1990). Charles Bonnet-syndrome bei einem Parkinson – patienten mit biedseitigem visusverlust. *Nervenarzt* **61**:52–6.

Post, F. (1982). The factor of ageing in affective illness. In A. Coppen & A. Walk, eds. *Recent Developments in Affective Disorders*. Ashford: Headley, pp. 105–16.

Post, F. (1966). *Persistent Persecutory States of the Elderly*. Oxford: Pergamon.

Preston, S., Hines, L., & Eggers, M. (1989). Demographic conditions responsible for populations ageing. *Demography* **26**:691–704.

Prince, M. (1997). The need for research in dementia in developing countries. *Trop Med Int Health* **2**:993–1000.

Pritchard, C. (1992). Changes in elderly suicides in the USA and the developing world 1974–1987. Comparison with current homicide. *Int J Geriatr Psychiatry* **7**:125–34.

Purandare, N. B., Berry, K., Stewart, C., *et al.* (2003). Tardive dyskinesia in older people with psychosis. *Psychogeriatrics* **15**(Suppl 2):163–4.

Rabins, P., Perlson, G., Jayram, G., *et al.* (1987). Increased VBR in late onset schizophrenia. *Am J Psychiatry* **144**:1216–18.

Rabins, P. V., & Lavrisha, M. (2003). Long-term follow-up and phenomenologic differences distinguish among late-onset schizophrenia, late-life depression, and progressive dementia. *Am J Geriatr Psychiatry* **11**:589–94.

Reynolds, C. F., Frank, E., Perel, J. M., *et al.* (1999). Nortriptyline and interpersonal psychotherapy as maintenance therapies for recurrent major depression. *JAMA* **281**:39–45.

Richman, A., Wilson, K., Scally, I., *et al.* (2003). Service intervention: an outreach support team for older people with mental illness *Psychiatr Bull* **27**:348–51.

Riecher-Rossler, A., Hafner H., Hafner Ranabauer, W., *et al.* (2003). Late-onset schizophrenia versus paranoid psychoses: a valid diagnostic distinction? *Am J Geriatr Psychiatry* **11**:595–604.

Robillard, M., & Conn, D. K. (2004). Lamotrigine use in geriatric patients with bipolar depression. *Can J Psychiatry* **47**:767–70.

Rolfson, D. The causes of delirium. (2002). In J. Lindesay, K. Rockwood & A. Macdonald, eds. *Delirium in the Old Age*. Oxford: Oxford University Press, Oxford, pp. 101–22.

Roose, S. P., Sackeim, H. A., Krishnan, K. R., *et al.* (2004). Old-Old Depression Study Group. Antidepressant pharmacotherapy in the treatment of depression in the very old: a randomized, placebo-controlled trial. *Am J Psychiatry* **161**:2050–9.

Rosin, A. J., & Glatt, M. M. (1971). Alcohol excess in the elderly. *Q J Stud Alcohol* **32**:53–9.

Roth, M. (1955). The natural history of mental disorders in old age. *J Ment Sci* **101**: 201–301

Rovner, B. W., Kafonek, S., Fillipp, L., *et al.* (1986). The prevalence of mental illness in a community nursing home. *Am J Psychiatry* **143**:1446–9.

Sajatovic, M., Sultana, D., Bingham, C. R., *et al.* (2002). Gender related differences in clinical characteristics and hospital based resource utilization among older adults with schizophrenia. *Int J Geriatr Psychiatry* **17**:542–8.

Salib, E., & Green, L. (2003). Gender in elderly suicide: analysis of coroners inquests of 200 cases of elderly suicide in Cheshire 1989–2001. *Int J Geriatr Psychiatry* **18**: 1082–7.

Salokangas, R. K., Honkonen, T., & Saarinen, S. (2003). Women have later onset than men in schizophrenia – but only in its paranoid form. Results of the DSP project. *Eur Psychiatry* **18**:274–81.

Salzman, C. (1983). Electroconvulsive therapy in the elderly patient. *Psychiatr Clin N Am* **5**:191–7.

Salzman, C., Wong, E., & Wright, B. C. (2002). Drug and ECT treatment of depression in the elderly, 1996–2001: a literature review. *Biol Psychiatry* **1**:52:265–84.

Saz, P., Copeland, J. R., de la Camara, C., *et al.* (1995). Cross-national comparison of prevalence of symptoms of neurotic disorders in older people in two community samples. *Acta Psychiatr Scand* **91**:18–22.

Schofield, I. (1997). A small exploratory study of the reaction of older people to an episode of delirium. *J Adv Nurs* **25**:942–52.

Scogin, F., & McElreath, L. (1994). Efficacy of psychosocial treatments for geriatric depression: a quantitative review. *J Consult Clin Psychol* **62**:69–74.

Scott, J., Fairbairn, A., & Woodhouse, K. 1998. Referrals to a psychogeriatric consultation – liaison service. *J Int Geriatr Psychiatry* **3**:131–5.

Shah, R., McNiece, R., & Majeed, A. (2001). General practice consultation rates for psychiatric disorders in patients aged 65 and over: prospective cohort study. *Int J Geriatr Psychiatry* **16**:57–63.

Shah, R., Uren, Z., Baker, A., & Majeed, A. (2002). Trends in suicide from drug overdose in the elderly in England and Wales, 1993–1999. *Int J Geriatr Psychiatry* **17**:416–21.

Shulman, K., & Post, F. (1980). Bipolar disorder in old age. *Br J Psychiatry* **136**:26–32.

Shulman, K., Shedletsky, R., & Silver, I. (1986). the challenge of time. Clock drawing and cognitive function in the elderly. *Int J Geriatr Psychiatry* **1**:135–40.

Shurr 1991 PTSD in vetsSteffens, D. C., & Krishnan, K. R. (1998). Structural neuroimaging and mood disorders: recent findings, implications for classification, and future directions. *Biol Psychiatry* **43**:705–12.

Stone, K. (1989). Mania in the elderly. *Br J Psychiatry* **155**:220–4.

Strain, J. J., Lyons, J. S., Hammer, J. S., *et al.* (1991). Cost off-set from a psychiatric consultation – liaison intervention with elderly hip fracture patients. *Am J Psychiatry* **148**:1044–9.

Symonds, L. L., Olichney, J. M., Jernigan T. L., *et al.* (1997). Lack of clinically significant gross structural abnormalities in MRIs of older patients with schizophrenia and related psychoses. *J Neuropsychiatry Clin Neurosci* **9**:251–8.

Taylor, D., & Lewis, S. (1993). Delirium. *J Neurol Neurosurg Psychiatry* **56**:742–751.

Teri, L., Gibbons, L., & McCurry, S. (2003). Exercise plus behavioural management in patients with Alzheimer's disease. *JAMA* **290**:2012–22.

Tew, J. D., Jr., Mulsant, B. H., Haskett, R. F., *et al.* (1999). Acute efficacy of ECT in the treatment of major depression in the old-old. *Am J Psychiatry* **156**:1865–70.

Thase, M. E., Sloan, D. M., & Kornstein, S. G. (2002). Remission as the critical outcome of depression treatment. *Psychopharmacol Bull* **36**(Suppl 4):12–25.

Thomas, R. K., Cameron, D. J., & Fahs, M. (1988). A prospective study of delirium and prolonged hospital stay. *Arch Gen Psychol* **45**:937–40.

Thomas, S. A., Chapa, D. W., Friedmann, E., *et al.* (2008). Depression in patients with heart failure: prevalence, pathophysiological mechanisms, and treatment. *Crit Care Nurse* **28**:40–55.

Tomassini, C. (2004). Demographic data needs for an ageing population. *Population Trends* 118;23–9.

Tuma, T. A. (2000). Outcome of hospital-treated depression at 4.5 years. An elderly and a younger adult cohort compared. *Br J Psychiatry* **176**:224–8.

Tyrer, P. (1985). Neurosis divisible. *Lancet* **1**:685–8.

van Zelst W. H., de Beurs, E., Beekman, A. T., *et al.* (2003). Prevalence and risk factors of posttraumatic stress disorder in older adults. *Psychother Psychosom* **72**:333–42.

Walstra, G. J., Teuaisse, S., Van Gool, W. A., & Van Crevel, H. (1997). Reversible dementia in elderly patients referred to a memory clinic. *J Neurology* **244**:17–22.

Wattis, J. P., Butler, A., Martin, C., & Sumner, T. (1994). Outcome of admission to an acute psychiatric facility for older people: a pluralistic evaluation. *Int J Geriatr Psychiatry* **9**:835–40.

Whittaker, J. J. (1989). Postoperative confusion in the elderly. *Int J Geriatr Psychiatry* **4**:321–6.

Wijeratne, C., Brodaty, H., & Hickie, I. (2003). The neglect of somatoform disorders by old age psychiatry: some explanations and suggestions for future research. *Int J Geriatr Psychiatry* **18**:812–19.

Wilkinson, D., Lilienfeld, S., & Truyen, L. Galantamine improves activities of daily living in patients with Alzheimer's disease: a 3-month placebo-controlled study. GAL-INT-2 study report. Janssen Research Foundation; data on file.

Wilkinson, D. G. (1997). Galantamine hydrobromide – results of a group study. 8th Congress International Psychogeriatric Association Jerusalem, abstract P70.

Wilkinson, D. G. (1999). The pharmacology of donepezil: a new treatment for Alzheimer's disease. *Ex Opin Pharmacother* **1**:1–15.

Wilkinson, D., Holmes, C., Woolford, J., *et al.* (2002). Prophylactic therapy with lithium in elderly patients with unipolar major depression. *Int J Geriatr Psychiatry* **17**:619–22.

Williams, J. W., Jr., Barrett, J., Oxman, T., *et al.* (2000). Treatment of dysthymia and minor depression in primary care: a randomized controlled trial in older adults. *JAMA* **284**:1519–26.

Wilson, K., Mottram, P., Sivanranthan, A., & Nightingale, A. (2001). Antidepressant versus placebo for depressed elderly. Cochrane Database Syst Rev **2**:CD000561.

World Health Organisation (1992). *International Classification of Impairments, Disabilities and Handicaps*, 10th revision. Geneva: World Health Organisation.

Yassa, R., Nair, V., Nastase, C., *et al.* (1988). Prevalence of bipolar disorder in a psychogeriatric population. *J Affect Disorders* **14**:197–201.

Yost, E. B., *et al.* (1986). *Group Cognitive Therapy: A Treatment Approach for Older Depressed Adults*. New York: Pergamon Press.

16

The psychiatry of intellectual disability

Anthony Holland

This chapter covers psychiatric aspects of intellectual disability; the overlap between psychiatric and intellectual disorders is sometimes referred to as *dual disability*. This chapter reviews various theoretical perspectives relevant to practice in the context of emerging research in this area. This research has progressed from epidemiological studies to investigations into the causation of problem behaviours and comorbid mental disorders. In this context, different terminologies and conceptual models have at times resulted in confusion. However, the state of the art at present is one of integrating these various theoretical perspectives into an overarching biopsychosocial model that is concerned with identifying and addressing predisposing, precipitating and maintaining factors that result in mental ill health or maladaptive behaviours.

Background

The term *intellectual disability* is used to describe a group of people who have in common early developmental delay and evidence of intellectual and functional impairments. This term is synonymous with others used in different countries and statutes, including *mental handicap, mental retardation* and *learning disabilities* (American Psychiatric Association, 1994; World Health Organisation [WHO], 1992). As a group, people with developmental intellectual disabilities are very heterogeneous. Those with severe and profound intellectual disabilities are likely to have a history of significant developmental delay and functional impairments, such that they require care throughout their lives. Those with milder intellectual disabilities may be able to live independent, or relatively independent, lives and require additional support only through their school years or at times of particular difficulties.

No single term fully encapsulates the complexity of need. The World Health Organisation's classification system of impairments, disabilities and handicaps helps to address this issue (WHO, 1980) This has been revised in the form of the *International Classification of Functioning, Disability and Health* (WHO, 2001). In the earlier WHO model, in the case of intellectual disabilities, the "impairment" reflects dysfunction of the brain; "disability", the extent to which the individual has limited functional and social skills as would be expected for his or her age; and the "handicap", the disadvantage that follows.

The extent of disadvantage at least partly depends on whether society invests in strategies that might compensate for such disability, such as the level of the support offered. Given the distribution and properties of formal IQ assessments, approximately 2% of the population can be said to have a significant intellectual impairment, and 3 to 5 per 1,000 of the population have been reported to have severe or

Essential Psychiatry, ed. Robin M. Murray, Kenneth S. Kendler, Peter McGuffin, Simon Wessely, David J. Castle.
Published by Cambridge University Press. © Cambridge University Press 2008.

profound intellectual disabilities. The reported age-specific prevalence rates for intellectual disability is influenced by problems associated with ascertainment across the age range and, because of differential effects on age-related mortality rates, by those with more severe disabilities having a reduced life expectancy (see Fryers, 2000, for review; McConkey *et al.*, 2006).

Causation and the heterogeneity of dual disability

The possible reasons for significant developmental delay and subsequent intellectual disabilities are multiple and include the presence of chromosome abnormalities and single gene disorders, as well as environmental factors such as perinatal trauma or intrauterine infections, and maternal and early childhood nutritional deficiencies, maternal alcohol abuse or severe childhood neglect and deprivation (Kaski, 2000). There are other, as yet unidentified presumed genetic causes (Thapar *et al.*, 1994). The presence of mild intellectual disability rarely has a single identifiable cause but is a consequence of both polygenic and social/environmental influences. The extent to which a particular cause predominates in any country will vary depending on the social, political and economic status of that country and the resultant health and nutritional status of the general population, particularly that of mothers and newborn children. Other factors contributing to the extent of a person's disability and "handicap" (disadvantage) include educational, social and health resources that might maximise abilities and determine the extent of available opportunities.

The heterogeneity of this group of people is therefore characterised by the fact that some will have genetically or environmentally determined disorders that have had a marked effect on brain development and therefore on intellectual, social and functional abilities. Others may develop adequate living skills, are able to make their needs and wishes known through spoken language and lead relatively independent lives, but may have poor

---

> **Box 16.1** Key issues in service provision for people with dual disability
>
> - Changing societal attitudes and more enlightened national and international policies have led to major changes in the nature of service provision with a commitment to community non-institutionally based support.
> - People with intellectual disabilities have in common the presence of early developmental delay and impairments in intellectual and functional abilities but differ very significantly in the cause, nature and extent of these impairments and disabilities.
> - Interdisciplinary and community-based services are required to provide expertise to work alongside people with intellectual disabilities and those that support them to ensure an optimal and appropriate social care environment according to need.

psychological resources and are also often disadvantaged in society. Some sensory, physical or developmental disabilities such as cerebral palsy and autism spectrum disorders are considered related to intellectual disability in that many individuals with these other conditions also have evidence of significant intellectual disability. The mental health needs of this heterogeneous group of people are therefore varied and complex, and mental health problems and behavioural disorders can present in both typical and atypical ways, often depending on the developmental level and communication skills (in particular, verbal skills) of the person concerned (Holland & Koot, 1998). All aspects from the biological functioning of the brain to the manifestations of disability to societal responses can play a part in the emergence of dysfunction and mental ill health during the course of development and over the lifespan. Key points relevant to this area are shown in Box 16.1.

Psychiatric and behaviour disorders in people with intellectual disabilities

In accepted systems of classification, such as the 10th revision of the International Classification of

Diseases (ICD-10; WHO, 1992) or the 4th edition of the *Diagnostic and Statistical Manual of Mental Disorders* (DSM-IV; American Psychiatric Association, 1994), intellectual disability (mental retardation) along with personality disorder are seen as disorders of development. For example, in DSM-IV, mental retardation is under Axis II and acquired clinical disorders under Axis I. Thus it is accepted that comorbidity can occur, and people with intellectual disabilities can, like the rest of the population, acquire other mental disorders. However, in the field of intellectual disability, there has been confusion in the terminology used with respect to mental health and behaviour disorders. It is clear that mental illnesses (such as depression) may present in people with intellectual disabilities as changes in behaviour (Meins, 1995; Tsiouris, 2001), but not all maladaptive behaviour should be seen as due to problems within the individual and therefore as a "mental health" problem.

Some terms are used diagnostically and others descriptively. In this chapter, therefore, the use of a term defining a specific comorbid mental disorder (e.g. bipolar disorder) is taken to imply some understanding as to aetiology and a distinguishable composite of affective, behavioural and cognitive characteristics. The diagnosis of such a mental disorder thereby provides a guide to empirically validated and effective treatment.

In contrast, terms such as *maladaptive, problem, aberrant* or *challenging behaviour or behaviour disorders* have also been used in the field of intellectual disability. These include such behaviours as aggression, self-injury, smearing and severe stereotype behaviours. These terms are generally descriptive and do not in themselves imply any understanding as to cause. For example, the basis of self-injurious behaviour is likely to be different in people with Lesch-Nyhan syndrome compared with self-injury in those with autism or to the skin picking associated with having Prader-Willi syndrome. However, the severity of such behaviours are often such that they threaten the person's physical health or may have a marked effect on his or her quality of life and opportunities, as well as that of family members and other caregivers. The task

---

Box 16.2 Conceptual models for maladaptive behaviours in people with intellectual disability

- Learning theory
- The consequences of developmental arrest
- The presence of comorbid physical or psychiatric disorders
- The presence of specific risks in association with particular syndromes (referred to as *behavioural phenotypes*)

---

in each individual case is to identify the reasons for such maladaptive behaviours so that interventions likely to be effective can be put in place.

Different conceptual models can be helpful when trying to explain the occurrence of particular maladaptive behaviours, shown in Box 16.2. The recognition that such varied models can all, individually or in combination, help explain the occurrence of such behaviours has been a significant advance. Thus in the case of both the presence of an additional mental disorder or of behaviour problems, a combination of developmental, biological, social or psychological factors interact and influence the occurrence of such behaviours. It is therefore important in the field of intellectual disability to consider how these different processes might have predisposed to, precipitate or be maintaining such problem behaviours or abnormal mental states.

Epidemiology

A number of studies in different countries have attempted to investigate the extent to which people with intellectual disabilities manifest additional mental or behaviour disorders. Such studies have proved methodologically difficult for several reasons. First, the definition of intellectual disability is in itself imprecise. Although measures of intellectual ability can provide a guide, there may be uncertainty whether someone should or should not be considered to meet the criteria. This is particularly so when cognitive function is superficially average but social function is markedly impaired. Second, although identification of children with an intellectual disability may be possible when they are receiving statutory education, identification of all adults with a possible intellectual difficulty is much more problematic, and most studies include only those people with intellectual disabilities known to services (an administrative sample). People with additional needs, such as people with both intellectual disabilities and mental or behavioural disorders, are likely to be overrepresented in this group. Third, the diagnosis of mental disorder relies heavily on the ability of the person to describe his or her own mental experiences and feelings. For some people with intellectual disabilities, this is not possible, and mental states may have to be inferred from observations made by family members or other carers. Fourth, the use of diagnostic criteria for different mental disorders entails determining the presence or lack of specific mental experiences, and these criteria in people with intellectual disabilities may need some modification. However, if they are broadened too much, they may no longer be valid (Einfeld & Aman, 1995; Royal College of Psychiatrists, 2001). Finally, different terminology and diagnostic criteria have been used across studies, and direct comparisons between studies may not be possible.

Despite the methodological problems just listed, studies undertaken in Australia, Europe and the United States using varied methodologies have arrived at broadly similar results. There is a general consensus that rates of mental disorder (including behaviour disorders) are high, with a prevalence of nearly 50% in people with severe or profound intellectual disabilities and of about 20% to 25% in people with milder intellectual disabilities (see Birch *et al.,* 1970; Borthwick-Duffy & Eyman, 1990; Cooper, 1997; Einfeld & Tonge, 1996; Jacobson, 1982; Lund, 1985; Robertson *et al.,* 2004; Rutter *et al.,* 1970; Taylor *et al.,* 2004). Overall, prevalence rates of "behaviour disorders" may be as high as 20% and occur more commonly among people with severe intellectual disabilities and in particular among those meeting criteria for autistic spectrum disorder and those with sensory impairments (see Emerson, 2001, for a full review). In a recent study of an administrative sample of people with intellectual disabilities, rates of specific psychiatric disorders have been shown to be increased, particularly the rates of schizophrenia and anxiety disorders (Deb *et al.,* 2001) Also, for those with mild intellectual disabilities, affective disorder may be both common and chronic (Richardson *et al.,* 2001).

Research has also shown that particular psychiatric disorders or behaviour problems may cluster in groups of people with specific causes for their intellectual disabilities. This relationship between a genetic syndrome and an increased propensity to a specific behaviour or psychiatric disorder has been referred to as *behavioural phenotypes.* An example of these are the relationship between Down's syndrome and the very high risk of Alzheimer's disease in midlife (Holland *et al.,* 2000; Lai & Williams, 1989), with rates of clinical dementia starting at 1% or 2% in the 30s and reaching between 40% and 75% in the 50s. Another very different example is the overeating and other behaviour problems, such as skin picking and repetitive behaviours, that occur in people with Prader-Willi syndrome (Holland *et al.,* 2003). Most striking is the high risk of psychotic illness in people with one genetic subtype of Prader-Willi syndrome due to uniparental disomy (UPD) (Boer *et al.,* 2002), with rates of psychosis in this subgroup reaching 100% in the mid to late 20s. Other associations include the high rates of social anxiety experienced by those with fragile X syndrome (Einfeld *et al.,* 1999) and of schizophrenia in those with velo-cardio-facial syndrome (Shprintzen *et al.,* 1992). For some, such as those people with tuberose sclerosis, rates of autism spectrum disorder are reported to reach 80% and are associated with the brain tubers in the temporal lobe (Bolton & Griffiths, 1997).

Although the epidemiological evidence indicates that the full range of acquired mental disorders can be found affecting people with intellectual disability, together with a range of maladaptive behaviours, the picture is complex, with vulnerabilities for specific disorders varying according to the cause, nature and severity of a person's intellectual disability. This would suggest that intellectual disability is in itself a risk factor for the development of mental ill health and behaviour disorders, but the mechanisms that link the presence of intellectual disability and these increased vulnerabilities are less clear. Again, such mechanisms are best conceptualised by considering the issue from a developmental perspective and identifying the biological, psychological and social factors and their respective roles in predisposing to, precipitating or maintaining the presence of an acquired mental or behavioural disorder.

Biological factors

There are various strands of evidence supporting the view that impairment of brain function, which is highly likely to be present in people with intellectual disability, may itself increase the vulnerability to mental ill health. First, there is the evidence that the vulnerability to major mental illnesses, such as schizophrenia, may not only relate to genetic factors but also to the presence of brain abnormalities (Sommer et al., 2001). Second is the observation that people with intellectual disabilities due to specific syndromes may have particular risks (as described earlier). Third, some biological factors may explain the onset of mental disorder. For example, severe epilepsy, which is common in people with intellectual disability, may be associated with aberrant behaviours in the prodromal, ictal or post-ictal phases, to psychotic-like experiences or mood disorder and the effects of anticonvulsants on mental states (Bowley & Kerr, 2000). Finally, when brain development is severely arrested, there may be a pattern of behaviour that reflects the level of development and coping skills of that person, irrespective of his or her chronological age – for example, the continuation of incidental self-stimulatory or repetitive movements, severe temper outbursts or checking behaviours that are characteristic of normal early childhood (Holland et al., 2003).

Psychological factors

A substantial body of work based on principles of applied behaviour analysis supports a view that particular behaviours may be shaped and learned

and acquire functional relationships within the context of environmental setting events that may be interpreted by observers as a form of communication (see Emerson, 2001, for a review). For example, aggressive or self-injurious behaviour may be reinforced through the response of others in the environment and its occurrence affected by different settings, events and environmental contingencies. The behaviour may be instrumental in escaping or avoiding certain tasks. From this perspective, such behaviours are not conceptualised as a mental disorder but rather as the result of a naturally occurring process through which specific behaviours are inadvertently shaped over time. These models are being elaborated further, and the significance of specific developmental disorders, such as those in the autistic spectrum, and different biological states or mental ill health has been recognised as important contributory variables. This is well illustrated by studies of the relationship between particular behaviours and a specific genetic cause for the person's intellectual disability, such as Angelman syndrome (Horsler & Oliver, 2005). Interaction between factors that are predominantly cognitive, affective or developmental in nature and environmental contingencies are likely to be common, and although these relationships are complex and not well understood, these interactions influence the behavioural expression of mental disorders. It is also important to recognise the importance of having an intellectual disability in terms of functioning effectively in a cognitively complex and demanding society given the limited opportunities for a satisfying and productive lifestyle that may be available to people with intellectual disabilities. Here, the mediating mechanisms may include reinforcement of feelings of worthlessness through the impact of negative life experience, lack of emotional support and limited life opportunities.

Social factors

In most cultures, the importance of family life and other cultural equivalents, an appropriate living environment, social networks, meaningful employment and the right to privacy are taken for granted (see Parmenter, 2001, for discussion). The social milieu in which people live constitutes an important contribution to resilience and the development of practical, social and coping skills that may provide protection against the development of mental ill health in both individuals with intellectual disabilities and their carers (Cummins, 2001). More recent research involving children with learning disabilities and their families has suggested that socioeconomic factors can explain some of the increased risk for mental health problems that is observed (Emerson *et al.,* 2006). The quality of social care and employment or occupational opportunities commensurate with individual abilities and, most importantly, freedom from exploitation and abuse are prerequisites for enhancing mental health and minimising the occurrence of behaviour disorders, as it would be for any group (Balogh *et al.,* 2001).

In addition, for people with impaired understanding and expressive communication, the use of augmented forms of communication, such as signing and objects of reference, are also important to maximise instrumental use of the environment to communicate needs and wishes and to help make life more meaningful and predictable. Box 16.3 summarises key points in considering correlations between intellectual disability and mental illness.

The prevention and detection of mental ill health and its treatment

In the beginning of this chapter, the considerable heterogeneity of the group of people covered by the term *intellectual disability* was emphasised. Some will have clearly biologically determined disorders of brain development and associated severe intellectual disabilities, whereas other people will have milder intellectual disabilities and may well have experienced social, educational or economic disadvantage and the related consequences of such problems. It is therefore difficult to generalise across this group because there are likely to be a very

---

Box 16.3 Key points in the relationship between intellectual disability and mental illness

- Difficulties relating to definitions and ascertainment make true population-based studies of the relationship between the presence of intellectual disabilities and the occurrence of behavioural and psychiatric disorder problematic.
- Rates of psychiatric and behavioural problems are high among people with intellectual disabilities, with the exact nature of the problem depending on the nature and extent of the intellectual disability of the population surveyed.
- Specific studies of people with particular syndromes known to be associated with intellectual disabilities indicate that the profile of mental ill health and/or problem behaviours may, in some circumstances, be strongly influenced by the cause of the person's intellectual disability.

---

diverse range of factors that contribute to mental ill health. Although there has been considerable research regarding behaviour disorders, there has been limited work investigating the vulnerabilities that contribute to psychiatric disorders, such as mental illness, among people with intellectual disabilities. It is likely that there will be both protective and preventative factors that increase the resilience to the psychosocial impacts of adverse effects and life events (Esbensen & Benson, 2006; Hastings *et al.,* 2003), as well as other factors that increase the risk for the future development of mental disorder. Many may be similar to that which has been observed in the general population.

Maintenance of mental health and prevention of mental ill health

The complexity of this group of people and the interrelationships among developmental, biological, psychological and social factors are likely to be complex. Furthermore, different factors may predispose to mental ill health, and other factors may be responsible for precipitating a particular episode

Box 16.4 Factors maintaining or ameliorating mental health problems in intellectual disability

- The physical environment and whether it is free from exploitation and abuse
- The quality of the communication that enables individual wishes and needs to be understood and appropriately met
- The nature of neuropsychological and other psychological behavioural strengths and weaknesses
- The extent of support to families and individuals that alleviate the carer's stress and enhance the quality of the home environment (Cummins, 2001)
- Relevant educational and meaningful life opportunities that help maintain life satisfaction through the performance of valued roles, albeit with supportive services
- The availability of leisure opportunities and appropriate social networks
- The presence of nondiscriminatory attitudes towards the person's specific disability or from beliefs about their gender, ethnicity and culture

of ill health and maintaining such problems over time. From a biological perspective, these include the vulnerability that might be directly associated with a specific syndrome, or, indirectly, because of the general impairment in brain function, the person's physical health and presence of other physical and sensory impairments or the effective management of epilepsy, if present. From the psychological, behavioural and social perspectives, the key issues will vary according to individual circumstances and the degree of impairment and disability but may include, inter alia, the issues shown in Box 16.4.

Detection of mental ill health

Acknowledging that people with intellectual disabilities may develop comorbid mental disorders or that particular patterns of behaviour may be the consequence of inappropriate support strategies has been a major advance in the field. There are, however, several problems that mitigate against the early and appropriate detection of such difficulties and

the development of meaningful interventions. The first, perhaps the most striking, is often referred to as *diagnostic overshadowing* (Reiss *et al.*, 1982). This is the phenomenon in which the development of a particular abnormal mental state or pattern of behaviour is attributed to the person's intellectual disability, and the possibility that there may be an underlying comorbid disorder is not considered. In addition, it may be difficult for people with intellectual disability to recognise themselves that they need help, and they often depend on others to identify the potential significance of such change. Thus the key to the detection of potential mental ill health is acknowledgement that it can and does occur among people with intellectual disabilities. A further confounding factor is the belief, on the part of carers, that such behaviour problems are inevitable and unchangeable, and therefore that it is not appropriate to seek advice. Also having identified the possibility of an underlying comorbid mental disorder, it may be difficult to obtain information from the person who has either limited or no language, and there may be a lack of good longitudinal data from informants demonstrating that there has been a change in mental or behavioural status. To aid the process of detection and of subsequent diagnosis, the Psychiatric Assessment Schedule for Adults with Developmental Disabilities (PAS-ADD) checklist and informant and patient/participant assessments have been developed (Moss *et al.*, 1996, 1998).

Assessment and treatment

Assessment, and subsequent treatment, is only possible if it is recognised that a problem exists and that an understanding of that problem can lead to interventions that may be effective. Having recognised that there is a problem, a comprehensive assessment is essential. The onset of superficially similar maladaptive behaviours (e.g. aggression or self-injurious behaviour) in one person as opposed to another may have very different causes. What predisposes to such behaviour may be different from

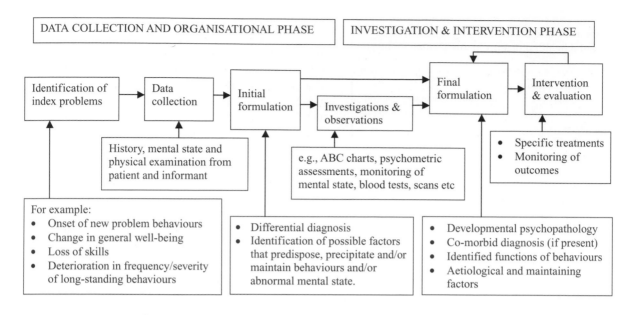

Figure 16.1 The process of assessment of the individual with dual disability.

what actually results in its manifestation, at a given point in time in a particular environment. Because of the potential complexity, it is likely that the perspectives of different disciplines will be required, and, in addition to a detailed history and mental and physical assessments, those supporting the person concerned will need to make structured observations over time. Such observations could include daily mood monitoring, records of seizures and the use of ABC charts to record the frequency of any maladaptive behaviours and what was observed prior to, during and after an incident. This information is then used to develop a detailed formulation of the index problem.

A psychiatric formulation includes an evaluation of the cause of the person's intellectual disability, a developmental history particularly exploring the possibility of autism, the diagnosis of any comorbid physical or psychiatric disorders and the identification of social or psychological factors (e.g. recent bereavement) that might account for a change in vulnerability or, as a life event, precipitated a change in mental state. A psychological perspective might focus on the identification of cognitive strengths

and weaknesses, on the identification of any pattern to the occurrence of such maladaptive behaviours and ultimately on identifying any functional component to the behaviours. In the case of depression, assessment would help determine the potential value of cognitive-behavioural therapy (Esbensen & Benson, 2005).

As the members of other disciplines, such as speech and language therapy experts, undertake their own assessments, a comprehensive picture of the developmental profile and present abilities of that person and of how identified problems can best be explained arises. Although in some cases the recent onset of a problem can be linked fairly easily to some life stress or the onset of a mental disorder, such as depression, in others the reasons for the occurrence of particular problems are not obvious, and as such extensive assessments are essential. Often the understanding that emerges is multifaceted. This process is illustrated in Figure 16.1.

It follows from this discussion that interventions are dictated by the results of the assessment. The bringing together of an understanding of a particular problem, through the process of formulation, can in itself result in improvement, perhaps because it brings some order to what are often very stressful and increasingly chaotic situations. The psychiatrist will have a role, along with other disciplines, in the development of the formulation. Some information encapsulated in the formulation will be important knowledge, but it does not in itself lead to an intervention. Other information (e.g. identification of a comorbid psychiatric or physical illness) may have an obvious and well-tested treatment. For example, knowing that a person has Lesch Nyhan, Smith Magenis or Cornelia de Lange syndrome, all known to be associated with self-injurious behaviour, does not immediately result in a specific targeted treatment for such behaviour; however, it is part of picture and may guide further investigation and then intervention. In the case of people with Cornelia de Lange syndrome, oesophageal reflux is common, and the associated pain may well result in nonspecific problem behaviours (Luzzani *et al.*, 2003).

Thus, assessment and intervention is an iterative process and needs to follow a logical progression, often with one intervention at a time so that success or poor results can be properly evaluated. As a general rule, the initial treatment of comorbid disorders followed by psychological and other interventions is the most appropriate course of action. If a person has severe depression, a psychotic illness, uncontrolled epilepsy, or a physical illness, until this is rectified, other interventions, particular ones that require engagement from the person concerned, are less likely to be successful. Furthermore, many of these disorders may be associated with mental and physical suffering; indeed, the sooner they are treated, the better, and treatment may also result in a complete resolution of the index problem.

Psychotropic medication

This section devoted to psychotropic medications has been included primarily because of concerns about their use in this population. Many studies have reported the high rates of psychotropic medication being given to people with intellectual disabilities for their "challenging behaviour"

(Kiernan *et al.*, 1995; Linaker 1990). As this chapter indicates, many causes may lead to such behaviour, and therefore the simplistic view that challenging behaviour, such as aggression, equates to the use of a major tranquiliser, is not sustainable (Brylewski & Duggan, 1999). A starting point is that psychotropic medication can be used to treat a diagnosed psychiatric disorder (such as bipolar disorder, depression or schizophrenia) that sound evidence has shown responds to this treatment. This evidence is usually from double-blind placebo-controlled trials undertaken in the nonintellectually disabled population, but there is no indication that that knowledge is not transferable to the treatment of people with intellectual disability (with some conditions).

First, an accurate psychiatric diagnosis is essential, and if a person does not respond to the treatment, a re-evaluation of the comorbid diagnosis is indicated. Second, particularly for those with genetically determined neurodevelopmental disorders, the use of medications that act on the central nervous system needs to be undertaken with caution because both the response and the risk of side effects may be atypical. Thus starting dosages are usually lower and increased with care. The use of atypical rather than typical neuroleptics is generally recommended. Third, making a diagnosis and determining response to the treatment of a suspected comorbid illness may be problematic, particularly in those with limited spoken language ability. It may be the case that treatments are given and monitored in situations of greater uncertainty than would be the case in the treatment of a similar disorder in a person without an intellectual disability. For this reason, the identification of possible markers of the illness (e.g. particular behaviours or mood states) and recording the nature, frequency and severity of such behaviours before starting and after the commencement of treatment is advisable. If there appears to be no response, further evaluation is indicated with respect to the original diagnosis, specifically regarding whether this suggests nonresponse to treatment or whether it is the wrong treatment because the diagnosis is incorrect (see Reiss & Aman, 1998).

Although such an approach (i.e. diagnosis informs choice of treatment) to the use of psychotropic medication is the standard, there are concerns that too rigid a diagnostic approach may result in people not receiving medication who would have otherwise benefited from it. The two main reasons for this are as follows: first, a recognition that the diagnosis of a comorbid psychiatric disorder may be difficult because of an atypical presentation or the lack of any description from the person of his or her mental state and, as described earlier, it may not be possible to make a definitive comorbid diagnosis, but there may be a high index of suspicion. Second, high levels, for example, of arousal, anxiety, or obsessiveness may all contribute to problematic behaviours, and although such phenomena may not meet formal diagnostic criteria for specific psychiatric disorders, they may respond to the use of neuroleptic, sedative or antidepressant medications. This is best illustrated with the reported benefits from the use of atypical antipsychotic medication and selective serotonergic reuptake inhibitors (SSRIs) in people with autistic spectrum disorders (Bodfish & Madison, 1993). For example, persistent or intermittent high levels of anxiety associated with unexpected changes in routine in a person with autism may be ameliorated through the use of specific neuroleptic or SSRI medication (or both) in conjunction with improving the communication environment (e.g. use of signs and symbols) and other strategies to bring predictability into that person's life. Such an approach may well be indicated in the context of the broader formulation and in the understanding of how the use of such medication might, for example, reduce a person's predisposition to problematic behaviours by raising the threshold for responding to unexpected environmental changes.

Conclusions

People with intellectual disabilities are a highly heterogeneous group with often complex, multiple and changing needs. Behavioural and psychiatric disorders have a high prevalence, and different approaches are required depending on an understanding of the index problem. For these reasons, interdisciplinary assessment is frequently needed that draws on different theoretical approaches and models of understanding. Intervention is often an iterative process informed by proper record keeping and by a combination of interventions. These may range from the treatment of an underlying physical or psychiatric comorbid illness, improvements in communication strategies, positive behaviour support and establishing structured, meaningful and appropriate social care.

For those with more severe intellectual disabilities, establishing the nature of any abnormal mental state or of an underlying physical illness may be problematic. For this reason, a high index of suspicion is required, and knowledge of syndrome-specific risks can be particularly helpful. Uncertainties that result because of problems with communication with respect to those with more severe intellectual disabilities means that knowledge held by families and paid carers, particularly about change in functioning or behaviour over time, is often of great value. Interventions may be further complicated with respect to the capacity of people with intellectual disabilities to consent. Legislation in different countries provides a framework for resolving this issue. However, the responsibility of clinicians is to engage the person in the assessment and intervention process as far as that is possible.

REFERENCES

American Psychiatric Association (1994). *Diagnostic and Statistical Manual of Mental Disorders*, 4th edn. Washington, DC: American Psychiatric Association.

Balogh, R., Bretherton, K., Whibley, S., *et al.* (2001). Sexual abuse in children and adolescents with intellectual disability. *J Intellect Disabil Res* **45**:202–11.

Birch, H., Richardson, S., Baird, D., *et al.* (1970). *Mental Subnormality in the Community: A Clinical and Epidemiological Study.* Baltimore: Williams & Wilkins.

Bodfish, J., & Madison, J. (1993). Diagnosis and fluoxetine treatment of compulsive behavior disorder of adults with mental retardation. *Am J Ment Retard* **98**: 360–7.

Boer, H., Holland, A., Whittington, J., *et al.* (2002). Psychotic illness in people with Prader-Willi syndrome due to chromosome 15 maternal uniparental disomy. *Lancet* **359**:135–6.

Bolton, P., & Griffiths, P. (1997). Association of tuberous sclerosis of temporal lobes with autism and atypical autism. *Lancet* **349**:392–5.

Borthwick-Duffy, S., & Eyman, R. (1990). Who are the dually diagnosed?. *Am J Ment Retard* **94**:586–95.

Bowley, C., & Kerr, M. (2000). Epilepsy and intellectual disability. *J Intellect Disabil Res* **44**:529–43.

Brylewski, J., & Duggan, L. (1999). Antipsychotic mediation for challenging behaviour in people with intellectual disability: a systematic review of randomised controlled trials. *J Intellect Disabil Res* **43**:360–71.

Cooper, S.-A. (1997). Epidemiology of psychiatric disorders in elderly compared with younger adults with learning disabilities. *Br J Psychiatry* **170**:375–80.

Cummins, R. (2001). The subjective well-being of people caring for a family member with severe disability at home: a review *J Intellect Disabil Res* **26**:83–100.

Deb, S., Thomas, M., Bright, C., *et al.* (2001). Mental disorder in adults with intellectual disability. 1: prevalence of functional psychiatric illness among a community - based population aged between 16 and 64 years. *J Intellect Disabil Res* **45**:495–505.

Einfeld, S. L., & Aman, M. (1995). Issues in the taxonomy of psychopathology in mental retardation. *J Autism Dev Disord* **25**: 143–67.

Einfeld, S. L., & Tonge, B. (1996). Population prevalence of psychopathology in children and adolescents with intellectual disability II: epidemiological findings. *J Intellect Disabil Res* **40**:99–109.

Einfeld, S., B. Tonge, Turner, G., *et al.* (1999). Longitudinal course of behavioural and emotional problems of young persons with Prader-Willi, Fragile X, Williams and Down syndromes. *J Intellect Disabil Res* **24**:349–54,

Emerson, E. (2001). *Challenging Behaviour: Analysis and Intervention in People with Severe Intellectual Disabilities.* Cambridge: Cambridge University Press.

Emerson, E., Hatton, C., Blacher, J., *et al.* (2006). Socioeconomic position, household composition, health status and indicators of the well-being of mothers of children with and without intellectual disabilities. *J Intellect Disabil Res* **50**:862–73.

Esbensen, A., & Benson, B. (2005). Cognitive variables and depressed mood in adults with intellectual disability. *J Intellect Disabil Res* **49**:481–9.

Esbensen, A., & Benson, B. (2006). A prospective analysis of life events, problems behaviours and depression in adults with intellectual disability. *J Intellect Disabil Res* **50**:248–58.

Fryers, T. (2000). Epidemiology of mental retardation. In M. Gelder, J. Lopes-Ibor & N. Andreasen, eds. *New Oxford Textbook of Psychiatry*, Vol. **2**. Oxford: Oxford University Press, p. 10.2.

Hastings, R., Hatton, C., Taylor, J. L., *et al.* (2003). Life events and psychiatric symptoms in adults with intellectual disability. *J Intellect Disabil Res* **48**:42–6.

Holland, A., Hon, J., Huppert, F. A., *et al.* (2000). Incidence and course of dementia in people with Down's syndrome: findings from a population-based study. *J Intellect Disabil Res* **44**:138–46.

Holland, A., & Koot, H. (1998). Mental Health and Intellectual Disabilities: an international perspective. *J Intellect Disabil Res* **42**:505–12.

Holland, A., Whittington, J., Butler, T., *et al.* (2003). Behavioural phenotypes associated with specific genetic disorders: evidence from a population-based study of people with Prader-Willi syndrome. *Psychol Med* **33**:141–53.

Horsler, K., & Oliver, C. (2005). Behavioural phenotype of Angelman syndrome. *J Intellect Disabil Res* **50**:33–53.

Jacobson, J. (1982). Problem behaviour and psychiatric impairment within a developmentally disabled population. Behaviour frequency. *J Appl Res Ment Retard* **3**:121–39.

Kaski, M. (2000). Aetiology of mental retardation: general issues and prevention. In M. Gelder, J. Lopes-Ibor & N. Andreasen, eds. *New Oxford Textbook of Psychiatry*. Oxford: Oxford University Press.

Kiernan, C., Reeves, D., Alborz, A., *et al.* (1995). The use of anti-psychotic drugs with adults with learning disabilities and challenging behaviour. *J Intellect Disabil Res* **39**:263–74.

Lai, F., & Williams, R. (1989). A prospective study of Alzheimer disease in Down syndrome. *Arch Neurol* **46**:849–53.

Linaker, O. (1990). Frequency and determinants for psychotropic drug use in an institution for the mentally retarded. *Br J Psychiatry* **156**:525–30.

Lund, J. (1985). The prevalence of psychiatric morbidity in mentally retarded adults. *Acta Psychiatr Scand* **7**:563–70.

Luzzani, S., Macchini, F., Valadè, F., *et al.* (2003). Gastroesophageal reflux and Cornelia de Lange syndrome: typical and atypical symptoms. *Am J Med Genet* **119**:283–7.

McConkey, R., Mulvany, F., Barron, S., *et al.* (2006). Adult persons with intellectual disabilities on the island of Ireland. *J Intellect Disabil Res* **50**:227–36.

Meins, W. (1995). Symptoms of major depression in mentally retarded adults. *J Intellect Disabil Res* **39**:41–6.

Moss, S., H. Prosser, Costello, H., *et al.* (1996). *PAS-ADD Checklist.* Manchester Hester Adrian Research Centre, University of Manchester.

Moss, S., Prosser, H., Costello, H., *et al.* (1998). Reliability and validity of the PAS-ADD Checklist for detecting psychiatric disorders in adults with intellectual disability. *J Intellect Disabil Res* **42**:173–83.

Parmenter, T. (2001). The contribution of science in facilitating the inclusion of people with intellectual disability into the community. *J Intellect Disabil Res* **45**: 183–93.

Reiss, S., & Aman, M. (1998). The international consensus process on psychopharmacology and intellectual disability. *J Intellect Disabil Res* **41**:448–55.

Reiss, S., Levitan, G., & Szyszko J. (1982). Emotional disturbance and mental retardation: diagnostic overshadowing. *Am J Ment Defic* **86**:567–74.

Richardson, S., Maughan, B., Hardy, R., *et al.* (2001). Long-term affective disorder in people with mild learning disability. *Br J Psychiatry* **179**:523–7.

Robertson, J., Emerson, E., Pinkney, L., *et al.* (2004). Treatment and management of challenging behaviours in congregate and noncongregate community-based supported accommodation. *J Intellect Disabil Res* **49**: 63–72.

Royal College of Psychiatrists (2001). *Guidelines for Researchers and for Research Ethics Committees on Psychiatric Research Involving Human Participants* (Council Report CR82). London: Gaskell.

Rutter, M., Tizard, J., & Whitmore, K. (1970). *Education, Health and Behaviour.* London: Longman.

Shprintzen, R., Goldberg, R., Shprintzen, R. J., *et al.* (1992). Late onset psychosis in the velo-cardio-facial syndrome. *Am J Med Genet* **42**:141–2.

Sommer, I., Ramsey, N., Aleman, A., *et al.* (2001). Handedness, language lateralisation and anatomical asymmetry in schizophrenia. Meta-analysis. *Br J Psychiatry* **178**:344–51.

Taylor, J., Hatton, C., Dixon, L., *et al.* (2004). Screening for psychiatric symptoms: PAS-ADD Checklist norms for adults with intellectual disabilities. *J Intellect Disabil Res* **48**:37–41.

Thapar, A., Gottesman, I., Owen, M., *et al.* (1994). The genetics of mental retardation. *Br J Psychiatry* **164**:747–58.

Tsiouris, J. (2001). The diagnosis of depression in people with severe/profound intellectual disability. *J Intellect Disabil Res* **45**:115–20.

World Health Organisation (1980). *International Classification of Impairments, Disabilites and Handicaps (10th revision)* Geneva, WHO.

World Health Organisation (1992). *International Statistical Classification of Disease and Related Health Problems (10th revision).* Geneva: World Health Organisation.

World Health Organisation (2001). *International Classification of Functioning, Disability and Health.* Geneva: World Health Organisation.

17

Sexual problems

John Bancroft

Sexuality plays a central role in most of our lives. It is a key factor in our principal relationships and the formation of our families. It is also a common source of problems. This chapter examines the relationship between mental health and sexuality: how mental health affects sexuality and, conversely, what effects sexual experiences can have on mental health. The more common sexual problems and their clinical management are reviewed. As a background, we first consider sexual development and the psychosomatic interface between psychological processes and physiological sexual response.

Sexual development

Normal sexual development results from the integration of three developmental "strands": gender identity, the capacity for close dyadic relationships and sexual responsiveness (Bancroft, 2005a). Both gender identity and the capacity for close dyadic relationships are fundamental to childhood development in a more general sense. In contrast, the sexual response strand has a much more variable role during childhood, with some children having clear sexual awareness and associated experiences, such as masturbation, and others remaining relatively unaware. The extent to which this variability results from early learning and family environment or is genetically or prenatally determined

remains unknown, and it is not clearly related to either gender identity or dyadic relationships prior to puberty. As the child approaches adolescence, all three strands become increasingly interactive and interdependent. Gender identity is thrown into a transient state of confusion. Hierarchies of relationships between peers can be disrupted. The newly organizing sense of masculinity or femininity will influence how dyadic relationships, both sexual and nonsexual, are formed and experienced. The emerging adolescent "scripts" for male and female behaviour will now have a clearer sexual component, and sexual response will have an impact on new relationships, leading to an evolving distinction between sexual and nonsexual relationships. The sexual response strand may make an early entry in the developmental process for some and a late entry for others, neither having clear implications for normal adult sexual development.

Factors influencing the integration of these three strands in early adolescence can be considered under three headings:

- *The "peri-pubertal" pattern.* The emerging sexual responsiveness in late childhood and early adolescence has a substantial hormonal basis and should be regarded as central to normal sexual development. Similarly, peri-pubertal changes in body shape, breast and hair growth, voice breaking and menarche all contribute to the upheaval of gender identity and related self-esteem around

Essential Psychiatry, ed. Robin M. Murray, Kenneth S. Kendler, Peter McGuffin, Simon Wessely, David J. Castle.
Published by Cambridge University Press. © Cambridge University Press 2008.

that time. Here we are dealing with processes relatively independent of the child's social and family context at this age.

- The *"parent versus peer group" pattern*. One aspect of adolescence is the process of developing a "separate identity", which in part is achieved by rejecting, often transiently, some of the values or norms or expectations that one's parents uphold, and in part by identifying with a "peer group". We need to understand the balance between parental influences, which tend to predominate during pre-pubertal childhood, and peer group influences, which are increasingly important during adolescence.
- The *"maladaptive" pattern*. Sexual behaviour is one of the adolescent "externalizing" behaviours which are often part of a pattern of maladaptive behaviour beginning in childhood and associated with a range of negative developmental influences. Sexual "acting out" gets added to the list of such behaviours as the child enters adolescence.

Gender identity

For the large majority of individuals, gender identity develops in a non-problematic way. Nonconformity in gender role behaviour, particularly for boys, can result in stigmatization and relative isolation from one's peer group. This, in itself, can have substantial effects on the integration of our three strands during adolescence. Thus Kagan and Moss (1962), in a unique longitudinal study from birth to early adulthood, found that boys who showed gender nonconformity between the ages of 3 and 10 years were more likely to report high sexual anxiety, less likely to engage in early dating and more likely to show avoidance of erotic behaviour in adolescence. Boys who avoided dating between 10 and 14 years were less likely to establish intimate heterosexual relationships or engage in erotic activity during late adolescence and adulthood. The inability to identify similar predictors in girls is noteworthy.

Reasons for gender nonconformity in childhood are usually unclear. Girls with adrenal cortical hyperplasia, exposed to high levels of androgens during foetal development and after birth until the condition is treated, typically show some masculinization of behaviour (Ehrhardt & Meyer-Balhburg, 1981). However, such cases with an obvious hormonal explanation are the exception. In general, gender nonconformity in boys is more problematic, with stigmatization both by adults and other children more marked than with masculinised behaviour in girls. Gender dysphoria in adolescence and later is usually preceded by gender nonconformity in childhood.

Sexual behaviour

The majority of males and females probably experience their first sexual arousal before puberty (Reynolds *et al.*, 2003), but there is considerable variability. Masturbation is an interesting marker of sexual development. Comparison of two samples of students collected around 50 years apart (Bancroft, Herbenick & Reynolds, 2003) showed some striking similarities, including interesting gender differences. In both samples, approximately 80% of males reported onset of masturbation within a 2-year period on either side of puberty. A substantially higher proportion of females reported masturbation in the recent sample, but of those in the two samples who had masturbated, a very similar pattern of age of onset was found, with a much wider age distribution than in the males. Some females started earlier than most boys and others much later in adolescence, if at all. The male pattern suggested a powerful organizing effect of puberty. The female pattern indicated much greater variability; it has been postulated that females vary much more in their sensitivity to androgens (discussed later). Thus early onset in highly sensitive females may result from hormonal stimulation around adrenarche; those who are moderately sensitive to androgens are stimulated around puberty, and those relatively insensitive to androgens show a much later onset (Bancroft, 2005b).

There is substantial evidence on age at first sexual intercourse in girls and more limited evidence for boys. A series of studies during the 1970s and 1980s showed a steady reduction in the age at first sexual intercourse, an increase in the proportion of girls who engaged in sexual intercourse and an associated increase in the average number of sexual partners. This trend levelled out during the late 1980s and 1990s. Sequential surveying of teenage boys did not start until 1988, and since then there has been a modest decline in the proportion of boys who had experienced intercourse (Santelli *et al.*, 2000). Overall, however, boys tend to start sexual intercourse earlier and have more sexual partners than girls. Given the emphasis that has been placed on the age at first intercourse, we understand surprisingly little about how the timing of this seemingly pivotal event affects the developmental process (Bancroft, 2005a). In contrast, we have very limited evidence on what sexual behaviour young teenagers engage in apart from sexual intercourse (e.g. genital touching, oral sex)

Sexual identity, sexual orientation and sexual preferences

As the three strands start to integrate in the transitional stage between childhood and adolescence, a key element is an emerging "sexual identity" "What kind of sexual person am I?" Sexual orientation (i.e. same sex or opposite sex attraction) is an important component of sexual identity, but its development is not understood. It is reasonable to assume that the basic developmental mechanisms will be the same for those with heterosexual and homosexual orientations. First is a "pre-labelling" stage, when childhood and early adolescent sexual experiences occur, including feelings of attraction, without the need to categorise them as either heterosexual or homosexual. At some stage, which is likely to be socially determined, the individual asks the question, "Am I straight or gay?" (the "self-labelling stage") and later the social world, in particular the peer group, starts asking the same questions about the individual ("social labelling stage"),

reinforcing the idea that "you are either one thing or the other" (Bancroft, 1989). The adolescent who is experiencing cross-gender attraction, will progress, almost without consideration, into a heterosexual identity, contrasting with one who is experiencing same-gender attraction, who will be either struggling in a sociocultural vacuum or, more likely, experiencing the impact of social stigmatization. Integration of our three developmental strands will take substantially longer in some who emerge with a homosexual identity, rendering them more psychologically vulnerable in the process. Early identification with a gay subculture is likely to be beneficial in this respect. (For recent discussions of determinants of sexual orientation, see Bem, 2000; Herdt, 2000; and Meyer-Bahlburg, 2000.) Biological factors, both genetic and prenatal hormonal, are likely to play an important role, probably more so in males than in females (see Mustanski *et al.*, 2002, for a review). However, there are also good grounds for concluding that "sexual identity" is socially constructed, reflecting the ways that different societies at different historical periods have made sense of variability in sexual preference. There is extensive evidence of an association between gender nonconformity in male children and subsequent homosexual orientation (Mustanski *et al.*, 2002). However, gender nonconformity is not a necessary prerequisite for homosexual orientation, and we remain uncertain whether the impact of biological or genetic factors is more directly on gender identity and secondarily on sexual orientation, or whether both are manifestations of a common biological basis.

Beyond sexual orientation, we also need to consider the extraordinary individual variability in more specific sexual preferences. Unusual sexual preferences, including most of the paraphilias, are more likely to be established in those relatively isolated from a "normalizing" peer group. Given the almost exclusive restriction of fetishes to males, the erectile response probably plays a crucial role in this discriminatory learning process, associated with increased arousability around puberty. In most respects, however, we understand very little about why some individuals develop preferences which are outside "normative" sexual interaction. Some abnormal types of sexual learning, particularly the more bizarre fetishes, are sometimes associated with abnormal brain function, such as temporal lobe epilepsy (Bancroft, 1989). Are there specific mechanisms in the brain relevant to sexual learning, which, although fundamental to normal sexual development, sometimes go wrong? At present we can only speculate.

Dyadic relationships

The key issue here is the extent to which sexual expression becomes established as something in its own right rather than one component of an ongoing dyadic relationship. Variability in this respect is not easily explained. Some individuals may pursue relatively uncommitted sexual interactions for many years, primarily for the sake of sexual pleasure and potential benefits to one's self-esteem from making sexual conquests. Others may see sex as one component of a relationship, which is what they primarily seek, whether as a series of monogamous relationships or a long-term one, as in marriage. Clearly moral and religious values are relevant here, but other factors relating to both personality and sexual responsiveness are also important. In a recent study of women, the ability to become sexually aroused depended, for some women (but not for others), on how the partner felt about them; those for whom it was not important reported higher numbers of casual sexual partners (Sanders *et al.*, unpublished data). The origins of such variance between women have not yet been explained.

Sexual intimacy

The incorporation of our emerging sexuality into intimate dyadic relationships can be adversely affected in a variety of ways. Less specific problems in coping with emotional intimacy, which may arise during childhood, may present barriers to establishing a rewarding sexual, as well as other types of close relationships. The establishment of negative attitudes or values about sex, or a tendency to

impaired sexual responsiveness, can make sexual intimacy difficult. Alternatively, the development of certain types of sexual preference may also provide barriers; many types of paraphilia have this effect. In general, the effect of sexuality on intimacy will depend to a considerable extent on the personalities of the partners involved.

The psychophysiology of sexual arousal

Sexual arousal can be conceptualised as a state motivated towards the experience of sexual pleasure and possibly orgasm, and involving (1) information processing of relevant stimuli, (2) arousal in a general sense, (3) incentive motivation and (4) genital response. *Sexual arousal* applies to the state, and *sexual arousability* to the capacity for experiencing sexual arousal, which varies across individuals and within individuals across time. Sexual interest or desire is an aspect of sexual arousal, when all four components may be involved to some extent, but where at least sexual information processing (e.g. sexual thoughts) is associated with some degree of incentive motivation. This is essentially a psychosomatic process in which psychological mechanisms interact with physiological responses, with the added "feedback effect" that awareness of physiological processes can enhance or inhibit further arousal (Bancroft, 1989).

A dual control model has been developed to deal with this complexity, postulating that there are sexual excitatory and sexual inhibitory systems within the brain which are independent of each other but which interact to determine whether sexual arousal occurs. The model further postulates that individuals vary in their propensity for both sexual excitation and sexual inhibition (Bancroft, 1999; Bancroft & Janssen, 2000). Questionnaire methods have been established to measure these propensities in men (Janssen *et al.*, 2002) and in women (Graham, Sanders & Milhausen, 2006). A basic premise of this model is that inhibition of sexual response is a normal, adaptive mechanism across species which reduces the likelihood of

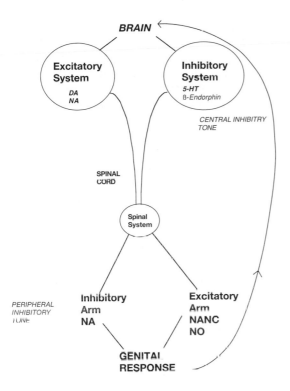

Figure 17.1

sexual arousal in circumstances when this would be disadvantageous. There are also likely to be sex differences, with inhibition having a greater adaptive role in females. Some individuals have a high propensity for inhibition, which makes them vulnerable to sexual dysfunction, and others have a low propensity, which increases the likelihood of engaging in high-risk or otherwise inappropriate sexual behaviour. This model is used as the framework for considering problematic sexual behaviour and is presented schematically in Figure 17.1, which shows both central and peripheral components of the two systems.

An important distinction needs to be made between inhibitory tone and reactive inhibition. A level of inhibitory tone appears necessary to maintain nonaroused states. Thus flaccidity of the penis depends on inhibitory tone, at least in the periphery. Erection may depend on a reduction in this tone,

or at least in a sufficient increase in excitation to overcome it (Bancroft & Janssen, 2000). Early studies of spinal cord transection resulting in enhanced reflexive sexual responses indicated inhibitory tone from the brain (McKenna, 2000). Brain imaging studies of response to visual sexual stimuli show areas of deactivation, mainly in the temporal lobes, which are also consistent with deactivation of *central inhibitory tone* (Mouras & Stoleru, 2007). Reactive inhibition implies an increase in the level of inhibition in response to a threatening situation.

Central mechanisms

The *excitation system* has three components to it:
1. central arousal of a relatively nonspecific kind, which is mainly dependent on the central noradrenergic system, originating in the locus coeruleus of the brainstem;
2. incentive motivation or "appetite" involves the mesolimbic tract, one component of the central dopaminergic system, which is involved in most kinds of "appetite"; and
3. genital response – at a central level, various mechanisms are involved, including the dopaminergic input to the medial preoptic area (MPOA) in the hypothalamus from the A14 periventricular system (Hull *et al.*, 1999).

Thus both noradrenaline (NA) and dopamine (DA) are key neurotransmitters in the central part of our *sexual excitatory system*, although the role of DA at the MPOA may depend on disinhibition of inhibitory tone.

The *inhibition system* is less easily defined, involves less discrete anatomical brain structures and probably a variety of neurotransmitters and mediators, including serotonin (5-HT), and neuropeptides such as beta-endorphin. The serotonergic system, which originates mainly in the raphe nuclei of the brainstem, is widely distributed, including descending neurons to the spinal cord. This system is generally inhibitory; more specific inhibition of sexual responses has been linked to the lateral hypothalamus (where there is an increase in 5-HT in the post-ejaculatory interval), and the nucleus para-gigantocellularis in the brainstem, which is linked to sympathetic and parasympathetic neurons in the penis by serotonergic neurons (McKenna, 2000) (see Figure 17.1).

Peripheral mechanisms

In addition to more general, nonspecific manifestations of arousal in the periphery (e.g. blood pressure and heart rate increase) the principal sexual responses are genital. Penile erection in the male results from relaxation of smooth muscle of the corpus cavernosum, resulting in increased blood flow into the erectile tissues, which, because of the relatively inelastic tunica albuginea, results in increased arterial pressure and associated compression of venous outflow. As indicated in Figure 17.1, the neurotransmitters involved are subsumed under the heading *nonadrenergic-noncholinergic* (NANC) and have not all been precisely identified (Levin, 2007). However, one key factor is the nitric oxidase-arginine-NO-cyclic GMP pathway (nitrergic transmission). It is the cyclic GMP which is responsible for smooth muscle relaxation and which is catabolised by phosphodiesterase V; hence the erection augmenting effect of phosphodiesterase V inhibitors such as sildenafil. The flaccid state of the erectile tissues depends on inhibitory tone, probably maintained by noradrenaline. Erection results when there is reduction of the inhibitory tone combined with the excitatory effect of the nitrergic pathway.

In the female, there are two key structures to consider, the clitoris and the vagina. The clitoris is the homologue of the penis and is an important source of erotic stimulation. Apart from the absence of the tunica albuginea, which means that the clitoral tissues become engorged without becoming rigid, the mechanisms of control are basically the same as in the penis. The vagina, on the other hand, has no equivalent in the male. The vaginal response during sexual arousal includes increased pulsatile blood flow in the vaginal wall, leading to vaginal transudation and lubrication, important for coitus.

Vasoactive intestinal polypeptide (VPI) may be involved, whereas the nitrergic pathway is probably not (Levin, 2007). The vaginal response may be part of a wider vascular response in the pelvis, with different patterns of central control than the clitoral (and penile) response.

There is an important gender difference in awareness of genital response. Penile erection in the male plays a central role in a man's subjective experience of sexual arousal; most women are not as aware of their vaginal and clitoral responses, and there is a less predictable relationship between their subjective experience of sexual arousal and genital response.

Orgasm, seminal emission and ejaculation

The phenomenon of orgasm, which entails some pervasive pattern of neurophysiological response in the brain as well as in the periphery, remains a mystery. Orgasm per se is probably basically the same in men and women. What is different is the associated response of seminal emission in the male, resulting from contraction of smooth muscles in the vas and urethra, which, together with orgasm, result in the experience of ejaculation. The rhythmic expulsion of semen at ejaculation depends on orgasm-related contractions of the striated muscles in the penis, and comparable contractions in the pelvic floor muscles are associated with orgasm in women. The neurophysiological relationship between orgasm and seminal emission, however, remains obscure.

The post-ejaculatory refractory period, when profound inhibitory mechanisms make further arousal difficult for a time, is possibly triggered by the mechanisms underlying seminal emission, because women do not experience the same predictable post-orgasmic refractory state.

The role of hormones in sexual arousal

Testosterone (T) is clearly necessary for normal sexual arousal and interest in men, as shown consistently by studies of hormone replacement in hypogonadal men and hormone manipulation in eugonadal men. The role of T during peripubertal development and changes in T responsiveness in the aging male are less well understood (Bancroft, 2005b). Nocturnal penile tumescence (NPT) or erection during REM sleep is androgen dependent. The precise explanation of NPT is still disputed, but noradrenergic neurons in the locus coeruleus "switch off" during REM sleep, consistent with descending inhibitory signals to the penis being switched off at that time, allowing existing "excitatory tone" to be expressed as erection. It is this "excitatory tone" which appears to be androgen dependent.

T and sexual arousal in women presents us with a contrasting picture (Bancroft, 2005b). T is associated with sexual arousal in a proportion of women, but at much lower concentrations than are necessary for men. In men there is a threshold level for T, and increasing levels above this has little effect on brain mechanisms. Such a threshold is not evident in women, and furthermore, exposing women to supraphysiological levels of T, as is often done with T replacement, results in tolerance.

To account for these striking gender differences, a *desensitization hypothesis* has been proposed (Bancroft, 2002). This postulates that early during normal male development, the brain is desensitised to T. As a result, the adult male brain can tolerate the high levels of T necessary for male differentiation and somatic characteristics, and genetic differences in sensitivity to T are obscured. The female is not desensitised, and consequently not only are females more sensitive to testosterone, but genetically determined variations in T sensitivity are also evident, accounting for the very variable picture in women.

Oestrogens are clearly important for normal vaginal lubrication, as evident in many postmenopausal women. However, their role in sexual arousal is uncertain. It is also unclear the extent to which T effects sexual arousal in women by increasing the availability of E, both as a result of aromatization and reduced binding of E by SHBG.

A further complicating aspect of gonadal steroid action is that T, and to some extent E, can have nonspecific enhancing effects on mood and energy, particularly in women. Hence some of the sexual-enhancing effects of T may result from mood and energy-enhancing effects.

Impact of mental health on sexuality

Mood

Reduction in sexual interest, and to some extent sexual arousability, is generally accepted as a common symptom of depressive illness (Beck, 1967; Cassidy *et al.*, 1957; Kennedy *et al.*, 1999) with a tendency for sexual interest to be increased in states of elevated mood such as hypomania (Segraves, 1998). Thus Beck (1967) reported that 61% of severe depressives experienced loss of sexual interest, compared with 27% of his nondepressed control group. He also found this symptom to be associated with fatigability, loss of appetite, weight loss and insomnia, suggesting that it was part of a biological syndrome. Schreiner-Engel and Schiavi (1986), in a study of men and women with primary loss of sexual interest, found that the large majority had suffered previous depressive illness, with loss of sexual desire being established during and persisting after one of these earlier depressive episodes.

With anxiety, the clinical evidence is much more limited. Ware, Emmanuel and colleagues (1996) found higher rates of sexual dysfunction in patients with anxiety disorders, whereas Angst (1998), in the Zurich Cohort Study, found that loss of sexual interest was more likely in generalised anxiety disorder but was not associated with panic disorder, agoraphobia or social phobia. Figueira *et al.* (2001) found that panic disorder patients were more likely to report sexual problems, particularly sexual aversion, than social phobics, whereas premature ejaculation was the most common sexual problem in men with social phobia. Considerable attention has been paid to the idea that anxiety about the sexual situation, in particular, anxiety about failure to respond sexually, may cause or at least aggravate impairment of sexual responsiveness, although this assumed relationship, which is central to much of sex therapy, has received remarkably little research attention.

The effects of mood and anxiety on orgasmic function is less clear. Insofar as negative mood states impair sexual arousal, orgasm is likely to be delayed in both men and women. There is no clear evidence, however, of specific inhibition of orgasm by negative mood. Premature ejaculation is not obviously affected by depression one way or the other. Anxiety, on the other hand, may aggravate premature ejaculation, possibly by activating the peripheral sympathetic mechanisms (Rowland *et al.*, 2007).

Nonclinical, community-based studies have also shown a relationship between mood and sexuality. In the Massachusetts Male Aging Study, Araujo *et al.* (1998) reported an association between erectile dysfunction and depressive symptoms, after controlling for other potentially confounding factors such as age and physical health. In the Zurich Cohort Study, a longitudinal study of men and women between the ages of 20 and 35 years, an association between depression and loss of sexual interest was found in both men and women, although more marked in the women (Angst, 1998). Laumann *et al.* (1999) found that men and women who reported emotional problems were also more likely to report sexual problems. In a survey of women in heterosexual relationships, the Mental Component Summary (MCS) 12, a measure of mental health from the widely used Short Form (SF) 12 (Ware, Kosinski & Keller 1996), was strongly predictive of distress about the sexual relationship and the woman's own sexuality (Bancroft *et al*,, 2003). The direction of causality in such studies is not always clear; depression may occur as a result of sexual difficulties or vice versa.

Most relevant studies have restricted their attention to negative effects of mood disorders on sexual interest and response. However, when questions have been asked about increased sexual interest in negative mood states, an interesting minority report this paradoxical pattern. Thus Mathew and Weinman (1982) found in a mixed-gender group of 57 depressives that, whereas 31% had loss of sexual interest, 22% reported increased sexual interest. Similarly, Angst (1998) found that among depressed men, 25.7% reported decreased and 23.3% increased sexual interest, compared with 11.1% and 6.9%, respectively, of a nondepressed group. In contrast, only 8.8% of their female participants reported increased interest when depressed compared with 35.3% decreased sexual interest (with 1.7% and 31.6%, respectively, of their nondepressed group). In an interesting study of depressed men receiving cognitive-behavioural therapy, Nofzinger *et al.* (1993) found that those who failed to respond to treatment had significantly higher levels of sexual interest than both those who remitted and their nondepressed control group. In addition, members of this high sexual interest, non-remitting group were more anxious and had more intermittent depression. There is also recent evidence of comorbidity between compulsive sexual behaviour or "sexual addictions" and mood disorders (Black *et al.*, 1997).

To explore the varied relationship between mood and sexuality more closely, a simple questionnaire (Mood & Sexuality Questionnaire [MSQ]; Bancroft, Janssen, Strong, *et al.*, 2003a) was devised which asks the respondent to indicate what typically happens to sexual interest and sexual responsiveness when in states of depression and anxiety. The subject can indicate that he or she has not experienced sufficient depression or anxiety to recognise any predictable pattern (i.e. an excluder). In a study of heterosexual men ($n = 919$), of the 574 who reported experience with depression, 42% reported decreased sexual interest and 9.4% increased interest (the remainder indicating no obvious change). For anxiety, 714 reported relevant experience, and of these 28.3% reported decreased and 20.6% increased sexual interest. The paradoxical patterns of increased sexual interest were less likely in older men (Bancroft *et al.*, 2003a). In a study of gay men ($n = 662$), 47% reported decreased and 16% increased sexual interest when depressed ($n = 455$), and 39% decreased and 24% increased sexual interest when anxious ($n = 506$); no association with age was found (Bancroft *et al.*, 2003b). In a study of heterosexual college women ($n = 663$), 50.5% reported decreased and 9.5% increased sexual interest when depressed, and 33.5% decreased and 22.9% increased sexual interest when anxious (Lykins *et al.*, 2006). Compared with a group of college men, the women were significantly less likely to report increased sexual interest in negative mood states.

The relevance of these paradoxical patterns to high-risk sexual behaviour have been explored in men. Heterosexual men who experienced increased sexual interest in states of depression, as measured by the MSQ, reported more partners in the previous year and more one-night stands (Bancroft *et al.*, 2004). In a similar fashion, gay men with this paradoxical pattern reported higher numbers of casual partners and more frequent "cruising" (Bancroft *et al.*, 2003c). Increased sexual interest in states of anxiety was not clearly related to these behaviours in either group. Comparable studies in women have yet to be conducted.

In a small study of self-defined "sex addicts" (Bancroft & Vukadinovic, 2004; $n = 29$ men and 2 women), these paradoxical mood sexuality relationships were highly relevant. Only 4 (13%) participants, all male, indicated that their sexual "acting out" was not predictably affected by their mood, whereas 17 (55%) reported it more likely when depressed and 19 (61%) when anxious, with 11 (35%) reporting the association with both depression and anxiety.

Overall, therefore, we find depression being most predictably associated with reduction or no change in sexual interest and response, with a minority, smaller in women, reporting a "paradoxical" increase. With anxiety, we find comparable variability, but with the paradoxical effect more likely in both men and women. What mechanisms underlie these various patterns?

The negative effects of depression have at least three possible explanations. When depression is part of a more generalised biological pattern, as identified by Beck (1967) in the associations with

fatigability, loss of appetite, weight loss and insomnia, a reduction in sexual arousability could be the main effect. This is supported by the impairment of NPT in depressive illness (Thase *et al.*, 1987). In addition, reactive inhibition of sexual interest and response may occur as part of the reaction to depressing circumstances. The negative effects of anxiety are most readily explained by associated inhibitory responses.

Positive "paradoxical" sexual effects of anxiety could be explained as *excitation transfer* (Zillmann, 1983); that is, the arousal evoked in a state of anxiety is transferred to heighten the arousal in response to sexual stimulation. The dual control model postulates that this pattern would be more likely in individuals with low inhibition and high excitation proneness, and support for this has been obtained (Bancroft *et al.*, 2003a, 2003b). The paradoxical effects of depression are more difficult to explain. Qualitative studies of straight and gay men shed some light on this. Descriptions of the effects of anxiety or stress show two fairly clear and contrasting patterns; either the anxious/stressed state leads to the need to focus on the cause of the distress (presumably with appropriate inhibition of sexual interest/response at the time) or it is associated with the use of sexual arousal and orgasm as a transient method of stress or anxiety relief. With depression a variety of patterns were described. When depressed, being sexual may allow one to connect with another person or feel closer to a partner or to feel validated when one's self-esteem is otherwise low. For some, being sexually active simply improves their mood, if only briefly. Sexual risk taking may be more likely because, when depressed, the risks don't matter so much (Bancroft *et al.*, 2003a, 2003b). All of these paradoxical patterns require either that there is no reduction in sexual interest or responsiveness in the negative mood state, so other benefits of sex can be obtained or there is reduced inhibition and high excitation proneness. A paradoxical effect of depression might also be due to anxiety being part of the depressive mood state, as found by Nofzinger and colleagues (1993).

Side effects of antidepressants and antianxiety drugs

There is now an extensive literature on sexual side effects of antidepressants (e.g. Rosen *et al.*, 1999), although much of it is inconclusive because of methodological shortcomings and inadequate distinction between different types of adverse sexual effects (Montgomery *et al.*, 2002). Sexual side effects are commonly reported with most types of tricyclic antidepressants and serotonin reuptake inhibitors (SSRIs). They are less often reported with pharmacologically atypical antidepressants such as bupropion, moclobemide, reboxetine, mirtazapine and nefazadone, but as Montgomery *et al.* (2002) pointed out, such drugs have been much less widely used, and sexual side effects were not so well recognised with more conventional antidepressants until they had been in use for many years. Bupropion, which is metabolised into an NA and DA reuptake inhibitor, has been associated with fewer sexual side effects in direct comparison with sertraline (Croft *et al.*, 1999) and various other SSRIs (Modell *et al.*, 1997). This is consistent with bupropion having a dopaminergic and central noradrenergic effect. Nefadazone, which is related to trazodone without the histaminergic sedative effect but with a clear 5-HT2 antagonist effect, has been shown to have fewer sexual side effects than SSRIs (Gregorian *et al.*, 2002).

Delayed ejaculation or orgasm is the most commonly reported sexual side effect in men and women. Across studies, 30% to 60% of patients on SSRIs report orgasmic or ejaculatory difficulty. It is more likely with SSRIs than with tricyclic antidepressants and is sufficiently predictable that it is now being exploited as a pharmacological treatment of premature ejaculation (Abdel-Hamid, 2004).

Sexual side effects of benzodiazepines, whether used as antianxiety drugs or hypnotics, have not been well studied. This class of compound, which acts through gamma-aminobutyric acid (GABA) receptors, is likely to have widespread inhibitory effects, but these are nonspecific and may involve inhibition of inhibitory mechanisms. The limited clinical evidence, largely dependent on case reports, indicates a range of effects both negative and positive (Crenshaw & Goldberg, 1996)

Personality problems

It is reasonable to assume that personality factors will influence sexual development, and in particular the establishment of sexual intimacy. "Neuroticism" was regarded as relevant to sexuality in early studies, but results were inconsistent (e.g. Cooper, 1968; Eysenck, 1976; Slater, 1945). Costa *et al.* (1992) used the NEO Personality Inventory to measure the five personality factors in men and women attending a "sexual behaviour consultation clinic." They found neuroticism to be correlated with lower sexual satisfaction and extraversion with sexual drive, but they did not report on associations with specific sexual dysfunctions.

Obsessive-compulsive personality warrants consideration. Compulsive thoughts of obsessive-compulsive disorder type often have sexual content, but these are typically accompanied by negative mood and no sexual arousal. Warwick and Salkovskis (1990) described two men whose obsessive-compulsive symptoms included intrusive sexual thoughts accompanied by penile erection. The awareness of the erection intensified the anxiety and, hence, reinforced the process. It is possible that a combination of obsessive-compulsive tendencies and a low propensity for inhibition or high propensity for excitation of sexual response leads to an atypical, sexualised type of compulsive behavioural pattern in some cases. Studies of "sex addicts" usually find a small minority with obsessive-compulsive personalities (e.g., Bancroft & Vukadinovic, 2004, 6%; Black *et al.*, 1997, 15%; Shapira *et al.*, 2000, 15%).

Schizophrenia

Assessing the effects of schizophrenia on sexuality is difficult. Although this illness can occur in people with previously normal personalities, many have "pre-schizophrenic personalities" which are likely to be associated with impaired, or in some way abnormal, sexual development.

Given that the florid positive symptoms of schizophrenia (e.g. hallucinations, delusions, aggressive behaviour) are believed to result from either increased DA activity or increased DA receptors in the mesolimbic system, one might expect that an increase in sexually motivated behaviour is a feature of the acute illness, at least before "negative" symptoms become established. Sexual thoughts and behaviours are common in schizophrenia, and there may be a relative increase in sexual activity. However, this is typically autoerotic or "compulsive" without any real object-relational quality (Lilleleht & Leiblum, 1993). Given the distortion of the ability to relate to others that occurs in this illness, this is not surprising. It is nevertheless difficult to assess whether there is a decline or an increase in the level of sexual interest or, alternatively, a dysfunctional pattern. Early studies suggested that loss of sexual interest was less likely in schizophrenia than in other types of psychiatric illness, although female schizophrenia patients were more likely to report a decline in sexual interest than their male counterparts (Gittleson & Dawson-Butterworth, 1967; Gittleson & Levine, 1966).

Side effects of psychotropic drugs

Sexual side effects of antipsychotic drugs are of particular interest because of the central role that DA is believed to play in the illness. The common factor in most antipsychotics is DA antagonism, particularly at the D2 receptor, and it is DA antagonism in the mesolimbic system which is believed to be most relevant to reduction of psychotic symptoms. The mesolimbic system is involved in a range of "motivated" behaviours, including sexual behaviour.

The prevalence of sexual dysfunction in patients treated with antipsychotic medication is reported to be approximately 60% in men and from 30% to 93% in women (Smith *et al.*, 2002), and these problems are generally assumed to be side effects of the medication. Smith *et al.* (2002), recognizing

the limited extent to which schizophrenic patients, treated or not, were able to engage in sexual relationships, developed a method of assessing sexual function that did not depend on such relationships. They found that the level of sexual interest did not differ from normal control subjects, whereas erectile dysfunction and ejaculatory dysfunction in men and orgasmic dysfunction in women were substantially more prevalent than in control subjects. In the men, ejaculatory problems were much more common than erectile problems. They interpreted the normal levels of sexual interest as possibly resulting from the normalizing effects of the treatment, although they did not speculate on whether this was due to an increase or a reduction of sexual interest to normal levels. They found some relationship between prolactin levels and problems with sexual arousal (erection in men, vaginal response in women) and sexual interest in women. From this they concluded that the principal sexual side effects of the medication resulted from the drug-induced hyperprolactinaemia. It is widely assumed in the literature (e.g. Cutler, 2003; Halbreich *et al.*, 2003; Kruger *et al.*, 2002) that prolactin has a negative effect on sexuality. However, it can be argued that, except for the extremely high levels of prolactin that result from prolactin-secreting tumours, the plasma level of prolactin is better seen as a marker of the dopaminergic-serotonergic balance in the tubero-infundibular system and quite possibly in other dopaminergic systems as well (Bancroft, 2005b).

Antipsychotic drugs, while having in common a DA antagonist effect, tend to have 5-HT effects as well. This is particularly the case with clozapine; here the relative absence of extrapyramidal side effects, which are important in the management of schizophrenia, is believed to result from the serotonergic effects of the drug within the mesostriatal system. The role of DA in the incerto-hypothalamic periventricular system, which projects to the MPOA, and the lack of evidence of any alteration of DA in this system in schizophrenia, makes the drug-induced sexual side effects of erectile problems in men and arousal problems in women easier to understand. Drugs such as these cannot be targeted on any one of the specific DA systems. It remains more difficult to explain the most prevalent side effect, orgasmic or ejaculatory suppression, as a result of DA antagonism, unless this is a result of a shift in the DA/5HT balance to a more serotonergic state.

Impact of sexual life on mental health

There are many possible ways for sexual experiences to influence our mental health, but two issues have received particular attention in recent years, homosexuality and child sexual abuse.

Homosexuality

As discussed earlier, the emergence of a homosexual identity during adolescence often leads to vulnerability in personality development; in many social contexts, there is still considerable stigma associated with homosexuality. Obviously, there are various ways to cope with this, and some individuals may well react by strengthening their coping resources, resilience and self-esteem (Savin-Williams, 2001). Nevertheless, recent studies have consistently shown that involvement in same-sex sexual behaviour is associated with increased psychiatric morbidity, particularly in terms of depression, anxiety disorders and suicidal behaviour (Bagley & Tremblay, 1997; Cochran *et al.*, 2003; Fergusson *et al.*, 1999; Garofalo *et al.*, 1998; Gilman *et al.*, 2001; Herrell *et al.*, 1999; Remafedi *et al.*, 1998; Sandfort *et al.*, 2001; Skegg *et al.*, 2003; Wichstrom & Hegna 2003). It is not yet clear to what extent this association results from the stigma, social stress or, in the case of men who have sex with men, the threat of AIDS that many experience from an early age, or from some vulnerability which is linked more directly to the determinants of sexual orientation (Bailey, 1999).

Child sexual abuse and sexual assault

It is widely assumed that being sexually abused as a child leads to a variety of mental health as well as sexual problems in adulthood. Depression, anxiety, low self-esteem, posttraumatic stress disorder (PTSD), borderline personality disorder, self-destructive behaviour, eating disorders and social maladjustment have all been found more prevalent in women and men with a history of childhood sexual abuse (CSA; Heiman *et al.*, 2003). Negative sexual consequences have also been reported, although evidence from community-based surveys indicates "sexualization", or the increased likelihood of inappropriate or problematic sexual interactions, as being more common than sexual avoidance. In the National Health and Social Life Survey in the United States, 12% of women and 6% of men reported that they had been sexually touched before age 14 by someone at least 4 years older and older than 14 (Browning & Laumann, 1997). Other studies have shown higher and lower incidence rates. The evidence is variable and inconsistent for a variety of reasons, including the following:

- the definition of what constitutes CSA, which can vary from a single experience of noncontact genital exposure to long-standing coercive vaginal or anal penetration by a family member;
- variations in how samples are obtained and how representative they are; and
- definitions of "child" (Loeb *et al.*, 2002).

There have been various explanations for the adverse effects of CSA, although most are based on the idea that CSA is sufficiently traumatic that the adverse effects are long lasting (e.g. PTSD). Intrafamilial abuse is particularly likely to be traumatic, and, to account for this, Summit (1983) described the child sexual abuse accommodation syndrome, which has five components, as shown in Box 17.1.

Finkelhor (1988) proposed a traumagenic dynamics model, which postulates that adverse effects of CSA depend on the presence or absence of four key factors, powerlessness, betrayal, traumatic sexualization and stigmatization. Browning and Laumann (2003) take a life course perspective which sees the CSA as having more immediate consequences, which in turn lead to other transitional patterns of behaviour, which may increase the likelihood of other, later maladaptive outcomes. Obviously such

Box 17.1 Elements of the child abuse accommodation syndrome

1. *Secrecy* – the need to keep quiet about the abuse for fear of the consequences of revealing it
2. *Helplessness* – with the need for secrecy, the difficulty in avoiding further abuse
3. *Entrapment and accommodation* – development of maladaptive behaviours which have a destructive effect on personality development
4. *Delayed and unconvincing disclosure* – usually at times of conflict with the family, resulting in rejection of the child's story and damaging sense of being "unbelieved"
5. *Retraction* – threat of disintegration of the family following disclosure, leading to retraction of the child's story, and further "invalidation" of the child

a perspective allows for variable intervening influences, which make later negative outcomes more or less likely.

A fundamental point with any of these perspectives is that not only does the degree of trauma from the CSA vary from case to case, but also individuals vary in how they react to the trauma, depending on a range of personality, family and other support factors. Thus although it is reasonable to assume that most if not all CSA experiences are distressing to the child at the time, some will end up with severe consequences, whereas others will have little or none. Clearly we need to understand better the determinants of this variable outcome, and this is of particular relevance to how incidents of CSA should be managed to minimise long-term effects.

Clinical management of sexual problems

Sexual response problems

Men

The most common problems presented by men are erectile dysfunction (ED) and premature ejaculation (PE). Delayed or absent ejaculation (DE) is a relatively infrequent complaint. Low sexual desire (LSD) may be the presenting problem, although in most cases, this is combined with ED or PE, and it is not always clear which came first. In a community-based sample, problems lasting for *at least 6 months* in the previous year were reported by 0.8% for ED, 2.9% for PE, 0.7% for DE and 1.8% for LSD. When asked about problems lasting for *at least a month*, the prevalence rates were 5.8%, 11.7%, 5.3% and 17.1%, respectively (Mercer *et al.*, 2003). These figures indicate that relatively transient problems are substantially more common than persistent ones.

Women

The conventional methods of categorizing sexual dysfunction, in particular the *Diagnostic and Statistical Manual of Mental Disorders* (4th edition) approach, although comparatively straightforward for men, have been criticised as arbitrary and of limited clinical value for women (Graham & Bancroft, 2006). This can be seen as a consequence of conceptualizing women's problems in male terms, which is problematic in part because of the very different role that genital response plays in the sexual experience of men and women and in part because of the more complex interaction between interpersonal, subjective and physiological factors in women. This has become particularly evident in relation to "disorders of sexual desire", the commonest type of complaint in women. The distinction between "sexual desire" and "sexual arousal" is difficult for many women, which may reflect the fact that genital response is less central to the subjective state of "sexual arousal" than it is in men.

Difficulty in achieving orgasm is not uncommon in women, and often this is situational in that orgasm is possible with masturbation, but not during sexual interaction with the partner. A more specific, and essentially female, complaint is vaginismus, in which vaginal penetration either by the partner's penis or finger is difficult, painful or impossible. Until recently, this condition has been regarded as a problem of spasm in the pelvic floor muscles surrounding the vagina. This concept, however, has now been challenged, and vaginismus explained as either a genital pain disorder or a "vaginal penetration aversion/phobia" (Reissing *et al.,* 1999). Other types of pain during sexual activity may present. Vulvodynia or vulvo-vestibulitis (pain in the vulvar vestibule), presents a particular clinical challenge because of the ill-understood interaction between local and more psychosomatic factors (Bergeron *et al.,* 2001).

Prevalence rates for women reported by Mercer *et al.* (2003) were as follows: *for at least 6 months in the previous year,* LSD, 10.2%; unable to experience orgasm, 3.7%; trouble lubricating, 2.6%; and painful intercourse, 3.4%. For *at least 1 month,* the rates were 40.6%, 14.4%, 9.2% and 11.8%, respectively.

Problems of sexual response from the dual control perspective

To what extent is reduced sexual response a result of increased inhibition, reduced excitation or a combination of the two? We can postulate three patterns: (1) low excitation which may result from physiological factors, such as hormonal deficiency or peripheral impairment of genital response; (2) reactive inhibition, induced by a variety of current circumstantial factors; and (3) high inhibitory tone, difficult to reduce sufficiently to allow a response to occur. The instrument developed to measure excitation and inhibition proneness in men (Janssen *et al.,* 2002) comprises three scales – SES, a measure of sexual excitation proneness, and two inhibition scales – SIS1, described as "inhibition due to the threat of performance failure" and SIS2, "inhibition due to threat of performance consequences". High SIS1 may reflect high inhibitory tone as well as a tendency to react to sexual situations with "reactive inhibition" because of the threat of failure. Some questions in SIS1 also reflect the impact of distraction on sexual response. SIS2 reflects the likelihood of reactive inhibition in a variety of contextual situations, such as a problematic relationship or when there is potential for sexually transmitted infection, unwanted pregnancy or breaking the law (see Bancroft & Janssen, 2001, for more comprehensive

consideration of these postulates). Reactive inhibition, most clearly assessed by SIS2, could be associated with relatively transient, context-specific reduction in sexual interest or responsiveness. This is likely to be relevant to the striking differences in prevalence of sexual problems "for at least a month" and "for at least 6 months" reported by Mercer *et al.* (2003) reported earlier. Many of these more transient changes are likely to be adaptive or at least understandable cases of "reactive inhibition", which do not involve "malfunction" of the sexual response system.

A clear relationship between low SES, high SIS1 and ED has been found in nonclinical and clinical samples of men. In the clinical context, "organic" aetiology is most predictably associated with low SES. Although this remains to be demonstrated, it is possible that men with high SIS1 and/or SIS2 will respond to psychological treatment, whereas men with low SES may need response-enhancing medication such as sildenafil. No association has been found between SES or SIS scores and PE or DE.

The instrument for assessing excitation and inhibition in women (SESI-W; Graham *et al.,* 2006) produces two higher-order scales – sexual excitation and sexual inhibition, and a range of subscales. Examination of these scales in relation to female sexual dysfunction is at an early stage. However, one subscale, labelled "arousal contingency", was strongly predictive of LSD in a nonclinical sample of women. The three questions making up this subscale conveyed difficulty in remaining sexually aroused, with the "slightest thing" reducing arousal and "the need for everything to be just right" for arousal to occur (i.e. "fragility" of sexual response and "easy distractibility"). This finding warrants closer examination.

Clinical management

In recent years, there have been significant breakthroughs in the pharmacotherapy of sexual dysfunction, particularly for men, with the discovery that phosphodiesterase V inhibitors such as sildenafil can improve erectile function and more recently with the use of short-acting SSRIs to treat premature ejaculation. Psychological methods of treatment are still important, but we are now faced with the challenge of deciding whether to use psychological or pharmacological methods or a combination of the two. Each case should be assessed through three windows:

1. *The current situation* – can the sexual response problem be understood as a reaction to current circumstances? Problems stemming from relationship difficulties, poor communication between the couple and misinformation about normal sexual response are in this category. Sex therapy, as we define it here, may reduce "reactive inhibition" by identifying factors relevant to the individual or the couple, which invoke inhibition, and finding ways to make them less threatening.

2. *Long-term history* – has either partner encountered problems of this kind earlier in their lives, or earlier within this relationship? Is there a history of either chronic or recurrent difficulty, and if so, how far does it go back? With such a history, whether or not aggravated by current circumstances, sex therapy may still be helpful but may need to focus on changing expectations as much as changing sexual response patterns. In such cases, high "inhibitory tone" may be a significant factor, and inhibition-reducing drugs, such as phentolamine, might be usefully combined with sex therapy (Bancroft & Janssen, 2000).

3. Are there any *physical health issues or medications* which could be having an adverse effect on sexual responsiveness? Sexual side effects of medications were discussed earlier and in some cases may involve activation of inhibitory mechanisms (e.g. SSRIs). Obviously withdrawal or change of medication is the first consideration. Most physical disease effects produce impaired arousability (low SES) and may be more difficult to modify with sex therapy. Drugs such as sildenafil (which acts peripherally to enhance genital response) and apomorphine (which acts centrally to enhance sexual desire) may be helpful and, when there are other factors in the

> **Box 17.2** Key elements of the therapeutic process in sex therapy
>
> - Clearly defined tasks are given, and the couple is asked to attempt them before the next therapy session.
> - Those attempts, and any difficulties encountered, are examined in detail.
> - Attitudes, feelings and conflicts that make the tasks difficult to carry out are identified.
> - These are modified or resolved so that subsequent achievement of the tasks becomes possible.
> - The next tasks are set, and so on.

sexual relationship which may be compounding the problem, may be usefully combined with sex therapy (Bancroft & Janssen, 2000).

Sex therapy

The most widely used form of sex therapy, based on the methods pioneered by Masters and Johnson (1970), does not aim to modify sexual response directly. Rather it aims to identify issues which may be invoking reactive inhibition and to find ways of resolving those issues, for example, by resolving current relationship difficulties or changing long-standing negative attitudes about sex. The assumption is that if such causative factors are resolved, the individuals basically normal sexual response system will act accordingly. Some components of sex therapy are focussed on improving specific sexual responses, for example, the "stop-start" technique for premature ejaculation or use of graded dilators for vaginismus. When appropriate, these are incorporated into the basic sex therapy program. The key elements of the therapeutic process are shown in Box 17.2.

The key is the nature of the tasks set. These are well suited to identifying relevant issues. The tasks are mostly behavioural in nature and, in some cases, sufficient in themselves to produce change. The behavioural program is in two parts; during the first part, the couple is asked to avoid any direct genital touching or stimulation and to focus on nongenital contact. These first, nongenital steps are effective in identifying important issues in the relationship, such as lack of trust or counter-productive stereotypical attitudes (e.g. once a man is aroused, he can't be expected not to have intercourse). Once these nongenital steps can be carried out satisfactorily and related problematic issues dealt with, the program moves on to the second part, which involves a graduated approach to genital touching and ultimately penile-vaginal intercourse. In this second part, more intrapersonal problems, such as long-standing negative attitudes about sex or the sequelae of earlier sexual trauma (e.g. CSA) are likely to be identified, and hopefully dealt with. (For a full discussion of this treatment approach, see Bancroft, 2006.)

Problems of LSD warrant particular attention. In couples in whom there is a disparity in levels of desire, the resulting pressure on the low-desire partner may suppress desire further. In this and some other ways, LSD can be understood as resulting from reactive inhibition. Such cases may benefit from sex therapy. LSD may also be a symptom of a depressive illness, and obviously treatment of the depression should be given priority. Other cases remain more difficult to understand. In men, LSD is occasionally found to be associated with low testosterone or high prolactin levels, both treatable conditions. In women, considerable attention has been paid to the use of testosterone as a treatment of LSD. This may be effective in those women who are particularly sensitive to the effects of testosterone (discussed earlier) but should not be regarded as a general panacea.

Other types of sexual problems in men and women

"Out of control" sexual behaviour

Problems of control over one's sexual behaviour can cause havoc for both men and women. This may lead to high-risk sexual behaviour or "out of control" sexual behaviour which is not necessarily risky but can be very damaging, either to one's relationships or work role, often referred to as "sexual addictions". The out of control behaviour may involve engagement with others (e.g. casual partners, voyeurism), or it may be solitary (e.g. masturbation or Internet use). The addiction concept is used more by analogy and has some heuristic value in methods of management. A culture of sex addicts has evolved to provide group support for those struggling with these behaviours, usually based on Alcoholics Anonymous (AA) principles. Because we don't understand the determinants of such behaviours, we should keep an open mind about the addiction concept as possibly having explanatory value. On the other hand, "compulsivity", from an obsessive-compulsive perspective, is only relevant in a small proportion of cases. In a small study of self-defined sex addicts, out of control sexual behaviour was more likely in men with high SES scores and, for those whose addictive pattern involved other people, low SIS2 (Bancroft & Vukadinovic, 2004).

In addition to the use of group support, such as the AA approach, individual therapy, both psychological and pharmacological, can be helpful. Understanding the typical sequence that leads to the out-of-control behaviour is important. Given that many with this problem are influenced by negative mood, with the sexual behaviour as a form of mood regulator, consideration should be given to establishing alternative, less problematic methods of mood regulation that can be initiated early enough in the sequence to avoid the overwhelming effects of sexual arousal. Pharmacologically, SSRIs are often helpful, although it is not clear to what extent benefits result from effects on mood or on drug-induced inhibition of sexual responsiveness – it is probably a combination of the two.

Problematic sexual preferences

Most paraphilic preferences, such as fetishism and sadomasochism, are seldom seen in a clinical setting. When they are, it is usually because of difficulties that the paraphilia causes in a relationship. A crucial distinction is between the person whose paraphilia is dominant, leading to persistent pursuit of paraphilic sexual gratification, and one for whom it is an occasional need, often in reaction to some problem in the primary relationship or some current emotional crisis. It is not unusual for a man to have shown paraphilic interests during adolescence, but once he has settled into a rewarding sexual relationship, his paraphilia becomes less important. However, if he then encounters problems within his sexual relationship, the paraphilic interest may return. In some cases, therefore, therapy should focus on improving the relationship or coping with the current emotional crisis.

Sexual offenders

Paedophilia, voyeurism and exhibitionism, because they are illegal, and at the same time are viewed by many as pathological, may be seen in the clinic. It is noteworthy that sexual abuse of a child may well lead to psychiatric referral by the court, whereas this seldom happens with sexual assault or rape of adults (Bancroft, 1991). Paedophilia is clearly the most serious of these paraphilias. This usually means being attracted to girls aged 8 to 11 years or boys aged 11 to 15 or, in some cases, both girls and boys. There is increasing evidence that a proportion of men with paedophilic tendencies were themselves sexually abused as children, which is an additional reason why we need a better understanding of the effects of CSA. Such men also tend to have problems establishing satisfactory adult relationships (Mohr *et al.*, 1964), although it is difficult to assess the extent that this is cause or effect.

Exhibitionism, or "indecent exposure", is also difficult to understand. Rooth (1971) concluded that the reaction of the "victim" was important; in his view, most exhibitionists want the full attention of the "victim" with some obvious emotional reaction, either negative or positive, but not indifference. Many exhibitionists are men who are otherwise timid and unassertive. It is tempting to wonder whether there is some link to the genital display shown by some primates, as an act of either aggression or asserting dominance (Dixson,

1998). Exhibitionism can be contrasted with voyeurism, which, although also offensive to the "victim", does not require the victim's awareness or response. Voyeurism often reflects a reluctance or lack of confidence in engaging in a sexual relationship and is a form of interaction which by avoiding the other person's participation is less threatening. This is sometimes manifested in an individual's fantasy life, when the preferred sexual image is of two other people engaging in sex, with the individual observing.

Whereas there have been attempts in the past to modify paraphilic preferences (e.g. by aversion therapy), such methods are now seldom used. Clinical interventions should focus on (1) improving self-control, using general principles of cognitive-behavioural therapy, and (2) improving the sexual relationship using sex therapy, in those cases where the paraphilia is a problem in the relationship or when relationship difficulties have led to a regression towards earlier paraphilic preoccupations. With illegal behaviours, such as CSA, when the consequences for the offender as well as the victim can be disastrous, the use of sexually inhibiting drugs may be justified. Most widely used are antiandrogens, such as cyproterone acetate; progestogens which have an antiandrogenic and a direct inhibitory effect (e.g. medroxyprogesterone acetate); or certain psychotropic drugs such as benperidol (see Bradford & Greenberg, 1996, for review). It is important to keep in mind, when considering such treatment, that some sexual offence behaviour is not driven by sexual desire, and in such cases suppressing sexual desire may not help and can sometimes aggravate the problem, leading to more aggressive behaviour.

Transvestism, transexuality and transgender

The interface between gender and sexuality is well illustrated by the range of gender identity problems which confront the psychiatrist. One theme runs across these various behavioural patterns – "cross-dressing", or dressing in the clothes of the opposite sex. Four types of cross-dresser can be

---

Box 17.3 Types of cross-dressing

- *The fetishistic transvestite:* This is a man (probably never a woman) who wears female clothes as fetish objects. The clothes are sexually arousing, and wearing them usually leads to masturbation. Once the man has ejaculated, he has no wish to keep the clothes on, often feeling guilty or ashamed for "having done it again". Cross-dressing in this case is a sexual act.

- *The transsexual:* A male (or female) who believes himself (herself) to be a woman (or man) or has a strong desire to be accepted as such in spite of his or her anatomy. For this person, cross-dressing is part of the process of expressing one's preferred gender. The term *transgender*, with its emphasis on gender rather than sexuality, is preferred by many such individuals.

- *The "double-role transvestite":* A male who lives most of his life as a normal heterosexual male (often married) and part dressing and "passing" as a woman. Although transgender role is a source of pleasure and comfort (not usually sexually arousing), there is no desire for a permanent gender change.

- *The homosexual transvestite:* A man (or occasionally a woman) who is sexually attracted to members of the same sex and who cross-dresses but with no clear intention of being considered of the opposite sex. Although possibly reflecting the individual's transgendered identity, there is also the benefit of appealing to a sexual partner who is ambivalent about homosexual activity and therefore finds a "transgendered" partner less confronting.

---

described, each emphasizing one particular aspect of this interface. These are outlined in Box 17.3.

These four examples demonstrate the three principal dimensions of the cross-dressing experience: a fetish component, cross-gender identity and role, and sexual orientation. Although most transgendered individuals claim a clear gender non-conforming childhood, children with such gender nonconformity are more likely to develop a homosexual orientation without out any interest in gender re-assignment. But we should also consider the interactions between these three dimensions. Many individuals with fetishistic transvestism move, over

a period of time, to a more transgendered identity. The cross-dressing loses its sexual quality and becomes more an aspect of gender identity, as if repeated wearing of women's clothes causes dissonance within the male identity, resolved by adopting a female identity. In other cases, this "transgendered shift" from the fetishistic pattern stops at the "dual-role transvestite" stage, at least for many years. Recently, we have been further confronted by the plasticity of gender identity with the impact of the Internet. There are now vigorous Internet transgender communities, and one apparent consequence is that we are seeing more varied patterns – males, for example, who like the idea of looking female without needing to change their gender identity. With the opportunities to engage with transgender subcultures, it seems that there is less need to pursue the clear gender dichotomy required by mainstream culture.

Clinical management

The fetishistic cross-dresser and the dual role transvestite are unlikely to seek psychiatric help unless problems are arising in their sexual relationships. The most likely reason for a transgendered individual to consult with a psychiatrist is to get support for gender reassignment. Within the professional community working with transgender, it is conventional to require psychiatric or psychological assessment by a clinician experienced in this field before considering any irreversible procedure such as gender-reassignment surgery. This usually involves a period of at least 1 year, living fully in the chosen gender role (the "real-life test"), before any surgical decision is taken. The psychiatrist's role is to ensure that the transgendered individual confronts himself or herself with the reality of living in the chosen gender; with many such individuals, their experiences have previously been restricted to private experimentation or very limited exposure. On the basis of physical appearances, voice and mannerisms, gender change is much easier for some individuals than others, and in most respects, such factors are not changeable by surgery. The individual therefore needs to be realistic about what to expect after surgery. In a review of the follow-up literature of gender-reassignment surgery, Green and Fleming (1990) identified the following favourable preoperative indicators: (1) psychological stability with no history of psychosis, (2) successful "real-life test", (3) sufficient understanding of the limitations and consequences of surgery, and (4) preoperative psychotherapy in the context of a gender-identity program.

Hormone therapy and facial electrolysis may be introduced at an earlier stage than surgery. For the male-to-female, oestrogens can be used to induce breast growth, a more female redistribution of body fat, some change in skin texture and slowing of facial and body hair growth. Oestrogens may also reduce sexual interest, which may or may not be acceptable to the patient. Progestogens are sometimes combined with oestrogens to augment breast growth but can have negative mood effects. For both steroids, risks of long-term use should be emphasised. For the female-to-male, androgens will increase muscle bulk, deepen the voice and increase facial and body hair growth. Clitoral enlargement is likely, often accompanied by an increase in sexual interest and response. Acne may be a problem. Again, long-term risks should be emphasised, and testosterone should be administered with gradually increasing dosage to minimise development of tolerance while achieving the desired effects with as small a dose as possible. With both oestrogens and androgens, the extent of the desired effects will depend on the target organ sensitivities, which vary across individuals and cannot be predicted.

Surgical reassignment procedures involve complex surgery and postoperative complications are not unusual. For the male-to-female, testes are removed and penile and scrotal skin usually retained to form the labia and vaginal opening, sometimes incorporating the corpora cavernosa to give an erectile base to the labia. Usually additional skin grafting is required to complete the surgically constructed vagina. For the female-to-male, mastectomy, hysterectomy and oophorectomy are usually involved. Phalloplasty presents more of a surgical challenge, particularly in ensuring urinary passage through the constructed penis. Surgical techniques are, however, improving.

Conclusions

This chapter has provided an overview of the development of sexuality in humans, outlined how mental illnesses can affect sexuality and detailed specific disorders of sexuality. As an important part of human functioning, sexuality should be an area of discussion between clinicians and their patients, and sexual problems dealt with in an appropriate and open manner.

REFERENCES

Abdel-Hamid, I. A. (2004). Phosphodiesterase 5 inhibitors in rapid ejaculation: potential use and possible mechanisms of action. *Drug* 64:13–26.

Angst, J. (1998). Sexual problems in healthy and depressed persons. *Int Clin Psychopharmacol* 13(Suppl. 6):S1–S4.

Araujo, A. B., Durante, R., Feldman, H. A., et al. (1998). The relationship between depressive symptoms and male erectile dysfunction: cross-sectional results from the Massachusetts Male Aging Study. *Psychosom Med* 60:450–65.

Bagley, C., & Tremblay, P. (1997). Suicidal behaviors in homosexual and bisexual males. *Crisis* 18:24–34.

Bailey, M. J. (1999). Homosexuality and mental illness. *Arch Gen Psychiatry* 56:883–4.

Bancroft, J. (1989). *Human Sexuality and Its Problems*, 2nd ed. Edinburgh: Churchill Livingstone.

Bancroft, J. (1991). The sexuality of sexual offending: the social dimension. *Crim Behav Ment Health* 1:181–92.

Bancroft, J. (1999). Central inhibition of sexual response in the male: a theoretical perspective. *Neurosci Biobehav Rev* 23:763–84.

Bancroft, J. (2002). Sexual effects of androgens in women: some theoretical considerations. *Fertil Steril* 77(Suppl 4):S55–S59.

Bancroft, J. (2005a). Normal sexual development. In H. L. Barbaree & W. M. Marshall, eds, *The Juvenile Offender*. New York: Guilford Press, pp. 19–57.

Bancroft, J. (2005b). Starling review: the endocrinology of sexual arousal. *J Endocrinol* **186**:411–27.

Bancroft, J. (2006). Sex therapy. In S. Bloch, ed. *An Introduction to the Psychotherapies*, 4th ed. Oxford: Oxford University Press.

Bancroft, J., Herbenick, D., & Reynolds, M. (2003). Masturbation as a marker of sexual development. In J. Bancroft, ed. *Sexual Development in Childhood*. Bloomington: Indiana University Press, pp. 156–85.

Bancroft, J., & Janssen, E. (2000). The dual control model of male sexual response: a theoretical approach to centrally mediated erectile dysfunction. *Neurosci Biobehav Rev* **24**:571–9.

Bancroft, J., Janssen, E., Carnes, L., *et al.* (2004). Sexual activity and risk taking in young heterosexual men: the relevance of personality factors. *J Sex Res* **41**:181–92.

Bancroft, J., Janssen, E., Strong, D., *et al.* (2003a). The relation between mood and sexuality in heterosexual men. *Arch Sex Behav* **32**:217–30.

Bancroft, J., Janssen, E., Strong, D., & Vukadinovic, Z. (2003b). The relation between mood and sexuality in gay men. *Archives of Sexual Behavior* **32**:231–42.

Bancroft, J., Janssen, E., Strong, D., *et al.* (2003c). Sexual risk taking in gay men: the relevance of sexual arousability, mood, and sensation seeking. *Arch Sex Behav* **32**:555–72.

Bancroft, J., Loftus, J., & Long, J. S. (2003). Distress about sex: a national survey of women in heterosexual relationships. *Arch Sex Behav* **32**:193–208.

Bancroft, J., & Vukadinovic, Z. (2004). Sexual addiction, sexual compulsivity, sexual impulse disorder or what? Towards a theoretical model. *J Sex Res* **41**:225–34.

Beck, A. T. (1967). *Depression: Clinical, Experimental and Theoretical Aspects*. London: Staples Press.

Bem, D. (2000). The exotic-becomes-erotic theory of sexual orientation. In J. Bancroft, *The Role of Theory in Sex Research*. Bloomington: Indiana University Press, pp. 67–80.

Bergeron, S., Binik, Y. M., Khalife, S., *et al.* (2001). Vulvar vestibulitis syndrome: reliability of diagnosis and evaluation of current diagnostic criteria. *Obstetr Gynecol* **98**:45–51.

Black, D. W., Kehrberg, L. L. D., Flumerfelt, D. L., & Schlosser, S. S. (1997). Characteristics of 36 subjects reporting compulsive sexual behavior. *Am J Psychiatry* **154**:243–9.

Bradford, J. M. W., & Greenberg, D. M. (1996). Pharmacological treatment of deviant sexual behaviour. *Annu Rev Sex Res* **7**:283–306.

Browning, C. R., & Laumann, E. O. (1997). Sexual contact between children and adults: a life course perspective. *Am Sociol Rev* **62**:540–60.

Browning, C. R., & Laumann, E. O. (2003). The social context of adaptation to childhood sexual maltreatment: a life course perspective. In J. Bancroft, ed. *Sexual Development in Childhood*. Bloomington: Indiana University Press, pp. 383–402.

Cassidy, W. L., Flanagan, N. B., Spellman, M., & Cohen, M. E. (1957). Clinical observations in manic depressive disease. *JAMA* **164**:1535–46.

Cochran, S. D., Sullivan, J. G., & Mays, V. M. (2003). Prevalence of mental disorders, psychological distress, and mental services use among lesbian, gay, and bisexual adults in the United States. *J Consult Clin Psychol* **71**:53–61.

Cooper, A. J. (1968). Hostility and male potency disorders. *Compre Psychiatry* **6**:621–6.

Costa, P. T., Fagan, P. J., Piedmont, R. L., *et al.* (1992). The five-factor model of personality and sexual functioning in outpatient men and women. *Psychiatr Med* **2**:199–215.

Crenshaw, T. L., & Goldberg, J. P. (1996). *Sexual Pharmacology: Drugs That Affect Sexual Functioning*. New York: Norton.

Croft, H., Settle, E., Jr., Houser, T., *et al.* (1999). A placebo-controlled comparison of the antidepressant efficacy and effects on sexual functioning of sustained-release bupropion and sertraline. *Clin Ther* **21**:643–58.

Cutler, A. J. (2003). Sexual dysfunction and antipsychotic treatment. *Psychoneuroendocrinology* **28**:69–82.

Dixson, A. F. (1998). *Primate Sexuality*. Oxford: Oxford University Press.

Ehrhardt, A. A., & Meyer-Bahlburg, H. F. L. (1981). Effects of prenatal sex hormones on gender-related behavior. *Science* **211**:1312–18.

Eysenck, H. J. (1976). *Sex and Personality*. London: Open Books.

Fergusson, D. M., Horwood, J. L., & Beautrais, A. L. (1999). Is sexual orientation related to mental health problems and suicidality in young people? *Arch Gen Psychiatry* **56**:876–80.

Figueira, I., Possidente, E., Marques, C., & Hayes, K. (2001). Sexual dysfunction: a neglected complication of panic disorder and social phobia. *Arch Sex Behav* **30**:369–77.

Finkelhor, D. (1988). The trauma of child sexual abuse: two models. In G. E. Wyatt & G. J. Powell, eds. *Lasting Effects* of Child Sexual Abuse. Newbury Park, CA: Sage, pp. 61–84.

Garofalo, R. A., Wolf, R. C., Kessel, S., et al. (1998). The associations between health risk behaviors and sexual orientation among a school-based sample of adolescents. Pediatrics 101:895–902.

Gilman, S. E., Cochran, S. D., Mays, V. M., et al. (2001). Risk of psychiatric disorders among individuals reporting same-sex sexual partners in the National Co-morbidity Survey. Am J Public Health 91:933–9.

Gittleson, N. L., & Dawson-Butterworth, K. (1967). Subjective ideas of sexual change in female schizophrenics. Br J Psychiatry 113:491–4.

Gittleson, N. L., & Levine, S. (1966). Subjective ideas of sexual change in male schizophrenics. Br J Psychiatry 112:779–82.

Graham, C., & Bancroft, J. (2006). Assessing the prevalence of female sexual dysfunction with surveys: what is feasible? In I. Goldstein, C. Meston, S. Davis & A. Traish, eds. Women's Sexual Function and Dysfunction: Study, Diagnosis and Treatment. London: Taylor & Francis, pp. 52–62.

Graham, C. A., Sanders, S. A., & Milhausen, R. (2006). The sexual excitation/inhibition inventory for women: psychometric properties. Arch Sex Behav 35:397–409.

Green, R., & Fleming, D. T. (1990). Transsexual surgery follow-up: status in the 1990's. Annu Rev Sex Res 1:163–74.

Gregorian, R. S., Jr., Golden, K. A., Bahce, A., et al. (2002). Antidepressant-induced sexual dysfunction. Ann Pharmacother 36:1577–89.

Halbreich, U., Kinon, B. J., Gilmore, J. A., & Kahn, L. S. (2003). Elevated prolactin levels in patients with schizophrenia: mechanisms and related adverse effects. Psychoneuroendocrinology 28:53–67.

Heiman, J. R., Verhulst, J., & Heard-Davison, A. R. (2003). Childhood sexuality and adult sexual relationships. In J. Bancroft, ed. Sexual Development in Childhood. Bloomington: Indiana University Press, pp. 404–20.

Herdt, G. (2000). Why the Sambia initiate boys before age 10. In J. Bancroft, ed. The Role of Theory in Sex Research. Bloomington: Indiana University Press, pp. 82–104.

Herrell, R., Goldberg, J., True, W. R., et al. (1999) Sexual orientation and suicidality: a co-twin control study in adult men. Arch Gen Psychiatry 56:867–74.

Hull, E. M., Lorrain, D. S., Du, J., Matuszewich, L., et al. (1998). Organizational and activational effects of dopamine on male sexual behavior. In L. Ellis & L. Eberty, eds. Male/Female Differences in Behavior: Toward Biological Understanding. New York: Greenwood Press.

Janssen, E., Vorst, H., Finn, P., & Bancroft, J. (2002). The Sexual Inhibition (SIS) and Sexual Excitation (SES) Scales: I. Measuring sexual inhibition and excitation proneness in men. J Sex Res 39:114–26.

Kagan, J., & Moss, H. A. (1962). Birth to Maturity: A Study in Psychological Development. New York: Wiley.

Kennedy, S. H., Dickens, S. E., Eisfeld, B. S., & Bagby, R. M. (1999). Sexual dysfunction before antidepressant therapy in major depression. J Affect Disord 56:201–208.

Kruger, T. H., Haake, P., Hartmann, U., et al. (2002). Orgasm-induced prolactin secretion: feedback control of sexual drive? Neurosci Biobehav Rev 26:31–44.

Laumann, E. O., Paik, A., & Rosen, R. C. (1999). Sexual dysfunctions in the United States: prevalence and predictors. JAMA 281:537–44.

Levin, R. (2007) The human sexual response – similarities and differences in the anatomy and function of the male and female genitalia: are they a trivial pursuit or a treasure trove? In E. Janssen, ed. The Psychophysiology of Sex. Bloomington: Indiana University Press, pp. 35–56.

Lilleleht, E., & Leiblum, S. R. (1993). Schizophrenia and sexuality: a critical review of the literature. Annu Rev Sex Res 4:247–76.

Loeb, T. B., Williams, J. M. K., Carmona, J. V., et al. (2002). Child sexual abuse: associations with the functioning of adolescents and adults. Annu Rev Sex Res 13:307–45.

Lykins, A. D., Janssen, E., & Graham, C. A. (2006). The relationship between negative mood and sexuality in heterosexual college women and men. J Sex Res 43:136–43.

Masters, W. H., & Johnson, V. E. (1970). Human Sexual Inadequacy. Boston: Little, Brown.

Mathew, R. J., & Weinman, M. L. (1982). Sexual dysfunction in depression. Arch Sex Behav 11:323–8.

McKenna, K. E. (2000). Some proposals regarding the organization of the central nervous system control of penile erection. Neurosci Biobehav Rev 24:535–40.

Mercer, C. H., Fenton, K. A., Johnson, A. M., et al. (2003). Sexual function problems and help seeking behaviour in Britain: national probability sample survey. BMJ 327:426–7.

Meyer-Bahlburg, H. F. L. (2000). Discussion paper: sexual orientation—discussion of Bem and Herdt from a psychobiological perspective. In J. Bancroft, ed. The Role of

Theory in Sex Research Bloomington: Indiana University Press, pp. 110–24.

Modell, J. G., Katholi, C. R., Modell, J. D., & DePalma, R. L. (1997). Comparative sexual side effects of bupropion, fluoxetine, paroxetine, and sertraline. *Clin Pharmacol Ther* **61**:476–87.

Mohr, J. W., Turner, R. E., & Jerry, M. B. (1964). *Paedophilia and Exhibitionism*. Toronto: University of Toronto Press.

Montgomery, S. A., Baldwin, D. S., & Riley, A. (2002). Antidepressant medications: a review of the evidence for drug-induced sexual dysfunction. *J Affect Disord* **69**: 119–40.

Mouras, H., & Stoleru, S. (2007). Functional neuroanatomy of sexual arousal. In F. Kandeel, T. Lue, J. Pryor, & R. Swerdloff, eds. *Male Sexual Dysfunction: Pathophysiology and Treatment*. New York: Marcel Dekker, pp. 39–54.

Mustanski, B. S., Chivers, M. L., & Bailey, J. M. (2002). A critical review of recent biological research on human sexual orientation. *Annu Rev Sex Res* **13**:89–140.

Nofzinger, E. A., Thase, M. E., Reynolds, C. F., *et al.* (1993). Sexual function in depressed men: assessment by self-report, behavioral, and nocturnal penile tumescence measures before and after treatment with cognitive behavior therapy. *Arch Gen Psychiatry* **50**:24–30.

Reissing, E. D., Binik, Y. M., & Khalife, S. (1999). Does vaginismus exist? A critical review of the literature. *J Nerv Ment Dis* **187**:261–74.

Remafedi, G., French, S., Story, M., *et al.* (1998). The relationship between suicide risk and sexual orientation: results from a population-based study. *Am J Public Health* **88**:57–60.

Reynolds, M. A., Herbenick, D. L., & Bancroft, J. (2003). The nature of childhood sexual experiences: two studies 50 years apart. In J. Bancroft, ed. *Sexual Development in Childhood*. Bloomington: Indiana University Press, pp. 134–55.

Rooth, F. G. (1971). Indecent exposure and exhibitionism. *Br J Sex Med* **April:** 521.

Rosen, R. C., Lane, R. M., & Menza, M. (1999). Effects of SSRIs on sexual function: a critical review. *J Clin Psychopharmacol* **19**:67–85.

Rowland, D. L., Tai, W., & Brummett, K. (2007). Interactive processes in ejaculatory disorders: psychophysiological considerations. In E. Janssen, ed. *The Psychophysiology of Sex*. Bloomington: Indiana University Press, 227–243.

Sandfort, T. G. M., de Graaf, R., Bijl, R. V., & Schnabel, P. (2001) Same-sex sexual behavior and psychiatric disorders. *Arch Gen Psychiatry* **58**:85–91.

Santelli, J., Lindberg, L. D., Abma, J., *et al.* (2000). Adolescent sexual behavior: estimates and trends from four nationally representative surveys. *Fam Plann Perspect* **32**:156–66.

Savin-Williams, R. C. (2001). A critique of research on sexual-minority youths. *J Adolesc* **24**:5–13.

Schreiner-Engel, P., & Schiavi, R. C. (1986). Lifetime psychopathology in individuals with low sexual desire. *J Nerv Ment Dis* **174**:646–51.

Segraves, R. T. (1998). Psychiatric illness and sexual function. *Int J Impot Res* **10**(Suppl 2):S131–S133.

Shapira, N. A., Goldsmith, T. D., Keck, P. E., *et al.* (2000). Psychiatric features of individuals with problematic Internet use. *J Affect Disord* **57**:267–72.

Skegg, K., Nada-Raja, S., Dickson, N., *et al.* (2003). Sexual orientation and self-harm in men and women. *Am J Psychiatry* **160**:541–6.

Slater, E. (1945). Neurosis and sexuality. *J Neurol Neurosurg Psychiatry* **8**:12–14.

Smith, S. M., O'Keane, V., & Murray, R. (2002). Sexual dysfunction in patients taking conventional antipsychotic medication. *Br J Psychiatry* **181**:49–55.

Summit, R. C. (1983). The child sexual abuse accommodation syndrome. *Child Abuse Neglect* **7**:177–193.

Thase, M. E., Reynolds, C. F., Glanz, L. M. *et al.* (1987). Nocturnal penile tumescence in depressed men. *Am J Psychiatry* **144**:89.

Ware, J. E., Kosinski, M., & Keller, S. (1996). A 12-tem Short-Form Health Survey (SF-12): construction of scales and preliminary tests of reliability and validity. *Med Care* **34**:220–33.

Ware, M. R., Emmanuel, N. P., Johnson, M. R., *et al.* (1996). Self-reported sexual dysfunctions in anxiety disorder patients. *Psychopharmacol Bull* **32**:530.

Warwick, H. M. C., & Salkovskis, P. M. (1990). Unwanted erections in obsessive-compulsive disorder. *Br J Psychiatry* **157**:919–21.

Wichstrom, L., & Hegna, K. (2003). Sexual orientation and suicide attempt: a longitudinal study of the general Norwegian adolescent population. *J Abnorm Psychol* **112**:144–51.

Zillman, D. (1983). Transfer of excitation in emotional behavior. In J. T. Cacioppo & R. E. Petty, eds. *Social Psychophysiology: A Sourcebook*. New York: Guilford Press, pp. 215–40.

SECTION 3

Special Topics

18

Social and cultural determinants of mental health

Vikram Patel, Alan J. Flisher and Alex Cohen

This chapter considers the evidence regarding the social and cultural determinants of mental health. It has an explicit international population mental health perspective. The chapter must be interpreted in light of the consensus that most psychiatric disorders are multifactorial in origin. Furthermore, effective clinical management is most likely to occur if an aetiological formulation considers the interaction of factors in the biological, psychological, social and cultural domains. The chapter is divided into two sections. The first examines the role of culture in psychiatry and begins with an examination of the historical evolution of research on the cultural influences on psychiatric concepts and classification. It ends with a critical evaluation of the contemporary understanding of the role of cultural influences on the aetiology, clinical presentation, treatment and outcome of mental disorders. The second section considers the evidence for social determinants of mental disorders and the implications for prevention.

Culture and mental health

Prince et al. (1998) defined culture as "the totality of habits, ideas, beliefs, attitudes and values, as well as the behaviors that spring from them (language, art, marriage patterns, eating habits and so forth)" (p. 15). The study of psychiatric disorders across cultures is of value for several reasons. First, such study can help inform clinical practice in different cultures, for example, by providing guidelines on diagnosis and management that are valid for a particular culture. For example, the diagnostic significance of hallucinations varies across cultures (Johns et al., 2002). Second, such study can help the growth of academic psychiatry by informing the validity of classification systems so that these evolve into truly international systems. It will become clear which disorders are universal in their aetiology and manifestations and ensure that culture-specific manifestations of disorders are included in such international systems. Third, cross-cultural studies may reveal therapeutic factors that operate in one or more settings but which may be applicable to a much wider context. Thus the range of available interventions will increase. Finally, because psychiatric disorders are multifactorial in aetiology, the study of disorders in populations in different geographical settings may help to elucidate the role of genetic and environmental factors in their causation. This is illustrated by cross-national studies of the risk factors for dementia (Hendrie et al., 1995).

Several terms have been used to describe the study of psychiatric disorders across cultures, such as *transcultural psychiatry, cross-cultural psychiatry, ethnopsychiatry, comparative psychiatry* and, simply, *cultural psychiatry*. Cultural psychiatry is, perhaps, the most appropriate term, originating from

Essential Psychiatry, ed. Robin M. Murray, Kenneth S. Kendler, Peter McGuffin, Simon Wessely, David J. Castle.
Published by Cambridge University Press. © Cambridge University Press 2008.

Wittkower's definition "that it concerned itself with the mentally ill in relation to their cultural environment within the context of a given cultural unit" (cited in Prince *et al.*, 1998, p. 12). Murphy (1982) proposed the term *comparative psychiatry* by which he meant "the study of the relations between mental disorder and the psychological characteristics which differentiate people, nations, or cultures. Its main goals are to identify, verify, and explain the links between mental disorder and these broad psychosocial characteristics" (p. 2). This term is useful because it does not seek to define the comparative groups exclusively according to a predetermined criterion such as culture. In this sense, the term comes closest to the concept of an "international psychiatry" described later.

Apart from culture, other groupings such as race and ethnicity have been used to define subgroups of human beings. Race is, technically, a biological category that refers to a group of persons who share a distinct genotype. However, on close inspection, the term *race* is not applicable to any human groups because genetic similarities are the rule across all the peoples of the world. Nevertheless, race has become a descriptive term by which people are grouped according to superficial physical characteristics (e.g. skin colour and facial features) that are often incorrectly presumed to reflect a host of genetic, biological or psychological characteristics (US Department of Health and Human Services, 2001). The term *ethnicity* is used to describe a group of people who share a common identity (i.e. how they describe their origins), a common ancestry (both historically and geographically) and, to some extent, shared beliefs and history. This term does not, however, describe either a single type of people or a single nation. Thus people from the Indian subcontinent living in the United Kingdom may be defined as "ethnic Asians", but this does not capture the fact that this apparently homogenous ethnic grouping is at least as internally diverse as an ethnic grouping of "Europeans". Despite its limitations, the term *ethnicity* is the most useful one for describing subgroups of people; it is routinely

ascertained in the collection of national statistics such as censuses and is also used in the study of the epidemiology of diseases. Studies based on either racial or ethnic distribution of mental disorder should be interpreted with caution because social or economic differences may explain much more of the differences reported than racial, ethnic or cultural effects (Isaacs & Schroeder, 2004).

The evolution of the discipline

The view that psychiatric phenomena can vary from one culture to another has existed for more than 200 years and probably first appeared at around the same time as the general acceptance that abnormal behaviour is caused by illness (as opposed to, for example, evil spirits). In keeping with this change in belief systems in the Western world, the doctors who treated mental disorders considered one of the causes to be the higher level of intellectual attainment of the civilization in Western societies. Thus, Sir Andrew Halliday in a survey of British mental hospitals referred to "the rarity of insanity among savage tribes of men, the contented peasantry of the Welsh mountains and those dwelling in the wilds of Ireland" (cited in Prince *et al.*, 1998, p. 3), and, in the same report he wrote "not one of our African travellers remark their having seen a single madman" (cited in Murphy, 1982, p. 4). White colonial psychiatrists thought that certain mental disorders were rare in Africans because their brains were considered too primitive to experience sophisticated emotional states (e.g., Le Roux, 1973). Much of the earlier literature written mainly during the colonial era is replete with terms such as "primitive" or "savages", as well as tainted by connotations of racism. The introduction of a scientific quality to the investigations of comparative psychiatry can be attributed to Kraepelin who studied patients in the Buitenzorg Asylum (currently the State Hospital of Bogor outside Jakarta) in Java in 1903. Kraepelin wrote, "Reliable comparison is, of course, only possible if we are able to draw clear distinctions between identifiable illnesses, as well as between clinical states" (Kraepelin, 2000 [1904], p. 38) and went on to note that, although it was possible to recognize schizophrenia and bipolar disorder among the Javanese, "comparison between the native and the European populations is made more difficult by the fact that the clinical symptomatology, while broadly in agreement with that seen [in Europe], presents certain very noteworthy differences in individual instances" (Kraepelin, 2000 [1904], p. 40).

Although Kraeplin's essay proved to be a seminal text for comparative psychiatry, it must be noted that his explanation for the variation was racial, claiming that, for example, the low incidence of delusions among the Javanese was the result of their "lower stage of intellectual development".

E. D. Wittkower made one of the most important contributions to the scientific study of cultural psychiatry when he set up the first academic unit devoted to this field at McGill University in 1955. Another historic milestone in the field was the work of Leighton and colleagues among the Navajo peoples of North America. These authors were later involved in one of the first cross-national collaborations (with Lambo and colleagues) in their pioneering comparative studies of mental illness in Canada and Nigeria. The study provided extensive information on symptoms, indigenous models and the prevalence of mental disorders (Leighton et al., 1963). The most important contributions to culture and mental disorders have been made in the past three decades, as a result of the debate on the influence of culture on the classification of mental disorders and the methodology for cross-cultural psychiatric epidemiological research. The growth of the scientific discipline of medical anthropology, led by authors such as Kleinman and Littlewood (e.g. Kleinman 1987; Littlewood, 1990), has also been a major contributor to the establishment of cultural psychiatry as a key discipline within psychiatry. It is not accidental that the recent surge of interest in culture as an independent variable in the design and interpretation of psychiatric research coincides with the spectacular demographic change

in the ethnic composition of many developed countries.

Culture and the classification of mental disorders

A key characteristic that differentiates the process of classification of mental disorders from that for physical pathology is that, for most mental disorders, there are no specific and replicable pathophysiological changes which can be identified in a clinical setting (see also Chapter 2). Virtually all the diagnostic categories used in psychiatry are essentially those of "illnesses" compared with "diseases". This distinction implies that classification is based on the nature of symptoms and syndromes rather than their aetiology (as, for example, in the case of infectious diseases) or their pathology (as, for example, in the case of vascular disease). The classification of mental disorders is thus influenced by cultural factors, such as the language of emotional distress, and the ways in which these are conceptualised by a particular culture. In the absence of demonstrable disease processes, a variety of explanations are likely to arise which are heavily influenced by other belief systems, notably religious beliefs. Historically, a number of classifications of mental disorders have coexisted in different cultures, each with its own taxonomy and causal models for various disorders.

The process of standardization has been driven largely by psychiatric classification systems originating in Euro-American societies (see Chapter 2). After standardizing the classification and associated interview schedules in Euro-American cultures, the systems and methods were subsequently used in other cultures. Most of the subsequent cross-cultural psychiatric investigations relied on implicit, largely untested assumptions (Beiser et al., 1994):

1. the universality of mental illnesses, implying that regardless of cultural variations, disorders as described in Euro-American classifications occur everywhere;

2. invariance, implying that the core features of psychiatric syndromes are invariant between cultures; and

3. validity, implying that although refinement is possible, the diagnostic categories of current classifications are valid clinical constructs.

Termed as the *etic* or *universalist* approach, this became the most popular method for epidemiological investigations of mental illness across cultures. The etic approach offered a perspective that because mental illness was similar throughout the world, psychiatric taxonomies, their measuring instruments and models of healthcare were also globally applicable.

Many researchers have cautioned that there is a risk of confounding culturally distinctive behaviour with psychopathology on the basis of superficial similarities of behaviour patterns or phenomena in different cultures (Kleinman, 1987). It was argued that classification of psychiatric disorders largely reflected American and European concepts of psychopathology based on implicit cultural concepts of normality and deviance. Critics accused the etic approach of contributing to a worldview that "privileges biology over culture" (Eisenbruch, 1991) and ignores the cultural and social contexts of psychiatric disorders.

In contrast, the *emic* approach argues that the culture-bound aspects of biomedicine, such as its emphasis on medical disease entities, limited its universal applicability. More specifically, it was argued that culture played such an influential role in the presentation of psychiatric disorders that it was wrong to presume a priori that Euro-American psychiatric categories are applicable throughout the world (Littlewood, 1990). The emic approach proposed to evaluate phenomena from within a culture and its context, aiming to understand its significance and relationship with other intracultural elements. This approach has also drawn its share of criticism. The studies are mostly small in scale and are unable to resolve questions of the long-term course and treatment outcome. Moreover, the approach has been criticised for not suggesting plausible alternatives, such as a set of

---

Box 18.1 Comparing the etic and emic approaches

	Etic	Emic
Presentation of mental disorders	Similar in all cultures, at least for core symptoms	Determined by language and culture, and thus varies between cultures
Classification of mental disorders	A common universal system such as ICD or DSM	Locally derived classifications of disorders
Measurement of mental disorders	Similar measures can be used in different cultures to identify similar disorders	Measures must be developed from within the culture
Research study methods	Quantitative measures preferred with emphasis on reliability	Qualitative measures preferred with emphasis on cultural validity
Treatment of mental disorders	Biomedically derived, evidence-based treatments most effective	Treatments consonant with local beliefs most effective
Help-seeking behaviour	Primarily determined by provision of health services	Primarily determined by belief systems

DSM = *Diagnostic and Statistical Manual of Mental Disorders*; ICD; *International Classification of Diseases.*

---

principles which would help ensure cultural sensitivity or models on which to fashion culturally sensitive nosologies (Beiser *et al.*, 1994). Another critique is that the emic approach has been unable to provide data which can be compared across cultures.

Thus there are strengths and weaknesses of both the etic and emic approaches in cross-cultural psychiatry (see Box 18.1). It is widely accepted that the integration of their methodological strengths is essential for the development of a culturally sensitive or "new cross-cultural psychiatry" (Kleinman, 1987; Littlewood, 1990). Value must be given to both folk perspectives about mental illness as well as those of biomedical psychiatry. It is important to investigate patients' "explanatory models", that is, how patients understand their problems, their nature, origins, consequences and remedies, because these can radically assist patient-doctor negotiations over appropriate treatment (Kleinman, 1987). Similarly, researchers should examine the psychiatric symptoms of people who are considered by the local population to be mentally ill and determine the relationship of the diagnostic system used by local health care providers with established psychiatric diagnostic categories. In essence, the central aim of the "new" cross-cultural psychiatry is to describe mental illness in different cultures using methods which are sensitive and valid for the local culture and resulting in data which are comparable across cultures. To tackle this difficult task, psychiatric research needs to blend both ethnographic and epidemiological methods, emphasizing the unique contribution of both approaches to the understanding of mental illness across cultures.

Both major international classifications of mental disorders have attempted to improve their cross cultural and international validity. The tenth revision of the *International Classification of Impairments, Disabilities and Handicaps* (ICD-10) was developed with the explicit purpose of being an international standard. Thus those drafting ICD-10 were drawn from as many countries as was feasible. The classification itself was field tested by more than 700 clinicians in 39 countries from all continents, although the largest number of centres were in European or developed countries. The vast majority of ICD-10 conditions had reasonable cross-cultural reliability (Sartorius *et al.*, 1993). Certain syndromes were, however, considered more

---

Box 18.2 Culture-bound syndromes

The ICD-10 defines culture-specific disorders as sharing two cardinal characteristics:

1. They are not "easily" accommodated by the categories in established and internationally used psychiatric classifications.
2. They were first described in, and subsequently closely or exclusively associated with, a particular population or cultural area.

Examples of culture-bound categories include the following:

Amok is an indiscriminate, unprovoked episode of severely aggressive behaviour, which may culminate in multiple homicide or suicide (Asia).

Dhat is an anxiety disorder in young men characteristically presenting with a complaint of a whitish discharge in the urine, which is believed to be semen (Asia).

Koro presents as an acute panic reaction in men associated with a strong fear of death as a result of the patient's firm conviction that his penis is retracting and shrinking into his abdomen (Asia).

Latah is a highly exaggerated stereotyped response to fright or trauma, followed by echolalia, echopraxia, coprolalia, automatic obedience or trancelike states (Indonesia, Malaysia).

Susto is a syndrome with diverse neurotic and somatic symptoms attributed to a frightening event that causes the soul to leave the body (Latin America).

Windigo is an acute presentation of bizarre behaviour and development of homicidal impulses usually directed at members of the immediate family (indigenous peoples of North America).

Taijin kyofusho is a neurotic condition characterised by a severe obsession of shame and fear of social contact and extreme self-consciousness regarding appearance (Japan).

ICD-10, *International Classification of Diseases*, 10th revision.

---

or less "specific" to certain cultures or subcultures, and these are labelled "culture-bound syndromes" in ICD-10 (see Box 18.2).

None of the culture-specific syndromes resemble severe mental disorders; all occur in the context of severe stress and are phenomenologically closest to the neurotic and dissociative disorders. Many conditions bear considerable similarity with one another and with a multitude of other conditions described in diverse cultures. *Susto* and *nervios* are folk idioms of distress, Artic hysteria and *windigo* are culturally stereotyped reactions to extreme environmental conditions, *koro* and *dhat* are related to a cultural concern regarding fertility and procreation, *latah* and *amok* are related to a cultural emphasis on learned dissociation and *brain fag* is an example of syndromes related to acculturative stress on adolescents (the pressure of academic performance of some cultures). A culture bound-syndrome should not in itself comprise a complete psychiatric diagnosis. Just as a diagnosis of anxiety disorder can signify anything from a hidden malignancy to a marital problem, all patients must be fully investigated to clarify any underlying pathology.

Alternative worldviews of mental illness

Indigenous classifications, by and large, are based on spiritual, supernatural or humoral aetiological theories (Murdock *et al.*, 1980) which are not tenable in the practice of biomedicine. Broadly, there is a general classification of illness into two categories, "normal" and "abnormal". The former is perceived to be caused by physical agents (such as infections and climactic changes) and considered to be treated effectively by either biomedical or traditional approaches. The latter is perceived to be caused by spiritual or supernatural causes, and is thus brought principally to traditional healers. "Abnormal" or "unnatural" causes of sickness and misfortune include causation by both supernatural forces or other human beings, and may be brought on as a consequence of specific actions or behaviours of an individual or their family. The classifications used are typically flexible and patient-dependent; thus even though phenomenology may be used by a healer to understand the nature of the illness, an aetiological model is almost always provided because it gives the illness experience meaning for the patient.

There is evidence that with the influence of urbanization and other changes in society, views about illness are also changing. Biomedical diagnostic systems are increasingly being used in non-Western settings, and multiple illness models are held simultaneously. It is therefore not uncommon for a person with a mental illness to consult both traditional/religious and biomedical healthcare providers. Most often, persons associate mental illness only with psychotic disorders. For these disorders, there is a striking similarity in the behavioural symptoms across cultures, with some behaviours such as incoherent speech, talking to oneself, disrobing, wandering and aggression being particularly common (Patel, 1995). However, there is much less emphasis on cognitive features such as delusions, which are central to diagnosis in the biomedical model. Disorders resembling depression and anxiety, although not often perceived to be mental disorders, are still recognised by local people and traditional healers as being sources of illness, suffering and misfortune.

Although the ICD-10 is an international system, it was not, at least initially, intended to supplant local classificatory systems. However, many countries have gradually shed their national classification schemes, and, of the few that remain, attempts have been made to make them as closely as possible to the ICD. China is possibly the only low and middle income country (LAMIC) which has its own, discrete classification of mental disorders. The first Chinese Classification of Mental Disorders (CCMD) appeared in 1979. Its third and most recent version has been heavily influenced by the ICD-10 and *Diagnostic and Statistical Manual of Mental Disorders* (4th edition; DSM-IV) systems but still retains certain local features. The main differences between the ICD-10 and the CCMD-3 are summarised by Lee (2001). Notable among these are the retention of the term *neurosis* and some specific categories of neurotic disorder, such as neurasthenia. Personality disorder is less often diagnosed in Chinese populations possibly because deviant behaviour is dealt with by the penal system. Two categories of personality disorder, borderline personality disorder and avoidant personality disorder, are excluded from the Chinese scheme. The Chinese task force excluded borderline personality disorder because impulsivity and emotional instability were viewed as character traits that should not be medicalised.

The CCMD also includes its own section of culture-related mental disorders such as *qigong*-induced mental disorder. *Qigong* is a trance-based form of a traditional Chinese healing system. The disorder is similar to a dissociative state with identity disturbance, irritability, hallucinations and aggressive and bizarre behaviours. These are often acute, brief episodes and are linked to excessive practise of *qigong* meditation by physically or psychologically ill subjects.

The contemporary relevance of cross-cultural psychiatry

The study of cultural influences on psychiatry has to a large extent focused on non-European cultures. There is the assumption that psychiatric syndromes and disorders as described in white European populations form the basis of a universal categorization of mental illness. The contribution of cultural factors to the aetiology and manifestation of mental illness in the West is generally overlooked and implicitly denied. An important thrust of the new cross-cultural psychiatry should be to understand the interaction of culture and psychopathology among people everywhere, not just among those in non-European cultures. Another anomaly of cross-cultural psychiatry is that although Western societies are considered "multicultural" such that studies need to be conducted for different ethnic groups to ensure findings are "culturally correct", the multicultural nature of developing societies is not recognised. It is not uncommon to read conclusions about all people in vast and diverse countries such as India or China being based on a sample from one site with people from a single culture or class. Cultural psychiatrists need to be less sweeping in their generalizations and more sensitive to the diversity of people everywhere.

Furthermore, there is often an implicit assumption that non-Western cultures are "traditional" or "nonscientific" in their explanatory models. A consequence of this is that research from Western cultures is automatically considered to be of international significance. Research from developing countries is undervalued, with its international significance being confined to its demonstration of the influence of culture on psychiatric disorders.

The main limitation of cross-cultural psychiatry, of course, is that it fails to recognise that cultures are dynamic, complex social constructs that defy easy definition or measurement. Globalization has had a pervasive impact on culture; no longer do cultures exist in relative isolation from one another. Instead, cultures are integrating, with attitudes, beliefs and practises from one culture finding new homes in others. Although the process of globalisation may work in diverse ways, in reality the dominant cultures are those of industrialised societies because many mechanisms of globalisation, such as the media, are largely controlled by these societies. The homogenization of cultures across the developing world in the past decade is a marker of the vulnerability of cultures to the onslaught of modern marketing and global media networks. For example, Becker *et al.* (2002) have shown how the introduction of Western television is associated with a rise in disordered eating behaviours in school-going Fijian adolescent girls, who were previously media-naïve (see discussion later in this chapter).

Despite these limitations, it is worth noting that cross-cultural research on the epidemiology of mental disorders has contributed to public mental health and clinical practise. Several important conclusions can be drawn. First, mental disorders are found in all cultures and societies. Second, the prevalence of mental disorders varies greatly across cultures, which suggests that social factors are crucial determinants of prevalence or that international diagnostic instruments and survey methods are not uniformly reliable and valid. Third, the clinical presentation of common mental disorder is often somatic, and such presentations tend to be more common in non-Western settings. Fourth, the prevalence and incidence of severe mental disorders also vary across a wide range, and the well-known World Health Organisation (WHO) multinational studies have found an apparently more favourable prognosis in developing countries, suggesting a sociocultural influence on the course of these disorders (Jablensky *et al.*, 1992). Fifth, cultural factors, notably language, can influence the clinical features of mental disorders. This can occur through unique idioms for common mental disorders such as "thinking too much" in many African languages, or the content of delusions and hallucinations. Sixth, the diagnostic specificity of some psychopathological phenomena such as hallucinations also varies across cultures. However, the core symptoms of severe and common mental disorders can be recognised in all cultures studied. Finally, cultural and ethnic factors influence the acceptability and clinical response to psychiatric treatments; for example, drug metabolism variations may influence the effective dosage ranges for psychotropic drugs, and psychological "talking" treatments may be less acceptable as interventions in societies in which patients are accustomed to receiving physical treatments.

The study of culture on mental health has been profoundly influential in guiding the clinician in managing psychiatric disorders in persons of different culture. This is best exemplified by the DSM-IV guidelines for clinicians to make a "cultural formulation" of a person's mental health problem (see Box 18.3).

Social determinants of mental disorders

This section considers four major social determinants of mental disorders: poverty, gender, conflict and the marginalisation experienced by indigenous communities across the world.

Poverty

Substantial evidence now confirms the relationship between poverty and socioeconomic

---

> **Box 18.3** Cultural formulation in the DSM-IV
>
> This formulation implies that the clinician provides a narrative summary on the following:
>
> - the cultural identity of the individual (e.g. language abilities, cultural preference group, degree of involvement with other cultures in community)
> - cultural explanations of the illness (similar to the explanatory models described earlier and including prominent idioms of distress, causal models and treatment preferences)
> - cultural factors related to the psychosocial environment and functioning (culturally relevant interpretations of social stressors, available social support and disability)
> - cultural elements of the relationship between the individual and the clinician (identify differences and similarities in cultural and social status that might influence diagnosis and treatment)
> - overall cultural assessment: a conclusion formulating how these cultural considerations influence diagnosis and treatment decisions
>
> DSM-IV = Diagnostic and Statistical Manual of Mental Disorders, 4th edn.

---

inequalities for both common and severe mental disorders. In the United Kingdom, for example, there is good evidence for an association between low standard of living and depression (Weich & Lewis, 1998). Evidence is also beginning to accumulate demonstrating a similar association between economic disadvantage and the presence of depression in developing countries. A recent review of 11 community-based epidemiological studies from six countries – in Latin America (Brazil, Chile), Africa (Lesotho, Zimbabwe) and Asia (Pakistan, Indonesia) – found that 10 studies showed a statistically significant relationship between prevalence of common mental disorder and indicators of low socioeconomic status. The most consistent relationship was between low education and mental disorder. Significant associations were evident for a number of other socioeconomic indicators, such as being in debt, and common mental disorders (Patel & Kleinman, 2003).

Studies in developed countries have shown that mortality and morbidity rates are affected by relative, rather than absolute, living standards. A survey in the United States, for example, showed an independent association between low income and living in "income-unequal states", with depression in women (Kahn *et al.*, 2000). The association between racial and economic inequality and poor mental health may be mediated by both individual psychological factors, such as low self-esteem and frustration, as well as a breakdown in structural factors in the community, such as social cohesion and infrastructure. The lack of social support and the breakdown of kinship structures is probably the key stressor for the millions of migrant labourers in the urban centres of Asia, Africa and South America, as well as the millions of dependants who are left behind in rural areas and whose only hope of survival is the remittances relatives send from distant cities. In developed countries, increased mobility of labour has reduced family ties and also led to the decline of the extended family.

The social consequences of low education are obvious, especially in developing countries that are facing a growing lack of security for employees as economies are reformed. Lack of secondary education may represent a diminished opportunity for persons who are depressed to access resources to improve their situation (Patel *et al.*, 1999). People living in conditions of poverty are at greater risk for physical health problems, and there is abundant evidence demonstrating a high degree of comorbidity between physical and mental illnesses.

Gender

Whereas *sex* is a term used to distinguish men and women on the basis of their biological characteristics, *gender* refers to the distinguishing features which are socially constructed. Gender is a crucial element in health inequities in developing countries. Gender influences the control men and women have over the determinants of their health, including their economic position and social status and access to resources and treatment. The female

excess for depression has been demonstrated in most community-based studies in all regions of the world (Patel *et al.*, 1999). The social gradient in health is heavily gendered, and women are disproportionately affected by the burden of poverty that, in turn, may influence their vulnerability for depression. Women are far more likely to be victims of violence in their homes, and women who experience physical violence by an intimate partner are significantly more likely to suffer depression, abuse drugs or attempt suicide.

Women who were sexually abused as children are significantly more likely to suffer depression in adulthood. Sexual and other forms of violence in youth are associated with depression in adolescence (Astbury, 2001). A study from Ghana investigating women's perceptions of their health found that the most important health concern was "thinking too much"; the explanations given included heavy workloads, financial insecurity and the burden of caring for children, duties which were heavily gendered in their distribution (Avotri & Walters, 1999).

Examples of the cultural context of some of these gendered stressors are illustrated by several recent studies. Research on depression in women in low-income townships of Harare, Zimbabwe, reported that nearly 18% women had a current episode of depression compared with only 9% of their counterparts in Camberwell, a deprived inner-London district thought to have a relatively high rate of depression (Broadhead & Abas, 1998). More women in Harare had experienced a severe life event (54%) in the preceding 12 months compared with women in Camberwell (31%). A notable finding in Harare was the high proportion of events involving humiliation and entrapment that were related to marital crises such as being deserted by husbands and left to care for several children, premature death, illness in family members and severe financial difficulties occurring in the absence of an adequate welfare safety net. Studies in South Asia have shown that marital violence and the culturally determined value placed on boys (compared with girls) adversely influence maternal mental health. Studies from India and

Pakistan have demonstrated the greater risk for postnatal depression in mothers who have a female child, especially if the desired sex was a boy or if the mother already had living girl children (Patel *et al.*, 2004).

The male excess for alcohol abuse has been demonstrated in almost every community study from every region of the world, although the disparities are greatest in developing countries. The wide sex differences in alcohol abuse in Latin American countries and the Caribbean have been attributed to a number of gender factors (Pyne *et al.*, 2002). Women, for example, face strict social scrutiny about many behaviours, drinking among them. Men's consumption of alcohol mostly takes place in the public realm, whereas women's more often occurs in private. Drinking among men has social meanings such as maintaining friendships, and refusing a drink can imply lack of trust and denial of mutual respect. At the other extreme, intoxication of men is more socially acceptable than that of women; indeed, women often tolerate their male partners' intoxication as being a "natural" condition of manhood. Drinking and drunkenness are more often perceived to be consistent with gendered notions of masculinity, and thus men who conform closely to cultural norms are more likely to drink. Drinking may also be a coping strategy when men are faced with serious life difficulties, such as unemployment and are unable to live up to the traditional expectations. Finally, in many cultures (but perhaps most well-recognised in Latin America), is the role of *machismo*, that is, the importance of male sexuality, in shaping alcohol consumption. Thus young men may consume excess alcohol with the deliberate intent of getting drunk because excessive drinking "celebrates male courage, sexual prowess, maturity and the ability to take risks, including sexual risks" (Pyne *et al.*, 2002, p. 23).

The evidence that gender plays a role in eating disorders stems from two observations: first, the enormous sex difference (females outnumbering men) and the fact that cultures which have been relatively immune to the media-driven creation of an ideal body image for women have very low rates of these disorders. Recently, a study from Fiji demonstrated that the introduction of television in a media-naïve non-Westernised population was associated with a rise in attitudes favouring thinner body image and self-induced vomiting in girls (Becker *et al.*, 2002). This finding adds credence to the theory that the emphasis on women's thinness by the media and fashion industries is contributing to a rise in disordered eating in societies that, through the forces of globalisation, are being increasingly influenced by Western imagery and values.

Conflict and displacement

Globally, there are an estimated 17 million refugees and asylum seekers who have fled their own countries and another 25 million who are internally displaced. Many of these persons will have experienced enormous trauma in the form of violence, crime or other humiliations; physical injury; economic dispossession; and disruption of family and community structures. Thus the rates of mental disorder among these people would be expected to be at least as high and probably higher than for migrants in general. A recent study of more than 3,000 respondents from post-conflict communities in Algeria, Cambodia, Ethiopia and Palestine found that post-traumatic stress disorder (PTSD), a psychiatric disorder which is considered a specific response to trauma, was the most common disorder in individuals exposed to violence associated with armed conflict (de Jong *et al.*, 2003).

A number of other factors may predispose refugees and immigrants to mental disorders. These include marginalisation and minority status, socioeconomic disadvantage, poor physical health, the loss of social support systems and cultural alienation in the new society. For illegal immigrants, there is also the constant fear of being found out and repatriated, and therefore access to possible sources of help is severely limited. Here it is relevant to note that the universal application of trauma-related mental disorders, in particular PTSD, has been criticised because it is itself based on culturally influenced notions of how a person is supposed to react to trauma. Thus, in narrating the experience of Cambodian refugees, Eisenbruch (1991, p. 673) described patients who were "possessed by spirits, troubled by visitations of ghosts from the homeland . . . and feel he or she is being punished for having survived". The cultural construction of symptoms is also an important determinant of help-seeking behaviour; thus, Buddhist monks might work as "allies to the clinician in clarifying the diagnosis of cultural bereavement" in Cambodia. Although there is consensus that trauma can negatively affect a person's mental health, the question of whether this negative impact should be conceptualised in psychiatric terms (with the concomitant implications of diagnosis and treatment) or in social and cultural terms remains unresolved. On the other hand, there is no doubt that trauma can have negative effects that can be conceptualised in psychiatric terms. Studies in a number of settings have clearly demonstrated that symptoms characteristic of PTSD can be identified in individuals who have been exposed to trauma and that these do cluster in the form typical of PTSD and are associated with suffering and disability (de Jong *et al.*, 2003; Silove *et al.*, 2002)

Indigenous communities

It is estimated that there are between 220 and 300 million indigenous persons living in 5,000 to 6,000 distinct groups in more than 70 countries. They exhibit a wide diversity of lifestyles, cultures, social organization, histories and political backgrounds. Nevertheless, they may share certain historical and political realities, including being subject to violence and genocide, depopulation from infectious diseases such as smallpox and measles, dislocation from traditional lands, extreme poverty due to the destruction of their subsistence economies and state-organised attempts to repress and eradicate their cultures. Given this scenario, it is not surprising that the indigenous peoples of the world experience high rates of depression, alcoholism and suicide (Cohen, 1999).

The case of the indigenous communities of Australia serves to illustrate the confluence of these historical, political, social and economic forces and to provide insights into why the rates of mental disorders are high among indigenous peoples. The indigenous peoples of Australia had a diversity of cultures dating back at least 40,000 years before the arrival of European settlers just over 200 years ago. The societies had rich cultural belief systems which attributed spiritual importance to the land and the environments in which they lived. Social relationships were governed by codes of behavior, and local taxonomies of illness guided the treatment of health problems. The brutal history of colonization which ultimately led to the destruction and devastation of hundreds of indigenous nations, each with a distinct language, lineage and culture, was marked by a number of severe social adversities. Notable among these were exposure to new diseases, removal from traditional lands, enslavement on the farms of European settlers, imprisonment without trial, denial of basic political rights, sexual abuse of women and, perhaps most tragic of all, the "stolen generations", that is, the children who were forcibly removed from their parents and fostered by white families in an effort to "breed out" the native population. The consequences of this history are reflected in socioeconomic, psychosocial and health indicators of all kinds including high rates of unemployment, low levels of income, and poor educational status; age-specific mortality rates 2 to 7 times higher and life expectancies that are more than 15 years shorter than those of the non-indigenous Australian population; and high levels of alcoholism and suicide (Cohen, 1999).

Implications for population mental health

An important implication of the association between poverty and mental disorders in developing countries is to place mental disorders alongside other diseases which attract considerable attention from health policy makers and donors because of their association with poverty. There is a need

to educate policy makers regarding the association between poverty and mental disorders and
to combat the myth (sometimes perpetuated by
media catering to the middle class in developing
countries) that depression and anxiety are disorders
of affluence or "Westernization". The impact of
research on policy is evident in the recent decision
by the Department of Foreign and International
Development (DFID), the principal overseas development and aid arm of the British government,
to include mental health as one funding priority
among other key poverty- and development-related
health issues. Mental health professionals will need
to confront global poverty, its relation to the current
phase of political and economic development and
its consequences for mental disorders.

From a public health perspective, an understanding of mechanisms of the relationship between
social adversity and mental health can inform primary and secondary preventive strategies. However,
evidence to support the efficacy of specific interventions in this field is weak, mainly because few
if any have been tried or evaluated in terms of
their impact on mental disorders. There is evidence
that interventions aimed at improving child development and educational outcomes in children living in poverty have had success. A recent review
of interventions aimed at improving nutrition and
development in socioeconomically disadvantaged
children found strong evidence for the benefit
of psychosocial and nutritional interventions for
cognitive development and improved educational
outcomes (WHO, 1999). Although mental health
outcomes have not been reported as yet, we may
speculate that the benefits evident in educational
outcomes may also translate to better mental
health. The emphasis on education will need to
focus on girls and on ensuring education beyond
primary schooling. Anecdotal findings from literacy
programs in India suggest that such programs may
have an unanticipated benefit on mental health by
reducing hopelessness and providing greater economic security (Cohen, 2002).

In many developing countries, indebtedness to
loan sharks is a consistent source of stress and
worry, demonstrated by the recent suicides of farmers in India (Sundar, 1999). Provision of low-interest
loans may reduce mental disorders by removing the
key cause of stress: the threat posed by the informal moneylender. Development, if implemented to
promote social capital, equity and basic infrastructure, may be associated with better mental health.
A study in Indonesia, for example, described rates
of depression according to levels of economic development (Bahar *et al.*, 1992). Villages which achieved
an improvement in development status and those
which were already at the highest level of development had the lowest rates of depression. The key
to secondary prevention is to strengthen the treatment of mental disorders in primary health care (see
Chapter 21 and Box 18.4).

The association of gender disadvantage with
mental health problems presents tremendous
opportunities for mental health research in terms of
allying with other public health research programs
which have an emphasis on gender issues and vice
versa. There is no better example than maternal
and reproductive health, one of the Millennium
Development Goals. The areas of intersection of
reproductive and mental health are considerable in
scope and include postnatal depression, the mental
health consequences of rape and adverse maternal outcomes such as stillbirths and miscarriage,
infertility, surgery on the reproductive organs, ster-
ilisation, adolescent reproductive and sexual health,
HIV/AIDS, gynaecological morbidities and menstrual health (Patel & Oomman, 1999). The growing
global concern regarding violence in families and
in communities, a significant proportion of which
is fuelled by alcohol abuse, provides an opportunity
for mental health programs on depression and alcohol use to integrate their work (WHO, 2002). There
is a need for gender sensitisation of mental health
policies and programs. Policies and programs must
be planned in consultation with key stakeholder
groups, including representatives of women and
men in the community. Gender barriers should be
explicitly addressed in the planning of programs,
in particular for mental health promotion, such
as challenging gender stereotypes of drinking in

Box 18.4 Poverty and psychopathology: a natural experiment (Costello *et al.*, 2003)

The association between poverty and increased rates of mental disorders has been recognized for many years. However, the debate continues over the direction of causality. On the social causation side, it is hypothesised that the stresses of living in poverty are the reason for high rates of psychopathology; on the social selection side, the reasoning is that the functional disabilities which are characteristic of mental disorders are the reason individuals drift into poverty. Resolving this debate is difficult because it requires evidence from natural experiments in which one can examine how changes in economic status effect the prevalence of mental disorders. Such a natural experiment arose during a community study (1993–2000) of the development of mental illness in children who lived in North Carolina in the United States. A total of 1,420 children were interviewed; of these, 350 were from the Eastern Band of Cherokee Indians. In 1996, a casino opened that gave tribal members a share of its profits. In addition, the opening increased employment in the region, especially for tribal members because of preferential hiring practices at the casino. These economic opportunities meant that a significant percentage (14%) of Indian families were raised out of poverty by the end of the study; 53% of Indian families remained poor and 32% were never poor.

Throughout the study (4 years before the casino opened and 4 years afterwards), surveys were administered to the children in the sample to collect information about psychiatric symptoms in two broad categories: emotional disorders (depression and anxiety) and behavioral disorders (conduct and oppositional disorders). The mean number of psychiatric symptoms maintained a steady, low rate in the "never-poor" children, but persistently poor children maintained a steady, high rate. In contrast, children whose families emerged from poverty experienced a significant decrease in rates: before the casino opened, these children had the same rate of psychiatric symptoms as the persistently poor children, but after the casino opened they had the same rate as never-poor children. However, the formerly poor children only experienced reductions in symptomatology for behavioral disorders, apparently because once out of poverty, parents were able to provide adequate supervision to them; rates of emotional symptoms did not decrease.

This natural experiment suggests that poverty is a causal factor in the aetiology of behavioral disorders among children. The explanation for the constant rate of emotional disorders among the formerly poor children is not so clear. The authors suggest that the lack of an association indicates that genetics have a greater role than environments in the aetiology of emotional disorders. It is also possible that poverty is a cause of emotional disorders among children, but, once established, such disorders are not easily resolved even by positive changes in the environment.

young men and women. Gender-based risk factors such as violence and restriction of opportunities must be tackled as potential prevention strategies for mental disorders. Gender biases which may operate in healthcare itself should be examined and minimised. Ultimately, the recognition and incorporation of gender as a key variable in mental health research and services will ensure that research findings and services are more sensitive to the social realities in which mental disorders occur in men and women in developing countries. An explicit recognition of the vulnerability of populations such as indigenous communities and persons affected by conflict is an important advocacy tool for mental health practitioners to lobby against conflict and the deliberate marginalisation faced by indigenous peoples across the world. The strong influence of social determinants on the risk for, and outcome of, mental disorders argues for the need for a greater focus on equity in the distribution of affordable and evidence-based mental health services.

Conclusions

Mental illness has achieved considerable global public health attention as a result of recent reports which have focused on the high prevalence and associated disability of mental disorders (WHO, 2001). However, much of the research on mental illness is derived from a small fraction of the world's population in developed countries (Patel & Sumathipala, 2001). This situation is gradually changing and is reflected in the changing content of cross-cultural studies. Over the past two decades there has been a shift away from examining the minutiae of obscure mental disorders in exotic (i.e. non-Western) societies towards an attempt to generate a practical understanding of the implications of the high prevalence and impact of psychiatric morbidity in developing nations or among specific, and often disadvantaged, ethnic communities or subgroups in the population. The future of a truly international psychiatry should be to establish psychiatry as a relevant medical discipline with strong public health roots in all nations of the world. A key to achieving this goal is the recognition that culture and social determinants play roles that are at least as great as biological factors in influencing the aetiology, frequency, outcome and treatment responsiveness of most psychiatric disorders.

REFERENCES

Astbury, J. (2001). Gender disparities in mental health. In *Mental Health: A Call for Action by World Health Ministers.* Geneva: World Health Organisation, pp. 73–92.

Avotri, J. Y., & Walters, V. (1999). You just look at our work and see if you have any freedom on earth: Ghanaian women's accounts of their work and health. *Soc Sci Med* **48**:1123–33.

Bahar, E., Henderson, A. S., & Mackinnon, A. J. (1992). An epidemiological study of mental health and socioeconomic conditions in Sumatera, Indonesia. *Acta Psychiatr Scand* **85**:257–63.

Becker, A. E., Burwell, R. A., Gilman, S. E., *et al.* (2002). Disordered eating behaviors and attitudes follow prolonged exposure to television among ethnic Fijian adolescent girls. *Br J Psychiatry* **180**:509–14.

Beiser, M., Cargo, M., & Woodbury, M. (1994). A comparison of psychiatric disorder in different cultures: depressive typologies in South-East Asian refugees and resident Canadians. *Int J Meth Psychiatr Res* **4**:157–72.

Broadhead, J. C., & Abas, M. A. (1998). Life events, difficulties and depression among women in an urban setting in Zimbabwe. *Psychol Med* **28**:29–38.

Cohen, A. (1999). *The Mental Health of Indigenous People: An International Overview.* Geneva: World Health Organisation.

Cohen, A. (2002). Our lives were covered in darkness. The work of the National Literary Mission in Northern India. In A. Cohen, A. Kleinman & B. Saraceno, eds. *World Mental Health Casebook: Social and Mental Health Programs in Low-Income Countries.* New York, London, Dordrecht: Kluwer Academic/Plenum, pp. 153–90.

Costello, E. J., Compton, S. N., Keeler, G., *et al.* (2003). Relationships between poverty and psychopathology: a natural experiment. *JAMA* **290**:2023–9.

de Jong, J. T. V. M., Komproe, I. H., & Ommeren, M. V. (2003). Common mental disorders in postconflict settings. *Lancet* **361**:2128–30.

Eisenbruch, M. (1991). From post-traumatic stress disorder to cultural bereavement: diagnosis of Southeast Asian refugees. *Soc Sci Med* **33**:673–80.

Hendrie, H., Osuntokun, B., Hall, K., *et al.* (1995). Prevalence of Alzheimer;s disease and dementias in two communities: Nigerian Africans and African Americans. *Am J Psychiatry* **152**:1485–92.

Isaacs, S. L., & Schroeder, S. A. (2004). Class – the ignored determinant of the nation's health. *N Engl J Med* **351**:1137–42.

Jablensky, A., Sartorius, N., Ernberg, G., *et al.* (1992). Schizophrenia: manifestations, incidence and course in different cultures: a World Health Organization ten-country study. *Psychological Medicine Monograph, Supplement 20.* Cambridge: Cambridge University Press.

Johns, L., Nazroo, J. Y., Bebbington, P., *et al.* (2002). Occurrence of hallucinatory experiences in a community sample and ethnic variations. *Br J Psychiatry* **180**:174–8.

Kahn, R. S., Wise, P. H., Kennedy, B. P., *et al.* (2000). State income inequality, household income, and maternal mental and physical health: cross-sectional national survey. *BMJ* **321**:1331.

Kleinman, A. (1987). Anthropology and psychiatry: the role of culture in cross-cultural research on illness. *Br J Psychiatry* **151**:447–54.

Kraepelin, E. (2000). Comparative psychiatry. In R. Littlewood & S. Dein, eds. *Cultural Psychiatry & Medical Anthropology: An Introduction and Reader.* London: Athlone Press, pp. 38–42. Original work published 1904.

Le Roux, A. G. (1973). Psychopathology in Bantu culture. *S Afr Med J* **47**:2077–2083.

Lee, S. (2001). From diversity to unity: the classification of mental disorders in 21st-century China. *Psychiatr Clin North Am* **24**:421–31.

Leighton, A. H., Lambo, T. A., Hughes, C. C., *et al.* (1963). *Psychiatric Disorder Among the Yoruba.* Ithaca, New York: Cornell University Press.

Littlewood, R. (1990). From categories to contexts: a decade of the new cross-cultural psychiatry. *Br J Psychiatry* **156**:308–27.

Murdock, G. P., Wilson, S. F., & Frederick, V. (1980). World distribution of theories of illness. *Transcultural Psychiatry Res Rev* **17**:37–64.

Murphy, H. B. M. (1982). *Comparative Psychiatry: The International and Intermittent Distribution of Mental Illness*. New York: Springer-Verlag.

Patel, V. (1995). Explanatory models of mental illness in sub-Saharan Africa. *Soc Sci Med* **40**:1291–8.

Patel, V., Araya, R., de Lima, M., *et al.* (1999). Women, poverty and common mental disorders in four restructuring societies. *Soc Sci Med* **49**:1461–71.

Patel, V., & Kleinman, A. (2003). Poverty and common mental disorders in developing countries. *Bull WHO* **81**:609–15.

Patel, V., & Oomman, N. M. (1999). Mental health matters too: gynecological morbidity and depression in South Asia. *Reprod Health Matters* **7**:30–8.

Patel, V., Rahman, A., Jacob, K. S., *et al.* (2004). Effect of maternal mental health on infant growth in low income countries: new evidence from South Asia. *BMJ* **328**:820–3.

Patel, V., & Sumathipala, A. (2001). International representation in psychiatric journals: a survey of 6 leading journals. *Br J Psychiatry* **178**:406–9.

Prince, R., Okpaku, S. O., & Merkel, R. L. (1998). Transcultural psychiatry: a note on origins and definitions. In S. O. Okpaku, ed. *Clinical Methods in Transcultural Psychiatry*. Washington, DC: American Psychiatric Association, pp. 3–17.

Pyne, H. H., Claeson, M., & Correia, M. (2002). *Gender Dimensions of Alcohol Consumption and Alcohol-Related Problems in Latin America and the Caribbean*. Washington, DC: World Bank.

Sartorius, N., Kaelber, C. T., Cooper, J. E., *et al.* (1993). Progress toward achieving a common language in psychiatry. *Arch Gen Psychiatry* **50**:115–24.

Silove, D., Steel, Z., McGorry, P., *et al.* (2002). The impact of torture on post-traumatic stress symptoms in war-affected Tamil refugees and immigrants. *Compr Psychiatry* **43**:49 55.

Sundar, M. (1999). Suicide in farmers in India [letter]. *Br J Psychiatry* **175**:585–6.

US Department of Health and Human Services (USDHHS). (2001). *Mental Health: Culture, Race, and Ethnicity*. Rockville, Maryland: Office of the Surgeon General, Public Health Service, USDHHS.

Weich, S., & Lewis, G. (1998). Poverty, unemployment and the common mental disorders: a population based cohort study. *BMJ* **317**:115–19.

World Health Organisation (1999). *A Critical Link: Interventions for Physical Growth and Child Development*. Geneva: World Health Organisation.

World Health Organisation (2001). *The World Health Report 2001: Mental Health: New Understanding, New Hope*. Geneva: World Health Organisation.

World Health Organisation (2002). *World Report on Violence and Health: Summary*. Geneva: World Health Organisation.

19

Psychiatric disorders of menses, pregnancy, postpartum and menopause

Anne Buist, Kimberly Yonkers and Michael Craig

Women's mental health issues have become increasingly prominent both politically and at a research level over the past 20 years. Although the reasons for this are many, the key driving factor is the higher prevalence of various mental illnesses in women; depression, predicted by the World Health Organisation (WHO) to be the leading cause of disability in 2020, is twice as common in women. In addition, women as the carer for the infant both in utero and infancy has a potentially highly significant influence both biologically and psychologically on the subsequent generation. This chapter summarises the current understanding of women's mental health issues related to three key time periods.

Aetiology and risk factors

Biological

Genetic

Risk of depression is due to a contribution of both inherited and environmental factors. Heritability accounts for anything from 33% to 45% of the risk (Kendler, Neale, *et al.*, 1992). A study of 1,000 twin pairs concluded that 60% of the genetic risk was direct, with psychosocial factors acting as mediators (Kendler, *et al.*, 1993).

The genetic contribution holds for depression perinatally (O'Hara & Swain, 1996). Premenstrual

mood disorders may also be mediated through a genetic predisposition to depression, but in addition there may be an independent familial vulnerability (Kendler, Silberg, *et al.*, 1992), as has been found in some studies of depression perinatally (Dennerstein *et al.* 1989) and at menopause (Dennerstein *et al.*, 1999).

Neuroendocrine

An understanding of hormonal influences on mood is important in trying to tie together those women who appear to be an increased risk of depression premenstrually, postnatally and at menopause.

At *menopause*, hormonal changes do not appear to have a major role. An Australian study of 354 women found no relationship between negative mood and gonadal hormone levels, although there was a relationship between more depressed mood in response to stressors occurring during the menopausal transition, suggesting that hormonal changes may make women vulnerable to stressors (Dennerstein *et al.*, 1999). An 11-year follow up of 438 of these women also found hormone therapy not to affect rates of depression, although a surgical menopause was associated with an increased rate of depression (Dennerstein *et al.*, 2004).

The pathophysiology of *premenstual dysphoric disorder* (PMDD) is not known. It was originally felt that some type of alteration in the hormonal milieu caused the illness. However, studies do not

Essential Psychiatry, ed. Robin M. Murray, Kenneth S. Kendler, Peter McGuffin, Simon Wessely, David J. Castle. Published by Cambridge University Press. © Cambridge University Press 2008.

consistently document abnormalities in levels of either progesterone or oestrogen or the relative ratio of these hormones. Current hypotheses posit that symptoms result from abnormal signalling to the central nervous system during usual menstrual cycles (Steiner & Pearlstein, 2000). This theory is consistent with findings showing dysregulation in neurotransmitters systems, including serotonin and gamma-aminobutyric acid (GABA) as hypothesised for other mood disorders (see Halbreich & Tworek, 1993, for a review).

Dysregulation in the serotonin system is suggested by studies that have found the following:

1. Altered binding to imipramine receptors is seen in PMDD women compared with control subjects (Rojansky *et al.*, 1991; Steege *et al.*, 1992).

2. Symptoms can be provoked during the follicular phase or worsened during the premenstrual phase if subjects are depleted of the serotonin (5-HT) precursor tryptophan (Heath *et al.*, 1998; Menkes, 1994) or administered the 5-HT receptor antagonist methergoline (Roca *et al.*, 2002).

3. Abnormal prolactin or cortisol responses (or both) occur after administration of a number of serotonergic probes, including L-tryptophan (Bancroft *et al.*, 1991; Rasgon *et al.*, 2000), buspirone (Yatham 1989), m-CPP (Su *et al.*, 1997) and fenfluramine (Fitzgerald *et al.*, 1997; Steiner *et al.*, 1999). Studies also find abnormalities in the GABA system (Epperson *et al.*, 2002; Halbreich *et al.*, 1996) and in allopregnanolone, a progesterone metabolite that binds to the GABA receptor and has agonist properties (Bicikova *et al.*, 1998; Girdler *et al.*, 2001; Montelone *et al.*, 2000; Rapkin *et al.*, 1997; Sundstrom, Ashbrook & Backstrom, 1997; Sundstrom & Backstrom, 1998; Sundstrom, Nyberg & Backstrom, 1997). Preclinical studies show that serotonin reuptake inhibitors (SSRIs) acutely change neurotransmission in serotonergic neurons but also alter progesterone metabolism and increase allopregnanolone (Uzunova *et al.*, 1998).

Perinatally, evidence has been inconsistent. In one study, Bloch *et al.* (2003) simulated pregnancy by giving and then withdrawing hormones in 16 women, half with a history of postpartum depression and half without. Five of those with a history – and none of those without – had significant mood symptoms in response to withdrawal. This suggests that there may be a differing response to oestrogen and progesterone change in those with and without a history of depression, giving weight to a hormonal contribution to mood disorders at this time, at least in some women.

Maternal anxiety and depression in *pregnancy* may have particular effects on the foetus. Recent studies (Glover & O'Connor, 2002; Wadhwa *et al.*, 2001) have suggested that these infants are exposed to high levels of corticosteroids, which may continue postpartum. It is postulated that the changes in the neuroendocrine axis – mediated by such parameters as levels of social support – may have effects on foetal development and growth, with implications for later reaction to stress and development of mental illness (O'Connor *et al.*, 2002; Wadhwa *et al.*, 2001). Later exposure to a depressed mother might also have an effect, increasing cortisol levels in these children (Ashman *et al.*, 2002).

Psychosocial

At all life stages, stressful life events and lack of social supports are closely correlated with an increased risk of depression (Dennerstein *et al.*, 1999; O'Hara & Swain, 1996). Perinatally, a stable relationship and social supports are particularly important for the woman's smooth transition to motherhood. Other factors, such as perfectionistic personality style (Boyce *et al.*, 1991) and a childhood abuse history (Buist, 1998), are also key factors that contribute to difficulties in adapting to being a mother. In cultures other than Western ones, the incidence of perinatal depression is increasingly recognised, although it is possibly lower when traditional societies have supported the mother physically and valued her role. In some cultures additional risks are relevant, including economic hardship and gender of the infant (Patel *et al.*, 2002).

Table 19.1 Relative importance of aetiological factors from current research

Factor	PMDD	PND	Menopause
Genetic	++	++	++
Sensitivity to hormonal change	+	+	–
Childhood trauma	–	++	+ (as risk to previous depression)
Social supports	++	+++	+++
Marital relationship	++	+++	+++
Poor health	–	–	++

At menopause, poor physical health becomes important in increasing the risk of depression (Dennerstein *et al.,* 1999; Dennerstein & Spencer-Gardner, 1983), as does a negative attitude to the menopause change (Dennerstein, 2001).

Summary

The most likely model that explains depression in women related to times of hormonal changes is one that incorporates the complex interplay of biological, psychological and social factors (see Table 19.1). Genetic loading has a clear influence. In addition, maternal biological factors may be important in the early development of the foetus' later ability to adapt and development of illness. The mother's social support and psychological stressors appear to mediate this process, as will the child's later experiences, including that of being raised by a depressed parent. These experiences help mould personality, which in turn will influence experiences and responses. These will be important in attitude to menopause, both physically and mentally, as well as possible accompanying psychological stress related to relationship difficulties and poor health.

Premenstrual disorders

Diagnostic considerations

Premenstrual syndrome and premenstrual dysphoric disorder

PMDD, which is a carefully codified and studied condition, is characterised by depressed mood, mood swings, flashes of anger and irritability, changes in sleep and appetite, as well as disturbances in functioning at home or at work (American Psychiatric Association, 1996). It can be distinguished from milder forms of premenstrual syndrome (PMS) in that mood or anxiety complaints are a requisite component of PMDD. Further, a woman suffering from PMDD must experience at least five premenstrual symptoms and functional impairment due to the symptoms. These symptoms should not be "merely an exacerbation" of another psychiatric or general medical condition. Symptoms need to be confirmed through daily ratings during two menstrual cycles.

PMDD has a lifetime prevalence of approximately 2% to 4% in menstruating women (Johnson *et al.,* 1988; Ramacharan, *et al.,* 1992; Rivera-Tovar & Frank, 1990), a rate lower than that estimated for the less restrictive category of moderate PMS (approximately 20%–50%; Borenstein *et al.,* 2003; Deuster, Adera, South-Paul *et al.,* 1999; Hargrove & Abraham, 1982; Kessel & Cantab, 1963; Woods *et al.,* 1982), but still encompassing a large proportion of the female population. Although it is common to trivialise premenstrual disturbances such as PMDD, the illness is serious for the women who are afflicted. Morbidity of the disorder is due to its severity, chronicity and resulting impairment in interpersonal relationships. Given an estimated mean age for illness onset of 16 years (Wittchen *et al.,* 2002), if women experience symptoms 7 to 10 days each cycle and if symptoms continue unabated until menopause, a woman with PMDD is expected to have more than 400 potentially symptomatic cycles or 2,800 to 4,300 symptomatic days (7–11 years) before she stops menstruating.

The temporal pattern of symptom expression varies, with some women experiencing only a few days of distress, whereas others have a symptomatic period of up to 2 weeks. Usually, symptoms peak within 2 days of the onset of menses and often linger a day or two into the next menstrual cycle (Sternfeld et al., 2002). When a woman has mild symptoms all the time with worsening during the week before menses, she is said to have premenstrual worsening or premenstrual magnification.

Treatment issues

Studies on the treatment of PMDD show that progesterone (Wyatt et al., 2001) has little benefit beyond placebo. Similarly, the few existing oral contraceptive studies (Freeman et al., 2001; Graham & Sherwin, 1992) have been negative. However, unlike studies testing progesterone, the oral contraceptive trials had sample sizes too small to address the issue of efficacy definitively. A role for vitamin B_6 in the treatment of PMS or PMDD is also unsupported (Wyatt et al., 1999). There is limited support for a number of other therapeutic interventions, including spironolactone (Burnet et al., 1991; Hellberg 1991; O'Brien et al., 1979), calcium (Alvir & Thys-Jacobs, 1991; Thys-Jacobs & Alvir, 1995; Thys-Jacobs et al., 1989, 1998), alprazolam (Freeman et al., 1995; Harrison, et al., 1987; Smith et al., 1987), buspirone (Rickels et al., 1989) and a complex carbohydrate drink (Freeman et al., 2002; Sayegh et al., 1995). Psychotherapy has enjoyed limited investigation, but no specific behavioural treatment has been shown superior to nonspecific treatment (Morse et al., 1991).

On the other hand, data showing the efficacy of acute-phase treatment are strong (Cohen et al., 2002; Eriksson et al., 1995; Freeman et al., 1999, 2000; Halbreich & Smoller, 1997; Jermain et al., 1999; Landen et al., 2002; Menkes et al., 1992; Miner et al., 2002; Ozeren et al., 1997; Pearlstein et al., 1997; Steiner et al., 1995; Stone et al., 1991; Su et al., 1997; Sundblad et al., 1992, 1993; Wikander et al., 1998; Wood et al., 1992; Yonkers et al., 1996; Young

et al., 1998). A meta-analysis of 15 SSRI trials found that the odds of improving were 6.9 (confidence interval = 3.9–12.2) times higher with an SSRI than with placebo (Dimmock et al., 2000; Wyatt et al., 2003). Approximately 70% of women with moderate to severe PMS can expect to feel well or nearly well after SSRI treatment, compared with 30% to 35% given placebo (Yonkers et al., 1997). The effect of antidepressant type is discriminating in that SSRIs are more effective in treating PMDD than antidepressants not active at the serotonin transporter (Eriksson et al., 1995; Freeman et al., 1999; Pearlstein et al., 1997).

The initial studies showing SSRIs to be effective in PMDD stipulated daily medication administration throughout the menstrual cycle. Recent work (Cohen et al., 2002; Halbreich & Smoller, 1997; Halbreich et al., 2002; Jermain et al., 1999; Landen et al., 2002; Miner et al., 2002; Steiner et al., 1997; Sundblad et al., 1993; Wikander et al., 1998; Young et al., 1998) also demonstrates the efficacy of luteal phase dosing (i.e. commencing treatment at ovulation with discontinuation on the first day of menses). Despite the efficacy of this modality when compared with placebo, daily treatment has been shown to be superior to luteal phase treatment in several studies (Landen et al., 2002). One study failed to find a difference in efficacy between the two platforms but did not differentiate active treatment from placebo (Freeman et al., 2004). Luteal phase dosing may be more difficult to implement because it is not common for women to monitor ovulation, and around a third of women have irregular cycles (Weller & Weller, 1998). Although some women may prefer luteal phase dosing, it is probably best reserved for those who have no anxious or depressive symptoms during the follicular (postmenstrual) phase of the cycle because they would be untreated during this interval. The last consideration merits emphasis because many women with premenstrual complaints have mild symptoms during the follicular phase, and as noted symptoms often linger into the menstrual week. Daily dosing as first-line treatment, especially in women who have more severe symptoms, is recommended by recently published expert guidelines (Altshuler *et al.,* 2001); calcium and spironolactone may be useful adjuncts.

Perinatal psychiatry

Diagnostic considerations

Mood and anxiety disorders

Characteristics

Postnatal depression (PND), since it was first coined as a term, has been poorly defined; now with the increasing evidence that at least some cases commence antenatally, it is also misleading. Both are perhaps better referred to as perinatal depression, although in many cases anxiety is a major feature. In most research, postnatal depression is restricted to those depressive illnesses commencing within 3 months postpartum, but other criteria include the whole first postnatal year.

Interest in this disorder originated from a belief that depression had a marked increase in prevalence at this time (Kendall *et al.,* 1987), of the order of 13% (O'Hara & Swain, 1996). More recently it has been noted that mood and anxiety disorders may actually begin antenatally, with a similar prevalence (12%; Bennett *et al.,* 2004). This has particular relevance because depression and anxiety in pregnancy have been linked to an increase in preterm deliveries and other obstetric complications (Dayan *et al.,* 2002) as well as high cortisol levels in infants at birth (O'Connor *et al.,* 2002).

It is important to differentiate PND from the more common adjustment symptoms, affecting some 30% of women (Dennerstein *et al.,* 1989); blurring of these disorders is frequent both clinically and in research, particularly if only a screening tool is used rather than a diagnostic interview.

In practice the presentation of PND is similar to depression at other times, but with an arguably greater difficulty of recognition because of symptoms being put down to those of pregnancy or sleep deprivation, as well as the reluctance of women to accept this diagnosis at a time that is expected to be positive. Presentation may thus be for infant-related concerns such as colic or sleep problems rather than maternal mood per se. In addition, anxiety is a common and often dominant symptom and again may be infant focused. This infant focus is thought to be somewhat protective against suicide, which is lower than in depressed patients who are not postpartum (Appleby, 1991).

Those women with pre-existing disorders—particularly affective and bipolar disorders—are at risk for exacerbation and recurrence of their illness in the postpartum period, and extra vigilance is required on the part of clinicians involved with their care.

Psychosis

Characteristics

One in 600 women will suffer a psychotic episode postpartum, known as puerperal or postpartum psychosis. This usually occurs within the first week to month postpartum and is classically described as an affective psychosis but with confusion commonly associated. It is thought to be a variant of bipolar disorder, with a risk of developing a recurrence of 50% to 70% (Pfuhlmann *et al.,* 2002). Unlike postnatal depression, there is a significant risk of suicide, and the infant might also be at risk.

Those women with pre-existing bipolar disorder are at a high risk of relapse postpartum, even if treatment with mood stabilisers is maintained (Yonkers *et al.,* 2004). This risk is probably also higher for those women with schizoaffective disorder but not in schizophrenia, providing medication is maintained.

Women with active psychotic illnesses may not recognise their pregnancy or signs of labour. Incorporating their unborn children into delusions is not uncommon. Women with schizophrenia are also reported to have higher rates of domestic violence oriented towards the abdomen, high rates of smoking and are less likely to seek antenatal care (Mowbray *et al.,* 1995).

Treatment issues

Issues for the mother

Biological

There are a few studies looking specifically at the use of biological treatments in postnatal illnesses; in general, treatment is the same as for depression, anxiety and psychosis at other times. The effect on the infant must be considered in pregnant and lactating women, considered later in the chapter. This is of considerable concern to many women, who are reluctant to consider medication at this time (Buist, 2004; Buist *et al.*, 2002) and may affect recognition and willingness to seek treatment, as well as compliance.

When medication is required through pregnancy, metabolic rate and renal clearance alter, and thus doses of medication may need to be altered accordingly. Of those antidepressants studied in perinatal depression, fluoxetine, sertraline and venlafaxine appear to be effective (Appleby *et al.*, 1997; Cohen *et al.*, 2001; Stowe & Nemeroff, 1995). Of note, possibly because of the high level of anxiety or the ongoing nature of the stress of child care postpartum, it may be that response is slower, and higher dosages may be required (Hendrick *et al.*, 2000). Reed *et al.* (1999) reviewed the use of electroconvulsive therapy in postpartum psychosis and found it to be an effective treatment.

Postpartum psychosis as a variant of bipolar disorder may require a mood stabiliser. Ideally for those with a previous history, the pregnancy will be planned carefully and an individual plan made with the woman and her partner, balancing the risks and benefits to mother and child. Sleep deprivation may be particularly important as a precipitant and should where possible be avoided in the early postpartum phase, by use of sedation and a family member caring for the child overnight.

Psychosocial

Whether causal, precipitant or perpetuating, the woman's psychosocial world changes markedly after having a baby, and her psychological response to these changes is important to explore. Women from abusive backgrounds and poor parenting role models may have particular struggles and anxieties that medication alone will not deal with. Common themes include awareness of their own vulnerability as experienced via the child, loss of control and feelings of failure; levels of support and whether the infant was wanted will have significant impact on this transition. Supportive therapy, cognitive-behavioural therapy and groups have all been shown to be effective (Newport *et al.*, 2002); some women will need intensive longer-term input.

Practical supports such as child care are particularly important; many women feel guilty, but this break can allow them time and space to recover parts of themself that often feel lost.

Issues for the father

In the Western world, men who become fathers are at increased risk for stress; gender stereotypes have undergone considerable change, and as a result it seems that many men experience confusion (Morse *et al.*, 2000). They may be subject to the same stresses that have contributed to their wife's illness such as financial difficulties or a death in the family. If in addition their wife is depressed, this can increase stress levels and contribute to depression. If there were already marital problems, the birth of a child and depression escalate the difficulties. Involving the partner in treatment is important – at the minimum, helping him understand his wife's illness is essential. Dealing with his own issues or those of the relationship are also important to consider.

Issues for the foetus and infant

Perinatal mental illness has particular implications for the infant. These are summarised in Table 19.2.

The mother is traditionally responsible for child care; depressed mothers may have particular problems in mothering. Follow-up studies have suggested that these children are at an increased

Table 19.2 Issues for the foetus / infant

In utero

Maternal anxiety

– Effects on foetal neuroendocrine axis

Psychosis

– Decreased antenatal care
– Increased domestic violence
– Increased smoking

Medication

– First trimester: teratogenicity
– Third trimester: withdrawal at birth
– Any time: unknown effects, nb on neural
  development

Postpartum

Depression

– Restricted affect and play, role model of decreased
  ways of dealing with adversity

Psychosis

– incorporation into delusion
– inability to meet needs
– poor eye contact, decreased play

Medication in breast milk

– Side effects
– Anytime: unknown effects, notably on neural
  development

---

risk of cognitive delays and behavioural problems, although the relative importance of antenatal or early postnatal depression, ongoing or current depression is unclear (Beck, 1998; Murray & Cooper, 1997). This has potential ongoing importance for mental health, with differing gender implications. Boys appear to be at risk for attention-deficit/hyperactivity and conduct disorders, reacting to maternal unavailability with anger, whereas girls become withdrawn and appear to mirror their mother's illness (Grace *et al.,* 2003; Murray *et al.,* 1996). In both cases, the children appear to have impaired coping skills in dealing with adversity.

Psychotic illnesses at this time raise other considerations; initially the main concern is one of safety for the mother and child. In a majority of cases, women with active psychosis need hospitalization and assessment of risk in a secure setting, preferably a specialised mother-baby unit. With

the resolution of psychotic symptoms, women with postpartum psychosis often lack confidence, but with support they are generally able to parent normally.

Women with more chronic illnesses need special considerations regarding safety. Studies suggest a number of problems for parenting in women with schizophrenia, as outlined in Table 19.2. The infant's father and extended family are important to include in consideration of how best to meet the child's needs. Chronicity of illness, compliance and insight and supports are key indicators of whether women with schizophrenia will be able to parent safely and effectively. Lack of a partner and support with a maternal diagnosis of schizophrenia increases the chances of infants needing to be separated from their mother (Buist *et al.,* 2004). Infanticide is rare, but the first year – and particularly the first day of life – are the times of highest risk of murder and abuse (Craig, 2004).

A relatively rare denial of pregnancy and subsequent neonaticide has also been recorded. Although some of these cases are related to psychotic illnesses, a majority appear to be due to a dissociative disorder in young women who have often had poor sex education and come from somewhat rigid and moral families (Sadoft, 1995). Other parental issues that need consideration in cases of infanticide include drug abuse and personality disorders; with older children the de facto partners are the more frequent offenders.

Limited studies have looked at intervention for the mother-infant relationship; although maternal mood is improved by a number of modalities, changing the mother-infant interaction may be more resistant (Murray *et al.,* 1996), possibly because those women from abusive backgrounds and poor role models are most at risk and require more intensive reparenting themselves (Buist, 1998).

Particular risks of medication to the foetus are summarised in Table 19.3. As a general principle, risks of treatment versus nontreatment to infant and mother need to be weighed up and discussed with the parents and appropriate others. It is also

Table 19.3 Medications in pregnancy and lactation

Type of medication	Pregnancy	Lactation
SSRIs	• Possible heart defects (conflicting evidence) linked to paroxetine (Cole *et al.*, 2007; Einarson *et al.*, 2008) • Most information on fluoxetine; associated with increased risk of prematurity (Pastuszak *et al.*, 1993) • Increasing information on sertraline; lower placental transfer (Hendrick *et al.*, 2003) • Some irritability at soft neurological change at birth and early postpartum; unclear significance (Zeskind & Stephens, 2004) • Breastmilk has double the plasma levels but minimal absorbed • Possible pulmonary hypertension (Chambers *et al.*, 2006)	
Tricyclics	Not teratogenic, no apparent problems	• Case reports of sedation • No apparent long term implications
SNRIs	Inadequate data	• Appear to be significantly higher in breast milk than SSRIs (Ilett *et al.*, 1998)
Other newer generation antidepressants	Inadequate data	Inadequate data
Typical antipsychotics	Limited data; irritability at birth	Limited data, no known difficulties
Atypical antipsychotics	Inadequate data	• Reversible blood dyscrasia on clozapine • Others appear not to be actively excreted in breast milk with low exposure to infant
Benzodiazepines	High doses of diazepam associated with cleft palate	Sedation, potential learning difficulties
Mood Stabilisers	Lithium, carbamazepine and sodium valproate all teratogenic; lithium least (0.1%), valproate worst (>5%) (Yonkers *et al.*, 2004)	Infant needs close monitoring, advised not to breast-feed on lithium.

SNRI = serotonin and norepinephrine reuptake inhibitor; SSRI = selective serotonin reuptake inhibitor.

important to consider specific strategies, including minimizing medication dosage and reducing polypharmacy. Particular caution should be exerted in premature or unwell infants.

Psychiatric disorders associated with menopause

Women in the Western world are living longer and are consequently spending more of their lives postmenopause. By 2050, 30% of the population in Western Europe will be over 65 years old, and the majority will be women. *Menopause* is the point in women's lives when menstruation stops completely, attributable to the loss of ovarian function. It is preceded by the *perimenopause* during which menstrual cycles become irregular and frequently anovulatory. Physical symptoms associated with the menopause include hot flushes, night sweats and vaginal dryness. It is widely accepted that these are directly related to reduced levels of circulating ovarian steroids, especially oestrogen, and oestrogen therapy has become the first-line treatment over the past couple of decades. Oestrogen therapy has also been used in the management of psychological/psychiatric and cognitive symptoms associated with the menopause. However, it has been argued that these symptoms may be more related to comorbid physical and psychosocial factors rather than the effects of ovarian failure (McKinlay *et al.,* 1987).

Diagnostic considerations

Mood disorders

Characteristics

Cross-sectional studies carried out on small clinical samples in menopause clinics report high levels of depressive symptoms among postmenopausal women (Hay *et al.,* 1994; Stewart *et al.,* 1992). These findings have not, however, been supported by the majority of epidemiological studies in the general population, and some studies report that depression may be less common postmenopause (Dennerstein *et al.,* 1993; Gath *et al.,* 1987; Hallstrom & Samuelson, 1985; Holte, 1992; Hunter, 1992; Oldenhave *et al.,* 1993). The Massachusetts Women's Health Study (MWHS; Avis *et al.,* 1994), one of the largest population-based longitudinal studies of middle-aged women, found a transitory increase in depression around the time of the perimenopause, which declines postmenopause. It has been suggested that women who suffer from the effects of fluctuating ovarian steroid levels at other times (e.g. premenstruation) may be more vulnerable during the perimenopausal transition (Novaes *et al.,* 1998). One recent study, for example, reported that acute ovarian suppression led to hypomania or depression in women who had previously been diagnosed with postnatal depression (Bloch *et al.,* 2000). However, other authors argue that mood symptoms during this transition may be attributable to comorbid physical and psychosocial factors rather than the direct effects of ovarian failure (McKinlay *et al.,* 1987).

Schizophrenia

Characteristics

Onset of schizophrenia in women peaks between 15 and 30 years with a second peak at the time of perimenopause between 45 and 49 years. These findings have been replicated across a variety of cultures and in both rural and urban settings (Castle & Murray RM, 1993; Jablensky *et al.,* 1992). There is a high degree of overlap in the clinical symptoms of schizophrenia between the genders; however, women are generally reported to present with a less severe form of schizophrenia, with more affective symptoms but fewer negative symptoms and fewer hospitalisations (Leung & Chue, 2000). These issues are discussed in more detail in Chapter 13.

Alzheimer's dementia

Characteristics

The population of the Western world is aging, and if recent trends continue, the number of patients with Alzheimer's dementia (AD) will nearly quadruple in the next 50 years (Brookmeyer *et al.,* 1998). Being female is a risk factor for AD (Andersen *et al.,* 1999). The cumulative risk for 65-year-old women to develop AD at age 95 years is more than twice that of men (Leon *et al.,* 1998). Histopathologic diagnosis of AD requires identification of neurofibrillary tangles and β-amyloid plaques in excess of the amounts expected to occur in age-matched healthy individuals. Animal models suggest that loss of ovarian function at the time of menopause may contribute to the pathology of AD. Ovariectomy in guinea pigs, for example, has been associated with an average 1.5-fold increase in brain β-amyloid levels compared with levels in intact animals (Petanceska *et al.,* 2000).

Treatment issues

Mood disorders

Biological

Several studies report a lack of significant difference between oestrogen and placebo in treating perimenopausal or early postmenopausal mood symptoms (Campbell & Whitehead, 1977; Cooper, 1981; Pearce *et al.*, 1997). However, two recent studies report an improvement in perimenopausal depression in women prescribed oestrogen (Schmidt & Rubinow, 1991; Soares *et al.*, 2001). The largest of these studies (Soares *et al.*, 2001) investigated the use of transdermal 17β-estradiol in a double-blind, placebo-controlled study. At the end of the treatment period, symptoms of depression in the oestradiol group were significantly lower than those for the placebo group. However, at the end of the study, women in the oestradiol group also had a significant reduction in menopausal symptoms (e.g. vasomotor symptoms, joint pain, sleep disturbance, headache) than women in the placebo group. It is therefore unclear whether improvements in depressive symptoms were attributable to direct antidepressant effects of oestrogen or due to the indirect effect of improvements in menopausal symptoms. Despite some evidence that oestrogen may have beneficial effects in the treatment of perimenopausal depression, antidepressant medication is still recommended as the first line of pharmacological treatment in depressed peri- and postmenopausal women.

Psychosocial

The time of menopause frequently represents a time of change in women's lives (e.g. children leaving home, problems with physical health). Treatment of depression at this time therefore needs to maintain a holistic approach. Identifying psychosocial factors that may be precipitating or perpetuating the depressive episode is an important part of management.

Schizophrenia

Biological

Oestrogens have been reported to modulate the sensitivity of the dopaminergic system in animals (Di Paolo, 1994) and humans (Craig *et al.*, 2004). An early report suggested that premenopausal women required lower maintenance doses of antipsychotic medication than their male counterparts, whereas after the age of 40, women required higher dosages than men (Seeman, 1983). Although this finding was not replicated in a later study (Salokangas, 1995), a small community study of postmenopausal women with schizophrenia who either had received or had never received oestrogen therapy found that the former group required lower average daily dosages of antipsychotic medication and had significantly less severe negative symptoms (but not positive symptoms) than the control subjects, independent of differences in antipsychotic dosage (Lindamer *et al.*, 2001). Future studies need to assess whether there is a role of for adjunct oestrogen therapy in some women using larger prospective randomised controlled study designs.

Considering antipsychotic treatment itself, atypical antipsychotics are recommended as first line in older women with schizophrenia for similar reasons as in younger premenopausal women (e.g. fewer extrapyramidal side effects) and should be offered where possible (Bouman & Pinner, 2002).

Psychosocial

Cognitive-behavioural therapy, social skills training, case management and caregiver supports are as important in postmenopausal women as they are in younger women and should form part of the treatment package.

Alzheimer's disease

Drugs used to treat AD can be broadly divided into (1) cholinergic enhancing agents, (2) antioxidants, (3) anti-inflammatory agents, (4) oestrogens and (5) miscellaneous "natural" agents (e.g. *Ginkgo biloba* alkaloids) with at least 60 drugs currently estimated to be in development including vaccines against β-amyloid plaques (Leonard, 2004). Cholinergic-enhancing drugs remain the first line of treatment, as discussed in Chapter 15. However, oestrogen replacement has been an area of growing interest since the mid-1990s in the prevention and treatment of AD in postmenopausal women. Thus several small, short-duration studies (Asthana *et al.,* 2001) suggest that oestrogen might benefit AD symptoms. However, larger studies of longer duration (Henderson *et al.,* 2000; Mulnard *et al.,* 2000) evaluated the effect of oestrogen on cognition in women with mild to moderate dementia and did not show a beneficial effect.

The most recent meta-analysis of observational studies on use of combined oestrogen/progesterone or unopposed oestrogen therapy indicated a 34% decreased risk of AD for healthy postmenopausal women who used oestrogen compared with women who had not (Le Blanc *et al.,* 2001). These findings have, however, not been supported by the recent Women's Health Initiative Memory Study (WHIMS; Shumaker *et al.,* 2003, 2004). In that study, 7,510 women over age 65 were randomised depending on their uterine status; 4,563 women with an intact uterus were randomised to "combined" oestrogen (conjugated equine estrogens [CEE] plus medroxyprogesterone acetate [MPA]) or placebo. In contrast 2,947 women with a previous hysterectomy were randomised to receive "unopposed" oestrogen (CEE) or placebo. Among women with an intact uterus, 61 were diagnosed with probable dementia; 40 of 2,229 women (1.8%) in the CEE/MPA group and 21 of 2,303 women (0.9%) in the placebo group. Thus the rate of women experiencing probable dementia in the CEE/MPA group was double that of the placebo group (hazard ratio [HR]: 2.05; 95% confidence interval [CI]: 1.21–3.48; 45 vs. 22 per 10,000 person years, $p = 0.01$). There was, however, no statistically significant difference in the risk of being diagnosed with AD. The CEE alone arm did not show a significant increase in all-cause dementia or AD. After an average 5 years of treatment, there were 37 cases of all-cause dementia per 10,000 person years in the treatment group compared with 25 in the placebo group (HR = 1.49; 95% CI = 0.83–2.66, $p = 0.18$). Because early postmenopausal women were not included in the study, it is unclear whether these results can be applied to women who take hormone therapy earlier in their menopause. Furthermore, some studies suggest a time window during early menopause when hormone therapy must be started to have a neuroprotective effect against AD

(Zandi, *et al.,* 2002), and if therapy is started after this time (e.g. as in WHIMS), it may be less likely to have any benefit.

In summary, research suggests oestrogens may have some benefit in the prevention of AD if prescribed in the immediate period post-menopause.

Conclusions

Research has yet to provide conclusive evidence for any one factor as the key to the higher incidence of many mental illnesses in women. The reasons appear to be complex, with a multifactorial interplay of genetic predisposition, intrauterine exposure, exposure to stress in childhood and later psychosocial issues. For the treating clinician, the key factors to consider are those that can be ameliorated with biological or psychosocial interventions (or both), with particular consideration for the potential longitudinal course the illness may take and the impact it may have on a woman's children.

REFERENCES

Altshuler, L., Cohen, L., Moline, M., *et al.* (2001). *Treatment of Depression in Women 2001.* McGraw-Hill.

Alvir, J., & Thys-Jacobs, S. (1991). Premenstrual and menstrual symptom clusters and response to calcium treatment. *Psychopharmacol Bull* **27**:145–8.

American Psychiatric Association (1996). *Violence and the Family. Report of the American Psychological Presidential Task Force in Violence and the Family.* 10. Washington, DC: American Psychiatric Association.

Andersen, K., Nielsen, H., Lolk, A., *et al.* (1999). Incidence of very mild to severe Dementia and Alzheimer's Disease in Denmark: the Odense Study. *Neurology* **52**:85–90.

Appleby, L. (1991). Suicide during pregnancy and in the first postnatal year. *BMJ* **302**:137–40.

Appleby, L., Warner, R., Whitton, A., *et al.* (1997). A controlled study of fluoxetine and cognitive-behavioural counselling in the treatment of postnatal depression. *BMJ* **314**:932–6.

Ashman, S. B., Dawson, G., Panagiotides, H., *et al.* (2002). Stress hormone levels of children of depressed mothers. *Dev Psychopathol* **14**:333–49.

Asthana, S., Baker, L., Craft, S., *et al.* (2001). High-dose estradiol improves cognition for women with AD: results of a randomized study. *Neurology* 57:605–12.

Avis, N., Brambilla, D., McKinlay, S., *et al.* (1994). A longitudinal analysis of the association between menopause and depression. Results from the Massachusetts Women's Health Study. *Ann Epidemiol* 4:214–20.

Bancroft, J., Cook, A., Davidson, D., *et al.* (1991). Blunting of neuroendocrine responses to infusion of L-tryptophan in women with perimenstrual mood change. *Psychol Med* 21:305–12.

Beck, C. T. (1998). The effects of postpartum depression on child development: a meta-analysis. *Arch Psychiatr Nurs* 1:12–20.

Bennett, H. A., Einarson, A., Taddio, A., *et al.* (2004). Prevalence of depression during pregnancy: systematic review. *Obstet Gynecol* 103:698–709.

Bicikova, M., Dibbelt, L., Hill, M., *et al.* (1998). Allopreg nanolone in women with premenstrual syndrome. *Horm Metab Res* 30:227–30.

Bloch, M., Daly, R. C., & Rubinow, D. R. (2003). Endocrine factors in the etiology of postpartum depression. *Compr Psychiatry* 44:234–46.

Bloch, M., Schmidt, P. J., Danaceau, M., *et al.* (2000). Effects of gonadal steroids in women with a history of postpartum depression. *Am J Psychiatry* 157:924 30.

Borenstein, J., Dean, B., Endicott, J., *et al.* (2003). Health and economic impact of the premenstrual syndrome. *J Reprod Med* 48:515–24.

Bouman, W., & Pinner, G. (2002). Use of atypical antipsychotic drugs in old age psychiatry. *Adv Psychiatr Treat* 8:49–58.

Boyce, P., Parker, G., Barnett, B., *et al.* (1991). Personality as a vulnerability factor to depression. *Br J Psychiatry* 159:106–14.

Brookmeyer, R., Gray, S., & Kawas, C. (1998). Projections of Alzheimer's disease in the United States and the public health impact of delaying disease onset. *Am J Public Health* 88:1337–42.

Buist, A. (1998). Childhood sexual abuse, postpartum depression and parenting difficulties. *Aust N Z J Psychiatry* 32:479–87.

Buist, A. (2004). The use of antidepressants in pregnant and breastfeeding women. In preparation.

Buist, A., Barnett, B., Milgrom, J., *et al.* (2002). To screen or not to screen – that is the question in perinatal depression. *Med J Aust* 177(Suppl):S101–S105.

Buist, A., Minto, B., Szego, K., *et al.* (2004). Mother-baby psychiatric units in Australia – the Victorian experience. *Arch Women Health* 7:81–7.

Burnet, R., Radden, H., Easterbrook, E., *et al.* (1991). Premenstrual syndrome and spironolactone. *Aust N Z J Obstetr Gynaecol* 31:366–8.

Campbell, S., & Whitehead, M. (1977). Oestrogen therapy and the menopause syndrome. *Clin Obstetr Gynecol* 4:31–47.

Castle, D., & Murray, R. M. (1993). The epidemiology of late-onset schizophrenia. *Schizophr Bull* 19:691–700.

Chambers, C. D., Hernandez-Diaz, S., Van Marter, L. J., *et al.* (2006). Selective serotonin-reuptake inhibitors and risk of persistent pulmonary hypertension of the newborn. *N Engl J Med* 354:579–87.

Cohen, L., Miner, C., Brown, E., *et al.* (2002). Premenstrual daily fluoxetine for premenstrual dysphoric disorder. a placebo-controlled, clinical trial using computerized diaries. *Obstetr Gynecol* 100:135 44.

Cohen, L. S., Viguera, A. C., Bouffard, S. M., *et al.* (2001). Venlafaxine in the treatment of postpartum depression. *J Clin Psychiatry* 62:592–6.

Cole, J., Ephross, S., Cosmatos, I., & Walker, A. (2007). Paroxetine in the first trimester and the prevalence of congenital malformations. *Pharmacoepidemiol Drug Saf* 16:1075–85.

Cooper, J. (1981). Is oestrogen therapy effective in the treatment of menopausal depression. *J Royal Coll Gen Practit* 31:134–40.

Craig, M. (2004). Perinatal risk factors for neonaticide and infant homicide: can we identify those at risk? *J Royal Soc Med* 97:57–61.

Craig, M., Cutter, W., Wickham, H., *et al.* (2004). Effect of long-term estrogen therapy on dopaminergic responsivity in postmenopausal women. *Psychoneuroendocrinology* 29:1309–16.

Dayan, J., Creveuil, C., Herlicoviez, M., *et al.* (2002). Role of anxiety and depression in the onset of spontaneous preterm labour. *Am J Epidemiol* 155:292–301.

Dennerstein, L. (2001). Factors contributing to positive mood during the menopausal transition. *J Nerv Ment Dis* 189:84–9.

Dennerstein, L., Guthrie, J., Clark, M., *et al.* (2004). A population based study of depressed mood in middle-aged, Australian-born women. *Menopause* 11:563–8.

Dennerstein, L., Lehert, P., Burger, H., *et al.* (1999). Mood and the menopausal transition. *J Nerv Ment Dis* 187:685–91.

Dennerstein, L., Lehert, P., & Riphagen, F. (1989). Post-partum depression – risk factors. *J Psychosom Obstetr Gynaecol* (Suppl 10):53–65.

Dennerstein, L., Smith, A., Morse, C., *et al.* (1993). Menopausal symptoms in Australian Women. *Med J Aust* **159**:232.

Dennerstein, L., & Spencer-Gardner, C. (1983). The menstrual cycle and mood changes. In D. Burrows, ed. *Handbook of Psychosomatic Obstetrics and Gynaecology*. Melbourne: Elsevier Biomedical Press, pp. 149–70.

Deuster, P., Adera, T., South-Paul, J., *et al.* (1999). Biological, social and behavioural factors associated with premenstrual syndrome. *Arch Fam Med* **8**:122–8.

Di Paolo, T. (1994). Modulation of brain dopamine transmission by sex steroids. *Rev Neurosci* **5**:27–41.

Dimmock, P., Wyatt, K., Jones, P., *et al.* (2000). Efficacy of selective serotonin-reuptake inhibitors in premenstrual syndrome: a systematic review. *Lancet* **356**:1131–6.

Einarson, A., Pistellis, A., DeSantis, M., *et al.* (2008). Evaluation of the risk of congenital cardiovascular defects associated with use of Paroxetine during pregnancy. *Am J Psychiatry (Adv AiA)* (online: ajp.psychiatryonline.org): 1–5.

Epperson, N., Haga, K., Mason, G., *et al.* (2002). Cortical GABA levels across the menstrual cycle in healthy women and those with premenstrual dysphoric disorder: a proton magnetic resonance spectroscopy study. *Arch Gen Psychiatry* **59**:851–85.

Eriksson, E., Hedberg, M. A., Andersch, B., *et al.* (1995). The serotonin reuptake inhibitor paroxetine is superior to the noradrenaline reuptake inhibitor maprotiline in the treatment of premenstrual syndrome. *Neuropsychopharmacology* **12**:167–76.

Fitzgerald, M., Malone, K., Li, S., *et al.* (1997). Blunted serotonin response to fenfluramine challenge in premenstrual dysphoric disorder. *Am J Psychiatry* **154**: 556–8.

Freeman, E., Kroll, R., Rapkin, A., *et al.* (2001). Evaluation of a unique oral contraceptive in the treatment of premenstrual dysphoric disorder. *J Women Health Gender Based Med* **10**:561–9.

Freeman, E., Rickels, K., Sondheimer, S., *et al.* (1995). A double-blind trial of oral progesterone, alprazolam, and placebo in treatment of severe premenstrual syndrome. *JAMA* **274**:51–7.

Freeman, E., Rickels, K., Sondheimer, S., *et al.* (1999). Differential response to antidepressants in women with premenstrual syndrome/premenstrual dysphoric disorder: a randomized controlled trial. *Arch Gen Psychiatry* **56**:932–9.

Freeman, E., Rickels, K., Sondheimer, S., *et al.* (2004). Continuous or intermittent dosing with sertraline for patients with severe premenstrual syndrome or premenstrual dysphoric disorder. *Am J Psychiatry* **161**:343–51.

Freeman, E., Stout, A., Endicott J, *et al.* (2002). Treatment of premenstrual syndrome with a carbohydrate-rich beverage. *Int J Gynecol Obstetr* **77**:253–4.

Freeman, E. W., Sondheimer, S. J., Polansky, M., *et al.* (2000). Predictors of response to sertraline treatment of severe premenstrual syndromes. *J Clin Psychiatry* **61**:579–84.

Gath, D., Osborn, M., Bungay, G., *et al.* (1987). Psychiatric disorder and gynaecological symptoms in middle aged women: a community survey. *BMJ* **294**:213–18.

Girdler, S., Straneva, P., Light, K., *et al.* (2001). Allopregnanolone levels and reactivity to mental stress in premenstrual dysphoric disorder. *Biol Psychiatry* **49**:788–97.

Glover, V., & O'Connor, T. G. (2002). Effects of antenatal stress and anxiety. *Br J Psychiatry* **180**:389–91.

Grace, S. L., Evindar, A., & Stewart, D. E. (2003). The effect of postpartum depression on child cognitive development and behaviour: a review and critical analysis of the literature. *Arch Women Ment Health* **6**:263–74.

Graham, C., & Sherwin, B. (1992). A prospective treatment study of premenstrual symptoms using a triphasic oral contraceptive. *J Psychosom Res* **36**:257–66.

Halbreich, U., & Smoller, J. W. (1997). Intermittent luteal phase sertraline treatment of dysphoric premenstrual syndrome. *J Clin Psychol* **58**:399–402.

Halbreich, U., Bergeron, R., Yonkers, K., *et al.* (2002). Efficacy of intermittent, luteal phase sertraline treatment of premenstrual dysphoric disorder. *Obstetr Gynecol* **100**:1219–29.

Halbreich, U., Petty, F., Yonkers, K., *et al.* (1996). Low plasma y-aminobutyric acid levels during the late luteal phase of women with premenstrual dysphoric disorder. *Am J Psychiatry* **153**:718–20.

Halbreich, U., & Tworek, H. (1993). Altered serotonergic activity in women with dysphoric premenstrual syndromes. *Int J Psychiatry Med* **23**:1–27.

Hallstrom, T., & Samuelson, S. (1985). Mental health in the climacteric. The longitudinal study of women in Gothenburg. *Acta Obstetr Gynaecol Scand Suppl* **130**:13–18.

Hargrove, J., & Abraham, G. (1982). The incidence of premenstrual tension in gynecologic clinic. *J Reprod Med* **27**:721–4.

Harrison, W., Endicott, J., Rabkin, J., *et al.* (1987). *Treatment of Premenstrual Dysphoria with Alprazolam and Placebo*. Paper presented at the Psychopharmacology Bulletin.

Hay, A., Bancroft J., & Johnstone, E. (1994). Affective symptoms in women attending a menopause clinic. *Br J Psychiatry* **164**:513–16.

Heath, A., Yonkers, K., Orsulak, P., *et al.* (1998). *Tryptophan Depletion in Premenstrual Dysphoric Disorder*. Paper presented at the Society of Biological Psychiatry 1998 Annual Meeting and Scientific Program.

Hellberg, D., Claesson, B., & Nilsson, S. (1991). Premenstrual tension: a placebo-controlled efficacy study with spironolactone and medroxyprogesterone acetate. *Int J Gynaecol Obstetr* **34**:243–8.

Henderson, V., Paganini-Hill, A., Miller, B., *et al.* (2000). Estrogen for Alzheimer's disease in women. Randomized, double-blind, placebo-controlled trial. *Neurology* **54**:295–301.

Hendrick, V., Altshuler, L., Strouse, T., *et al.* (2000). Postpartum and nonpostpartum depression: differences in presentation and response to pharmacological treatment. *Depress Anxiety* **11**:66–72.

Hendrick, V., Stowe, Z. N., Altshuler, L. L., *et al.* (2003). Placental passage of antidepressant medications. *Am J Psychiatry* **160**:993–6.

Holte, A. (1992). Influences of natural menopause on health complaints: a prospective study of Norwegian women. *Maturitas* **14**:127–41.

Hunter, M. (1992). The South East England longitudinal study of the climacteric and postmenopause. *Maturitas* **14**:17–26.

Ilett, K. F., Hackett, L. P., Dusci, L. J., *et al.* (1998). Distribution and excretion of venlafaxine and O-desmethylvenlafaxine in human milk. *Br J Clin Pharmacol* **45**:459–62.

Jablensky, A., Sartorius, N., & Ernberg, G. (1992). Schizophrenia: manifestations, incidence and course in different cultures. A World Health Organisation Ten-Country Study. *Psychol Med Monogr* **20**.

Jermain, D., Preece, C., Sykes, R., *et al.* (1999). Luteal phase sertraline treatment for premenstrual dysphoric disorder: results of a double-blind, placebo-controlled, crossover study. *Arch Fam Med* **8**:328–32.

Johnson, S., McChesner, C., & Bean, J. (1988). Epidemiology of premenstrual symptoms in a nonclinical sample. I. Prevalence, natural history and help-seeking behaviour. *J Reprod Med* **33**:340–6.

Kendall, R. E., Chalmers, J. C., & Platz, C. (1987). Epidemiology of puerperal psychosis. *Br J Psychiatry* **150**:662–73.

Kendler, K., Kessler, R., Neale, M., *et al.* (1993). The prediction of major depression in women: toward an integrated etiopic model. *Am J Psychiatry* **150**:1139–48.

Kendler, K., Neale, M., Kessler, R., *et al.* (1992a). A population based twin study of major depression in women. *Arch Gen Psychiatry* **49**:257–66.

Kendler, K., Silberg, J., Neale, M., *et al.* (1992b). Genetic and environmental factors in the etiology of menstrual, premenstrual and neurotic symptoms: a population based twin study. *Pscyhol Med* **22**:85–100.

Kessel, N., & Cantab, M. (1963). The prevalence of common menstrual symptoms. *Lancet* 61–4.

Landen, M., Sorvik, K., Ysander, C., *et al.* (2002). *A Placebo-Controlled Trial Exploring the Efficacy of Paroxetine for the Treatment of Premenstrual Dysphoria*. Paper presented at the American Psychiatric Association meeting, Philadelphia, PA.

Le Blanc, E., Janowsky, J., Chan, B., *et al.* (2001). Hormone Replacement Therapy and cognition: systematic review and meta-analysis. *JAMA* **285**:1489–99.

Leon, J., Cheng, C., & Neumann, P. (1998). Alzheimer's disease care: costs and potential savings. *Health Affairs* **17**:206–16.

Leonard, B. (2004). Pharmacotherapy in the treatment of Alzheimer's disease: an update. *World Psychiatry* **3**:84–8.

Leung, A., & Chue, P. (2000). Sex differences in schizophrenia: a review of the literature. *Acta Psychiatr Scand Suppl* **401**:3–38.

Lindamer, L., Buse, D., Lohr, J., *et al.* (2001). Hormone replacement therapy in postmenopausal women with schizophrenia: positive effect on negative symptoms. *Biol Psychiatry* **49**:47–51.

McKinlay, J., McKinlay, S., & Brambilla, D. (1987). The relative contributions of endocrine changes and social circumstances to depression in mid-aged women. *J Health Soc Behav* **28**:345–63.

Menkes, D., Coates, D., & Fawsett, J. (1994). Acute tryptophan depletion aggravates premenstrual syndrome. *J Affect Disord* **32**:37–44.

Menkes, D., Taghavi, E., Mason, P., *et al.* (1992). Fluoxetine treatment of severe premenstrual syndrome. *BMJ* **305**:346–7.

Miner, C., Brown, E., McCray, S., *et al.* (2002). Weekly luteal phase dosing with enteric-coated fluoxetine 90 mg in premenstrual dysphoric disorder: a randomized, double-blind, placebo-controlled clinical trial. *Clin Ther* **24**:417–33.

Montelone, P., Luisi, S., Tonetti, A., *et al.* (2000). Allopregnanolone concentrations and premenstrual syndrome. *Eur J Endocrinol* **142**:269–73.

Morse, C., Buist, A., & Durkin, S. (2000). First time parenthood: influences on pre and postnatal adjustment in fathers and mothers. *J Psychosom Gynechol* **21**:109–20.

Morse, C., Dennerstein, L., Farrell, E., *et al.* (1991). A comparison of hormone therapy, coping skills training and relaxation for the relief of premenstrual syndrome. *J Behav Med* **14**:469–89.

Mowbray, C. T., Oyserman, D., Zemencuk, J. K., *et al.* (1995). Motherhood for women with serious mental illness: pregnancy, childbirth and the postpartum period. *Am J Orthopsychiatry* **65**:21–38.

Mulnard, R., Cotman, C., Kawas, C., *et al.* (2000). Estrogen replacement therapy for treatment of mild to moderate Alzheimer disease: a randomized controlled trial. *JAMA* **283**:1007–15.

Murray, L., & Cooper, P. J. (1997). Effects of postnatal depression on infant development. *Arch Dis Child* **77**:99–101.

Murray, L., Fiori, C., Hooper, R., *et al.* (1996). The impact of postnatal depression and associated adversity on early infant interactions and later infant outcome. *Child Dev* **67**:2512–16.

Murray, L., Hipwell, A., Hooper, R., *et al.* (1996). The cognitive development of five year old children of postnatally depressed mothers. *J Child Psychol Psychiatry* **37**:927–36.

Newport, D. J., Stowe, Z. N., & Nemeroff, C. B. (2002). Parental depression: animal models of an adverse life event. *Am J Psychiatry* **159**:1265–83.

Novaes, C., Almeida, O., & de Melo, N. (1998). Mental health among perimenopausal women attending a menopause clinic: possible association with premenstrual syndrome? *Climacteric* **1**:264–70.

O'Brien, P., Craven, D., Selby, C., *et al.* (1979). Treatment of premenstrual syndrome by spironolactone. *Br J Obstetr Gynaecol* **86**:142–7.

O'Connor, T., Ben-Shlomo, Y., Heron, J., *et al.* (2005). Prenatal anxiety predicts individual differences in cortisol in pre-adolescent children. *Biol Psychiatry* **58**:211–17.

O'Connor, T., Heron, J., Golding, J., *et al.* (2002). Antenatal anxiety predicts child behavioural/emotional problems independently of postnatal depression. *J Am Acad Child Adolesc Psychiatry* **41**:1470–7.

O'Connor, T. G., Heron, J., Golding, J., *et al.* (2002). Maternal prenatal anxiety and children's behavioural/emotional problems at 4 years. *Br J Psychiatry* **180**:502–8.

O'Hara, M. W., & Swain, A. M. (1996). Rates and risk of postpartum depression – a meta-analysis. *Int Rev Psychiatry* **8**:37–54.

Oldenhave, A., Jaszmann, L., Haspels, A., *et al.* (1993). Impact of climacteric on well-being. *Am J Obstetr Gynecol* **168**:772–90.

Ozeren, S., Corakci, A., Yucesoy, I., *et al.* (1997). Fluoxetine in the treatment of premenstrual syndrome. *Eur J Obstetr Gynecol Reprod Biol* **73**:167–70.

Pastuszak, A., Schick-Boshotto, B., Zuber, C., *et al.* (1993). Pregnancy outcome following first-trimester exposure to Fluoxetine (Prozac). *JAMA* **269**:2246–8.

Patel, P., Wheatcroft, R., Park, R. J., *et al.* (2002). The children of mothers with eating disorders. *Clin Child Fam Rev Psychol Rev* **5**:1–18.

Pearce, J., Hawton, K., Blake, F., *et al.* (1997). Psychological effects of continuation versus discontinuation of hormone replacement therapy by estrogen implants: a placebo-controlled study. *J Psychosom Res* **42**:177–86.

Pearlstein, T., Stone, A., Lund, S., *et al.* (1997). Comparison of fluoxetine, bupropion and placebo in the treatment of premenstrual dysphoric disorder. *J Clin Psychopharmacol* **17**:261–6.

Petanceska, S., Nagy, V., Frail, D., *et al.* (2000). Ovariectomy and 17B-estradiol modulate the levels of Alzheimer's amyloid B peptides in brain. *Neurology* **54**: 2212–17.

Pfuhlmann, B., Stoeber, G., & Beckmann, H. (2002). Postpartum psychoses: prognosis, risk factors and treatment. *Curr Psychiatry Reports* **4**:185–90.

Ramacharan, S., Love, E., Fick, G., *et al.* (1992). The epidemiology of premenstrual symptoms in a population-based sample of 2650 urban women: attributable risk and risk factors. *J Clin Epidemiol* **45**:377–92.

Rapkin, A., Morgan, M., Goldman, L., *et al.* (1997). Progesterone metabolite allopregnanolone in women with premenstrual syndrome. *Obstetr Gynecol* **90**:709–14.

Rasgon, N., McGuire, M., Tanavoli, S., *et al.* (2000). Neuroendocrine response to an intravenous L-tryptophan challenge in women with premenstrual syndrome. *Fertil Steril* **73**:144–9.

Reed, P., Sermin, N., Appleby, L., *et al.* (1999). A comparison of clinical response to electroconvulsive therapy in puerperal and non-puerperal psychoses. *J Affect Disord* **54**:255–60.

Rickels, K., Freeman, E., & Sondheimer, S. (1989). Buspirone in treatment of premenstrual syndrome. *Lancet* **4**:777.

Rivera-Tovar, A., & Frank, E. (1990). Late luteal phase dysphoric disorder in young women. *Am J Psychiatry* **147**:1634–6.

Roca, C., Schmidt, P., Smith, M., *et al.* (2002). Effects of methergoline on symptoms in women with premenstrual dysphoric disorder. *Am J Psychiatry* **159**:1876–81.

Rojansky, N., Halbreich, U., Zander, K., *et al.* (1991). Imipramine receptor binding and serotonin uptake in platelets of women with premenstrual changes. *Gynecol Obstet Invest* **31**:146–52.

Sadoft, R. (1995). Mothers who kill their children. *Psychiatr Ann* **25**:601–5.

Salokangas, R. (1995). Gender and the use of neuroleptics in schizophrenia. Further testing of the oestrogen hypothesis. *Schizophr Res* **16**:7–16.

Sayegh, R., Schiff, I., Wurtman, J., *et al.* (1995). The effect of a carbohydrate-rich beverage on mood, appetite and cognitive function in women with premenstrual syndrome. *J Am Coll Obstetr Gynecol* **86**:520–8.

Schmidt, P., & Rubinow, D. (1991). Menopause-related affective disorders: a justification for further study. *Am J Psychiatry* **148**:844–52.

Seeman, M. (1983). Interaction of sex, age and neuroleptic dose. *Compr Psychiatry* **24**:125–8.

Shumaker, S., Legault, C., Kuller, L., *et al.* (2004). Conjugated equine estrogens and incidence of probable dementia and mild cognitive impairment in postmenopausal women: Women's Health Initiative Memory Study. *JAMA* **291**:2947–58.

Shumaker, S., Legault, C., Rapp, S., *et al.* (2003). Estrogen plus progestin and the incidence of dementia and mild cognitive impairment in postmenopausal women: the Women's Health Initiative Study: a randomized controlled trial. *JAMA* **289**:2651–62.

Smith, S., Rinehart, J., Ruddock, V., *et al.* (1987). Treatment of premenstrual syndrome with alprazolam: results of a double-blind, placebo-controlled, randomized crossover clinical trial. *Obstetr Gynecol* **70**:37–43.

Soares, C., Almeida, O., Joffe, H., *et al.* (2001). Efficacy of estradiol for the treatment of depressive disorders in perimenopausal women: a double-blind, randomized, placebo-controlled trial. *Arch Gen Psychiatry* **58**:529–34.

Steege, J., Stout, A., Knight, B., *et al.* (1992). Reduced platelet tritium-labelled imipramine binding sites in women with premenstrual syndrome. *Am J Obstetr Gynecol* **167**:168–72.

Steiner, M., Korzekwa, M., Lamont, J., *et al.* (1997). Intermittent fluoxetine dosing in the treatment of women with premenstrual dysphoria. *Psychiatry Res* **87**:107–15.

Steiner, M., & Pearlstein, T. (2000). Premenstrual dysphoria and the serotonin system: pathophysiology and treatment. *J Clin Psychiatry* **61**(Suppl 12):17–21.

Steiner, M., Steinberg, S., Stewart, D., *et al.* (1995). Fluoxetine in the treatment of premenstrual dysphoria. *New Engl J Med* **332**:1529–34.

Steiner, M., Yatham, L. N., Coote, M., *et al.* (1999). Serotonergic dysfunction in women with pure premenstrual dysphoric disorder: is the fenfluramine challenge test still relevant? *Psychiatry Res* **87**:107–15.

Sternfeld, B., Swindle, R., Chawla, A., *et al.* (2002). Severity of premenstrual symptoms in a health maintenance organization population. *Obstetr Gynecol* **99**:1014–24.

Stewart, D., Boydell, K., Derzko, C., *et al.* (1992). Psychological distress during the menopausal years in women attending a menopause clinic. *Int J Psychiatry Med* **22**:213–20.

Stone, A., Pearlstein, T., & Brown, W. (1991). Fluoxetine in the treatment of late luteal phase dysphoric disorder. *J Clin Psychiatry* **52**:290–3.

Stowe, A., & Nemeroff, C. (1995). Women at risk of postpartum-onset major depression. *Am J Obstetr Gynecol* **173**:639–45.

Su, T.-P., Schmidt, P., Danaceau, M., *et al.* (1997). Effect of menstrual cycle phase on neuroendocrine and behavioural responses to the serotonin agonist m chlorophenylpiperazine in women with premenstrual syndrome and controls. *J Clin Endocrinol Metabol* **82**:1220–8.

Sundblad, C., Hedberg, M., & Erikson, E. (1993). Clomipramine administered during the luteal phase reduces the symptoms of premenstrual syndrome: a placebo-controlled trial. *Neuropsychopharmacology* **9**:133–45.

Sundblad, C., Modigh, K., Andersch, B., *et al.* (1992). Clomipramine effectively reduces premenstrual irritability and dysphoria: a placebo-controlled trial. *Acta Psychiatr Scand* **85**:39–47.

Sundstrom, I., Ashbrook, D., & Backstrom, T. (1997). Reduced benzodiazepine sensitivity in patients with premenstrual syndrome: a pilot study. *Psychoneuroendocrinology* **22**:25–38.

Sundstrom, I., & Backstrom, T. (1998). Citalopram increases pregnanolone sensitivity in patients with premenstrual syndrome: an open trial. *Psychoneuroendocrinology*, **23**:73–88.

Sundstrom, I., Nyberg, S., & Backstrom, T. (1997). Patients with premenstrual syndrome have reduced sensitivity to midazolam compared to control subjects. *Neuropsychopharmacology*, **17**:370–81.

Thys-Jacobs, S., & Alvir, M. (1995). Calcium-regulating hormones across the menstrual cycle: evidence of a secondary hyperparathyroidism in women with PMS. *J Clin Endocrinol Metab* **80**:2227–32.

Thys-Jacobs, S., Ceccarelli, S., Bierman, A., *et al.* (1989). Calcium supplementation in premenstrual syndrome: a randomized crossover trial. *J Gen Int Med* **4**:183–9.

Thys-Jacobs, S., Starkey, P., Bernstein, D., *et al.* (1998). Calcium carbonate and the premenstrual syndrome: effects on premenstrual and menstrual symptoms. *Premenstrual Syndrome Study Group. Am J Obstetr Gynecol* **179**:444–52.

Uzunova, V., Sheline, Y., Davis, J., *et al.* (1998). Increase in the cerebrospinal fluid content of neurosteroids in patients with unipolar major depression receiving fluoxetine or fluvoxamine. *Proc Nat Acad Sci USA* **95**:3239–44.

Wadhwa, P. D., Sandman, C. A., & Garite, T. J. (2001). The neurobiology of stress in human pregnancy: implications for prematurity and development of the fetal central nervous system. *Prog Brain Res* **133**:131–42.

Weller, A., & Weller, L. (1998). Assessment of menstrual regularity and irregularity using self reports and objective criteria. *J Psychosom Obstetr Gynaecol* **19**:111–16.

Wikander, I., Sundlad, C., Andersch, B., *et al.* (1998). Citalopram in premenstrual dysphoria: is intermittent treatment during luteal phases more effective than continuous medication throughout the menstrual cycle? *J Clin Psychopharmacol* **18**:390–8.

Wittchen, H., Becker, E., Lieb, R., *et al.* (2002). Prevalence, incidence and stability of premenstrual dysphoric disorder in the community. *Psychol Med* **18**:390–8.

Wood, S., Mortola, J., Chan, Y.-F., *et al.* (1992). Treatment of premenstrual syndrome with fluoxetine: a double-blind, placebo-controlled, crossover study. *Obstetr Gynecol* **80**:339–44.

Woods, N., Most, A., & Dery, G. (1982). Prevalence of perimenstrual symptoms. *Am J Public Health* **72**:1257–64.

Wyatt, K., Dimmock, P., Jones, P., *et al.* (1999). Efficacy of vitamin B6 in the treatment of premenstrual syndrome: systematic review. *BMJ Clin Res Ed* **318**:1375–81.

Wyatt, K., Dimmock, P., Jones, P., *et al.* (2001). Efficacy of progesterone and progestogens in management of premenstrual syndrome: a systematic review. *BMJ* **323**:776–81.

Wyatt, K., Dimmock, P., & O'Brien, P. (2003). Selective serotonin reuptake inhibitors for premenstrual syndrome. *Cochrane Database Syst Rev* **3**: CD001396.

Yatham, L., Barry, S., & Dinan, T. (1989). Serotonin receptors, buspirone and premenstrual syndrome. *Lancet* **1**:1447–8.

Yonkers, K., Clark, R., & Trivedi, M. (1997). The psychopharmacological treatment of nonmajor mood disorders. In A. Rush, ed. *Mood Disorders. Systematic Medication Management. Modern Problems of Pharmacopsychiatry*, Vol. 25. Basel: Karger, pp. 146–66.

Yonkers, K., Halbreich, U., Freeman, E., *et al.* (1996). Sertraline in the treatment of premenstrual dysphoric disorder. *Psychopharmacol Bull* **32**:41–6.

Yonkers, K. A., Wisner, K. L., Stowe, Z., *et al.* (2004). Management of bipolar disorder during pregnancy and the postpartum period. *Am J Psychiatry* **161**:608–20.

Young, S., Hurt, P., Benedek, D., *et al.* (1998). Treatment of premenstrual dysphoric disorder with sertraline during the luteal phase: a randomised, double-blind, placebo-controlled crossover trial. *J Clin Psychiatry* **59**:76–80.

Zandi, P., Carlson, M., Plassman, B., *et al.* (2002). Hormone replacement therapy and incidence of Alzheimer's disease in older women: the Cache County Study (comment). *JAMA* **288**:2123–9.

Zeskind, P. S., & Stephens, L. E. (2004). Maternal selective serotonin reuptake inhibitor use during pregnancy and newborn neurobehaviour. *Pediatrics* **113**:365–73.

20

Suicide and self-harm

Navneet Kapur and Louis Appleby

In this chapter, we consider suicide and self-harm separately, but the distinction may be an artificial one. These two aspects of suicidal behaviour are closely linked. As many as 1 in 10 of those who self-harm will eventually die by suicide, and at least half of those who complete suicide have a history of previous self-harm.

Suicide

Definitions and case ascertainment

Suicide describes an intentional self-inflicted act which has resulted in death (Maris, 2002). In many countries, suicide is determined by coroners and medical examiners. However, the criteria for recording a suicide verdict vary widely. In England, for example, cases of unnatural death are investigated by the coroner, and an inquest is held. The definition of suicide is a strict one which requires proof of intention to die. When there is doubt over the victim's intent, a coroner is obliged to record an open (undetermined) verdict. This contrasts with other countries, which require only that suicide was the most probable explanation for death (Pounder, 1991). Other countries use a more stringent definition and require a suicide note before a death can be registered as suicide. Even within the same countries, there may be marked variation in death certification practices (Neeleman & Wessley, 1997).

Undetermined deaths are often included in official statistics and research studies because the majority are likely to be suicides (Linsley *et al.*, 2001). The inclusion of accidental deaths is more controversial, although it is probable that a proportion of these are also suicides (Phillips & Ruth, 1993). Variations in definition and inclusion criteria mean that statistics recording the incidence of suicide need to be interpreted cautiously.

Epidemiology

Worldwide there are an estimated 1 million deaths per year from suicide. On the basis of current estimates, this will increase to 1.5 million deaths per year by 2020 (Bertolote & Fleischmann, 2002). Although overall suicide rates represent an important estimate of the burden of this phenomenon, another factor to consider is the effect of premature mortality. Measures of potential years of life lost can help to quantify the effect of early death (Gunnell & Middleton, 2003). This might be especially relevant given the recent increase in suicide among young people in many countries (Cantor, 2000).

International comparisons

Rates of suicide vary widely between countries (Table 20.1). This may reflect differences in death certification practices (perhaps influenced by legal, moral and cultural considerations). It may also be

Essential Psychiatry, ed. Robin M. Murray, Kenneth S. Kendler, Peter McGuffin, Simon Wessely, David J. Castle.
Published by Cambridge University Press. © Cambridge University Press 2008.

accounted for by the fact that it is often crude rates of suicide that are compared. These do not adjust for the different age structure of the national populations. However, it seems likely that at least some of the reported patterns of cross-national variation reflect genuine differences in rates.

There is a greater than 10-fold difference in rates between the countries with the highest rates (Hungary, Japan, Finland, the countries of the former Soviet Union and Sri Lanka) and the countries with the lowest rates (South America, Southern Europe and some Islamic countries; Levi *et al.*, 2003). Explanations for these differences remain speculative but include alcohol misuse, cultural differences in help-seeking behaviour, societal attitudes towards suicide, socioeconomic upheaval, the availability of highly lethal methods of suicide, and religion.

Trends in suicide rates

In most countries in the European Union, there has been a downward trend in the suicide rate in the past two decades (Chishti *et al.*, 2003). The suicide rate in the United States fell by almost 10% in the same time period (Mann, 2002). However, these overall rates may conceal different trends in specific subgroups of individuals. For example, the downward trends that have been observed in many countries may be largely due to reduced suicide in older men and women. They may mask rises in the rate of suicide among young males and, in some cases, young females (Cantor, 2000).

The suicide rate in the United Kingdom fluctuated throughout the twentieth century, although it fell, particularly in men, during both World Wars. Rises were recorded during the early 1930s, a time of high unemployment, and the late 1950s, one of relative prosperity. The rate fell in the mid-1960s after relatively nontoxic natural gas was introduced into the domestic gas supply (Kreitman, 1976) but rose gradually in the 1970s and 1980s. Over the last 20 years, the annual suicide rate in the United Kingdom has been around 10 to 12 per 100,000 population, but the rate has been falling since the late

Table 20.1 Suicide Rates (per 100,000) by country, year and gender; most recent year available as of May 2003

Country	Year	Males	Females
Australia	01	20.1	5.3
Austria	02	30.5	8.7
Belarus	01	60.3	9.3
Belgium	97	31.2	11.4
Brazil	95	6.6	1.8
Canada	00	18.4	5.2
China (selected rural and urban areas)	99	13.0	14.8
Czech Republic	01	26.0	6.3
Denmark	99	21.4	7.4
Egypt	87	0.1	0.0
Finland	02	32.3	10.2
France	99	26.1	9.4
Germany	01	20.4	7.0
Greece	99	5.7	1.6
Hungary	02	45.5	12.2
India	98	12.2	9.1
Ireland	00	20.3	4.3
Italy	00	10.9	3.5
Japan	00	35.2	13.4
Kuwait	01	1.9	0.9
Lithuania	02	80.7	13.1
Mexico	95	5.4	1.0
Netherlands	00	12.7	6.2
New Zealand	00	19.8	4.2
Norway	01	18.4	6.0
Paraguay	94	3.4	1.2
Peru	89	0.6	0.4
Portugal	00	8.5	2.0
Russian Federation	02	69.3	11.9
Spain	00	13.1	4.0
Sri Lanka	91	44.6	16.8
Sweden	01	18.9	8.1
Switzerland	00	27.8	10.8
Syrian Arab Republic	85	0.2	0.0
Thailand	94	5.6	2.4
Turkmenistan	98	13.8	3.5
Ukraine	00	52.1	10.0
United Kingdom	99	11.8	3.3
United States of America	00	17.1	4.0

Source: http://who.int/mental_health/prevention/suicide/suiciderates.

1990s. It is currently 9.1 per 100,000 per year in England (provisional 2003 figures based on 1-year rates, personal communication, National Confidential Inquiry into Suicide and Homicide). In recent years, there have been approximately 4,500 to 5,000 suicides and deaths from undetermined cause in England annually.

Methods of suicide

Men are more likely to use violent methods such as hanging or shooting, whereas women are more likely to poison themselves with antidepressants or analgesics. In the United Kingdom, the three most common methods of suicide are hanging, drug-related poisoning and "other poisoning" (including poisoning by motor vehicle exhaust gas) for men and drug-related poisoning, hanging and "other and unspecified cause of death" for women. There has been a large decline in deaths by inhalation of car exhaust fumes since the early 1990s with the introduction of catalytic converters (Amos et al., 2001) and a smaller decline in deaths from paracetamol poisoning since legislation restricting pack sizes (Brock & Griffiths, 2003). However, the rate of death by hanging has doubled over the last two decades, and this might partly reflect method substitution. There has also been a substantial increase in the number of suicides occurring on the railways (Abbott et al., 2003). Of course methods of suicide vary by country. Firearm suicides are common in the United States, where they account for approximately 60% of suicide deaths. Self-poisoning with agro-chemicals is the most important cause of death in Sri Lanka and rural China. Certain methods may be associated with specific groups of individuals, for example, self-burning in Asian women (Soni Raleigh et al., 1990) and violent methods in those with mental disorder.

Sociodemographic factors and suicide

A number of sociodemographic factors may influence the risk of suicide.

Age

In general, the suicide rate increases with age. This is true of both sexes, although the increase is more gradual in women. In the United Kingdom, suicide is rare in children under 12 and increases rapidly after the mid-teens. However, the effect of age has changed dramatically during the last three decades. Over this time, the suicide rate in men in their late teens and early 20s has doubled, most of the increase occurring since 1980, whereas there has been a 30% fall among people aged over 65. The reasons for the former trend are unknown, although possible factors include rising rates of alcohol and drug misuse, divorce and unemployment, as well as the increasing use of dangerous methods of self-harm (Gunnell et al., 2003). These changes mean that the highest rates of suicide in the United Kingdom now occur in males aged 25 to 44, and suicide is the most common cause of death in this age group. Very recent data suggest rates of suicide in young people in England and Wales are now falling (Biddle et al., 2008).

Sex

Suicide is considerably more common in men than women in most countries. In the United Kingdom, the rate in men is around 4 times higher than that in women in the younger age groups and around twice as high in older age groups (source: www.statistics.gov.uk 2004). An exception to the general preponderance of males among those who complete suicide occurs in China, where a male to female ratio of 0.8 to 1 has been reported (Pritchard, 1996).

Social class and employment

The suicide rate varies according to social class, with the highest rate being found in the lowest classes (social class V in the United Kingdom) and the lowest rate in the professional classes. Unemployment is a risk factor for suicide (Pritchard, 1988), as are certain forms of employment such as medicine, nursing and farming.

Ethnicity

The suicide rates of immigrant ethnic minorities often reflect the rates in their country of origin. Thus in the United Kingdom, the suicide rate may be lower among African-Caribbeans and higher in Eastern European immigrants than it is in the indigenous UK population (Soni Raleigh & Balarajan, 1992). Similar findings have been reported in Australia (Cantor & Neulinger, 2000). In the United States and Canada, high rates have been reported in native North Americans. Specific racial subgroups, such as young Asian women in the United Kingdom, appear to be at high risk (Soni Raleigh *et al.*, 1990).

Marital status and children

Suicide is more common in people who are single, separated or divorced, or widowed (Heikinen *et al.*, 1995). Recent widowhood is thought to be an important risk factor in the elderly, but one study of marital status and male suicide found that bereavement had the greatest effect on relatively young adults, whereas divorce was associated with the greatest risk in the elderly (Kreitman, 1988). Although depression in women has been linked to the presence of children in the home and is common after childbirth, children appear to be a protective factor with respect to suicide (Qin *et al.*, 2000). A study in the United Kingdom found the rate of suicide in the first postnatal year to be only one sixth the rate in the general female population (Appleby, 1991). A Norwegian study found an inverse relationship between the number of children in the family and the risk of suicide (Hoyer & Lund, 1993).

Environmental factors and suicide

Area level factors

The relative rates of suicide in urban and rural populations have varied over time. In the late 1980s in the United Kingdom, the suicide rate was highest in rural regions such as East Anglia and the South-West. Later cross-sectional studies reported high rates in urban areas. A recent analysis of trends in suicide rates in urban and rural areas of England and Wales between 1981 and 1998 found the biggest increases in suicide among 15 to 44 year olds in areas remote from the main centres of population (Middleton *et al.*, 2003).

Socioeconomic deprivation is associated with suicide, but lack of social integration may be a more important factor. Middleton and colleagues explored a number of census-derived measures of the social, health and economic characteristics of over 9,000 small areas in England and Wales (Middleton *et al.*, 2004). They found that indicators of social fragmentation (number of single-person households, households privately renting, unmarried adults, population mobility) were the factors most strongly associated with suicide risk, even after adjusting for other area characteristics. Deprivation scores were less consistently associated with suicide, and the associations weakened after adjustment for the other factors.

Seasonality

Just as the prevalence of depression shows seasonal variation, with higher rates in winter months, the suicide rate also follows a seasonal pattern. In the United Kingdom, the rate is highest between April and June, and other countries – including those in the Southern Hemisphere – have reported a similar rise in spring. Possible explanations include an increase in social activity in the spring (accompanied by increased alcohol use and conflict in relationships) or individuals externalising their misery (to the weather) in winter but internalising it in spring when the rest of society is at its most optimistic. There are also possible biological explanations, for example, the increase in daylight in the spring stimulating the pineal gland and contributing to the risk of affective disorders (Cantor, 2000). There is some evidence that the seasonal variation in suicide may be decreasing over time (Ajdacic-Gross *et al.*, 2005).

Biological factors and suicide

A family history of suicide increases the individual's risk of suicide (Shafii *et al.*, 1985; Tsuang, 1983), a finding that may be explained by observational learning or genetic predisposition. A genetic explanation is supported by twin studies that have shown an increased concordance for monozygotic compared to dizygotic twin pairs (Roy, 1990). A study of Danish adoptees who completed suicide found a high rate of suicide in their biological but not adoptive parents (Schulsinger *et al.*, 1979; Wender *et al.*, 1986).

What is inherited is unknown. One of the challenges for studies in this area is identifying the genetic factors that contribute to the risk of suicide independent of the genetic factors for psychiatric disorders. Candidate genes might include the gene for tryptophan hydroxylase (which is involved in the synthesis of serotonin) and the serotonin 5-HT2a receptor gene (Mann, 2002).

Altered serotonergic function is certainly implicated in suicidal behaviour. Biochemical studies have found reduced 5-HIAA in the cerebrospinal fluid of those who have completed suicide, reflecting reduced serotonin metabolism in the brain (Traskman *et al.*, 1981). These changes may be independent of psychiatric diagnosis. Serotonergic hypofunction may be associated with more lethal suicide attempts. Other changes that have been demonstrated include reduced serotonergic input to the orbital prefrontal cortex and altered serotonin receptor populations (e.g. decreases in presynaptic binding sites in the prefrontal cortex; Mann, 2002). It has been suggested that the apparent association between low cholesterol and suicidal behaviour is mediated through the serotonergic system (Muldoon *et al.*, 1990).

With respect to the noradrenergic system, studies have shown fewer noradrenergic neurones in the locus coeruleus of those who have completed suicide, increased levels of tyrosine hydroxylase in the brainstem and lower levels of postsynaptic adrenergic receptors in the cortex (Mann, 2002). These changes may also be consistent with an excessive stress response before suicide.

Although research examining the biological variables implicated in suicide is still at a relatively early stage, advances in brain imaging and other techniques may help our understanding of the biological processes underlying suicidal behaviour.

Clinical factors and suicide

Adverse life events

Adverse life events such as interpersonal loss or conflict, financial difficulty or serious physical illness can serve as important precipitants of suicide. In a study of young people, those who died by suicide had more interpersonal and life events relating to criminal behaviour than living age- and sex-matched control subjects (Cooper *et al.*, 2002). Cavanagh and colleagues (1999) matched case and control subjects on age, sex and diagnosis and found greater interpersonal family adversity as well as greater physical ill health in those who completed suicide.

Self-harm and medical history

There is a strong association between suicide and self-harm. Approximately half of suicides have a history of self-harm (Foster *et al.*, 1997) and this proportion increases to two thirds in younger age groups (Appleby, Cooper, *et al.*, 1999). Physical illness is also associated with the risk of suicide, especially in the elderly. A case control study of subjects aged 65 and over in Sweden found that visual impairment, neurological disorders and malignant disease increased the risk of suicide between 3 and 7 times (Waern *et al.*, 2002). Serious physical illness was an independent risk factor for suicide in a multivariate analysis.

Along with previous self-harm, one of the strongest risk factors for suicide is psychiatric disorder.

Suicide and psychiatric disorder

Patients with a psychiatric diagnosis are at increased risk of dying prematurely when compared with the general population. Much of this excess mortality is accounted for by suicide. It has been estimated that mental disorder is associated with an 11-fold increase in the risk of suicide (Harris & Barraclough,

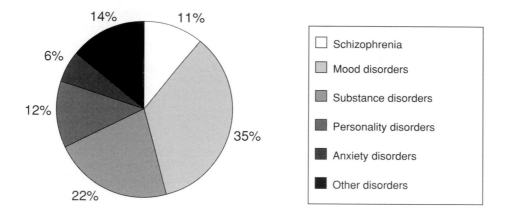

Figure 20.1 Suicide and mental disorders in 14,629 cases of suicide worldwide (Bertolote & Fleischmann, 2002).

1997). However, the risk is not uniform over time. For example, it is increased 30 times in the 6 months after hospital discharge (King & Barraclough, 1990; Qin & Nordentoft, 2005; Temoche *et al.*, 1964). Half of those who die by suicide have previously been referred to psychiatric services, and a quarter have been in contact with services in the year before their death (Appleby *et al.*, 2001). A recent review of 31 studies from around the world involving 14,629 cases of suicide reported that 98% of them had *International Classification of Diseases* (ICD) or *Diagnostic and Statistical Manual of Mental Disorders* (DSM) mental disorder at the time death (Bertolote & Fleischmann, 2002). Figure 20.1 shows the primary psychiatric diagnoses for these subjects.

The association of mental disorder with suicide is consistent across settings. Two main methodological approaches have been used to explore this relationship: the psychological autopsy study and the follow-up study.

Psychological autopsy studies

Many studies have involved *psychological autopsies,* or the collection of information on subjects who have completed suicide from interviews with family members, relatives, friends and healthcare staff.

This allows detailed collection of relevant information, but because of the retrospective nature of the investigation, the findings may be subject to recall bias. Studies using this approach suggest that the vast majority (more than 90%) of individuals who complete suicide are suffering from a psychiatric disorder at the time of their death (Appleby, Dennehy, *et al.*, 1999; Cavanagh *et al.*, 2003; Foster *et al.*, 1997). The population attributable fraction for mental disorder (the proportion of suicides in the population that would be prevented by eliminating mental disorder, assuming mental disorder and suicide were casually related) has been calculated to be in the region of 47% to 74% (Cavanagh *et al.*, 2003).

Cohort studies

An alternative method of investigating the association between psychiatric disorder and suicide is the *cohort study*. Individuals with a specified mental disorder are followed up over a period of (usually) several years, and mortality data are collected. A meta-analysis combined the results of 249 studies that had followed up subjects for at least 2 years (Harris & Barraclough, 1997); there were more than 7,000 deaths by suicide. Table 20.2 summarises the findings, which are presented as Standardised Mortality Ratios (SMRs). This statistic indicates the

Table 20.2 Common mental disorders and the risk of suicide

Disorder	SMR (95% CI)
Schizophrenia	845 (798–895)
Bipolar disorder	1505 (1225–1844)
Major depression	2035 (1827–2259)
Dysthymia	1212 (1150–1277)
Panic disorder	1000 (457–1898)
Alcohol misuse	586 (541–633)
Substance use: opioids	1400 (1079–1788)
Substance use: hypnotics	2034 (1425–2816)
Eating disorders	2314 (1538–3344)
Personality disorders	708 (477–1010)

From Harris & Barraclough, 1997.

CI = confidence interval; SMR = standardised mortality ratio, figures over 100 indicate increased risk of suicide.

mortality rate in the sample of interest compared with the mortality rate that would be expected in a "standard population" with a similar age and sex profile. An SMR of 100 indicates equivalent risk, whereas SMRs greater than 100 indicate increased risk of suicide. Most psychiatric disorders were associated with an increased risk of suicide. Schizophrenia was associated with an 8-fold increase in risk, bipolar disorder with a 15-fold increase and major depression with a 20-fold increase. All treatment settings (in-patient, community, forensic) were associated with greater risk of suicide, but most studies were carried out in secondary care. These results may therefore not be generalisable to patients receiving treatment for their mental disorder in primary care settings.

In a more recent study in Denmark involving 72,000 individuals followed for up to 20 years, there were nearly 13,000 cases of suicide (Hiroeh *et al.*, 2001). The SMR for those hospitalised with psychiatric disorder was 1,356 for women (or more than 13 times the expected rate) and 1,212 for men (or more than 12 times the expected rate). The risks associated with individual disorders in the Danish study were similar to those reported in the meta-analysis, with the exception of the SMRs for alcoholism

and personality disorder, both of which were higher in the Danish study (SMR for alcoholism: women 1,586, men 1,064; SMR for personality disorder: women 1,568, men 1,198).

The National Confidential Inquiry into Suicide and Homicide

Much of what we know about suicide in the UK psychiatric population is based on data collected by the National Confidential Inquiry into Suicide and Homicide by People with Mental Illness (Appleby *et al.*, 2001).

The Inquiry currently holds information on more than 9,000 suicides. The figures presented here refer to the 4,859 cases collected during the first 4 years of data collection (1996–2000). This represents 24% of the total number of suicides in the general population during this time period. These findings are based on a retrospective method. Because the Inquiry is essentially a descriptive study, firm aetiological conclusions regarding specific risk factors are difficult to draw. We therefore also refer to relevant case-control studies when appropriate.

Sociodemographic and clinical characteristics

What are the sociodemographic and clinical characteristics of patients with mental disorder who complete suicide? Table 20.3 presents data from the National Confidential Inquiry. As with suicides in the general population, males are overrepresented. There is also an apparent association with social isolation – high proportions of patients were unmarried, unemployed or living alone. They are a relatively morbid group – more than half of patients had a secondary psychiatric diagnosis, and 16% of patients had been admitted to a psychiatric bed on more than five occasions. Two thirds had a history of deliberate self-harm, and violence and substance misuse also featured prominently. With respect to aspects of clinical care, almost half had had contact with services within 7 days of death, and two thirds had active symptoms at their last contact. Almost one third of the sample was out of contact

Table 20.3 Sociodemographic characteristics, clinical characteristics and aspects of care for suicides in contact with mental health services (*N* = 4,859)

	Number (*n* = 4,859)	% (95% CI)
Sociodemographic characteristics		
Median age (range)	41 (13–95)	
Male	3,198	66 (64–67)
Ethnic minority	282	6 (5–7)
Not currently married	3,405	71 (70–73)
Unemployed/long-term sick	2,765	58 (58–60)
Living alone	2,006	43 (41–44)
Clinical characteristics		
Any secondary diagnosis	2,460	52 (51–54)
Over five previous admissions	712	16 (15–17)
History of previous self-harm	3,077	64 (63–66)
History of violence	920	19 (18–21)
History of alcohol misuse	1,899	40 (38–41)
History of drug misuse	1,348	28 (27–30)
Aspects of clinical care		
Last contact with services within 7 days	2,308	48 (47–50)
Symptoms at last contact	2,990	64 (63–65)
Out of contact with services	1,153	29 (27–30)
Noncompliant with treatment	929	22 (21–24)

From Appleby *et al.*, 2001.

with services, and a fifth were noncompliant with treatment.

A case-control study of 149 subjects who had died by suicide and 149 control subjects matched for age, sex, diagnosis and date of last admission carried out in Greater Manchester, United Kingdom (Appleby, Dennehy, *et al.*, 1999), suggested that the most important independent clinical predictors of suicide were a previous history of deliberate self-harm (odds ratio [OR]: 3.7, 95% confidence interval [CI]: 1.7–5.7) and expressing suicidal thoughts during aftercare (OR: 1.9, 95% CI: 1.0–3.5). The suicides were more likely to have had their level of care reduced at their final appointment before their death (OR: 3.7, 95% CI: 1.8–7.6), but no other aspects

of aftercare were independently associated with suicide risk.

In-patients and those recently discharged

Conventional clinical wisdom suggests that patients with psychiatric disorders who are at high risk of suicide should be admitted to a psychiatric hospital bed. The assumption is that admission will help to contain the risk and prevent suicide. Patients who complete suicide while in-patients or shortly after discharge from hospital are therefore a particularly important group because the circumstances of their death may highlight deficiencies in service provision.

A surprisingly high proportion of the Inquiry sample (16%) were in-patients at the time of their death. They were a more morbid group than the sample as a whole, with one third having had multiple admissions to hospital and three quarters having a history of previous deliberate self-harm. A quarter of in-patient suicides occurred during the first week of admission, and 31% occurred on the ward itself. The majority of ward suicides were by hanging. Forty percent of suicides occurring off the ward were in patients who had left the ward without staff permission. Almost one third of inpatient suicides were detained under the Mental Health Act. A quarter of wards reported problems observing patients because of ward design. A case-control study of 59 inpatient suicides and 106 control subjects matched for age, sex, diagnosis and admission date in one English region found seven independent risk factors for suicide (King *et al.*, 2001a); these were previous deliberate self-harm, admission under the Mental Health Act, involvement of the police in admission, depressive symptoms, violence towards property, going absent without leave and a significant care professional being on leave. The study was comparatively small, and thus estimates regarding the strength of the association between these factors and suicide were imprecise.

Almost a quarter of the Inquiry cases had died within 3 months of discharge from psychiatric inpatient care. Post-discharge suicides were most frequent in the 2 weeks after leaving hospital, with 30% of the post-discharge suicides occurring during this time period. Within the first 2 weeks, the highest number of suicides was on the day after discharge. The post-discharge group was more likely to have a history of self-harm than the Inquiry sample as a whole, and in 30% of cases, the final admission lasted less than 7 days. Patients had initiated their own discharge in one third of cases. Most patients (92% of the post-discharge group) had a follow-up appointment arranged. However, in 40% of cases, suicide took place before this appointment. A case-control study of 234 patients who completed suicide within 1 year of hospital discharge and 431 control subjects matched for age, sex, diagnosis and admission period found a number of independent risk and protective factors (King et al., 2001b). The 11 risk factors were as follows: non-white ethnic status, living alone, history of self harm, suicidal ideas precipitating admission, hopelessness, change of consultant since previous admission, relationship difficulties, loss of job, self harm while an inpatient, unplanned discharge and a significant care professional leaving or being on leave. The four protective factors were as follows: shared accommodation, delusions at admission, misuse of non-prescribed substances and continuity of contact. Thirty-two percent of suicides and 9% of control subjects had at least four risk factors; 3.4% of cases and 15% of control subjects had no risk factors.

Suicide in individual psychiatric disorders

Schizophrenia

Most estimates of the lifetime suicide rate in schizophrenia are in the region of 5% to 10%, slightly less than in major affective disorders, although one Swedish study found that those with schizophrenia were most at risk (Allebeck & Allgulander, 1990). The same Swedish group also studied a cohort of discharged in-patients with schizophrenia and found the rate of suicide over the following 10 years to be 3.9% (Allebeck & Wistedt, 1986). More recently there

has been a suggestion that many estimates of the lifetime risk for suicide in schizophrenia have been too high because of the comparatively short follow-up periods of most studies and their poor methodological quality (Inskip et al., 1998). A revised figure for lifetime risk in schizophrenia of 4% has been proposed.

A number of mental state features have been related to suicide in people with schizophrenia, particularly depressed mood (Cohen et al., 1990; Drake et al., 1984; Roy, 1982a), suicidal ideas (Drake et al., 1984; Roy, 1982b) and hallucinations with a suicidal content (Roy, 1982b; Crammer, 1984; Sims & O'Brien, 1979). A past history of depression has also been linked to later suicide (Cohen et al., 1990), underlining the importance of low mood, even when the primary diagnosis is not of an affective disorder. However, this is not a universal view. One study found that the relationship with depression per se disappeared once multivariate analysis had controlled for the symptom of hopelessness (Drake & Cotton, 1986). Another found no link to depression and concluded that for most of those with schizophrenia who completed suicide, it was an impulsive act rather than mood related (Allebeck et al., 1987).

Only one study has reported a relationship between suicide and aspects of insight, namely, an awareness of the effects of the illness and fear of further mental disintegration (Drake et al., 1984). However, several studies have found risk to be greatest during the period of clinical recovery (Copas et al., 1971; Gale et al., 1980).

Affective disorders

The long-term risk of suicide in primary affective disorder has been estimated at 15% (Guze & Robins, 1970), this widely quoted figure being based on the varying results of early studies. However, more recent cohort studies have reported lower rates: 8.5% in the case of in-patients with depression (Berglund & Nilsson, 1987) and 3.6% in a cohort of people with affective (including schizoaffective) disorders (Fawcett et al., 1987, 1990). A recent study in one English health district which modelled life-time rates of suicide pointed out that most estimates of mortality were based on hospitalised samples of depressed individuals (Boardman & Healy, 2001). The authors of this study proposed much lower rates for the lifetime risk of suicide: 2.4% for any affective disorder and 1.1% for individuals with uncomplicated affective disorder who had no history of mental health service contact.

A number of clinical features seem to be linked to suicide, and these appear to vary with time. The early deaths (within 1 year of initial assessment) are associated with anxiety, panic, insomnia, anhedonia, poor concentration and alcohol abuse, whereas longer-term risk is associated with hopelessness (Beck *et al.*, 1985; Fawcett *et al.*, 1990).

Alcohol and substance misuse

The long-term suicide rate in those with alcohol dependence who have been in-patients has been estimated to be between 3.4% (Murphy & Wetzel, 1990) and 6.7% (Berglund & Nilsson, 1987). Lifetime mortality is in the region of 2.2% for those with a history of out-patient treatment. A past history of depression is the most important clinical risk factor for those with alcohol problems (Berglund, 1984). Continued alcohol use is also important and the recent loss of a relationship, usually by separation, has been described in one third of suicides (Murphy *et al.*, 1979). Similarly, interpersonal loss or conflict has been reported as preceding many suicides by those who misuse substances (including alcohol; Rich *et al.*, 1988).

Models of suicidal behaviour

Suicide is a complex and multifaceted behaviour. Although risk factors may provide some clues to aetiology, they are unable to explain why suicide occurs. Explanatory models of suicidal behaviour may help us to understand the phenomena better, help to formulate testable hypothesis and ultimately facilitate the development of appropriate treatments.

Table 20.4 A sociological model of suicidal behaviour

	The individual's sense of community	The community's control of the individual
Too strong	Altruism	Fatalism
Too weak	Egoism	Anomie

From Bille-Brahe, 2000.

Sociological models of suicide

One of the earliest models of suicide was proposed by Durkheim (1897/1951). Suicidal behaviour in this model is not viewed as an individual phenomenon but as a function of the relationship between the individual and the wider community (i.e. a function of social integration; Bille-Brahe, 2000). The degree of social integration can be defined according to two dimensions: one referring to the individual's sense of community and the other to the degree of control the community exerts over the individual. On this basis, it is possible to describe four conditions in which the balance between individuality and collectivity may be disturbed, resulting in an increased risk of suicide (Table 20.4). It should be noted that these states are not necessarily independent of one another. Altruistic suicide describes ending one's life for the sake of the wider group, the greater good. Fatalistic suicide may occur as a consequence of the overly strict rules of a society impairing individual freedom. Egoistic suicide may occur in situations in which the individual no longer feels a sense of community and consequently does not feel bound by societal norms. Anomic suicide reflects a situation in which perhaps at a time of societal upheaval, the ability of the community to create and maintain social norms is inadequate and its ability to exercise social control insufficient. More recent sociological models of suicidal behaviour have considered socio-economic and cultural perspectives (Bille-Brahe, 2000).

Clinical models of suicide

One of the most influential models of suicidal behaviour is the stress-diathesis or stress-vulnerability model (Mann, 2002). This suggests that certain individuals carry with them a predisposition to suicidal behaviour (which may be related to sex, religion, familial and genetic factors, childhood experiences, psychosocial support systems, access to lethal methods or biological factors). The vulnerability only leads to suicidal behaviour when the individual encounters a stressor (which could be a mental disorder, alcohol or drug misuse, a medical illness or a psychosocial crisis). A refinement of the stress-diathesis model is the suicidal process model, which explains suicide as the endpoint of a long-term process which is subject to the balance between risk and protective factors (Van Heeringen, 2001). The concept assumes the existence of an underlying and persistent vulnerability that is made up of biological and psychological trait characteristics. The threshold for suicidal behaviour will vary from individual to individual. This model suggests that intervention at an early stage in the "suicidal career" (e.g. at the first suicide attempt) may be more fruitful than intervention later on (Van Heeringen, 2001). Other models of suicide again emphasise the role of risk and protective factors (which can be acute or chronic) but also point out that these factors may interact and feed back in complex ways (Appleby, 1992; Maris, 2002).

Preventing suicide

Suicide is a major public health problem around the world. The prevention of suicide is a health priority in many countries (Commonwealth Department of Health and Aged Care, 2000; Department of Health, 2002; US Public Health Service, 1999; Wilson, 2004), and some have taken the approach of setting targets for suicide reduction. For example, the current target in England is a reduction of the suicide rate by one fifth by 2010 (Department of Health, 2002). Suicide is a rare event and our ability to identify truly high-risk groups in whom to intervene is limited because of the poor predictive value of our screening tools. Equally, the relatively low incidence of suicide means that trials which aim to use it as an outcome measure require many thousands of patients in each treatment limb. It is therefore unsurprising that data regarding the effectiveness of measures designed to prevent suicide are lacking.

High risk and population approaches to prevention

There are, broadly speaking, two approaches to prevention: the high-risk strategy and the population-based strategy (Kapur & House, 1998; Rose, 1992).

The aim in the high-risk approach is to concentrate preventive actions on individuals or groups characterised by demographic and clinical variables predictive of suicide – for example, people with mental illness, a history of self-harm or those employed in certain occupations. The benefit of this approach is that it targets resources such as mental health services on those who are at greatest need. However, the difficulty is the low predictive value of most risk factors. Targeting high-risk groups can also create the assumption that people at lower degrees of risk are at no risk. It is notable that mental health patients who complete suicide have often been previously judged by professionals to be at relatively low risk (Appleby, Shaw, et al., 1999).

In the population-based strategy, the whole population is targeted, often by measures to tackle a social characteristic linked to suicide, such as alcohol consumption. The advantage of this approach is the potential for small changes in the population to have a major impact. The difficulty in relation to suicide prevention is that most population risk factors are not easily influenced.

Suicide prevention strategies

The National Suicide Prevention Project was set up in Finland in 1986 with the explicit aim of reducing the suicide rate. The initial research phase involved a national psychological autopsy study of nearly 1,400 individuals who had completed suicide. Since

---

Box 20.1 Approaches to preventing suicide

- Reduce risk in key high-risk groups
- Promote mental well-being in the wider population
- Reduce the availability and lethality of suicide methods
- Improve reporting of suicidal behaviour in the media
- Promote research in suicide and suicide prevention
- Improve monitoring of progress towards the *Saving Lives: Our Healthier Nation* target for reducing suicide

From the National Suicide Prevention Strategy for England (Department of Health, 2002).

Box 20.2 Specific strategies to reduce suicide in the mentally ill

- Regular staff risk management training
- Patients with severe mental illness and self-harm to receive the most intensive level of care
- Individualised care plans
- Prompt access to services for patients in crises
- Assertive outreach teams
- Availability of atypical antipsychotics
- Strategies for dual diagnosis
- Inpatient wards to remove all likely ligature points
- Prompt follow up after discharge from inpatient care
- Careful prescribing of medication
- Multidisciplinary post incident review

From Department of Health, 2001.

---

then a number of other countries have devised suicide prevention strategies of their own (Taylor *et al.*, 1997). These strategies have a number of common elements, and a detailed discussion of one of the more recent examples will help to illustrate some of the key principles of suicide prevention.

The National Suicide Prevention Strategy for England was published in 2002 (Department of Health, 2002). It is designed to be a long-term strategy which will evolve as new priorities and new evidence on prevention emerge. It involves both high-risk and population-based strategies for prevention. The strategy lists six goals to support a reduction in the death rate from suicide of at least 20% by 2010 (Box 20.1).

The first goal relates to reducing risk in key high-risk groups and the second to promoting mental well-being in the wider population. Key high-risk groups include those with a history of mental disorder and those with a history of self-harm. Specific measures include encouraging mental health services to implement "Twelve Points to a Safer Service" (developed from the work of the National Confidential Inquiry; Box 20.2) and guidelines and national monitoring for self-harm.

Suicide may be impulsive, and individuals may be ambivalent at the time of the act. There is fairly good evidence that reducing the availability and lethality of methods of suicide (Goal 3 of the strategy) will reduce suicide rates, although method substitution may occur in some cases (Gunnell & Frankel, 1994).

Examples of effective interventions include changes to the domestic gas supply in Japan and England (Gunnell *et al.*, 2000; Lester, 1989), the introduction of catalytic converters to car exhausts (Amos *et al.*, 2001), reductions in analgesic pack sizes (Hawton *et al.*, 2004) and tighter gun control (Boyd, 1983). Specific additional examples from the strategy include reducing access to ligature points in hospital wards and prisons, encouraging safer prescribing of toxic medication, and working with the relevant agencies to help prevent railway deaths and deaths by jumping from high places.

The fourth goal relates to media representation of suicide. This has been shown to be an important influence on suicidal behaviour. In the eighteenth century a book by Goethe which involved the suicide of a young man by shooting after a love affair led to a spate of suicides in Europe and the banning of the book in several countries. Television dramas featuring suicidal acts have resulted in increases in method-specific suicidal behaviour in Germany and Britain (Hawton, Simkin, *et al.*, 1999; Schmidtke & Hafner, 1988). The strategy suggests that the media should follow guidelines to ensure the responsible reporting of suicide with reduced sensationalism, avoiding reference to means of suicide, reporting of facts rather than speculation and improving awareness of the potential benefits of help seeking in times of crisis. The effect of new media such as the Internet and mobile phones on suicidal behaviour is largely unknown and warrants further investigation.

The final two goals of the strategy aim to promote research on suicide and the prevention of suicidal behaviour and to improve monitoring of progress towards achieving the targets for the reduction in suicide rates.

Treating depression

Suicidal thoughts often accompany serious depressive illness, and most clinicians would advocate treatment for depression (either pharmacological or psychological) as one strategy for reducing the risk of suicide. However, because suicide is a comparatively rare event, this is difficult to demonstrate at a population level in randomised trials. Meta-analyses show no difference in suicide rates between those treated with antidepressants and those treated with placebo (Khan et al., 2003), but study samples are not always representative of typical clinical populations (Gunnell & Ashby, 2004). Before and after studies have shown reductions in suicide rates following training for general practitioners in the assessment and treatment of suicidal patients (Rutz et al., 1992). Ecological studies have shown associations between increased rates of antidepressant prescribing and decreases in suicide rates in some countries (e.g. Sweden – Isaccson, 2000; Australia – Hall et al., 2003; Northern Ireland – Kelly et al., 2003) but not others (e.g. Italy – Barbui et al., 1999; Iceland – Helgason et al., 2004; Britain – Gunnell & Ashby, 2004). However, even in the presence of a positive result, ecological studies are unable to demonstrate that the observed associations are causal. The situation has been further complicated by assertions that one particular class of antidepressant (the selective serotonin reuptake inhibitors [SSRIs]) actually increases the risk of suicide, especially in adolescents. There is some uncertainty about the balance of risks and benefits for SSRIs in this regard (Geddes &

Cipriani, 2004). Nevertheless, appropriate treatment for depression probably still represents a very important strategy for reducing an individual's risk of suicide (Rihmer, 2001).

Pharmacological treatments

As well as antidepressant medication, lithium and clozapine have both been reported to have specific antisuicidal effects. A large randomised controlled trial comparing clozapine to olanzapine in patients with schizophrenia found a 25% reduction in all key measures of suicidality in favour of clozapine (Meltzer et al., 2003). In the United Kingdom, it has been estimated that 50 lives per year (or 5% of the overall national target for suicide prevention) could be saved by increased prescribing of clozapine (Duggan et al., 2003). It has been suggested, mostly on the basis of nonrandomised cohort studies, that long-term treatment with lithium reduces suicide risk in those with affective disorders to levels close to those in the general population (Baldessarini et al., 2003). In a recent retrospective cohort study of more than 20,000 individuals with bipolar disorder, the suicide risk in those taking divalproex was nearly 3 times higher than in those taking lithium (Goodwin et al., 2003). A recent systemic review of randomized trials also suggests that lithium can prevent suicidal behaviour (Cipriani et al., 2005).

Self-harm

Terminology

A number of terms have been used to describe this aspect of suicidal behaviour. *Attempted suicide* is not ideal because many self-harming patients do not wish to die or are too distressed to have formed a clear intent at the time of the episode. *Parasuicide* describes an act of deliberate self-injury or poisoning which mimics the act of suicide but does not result in a fatal outcome (Kreitman, 1977). However, the term still contains a reference to suicide. *Deliberate self-harm* can be defined as an act of intentional self-poisoning or injury irrespective of the apparent purpose of the act (National Health Service Centre for Reviews and Dissemination, 1998). Recently, the prefix *deliberate* has been dropped from *self-harm* in response to the heterogeneous nature of the phenomenon and the concerns of service users (National Collaborating Centre for Mental Health, 2004; Royal College of Psychiatrists, 2004). *Self-harm* is the term that will be used throughout this chapter.

Epidemiology

National statistics on self-harm are difficult to obtain, and much of the epidemiological data come from hospital attendances for self-harm in selected centres. It is estimated that there are at least 170,000 episodes of self-harm presenting to hospitals annually in the United Kingdom, and it is one of the commonest reasons for admission to a general medical bed (Kapur *et al.,* 1998; National Collaborating Centre for Mental Health, 2004). In the United States, it has been suggested that 4% to 5% of the general population report a history of suicidal behaviour (Kessler *et al.,* 1999). Self-harm imposes a significant economic burden, with admission to a medical bed and admission to the intensive care unit accounting for the greatest proportion of direct costs (Kapur *et al.,* 2002).

International comparisons

In Europe, the United States and Australia, there was a substantial increase in the number of hospital-treated episodes of intentional overdose or self-injury in the 1960s and 1970s. Rates stabilised in the 1980s but increased in some countries in the 1990s (Kerkhof, 2000). One of the longest established self-harm monitoring systems in Oxford, United Kingdom, suggests that rates may currently be increasing (Hawton *et al.,* 2002).

In a comparison of rates from nine countries (United States, Canada, Puerto Rico, France, West Germany, Lebanon, Taiwan, Korea and New Zealand) using similar diagnostic criteria, the figure for the lifetime prevalence of suicidal ideation ranged from 2% in Lebanon to 18% in New Zealand (Weissmann *et al.,* 1999). The lifetime prevalence of suicide attempts ranged from 0.7% in Lebanon to 6% in Puerto Rico. Large epidemiological surveys have suggested that 13.5% of the population in the United States and 14.9% in the United Kingdom had experienced suicidal ideas at some point in their life, whereas 4.6% in the United States and 4.4% in the United Kingdom had harmed themselves (Kessler *et al.,* 1999; Meltzer *et al.,* 2002).

The World Health Organisation/Euro multicentre study on attempted suicide investigated incidence rates in well-defined catchment areas in 16 countries (Schmidtke *et al.,* 1996). Medical personnel were asked to fill out standardised monitoring forms on all those who were treated in general hospitals and other medical facilities. However, some episodes never came to medical attention, and so it is likely that the rates quoted in this study underestimate the true rates. For females the age-standardised rate of attempted suicide (1989–1992) ranged from 69 per 100,000 per year in Spain to 462 per 100,000 per year in France. For males the rates ranged from 45 per 100,000 per year in Spain to 314 per 100,000 per year in Finland.

The current rates of self-harm in the United Kingdom are likely to be among the highest in Europe. Recent estimates suggest rates between 300 and 500 per 100,000 per year (Kelly *et al.,* 2002). However, these figures are based on hospital attendances and may represent as few as one third of self-harm episodes overall (Meltzer *et al.,* 2002).

Methods of self-harm

Approximately 80% to 90% of episodes of self-harm are of self-poisoning, and most of the remainder are of self-laceration. Less common methods include burning, stabbing, hanging, self-battery and jumping from a height or in front of a moving vehicle.

The substances taken in overdose tend to reflect general availability or, in the case of prescription-only medication, prescribing trends. For example, barbiturate poisoning was relatively common in the 1960s in the United Kingdom, but this was largely replaced by benzodiazepine poisoning in the 1970s. Benzodiazepines in turn became a relatively uncommon method of poisoning by the 1990s. Recently there has been a substantial increase in the use of paracetamol-containing compounds (taken in 32% of overdoses in 1985 but 50% of episodes in 1997) and antidepressants (taken in 12% of overdoses in 1985 but 20% of episodes in 1997; Townsend, Hawton, Harriss, et al., 2001). Legislation to reduce paracetamol pack sizes in 1998 in the United Kingdom resulted in a 15% decrease in the number of presentations to hospital with paracetamol overdose (and a 29% decrease in the number of deaths) in 1999, but no further decrease in the ensuing 2 years (Hawton et al., 2004). The number of paracetamol tablets taken in overdose decreased in the 3 years after the legislation, as did the number of large paracetamol overdoses.

Sociodemographic factors and self-harm

Self-harm is more common in females than males, but in the United Kingdom, there has been a steady decrease in the female to male ratio over time. Whereas 3 times as many women as men harmed themselves 30 years ago, the current female to male ratio is in the region of 1.5 to 1 (Kelly et al., 2002). Peak ages are 15 to 24 for women and 25 to 34 for men. There is evidence suggesting an increased incidence in certain ethnic groups; for example, it has been reported that young women of South Asian origin are 2.5 times more likely to harm themselves than are white women (Bhugra et al., 1999).

There is a strong association with low social class and unemployment (Platt & Kreitman, 1985). Self-harm is more common among those who are socioeconomically disadvantaged; those who are single, divorced or live alone; those who are single parents; and those who lack social support (Meltzer et al., 2002). A recent study followed up more than 2,000 individuals for 18 months to investigate the factors associated with the development of suicidal thoughts in the general population (Gunnell et al., 2004). The annual incidence of

suicidal thoughts was 2.3%. Female sex, age 16 to 24, lack of a stable relationship, low levels of social support and being unemployed were the baseline factors associated with an increased risk of developing suicidal thoughts over the following 18 months.

Clinical factors and self-harm

Life events are common in the 6 months before self-harm (Paykel, 1975), and difficulties in interpersonal relationships are often the most important precipitating factors (Bancroft et al., 1977). There is also an association between self-harm and the number and type of adverse life events that an individual reports having experienced during his or her lifetime. Sexual abuse may be a particularly strong risk factor (Meltzer et al., 2002).

Although early studies suggested that only a minority of self-harming patients had clinically significant psychiatric illness (Newson-Smith & Hirsch, 1979), more recent work suggests as many as 90% may have an Axis I psychiatric disorder according to research criteria (Haw et al., 2001). The most common diagnosis in this study was affective disorder (70%). Almost half of subjects had psychiatric comorbidity. Personality disorder was identified in 46% of patients at 12- to 16-month follow-up. The authors suggested that patients should be carefully screened for psychiatric disorder at the time of assessment and treated appropriately. However, it is possible that psychiatric symptoms at the time of the episode are relatively transient and may remit spontaneously in a substantial proportion of cases.

A number of psychological characteristics are more common among those who self-harm; these include impulsivity, poor problem solving and hopelessness. It is possible to apply diagnostic labels to these characteristics (e.g. personality disorder), but this may not be particularly helpful because the label may be stigmatising, divert attention from enabling individuals to overcome problems or even lead to them being denied help (National Collaborating Centre for Mental Health, 2004).

Hospital services for self-harm

Service provision

Guidelines for the management of self-harm were published in the United Kingdom in 1994 (Royal College of Psychiatrists, 1994). Two years later, a survey of four teaching hospitals in England found that services for self-harm were in disarray (Kapur *et al.*, 1998). Almost half the patients did not receive the recommended psychosocial assessment. There were wide variations in service provision. For example, there was a fourfold difference in the proportion of patients discharged directly from the emergency department (18%–76%) and a twofold difference in the proportion of patients leaving hospital without a psychosocial assessment (32%–64%). More recent studies (Bennewith *et al.*, 2004; Kapur *et al.*, 2003) suggest that the differences in management are as wide as ever. This striking variability is not due to differences in patient characteristics, so what might account for these findings? Poor resources and a lack of research evidence could be contributing, but there may also be a perception among hospital staff and managers that individuals who burden the Health Service with self-inflicted problems deserve less comprehensive services than those with "serious" medical and psychiatric illnesses (James, 2004).

Guidelines for self-harm

Two sets of guidelines on the management of self-harm have been issued in the United Kingdom recently. The National Institute of Clinical Excellence (NICE)[1] guideline (National Collaborating Centre for Mental Health, 2004) considers the short-term physical and psychosocial management of self-harm. It also includes service users' experience of services and considers issues specific to young people and older adults. The guideline was developed following extensive literature reviews, two focus groups with users and a lengthy consultation process. The main recommendations

---

[1] NICE is a National Health Service body responsible for producing evidence-based clinical guidance in England and Wales.

> **Box 20.3:** Recommendations for the management of self-harm
>
> - People who self-harm should be treated with the same care, respect and privacy as any patient.
> - Clinical and non-clinical staff who have contact with people who self-harm should be provided with appropriate training.
> - Ambulance and emergency department services should ensure that activated charcoal is available to staff at all times.
> - All people who self-harm should be offered a preliminary psychosocial assessment at triage.
> - Consideration should be given to introducing the Australian Mental Health Triage Scale.
> - If a person who has self-harmed has to wait for treatment, he/she should be offered an environment that is safe, supportive and minimises any distress.
> - People who have self-harmed should be offered treatment for the physical consequences of self-harm regardless of their willingness to accept psychosocial or psychiatric treatment.
> - Adequate anaesthesia and/or an analgesia should be offered to people who have self-injured throughout the process of suturing or other painful treatments.
> - Staff should provide all information about treatment options.
> - All people who have self-harmed should be offered an assessment of needs.
> - All people who have self-harmed should be assessed for risk.
> - Following psychosocial assessment the decision regarding further treatment should be based on a comprehensive assessment.
>
> From NICE guidance (National Collaborating Centre for Mental Health, 2004).

are uncontroversial and will be regarded by many as simply components of good practice (Box 20.3). The first recommendation may appear self-evident but is particularly important given the attitudes of some professionals.

The Royal College of Psychiatrists (2004) guideline describes the clinical competencies that might be expected of both nonspecialists and specialists. The guideline also describes standards for the organisation of services, clinical procedures and facilities and training and supervision in a variety of settings (the emergency department, the general hospital, the community setting and the psychiatric inpatient unit). Organisationally, the role of the self-harm services planning group is emphasised. Standards for clinical facilities include all patients being interviewed in private surroundings, emergency department staff having good access to psychiatrists (ideally within 30 minutes in urban areas), swift liaison with general practitioners following discharge and removal of ligature points from in-patient settings.

The outcome of self-harm

Fatal and nonfatal repetition

The 1-year repetition rate for deliberate self-harm is in the region of 15% (Owens *et al.*, 2002). Repetition tends to occur quickly – one third of those who repeat within a year do so within 4 weeks, and the median time to repetition is only around 10 weeks (Kapur *et al.*, 2007). Follow-up studies have shown rates of suicide to be 0.5% to 2% in the year after a deliberate self-harm episode (or 50–200 times the general population rate). It is important to note that this risk persists, with rates of suicide of 3% at 5 years and around 7% for periods longer than 10 years (Owens *et al.*, 2002). A recent UK study suggested a somewhat lower long-term risk, with rates of suicide of 2.4% at 10 years and 3% at 15 years (Hawton *et al.*, 2003). Men and older adults were at greatest risk of suicide. Repeated episodes of self-harm also increased the likelihood of suicide (Zahl & Hawton, 2004). There is also a suggestion that those who cut themselves are at particularly increased risk of suicide (Cooper *et al.*, 2005).

Much has been made of so-called risk factors for repetition and suicide. Some of the most widely reported are listed in Box 20.4. Such risk factors may be of only limited usefulness in everyday practice because of their poor predictive value.

Mortality from natural causes

A British study (Hawton & Fagg, 1988) found twice the expected number of deaths from natural

> **Box 20.4** Risk factors for repetition of self-harm and completed suicide
>
> **Risk factors for repetition of self-harm**
> * Previous history of self-harm
> * Psychiatric history
> * Unemployment
> * Lower social class
> * Alcohol or drug problems
> * Criminal record
> * Antisocial personality
> * Lack of co-operation with treatment
> * Hopelessness
> * High suicidal intent
>
> **Risk factors for completed suicide**
> * Older age
> * Male
> * Previous history of self-harm
> * Psychiatric history
> * Unemployment
> * Poor physical health
> * Social isolation

causes in a large cohort of self-harm patients. The increased risk was particularly associated with deaths from accidents, endocrine causes, nervous system disorders and respiratory disorders. Females were at greater risk than males. A Danish study reported a similar increase in natural deaths but found that men were at greater risk than women (Nordentoft *et al.*, 1993). It found higher than expected rates of death from alcohol-related conditions, digestive disorders, nervous system disorders, respiratory disorders and neoplasms.

Management of self-harm

General principles

The clinical evaluation of patients following self-harm has been referred to as one of the most complex assessments in psychiatry (Isacsson & Rich, 2001). A number of basic principles can be applied to all patients after a self-harm episode.

The initial priority is to ensure that the individual's physical condition is thoroughly assessed and appropriately managed. Thereafter a psychosocial

---

Box 20.5 Information to be recorded in a psychosocial assessment

- Conscious level
- Psychiatric history and Mental State Examination
- Social situation and recent life events
- Risk assessment
- Alcohol and drug use
- Decisions taken
- Specific arrangements for follow-up

Box 20.6 Risk assessment following self-harm

Suicidal intent of current episode
- Premeditation
- Risk of discovery
- Calls for assistance
- Stated intent
- Actual and perceived lethality of method

Psychiatric state
- Depressive features
- Guilt and hopelessness
- Continued suicidal thoughts
- Alcohol and drug misuse
- Impulsive or aggressive personality traits

Social support
- Housing
- Employment
- Family support
- Social isolation
- Involvement of statutory or non statutory organisations

Epidemiological risk factors
- (See Box 20.4)

---

assessment needs to be carried out in all patients to identify and manage those with significant mental health problems and those at high risk of suicide. Box 20.5 lists some of the key components of psychosocial assessment.

Risk assessment, that is, assessing the risk of future self-harm or suicide, is an important clinical skill. It is probably helpful to focus on four areas when carrying out a risk assessment: intent, current psychiatric state, social support and epidemiological risk factors (Box 20.6).

However, risk is not easy to quantify. A recent review of the worldwide literature concluded that there was no evidence that screening for suicide risk reduced suicide attempts or mortality (US Preventive Services Task Force, 2004). There seems to be growing recognition of this fact, with a change in emphasis from "risk assessment" to "needs assessment" in current guidance (National Collaborating Centre for Mental Health, 2004). A needs assessment aims to identify psychosocial factors that might explain an act of self-harm. This will lead to a formulation (describing short- and long-term vulnerability factors and precipitating factors) which will directly inform future management.

After a psychosocial assessment has been carried out, patients should ideally have an individualised management plan. This might involve treatment for psychiatric disorder, the development of skills to solve external problems or admission to a psychiatry in-patient facility.

Compulsory treatment

The issues of compulsory treatment following self-harm are complex. Often the clinician is confronted with an individual who sees no way out of his or her current difficulties, is ambivalent about future suicidal intent and is hostile to the involvement of professionals. A full discussion of these issues is beyond the scope of this chapter, but further guidance is available from both the published literature and medical defence organisations. There are two aspects of treatment which need to be considered: treatment for the physical consequences of the self-harm episode and treatment for any underlying psychiatric disorder. They may be covered by different legislative frameworks (National Collaborating Centre for Mental Health, 2004).

Overnight admission facilities

One important issue is whether patients should routinely be admitted to a medical bed after deliberate self-harm or only if their physical condition warrants it. One randomised controlled trial suggested that admission made no difference to outcome (Waterhouse & Platt, 1990), but the study used a small sample which was not representative of the self-harming population as a whole. Admission has several potential benefits: it makes subsequent psychiatric assessment much easier, especially when (as in half of cases) alcohol consumption is part of the act; it makes it possible to obtain information from other informants; it provides temporary respite; and it allows time to organise follow-up services. Despite these practical advantages, scarce resources mean that some screening of self-harm patients in the emergency department is inevitable in most hospitals. Those who are admitted should ideally go to a single assessment ward. This enables staff on these wards to acquire expertise in dealing with the complex problems of this patient group. It also helps facilitate the referral process to the specialist teams. However, a single assessment facility is unlikely to be widely available in smaller hospitals.

Multidisciplinary teams

There is evidence that health professionals other than psychiatrists can carry out adequate assessments following self-harm attempts (Catalan et al., 1980; Newson-Smith & Hirsch, 1979). The key determinants for successful involvement of other professionals are appropriate training, continuing clinical supervision and easy access to a psychiatric opinion when there is doubt. Self-harm teams might include psychiatric nurses, social workers, junior doctors, clinical psychologists, occupational therapists or emergency department staff. Multidisciplinary approaches have several advantages: the range of available interventions is increased, a wide range of skills can be shared, administrative efficiency and speed of response may be increased and the team approach helps to maintain morale in a service dealing with a difficult patient group.

Aftercare and interventions

Aftercare should be provided promptly in view of the fact that one third of patients who repeat self-harm in the year following an episode do so within 4 weeks. However, this patient group is notoriously difficult to engage. Strategies that could be used to improve uptake of treatment include outreach programmes, home visits, the use of written prompts and aftercare being provided by the health professional who carried out the initial assessment.

What form should intervention take? Psychiatric disorder and continued suicidal intent need to be managed appropriately, perhaps by pharmacological means or admission to psychiatric hospital. Although it is widely reported that no treatments reduce repetition rate, this is principally because studies to date have been too small (Hawton, Townsend, et al., 1999). There are a number of promising interventions. Problem-solving therapy is a brief problem-orientated, cognitively based treatment. Controlled clinical trials have suggested it results in clinically significant improvements following deliberate self-harm (Townsend, Hawton, Altman, et al., 2001). Brief psychodynamic interpersonal therapy involves exploring interpersonal problems which cause or exacerbate psychological distress. The patient–therapist relationship is considered a valuable tool for identifying and helping to resolve interpersonal difficulties. It has been shown to reduce suicidal intent and self-reported deliberate self-harm (Guthrie et al., 2001). For the difficult subgroup of "multiple repeaters", dialectical behaviour therapy is also a possibility (Linehan et al., 1993). It was devised in the United States and combines treatment strategies from supportive, cognitive and behavioural approaches. It involves weekly group and individual sessions for a year, concentrating initially on the suicidal behaviours themselves. Linehan and colleagues' (1993) study showed that this treatment reduced further self-harm in women who had repeatedly harmed themselves. However, the intensity and expense of the treatment means that is unlikely to be suitable for widespread use in centrally managed health services.

The benefit of suicide prevention help lines, such as those run by the Samaritans in the United Kingdom, has not been proved. They provide valuable support to people in crisis and may dissuade individuals from killing themselves, but there is no clear evidence that their impact is sufficient to reduce self-harm or suicide rates (Jennings *et al.*, 1978). However, one naturalistic study did suggest a telephone support and assessment intervention for those over 65 reduced the rate of suicide, especially in elderly women (De Leo *et al.*, 2002).

There is limited evidence that "crisis cards" (which carry advice about seeking help in the event of a crisis and provide contact details) may be beneficial in certain groups of patients. The original Bristol Green Card study showed a significant decrease in repetition in those who received the card compared with those who did not (Morgan *et al.*, 1993). However, this study only included those for whom the index episode was their lifetime first. A later study of the same intervention in a larger sample found no overall benefit (Evans *et al.*, 1999). There was a small decrease in repetition among first-time presenters but a significant increase in those who had made previous attempts. Sending regular postcards to individuals after hospital attendance for self-poisoning may reduce repetition in sub-groups of patients (Carter *et al.*, 2005).

The largely negative results of some of the recent larger trials (Tyrer *et al.*, 2003) have led some investigators to argue that perhaps we should concentrate either on very large trials of low-intensity interventions (such as emergency cards) or smaller trials of longer-term, more intensive psychological treatments (Williams, 2004). However, because one of the difficulties in this area of research is ensuring that patients receive the assigned treatment, an alternative might be a large-scale evaluation of a brief psychological intervention which specifically addresses issues related to engagement early in the therapy. We should probably consider outcomes other than repeat presentation to hospital (such as self-reported self-harm, depression, hopelessness, loss from services, quality of life and user satisfaction). Alternative methodological approaches may also be of benefit, such as qualitative or cohort study designs.

Conclusions

Suicide and self-harm are important health problems worldwide and an important cause of premature mortality. Advances in epidemiology, neuroimaging and genetics may help to improve our understanding of these complex behaviours. Research in this area is difficult because outcomes related to suicide or repetition of suicidal behaviour are comparatively rare. Suicide prevention has become a priority in many countries, and suicide prevention strategies need to be comprehensive and involve a wide range of agencies. Large-scale intervention studies are required to inform specific treatment approaches.

REFERENCES

Abbott, R., Young, S., Grant, G., Goward, P., Seager, C., & Ludlow, J. (2003). *Railway Suicide: An Investigation of Individual and Organisational Consequences.* Doncaster: Doncaster and South Humber Healthcare NHS Trust.

Ajdacic-Gross, V., Bupp, M., Sansossic, R., *et al.* (2005). Diversity and change in suicide seasonality over 125 years. *J Epidemiol Community Health* 59:967–72.

Allebeck, P., & Allgulander, C. (1990). Suicide among young men: psychiatric illness, deviant behaviour and substance abuse. *Acta Psychiat Scand* 81:565–70.

Allebeck, P., Varla, A., Kristjansson, E., & Wistedt, B. (1987). Risk factors for suicide among patients with schizophrenia. *Acta Psychiat Scand* 81:565–70.

Allebeck, P., & Wistedt, B. (1986). Mortality in schizophrenia. A ten year follow-up based on the Stockholm county in-patient register. *Arch Gen Psychiaty* 43:650–3.

Amos, T., Appleby, L., & Kiernan, K. (2001). Changes in rates of suicide by car exhaust asphyxiation in England and Wales. *Psychol Med* 31:935–9.

Appleby, L. (1991). Suicide during pregnancy and in the first postnatal year. *BMJ* 302(6769):137–40.

Appleby, L. (1992). Suicide in psychiatric patients: risk and prevention. *Br J Psychiatry* 161:749–58.

Appleby, L., Cooper, J., Amos, T., & Faragher, B. (1999). Psychological autopsy study of suicides by people aged under 35. *Br J Psychiatry* **175**:168–74.

Appleby, L., Dennehy, J. A., Thomas, C. S., *et al.* (1999b). Aftercare and clinical characteristics of people with mental illness who commit suicide: a case-control study. *Lancet* **353**:1397–1400.

Appleby, L., Shaw, J., Amos, T., *et al.* (1999). Suicide within 12 months of contact with mental health services: national clinical survey. *BMJ* **318**:1235–9.

Appleby, L., Shaw, J., Meehan, J., *et al.* (2001). *Safety First. Five year report of the National Confidential Inquiry into Suicide and Homicide by People with Mental Illness.* London: Department of Health.

Baldessarini, R. J., Tondo, L., & Hennen, J. (2003). Lithium treatment and suicide risk in major affective disorders: update and new findings. *J Clin Psychiatry* **64**(suppl 5): 44–52.

Bancroft, J., Skrimshire, A., Casson, J., *et al.* (1977). People who deliberately poison or injure themselves: their problems and their contacts with helping agencies. *Psychol Med* 77:289–303.

Barbui, C., Campomori, A., D'Avanzo, B., *et al.* (1999). Antidepressant drug use in Italy since the introduction of the SSRIs: national trends, regional differences and impact on suicide rates. *Soc Psychiatry Psychiatr Epidemiol* 34:152–6.

Beck, A. T., Emery, G., & Greenberg, R. L. (1985). *Anxiety Disorders and Phobias: A Cognitive Perspective.* New York: Basic Books.

Bennewith, O., Gunnell, D., Peters, T. J., *et al.* (2004). Variations in the hospital management of self harm in adults in England: observational study. *BMJ* **328**:1108–9.

Bertolote, J. M., & Fleischmann, A. (2001). Suicide and a psychiatric diagnosis: a world-die perspective. *World Psychiatry* 1:181–5.

Berglund, M. (1984). Suicide in alcoholism. A prospective study of 88 suicides: I. The multidimensional diagnosis at first admission. *Arch Gen Psychiatry* 41:888–91.

Berglund, M., & Nilsson, K. (1987). Mortality in severe depression. A prospective study including 103 suicides. *Acta Psychiatr Scand* **76**:372–80.

Bhugra, D., Desai, M., & Baldwin, D. (1999). Attempted suicide in West London 1: rates across ethnic communities. *Psychol Med* 29:1125–30.

Biddle, L., Brook, A., Brookes, S. T., & Gunnell, D. (2008). Suicide rates in young men in England and Wales in the 21st century: time trend study. *BMJ* **336**:539–42.

Bille-Brahe, U. (2000). Sociology and suicidal behaviour. In K. Hawton & K. Van Heeringen, eds. *N Suicide and Attempted Suicide.* Chichester: Wiley, pp. 193–207.

Boardman, A. P., & Healy, D. (2001). Modelling suicide risk in affective disorders. *Eur Psychiatry* **16**:400–5.

Boyd, J. H. (1983). The increasing rate of suicide by firearms. *N Engl J Med.* **308**:872–4.

Brock, A., & Griffiths, C. (2003). Trends in suicide by methods in England and Wales, 1979 to 2001. *Health Stat Q* **20**:7–18.

Cantor, C. H. (2000). Suicide in the Western world. In K. Hawton & K. Van Heeringen, eds. *Suicide and Attempted Suicide.* Chichester: Wiley, pp. 9–28.

Cantor, C., & Neulinger, K. (2000). The epidemiology of suicide and attempted suicide among young Australians. *Aust N Z J Psychiatry.* 34:370–87.

Carter, G. L., Clover, K., Whyte, I. M., Dawson, A. H., & D'Este, C. (2005). Postcards from the EDge project: randomised controlled trial of an intervention using postcards to reduce repetition of hospital treated deliberate self poisoning *BMJ* 331:805–7.

Catalan, J., Marsack, P., Hawton, K., *et al.* (1980). Comparison of doctors and nurses in assessment of deliberate self-poisoning patients. *Psychol Med* 10:483–91.

Cavanagh, J. T. O., Carson, A. J., Sharpe, M., & Lawrie, S. M. (2003). Psychological autopsy studies of suicide: a systematic review. *Psychol Med* 33:395–405.

Cavanagh, J. T. O., Owens, D. G. C., & Johnstone, E. C. (1999). Suicide and undetermined death in South East Scotland: a case control study using the psychological autopsy method. *Psychol Med* 29:1141–9.

Chishti, P., Stone, D. H., Corcoran, P., *et al.* (2003). Suicide mortality in the European Union. *Eur J Public Health* 13:108–14.

Cipriani, A., Pretty, H., Hawton, K., *et al.* (2005). Lithium in the prevention of suicidal behaviour and all-cause mortality in patients with mood disorders: a systematic review of randomized trials. *Am J Psychiatry* **162**:1805–19.

Cohen, L. J., Test, M. A., & Brown, R. L. (1990). Suicide and schizophrenia: data from a prospective community treatment study. *Am J Psychiatry* **147**:602–7.

Commonwealth Department of Health and Aged Care (2000). *Living Is for Everyone: A Framework for the Prevention of Suicide and Self-Harm in Australia.* Canberra: Commonwealth Department of Health and Aged Care.

Cooper, J., Appleby, L., & Amos, T. (2002). Life events preceding suicide by young people. *Soc Psychiatry Psychiatr Epidemiol* 37:271–5.

Cooper, J., Kapur, N., Webb, R., *et al.* (2005). Suicide in the first four years following self harm: a cohort study. *Am J Psychiatry* **162**:297–303.

Copas, J. B., Freeman-Browne, D. L., & Robin, A. A. (1971). Danger periods for suicide in patients under treatment. *Psychol Med* **1**:400–4.

Crammer, J. L. (1984). The special characteristics of suicide in hospital in-patients. *Br J Psychiatry* **145**:460–76.

De Leo, D., Buono, M. D., & Dwyer, J. (2002). Suicide among the elderly: the long-term impact of a telephone support and assessment intervention in northern Italy. *Br J Psychiatry* **181**: 226–9.

Department of Health (2002). *National Suicide Prevention Strategy for England.* London: Her Majesty's Stationery Office.

Drake, R. E., & Cotton, P. G. (1986). Depression, hopelessness and suicide in chronic schizophrenia. *Br J Psychiatry* **148**:554–9.

Drake, R. E., Gates, C., & Cotton, P. G., & Whittaker, A. (1984). Suicide among schizophrenics. Who is at risk? *J Nerv Ment Dis* **172**:613–17.

Duggan, A., Warner, J., Knapp, M., & Kerwin, R. (2003). Modelling the impact of clozapine on suicide in patients with treatment resistant schizophrenia in the UK. *Br J Psychiatry* **182**:505–8.

Durkheim, E. (1951). *Suicide.* New York: Free Press. Original work published 1897.

Evans, M., Morgan, H., Heywood, A., & Gunnell, D. (1999). Crisis telephone consultation for deliberate self harm patients: effects on repetition. *Br J Psychiatry* **175**:23–7

Fawcett, J., Scheftner, W., Clark, D., *et al.* (1987). Clinical predictors of suicide in patients with major affective disorders: a controlled prospective study. *Am J Psychiatry* **144**:35–40.

Fawcett, J., Scheftner, W. A., Fogg, L., *et al.* (1990). Time-related predictors of suicide in patients with major affective disorder. *Am J Psychiatry* **147**:1189–94.

Foster, T., Gillespie, K., & Mclelland, R. (1997). Mental disorders and suicide in Northern Ireland. *Br J Psychiatry* **170**:447–52.

Gale, S., W., Mesnikoff, A., Fine, J., *et al.* (1980). Study of suicide in state mental hospitals in New York City. *Psychiatr Q* **52**:201–13.

Geddes, J. R., & Cipriani, A. (2004). Selective serotonin reuptake inhibitors. *BMJ* **329**:809–10.

Gunnell, D., & Ashby, D. (2004). Antidepressants and suicide: what is the balance of benefit and harm. *BMJ* **329**:34–8.

Goodwin, F. K., Fireman, B., Simon, G. E., *et al.* (2003). Suicide risk in bipolar disorder during treatment with lithium and divalproex. *JAMA* **290**:1467–73.

Gunnell, D., & Frankel, S. (1994). Prevention of suicide: aspirations and evidence. *BMJ* **308**:1227–33.

Gunnell, D., Harbord, R., Singleton, N., *et al.* (2004). Factors influencing the development and amelioration of suicidal thoughts in the general population. *Br J Psychiatry* **185**:385–93.

Gunnell, D., & Middleton, N. (2003). National suicide rates as an indicator of the effect of suicide on premature mortality. *Lancet* **362**:961–2.

Gunnell, D., Middleton, N., & Frankel, S. (2000). Method availability and the prevention of suicide – a re-analysis of secular trends in England and Wales 1950–1975. *Soc Psychiatry Psychiatr Epidemiol* **35**(10):437–43

Gunnell, D., Middleton, N., Whitley, E., *et al.* (2003). Why are suicide rates rising in young men but falling in the elderly? – a time series analysis of trends in England and Wales 1959–1998. *Soc Sci Med* **57**:595–611.

Guthrie, E., Kapur, N., Mackway-Jones, K., *et al.* (2001). Randomised controlled trial of brief psychological intervention after deliberate self poisoning. *BMJ* **323**:135–8.

Guze, S. B., & Robins, E. (1970). Suicide and primary affective disorder. *Br J Psychiatry* **117**:437–8.

Hall, W. D., Mant, A., Mitchell, P. B., *et al.* (2003). Association between antidepressant prescribing and suicide in Australia, 1991–2000: trend analysis. *BMJ* **326**:1008–12.

Harris, E. C., & Barraclough, B. (1997). Suicide as an outcome for mental disorders. A meta-analysis. *Br J Psychiatry* **170**:205–28.

Haw, C., Hawton, K., Houston, K., & Townsend, E. (2001). Psychiatric and personality disorders in deliberate self-harm patients. *Br J Psychiatry* **178**:48–54.

Hawton, K., Casey, D., Simkin, S., *et al.* (2002). *Deliberate Self-Harm in Oxford.* Oxford: University of Oxford, Centre for Suicide Research.

Hawton, K., & Fagg, J. (1988). Suicide, and other causes of death, following attempted suicide. *Br J Psychiatry* **152**:359–66.

Hawton, K., Simkin, S., Deeks, J. J., *et al.* (1999). Effects of a drug overdose in a television drama on presentations to hospital for self-poisoning: time series and questionnaire study. *BMJ* **318**:972–7.

Hawton, K., Townsend, E., Arensman, E., *et al.* (1999b). Psychosocial and pharmacological treatments for deliberate self harm. *Cochrane Database of Syst Rev* **4**:CD001764.

Hawton, K., Zahl, D., & Weatherall, R. (2003). Suicide following deliberate self-harm: long term follow-up of patients who presented to a general hospital. *Br J Psychiatry* 182:537–42.

Hawton, K., Simkin, S., Deeks, J., *et al.* (2004). UK legislation on analgesic packs: before and after study of long term effect on poisonings. *BMJ* 329:1076.

Heikkinen, M. E., Isometsa, E. T., Marttunen, M. H., *et al.* (1995). Social factors in suicide. *Br J Psychiatry* 167:747–53.

Helgason, T., Tomasson, H., Zoega, T. (2004). Antidepressants and public health in Iceland. Time series analysis of national data, *Br J Psychiatry* 184:157–62.

Hiroeh, U., Appleby, L., Mortensen, P. B., & Dunn, G. (2001). Death by homicide, suicide and other unatural causes in people with mental illness: a population based study. *Lancet* 358:2110–12.

Hoyer, G., & Lund, E. (1993). Suicide among women related to number of children in marriage. *Arch Gen Psychiatry* 50.134–7.

Inskip, H. M., Harris, C. E., & Barraclough, B. (1998). Lifetime risk of suicide for affective disorder, alcoholism and schizophrenia. *Br J Psychiatry* 1721:35–7.

Isacsson, G. (2000). Suicide prevention – a medical breakthrough. *Acta Psychiatr Scand* 102:113–27.

Isacsson, G., & Rich, C. I. (2001). Management of patients who deliberately harm themselves. *BMJ* 322:213–15.

James, A. (2004). Psychiatrists rebuke colleagues over remarks on self harming patients. Available at http://www.psychminded.co.uk. Accessed 15 October 2004.

Jennings, C., Barraclough, B. M., & Moss, J. R. (1978). Have the Samaritans lowered the suicide rate? A controlled study. *Psychol Med* 8:412–22.

Kapur, N., Cooper, J., King-Hele, S., *et al.* (2006). The repetition of suicidal behaviour: a multicenter cohort study. *J Clin Psychiatry* 67:1599–1609.

Kapur, N., & House A. (1998). Against a high-risk strategy in the prevention of suicide. *Psychiatr Bull* 22:534–6.

Kapur, N., House, A., Creed, F., *et al.* (1998). Management of deliberate self-poisoning in adults in four teaching hospitals: descriptive study. *BMJ* 316:831–2.

Kapur, N., House, A., Dodgson, K., *et al.* (2002). Management and costs of deliberate self-poisoning in the general hospital: a multi-centre study. *J Ment Health* 11:223–30.

Kapur, N., House, A., May, C., & Creed, F. (2003). Service provision and outcome for deliberate self-poisoning in adults: results from a six centre descriptive study. *Soc Psychiatry Psychiatr Epidemiol* 38:390–5.

Kelly, C. B., Ansari, T., Rafferty, T., & Stevenson, M. (2003). Antidepressant prescribing and suicide rate in Northern Ireland. *Eur Psychiatry* 18:325–8.

Kelly, J., Cooper, J., Johnston, A., *et al.* (2002). *Manchester Self-Harm Project, 5th Year Report.* Manchester: University of Manchester.

Kerkhof, A. J. F. M. (2000). Attempted suicide: patterns and trends. In K. Hawton & K. Van Heeringen, eds. *Suicide and Attempted Suicide.* Chichester: Wiley, pp. 49–64.

Kessler, R. C., Borges, G., & Walters, E. (1999). Prevalence of and risk factors for lifetime suicide attempts in the national comorbidity survey. *Arch Gen Psychiatry* 56:617–26.

Khan, A., Khan, S., Kolts, R., & Brown, W. A. (2003). Suicide rates in clinical trials of SSRI's, other antidepressants, and placebo: analysis of FDA reports. *Am J Psychiatry* 160:760–92.

King, E., Baldwin D., Sinclair, J, *et al.* (2001a). The Wessex recent inpatient suicide study, 2. Case control study of 59 inpatient suicides. *Br J Psychiatry* 178:537–42.

King, E., Baldwin, D., Sinclair, J., *et al.* (2001b). The Wessex recent inpatient suicide study, 1. Case control study of 234 recently discharged psychiatric patient suicides. *Br J Psychiatry* 178:531–6.

King, E., & Barraclough, B. (1990). Violent death and mental illness. A study of a single catchment area over 8 years. *Br J Psychiatry* 156:714–20.

Kreitman, N. (1976). The coal gas story. *Br J Prevent Soc Med* 30:86–93.

Kreitman, N. (1977). *Parasuicide.* London: Wiley.

Kreitman, N. (1988). Suicide, age and marital status. *Psychol Med* 18:121–8.

Lester, D., & Abe, K. (1989). The effect of restricting access to lethal methods for suicide: a study of suicide by domestic gas in Japan. *Acta Psychiatr Scand* 80:180–2.

Levi, F., La Vecchia, C., & Saraceno, B. (2003). Global suicide rates. *Eur J Public Health* 13:97–8.

Linehan, M. M., Heard, H. L., & Armstrong, H. E. (1993). Naturalistic follow up of a behavioral treatment for chronically parasuicidal borderline patients. *Arch Gen Psychiatry* 50:971–4.

Linsley, K. R., Schapira, K., & Kelly, T. P. (2001). Open verdict vs. suicide – importance to research. *Br J Psychiatry* 178:465–8.

Mann, J. J. (2002). A current perspective of suicide and attempted suicide. *Ann Int Med* 136:302–11.

Maris, R. W. (2002). Suicide. *Lancet* 360:319–26.

Meltzer, H., Lader, D., & Corbin, T., *et al.* (2002). *Non-Fatal Suicidal Behaviour Among Adults Aged 16–74 in Great*

Britain. London: Office of National Statistics, The Stationary Office.

Meltzer, H. Y., Alphs, L., Green, A. I., *et al.* (2003). Clozapine treatment for suicidality in schizophrenia: International Suicide Prevention Trial (InterSePT). *Arch Gen Psychiatry* **60**:82–91.

Middleton, N., Gunnell, D., Frankel, S., *et al.* (2003). Urban-rural differences in suicide trends in young adults: England and Wales, 1981–1998, *Soc Sci Med* **57**:1183–94.

Middleton, N., Whitley, E., Frankel, S., *et al.* (2004). Suicide risk in small areas in England and Wales, 1991–1993. *Soc Psychiatry Psychiatr Epidemiol* **39**:45–52.

Morgan, H. E., Jones, E. M., & Owen, J. H. (1993). Secondary prevention of non fatal deliberate self harm: the green card study. *Br J Psychiatry* **163**:111–12.

Morgan, H. G. (1979). *Death Wishes? The Understanding and Management of Deliberate Self Harm*. Chichester: Wiley.

Muldoon, M., Manucks, S., & Matthews, K. (1990). Varying cholesterol concentration zone mortality: a quantitative view of primary prevention trials *BMJ* **301**:309–14.

Murphy, G. E., Armstrong, J. W., Hermele, S. L., *et al.* (1979). Suicide and alcoholism. Interpersonal loss confirmed as a predictor. *Arch Gen Psychiatry* **36**:65–9.

Murphy, G. E., & Wetzel, R. D. (1990). Lifetime risk of suicide in alcoholism. *Arch Gen Psychiatry* **47**:383–92.

National Collaborating Centre for Mental Health (2004). *Self-Harm: The Short Term Physical and Psychological Management and Secondary Prevention of Self-Harm in Primary and Secondary Care* (full guideline). Clinical Guideline 16. London: National Institute of Clinical Excellence.

Neeleman, J., & Wessely, S. (1997). Changes in classification of suicide in England and Wales: time trends and associations with coroners' professional backgrounds. *Psychol Med* **27**:467–72.

Newson-Smith, J. G. B., & Hirsch, S. R. (1979). A comparison of social workers and psychiatrists in evaluating parasuicide. *Br J Psychiatry* **134**:335–42.

National Health Service Centre for Reviews and Dissemination (1998). *Effect Health Care Bull* **4**:1–12.

Nordentoft, M., Breum, L., Munck, L., *et al.* (1993). High mortality by natural and unnatural causes: a 10 year follow up study of patients admitted to a poisoning treatment centre after suicide attempts. *BMJ* **306**:1637–41.

Owens, D., Horrocks, J., & House, A. (2002). Fatal and non-fatal repetition of self harm. *Br J Psychiatry* **181**:193–9.

Paykel, E. (1975). Suicide attempts and recent life events. *Arch Gen Psychiatry* **32**:327–33.

Phillips, D. P., & Ruth, T. E. (1993). Adequacy of official suicide statistics for scientific research and public policy. *Suicide Life-Threat Behav* **23**:207–19.

Platt, S., & Kreitman, N. (1985). Parasuicide and unemployment among men in Edinburgh *Psychol Med* **15**:113–23.

Pounder, D. J. (1991). Changing patterns of male suicide in Scotland. *Foren Sci Int* **51**:79–87.

Pritchard, C. (1996). Suicide in the People's Republic of China categorized by age and gender: evidence of the influence of culture on suicide. *Acta Psychiatr Scand* **93**:362–7.

Pritchard, C. (1988). Suicide gender and unemployment in the British Isles and the EEC 1974–85. *Soc Psychiatry Psychiatr Epidemiol* **23**:85–9.

Qin, P., Agerbo, E., & Westergard-Neilsen, N., *et al.* (2000). Gender differences in risk factors for suicide in Denmark. *Br J Psychiatry* **177**:546–50.

Qin, P., & Nordentoft, M. (2005). Suicide risk in relation to psychiatric hospitalization. Evidence based on longitudinal registers. *Arch Gen Psychiatry* **62**:427–32.

Rich, C. L., Fowler, R. C., Fogarty, L. A., & Young, D. (1988). San Diego suicide study. III. Relationship between diagnoses and stressors. *Arch Gen Psychiatry* **45**:589–92.

Rihmer, Z. (2001). Can better recognition and treatment of depression reduce suicide rates? A brief review. *Eur Psychiatry* **16**:406–9.

Rose, G. (1992). *The Strategy of Preventative Medicine*. Oxford: Oxford University Press.

Roy, A. (1990). Suicide in twins. *Arch Gen Psychiatry* **48**:29–31.

Roy, A. (1982a). Risk factors for suicide in psychiatric patients. *Arch Gen Psychiatry* **39**:1089–95.

Roy, A. (1982b). Suicide in chronic schizophrenia. *Br J Psychiatry* **141**:613–17.

Royal College of Psychiatrists. (1994). *The General Hospital Management of Adult Deliberate Self-Harm: A Consensus Statement on Standards for Service Provision* (Council Report Number 32). London: Royal College of Psychiatrists.

Royal College of Psychiatrists. (2004). *Assessment Following Self-Harm in Adults*. London: Royal College of Psychiatrists.

Rutz, W., Von Knorring, L., & Walinder, J. (1992). Long term effects of an educational program for general practitioners given by the Swedish committee for the prevention and treatment of depression. *Acta Psychiatrica Scand* **85**:83–8.

Schmidtke, A., Bille-Brahe, U., DeLeo, D., *et al.* (1996). Attempted suicide in Europe: rates, trends and sociodemographic characteristics of suicide attempters during the period 1989–1992. Results of the WHO/EURO multicentre study on parasuicide. *Acta Psychiatr Scand* **93**:327–38.

Schmidtke, A., & Hafner, H. (1988). The Werther effect after television films: new evidence for an old hypothesis. *Psychol Med* **18**:665–76.

Schulsinger, R., Kety, S., Rosenthal, D., & Wender, P. (1979). A family study of suicide. In M. Schow & E. Strongen, eds. *Origins, Prevention and Treatment of Affective Disorders*. New York: Academic Press.

Shafii, M., Carrigan, S., Whittinghilld, R., & Derrick, A. (1985). Psychological autopsy of completed suicides in children and adolescence. *Am J Psychiatry* **142**:1061–4.

Sims, A., & O'Brien, K. (1979). Autokabalesis: an account of mentally ill people who jump from buildings. *Med Sci Law* **19**:195–8.

Soni Raleigh, V., & Balarajan, R. (1992). Suicide levels and trends among immigrants in England and Wales. *Health Trends* **24**:91–4.

Soni Raleigh, V., Bulusu, L., & Balarajan, R. (1990). Suicides among immigrants from the Indian sub-continent. *Br J Psychiatry* **156**:46–50.

Taylor, S. J., King, D., Jenkins, R. (1997). Stop power nations trying to prevent suicide? An analysis of national suicide prevention strategies. *Acta Psychiatr Scand* **95**:457–63.

Temoche, A., Pugh, T. F., & McMahon, B. (1964). Suicide rates among current and former mental institution patients. *J Nerv Ment Dis* **138**:124–31.

Townsend, E., Hawton, K., Altman, D. G., et al. (2001). The efficacy of problem solving treatments after deliberate self-harm: meta analysis of randomized controlled trials with respect to depression, hopelessness and improvements in problems. *Psychol Med* **31**:979–88.

Townsend, E., Hawton, K., Harriss, L., et al. (2001). Substances used in deliberate self-poisoning 1985–1997: trends and associations with age, gender, repetition and suicide intent. *Soc Psychiatry Psychiatr Epidemiol* **36**:228–34.

Traskman, L., Asberg, M., & Birtleson, L. (1981). Monomine metabolites in CSF and suicidal behaviour. *Arch Gen Psych* **38**:631–6.

Tsuang, M. T. (1983). Risk of suicide in the relatives of schizophrenics, manics, depressives and controls. *J Clin Psychiatry* **44**:396–400.

Tyrer, P., Thompson, S., Schmidt, U., et al. (2003). Randomized controlled trial of brief cognitive behaviour therapy versus treatment as usual in recurrent deliberate self-harm: the POPMACT study. *Psychol Med* **33**:969–76.

US Preventative Services Task Force. (2004). Screening for Suicide Risk: Recommendation and Rationale. *Ann Int Med* **140**:820–37.

US Public Health Service (1999). *The Surgeon General's Call to Action to Prevent Suicide*. Washington, DC: US Public Health Service.

Van Heeringen, K. (2001). *Understanding Suicidal Behaviour*. Chichester: Wiley.

Waern, M., Rubenowitz, E., Runeson, B., et al. (2002). Burden of illness and suicide in elderly people: case control study. *BMJ* **324**:1355–7.

Waterhouse, J., & Platt, S. (1990). General hospital admission in the management of parasuicide: a randomized controlled trial. *Br J Psychiatry* **156**:236–42.

Weissman, M. M., Bland, R. C., Canino, G. J., et al. (1999). Prevalence of suicide ideation and suicide attempts in nine countries. *Psychol Med* **29**:9–17.

Wender, P., Kety, S., Rosenthal, D., et al. (1986). Psychiatric disorders in the biological and adoptive families of adopted individuals with affective disorders. *Arch Gen Psychiatry* **43**:923–9.

Williams, M. G. (2004). Psychological treatment for suicidal behaviour. Plenary presentation (PL04.2) at the 10th European Symposium on Suicide and Suicidal Behaviour, Copenhagen, Denmark 25–28 August 2004.

Wilson, J. F. (2004). Finland pioneers international suicide prevention. *Ann Int Med* **140**:853–6.

Zahl, D. L., & Hawton, K. (2004). Repetition of deliberate self-harm and subsequent suicide risk: long term follow-up study of 11583 patients. *Br J Psychiatry* **185**:70–5.

Psychiatry in Specific Settings

Psychiatry in primary care

Paul Walters, André Tylee and Sir David Goldberg

Primary care occupies a position of utmost importance in the management of mental health problems. This was recognised nearly 40 years ago when Shepherd *et al.* (1966) completed their seminal study *Psychiatric Illness in General Practice*. For the first time, mental health morbidity in primary care became quantifiable, and these researchers were able to show that mental health problems were among the more common reasons for consultation in general practice. Since then, research into mental health problems in primary care has increased. However, the findings remain largely similar: much of the psychiatric morbidity in primary care is missed and a significant proportion of patients suffering from mental health problems in primary care have a less-than-optimal outcome. Despite this, recent research exploring novel methods of service provision in primary care settings are showing encouraging results, confirming Shepherd and colleagues' views that improvements in the provision of mental health care would be achieved through "a strengthening of the family doctor in his therapeutic role" rather than directly through psychiatric services (Shepherd *et al*, 1966).

Epidemiology

Mental health problems are common in primary care. The World Health Organisation's (WHO) collaborative study, Psychological Problems in General Health Care, screened nearly 26,000 consecutive primary care patients for common mental disorders in 15 centres across 14 countries (Turkey, Greece, India, Germany, Netherlands, Nigeria, United Kingdom, Japan, France, Brazil, Chile, United States, China and Italy; Ustun *et al.*, 1995). Of these nearly 5,500 patients completed a baseline diagnostic assessment, and nearly 3,200 completed a 12-month follow-up. Overall the prevalence rates of current *International Classification of Diseases* (10th revision; ICD-10) disorders were as follows: depression 10.4%, generalised anxiety disorder 7.9%, harmful use of alcohol 3.3%, alcohol dependence 2.7%, somatisation disorder 2.7%, dysthymia 2.1%, panic disorder 1%, agoraphobia 1.5% and hypochondriasis 0.8%. Twenty-four percent had a current mental disorder as defined by ICD-10, and 9.5% had two or more disorders. Considerable variation in prevalence across centres was found, although depression, generalised anxiety disorder and alcohol problems were the commonest across all the centres. Women were almost twice as likely as men to suffer from depression, but men were more likely to suffer from alcohol problems. Overall the prevalence of common mental disorders was the same for men and women. Other studies of consecutive general practitioner (GP) attendees have found a similar prevalence of common mental disorders of between 25% and 50% with depression accounting for 5% to 15% of consecutive consultations (Blacker & Clare, 1987; Freeling *et al.*, 1985;

Essential Psychiatry, ed. Robin M. Murray, Kenneth S. Kendler, Peter McGuffin, Simon Wessely, David J. Castle.
Published by Cambridge University Press. © Cambridge University Press 2008.

Level	Prevalence of mental disorder (per 1000 adults per year)	Filter
1. Community	260–315	
		1. Illness behaviour
2. Primary Care – total prevalence of mental disorder	230	
		2. Ability of GP to recognise mental illness
3. Primary Care – prevalence of mental illness recognised by GP	100	
		3. Referral to specialist services
4. Referred to specialist services	24	
		4. Admission to psychiatric hospital
5. Psychiatric in-patient care	6	

Figure 21.1 Pathways to Psychiatric Care, rates per thousand population at risk, South Manchester 1992. Adapted from Goldberg & Huxley (page 4, Table 1.1 in *Common mental disorders. A biosocial model.* Goldberg & Huxley, 1992).

Tiemens *et al.*, 1996). In any one year, 14% of patients registered with a GP in the United Kingdom will consult for a mental health problem (Shepherd *et al.*, 1966). Psychotic disorders are much less common in primary care. In the United Kingdom, the prevalence of treated schizophrenia in primary care is about 0.2% (Office for National Statistics, 1998) and 0.3% to 0.4% for bipolar affective disorder (Strathdee & Jenkins, 1996).

Mental health problems are also common in the young and the elderly in primary care. Up to 25% of children in primary care suffer from a psychiatric disorder, emotional problems being the most common. Garralda *et al.* (1994) found 23% of consecutive child attendees aged between 7 and 12 had an emotional, conduct or mixed emotional and conduct disorder. Among older people, up to 16% of those aged over 65 and 10% of those over 75 in primary care suffer from depression (Copeland *et al.*, 1992; Livingston *et al.*, 1990). In an average list of 2,000 patients, 30 (10%) patients over age 65 could

be expected to suffer an organic brain syndrome and 93 (31%) from a functional disorder (Graham, 1991).

Goldberg and Huxley (1980) proposed a "pathways to care model" to conceptualise psychiatric morbidity in the community. Their model has five levels (see Figure 21.1). The first level corresponds to the prevalence of psychiatric disorder in the community; the second level, the prevalence of mental illness in those who attend their GP for any reason; the third level, the prevalence of mental disorder correctly identified by the GP; the fourth level, the prevalence of psychiatric morbidity referred to specialist mental health services; and the fifth level, the prevalence of patients with mental disorders admitted to hospital. Between each level, the authors conceptualised filters which determine the passage of patients from one level to the next. The first filter is the health-seeking behaviour of patients. The second is the ability of the GP to diagnose a mental disorder correctly, the third filter is referral to specialist mental health services and the fourth filter is the decision by specialist mental health services to admit the patient to hospital (Goldberg & Huxley, 1992).

Classification of mental disorders in primary care

Diagnosis in primary care is often more complex than in secondary care. Patients rarely present with discrete illnesses, and usually a mixture of physical and somatic symptoms are presented. Complicating diagnosis further, patients with chronic medical disorders are more likely to suffer from psychiatric illness. It can often be difficult to disentangle which symptoms are due to a physical and which to a psychiatric disorder. Any classification system for use in primary care therefore needs to be flexible and take these difficulties into consideration. It should also make clinical sense, be linked to clinical practice and be user-friendly to enable its use by any member of a multiprofessional primary care team.

A number of approaches have been taken to classify mental health problems in primary care. Broadly these can be divided into the following: systems designed by primary care professionals, systems derived from specialist classifications and systems designed jointly by GPs and specialists. All have merits and limitations, although those designed jointly may be better able to take into account the needs of both professional sectors.

The International Classification of Health Problems in Primary Care (ICHPCC-2) is a system developed by primary care professionals which allows the classification of 21 mental health conditions. However, a limitation of this system is that some of the conditions it recognises are overinclusive, whereas other important syndromes are not classified. (World Organisation of National Colleges Academies and Academic Associations of General Practitioners, 1988.)

The Read Code system is widely used by GPs in the United Kingdom and allows classification by diagnoses, symptoms and problems (Saint-Yves, 1992). Currently about 97% of UK practices use Read Codes, and they are also used for data collection within the National Health Service. A problem with this system is that its heterogeneity (which promotes its clinical utility) can give rise to great variation in how practices use it (Jenkins *et al.*, 1988).

Specialist classification systems (e.g. ICD-10 and *Diagnostic and Statistical Manual of Mental Disorders,* 4th edition [DSM-IV]) used in primary care can be problematic because they are devised for a very different population of patients from those seen in primary care, are too complicated and unwieldy for routine use in primary care and their clinical utility is limited because they are not linked to management. One solution has been to try to adapt these systems for use in primary care. The ICD-10 PHC (ICD-10 Primary Health Care Version) is a classification system derived from the ICD-10 but developed jointly by mental health specialists and GPs. It aims to provide a clinically useful classification system for use in primary care. The ICD-10-PHC is limited to 25 categories. The categories were chosen because of their public health importance, the availability of effective management strategies in the primary care setting, cross-cultural applicability and consistency with the main ICD-10 classification. Diagnostic and detailed management guidelines are provided for all the 25 conditions, including presenting complaints, diagnostic features, differential diagnosis, essential information for the patient and carer, counselling advice, advice on medications and guidelines for referral to specialist services. It has proved internationally reliable, and in England, GPs using the system expanded their concept of depressive illness and reduced their prescription of antidepressant medication (Goldberg *et al.*, 1995). GPs using this classification have also been found to make more use of psychological interventions (Upton *et al.*, 1999). The classification has been adapted for the WHO *Guide to Mental and Neurological Health in Primary Care*, which has been revised to include neurological conditions and psychiatric disorders of childhood relevant to primary care (World Health Organisation, 2004). In the United States, the DSM-IV has also been amended for use in primary care. Like the ICD-10-PHC, the DSM-IV-PC also focuses on a limited number of conditions prevalent in primary care, but it does not give advice on management or information to be given to patients and their families.

The burden of psychiatric disorder in primary care

Psychiatric illness in the primary care setting poses a considerable burden not only to the individual and his or her family but also to primary care services and economically to the wider society. By 2020, it has been estimated that depression will be the leading cause of disability after ischaemic heart disease (Murray & Lopez, 1996). Fifty-five percent of patients with a defined psychiatric disorder were found to have moderate or severe disability in the Manchester arm of the WHO collaborative study of Mental Disorders in General Medical Settings (Ustun *et al.,*1995). Disability increases linearly with increasing symptomatology, and the level of disability in patients with a psychiatric disorder in primary care is similar to that in psychiatric out-patients and that caused by physical ill health (Ormel, Van Korff, *et al.,* 1993; Wells, Stewart, *et al.,* 1989). Disability appears to resolve synchronously with symptom resolution, although partial remission is more common than full remission and is associated with residual disability (Ormel, Van Korff, *et al.,* 1993). Mental disorders in primary care also have a larger impact on quality of life than common medical disorders (Spitzer *et al.,* 1995). Patients suffering from depression consult their GP two to three times more often than the general population, and this may in part explain why up to 30% of consultations held in primary care concern such problems (Lepine *et al.,* 1997).

Prognosis of mental health problems in primary care

A significant proportion of patients with mental health problems in primary care have a poor prognosis. Mann *et al.* (1981) followed up primary care patients with neurotic illness and found 48% still met case criteria at 12 months. Twenty-four percent had recovered, 52% had an intermittent course, but another 25% had persistent symptoms throughout this time. Patients who reported continuous symptoms were older, physically ill and more likely to have received psychotropic medication. Similar figures for the 1-year outcome of psychiatric illness in primary care have been found in other studies (Wright & Anderson, 1995).

The same cohort of patients was re-assessed 11 years later (Lloyd *et al.,* 1996). Fifty-four percent still met case criteria by the General Health Questionnaire (GHQ), and 37% had a relapsing or chronic course. A psychiatric diagnosis at 11 years was associated with high GP attendance rates (more than 12 visits per year), whereas the severity of illness at outset predicted the GHQ score at 11-year follow-up. WHO Psychological Problems in General Health Care Study followed up depressed primary care patients for 12 months across its 15 international centres. This also demonstrated that persistence and severity at 12 months was strongly influenced by severity at baseline (Goldberg *et al.,* 1998). Forty-five percent of severely depressed patients recognised by their GP remained depressed at 12 months, and of these nearly 30% remained severely depressed. It appears that neurotic illness in primary care often becomes chronic and is associated with high use of services. The reasons for this may in part be due to factors concerning the recognition and management of mental health problems by primary care professionals.

The detection of psychiatric disorder in primary care

Recognition of psychiatric disorders by GPs varies widely. If standardised research interviews are compared with GP recognition, between 30% and 70% of patients with a psychiatric disorder, as determined by standardised interview, are missed by GPs (Blacker & Clare, 1987; Bridges & Goldberg, 1985; Dowrick & Buchan, 1995; Freeling *et al.,* 1985;

Goldberg & Huxley, 1980; Ronalds *et al.*, 1997; Rost *et al.*, 1998; Simon *et al.*, 1999; Simon & VonKorff, 1995; Tiemens *et al.*, 1996; Ustun *et al.*, 1995; Wells, Hays, *et al.*, 1989). However, these findings mainly derive from cross-sectional studies, and they conceal the enormous variation between individual clinicians in their ability to detect these disorders. Cross-sectional studies may overestimate the proportion of patients with psychiatric illness that are missed because they fail to take into account the longitudinal nature of primary care. In primary care, there are opportunities for a patient's mental illness to be identified in subsequent consultations (Freeling & Tylee, 1992; Ormel & Tiemens, 1995). When a longitudinal perspective is taken, Kessler *et al.* (2002) found only 14% of patients with depression or anxiety remained unrecognised after 3 years.

In primary care, psychiatric disorders tend to run along a continuum rather than present as discrete entities. A dimensional approach to diagnosis may therefore be more valid (Goldberg & Huxley, 1992). Thompson and colleagues (2001) calculated that GPs only missed one "probable case" of depression in every 28.6 consultations for any reason when a dimensional rather than categorical approach to diagnosis was used.

Patients who are not recognised tend to have less severe mental health problems, and failure to recognise them may not have a detrimental effect on outcome in the longer term (Dowrick, 1995; Gask *et al.*, 1998; Ronalds *et al.*, 1997; Simon *et al.*, 1999; Thompson *et al.*, 2001; Wittchen *et al.*, 2001). Goldberg *et al.* (1998) found that recognition of depression improved outcomes at 3 months but by 12 months there was no difference between those recognised and those that had gone unrecognised.

Factors affecting the recognition of psychiatric illness in primary care

Factors influencing recognition can be divided into those concerning the patient and those concerning the doctor.

Patient factors influencing recognition

Patient characteristics and the way in which a patient presents during the consultation are associated with recognition of mental health problems in primary care. Being middle-aged, unemployed, bereaved, separated or white make it more likely that mental health problems are accurately identified. On the other hand, patients with comorbid physical illness are more likely to have their psychiatric illness missed (Freeling *et al.*, 1985; Marks *et al.*, 1979; Thompson *et al.*, 2001; Tylee *et al.*, 1993). There is conflicting evidence regarding the role of gender and recognition although rates of diagnosing depression in men are lower than those in women (Gater *et al.*, 1998; Jenkins & Meltzer, 1995; Marks *et al.*, 1979; Thompson *et al.*, 2001).

Patients presenting with a psychological or social problem are more likely to have their mental health problems recognised, as are patients with more than one psychiatric illness and patients who have received a psychiatric diagnosis by their GP in the prior year (Ormel & Tiemens, 1995). These patients, however, are also more likely to receive a psychiatric diagnosis when not psychiatrically unwell (Ormel & Tiemens, 1995). Shiels *et al.* (2004) found men living in rural areas with chest pain, low energy and poor job satisfaction were more likely to be depressed. Patients often present psychosocial problems towards the end of the consultation, but symptoms presented at the end of the consultation are not given the same attention as those presented initially even though these problems are just as important (Beckman & Frankel, 1984; Burack & Carpenter, 1983; Tylee *et al.*, 1995).

GP factors influencing recognition

There is a large variation between GPs in their ability to recognise mental health problems (Goldberg & Huxley, 1980, 1992; Goldberg *et al.*, 1993; Marks *et al.*, 1979; Millar & Goldberg, 1991; Ustun *et al.*, 1995). An accurate conceptual model of mental health problems on the part of the GP is associated with improved recognition of mental health

> **Box 21.1** Consultation skills that improve detection of mental health problems
>
> - Open questions
> - Unhurried style
> - Frequent eye contact
> - Picking up and following verbal cues
> - Picking up and following nonverbal cues
> - Ability to listen empathically

problems (Goldberg & Huxley, 1980; Marks *et al.,* 1979; Millar & Goldberg, 1991). Empathy, an interest in psychiatry and asking about family and problems at home are also associated with an increased recognition of mental illness (Marks *et al.,* 1979). Poor knowledge about mental health problems and a preoccupation with organic illness together with a tendency to underrate the severity and treatability of mental health problems are associated with reduced recognition (Schulberg & McClelland, 1987).

Consultation skills have been shown to be a vital determinant in recognition of emotional distress. GPs with better communication skills allow patients to express more distress during their consultations, whereas GPs with poorer skills are more likely to collude with their patients in not discussing emotional problems. Using open questions, an unhurried style with frequent eye contact, listening skills and the ability to pick up on verbal, vocal and nonverbal cues have all been shown to improve the recognition of depression (Davenport *et al.,* 1987; Goldberg *et al.,* 1993). Importantly these skills can also be taught, and skills training has been shown to improve detection and outcomes for depressed patients in primary care (Gask *et al.,* 1987, 1988, 1989, 1991). Suggested interview techniques are shown in Box 21.1.

Somatisation

Somatisation has been described as the expression of psychological distress through physical symptoms, and it appears to be a universal phenomenon

that is ubiquitous across cultures (Gureje *et al.,* 1997; Reid & Wessely, 2001). Patients in primary care often present physical symptoms at the onset of a psychiatric illness (Bridges & Goldberg, 1985). Simon and Von Korff (1991) found that 50% of patients with five or more functional somatic symptoms met criteria for a current psychiatric diagnosis with strongest associations for depression and anxiety. Of patients suffering from depression or anxiety, 76% made somatic presentations in primary care (Kirmayer *et al.,* 1993). Patients who somatise are more likely to normalise the cause of their symptoms and are less likely to discuss emotional problems with their doctor (Kirmayer & Robbins, 1996).

Stigma associated with mental health problems also contributes to the widespread reluctance to consult and receive appropriate treatment in primary care (Priest *et al.,* 1996). Seventy-seven percent of patients with identified mental health problems did not present emotional problems to their GP, and in 45% of these, it was because of stigma (Cape & McCulloch, 1999).

Case finding in primary care

The use of case-finding tools has been advocated to improve recognition rates of mental health problems in primary care (US Preventive Services Task Force, 2002). Case-finding tools for depression in primary care have reasonable sensitivity (80%–90%) but a lower specificity (70%–85%; Mulrow *et al.,* 1995). In the elderly, screening instruments for depression have a sensitivity of between 67% and 100% and a specificity of 53% and 98% (Watson & Pignone, 2003). A two-question case-finding instrument for depression has been found to have 96% sensitivity (although only 57% specificity), and this may have the most clinical utility in primary care (Whooley *et al.,* 1997). The two questions are:

1. Over the past 2 weeks, have you felt down, depressed or hopeless?
2. Over the past 2 weeks, have you felt little interest or pleasure in doing things?

These could easily be asked by any member of the primary care team. A patient answering "yes" to both questions would then need to have a clinical interview to rule out a false-positive diagnosis. The two-question screen could be particularly useful for patients in high-risk groups.

The effects of case finding on the clinical outcomes of mental health problems in primary care remain uncertain. With regard to depression, case finding by and large has failed to improve outcomes when used alone (Gilbody, 2001; Pignone et al., 2002; Valenstein et al., 2001). However, in the United States, screening for depression has been recommended in practices that have the facilities to ensure effective management (US Preventive Services Task Force, 2002).

It is probable that using case-finding instruments for mental health problems routinely in primary care will only improve clinical outcomes when used as part of an overall comprehensive and structured management program and until practices have these in place there may be little to gain from their use (Pignone et al., 2002; Valenstein et al., 2001). Screening should therefore probably be limited to high-risk groups such as those with chronic physical illness, patients with other mental health problems, or those with ongoing psychosocial stressors such as unemployment or bereavement.

Improving outcomes of mental illness in primary care

A number of strategies have been used in an attempt to improve outcomes of patients with mental health problems in primary care. Most of these have been directed at improving the outcomes for patients with depression and were usefully reviewed by Gilbody et al. (2003). These strategies have included the use of clinical guidelines, education initiatives, and enhanced care packages (see Box 21.2).

The use of clinical guidelines in the primary care arena is complex. Since the 1990s, an increasing number of clinical guidelines have been produced, many of them specifically aimed at primary care.

> **Box 21.2** Improving the management of depression in primary care (from Gilbody et al., 2003)
>
> **Effective methods**
> - Collaborative care
> - Stepped collaborative care
> - Quality improvement programs
> - Case management
> - Academic detailing
>
> **Ineffective methods**
> - Use of guidelines alone
> - Educational strategies alone

Hibble et al. (1998) visited GP practices and asked them to produce copies of all the clinical guidelines they had received. They found 855 different guidelines; of these, 40% had been produced nationally. The use of guidelines alone for the management of depression in primary care has generally failed to have an impact on clinical outcome, as have stand-alone educational initiatives (Dowrick & Buchan, 1995; Gilbody et al., 2003; Ormel et al., 1990, Schulberg et al., 1987; Simon et al., 1999; Tiemens et al., 1996).

A number of studies in the United States have demonstrated improved clinical outcomes using enhanced depression management programs (Hunkeler et al., 2000; Katon et al., 1995, 1996, 1999; Katzelnick et al., 2000; Lin et al., 1997; Rost et al., 2001; Wells et al., 2000). These enhanced programs vary but generally combine educational initiatives, close follow-up, organisational restructuring to establish close relationships with specialist services, and case management.

Unfortunately a similar enhanced care package in the United Kingdom failed to demonstrate any difference in the outcomes of depressed primary care patients. The Hampshire Depression Project studied the effects of a clinical practice guideline and an educational program for depression on the detection and outcome of depression in the primary care setting. The guidelines were extensive and included advice on practice organisation, roles of nonmedical professionals and useful general and local information. The educational initiatives included seminars, video teaching and small-group discussions. No differences were found between the intervention and the control group in terms of recognition rates or patient outcomes (Thompson *et al.*, 2000).

Improving outcomes for primary care patients with mental health problems is therefore complex, and it remains to be seen whether successful programs can be generalised internationally. Von Korff and Goldberg (2001) reviewed the elements of enhanced care packages for depression in primary care and found the consistent elements of successful packages were case management and specialist support. They suggested that to improve the outcomes of primary care patients with depression the focus should be on low-cost case management with ease of access across the interface between specialist services, the case manger and primary care.

The interface between primary care and psychiatry

The interface between primary care and psychiatric services is of key importance in the delivery of mental health services. Traditionally this interface consisted of a referral letter from GP to psychiatrist and vice versa (Pullen, 1985). However, more recently, novel approaches have been developed (Strathdee & Williams, 1984). Gask *et al.* (1987) evaluated models of service provision across the primary-secondary care interface. They described four main models: the community mental health team, the shifted out-patient clinic, attached mental health professionals and consultation-liaison.

Community mental health teams (CMHT) are increasingly aligning themselves to primary care groups rather than by geographical region, allowing a closer relationship between primary and secondary care professionals responsible for the same population of patients. This also allows the primary care group and CMHT to develop referral pathways and care protocols jointly. Despite this, the relationship between a conventional CMHT and primary care is often unsatisfactory. New patients are usually assigned to community nurses depending on size of caseload and level of experience. Each community nurse is therefore responsible for patients under the care of many GPs, making close working relationships difficult.

The shifted out-patient model consists largely of psychiatrists conducting clinics in primary care. Within this model, the degree to which psychiatrists and GPs interact varies, and it has been argued that its major benefit to primary care is the informal "consultation-liaison" contacts it provides with primary care professionals (Darling & Tyrer, 1990; Gask *et al.*, 1997).

The attached mental health professional is another method to provide mental health care across the interface. Mental health professionals, such as community psychiatric nurses, counsellors, clinical psychologists and social workers, attach themselves to primary care practices. For instance, in the United Kingdom, an increasing number of practices have access to counsellors. As the expertise of mental health professionals working in primary care grows, so roles and relationships may change. Wilkin (2001) has documented the evolution of a new breed of mental health professional, the "primary mental health nurse" who has developed a unique set of skills and expertise in primary care liaison.

The consultation-liaison model has as its aim, and through the consultation-liaison process, the care of patients with severe mental health problems by psychiatric services, while primary care retains the management of less severe mental disorders. A potential problem with this model is that primary and secondary care's perception of severe mental health problems often differs, and common mental health problems encountered in primary care may be just as chronic and disabling as the more "serious" mental illnesses. This can lead to discord between services unless the consultation-liaison process is properly managed.

As Gask *et al.* (1997) pointed out, these models are not mutually exclusive but can complement one another as services develop to meet their own local needs. Models can also be adapted to take into account local workforce issues and staff availability. Some health trusts in the United Kingdom have created primary care mental health teams. These *primary care teams* often consist of a link-worker (usually a community psychiatric nurse), practice counsellor and/or psychologist, social worker, practice nurse and GP. Although based physically in the primary care environment, they act directly at the interface, with primary care professionals and specialist services being able to refer patients to them. Other primary care mental health teams focus on particular patient populations. One primary care trust has developed a primary care mental health team to promote the effective provision of psychiatric care in the primary care setting for patients with stable but enduring mental illness. Within this model mental health primary care workers are able to triage patients, assess their needs, provide care and ensure referral to the most appropriate service when needed (D. Fisher, personal communication, 2002). Other services have developed clinics in primary care for patients with mild to moderate mental health problems staffed by a multidisciplinary primary care team, managing patients whose problems are too complex or time consuming to be managed by a traditional primary care team (H. Raistrick, personal communication, 2002).

Shared care

Arguably primary care has a role to play in the management of all mental disorders. Patients with "severe" mental disorders (such as schizophrenia, bipolar illness and dementia) can benefit from having their care shared by mental health services and primary care, whereas other disorders are treated solely by primary care services unless there is a failure to respond to treatment from the GP (Hansen, 1987).

Traditionally shared care has been widely practiced on an informal basis, but increasingly shared care arrangements are being formalised with "shared care" plans. Mental health "link-workers" are being employed who are attached to specific practices and assigned the care of specific patients. In effect the link-workers facilitate the care of patients with severe mental health problems and are responsible for keeping shared care plans up to date and liaising between the two services. Having access to a specific link-worker has proved popular with GPs.

Shared care has developed in many areas of the United Kingdom from the use of shared care registers for patients with severe mental illness. Plans are developed for particular patients who meet shared care criteria. These plans document the key worker, psychiatrist, and GP; the management strategy; medication and who is responsible for prescribing; warning signs of a relapse and what to do in an emergency. These plans need to be mutually agreed upon by the patient, and the psychiatric and primary care teams. Shared care also lends itself to shared training opportunities which can further facilitate communication between teams.

Mental health skills training and education for primary care professionals

In the United Kingdom, few GPs have any higher professional training in mental health and only about 50% of GP trainees undertake a psychiatry rotation as part of their vocational training (Turton *et al.*, 1995; Tylee, 2001). GPs have been successfully trained in mental health skills such as depression management, re-attribution skills for patients who somatise, cognitive-behavioural skills, counselling skills and problem-solving skills. Some have been trained to teach these skills to other primary care professionals (Bowman *et al.*, 1992; Evans *et al.*, 2001; Gask, 1998; Gask *et al.*, 1989, 1991; Morriss & Gask, 2002; Naji *et al.*, 1986). Practice nurses, too, have been taught a wide range of mental health skills. They have been taught to assess and manage depression, use problem-solving techniques, administer depot antipsychotic medication, monitor compliance, and coordinate the care of patients with mental health problems. They have been found to improve outcome and patient satisfaction by using telephone follow-up and progress monitoring (Burns *et al.,* 1998; Hunkeler *et al.,* 2000; Mann *et al.,* 1998; Mynors-Wallis, 1997; Peveler *et al.,* 1999).

Training can be successfully delivered to the whole primary care team, rather than to particular professional groups. Tylee (1999) has advocated whole practice multi-professional mental health skills training and has found it to be successful and, in some instances, preferred to teaching for individual professional groups.

There is now an expanding range of teaching aids for use in primary care. For instance, the World Psychiatric Association has produced a mental health skills training pack specifically for primary care (Goldberg *et al.,* 2001). This training pack allows specific mental health skills to be taught through modelling those demonstrated on videos. It encourages the use of role-plays to allow professionals to practice the new skills they have been taught and has information on the planning and running of tutorials on mental health topics.

There are also innovative approaches to mental health education such as the Trailblazer programme in the United Kingdom and the Better Outcomes in Mental Health Care initiative in Australia. The Trailblazer programme was developed to improve the mental health skills of primary care professionals and facilitate the cascade of these skills to other members of the primary care team. It uses the novel approach of participants attending the course in pairs, each pair being made up of one person from primary care and one person from mental health services. During the courses, the learning needs of participants are defined, and each course is then designed around these specific learning needs. The courses consist of three modules over 6 to 8 months and use a wide variety of teaching methods. They take an adult learner–centred approach utilising the skills and experience of the participants. The courses are by definition multi-professional, and this joint training has been found to foster a close collaborative relationship between pairs and within the group, which continues after the courses have finished. To date more than 350 participants have already been through the courses in the United Kingdom, and they are being developed in New Zealand, Australia and the United States (Dwyer, 2002; Tylee *et al.,* 2004; Walters, 2003).

The Better Outcomes in Mental Health Care initiative has five major components designed to improve access to primary health services by providing education and training to GPs (www.mentalhealth.gov.au). The first component relates to the education and training of GPs and has three levels of training. It enables GPs to provide evidence-based, focussed psychological interventions and other evidence-based treatment strategies. This training also allows GPs to be remunerated for the mental health services they provide.

In Athens, Greece, an educational programme has been developed to train trainers in basic issues of psychiatric prevention and mental health promotion. The programme has theoretical and practical components. Course participants have included health professionals and community agents such as priests, police officers, jurists and journalists. One hundred and twenty people have completed the three-semester course, and it has been favourably received (Vassiliadou *et al.,* 2004). In the Russian Federation, GP trainers in Ekaterinburg now offer special training to GPs in mental health skills and plan to make this available to trainers in the Department of Family Medicine.

Management of mental disorders in primary care

Ninety percent of people with a mental illness are treated in primary care alone (Shepherd *et al.,* 1966). An increasing number of treatments have proved beneficial in the primary care setting. These include medication, cognitive-behavioural techniques, problem-solving techniques, reattribution skills for somatisation, counselling, self-help and bibliotherapy.

Treatment of depression in primary care

Antidepressant medication

Antidepressant medications are effective in primary care for the treatment of major depression of at least moderate severity, although there is less evidence for their efficacy in mild major depression (Anderson *et al.*, 2000; Judd *et al.*, 2004). There is a wide variation in prescribing practices of antidepressant medications in primary care with few patients receiving an adequate dose for an adequate length of time (Donoghue & Tylee, 1996; Dunn *et al.*, 1999; Goldberg *et al.*, 1998). Currently SSRIs are the most commonly prescribed antidepressants in primary care in the United Kingdom, making up 75% of all antidepressant prescriptions (Skevington & Wright, 2001). There is no evidence that one antidepressant class is more effective than another in the primary care setting, although newer antidepressants may be better tolerated and less likely to be prematurely discontinued by the patients (Barbui *et al.*, 2000).

Adherence to antidepressant medication remains a problem. Of patients prescribed an antidepressant, 30% to 50% fail to refill their initial prescriptions, and 50% to 80% stop taking antidepressant medication within 1.5 to 6 months of commencement (Lawrenson *et al.*, 2000; Lin *et al.*, 1995). Monitoring adherence, education about depression and antidepressant medications should therefore be a routine part of management (Lin *et al.*, 1995; Peveler *et al.*, 1999).

Psychological therapies

Cognitive-behaviour therapy (CBT; Appleby *et al.*, 1997; Scott *et al.*, 1997), interpersonal therapy (IPT; Schulberg *et al.*, 1996) and problem-solving therapy (Mynors-Wallis & Gath, 1997; Mynors-Wallis *et al.*, 2000) are as effective as antidepressant medication for the treatment of mild to moderate depression in primary care.

Availability of psychological therapies in primary care varies widely, and their use is often limited by lack of trained staff to deliver them. One way to increase access to psychological treatments is the use of computerised CBT (cCBT). cCBT has been found to be effective for the treatment of depression and anxiety in primary care and is well received by patients (Proudfoot *et al.*, 2003, 2004).

Counselling

Bower *et al.* (2004) reviewed the effectiveness of counselling in primary care for common mental disorders. They found that counselling was associated with modest improvements in short-term outcome compared with usual GP care and concluded that it may be a useful addition to the treatment strategies available in primary care. However, there are many different types of counselling. Probably the most beneficial is that which uses a problem-orientated framework. Counselling using a psychodynamic framework has not been found to be significantly better than routine GP care in patients with chronic depression (Simpson *et al.*, 2003). In the early 1990s, about a third of practices had access to counselling, and this is likely to be higher now (Sibbald *et al.*, 1993). Given the choice, patients seem to prefer it over usual care with antidepressant medication (Chilvers *et al.*, 2001).

Guided self-help and bibliotherapy

Guided self-help is the process whereby limited contact with professionals is used to facilitate and support the patient in the use of self-help literature, which often uses a cognitive-behavioural approach to treatment. Although some studies have shown self-help and bibliotherapy to be effective for depression in primary care, there is not enough evidence to be able to provide any firm conclusions regarding its efficacy (Bower *et al.*, 2001; Dowrick *et al.*, 2000; Williams, 2001). The use of websites offering information about depression or CBT has

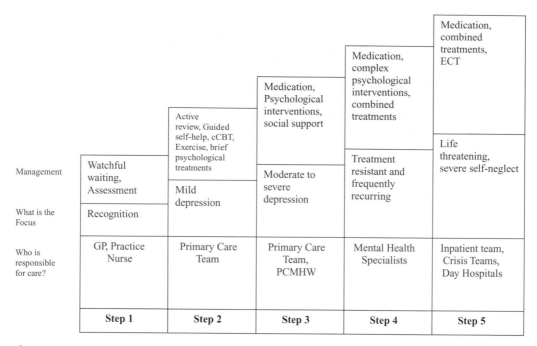

Figure 21.2. Stepped Care (Adapted from Depression: The Management of Depression in Primary and Secondary Care. National Collaborating Centre for Mental Health, 2003).

also been found to reduce the symptoms of depression (Christensen *et al.*, 2004). Self-help and bibliotherapy may prove useful for people with milder mental health problems and serve as important adjuncts to other treatments.

Other treatments

Exercise has been shown to improve significantly the symptoms of depression, especially for patients with mild to moderate depression; in the United Kingdom "Exercise on Prescription" has become increasingly popular (Biddle *et al.*, 1994).

Stepped care

Patients with depression differ in their needs. With limited resources in primary care, a stepped collaborative care approach may prove best to meet these needs with the available resources (see Figure 21.2).

Stepped care allows the interventions to be tailored to the individual. In this model, self-help, exercise, cCBT or another brief psychological intervention may be the first step in management for people with mild depression. People with moderate to severe depression may be prescribed an antidepressant and offered a psychological treatment and social support. This targets resources at those patients likely to gain the most benefit from them.

Katon *et al.* (1999) found that depressed patients in primary care who had not responded to antidepressant medication at 6 to 8 weeks were more likely to get adequate treatment, to adhere to it and to have better clinical outcomes if treated within a stepped-care collaborative model. The stepped-care model was associated with only modest increases in costs (Simon *et al.*, 2001). A similar stepped-care management program for depressed women in Chile was also found to improve outcomes (Araya *et al.*, 2003).

The role of primary care nurses

Practice nurses may well have an important part to play within stepped-care management, as well as more generally in managing patients with chronic mental health problems. As has been discussed, nurses have been successfully trained to deliver a number of mental health interventions. In the United Kingdom, practice nurses are frequently involved in chronic disease management programmes and often run "mini-clinics". These clinics can be modified for patients with chronic mental health problems, allowing the systematic assessment of symptoms, treatment, assessment of side-effects and assertive follow-up with outreach to nonattenders (Peveler & Kendrick, 2001). Nurse-led services for people suffering from depression have also been developed and appear to facilitate the access of a population of patients who may not have sought or received help form traditional primary care services (Symons et al., 2004).

Suicide and primary care

There are about 5,000 deaths from suicide annually in the United Kingdom. Nearly 80% of these are accounted for by men and, since the early 1990s, suicide has been commonest cause of death among young men (Brook & Griffiths, 2003). The most important factor associated with suicide, in men and women, is mental illness (Foster et al., 1997; Hawton, 2000; Henriksson et al., 1993; and see also Chapter 20). However, the major barrier to receiving appropriate care for a mental illness is a failure to consult health services (Stanistreet et al., 2004). Thus despite the prevalence of suicide, it is a relatively rare occurrence in primary care, and the average GP will have a patient commit suicide once every 4 to 7 years. Improved detection and risk assessment therefore offer only a partial solution to decreasing the suicide rate. Educational activities such as those in Gotland, Sweden, which demonstrated a decreased suicide rate following an

educational initiative for GPs, are unlikely to be generally effective, and subsequent research failed to replicate these findings (Rutz et al., 1989, 1992; Thompson et al., 2000). This may be because the Gotland study was small, and the findings likely to have been artefactual. Issues of improved and novel types of access to health services, especially for young men, need to be addressed, as does a more sophisticated understanding of the ways in which a depressive illness may manifest differently in men and women. Angst et al. (2002) suggested that men suffering from depression may show fewer classical symptoms but be just as functionally impaired as depressed women. If this is the case, diagnosis of depression in men may need to take into account a different set of factors than traditionally thought (Shiels et al., 2004).

Management of psychosis in primary care

Primary care plays a vital role in the management of patients with psychotic illnesses. Between 25% and 40% of patients with schizophrenia rapidly lose contact with psychiatric services, and the GP is the health professional most likely to keep in contact with them (Burns & Kendrick, 1997). GPs are therefore able to offer a continuity of care which can be difficult to achieve by mental health services for a substantial proportion of patients with psychotic illnesses. Patients with psychoses have greater physical and social needs than those of the general population. They have increased rates of death from infections and cardiovascular and respiratory diseases (Harris & Barraclough, 1998), and primary care is probably in the best position to monitor their physical health and provide a hub for communication between professionals and carers. Primary care is in a good position to monitor mental states allowing early recognition of relapse and monitor medication such as lithium. GPs are also important in the recognition of the early signs of a psychotic illness facilitating referral to early onset teams. The ideal for patients with a chronic psychotic illness is probably a well-defined shared care arrangement between primary care and specialist services.

Conclusions

Mental illness is a major public health problem. Primary care manages the vast majority of mental illness, and therefore optimising primary care management is vital if this problem is to be adequately addressed. The poor outcome for a substantial proportion of people suffering from a mental health problem in primary care appears to be international and has important implications for service delivery and training of primary care professionals. Communication skills training may be particularly important in this regard. It remains unclear, however, whether models of service delivery shown to improve the management of people with a mental illness can be generalised to settings other than those in which they were initially shown to be beneficial. Future research needs to be focused on low-cost methods of self-help for people with less severe problems, increased availability of problem-solving and computerised CBT treatments and the optimum forms of long-term care for those with chronic or frequently relapsing mental illnesses.

Part of the difficulty in generalising systems within primary care is that the structure of primary care around the world varies considerably. In some parts of the world, large multi-professional primary care teams are now the norm, whereas in other parts primary care consists of single-handed GPs working in relative isolation. This diversity in delivery of primary care services is likely to mean that no one system of mental health service provision will suit all. However, it may be possible for the factors important in improving recognition and outcomes to be incorporated into local service models. The challenge for the future is to define which components of these complex interventions are important and determine how well they can be incorporated into different models of primary care provision.

REFERENCES

Anderson, I. M., Nutt, D. J., & Deakin, J. F. (2000). Evidence-based guidelines for treating depressive disorders with antidepressants: a revision of the 1993 British Association for Psychopharmacology guidelines. British Association for Psychopharmacology. *J Psychopharmacol* **14**:3–20.

Angst, J., Gamma, A., Gastpar, M. (2002). Gender differences in depression. Epidemiological findings from the European DEPRES I and II studies. *Eur Arch Psychiatry Clin Neurosci* **252**:201–9.

Appleby, L., Warner, R., Whitton, A., & Faragher, B. (1997). A controlled study of fluoxetine and cognitive-behavioural counselling in the treatment of postnatal depression. *BMJ* **314**:932–6.

Araya, R., Rojas, G., Fritsch, R., *et al.* (2003). Treating depression in primary care in low-income women in Santiago, Chile: a randomised controlled trial. *Lancet* **361**:995–1000.

Barbui, C., Hotopf, M., Freemantle, N., *et al.* (2000). Selective serotonin reuptake inhibitors versus tricyclic and heterocyclic antidepressants: comparison of drug adherence. *Cochrane Database Syst Rev* **4**:CD002791.

Beckman, H. B., & Frankel, R. M. (1984). The effect of physician behavior on the collection of data. *Ann Int Med* **101**:692–6.

Biddle, S., Fox, K., & Edmund, L. (1994). *Physical Activity in Primary Care in England*. London: Health Education Authority.

Blacker, C. V., & Clare, A. W. (1987). Depressive disorder in primary care. *Br J Psychiatry* **150**:737–51.

Bower, P., Richards, D., & Lovell, K. (2001). The clinical and cost-effectiveness of self-help treatments for anxiety and depressive disorders in primary care: a systematic review. *Br J Gen Pract* **51**:838–45.

Bower, P., Rowland, N., & Hardy, R. (2003). The clinical effectiveness of counselling in primary care: a systematic review and meta-analysis. *Psychol Med* **33**:203–15.

Bowman, F. M., Goldberg, D. P., Millar, T., *et al.* (1992). Improving the skills of established general practitioners: the long-term benefits of group teaching. *Med Educ* **26**:63–8.

Bridges, K., & Goldberg, D. (1985). Somatic presentation of DSM-III psychiatric disorders in primary care. *J Psychosom Res* **29**:563–9.

Brook, A., & Griffiths, C. (2003). *Trends in the Mortality of Young Adults Aged 15–44 in England and Wales 1961–2001*. London: Office of National Statistics.

Burack, R. C., & Carpenter, R. R. (1983). The predictive value of the presenting complaint. *J Fam Pract* **16**:749–54.

Burns, T., & Kendrick, T. (1997). The primary care of patients with schizophrenia: a search for good practice. *Br J Gen Pract* **47**:515–20.

Burns, T., Millar, E., Garland, C., *et al.* (1998). Randomized controlled trial of teaching practice nurses to carry out structured assessments of patients receiving depot antipsychotic injections. *Br J Gen Pract* **48**:1845–8.

Cape, J., & McCulloch, Y. (1999). Patients' reasons for not presenting emotional problems in general practice consultations. *Br J Gen Pract* **49**:875–9.

Chilvers, C., Dewey, M., Fielding, K., *et al.* Counselling versus Antidepressants in Primary Care Study Group. (2001). Antidepressant drugs and generic counselling for treatment of major depression in primary care. randomised trial with patient preference arms. *BMJ* **322**:772–5.

Christensen, H., Griffiths, K. M., & Jorm, A. F. (2004). Delivering interventions for depression by using the internet: randomised controlled trial. *BMJ* **328**:265.

Copeland, J. R., Davidson, I. A., Dewey, M. E., *et al.* (1992). Alzheimer's disease, other dementias, depression and pseudodementia: prevalence, incidence and three-year outcome in Liverpool. *Br J Psychiatry* **161**:230–9.

Darling, C., & Tyrer, P. (1990). Brief encounters in general practice: liaison in general practice psychiatry clinics. *Psychiatr Bull* **14**:592–4.

Davenport, S., Goldberg, D., & Millar, T. (1987). How psychiatric disorders are missed during medical consultations. *Lancet* **2**:439–41

Donoghue, J. M., & Tylee, A. D. (1996). The treatment of depression: prescribing patterns of antidepressants in primary care in the UK. *Br J Psychiatry* **168**:164–8.

Dowrick, C. F. (1995). Case or continuum? Analysing GPs' ability to detect depression in primary care. *Primary Care Psychiatry* **1**:255–7.

Dowrick, C., & Buchan, I. (1995). Twelve month outcome of depression in general practice: does detection or disclosure make a difference? *BMJ* **311**:1274–6.

Dowrick, C., Dunn, G., Ayuso-Mateos, J. L., *et al.* (2000). Problem solving treatment and group psychoeducation for depression: multicentre randomised controlled trial. Outcomes of Depression International Network (ODIN) Group. *BMJ* **321**:1450–4.

Dunn, R. L., Donoghue, J. M., Ozminkowski, R. J., *et al.* (1999). Longitudinal patterns of antidepressant prescribing in primary care in the UK: comparison with treatment guidelines. *J Psychopharmacol* **13**:136–43.

Dwyer M. (2002). Trailblazers. *J Primary Care Ment Health* **6**:17.

Evans, A., Gask, L., Singleton, C., & Bahrami, J. (2001). Teaching consultation skills: a survey of general practice trainers. *Med Educ* **35**:222–4.

Foster, T., Gillespie, K., & McClelland, R. (1997). Mental disorders and suicide in Northern Ireland. *Br J Psychiatry* **170**:447–52.

Freeling, P., Rao, B. M., Paykel, E. S., *et al.* (1985). Unrecognised depression in general practice. *Br Med J Clin Res Ed* **290**:1880–3.

Freeling, P., & Tylee A. (1992). Depression in general practice. In E. S. Paykel, ed. *Handbook of Affective Disorders*. Edinburgh: Churchill Livingstone, Edinburgh, pp. 651–6.

Garralda, M. E. (1994). Primary care psychiatry. In M. Rutter, L. Hersov, & E. Taylor F, *Child and Adolescent Psychiatry*. Oxford: Blackwell Science.

Gask, L. (1998). Small group interactive techniques utilizing videofeedback. *Int J Psychiatry Med* **28**:97–113.

Gask, L., Goldberg, D., Boardman, J., *et al.* (1991). Training general practitioners to teach psychiatric interviewing skills: an evaluation of group training. *Med Educ* **25**:444–51.

Gask, L., Goldberg, D., Lesser, A. L., & Millar, T. (1988). Improving the psychiatric skills of the general practice trainee: an evaluation of a group training course. *Med Educ* **22**:132–8.

Gask, L., Goldberg, D., Porter, R., & Creed, F. (1989). The treatment of somatization: evaluation of a teaching package with general practice trainees. *J Psychosom Res* **33**:697–703.

Gask, L., McGrath, G., Goldberg, D., & Millar, T. (1987). Improving the psychiatric skills of established general practitioners: evaluation of group teaching. *Med Educ* **21**:362–8.

Gask, L., Sibbald, B., & Creed, F. (1997). Evaluating models of working at the interface between mental health services and primary care. *Br J Psychiatry* **170**:6–11.

Gask, L., Usherwood, T., Thompson, H., & Williams, B. (1998). Evaluation of a training package in the assessment and management of depression in primary care. *Med Educ* **32**:190–8.

Gater, R., Tansella, M., Korten, A., *et al.* (1998). Sex differences in the prevalence and detection of depressive and anxiety disorders in general health care settings: report from the World Health Organization Collaborative Study on Psychological Problems in General Health Care. *Arch Gen Psychiatry* **55**:405–13.

Gilbody, S., Whitty, P., Grimshaw, J., & Thomas, R. (2003). Educational and organizational interventions to improve the management of depression in primary care: a systematic review. *JAMA* **289**:3145–51.

Gilbody, S. M., House, A. O., & Sheldon, T. A. (2001). Routinely administered questionnaires for depression and anxiety: systematic review. *BMJ* **322**:406–9.

Goldberg, D., Gask, L., & Sartorius, N. (2001). *Training Physicians in Mental Health Skills*. Geneva: World Psychiatric Association.

Goldberg, D. P., Sharp, D., & Nanayakkara, K. (1995). The field trial of the mental disorders section of ICD-10 designed for primary care. *Fam Pract* **12**:466–73.

Goldberg, D., & Huxley, P. (1980). *Mental Illness in the Community. The Pathway to Psychiatric Care*. London: Tavistock.

Goldberg, D., & Huxley, P. (1992). *Common Mental Disorders. A Biosocial Model*. London: Routledge.

Goldberg, D., Privett, M., Ustun, B., Simon, G., & Linden, M. (1998). The effects of detection and treatment on the outcome of major depression in primary care: a naturalistic study in 15 cities. *Br J Gen Pract* **48**:1840–4.

Goldberg, D. P., Jenkins, L., Millar, T., & Faragher, E. B. (1993). The ability of trainee general practitioners to identify psychological distress among their patients. *Psychol Med* **23**:185–93.

Graham, H. J. (1991). General practice and the elderly mentally ill. In R. Jacoby & C. Oppenheimer, eds. *Psychiatry in the Elderly*. Oxford: Oxford Medical Publications, pp. 448–513.

Gureje, O., Simon, G. E., Ustun, T. B., & Goldberg, D. P. (1997). Somatization in cross-cultural perspective: a World Health Organization study in primary care. *Am J Psychiatry* **154**:989–95.

Hansen, V. (1987). Psychiatric services within primary care. *Acta Psychiatr Scand* **76**:121–8.

Harris, E. C., & Barraclough, B. (1998). Excess mortality of mental disorder. *Br J Psychiatry* **173**:11–53.

Hawton, K. (2000). Sex and suicide. Gender differences in suicidal behaviour. *Br J Psychiatry* **177**:484–5.

Henriksson, M. M., Aro, H. M., Marttunen, M. J., *et al.* (1993). Mental disorders and comorbidity in suicide. *Am J Psychiatry* **150**:935–40.

Hibble, A., Kanka, D., Pencheon, D., & Pooles, F. (1998). Guidelines in general practice: the new Tower of Babel? *BMJ* **317**:862–3.

Hunkeler, E. M., Meresman, J. F., Hargreaves, W. A., *et al.* (2000). Efficacy of nurse telehealth care and peer support in augmenting treatment of depression in primary care. *Arch Fam Med* **9**:700–8.

Jenkins, R., Smeeton, N., & Shepherd, M. (1988). Classification of mental disorders in primary care. *Psychol Med Suppl* **12**:1–59.

Jenkins, R., & Meltzer, H. (1995). The national survey of psychiatric morbidity in Great Britain. *Soc Psychiatry Psychiatr Epidemiol* **30**(1):1–4.

Judd, L. L., Rapaport, M. H., Yonkers, K. A., *et al.* (2004). Randomized, placebo-controlled trial of fluoxetine for acute treatment of minor depressive disorder. *Am J Psychiatry* **161**:1864–71.

Katon, W., Robinson, P., Von Korff, M., *et al.* (1996). A multifaceted intervention to improve treatment of depression in primary care. *Arch Gen Psychiatry* **53**:924–32.

Katon, W., Von Korff, M., Lin, E., *et al.* (1995). Collaborative management to achieve treatment guidelines. Impact on depression in primary care. *JAMA* **273**:1026–31.

Katon, W., Von Korff, M., Lin, E., *et al.* (1999). Stepped collaborative care for primary care patients with persistent symptoms of depression: a randomized trial. *Arch Gen Psychiatry* **56**:1109–15.

Katzelnick, D. J., Simon, G. E., Pearson, S. D., *et al.* (2000). Randomized trial of a depression management program in high utilizers of medical care. *Arch Fam Med* **9**:345–51.

Kessler, D., Bennewith, O., Lewis, G., & Sharp, D. (2002). Detection of depression and anxiety in primary care: follow up study. *BMJ* **325**:1016–17.

Kirmayer, L. J., & Robbins, J. M. (1996). Patients who somatize in primary care: a longitudinal study of cognitive and social characteristics. *Psychol Med* **26**:937–51.

Kirmayer, L. J., Robbins, J. M., Dworkind, M., & Yaffe, M. J. (1993). Somatization and the recognition of depression and anxiety in primary care. *Am J Psychiatry* **150**:734–41.

Lawrenson, R. A., Tyrer, F., Newson, R. B., & Farmer, R. D. (2000). The treatment of depression in UK general practice: selective serotonin reuptake inhibitors and tricyclic antidepressants compared. *J Affect Disord* **59**:149–57.

Lepine, J. P., Gastpar, M., Mendlewicz, J., & Tylee, A. (1997). Depression in the community: the first pan-European study DEPRES (Depression Research in European Society). *Int Clin Psychopharmacol* **12**:19–29.

Lin, E. H., Katon, W. J., Simon, G. E., *et al.* (1997). Achieving guidelines for the treatment of depression in primary care: is physician education enough? *Med Care* **35**:831–42.

Lin, E. H., Von Korff, M., Katon, W., *et al.* (1995). The role of the primary care physician in patients' adherence to antidepressant therapy. *Med Care* **33**:67–74.

Livingston, G., Hawkins, A., Graham, N., *et al.* (1990). The Gospel Oak Study: prevalence rates of dementia, depression and activity limitation among elderly residents in inner London. *Psychol Med* **20**:137–46.

Lloyd, K. R., Jenkins, R., & Mann, A. (1996). Long-term outcome of patients with neurotic illness in general practice. *BMJ* **313**:26–8.

Mann, A., Blizard, R., & Murray, J. (1998). An evaluation of practice nurses working with general practitioners to treat people with depression. *Br J Gen Pract* **48**:875–9.

Mann, A. H., Jenkins, R., & Belsey, E. (1981). The twelve-month outcome of patients with neurotic illness in general practice. *Psychol Med* **11**:535–50.

Marks, J. N., Goldberg, D., & Hillier, V. F. (1979). Determinants of the ability of general practitioners to detect psychiatric illness. *Psychol Med* **9**:337–53.

Millar, T., & Goldberg, D. P. (1991). Link between the ability to detect and manage emotional disorders: a study of general practitioner trainees. *Br J Gen Pract* **41**:357–9.

Morriss, R. K., & Gask, L. (2002). Treatment of patients with somatized mental disorder: effects of reattribution training on outcomes under the direct control of the family doctor. *Psychosomatics* **43**:394–9.

Mulrow, C. D., Williams, J. W. J., Gerety, M. B., *et al.* (1995). Case-finding instruments for depression in primary care settings. *Ann Int Med* **122**:12:913–21.

Mulrow, C. D. M., Williams, J. W. J., Chiquette, E. P., *et al.* (2000). Efficacy of newer medications for treating depression in primary care patients. *Am J Med* **108**:54–64.

Murray, C. J. L., & Lopez, A. D. (1996). *The Global Burden Of Disease: A Comprehensive Assessment of Mortality and Disability of Diseases, Injuries and Risk Factors in 1990 Projected to 2020*. Cambridge, Massachusetts: Harvard University Press.

Mynors-Wallis, L., Davies, I., Gray, A., *et al.* (1997). A randomised controlled trial and cost analysis of problem-solving treatment for emotional disorders given by community nurses in primary care. *Br J Psychiatry* **170**:113–19.

Mynors Wallis, L., & Gath, D. (1997). Predictors of treatment outcome for major depression in primary care. *Psychol Med* **27**:731–6.

Mynors-Wallis, L. M., Gath, D. H., Day, A., & Baker, F. (2000). Randomised controlled trial of problem solving treatment, antidepressant medication, and combined treatment for major depression in primary care. *BMJ* **320**:26–30.

Naji, S. A., Maguire, G. P., Fairbairn, S. A., *et al.* (1986). Training clinical teachers in psychiatry to teach interviewing skills to medical students. *Med Educ* **20**:140–7.

National Collaborating Centre for Mental Health. (2003). *Depression: The Management of Depression in Primary and Secondary Care* (draft for second consultation). National Institute for Clinical Excellence,

Office for National Statistics. (1998). *Key Health Statistics from General Practice 1998. Office for National Statistics.* London: Her Majesty's Stationery Service.

Ormel, J., & Tiemens, B. (1995). Recognition and treatment of mental illness in primary care. Towards a better understanding of a multifaceted problem. *Gen Hosp Psychiatry* **17**:160–4.

Ormel, J., Van Den Brink, W., Kocter, M. W., *et al.* (1990). Recognition, management and outcome of psychological disorders in primary care: a naturalistic follow-up study. *Psychol Med* **20**:909–23.

Ormel, J., Von Korff, M., Van Den Brink, W., *et al.* (1993). Depression, anxiety, and social disability show synchrony of change in primary care patients. *Am J Public Health* **83**:385–90.

Ormel, J., Oldehinkel, T., Brilman, E., & Van Den Brink, W. (1993). Outcome of depression and anxiety in primary care: a three-wave 3 1/2-year study of psychopathology and disability. *Arch Gen Psychiatry* **50**:759–66.

Peveler, R., George, C., Kinmonth, A. L., *et al.* (1999). Effect of antidepressant drug counselling and information leaflets on adherence to drug treatment in primary care: randomised controlled trial. *BMJ* **319**:612–15.

Peveler, R., & Kendrick, T. (2001). Treatment delivery and guidelines in primary care. *Br Med Bull* **57**:193–206.

Pignone, M. P. M., Gaynes, B. N. M., Rushton, J. L. M., *et al.* (2002). Screening for depression in adults: a summary of the evidence for the U.S. Preventive Services Task Force. *Ann Int Med* **136**:765–76.

Priest, R. G., Vize, C., Roberts, A., *et al.* (1996). Lay people's attitudes to treatment of depression: results of opinion poll for Defeat Depression Campaign just before its launch. *BMJ* **313**:858–9.

Proudfoot, J., Goldberg, D., Mann, A., *et al.* (2003). Computerized, interactive, multimedia cognitive-behavioural program for anxiety and depression in general practice. *Psychol Med* **33**:217–27.

Proudfoot, J., Ryden, C., Everitt, B., *et al.* (2004). Clinical efficacy of computerised cognitive-behavioural therapy for anxiety and depression in primary care: randomised controlled trial. *Br J Psychiatry* **185**:46–54.

Pullen, I. Y. A. (1985). Is communication improving between general practitioners and psychiatrists? *BMJ* **290**:31–3.

Reid, S., & Wessely, S. (2001). Somatisation and depression. In A. Dawson & A. Tylee, eds. *Depression: Social and Economic Timebomb*. London: BMJ Books for the World Health Organisation, pp. 55–61.

Ronalds, C., Creed, F., Stone, K., *et al.* (1997). Outcome of anxiety and depressive disorders in primary care. *Br J Psychiatry* 171:427–33.

Rost, K., Nutting, P., Smith, J., *et al.* (2001). Improving depression outcomes in community primary care practice: a randomized trial of the quEST intervention. Quality Enhancement by Strategic Teaming. *J Gen Int Med* 16:143–9.

Rost, K., Zhang, M., Fortney, J., *et al.* (1998). Persistently poor outcomes of undetected major depression in primary care. *Gen Hosp Psychiatry* 20:12–20.

Rutz, W., von Knorring, L., & Walinder, J. (1989). Frequency of suicide on Gotland after systematic postgraduate education of general practitioners. *Acta Psychiatr Scand* 80:151–4.

Rutz, W., von Knorring, L., & Walinder, J. (1992). Long-term effects of an educational program for general practitioners given by the Swedish Committee for the Prevention and Treatment of Depression. *Acta Psychiatr Scand* 85:83–8.

Saint-Yves, I. F. (1992). The Read Clinical Classification. *Health Bull* 50:422–7.

Schulberg, H. C., Block, M. R., Madonia, M. J., *et al.* (1996). Treating major depression in primary care practice. Eight-month clinical outcomes. *Arch Gen Psychiatry* 53:913–19.

Schulberg, H. C., & McClelland, M. (1987). A conceptual model for educating primary care providers in the diagnosis and treatment of depression. *Gen Hosp Psychiatry* 9:1–10.

Schulberg, H. C., McClelland, M., & Gooding, W. (1987). Six-month outcomes for medical patients with major depressive disorders. *J Gen Int Med* 2:312–17.

Scott, C., Tacchi, M. J., Jones, R., & Scott, J. (1997). Acute and one-year outcome of a randomised controlled trial of brief cognitive therapy for major depressive disorder in primary care. *Br J Psychiatry* 171:131–4.

Shepherd, M., Cooper, B., Brown, A. C., & Kalton, G. (1966). *Psychiatric Illness in General Practice*. London: Oxford University Press.

Shiels, C., Gabbay, M., Dowrick, C., & Hulbert, C. (2004). Depression in men attending a rural general practice: factors associated with prevalence of depressive symptoms and diagnosis. *Br J Psychiatry* 185:239–44.

Sibbald, B., Addington-Hall, J., Brenneman, D., & Freeling, P. (1993). Counsellors in English and Welsh general practices: their nature and distribution. *BMJ* 306:29–33.

Simon, G. E., Goldberg, D., Tiemens, B. G., & Ustun, T. B. (1999). Outcomes of recognized and unrecognized depression in an international primary care study. *Gen Hosp Psychiatry* 21:97–105.

Simon, G. E., Katon, W. J., VonKorff, M., *et al.* (2001). Cost-effectiveness of a collaborative care program for primary care patients with persistent depression. *Am J Psychiatry* 158:1638–44.

Simon, G. E., & VonKorff, M. (1991). Somatization and psychiatric disorder in the NIMH Epidemiologic Catchment Area study. *Am J Psychiatry* 148:1494–1500.

Simon, G. E. M. M. & VonKorff, M. S. (1995). Recognition, management, and outcomes of depression in primary care. *Arch Fam Med* 4:99–105.

Simpson, S., Corney, R., Fitzgerald, P., & Beecham, J. (2003). A randomized controlled trial to evaluate the effectiveness and cost-effectiveness of psychodynamic counselling for general practice patients with chronic depression. *Psychol Med* 33:229–39.

Skevington, S. M., & Wright, A. (2001). Changes in the quality of life of patients receiving antidepressant medication in primary care: validation of the WHOQOL-100. *Br J Psychiatry* 178:261–7.

Spitzer, R. L., Kroenke, K., Linzer, M., *et al.* (1995). Health-related quality of life in primary care patients with mental disorders. Results from the PRIME-MD 1000 Study. *JAMA* 274:1511–17.

Stanistreet, D., Gabbay, M. B., Jeffrey, V., & Taylor S. (2004). Missed opportunities? Preventing violent deaths in young men, an epidemiological study. *Br J Gen Pract* 54:254–8.

Strathdee, G., & Jenkins, R. (1996). Purchasing mental health for primary care. In G. Thornicroft & G. Strathdee, eds. *Commissioning Mental Health Services*. London: Her Majesty's Stationery Office, pp. 77–83.

Strathdee, G., & Williams, P. (1984). A survey of psychiatrists in primary care: the silent growth of a new service. *J Royal Coll Gen Pract* 34:615–18.

Symons, L., Tylee, A., Mann, A., *et al.* (2004). Improving access to depression care: descriptive report of a multidisciplinary primary care pilot service. *Br J Gen Pract* 54:679–83.

Thompson, C., Kinmonth, A. L., Stevens, L., *et al.* (2000). Effects of clinical-practice guideline and practice-based education on detection and outcome of depression in primary care: Hampshire Depression project randomised controlled trial. *Lancet* 355:185–91.

Thompson, C., Ostler, K., Peveler, R. C., *et al.* (2001). Dimensional perspective on the recognition of depressive symptoms in primary care: the Hampshire depression project 3. *Br J Psychiatry* **179**:317–23.

Tiemens, B. G., Ormel, J., & Simon, G. E. (1996). Occurrence, recognition, and outcome of psychological disorders in primary care. *Am J Psychiatry* **153**:636–44.

Turton, P., Tylee, A., & Kerry, S. (1995). Mental health training needs in general practice. *Primary Care Psychiatry* **1**:197–9.

Tylee, A. (1999). Training the whole primary care team in common mental disorders, In M. Tansella & G. Thornicroft. *Mental Disorders in Primary Care*. London: Routledge.

Tylee, A. (2001). Management of depression in primary care. In A. Dawson & A. Tylee, eds. *Depression: Social and Economic Timebomb*. London: BMJ Books for the World Health Organisation, pp. 85–92.

Tylee, A., Freeling, P., Kerry, S., & Burns, T. (1995). How does the content of consultations affect the recognition by general practitioners of major depression in women? *Br J Gen Pract* **45**:575–8.

Tylee, A., Walters, P., & Enright, A. (2004). Trailblazers. *Primary Care Ment Health* **2**:1–3.

Tylee, A. T. Freeling, P., & Kerry S. (1993). Why do general practitioners recognise major depression in one woman patient yet miss it in another? *Br J Gen Pract* **43**: 327–0.

US Preventive Services Task Force (2002). Screening for depression: recommendations and rationale. *Ann Int Med* **136**:760–4.

Upton, M. W., Evans, M., Goldberg, D. P., & Sharp, D. J. (1999). Evaluation of ICD-10 PHC mental health guidelines in detecting and managing depression within primary care. *Br J Psychiatry* **175**:476–82.

Ustun, T. B., Sartorius, N. Eds. (1995). *Mental Illness in General Health Care. An International Study.* Chichester: John Willey.

Valenstein, M. M., Vijan, S. M., Zeber, J. E. M., Boehm, K. M., & Buttar, A. M. (2001). The cost-utility of screening for depression in primary care. *Ann Int Med* **134**:345–60.

Vassiliadou, M., Goldberg, D., Tylee, A., & Christodoulou, G. (2004). The Athens Mental Health Promotion Educational Programme. *Primary Care Mental Health* **2**: 73–6.

Von Korff, M., & Goldberg, D. (2001). Improving outcomes in depression: the whole process of care needs to be enhanced. *BMJ* **323**:948–9.

Walters, P. (2003). Trailblazers – an update. *J Primary Care Ment Health* **7**:18

Watson, L. C., & Pignone, M. P. (2003). Screening accuracy for late-life depression in primary care: a systematic review. *J Fam Pract* **52**:956–64.

Wells, K. B., Hays, R. D., Burnam, M. A., *et al.* (1989). Detection of depressive disorder for patients receiving prepaid or fee-for-service care. Results from the Medical Outcomes Study. *JAMA* **262**:3298–3302.

Wells, K. B., Sherbourne, C., Schoenbaum, M., *et al.* (2000). Impact of disseminating quality improvement programs for depression in managed primary care: a randomized controlled trial. *JAMA* **283**:212–20.

Wells, K. B., Stewart, A., Hays, R. D., *et al.* (1989). The functioning and well-being of depressed patients. Results from the Medical Outcomes Study. *JAMA* **262**:914–19.

Whooley, M. A. M., Avins, A. L. M., Miranda, J. P., & Browner, W. S. M. M. (1997). Case-finding instruments for depression: two questions are as good as many. *Journal of General Internal Medicine*, **12**:439–45.

Wilkin, P. (2001). The primary care role of the community psychiatric nurse. *Primary Care Psychiatry* **7**:79–84

Williams, C. (2001). Use of written cognitive-behavioural therapy self-help materials to treat depression. *Adv Psychiatr Treat* **7**:233–40.

Wittchen, H. U., Hofler, M., & Meister, W. (2001). Prevalence and recognition of depressive syndromes in German primary care settings: poorly recognized and treated? *Int Clin Psychopharmacol* **16**:121–35.

World Health Organisation. (2004). *World Health Organisation Guide to Mental and Neurological Health in Primary Care*, 2nd edn. London: Royal Society of Medicine Press.

World Organisation of National Colleges Academies and Academic Associations of General Practitioners. (1988). *ICHPCC-2-Defined: International Classification of Health Problems in Primary Care*, 3rd edn. Oxford: Oxford Medical Publishers.

Wright, A. F., & Anderson, A. J. (1995). Newly identified psychiatric illness in one general practice: 12-month outcome and the influence of patients' personality. *Br J Gen Pract* **45**:83–7.

22

Community psychiatry and service delivery models

Michele Tansella, Graham Thornicroft and Ezra Susser

This chapter focuses on the following key questions for psychiatrists. What are the main mental health service delivery models, and how far are they evidence-based or ethics-based? Should mental health services be provided in community or hospital settings? What service components are necessary and which are optional? What are service development priorities for countries with low, medium and high levels of resources? This chapter discusses mental health services for adults of working age and does not directly address other important groups, including children, older people or those suffering primarily from alcohol or drug misuse. The reader is referred to Chapters 6, 15, 10 and 11, respectively, for coverage of those issues.

Definition of key terms

How does *community psychiatry* differ from *social psychiatry*? The latter has rarely been defined in formal terms, and Leff (1993) stated that "social psychiatry is concerned with the effects of the social environment on the mental health of the individual, and with the effects of the mentally ill person on his/her environment" (p. 5). Most texts on social psychiatry have focused on identifying social influences on the onset and course of mental disorders (Bebbington, 1990; Leff, 1993). Community psychiatry, by contrast,

focuses on interventions (Tyrer, 1995). Common to both is a dependency on epidemiological methods to identify risk factors for social psychiatry and to establish population-level needs for community psychiatry.

In our view, community psychiatry comprises the principles and practices needed to provide mental health services for a local population by (1) establishing *population-based needs* for treatment and care; (2) providing a service system linking a wide *range of resources* of adequate capacity, operating in *accessible locations*; and (3) *delivering evidence-based treatments* to people with mental disorders. In relation to this, we have defined a community-based mental health service as "one which provides a full range of effective mental health care to a defined population, and which is dedicated to treating and helping people with mental disorders, in proportion to their suffering or distress, in collaboration with other local agencies" (Thornicroft & Tansella, 1999, p. 12).

Historical background

The recent history of mental health services can be seen in terms of three periods: (1) the rise of the asylum, (2) the decline of the asylum, and (3) balancing mental health care (Thornicroft & Tansella, 1999).

Essential Psychiatry, ed. Robin M. Murray, Kenneth S. Kendler, Peter McGuffin, Simon Wessely, David J. Castle. Published by Cambridge University Press. © Cambridge University Press 2008.

Period 1. The rise of the asylum

Forerunners to asylum care can be traced back many centuries. It was not until the first half of the nineteenth century, however, that the asylum emerged as the main societal institution for care of the mentally ill. In France, England, the United States and other industrializing countries, some of the early asylums represented attempts to provide more humane care, sometimes termed *moral treatment* (Rothman, 1971; Susser *et al.*, 2005; Weiner, 1993). By the end of the nineteenth century, however, asylums had mainly become a form of unenlightened or merely custodial hospital care, with higher than expected mortality rates (Singer, 2001). In many of the more economically developed countries, the period from 1880 to approximately 1950 was characterised by the construction and enlargement of asylums, remote from their populations, offering mainly custodial containment and the provision of the basic necessities for survival to people with a wide range of clinical disorders and social abnormalities. Some remarkable attempts at care outside asylums have been documented, but they were the exception rather than the rule (Bartlett & Wright, 1999). There is now strong evidence that the asylum model produced overall poor standards of treatment and care (Leff, 1997). Despite this, in some countries, especially those which are less economically developed, almost all mental health service expenditure continues to pay for asylum care.

Period 2. The decline of the asylum

This has taken place in many economically developed countries since about 1950, when their manifest shortcomings were demonstrated. Perhaps the most profound of these failures were the effects asylums had on patients, including the progressive loss of life skills and the accumulation of "deficit symptoms" (institutionalism; Wing & Brown, 1970). Further concerns included repeated cases of ill treatment of patients, the geographical and professional isolation of the institutions and their staff, poor reporting and accounting procedures, failures of management and leadership, ineffective administration, poorly targeted financial resources, weak staff training and inadequate inspection and quality assurance procedures. In response to this, deinstitutionalisation proceeded. Deinstitutionalisation can be defined in terms of three essential components: (1) the prevention of inappropriate mental hospital admissions through the provision of community facilities, (2) the discharge to the community of long-term institutional patients who have received adequate preparation and (3) the establishment and maintenance of community support systems for noninstitutionalised patients.

Period 3. Balancing mental health care

During this period, the main goal has been to develop a range of *balanced care* within local settings. In this process, which has not yet begun in some regions and countries, it is important to ensure that all the positive functions of the asylum are fully reprovided, and the negative aspects of the institutions are not perpetuated. The balanced care approach aims to provide services which offer treatment and care with the following characteristics:

- services which are close to home, including modern hospital care for acute admissions and long-term residential facilities in the community;
- interventions related to disabilities as well as symptoms;
- treatment and care specific to the diagnosis and needs of each individual;
- services consistent with international conventions on human rights;
- services which reflect the priorities of service users themselves (Rose *et al.*, 2003; Faulkner & Thomas, 2002);
- services which are co-ordinated between mental health professions and agencies; and
- mobile rather than static services, including those which can offer home treatment.

Table 22.1 Overview of the matrix model

Geographical dimension	Temporal dimension		
	A. Input phase	B. Process phase	C. Outcome Phase
1. Country/ regional level	1A	1B	1C
2. Local level	2A	2B	2C
3. Individual level	3A	3B	3C

Contextual issues in developing mental health services

For planning, delivering and evaluating mental health services, there is a clear need for an overall conceptual framework. We have proposed such a framework (the matrix model), which uses two dimensions, the geographical/service organisation level (country, local and patient levels, identified by the numbers 1, 2 and 3) and the temporal (input, process and outcome phases, both short and long term outcomes, referred to by the letters A, B and C; Tansella & Thornicroft, 1998). Using these two dimensions a 3 × 3 matrix with nine cells is constructed to bring into focus critical issues for mental health services. The overall scheme is illustrated in Table 22.1.

Service models in low-, medium- and high-level resource areas

Table 22.2 presents a scheme to show models of mental health service delivery appropriate to the level of resources available locally. For simplicity, the table is organised along the lines proposed by the World Health Organisation (WHO) World Health Report (WHO, 2001, pp. 112–115). The table indicates that countries with a low level of resources

(Column 1) are likely to need to provide most or all of their formal mental health care in primary health care settings, delivered by primary care staff, with specialist backup to provide training, consultation for complex cases and in-patient assessment and treatment for cases which cannot be managed in primary care (Mubbashar, 1999). Because even these types of formal services are extremely limited in many settings, informal care by families, other community resources and care by traditional healers may assume central importance (Desjarlais *et al.*, 1995; Susser *et al.*, 1996). Accordingly, the interrelationships between the various formal and informal sectors need careful attention. There is enormous variation in the nature of care received both within and across low-resource countries. In the worst instances, apparent community care in fact represents widespread neglect of mentally ill people. Where asylums do exist, policy makers will face choices about whether to upgrade the quality of care offered (Njenga, 2002) or to use the resources of the larger hospitals to set up decentralised services instead (Alem, 2002).

It is important to recognise that the differences between the low- and the high-resource countries are vast. In Europe, for example, there are between 5.5 and 20.0 psychiatrists per 100,000 population, whereas the figure is 0.05 per 100,000 in African countries (Njenga, 2002); the average number of psychiatric beds is 87 per 100,000 in the European region and 3.4 per 100,000 in Africa (Alem, 2002). Furthermore, approximately 5% to 10% of the total health budget is spent on mental health in Europe (Becker & Vazquez-Barquero, 2001), whereas on the African continent 80% of countries spend less than 1% of their limited total health budget on mental health (World Bank, 2002). Further, for both Europe and Africa, there are huge variations between countries as well as between local areas within countries. As a consequence, the models of service provision relevant to low-resource areas will be substantially different from those required by medium- and high-resource countries. The scheme used in this chapter is that elaborated in the WHO World Health Report, which describes low, medium and high levels of

Table 22.2 Mental health service components relevant for countries with low, medium and high levels of resources

1. Low levels of resource countries	2. Medium levels of resource countries	3. High levels of resource countries
A. Primary care mental health with specialist back-up	**A. Primary care mental health with specialist back-up *and*** **B. Mainstream mental health care**	**A. Primary care mental health with specialist backup *and*** **B. Mainstream mental health care *and*** **C. Specialised/differentiated mental health services**
Screening and assessment by primary care staff	Out-patient/ambulatory clinics	Specialised clinics for specific disorders or patient groups, including: – eating disorders – dual diagnosis – treatment-resistant affective disorders – adolescent services
Talking treatments, including counselling and advice	Community mental health teams	Specialised community mental health teams, including: – early inventions teams – assertive community treatment
Pharmacological treatment Liaison and training with mental health specialist staff, when available	Acute in-patient care	Alternatives to acute hospital admission, including: – home treatment/crisis resolution teams – crisis/respite houses – acute day hospitals
Limited specialist backup available for: – training – consultation for complex cases – in-patient assessment and treatment for cases which cannot be managed in primary care, for example, in general hospitals	Long-term community-based residential care Occupation/day care	Alternative types of long-stay community residential care, including: – intensive 24-hour staffed residential provision – less intensively staffed accommodation – independent accommodation Alternative forms of occupation and vocational rehabilitation: – sheltered workshops – supervised work placements – cooperative work schemes – self-help and user groups – clubhouses/transitional employment programmes – vocational rehabilitation – individual placement and support service

resource countries in relation to their "resource realities" (WHO, 2001), although it is recognised that as yet there are no agreed and standardised criteria in terms of socioeconomic indicators (such as gross national product per capita) to define which countries can be classified in each of these three resource groups.

Countries with a medium level of resources (Column 2 of Table 22.2) may first establish the service components shown and later, as resources allow, chose to develop some of the wider range of more differentiated services, which are indicated in Column 3. The choice of which of these more specialised services to develop first depends on local factors, including services traditions and specific circumstances; consumer, carer and staff preferences; existing services' strengths and weaknesses; and the way in which evidence is interpreted and used. Policy makers will need to decide which service components to commission and also which services to decommission according to the resources available and according to the local priorities and guiding principles adopted. The scheme also indicates that the models of care relevant and affordable to countries with a high level of resources (Column 3) may be entirely different to those with low levels of resources.

Primary care mental health with specialist backup

From the research literature, there is a consensus that well-defined psychological problems are common in general health care and primary health care settings in every country, with an average prevalence of 24% attending these settings. Marked disability is often associated with these disorders, and disability is usually in proportion to the number of symptoms present (Goldberg, 2000; Ormel *et al.*, 1994). The main results of studies conducted so far are the following:

- In high-, moderate- and low-resource countries, most people with mental disorders are not seen in specialist services.

- Psychological disorders can affect people's perceptions of their physical health status.
- Most primary care staff are aware of psychological disorders, but the agreement between clinician recognition and the actual occurrence of these problems (assessed by research measures) is only low to moderate.
- Mental disorders seen in primary care settings are a major public health problem and cause a substantial burden to society.
- Mental health treatments should therefore be an integral part of primary care.
- The training of staff in the recognition and treatment of these disorders should therefore be given a high priority so that these skills are a part of their core expertise (Tansella & Thornicroft, 1999; Ustun & Sartorius, 1995; Von Korff *et al.*, 2001).

In relation to countries with a low level of resources with specialist backup (Column 1 in Table 22.2), the large majority of cases of mental disorders should be recognised and treated within primary health care (Desjarlais *et al.*, 1995; WHO, 2001). The WHO has shown that integration of essential mental health treatments within primary health care in such countries is feasible (WHO, 2001).

Mainstream mental health care

Mainstream mental health care refers to a range of service components, which may be necessary in countries that can afford more than a primary care–based system with specialist backup alone. However, the recognition and treatment of the majority of people with mental illnesses, especially depression and anxiety-related disorders, remains a task which falls mostly to primary care. Von Korff and Goldberg (2001) reviewed 12 randomised controlled trials of enhanced care for major depression in primary care settings, showing that disorders often remit with time without any intervention and that interventions should focus on low-cost case management coupled with fluid and accessible working relationships between the case manager, the primary care doctor and the mental health specialist (see also Chapter 21). In other words, the whole process of care needs to be enhanced with the following elements: active follow up by the case manager (who is often a primary care nurse), monitoring treatment adherence and patient outcomes, adjustment of treatment plan if patients do not improve and referral to a specialist when necessary (Gask *et al.*, 1997; Von Korff & Goldberg, 2001). The evidence therefore supports a multimodal approach, and interventions directed solely towards training and supporting GPs have not been shown to be effective (Simon, 2002; Wells *et al.*, 2000).

As specialist services are scarce and expensive, they should target
* assessment and diagnosis of complex cases, and those requiring an expert second opinion;
* treating people with the most severe symptoms (Ruggeri *et al.*, 2000);
* providing care for those with the greatest degree of disability consequent from mental illness; and
* making treatment recommendation for those conditions which have proved nonresponsive to initial treatment.

To achieve this consistently, a service will need to identify priority groups of those who should receive access to specialist care, from among the 25% of the whole population who suffer from a mental disorder in any given year. Well targeted services are those in which specialist care concentrates on providing direct services to people with the most severe degrees of symptoms and disability (often called *severe mental illness*). This means treating, to a high clinical standard of evidence-based care, both psychotic and nonpsychotic severe disorders, in the acute and post-acute phases. Moreover, they should also offer consultation, liaison and advice to primary care and other services which treat the more common mental disorders, with a special responsibility for the treatment-resistant and more chronically disabling mental disorders seen in those settings. Sufficient services will need to be provided in all of the five categories included in column 2 of Table 22.2. One therefore has to address the capacity needed for each of these categories, taking into account the services that are available in all the other categories, and this orientation is sometimes called *whole system planning* (Thornicroft & Tansella, 1999).

Out-patient and ambulatory clinics

Such clinics can be seen as clinical services provided in various settings (such as primary care health centres, general hospitals or community mental health centres) in which trained mental health staff offer assessment and treatment, including pharmacological, psychological and social interventions. These components include huge variations in practice, for example, in relation to whether (1) patients can self-refer or need to be referred by other agencies such as primary care; (2) there are fixed appointment times or open access assessments; (3) doctors, alone or with other disciplines, also provide clinical contact; and (4) direct or indirect payment is made. Other considerations include methods to enhance attendance rates, how to respond to nonattenders and the frequency and duration of clinical contacts. There is surprisingly little evidence on all of these key characteristics of out-patient care (Becker, 2001). Even so, there is a strong clinical consensus in many countries that they are a relatively efficient way to organise the provision of assessment and treatment of mental health care providing that the clinic sites are accessible to local populations. Nevertheless, these clinics are simply methods of arranging clinical contact between staff and patients, and thus the key issue is the *content* of the clinical interventions, namely, to deliver only treatments which are known to be evidence-based (Nathan & Gorman, 2002).

Community mental health teams

Community mental health teams (CMHTs) are the basic building block for community mental health services. The simplest model of provision of community care is for generic (meaning nonspecialised) CMHTs to provide the full range of interventions, prioritising adults with severe mental illness, in a local defined geographical catchment area. Evidence from the United Kingdom (Simmonds *et al.,* 2001; Thornicroft *et al.,* 1998; Tyrer *et al.,* 1995, 1998, 2003) suggests that there are clear benefits to the introduction of generic community-based multidisciplinary teams. They may improve engagement with services, enhance user satisfaction and increase met needs, although they do not have significant benefits for symptomatic or social improvement. The central advantages of generic CMHTs are in continuity of care and in flexibility, which have been shown to be more developed where a more community-based model is in place (Sytema *et al.,* 1997). Patients may benefit from seeing the same staff long-term, and when in crisis the relationships staff members have already established may be invaluable. The ability of mobile CMHTs to contact patients at home, at work, in neutral settings such as local cafes or in other institutions means that early relapse identification and treatment is more often achieved and that adherence to treatment may be more often maintained (McDonald *et al.,* 2002).

The generic CMHT is flexible in that intensity of input may be varied according to the patient's current needs, without requiring transfer to another team. There may be patients who will benefit from frequent contact and outreach – for example, during a relapse – but who at other times require relatively low levels of input. The scope for providing such flexibility may be diminished with discrete, specialised teams, which have a remit only to provide intensive support (Burns, 2001; Mueser *et al.,* 1998).

Case management has been described as the "co-ordination, integration and allocation of individualised care within limited resources" (Thornicroft, 1991, p. 141). There is now a considerable literature to show that this style of working can be moderately effective in improving continuity of care, quality of life and patient satisfaction, but there is conflicting evidence on whether case management has any impact on the use of in-patient services (Hansson *et al.,* 1998; Mueser *et al.,* 1998; Saarento *et al.,* 1996; Ziguras & Stuart, 2000; Ziguras *et al.,* 2002). Case

management needs to be carefully distinguished from the more specific and more intensive *assertive community treatment* (discussed later). At this stage, the evidence suggests that the practice of case management can most usefully be implemented within the context of community mental health teams and is a method of delivering care rather than being a particular type of clinical intervention in its own right (Holloway & Carson, 2001).

Acute in-patient care

There is no evidence for countries with medium or high levels of resources that a balanced system of mental health care can be provided without some acute psychiatric in-patient care. Some services (such as home treatment teams, crisis house and acute day hospital care) may be able to offer realistic alternative care to some voluntary patients. Nevertheless, those who need urgent medical assessment, or with severe and comorbid medical and psychiatric conditions, severe psychiatric relapse and behavioural disturbance, high levels of suicidality or assaultativeness, acute neuropsychiatric conditions, or elderly patients with concomitant severe physical disorders, will usually require high-intensity immediate support in acute in-patient hospital units, sometimes on a compulsory basis (Department of Health, 2002).

There is a relatively weak evidence base on many aspects of in-patient care, and most studies have been descriptive accounts (Szmukler & Holloway, 2001). There have been few systematic reviews in this field, one of which found that there were no differences in outcomes between routine admissions and planned short hospital stays (Johnstone & Zolese, 1999). More generally, it is possible to say that although there is a consensus that acute in-patient services are necessary, the number of beds required is highly contingent on which other services exist locally and on local social and cultural characteristics, including the degree of tolerance of disturbed behaviour (Thornicroft & Tansella, 1999). Acute in-patient care commonly absorbs most of the mental health budget (Knapp *et al.,* 1997).

Therefore, realistically minimising the use of bed-days – for example, by reducing the average length of stay – may be an important policy goal, *if* the resources released in this way can be used for other mental health service components. Given the need for some in-patient services in medium- and high-resource countries, a second pressing policy issue concerns measures to provide these in a humane way that is acceptable to patients – for example, in general hospital units (Quirk & Lelliott, 2001; Tomov, 2001).

Long-term community-based residential care

Larger psychiatric hospitals, where they exist, usually provide more long-term than acute care. From a policy perspective, it is important to know whether long-term patients should continue to be cared for in such institutions or whether they should be transferred to long-term community-based residential care. The evidence here, for medium- and high-resource level countries, is clear. When deinstitutionalisation is carefully planned and managed, the outcomes will be more favourable for most patients who are discharged to community care (Shepherd & Murray, 2001; Tansella, 1986; Thornicroft & Bebbington, 1989). The TAPS study in London (Leff, 1997), for example, completed a 5-year follow up on more than 95% of 670 discharged long-stay nondemented patients and found the following:

- At the end of 5 years, two thirds of the patients were still living in their original residence.
- The new form of service did not increase the death rate or the suicide rate.
- Fewer than 1 in 100 patients became homeless, and no patient was lost to follow-up from a staffed home.
- More than one third were readmitted during the follow-up period, and at the time of follow-up 10% of the sample were in hospital (a Nordic multicentre study has also emphasised this point; Oiesvold *et al.*, 2000).
- Overall, the patient's quality of life was greatly improved by the move to the community, but

disabilities remained due to the nature of severe psychotic illnesses (Leff, 1997).
- There was little difference overall between hospital and community costs, and the economic evaluation suggested that community care is more cost-effective than long-stay hospital care.

The range and capacity of community residential care that will be needed in any particular area is highly dependent on two key factors: the nature of the other mental health service components which are available locally and social and cultural factors such as the amount of family/carer which is usually provided (van Wijngaarden *et al.*, 2003).

Occupation and day care

Rates of unemployment among people with mental disorders are usually much higher than in the general population (Warner, 1994; Warr, 1987). Traditional methods to offer occupation, especially to people with longer-term and more disabling mental disorders, have been day centres or a variety of nonstandardised psychiatric rehabilitation centres (Rosen & Barfoot, 2001; Shepherd, 1990). There is little scientific research of these traditional forms of day care, and a recent review of more than 300 papers, for example, found no relevant randomised controlled trials. Nonrandomised studies have given conflicting results and for countries with medium levels of resources, it is reasonable at this stage to make pragmatic decisions about the provision of rehabilitation and day care services if the options discussed later are not affordable (Catty *et al.*, 2003).

It is important to ensure that the interfaces between the services are functioning properly, as a condition for successful implementation of the service as a whole. Such interfaces will operate across the whole range of statutory and voluntary/community organisations. Communication of information and transfer of patients may need to be arranged, for example, between *health services* (general physical and dental health, primary care and, when available, forensic, old age, learning disability/mental handicap/mental retardation, psychotherapies), *social services/welfare benefits* (income support, domiciliary care, respite care), *housing agencies* (staffed and unstaffed accommodation and residential care), *other governmental agencies* (police, prison) and *non-governmental agencies* (religious organisations, voluntary groups, for-profit private organisations) (Goldberg & Jackson, 1992). This degree of integration implies that a planning authority/agency is required at the local level to co-ordinate the commissioning and provision of services so that the service components work effectively together in an integrated way, although the degree of service integration has not itself been formally tested for in systematic reviews of randomised controlled trials (Gask *et al.,* 1997; Tyrer *et al.,* 1989).

Specialised/differentiated mental health services

The approach adopted in this chapter is that a balanced approach to community-based mental health services requires a mixed portfolio of service components and that this blend will in large part depend on the level of resources available. In countries which have a high level of resources, it maybe possible to develop, in addition to the primary care mental health with specialised backup services and also in addition to the mainstream services, more specialised and more differentiated services dedicated to particular subgroups of patients or to specific goals. Where these are well implemented, they may reduce part of the demand for the mainstream services, for instance, the substitution of acute in-patient care by home treatment teams or services to help homeless persons with mental illness adjust to community living and integrate into the care system (Susser *et al.,* 1997). Interestingly the evidence base for these more recent and more innovative forms of care is far wider and more scientifically rigorous than for *any* of the service components described earlier in relation to lower-resource countries, and indeed few high-quality scientific studies have been carried out in low-income countries, across all fields of health (Isaakidis *et al.,* 2002; Patel & Sumathipala, 2001).

Specialised out-patient and ambulatory clinics

Specialised out-patient facilities for specific disorders or patient groups are common in many high-resource countries and may include the following services, dedicated to:
• patients with eating disorders;
• patients with dual diagnosis (psychotic disorders and substance abuse);
• cases of treatment-resistant affective or psychotic disorders;
• individuals requiring specialised forms of psychotherapy;
• mentally disordered offenders;
• mentally ill mothers and their babies; and
• those with other specific disorders (such as post-traumatic stress disorder).

Local decisions about whether to establish such specialist clinics will depend on a number of factors, including their relative priority in relation to the other specialist services described later, identified services gaps, and the financial opportunities available (Dixon *et al.,* 2001; Olfson *et al.,* 1998; Rosenheck *et al.,* 2000).

Specialised community mental health teams

Specialised mental health teams are by far the most researched of all the possible components of balanced mental health service, and most recent randomised controlled trials and systematic reviews in this field refer to such teams (Mueser *et al.,* 1998). Two types of specialist community mental health team have been particular well developed as adjuncts to the generic community mental health team: assertive community treatment (ACT) teams and early intervention teams.

Assertive community treatment teams

These teams provide a form of specialised mobile outreach treatment for people with more disabling mental disorders and have been characterised (Deci *et al.,* 1995; Scott & Lehman, 2001; Teague *et al.,* 1998) as requiring the following features:

- small caseloads (the number of patients cared for by the programme should be in the region 100 patients with 10 core staff);
- continuous services (provided 24 hours a day, 7 days a week);
- medication delivered by team members daily, if necessary;
- ability for patients to graduate to less intensive interventions;
- a team approach, including the contributions of psychiatrists, nurses and other professionals;
- the team arranges or directly manages patients' finances; and
- the average proportion of team activity which takes place in the community is targeted at 80%.

There is now strong evidence that ACT, offered to people with severely disabling psychotic disorders in high-resource level countries can produce the following advantages: (1) reductions in admissions to hospital, and in the use of acute in-patient bed-days; (2) improvements in accommodation status and occupation; and (3) increase of service satisfaction. ACT has not been shown to produce improvements in mental state or social behaviour. Compared with usual services, the costs of in-patient services were reduced, but ACT did not change the overall costs of care (Latimer, 1999; Marshall & Lockwood, 2003; Phillips et al., 2001; Rosenheck & Neale, 1998). Nevertheless, the extent to which ACT is cross-culturally relevant is not yet established, and there is evidence that ACT may be less effective where usual services have been already well developed to offer high levels of continuity of care (Burns et al., 1999, 2001; Fiander et al., 2003).

Early intervention teams

There has been considerable interest in recent years in the prompt identification and treatment of first or early episode cases of psychosis. Much of the research in this field has focussed on the time between first clear onset of symptoms and the beginning of contact with treatment services, referred to as the *duration of untreated psychosis* (DUP). Emerging evidence now suggests that longer DUP is a strong predictor of worse outcome for psychosis; in other words, if patients wait a long time after developing a psychotic condition before they begin to receive treatment, they may take longer to recover and may have a less favourable long-term prognosis. So far few controlled trials have been published of interventions in this field, and no Cochrane systematic review has been completed. Thus it is premature to judge, at this stage, whether specialised early intervention teams should be seen as a high priority (Friis et al., 2003; Harrigan et al., 2003; Larsen et al., 2001; McGorry & Killackey, 2002; McGorry et al., 2002; Warner & McGorry, 2002).

Alternatives to acute in-patient care

In recent years three main alternatives to acute in-patient care have been developed: acute day hospitals, crisis houses and home treatment/crisis resolution teams. *Acute day hospitals* are facilities which offer programmes of day treatment for those with acute and severe psychiatric problems, as an alternative to admission to in-patient units. A recent systematic review of nine randomised controlled trials established that acute day hospital care is suitable for between a quarter and a third of those who would otherwise be admitted to hospital. Day hospital care offers advantages in terms of faster clinical improvement, and it is less expensive. It is reasonable to conclude that acute day hospital care is an effective option when demand for in-patient beds is high (Harrison et al., 1999; Marshall et al., 2001; Wiersma et al., 1995).

Crisis houses are houses in community settings which are staffed by trained mental health professionals and which offer admission for some patients who would otherwise need in-patient care because of their acute and severe mental health condition. A wide variety of respite houses, havens and refuges have been developed – for example, for women escaping from scenes of domestic violence, but *crisis house* is used here only to refer to facilities which may be alternatives to noncompulsory hospital admission. There is relatively little research evidence about such houses at present. Where they have been established they are very acceptable to their residents (Davies *et al.*, 1994; Sledge, Tebes, & Rakfeldt, 1996a; Szmukler & Holloway, 2001), may be able to offer an alternative to hospital admission for about a quarter of otherwise admitted patients and may be more cost-effective than hospital admission (Sledge, Tebes, & Rakfeldt, 1996a, 1996b). A particular type of crisis house for psychotic patients is the Soteria experience in the United States, which was shown to have advantages over usual hospital treatment (Mosher, 1999).

Home treatment/crisis resolution teams are mobile community mental health teams which aim to offer assessment of patients in psychiatric crises and then provide intensive treatment and care at home to avoid or minimise the use of acute hospital admission. A recent Cochrane systematic review (Catty *et al.*, 2002) has found that most of the research evidence is from the United States or United Kingdom and concluded that home treatment teams reduce the days spent in hospital for people in mental heath crises, especially if the teams make regular home visits and have responsibility for both health and social care (Department of Health, 2001; Harrison *et al.*, 2001; Joy *et al.*, 2002; Rosen, 1997).

Alternative types of long-stay community residential care

Mental health services which are reducing the scale of large psychiatric institutions commonly provided long-stay residential care in the community to receive patients transferred from asylums (Shepherd *et al.*, 1996, 2001; Trieman *et al.*, 1998). Such residential care usually acts as a direct substitute for long-stay hospital wards and includes both nursing homes and residential care homes which have a combination of trained nurses, nursing assistants or care assistants present 24 hours a day. More specialised forms of residential care are commonly developed at a later stage to provide graded levels of support for mentally ill people who are not able to cope in independent accommodation without assistance. Three categories of such residential care can be identified, namely:

1. *24-hour staffed residential care:* a high-staffed hostel, residential care home or nursing home, depending on whether the staff have professional qualifications;
2. *day-staffed residential places:* s day-staffed hostel or residential home which has staff attending regularly for fixed hours, several days a week;
3. *lower supported accommodation:* minimally supported hostels or residential homes with visiting staff, including any supported, self-contained flats with one or several staff on call in separate accommodation.

There is somewhat limited evidence on the cost-effectiveness of these various levels of residential care, and there are no completed systematic reviews (Chilvers *et al.*, 2003), so it is reasonable for policy makers to decide on the need for such services with local stakeholders (Hafner, 1987; Nordentoft *et al.*, 1992; Rosen & Barfoot, 2001; Thornicroft, 2001).

Alternative forms of occupation and vocational rehabilitation

Work represents an important goal for many people with severe mental illnesses. Gainful employment addresses practical needs through improved economic independence, as well as therapeutic needs by enhancing self-esteem and overall functioning (Lehman, 1995; Wiersma *et al.*, 1997). Although vocational rehabilitation has been offered in various forms to people with severe mental illnesses for more than a century, its role has weakened because of discouraging results from earlier vocational rehabilitation efforts, financial disincentives to work, and a general pessimism about outcomes for these patients (Polak & Warner, 1996). However, several recent developments have again raised employment as an outcome priority. The advent of new pharmacological agents has raised hopes that overall outcomes may improve and that patients may be better able to take advantage of rehabilitation efforts (Lehman, 1999). Consumer and carer advocacy groups have set work and occupation as

---

Box 22.1 A stepwise approach to delivering mental health services

It may facilitate the implementation and delivery of mental health services to break down tasks into seven specific steps: (1) establishing the service principles, (2) setting the boundary conditions, (3) assessing population needs, (4) assessing current provision, (5) formulating a strategic plan, (6) implementing the service components at the local level and (7) a monitoring and review cycle (Reynolds & Thornicroft, 1999; Thornicroft & Tansella, 1999). This last step means that the consequences of care need to be assessed on a regular basis. In relation to the matrix model, it is our view that the main focus of such evaluations should be the outcomes of care for individual patients, for example, through the routine implementation of standardised outcome measures (Dash *et al.*, 2003; Ruggeri *et al.*, 2002; Gilbody *et al.*, 2002; Slade *et al.*, 1999).

---

one of their highest priorities to enhance both functional status and quality of life (Becker *et al.*, 1996; Thornicroft *et al.*, 2002).

There are recent indications from the United States that it is possible to improve vocational and psychosocial outcomes greatly with supported employment models. These models emphasise rapid placement in competitive jobs and support from employment specialists within a mental health treatment team (Drake *et al.*, 1999). The *individual placement and support* (IPS) model is a supported employment programme that emphasises competitive employment in integrated work settings with follow-up support, thereby bypassing the traditional stepwise approaches to vocational rehabilitation (Priebe *et al.*, 1998). Studies of IPS programmes have been encouraging in terms of increased rates of competitive employment (Lehman *et al.*, 2002; Marshall *et al.*, 2001). The traditional model uses a "train and place" approach, offering training in sheltered workshops and then placing individuals in real-life work settings. The IPS programme is the reverse, that is, "place and train", so that clients are placed in real jobs and then offered variable amounts of direct personal support to be able to retain their work positions.

The ethical base of mental health care

The ethical codes and declarations relevant to medicine include several which relate specifically to mental health care (Amnesty International, 2000). The United Nations Principles for the Protection of Persons with Mental Illness and the Improvement of Mental Health Care was adopted by General Assembly in 1991 (available at www.unhchr.ch/html/menu3/b/68.htm), and stressed the inherent humanity of persons with mental illness. By the same token, the 1996 World Psychiatric Association Declaration of Madrid (available at www.wpanet.org/generalinfo/ethic1.html) seeks to reverse the process of segregation and discrimination. Both of these provisions are a blend of positive and negative rights. The positive rights seek to guarantee to persons with mental illness the best available mental health care. The negative rights emphasise that mental illness per se should not result in the loss of right to self-determination and should accord recognition to the autonomy of persons with mental illness and guarantee their protection from exploitation and discrimination.

After the declaration of such principles, has the transition from rhetoric to reality really taken place? Unfortunately the worldwide evidence is that there are violations of even the most basic human rights of mentally ill people (Desjarlais *et al.*, 1995; Sartorius, 2001; WHO, 2001). For example, the Mental Disability Advocacy Centre has recently published concerns about the use of caged beds in several central and eastern European countries, including the Czech Republic, Hungary, Slovakia and Slovenia, all of which joined the European Union in 2004 (see http://www.mdac.info/cagebeds.htm). Similarly, the family members' organisation Zenkaren in Japan has published details of how, until recently, mentally ill persons have been excluded by local statue from such local amenities as public swimming baths in many parts of Japan (Takizawa, 1993). In India, a report by the National Human Rights Commission exposed the gross violations of human rights in many mental hospitals of the country (National Human Rights Commission, 1999).

It is therefore impossible to resist the conclusion that basic human rights of people with mental illness are systematically disregarded in some settings.

How can this be the case? It is helpful to consider the conceptual model of stigma developed by Link and colleagues (Link, 2001; Link & Phelan, 2001), in which the key aspects of stigmatisation are as follows: labelling, stereotyping, separation, status loss and discrimination and that for stigmatisation to occur, power must be exercised. Seen in this context, persons with mental illness have traditionally had little power to challenge the labels attached to them by others or to resist the social processes (rather similar in many ways to institutional racism) that have severely limited their life opportunities.

Conclusions

This chapter makes clear that there is no compelling argument and no scientific evidence which favours a model of mental health services that is based in hospitals alone (Drake *et al.*, 2001). However, there is also no scientific evidence that community services alone can provide satisfactory comprehensive care. Both the evidence available so far and accumulated clinical experience in many countries support a balanced model, which includes both elements of hospital and community care (Thornicroft & Tansella, 2002).

In terms of financial resources, the evidence from cost-effectiveness studies, when they have been applied in relation to deinstitutionalisation and the provision of community mental health teams, is that the quality of care is closely related to the expenditure on services – community-based models of care have been shown to be largely equivalent in cost to the services which they replace. They cannot be considered as primarily cost-saving or cost-containing measures. Nevertheless the material resources available will constrain how the balanced model is applied, and one may need to take a long-term perspective so that the components of the balanced care model are implemented over

time, as resources allow, increasingly to offer more choice to patients and consumers between services which are based on increasingly strong evidence of cost-effectiveness.

Acknowledgements

We are pleased to acknowledge the constructive contributions of Professor Sir David Goldberg and the WHO Health Evidence Network review on which this chapter is based.

REFERENCES

Alem, A. (2002). Community-based vs. hospital-based mental health care: the case of Africa. *World Psychiatry* **1**:99–100.

Amnesty International (2000). *Ethical Codes and Declarations Relevant to the Health Professions.* London: Amnesty International.

Bartlett, P., & Wright, D. (1999). *The History of Care in the Community 1750–2000.* London: Athlone Press.

Bebbington, P. (1990). *Social Psychiatry: Theory, Methodology and Practice.* New Brunswick, New Jersey: Transaction Publishers.

Becker, D. R., Drake, R. E., Farabaugh, A., *et al.* (1996). Job preferences of clients with severe psychiatric disorders participating in supported employment programs. *Psychiatr Serv* **47**:1223–6.

Becker, T. (2001). Out-patient psychiatric services. In G. Thornicroft & G. Szmukler, eds. *Textbook of Community Psychiatry.* Oxford: Oxford University Press, pp. 277–82.

Becker, T., & Vazquez-Barquero, J. L. (2001). The European perspective of psychiatric reform. *Acta Psychiatr Scand Suppl* 8–14.

Burns, T. (2001). Generic versus specialist mental health teams. In G. Thornicroft & G. Szmukler, eds. *Textbook of Community Psychiatry.* Oxford: Oxford University Press, pp. 231–41.

Burns, T., Creed, F., Fahy, T., *et al.* (1999). Intensive versus standard case management for severe psychotic illness: a randomised trial. UK 700 Group. *Lancet* **353**:2185–9.

Burns, T., Fioritti, A., Holloway, F., *et al.* (2001). Case management and assertive community treatment in Europe. *Psychiatr Serv* **52**:631–6.

Catty, J., Burns, T., & Comas, A. (2003). Day centres for severe mental illness [Cochrane review]. *The Cochrane Library, 1.* Oxford: Update Software.

Catty, J., Burns, T., Knapp, M., *et al.* (2002). Home treatment for mental health problems: a systematic review. *Psychol Med* 32:383–401.

Chilvers, R., Macdonald, G., & Hayes, A. (2003). *Supported housing for people with severe mental disorders* [Cochrane Review]. Oxford: Update Software.

Dash, P., Gowman, N., & Traynor, M. (2003). Increasing the impact of health services research. *BMJ* 327:1339–41.

Davies, S., Presilla, B., Strathdee, G., *et al.* (1994). Community beds: the future for mental health care? *Soc Psychiatry Psychiatr Epidemiol* 29:241–3.

Deci, P. A., Santos, A. B., Hiott, D. W., *et al.* (1995). Dissemination of assertive community treatment programs. *Psychiatr Serv* 46:676–8.

Department of Health (2001). Crisis resolution/home treatment teams. In *The Mental Health Policy Implementation Guide.* London: Department of Health.

Department of Health (2002). *Acute Adult In-Patient Care: Policy Implementation Guide.* London: Department of Health.

Desjarlais, R., Eisenberg, L., Good, B., *et al.* (1995). *World Mental Health. Problems and Priorities in Low Income Countries.* Oxford: Oxford University Press.

Dixon, L., Lyles, A., Smith, C., *et al.* (2001). Use and costs of ambulatory care services among Medicare enrollees with schizophrenia. *Psychiatr Serv* 52:786–92.

Drake, R. E., Goldman, H. H., Leff, H. S., *et al.* (2001). Implementing evidence-based practices in routine mental health service settings. *Psychiatr Serv* 52:179–82.

Drake, R. E., McHugo, G. J., Bebout, R. R., *et al.* (1999). A randomized clinical trial of supported employment for inner-city patients with severe mental disorders. *Arch Gen Psychiatry* 56:627–33.

Faulkner, A., & Thomas, P. (2002). User-led research and evidence-based medicine. *Br J Psychiatry* 180:1–3.

Fiander, M., Burns, T., McHugo, G. J., *et al.* (2003). Assertive community treatment across the Atlantic: comparison of model fidelity in the UK and USA. *Br J Psychiatry* 182:248–54.

Friis, S., Larsen, T. K., Melle, I., *et al.* (2003). Methodological pitfalls in early detection studies – the NAPE Lecture 2002. Nordic Association for Psychiatric Epidemiology. *Acta Psychiatr Scand* 107:3–9.

Gask, L., Sibbald, B., & Creed, F. (1997). Evaluating models of working at the interface between mental health services and primary care. *Br J Psychiatry* 170:6–11.

Gilbody, S. M., House, A. O., & Sheldon, T. A. (2002). Outcomes research in mental health. Systematic review. *Br J Psychiatry* 181:8–16.

Goldberg, D. (2000). Distinguishing mental illness in primary care. Mental illness or mental distress? *BMJ* 321:1412.

Goldberg, D., & Jackson, G. (1992). Interface between primary care and specialist mental health care. *Br J Gen Pract* 42:267–9.

Hafner, H. (1987). Do we still need beds for psychiatric patients? An analysis of changing patterns of mental health care. *Acta Psychiatr Scand* 75:113–26.

Hansson, L., Muus, S., Vinding, H. R., *et al.* (1998). The Nordic Comparative Study on sectorized psychiatry: contact rates and use of services for patients with a functional psychosis. *Acta Psychiatr Scand* 97:315–20.

Harrigan, S. M., McGorry, P. D., & Krstev, H. (2003). Does treatment delay in first-episode psychosis really matter? *Psychol Med* 33:97–110.

Harrison, J., Alam, N., & Marshall, J. (2001). Home or away: Which patients are suitable for a psychiatric home treatment service? *Psychiatr Bull* 25:England, www.

Harrison, J., Poynton, A., Marshall, J., *et al.* (1999). Open all hours: extending the role of the psychiatric day hospital. *Psychiatr Bull* 23:400–4.

Holloway, F., & Carson, J. (2001). Case management: an update. *Int J Soc Psychiatry* 47:21–31.

Isaakidis, P., Swingler, G. H., Pienaar, E., *et al.* (2002). Relation between burden of disease and randomised evidence in sub-Saharan Africa: survey of research. *BMJ* 324:702.

Johnstone, P., & Zolese, G. (1999). Systematic review of the effectiveness of planned short hospital stays for mental health care. *BMJ* 318:1387–90.

Joy, C. B., Adams, C. E., & Rice, K. (2002). Crisis intervention for people with severe mental illnesses. *Cochrane Database Syst Rev* Release 2.

Knapp, M., Chisholm, D., Astin, J., *et al.* (1997). The cost consequences of changing the hospital-community balance: the mental health residential care study. *Psychol Med* 27:681–92.

Larsen, T. K., Friis, S., Haahr, U., *et al.* (2001). Early detection and intervention in first-episode schizophrenia: a critical review. *Acta Psychiatr Scand* 103:323–34.

Latimer, E. A. (1999). Economic impacts of assertive community treatment: a review of the literature. *Can J Psychiatry* 44:443–54.

Leff, J. (1993). Principles of social psychiatry. In D. Bhugra & J. Leff, eds. *Principles of Social Psychiatry.* Oxford: Blackwell Scientific.

Leff, J. (1997). *Care in the Community. Illusion or Reality?* London: Wiley.

Lehman, A. F. (1995). Vocational rehabilitation in schizophrenia. *Schizophr Bull* **21**:645–56.

Lehman, A. F. (1999). Quality of care in mental health: the case of schizophrenia. *Health Aff (Millwood)* **18**:52–65.

Lehman, A. F., Goldberg, R., Dixon, L. B., *et al.* (2002). Improving employment outcomes for persons with severe mental illnesses. *Arch Gen Psychiatry* **59**:165–72.

Link, B. G. (2001). Stigma: many mechanisms require multifaceted responses. *Epidemiol Psichiatr Soc* **10**:8–11.

Link, B. G., & Phelan, J. C. (2001). Conceptualizing stigma. *Annu Rev Sociol* **27**:363–85.

Marshall, M., Crowther, R., Almaraz-Serrano, A., *et al.* (2001). Systematic reviews of the effectiveness of day care for people with severe mental disorders: (1) acute day hospital versus admission; (2) vocational rehabilitation; (3) day hospital versus outpatient care. *Health Technol Assess* **5**:1–75.

Marshall, M., & Lockwood, A. (2003). Assertive community treatment for people with severe mental disorders (Cochrane Review). *Cochrane Library,* Issue 1. Oxford: Update Software.

McDonald, H. P., Garg, A. X., & Haynes, R. B. (2002). Interventions to enhance patient adherence to medication prescriptions: scientific review. *JAMA* **288**:2868–79.

McGorry, P. D., & Killackey, E. J. (2002). Early intervention in psychosis: a new evidence based paradigm. *Epidemiol Psichiatr Soc* **11**:237–47.

McGorry, P. D., Yung, A. R., Phillips, L. J., *et al.* (2002). Randomized controlled trial of interventions designed to reduce the risk of progression to first-episode psychosis in a clinical sample with subthreshold symptoms. *Arch Gen Psychiatry* **59**:921–8.

Mosher, L. R. (1999). Soteria and other alternatives to acute psychiatric hospitalization: a personal and professional review. *J Nerv Ment Dis* **187**:142–9.

Mubbashar, M. (1999). Mental health services in rural Pakistan. In M. Tansella & G. Thornicroft, eds. *Common Mental Disorders in Primary Care.* London: Routledge, pp. 67–80.

Mueser, K. T., Bond, G., Drake, R. E., *et al.* (1998a). Models of community care for severe mental illness: a review of research on case management. *Schizophr Bull* **24**:37–74.

Nathan, P., & Gorman, J. (2002). *A Guide to Treatments That Work,* 2nd edn. Oxford: Oxford University Press.

National Human Rights Commission (1999). *Quality Assurance in Mental Health.* New Delhi: National Human Rights Commission.

Njenga, F. (2002). Challenges of balanced care in Africa. *World Psychiatry* **1**:96–8.

Nordentoft, M., Knudsen, H. C., & Schulsinger, F. (1992). Housing conditions and residential needs of psychiatric patients in Copenhagen. *Acta Psychiatr Scand* **85**:385–9.

Oiesvold, T., Saarento, O., Sytema, S., *et al.* (2000). Predictors for readmission risk of new patients: the Nordic Comparative Study on Sectorized Psychiatry. *Acta Psychiatr Scand* **101**:367–73.

Olfson, M., Mechanic, D., Boyer, C. A., *et al.* (1998). Linking inpatients with schizophrenia to outpatient care. *Psychiatr Serv* **49**:911–17.

Ormel, J., Von Korff, M., Ustun, B., *et al.* (1994). Common mental disorders and disability across cultures. Results from the WHO Collaborative Study on Psychological Problems in General Health Care. *JAMA* **272**:1741–8.

Patel, V., & Sumathipala, A. (2001). International representation in psychiatric literature: survey of six leading journals. *Br J Psychiatry* **178**:406–9.

Phillips, S. D., Burns, B. J., Edgar, E. R., *et al.* (2001). Moving assertive community treatment into standard practice. *Psychiatr Serv* **52**:771–9.

Polak, P., & Warner, R. (1996). The economic life of seriously mentally ill people in the community. *Psychiatr Serv* **47**:270–4.

Priebe, S., Warner, R., Hubschmid, T., *et al.* (1998). Employment, attitudes toward work, and quality of life among people with schizophrenia in three countries. *Schizophr Bull* **24**:469–77.

Quirk, A., & Lelliott, P. (2001). What do we know about life on acute psychiatric wards in the UK? A review of the research evidence. *Soc Sci Med* **53**:1565–74.

Reynolds, A., & Thornicroft, G. (1999). *Managing Mental Health Services.* Buckingham: Open University Press.

Rose, D., Wykes, T., Leff, H. S., *et al.* (2003). Patients' perspectives on electroconvulsive therapy: systematic review. *BMJ* **326**:1363–6.

Rosen, A. (1997). Crisis management in the community [review]. *Med J Aust* **167**:633–8.

Rosen, A., & Barfoot, K. (2001). Day care and occupation: structured rehabilitation and recovery programmes and work. In G. Thornicroft & G. Szmukler, eds. *Textbook of Community Psychiatry.* Oxford: Oxford University Press, pp. 296–308.

Rosenheck, R. A., Desai, R., Steinwachs, D., *et al.* (2000). Benchmarking treatment of schizophrenia: a comparison of service delivery by the national government and by state and local providers. *J Nerv Ment Dis* **188**:209–16.

Rosenheck, R. A., & Neale, M. S. (1998). Cost-effectiveness of intensive psychiatric community care for high users of inpatient services. *Arch Gen Psychiatry* **55**:459–66.

Rothman, D. (1971). *The Discovery of the Asylum*. Boston: Little, Brown.

Ruggeri, M., Gater, R., Bisoffi, G., *et al.* (2002). Determinants of subjective quality of life in patients attending community-based mental health services. The South-Verona Outcome Project 5. *Acta Psychiatr Scand* **105**:131–40.

Ruggeri, M., Leese, M., Thornicroft, G., *et al.* (2000). Definition and prevalence of severe and persistent mental illness. *Br J Psychiatry* **177**:149–55.

Saarento, O., Hansson, L., Sandlund, M., *et al.* (1996). The Nordic comparative study on sectorized psychiatry. Utilization of psychiatric hospital care related to amount and allocation of resources to psychiatric services. *Soc Psychiatry Psychiatr Epidemiol* **31**:327–35.

Sartorius, N. (2001). Reducing the stigma of mental illness. *Lancet* **357**:1055.

Scott, J., & Lehman, A. (2001). Case management and assertive community treatment. In G. Thornicroft & G. Szmukler, eds. *Textbook of Community Psychiatry*. Oxford: Oxford University Press, pp. 253–64.

Shepherd, G. (1990). *Theory and Practice of Psychiatric Rehabilitation*. Chichester: Wiley.

Shepherd, G., Muijen, M., Dean, R., *et al.* (1996). Residential care in hospital and in the community – quality of care and quality of life. *Br J Psychiatry* **168**:448–56.

Shepherd, G., & Murray, A. (2001). Residential care. In G. Thornicroft & G. Szmukler, eds. *Textbook of Community Psychiatry*. Oxford: Oxford University Press, pp. 309–20.

Simmonds, S., Coid, J., Joseph, P., *et al.* (2001). Community mental health team management in severe mental illness: a systematic review. *Br J Psychiatry* **178**:497–502.

Simon, G. E. (2002). Evidence review: efficacy and effectiveness of anti-depressant treatment in primary care. *Gen Hosp Psychiatry* **24**:213–24.

Singer, R. B. (2001). The first mortality follow-up study: the 1841 Report of William Farr (physician) on the mortality of lunatics. *J Insur Med* **33**:298–309.

Slade, M., Thornicroft, G., & Glover, G. (1999). The feasibility of routine outcome measures in mental health. *Soc Psychiatry Psychiatr Epidemiol* **34**:243–9.

Sledge, W. H., Tebes, J., Rakfeldt, J., *et al.* (1996a). Day hospital/crisis respite care versus inpatient care, part I: clinical outcomes. *Am J Psychiatry* **153**:1065–73.

Sledge, W. H., Tebes, J., Rakfeldt, J., *et al.* (1996b). Day hospital/crisis respite care versus inpatient care, Part II: service utilization and costs. *Am J Psychiatry* **153**:1074–83.

Susser, E., Collins, P., Schanzer, B., *et al.* (1996). Topics for our times: can we learn from the care of persons with mental illness in developing countries? *Am J Public Health* **86**:926–8.

Susser, E., Schwartz, S., Morabia, A., *et al.* (2006). *Psychiatric Epidemiology: Searching for the Causes of Mental Disorders*. New York: Oxford University Press.

Susser, E., Valencia, E., Conover, S., *et al.* (1997). Preventing recurrent homelessness among mentally ill men: a "critical time" intervention after discharge from a shelter. *Am J Public Health* **87**:256–62.

Sytema, S., Micciolo, R., & Tansella, M. (1997). Continuity of care for patients with schizophrenia and related disorders: a comparative south Verona and Groningen case-register study. *Psychol Med* **27**:1355–62.

Szmukler, G., & Holloway, F. (2001). In-patient treatment. In Thornicroft & G. Szmukler, eds. *Textbook of Community Psychiatry*. Oxford: Oxford University Press, pp. 321–37.

Takizawa, T. (1993). Patients and their families in Japanese mental health. *New Dir Ment Health Serv* **25**:34.

Tansella, M. (1986). Community psychiatry without mental hospitals – the Italian experience: a review. *J R Soc Med* **79**:664–9.

Tansella, M., & Thornicroft, G. (1998). A conceptual framework for mental health services: the matrix model. *Psychol Med* **28**:503–8.

Tansella, M., & Thornicroft, G. (Ed.). (1999). *Common Mental Disorders in Primary Care*. London: Routledge.

Teague, G. B., Bond, G. R., & Drake, R. E. (1998). Program fidelity in assertive community treatment: development and use of a measure. *Am J Orthopsychiatry* **68**:216–32.

Thornicroft, G. (1991). The concept of case management for long-term mental illness. *Int Rev Psychiatry* **3**:125–32.

Thornicroft, G. (2001). *Measuring Mental Health Needs*, 2nd edn. London: Royal College of Psychiatrists, Gaskell.

Thornicroft, G., & Bebbington, P. (1989). Deinstitutionalisation – from hospital closure to service development. *Br J Psychiatry* **155**:739–53.

Thornicroft, G., Rose, D., Huxley, P., *et al.* (2002). What are the research priorities of mental health service users? *J Ment Health* **11**:1–5.

Thornicroft, G., & Tansella, M. (1999). *The Mental Health Matrix: a Manual to Improve Services*. Cambridge: Cambridge University Press.

Thornicroft, G., & Tansella, M. (2002). Balancing community-based and hospital-based mental health care. *World Psychiatry* 1:84–90.

Thornicroft, G., Wykes, T., Holloway, F., *et al.* (1998). From efficacy to effectiveness in community mental health services. PRiSM Psychosis Study. 10. *Br J Psychiatry* 173:423–7.

Tomov, T. (2001). Central and Eastern European Countries. In G. Thornicroft & M. Tansella, eds. *The Mental Health Matrix. A Manual to Improve Services*. Cambridge: Cambridge University Press, pp. 216–27.

Trieman, N., Smith, H. E., Kendal, R., *et al.* (1998). The TAPS Project 41: homes for life? Residential stability five years after hospital discharge. Team for the Assessment of Psychiatric Services. *Commun Ment Health J* 34:407–17.

Tyrer, P. (1995). Essential issues in community psychiatry. In *Community Psychiatry in Action. Analysis and Prospects*. Cambridge: Cambridge University Press.

Tyrer, S., Coid, J., Simmonds, S., *et al.* (2003*). Community mental health teams (CMHTs) for people with severe mental illnesses and disordered personality* [Cochrane Review]. Oxford: Update Software.

Tyrer, P., Evans, K., Gandhi, N., *et al.* (1998). Randomised controlled trial of two models of care for discharged psychiatric patients. *BMJ* 316:106–9.

Tyrer, P., Morgan, J., Van Horn, E., *et al.* (1995). A randomised controlled study of close monitoring of vulnerable psychiatric patients. *Lancet* 345:756–9.

Tyrer, P., Turner, R., & Johnson, A. L. (1989). Integrated hospital and community psychiatric services and use of inpatient beds. *BMJ* 299:298–300.

Ustun, T. B., & Sartorius, N. (1995). *Mental Illness in General Health Care. An International Study*. Chichester: Wiley.

van Wijngaarden, G. K., Schene, A., Koeter, M., *et al.* (2003). People with schizophrenia in five European countries: conceptual similarities and intercultural differences in family caregiving. *Schizophr Bull* 29:573–6.

Von Korff, M., & Goldberg, D. (2001). Improving outcomes in depression. The whole process of care needs to be enhanced. *BMJ* 323:948–9.

Von Korff, M., Unutzer, J., Katon, W., *et al.* (2001). Improving care for depression in organized health care systems. *J Fam Pract* 50:530–1.

Warner, R. (1994). *Recovery from Schizophrenia*, 2nd edn. London: Routledge.

Warner, R., & McGorry, P. D. (2002). Early intervention in schizophrenia: points of agreement. *Epidemiol Psichiatr Soc* 11:256–7.

Warr, P. (1987). *Work, Unemployment and Mental Health*. Oxford: Oxford University Press.

Weiner, D. B. (1993). *The Citizen-Patient in Revolutionary and Imperial Paris*. Baltimore: Johns Hopkins University Press.

Wells, K. B., Sherbourne, C., Schoenbaum, M., *et al.* (2000). Impact of disseminating quality improvement programs for depression in managed primary care: a randomized controlled trial. *JAMA* 283:212–20.

Wiersma, D., Kluiter, H., Nienhuis, F. J., *et al.* (1995). Costs and benefits of hospital and day treatment with community care of affective and schizophrenic disorders. *Br J Psychiatry Suppl* 52–9.

Wiersma, D., Nienhuis, F. J., Slooff, C. J., *et al.* (1997). Assessment of needs for care among patients with schizophrenic disorders 15 and 17 years after first onset of psychosis. *Epidemiol Psichiatr Soc* 6:21–8.

Wing, J. K., & Brown, G. (1970). *Institutionalism and Schizophrenia*. Cambridge: Cambridge University Press.

World Bank (2002). *World Development Report 2002. Building Institutions for Markets*. Washington, DC: World Bank.

World Health Organisation (2001). *World Health Report 2001. Mental Health: New Understanding, New Hope*. Geneva: World Health Organization. Available at www.who.int/whr2001/2001/main/en/.

Ziguras, S. J., & Stuart, G. W. (2000). A meta-analysis of the effectiveness of mental health case management over 20 years. *Psychiatr Serv* 51:1410–21.

Ziguras, S. J., Stuart, G. W., & Jackson, A. C. (2002). Assessing the evidence on case management. *Br J Psychiatry* 181:17–21.

23

General hospital psychiatry

Matthew Hotopf and Simon Wessely

General hospital psychiatry (also known as *consultation-liaison psychiatry*, *liaison psychiatry* and *psychological medicine*) arguably encompasses a wider range of clinical problems and presentations than any other branch of adult psychiatry. The problems seen by psychiatrists and other mental health professionals do not necessarily fit within the bounds of psychiatric classifications but include:

- Medically unexplained symptoms and syndromes (also known as somatoform disorders, functional symptoms, or "overlay")
- Factitious disorders and malingering
- Deliberate self-harm and other psychiatric emergencies (Chapter 20)
- Organic disorders (Chapter 14)
- Problems with adjustment to physical disease, including anxiety and depression
- Alcohol and other substance use disorders (Chapters 10 and 11)
- Problems with mental incapacity
- Postpartum mental disorders (Chapter 19)

This chapter begins with a description of some of the general themes that are pertinent across all disorders in their presentation within general hospitals. We then discuss two central groups of disorder in some depth – medically unexplained symptoms and the relationship between common mental disorders and physical diseases. We then briefly consider the aspects specific to general hospital psychiatry for various topics which are covered in more depth in other chapters.

General themes in general hospital psychiatry

Psychiatric disorders are common

Studies of general hospital inpatients (Table 23.1) show that approximately 20% to 40% have a *Diagnostic and Statistical Manual of Mental Disorders* (DSM) or *International Classification of Diseases* (ICD) diagnosis, the most common groups being common mental disorders (depression and anxiety), alcohol and drug dependence and organic disorders (delirium and dementia). Accident and emergency departments in the United Kingdom see around 170,000 presentations with deliberate self-harm per year, and this remains one of the commonest causes of medical admission in younger adults. Other psychiatric emergencies (e.g. acute psychotic illness) also present to accident and emergency departments. Outpatient departments also see a high rate of patients with common mental disorders and cognitive impairment (Carson *et al.*, 2000; Van Hemert *et al.*, 1993) but also a large number of patients with medically unexplained symptoms – which account for up to 50% of new patient referrals to medical and gynaecology clinics,

Essential Psychiatry, ed. Robin M. Murray, Kenneth S. Kendler, Peter McGuffin, Simon Wessely, David J. Castle.
Published by Cambridge University Press. © Cambridge University Press 2008.

Table 23.1 Frequency of psychiatric disorders in general hospital inpatients

Study	Setting/population	Prevalence
Silverstone (1996)	343 emergency medical admissions United Kingdom	343 full sample: 8.7% cognitive impairment 6.1% delirium 2.6% dementia Cognitive impairment excluded from SCAN interview 313 sample: 27.2% DSM-IV diagnosis 7.7% major depression 6.7% anxiety disorder 5.1% alcohol dependence or abuse 13.7% adjustment disorder
Hansen *et al.* (2001)	294 internal medicine patients, Denmark	38.7% any mental disorder 8.3% depression 16.3% anxiety 17.6% somatoform 10.9% substance use 3.7% other
Diez-Quevedo *et al.* (2001)	1,003 medical and surgical inpatients in university hospital, Spain; cognitive impairment excluded	41.5% any disorder 20.5% "threshold disorders only" 26.2% any mood disosder 14.8% major depression 14.1% anxiety disorder 13.2% alcohol abuse/dependence 6.5% any eating disorder 1.2% bulimia
Martucci *et al.* (1999)	1,039 general medical and surgical patients in Italy; two-phase design	ICD-10 26.1% any diagnosis 12.8% current depression 1.0% dysythmia 10.8% GAD 2.6% harmful use of alcohol 2.4% alcohol dependence 0.7% agoraphobia 0.3% panic disorder 1.5% neurasthenia 0.4% hypochondria 1.0% somatisation disorder
Nair & Pillay (1997)	230 general hospital patients South Africa	12% substance dependence 7% depressive disorder 2% adjustment disorder 1% organic mood disorder

(cont.)

Table 23.1 *(cont.)*

Study	Setting/population	Prevalence
Booth, Blow, & Loveland Cook (1998)	1,007 general hospital patients, United States	17.8% any disorder 10.9% anxiety disorders 7.6 mood disorders 7% depression 5.6% substance abuse 0.8% schizophrenia
Feldman *et al.* (1987)	382 medical inpatients United Kingdom	14.6% affective disorder 8.8% had major cognitive impairment (half delirium, one quarter dementia, one quarter both) 15% men and 3% women +ve on CAGE 4% men and 1% women excess alcohol consumption
Wancata *et al.* (2000)	505 general hospital inpatients Austria	All diagnoses 37.3% 12.1% minor depression 9.7% dementia 6.2% substance misuse 2.5% major depressive disorder 3.3% anxiety disorders 2.7% personality disorder
Koenig (1997)	542 general medical, cardiology and neurology inpatients aged over 60; United States	15% impaired on MMSE 21.6% major depressive disorder 27.8% minor depression
Maguire *et al.* (1974)	230 medical inpatients United Kingdom	16% affective disorders 3% "organic psychoses" 1% severe personality disorder or alcohol dependence

DSM-IV = *Diagnostic and Statistical Manual of Mental Disorders*, 4th edition; GAD = generalised anxiety disorder; ICD-10 = *International Classification of Diseases* MMSE = Mini-Mental State Examination.

making this the largest "diagnostic" group in secondary medical care (Nimnuan, Hotopf, & Wessely, 2001).

Psychiatric disorders are frequently unrecognised and untreated

Mental health services in general hospitals see only a tiny minority of all those with psychiatric disorders. Obviously the figure depends on the availability of services, but even in hospitals with established liaison psychiatric services, only 12% of those identified as having a psychiatric disorder were referred in one cross-sectional study (Hansen *et al.*, 2001). Similarly only around one quarter to one half of those with a psychiatric diagnosis are recognised to have a problem by the clinical teams responsible for their medical care (Chen *et al.*, 2004, Diez-Quevedo *et al.*, 2001; Martucci *et al.*, 1999; Silverstone, 1996).

Psychiatric disorders have significant consequences

Patients with comorbid physical disease and psychiatric disorder have a worse outcome in several respects. First, symptoms of the physical disease may be more marked when there is comorbid psychiatric disorder. Second, the combination of psychiatric disorder and physical disease has a negative impact on quality of life (Wells & Sherbourne, 1999). Third, prognosis of physical disease may be worse when there is comorbid psychiatric disorder – this may be in part because organic psychiatric disorders are more common in more severe and advanced physical illness (Van Hemert *et al.*, 1994); and when physical disease is a consequence of substance misuse, it is obvious that continued and untreated substance misuse will worsen the outcome of the physical disease. However, there is also evidence that mood disorders are associated with higher mortality in patients with physical disease, and this association (explored later in this chapter) is not simply due to uncontrolled confounders. Fourth, psychiatric disorders impact on healthcare costs, principally by the association with more and longer admissions and more investigations (Koopmans *et al.*, 2005). Finally, psychiatric disorders may disrupt the doctor-patient relationship (Hahn *et al.*, 1994; Jackson & Kroenke, 1999; Sensky *et al.*, 1989; Sharpe *et al.*, 1994) being a strong risk factor for interactions which the (nonpsychiatrist) doctor rates as "difficult".

Psychiatric disorders are treatable, but services are often inadequate

Psychiatric disorders are underrecognised in the general medical sector. If recognition of a psychiatric disorder did not change management, it might not matter, but there is increasing evidence that common mental disorders, when occurring with physical illness, can be treated effectively (discussed later), as can medically unexplained symptoms. However, psychiatric provision for the general hospital sector is poor, and although there is evidence that the speciality of liaison psychiatry has grown in the last 20 years in the United Kingdom (Swift & Guthrie 2003), mental health policy has tended to ignore the needs of general hospital patients.

Comorbid depression and anxiety in physical disease

Diagnostic concerns

Depression and anxiety are common in general hospital patients, and there is a strong epidemiological association between physical disease and common mental disorders in the wider population. A key problem in interpreting this association is the nature of symptoms of anxiety and depression in physical disease. It is normal for patients experiencing what may be a life-threatening illness or one which severely limits previous activities, to feel sad and anxious about the future. Further, many of the somatic symptoms of depression and anxiety may overlap with symptoms caused directly by physical illness. Thus fatigue may be a direct result of most diseases, sleep disturbance is a prominent problem in hospitals due to a noisy environment or pain, and appetite and weight loss may be a feature of diseases such as cancer. How should clinicians take account of these symptoms which overlap with those of depression?

One approach is to emphasise cognitive or affective symptoms rather than physical ones when making the diagnosis of mood disorder in this population. Thus the Endicott substitution criteria (Endicott, 1984) replace symptoms like change in appetite or weight with mental state changes such as tearfulness and depressed appearance. Likewise the Hospital Anxiety and Depression Scale (HADS), designed as the name implies, for use in patients with physical illness, avoids somatic symptoms of both depression and anxiety. Yet using this approach makes surprisingly little difference to the detected prevalence of depression in physically ill patients (Chochinov *et al.*, 1994). Another approach is to "raise the bar" and not to make a psychiatric diagnosis on standard criteria but increase the number or severity of symptoms required. This approach predictably reduces detected prevalence rates (Chochinov *et al.*, 1994), but there is no a priori reason for thinking that one prevalence estimate is more valid than another. Perhaps more important is the degree to which symptoms alter function and interfere with quality of life.

Ultimately depression and anxiety are syndromal diagnoses, defined in a somewhat artificial manner, and with many causes (House, 1988). One argument is to ignore the problem of definition but instead to focus on the predictive validity of these disorders (i.e. what are their consequences?) and whether they can be treated (e.g. what are the features of depression in this population which make it most amenable to antidepressant medication or psychotherapy?). If depression and anxiety are associated with a poor outcome in terms of disability, symptoms and survival and can be treated, then there seems little point in tampering with diagnostic thresholds.

Frequency of depression and anxiety

It is difficult to find studies which do not find associations between physical disease and common mental disorders. The association is observed in community studies (Black *et al.*, 1998), where, for example, there is a near fourfold increase in significant depressive symptoms in the 2 years following cancer diagnosis and smaller but significant increases following heart disease, arthritis and chronic lung disease (Polsky *et al.*, 2005). Similarly, medical illnesses as a whole are associated with an increased risk of suicidal ideation and attempts (Druss & Pincus, 2000).

Among medical patients, rates of depression vary widely depending on the definition and measures used and the population studied. Table 23.1 demonstrates that many studies estimate the prevalence of affective disorders in the range from 7% to 20%, with major depressive disorder being somewhat less common than minor depressions. In specialist settings depressive disorders may be considerably more common; for example, in a systematic review of patients with advanced disease receiving palliative care, the median prevalence of major depressive disorder was 15% (Hotopf *et al.*, 2001). Anxiety disorders have not been studied to the same extent

and are generally reported to be less common than affective disorders in this population. The pattern repeats itself among medical outpatients, with 15% having a depressive illness and a further 10% an anxiety disorder (Van Hemert *et al.*, 1993). When clinical samples of patients with specific diseases are studied, there is again a high prevalence, with 11% of patients with diabetes having depression (and nearly a third reporting significant depressive symptoms; Anderson *et al.*, 2001). Similarly depression is found in 40% of those with Parkinson's disease (Cummings, 1992), 8% of stroke survivors (Sharpe *et al.*, 1990), and 15% to 20% of patients following myocardial infarction (Musselman *et al.*, 1998b).

Associations of depression

Which patients with physical disease get depression and anxiety? Most risk factors are similar to those in the general population. Women, the young, those with previous episodes of depression, people with low social support and more life events are all at higher risk (Burgess *et al.*, 2005; Mayou & Hawton, 1986).

The relationship between the specific nature of the physical disease and depression is not as clear-cut as might be expected. Much depends on the context, and in particular on the relationship between severity and duration of disease. In cancer, for example, it is probable that depression is highest at certain key points in the "cancer journey", such as at diagnosis, following a recurrence and during the most advanced stages. At each point, the patient has to make radical adjustments, and it is not surprising that – following diagnosis – the prevalence of depression slowly diminishes (Burgess *et al.*, 2005). Thus taking a mixed clinical population of patients with cancer may not show a strong relationship between depression and *severity* of disease, because those with more severe disease will often have had longer to make psychological and practical adaptations to their predicament. Chronic pain and other unremitting symptoms, disfigurement and severe limitations imposed by the disease all increase the risk of depression.

There is no doubt that another reason for the link between physical disease and depression is via direct specific biological mechanisms related to the disease process. Factors which might be associated with depression are described in Chapter 14 and include endocrine disorders, exogenous steroids, neurological disorders and some infectious diseases. Many different potential biological mechanisms exist. The association between depression and corticosteroids has long been recognised. More recent work has also shown strong associations with immune variables such as the illness behaviour cytokines, the effects of which strongly overlap with depression (Dunlop & Campbell, 2000).

The association between depression and physical disease is therefore explained partly by various organic factors and partly by the impact of physical disease as a life event which has serious implications for the sufferer. These range from the imminent loss of life, serious loss of function and loss of role at work or home. Many chronic physical diseases impose ongoing restrictions to lifestyle and although less acute and severe than a life event, none the less qualify as ongoing difficulties.

However, the association between depression and physical disease may in part be explained by the effects of depression on physical health. It has long been observed that many psychiatric disorders are associated with elevated mortality, and this excess is not exclusively through suicide (Harris & Barraclough, 1998). This association may be mediated by numerous factors – for example, patients with depression have increased rates of smoking and obesity and participate less in physical exercise (Hasler *et al.*, 2005; Ismail *et al.*, 2000). There may also be direct biological mechanisms which may be general or specific to certain diseases. For example, the relative hypercortisolaemia present in depression may lead to type 2 diabetes by causing insulin resistance (Musselman *et al.*, 2003). Increasing evidence suggests that depression raises the risk of incident ischaemic heart disease, and this may be via changes to blood coagulability or to altered autonomic function, manifested for example via changes in heart rate variability (indicating reduced vagal tone on the heart; Musselman, Evans, & Nemeroff, 1998a).

Prognosis of depression and anxiety

Few studies have described the natural history of depression and anxiety in medically ill patients. A significant proportion (between one and two thirds) of those with established disorders will have persistent symptoms over the next year (Balestrieri *et al.*, 2000; Zung *et al.*, 1990). Most episodes of depression in this population are prolonged (over 3 months; Burgess *et al.*, 2005).

Consequences of depression and anxiety

There is growing epidemiological evidence to show that depression is a risk factor for poor prognosis of physical diseases. This may be related to reduced adherence to treatment, and there is certainly evidence that depression, although not anxiety, has a major and consistent impact on adherence across a range of medical diagnoses (DiMatteo *et al.*, 2000). Both depression and anxiety are associated with poorer functioning across a range of quality of life domains (Booth, Blow, & Cook, 1998).

One striking association is the apparent impact of depression on mortality for many physical diseases. Associations have been reported across diagnostically mixed groups of physically ill patients (Arfken *et al.*, 1999; Herrmann *et al.*, 2000; Silverstone, 1990), as well as following myocardial infarction (Frasure-Smith *et al.*, 1993), heart failure (Freedland *et al.*, 1991; Jiang *et al.*, 2001), stroke (House *et al.*, 2001; Morris *et al.*, 1993), HIV/AIDS (Patterson *et al.*, 1996), renal disease (Peterson *et al.*, 1991) and cancer (Schulz *et al.*, 1996). A good example of this literature is the series of studies by Frasure-Smith (Frasure-Smith *et al.*, 1993, 2000), who found that six months following a myocardial infarction, patients who had high depression scores had a threefold

Table 23.2 Physical illness and physical treatment of depression

Disease	Treatment
Cardiovascular disease	
Recent myocardial infarction	Tricyclics contraindicated
Heart block	MAOIs contraindicated
Congestive cardiac failure	Tricyclic: risk postural hypotension – avoid
	Lithium excretion lowered by ACE inhibitors and diuretics
Aortic or cerebral aneurysm	ECT contraindicated
Hypertension	Lithium excretion reduced by diuretics
	MAOIs enhance antihypertensives
	Avoid venlafaxine
Eye disease: glaucoma	Tricyclics, duloxetine, mirtazapine contraindicated
Genito-urinary disease	
Prostatic hypertrophy	Tricyclics worsen symptoms – risk of retention of urine
Renal failure	Risk of toxicity from lithium
Neurological disease	
Epilepsy	All antidepressants lower seizure threshold
	Maprotiline contraindicated
	Interactions between SSRIs and anticonvulsants (raised levels of phenytoin, carbamazepine)
	Avoid carbamazepine with MAOIs
Intracranial-space-occupying lesion	ECT contraindicated
Raised intracranial pressure	ECT contraindicated
Cerebrovascular accident	ECT potentially dangerous
	MAOIs contraindicated
Parkinson's disease	Interaction between fluoxetine and selegiline (confusional state)
Migraine	Interaction between fluoxetine and selegiline (confusional state)
Liver failure	Decrease dose of all antidepressants
	If severe, tricyclics contraindicated
Gastro-intestinal (GI) disease	
Upper GI tract disease	SSRIs may worsen nausea
	SSRIs may cause GI bleeding in at risk individuals.
Lower GI tract disease	Tricyclic levels raised by cimetidine
Severe diarrhoea	Tricylics may worsen constipation
	Lithium contraindicated
Endocrine disease	
Addison's syndrome	Lithium contraindicated
Hypothyroidism	Lithium contraindicated
Phaeochromocytoma	MAOIs and moclobemide contraindicated
Hyperthyroidism	Tranylcypromine and moclobemide contraindicated. Caution with venlafaxine
Blood disorders	
Agranulocytosis	Tricyclics and mianserin contraindicated
Sickle cell disease	Caution with ECT, anaesthetic risk
Warfarin treatment	Avoid mirtazapine
Porphyria	Avoid tricyclics

ACE = angiotensin-converting enzyme; ECT = electroconvulsive therapy; MAOI = monoamine oxidase inhibitor; SSRI = selective serotonin reuptake inhibitors.

increased death rate, which was independent of both disease severity and lifestyle factors such as smoking, and as strong a risk factor as any other. In heart disease various direct mechanisms have been proposed, including increased coagulability of platelets and decreased heart rate variability indicating reduced vagal tone (Musselman *et al.*, 1998).

Identification of depression and anxiety

Epidemiological studies (e.g. Diez-Quevedo *et al.*, 2001; Martucci *et al.*, 1999; Silverstone, 1996) suggest that only 25% to 50% of hospital patients with depression are identified. As in primary care (see Chapter 21), there are many reasons why depression and anxiety are overlooked in general hospitals, including lack of time, poor skills in evaluating psychological symptoms and a sense that depression is "understandable" in the face of medical illness. Given the importance of depression as a risk factor for poor prognosis related to physical disease, a major public health question is whether improving the identification and treatment of patients with depression would improve physical health as well as mental health outcomes. Although the question is not resolved, recent guidelines by the British National Institute of Clinical Excellence (NICE) suggest that the physically ill should be screened for depression (National Institute for Clinical Excellence, 2004). There have been numerous studies on use of screening tools in general hospital settings, often in specific diagnostic groups (see Box 23.1). Much has been written on the benefits of one measure over others, and measures exist (e.g. the Hospital Anxiety and Depression Scale [HADS]; Zigmond & Snaith, 1983) which have been specifically designed for the medically ill. Whichever instrument is used, it is necessary to ensure that the cut-point at which a patient is labelled as a "case" is appropriate for the setting – cut-points developed in community studies will generate an unacceptable number of "false positives" in a physically ill group. The measures must be appropriate given the potential frailties of the population studied and must therefore be simple. Finally those using the measure must receive adequate instruction and

---

> **Box 23.1** Questionnaires to screen for depression
>
> Hospital anxiety and depression scale (Zigmond & Snaith, 1983): 14 items. Widely used. Can be scored as depression and anxiety separately or as a combined scale. Emphasises affective and cognitive symptoms. Designed for hospital settings.
>
> Center for Epidemiological Studies – Depression scale (Radloff, 1977): 20-item scale. Freely available. Designed for general population studies. Specific to depression.
>
> Edinburgh Postnatal Depression Scale (Cox *et al.*, 1987): 10-item scale designed to detect postnatal depression. Emphasises affective and cognitive symptoms. Some evidence that it is an effective measure in cancer. Specific to depression. Freely available.
>
> Patient Health Questionnaire-9 (Kroenke *et al.*, 2001): 9-item scale designed to detect depression in primary and secondary medical care. Freely available.
>
> General Health Questionnaire (GHQ)-12 (Goldberg & Williams, 1988): the shortest of GHQ questionnaires – designed to detect common mental disorders in community or primary care settings. Has been used successfully in general hospital settings.

---

support in how to manage patients who score "positive". Unless clear guidance is available on how to manage depression and anxiety, there is little point in identifying it.

Treatment

Drug treatment

Antidepressants are widely used to treat depression in patients with physical illnesses, but are they effective? A relatively small number of small placebo controlled randomised controlled trials were reviewed in a meta-analysis (Gill & Hatcher, 2000). This showed an overall benefit of antidepressants which was slightly less impressive than the results of randomised controlled trials in patients without physical disease but nonetheless indicated that for every four patients whose depression was treated with an antidepressant one person would gain a useful benefit (number needed to treat). A subsequent large randomised trial of sertraline versus placebo in patients with heart disease found that although sertraline was well tolerated, it had only a modest impact on depressive symptoms. However, a subgroup analysis indicated that it was more emphatically effective in recurrent and more severe depressive episodes (Glassman *et al.*, 2002).

It is still unclear what the threshold of severity of chronicity of depression should be before antidepressants are used. There is little evidence from comparative studies on which are the most effective antidepressants in the medically ill. Selective serotonin reuptake inhibitors (SSRIs) are slightly better tolerated than tricyclics (Hotopf *et al.*, 1997), although there is a small amount of evidence that the tricyclics are slightly more effective in those who can tolerate them (Barbui & Hotopf, 2001). Choice of antidepressant may reflect the symptom profile of the patient and the nature of the physical disease. Certain specific diseases may contraindicate antidepressants (see Table 23.2). There are relatively few serious interactions between antidepressants and other medications. The patient's symptom profile may be the strongest influence of the type of antidepressant chosen. For example, the SSRIs can cause nausea and anorexia, which may be an unpopular side effects in patients who have recently completed chemotherapy for cancer.

Psychological treatment

A distinction should be drawn between psychological interventions which have been proposed to assist adjustment among patients with physical disease in general and those which have been specifically designed with the aim of improving depression. For example, psychoeducational interventions have been used with some success to improve treatment adherence in diabetes mellitus (Ismail *et al.*, 2004). Similar interventions have been tried with varying success to improve coping in people with sickle cell disease (Anie & Green, 2000) and cancer (Meyer & Mark, 1995), for example. In public health terms, these interventions may be important if they improve treatment adherence and reduce the incidence of depression among vulnerable populations, but their principal aim is not to treat depression.

There is less evidence that specific psychological interventions are effective for depression in the context of physical disease. Most studies have used cognitive-behavioural psychotherapy (CBT) or components thereof. An early study in cancer patients showed that six sessions of adjuvant psychological therapy for those with anxiety or depression improved adjustment to cancer but had only modest effects on anxiety and no statistically significant effect on depression at follow up (Greer *et al.*, 1992). A large randomised controlled trial of cognitive-behavioural therapy for patients with depression following myocardial infarction showed a modest improvement in depression scores at 6 months (Writing Committee for the ENRICHD Investigators, 2003). The primary outcome the study aimed to address was reoccurrence of myocardial infarction and no benefit of CBT was found for this.

Conclusions

Physical disease is an important risk factor for depression and anxiety, and these disorders have a range of negative effects on the course of the physical disease. The nature of the public health problem is clear. Although conventional treatment for depression appears effective on an individual basis, unlike in primary care, it has yet to be demonstrated that a more systematic approach to the detection and treatment of depression improves function and morbidity related to the comorbid physical disease.

Medically unexplained symptoms

Definitions and terminology

Patients who report physical symptoms that resist a conventional biomedical explanation are common in both primary care and the general hospital setting and make up the largest single "diagnostic problem" encountered in these settings. Despite this, definition and classification remains a perennial problem, and there is still no consensus or common approach. The primary care literature tends to emphasise the presentation of medically unexplained symptoms as a process, which is often labelled *somatisation* (Bridges *et al.*, 1991; Lipowski 1988, 1990). The underlying assumption is that patients with anxiety or depression present with physical rather than emotional symptoms, and it is the doctor's job to identify and treat the mental disorder. The problem with this formulation is that although physical symptoms may be the most common presentation for mental disorders, not all medically unexplained symptoms can be explained by psychological processes or mental disorders. For example Kroenke and Mangelsdorff (1989), in their classic study of 1,000 primary care patients, found that although the vast majority of physical symptoms presenting were not explained by physical disease, many were also not attributable to depression or anxiety either.

The second approach which has developed in secondary medical care is via the so-called *functional somatic syndromes* (Wessely *et al.*, 1999). Each medical specialty has created a functional somatic syndrome to deal with patients who have symptoms but no clear diagnosis. The symptom profile of functional somatic syndromes differs in accordance of the specialty which has invented it. For example, irritable bowel syndrome (gastroenterology) is dominated by abdominal pain and change in bowel habit, whereas fibromyalgia (rheumatology) is characterised by joint and muscle pain and tenderness. The difficulty with this approach is that the subdivision of functional somatic syndromes ignores important commonalities and thereby stifles research. There is considerable overlap between these syndromes, not only in the constellation of syndromes but also in terms of risk factors (Nimnuan, Rabe-Hesketh, *et al.*, 2001).

The third approach – that adopted in psychiatry – is the least satisfactory of all. ICD-10 and DSM-IV have both created the somatoform disorders which include entities such as hypochondriasis, somatisation disorder, chronic pain syndrome and

conversion disorder. This grouping has been criticised as arbitrary, insufficient to describe the clinical problems as they present in everyday practice and creating labels which patients find pejorative. There have been calls for the somatoform disorders to be abandoned in future versions of ICD and DSM (Mayou *et al.*, 2005).

Epidemiology

The prevalence of medically unexplained symptoms depends on the population studied and the way in which the symptoms are defined. Troublesome fatigue is present in about 20% of men and 30% of women in the general population. Chronic fatigue syndrome (defined by persistent fatigue, present for at least 6 months and causing disability) is present in approximately 1% of the population (Afari & Buchwald, 2003; Wessely *et al.*, 1998). Chronic pain is present in between 7% and 13% of the population, but the prevalence of fibromyalgia (characterised by chronic widespread pain plus tender points) is present in between 0.5% to 5% (MacFarlane *et al.*, 1996; Neumann & Buskila, 2003). Abdominal symptoms are extremely common with as many as 60% to 70% of the population reporting one or more troublesome gastrointestinal symptom at a point in time, and the prevalence of irritable bowel syndrome varies from 3% to 20% depending on the criteria used (Brandt *et al.*, 2002). Reliable estimates for somatoform disorder prevalence in the general population are far more difficult to come by, but the most severe form, somatisation disorder, is present in less than 1% (Faravelli *et al.*, 1997).

Given how common symptoms and functional somatic syndromes are in the general population, it is not surprising that these are common presentations in clinical settings. In a classic paper, Kroenke and Mangelsdorff (1989) found that in only 16% of new presentations to primary care was a physical cause found for physical symptoms. Studies in secondary care indicate that approximately 50% of patients presenting with a new physical symptom have unexplained symptoms (Nimnuan

Hotopf, & Wessely, 2001). Although this may indicate an appropriate referral from general practice, the finding that approximately 20% of consultation episodes in frequent attenders at general medical clinics of medically unexplained symptoms suggests that a proportion of such problems are never properly identified and addressed, and this group of patients may lead to excessively high healthcare costs and risks of iatrogenic harm (Reid *et al.*, 2001).

Relatively little longitudinal data exist on the outcome of medically unexplained symptoms, but that which does exist suggest that they are chronic disorders, which often are present for many years. Kroenke and Mangelsdorff (1989) followed their sample and found that (where information was available) only about half of all symptoms got better, and having an organic cause for the symptom was associated with it recovering. In more established functional somatic syndromes, the course is often persistent: the majority of patients with chronic fatigue syndrome neither deteriorate nor improve over the course of a follow-up of months or years (Cairns & Hotopf, 2005); however, most such studies have been performed only in specialist centres, and the evidence is that symptoms presenting in primary care tend to resolve more rapidly. A similar pattern is seen in samples of patients with chronic pain (MacFarlane *et al.*, 1996).

Associations and aetiology

Predisposing factors

The most consistent association with unexplained symptoms is female gender (Kroenke & Price, 1993; Kroenke & Spitzer, 1988). The difference in prevalence between genders is particularly pronounced for more severe presentations of unexplained symptoms, for example, somatisation disorder, for which only approximately 20% of sufferers are male (Golding *et al.*, 1991). This excess is greatest in specialist settings, but is also present in population-based samples and thus is not solely due to gender differences in help-seeking behaviour.

There is a close association between psychiatric disorders and unexplained symptoms (Hotopf *et al.*, 1998). There is a direct correlation between number of symptoms of depression and anxiety and number of physical symptoms – the more of the former, the more of latter (which incidentally speaks powerfully against the concept of alexithymia – that physical symptoms are a defence against the experience of psychological symptoms). Likewise, patients with medically unexplained syndromes are considerably more likely to fulfil criteria for psychiatric disorders than normal control subjects. Indeed it has been demonstrated that medically unexplained syndromes are associated with higher rates of psychiatric disorder than many physical diseases, suggesting a causal relationship.

Twin studies of somatisation symptoms (Kendler *et al.*, 1995), chronic fatigue syndrome (Buchwald *et al.*, 2001) and irritable bowel syndrome (Morris-Yates *et al.*, 1998) suggest evidence for heritability. Clinical studies have shown that patients presenting with unexplained symptoms have considerably higher rates of childhood sexual abuse and other aversive experiences than comparison groups of patients with physical disease (Walker *et al.*, 1995). A second, more specific childhood risk factor is the experience of physical disease in a close family member. Craig and colleagues (1993) studied somatisers presenting to primary care and found they were considerably more likely to report either having had a chronic physical illness during their own childhood or growing up with a family member who had an illness than were patients with physical disease. In a prospective study (Hotopf *et al.*, 1999), children whose parents rated their health as poor were considerably more likely to develop unexplained symptoms.

Precipitating factors

There is often a history of a specific precipitant, the nature of which may influence subsequent symptomatology. For example, gastrointestinal infections are associated with irritable bowel syndrome (Talley & Spiller, 2002), and glandular fever can precipitate chronic fatigue syndrome (White *et al.*, 1998). However, although infections can precipitate such syndromes, there are few specific links between the nature of the infection and the degree of risk, and previous psychosocial factors such as psychiatric morbidity, female gender and prolonged convalescence following the infectious illness are the most important predictors of developing a medically unexplained syndrome such as irritable bowel syndrome or chronic fatigue syndrome following an infection (Hotopf *et al.*, 1996).

Acute and chronic stresses are also associated with the onset of physical symptoms. In a study which compared life events in patients who presented with symptoms of acute appendicitis, those with a noninflamed appendix were more likely to have had a recent severe stressful life event than those in whom histological evidence of inflammation was found (Creed *et al.*, 1988). Life events have also been related to presentations with somatisation in primary care settings (Craig *et al.*, 1994).

Maintaining factors

Many medically unexplained symptoms are strongly associated with easy fatigue and fatigability and/or muscle pain. Consequently many sufferers use rest as a coping strategy and avoid activity, both of which are firm associations of disability. It is inevitable that this will lead to diminished physical fitness and sometimes observable physiological deconditioning. Cognitive-behavioural formulations of unexplained syndromes such as chronic fatigue syndrome or chronic low back pain suggest that this is one factor that maintains disability, perhaps by a vicious circle of avoidance, deconditioning, catastrophic interpretations of symptomatology and hence further avoidance. There is evidence that patients with fibromyalgia who have high levels of physical activity have a comparatively good outcome (Wigers, 1996), and conversely those who respond to symptoms of chronic fatigue by changing their lifestyle (e.g. giving up work) are more likely to remain ill for

protracted periods (Cairns & Hotopf, 2005). Such effects may be explained by the severity of illness in some individuals, but irrespective of causation, there is good evidence that interventions which increase exercise are beneficial (Fulcher & White, 1997).

Biological mechanisms

The extent to which unexplained symptoms will in the future will be "explained" by a more sophisticated understanding of pathophysiology remains an open question. To state that a symptom is unexplained only means that it is currently unexplained, and of course this may change in the future. Many historically unexplained illnesses have had their pathological basis elaborated by advances in medical science. This is, however, not one-way traffic – many apparently medically explained syndromes, such as neurasthenia, visceral proptosis, autointoxicated colon and chronic appendicitis, have lost their medical legitimacy in the light of similar advances. Likewise, "medically unexplained" does not imply that it is inexplicable by biological mechanisms, and indeed there are many normal physiological processes which are responsible for symptoms and often provide a helpful way to explain these to patients (Sharpe & Bass, 1992).

Numerous studies have also shown demonstrable differences in biological variables between patients with unexplained symptoms and healthy control subjects. These include neuroendocrine functioning in chronic fatigue syndrome (Cleare *et al.*, 1995), central nervous system changes in chronic pain (Cook *et al.*, 2004) and changes in gut physiology in irritable bowel syndrome. A detailed discussion of such changes is beyond the scope of this chapter, but it is important to note that many such changes may still be secondary to alterations in lifestyle which patients with unexplained symptoms show. An example comes from the body of literature linking a relative underactivity of the hypothalamic pituitary axis to chronic fatigue syndrome (Parker *et al.*, 2001). Although this finding seems robust, it does not imply a causal association – all studies finding the association are cross-sectional. Prospective studies which have measured corticosteroids in groups at high risk of developing chronic fatigue syndrome do not find any association (Candy *et al.*, 2003; Rubin *et al.*, 2005). It may be, therefore, that such changes are a result of behavioural changes related to the disorder, such as reduced activity and sleep disturbance, rather than a primary cause.

Illness beliefs

Barsky and Borus (1999) have described *symptom amplification* whereby innocuous bodily sensations become misattributed to a more serious underlying condition and incorporated into an illness label. As further symptoms arise, they too are incorporated into this label. Such beliefs and attributions may lead to a range of compensatory behaviours including avoidance. Individuals with chronic pain may attribute pain as evidence that they are doing too much, leading to a reduction in activity. Patients may become increasingly sensitive to such symptoms and respond to them in a catastrophic fashion, which may greatly reduce activity and lead to deconditioning. The most compelling evidence for this process comes from chronic fatigue syndrome in which studies have consistently found that holding a strong physical attribution for the symptom of fatigue is associated with a poor outcome (Cairns & Hotopf, 2005).

Social factors

Numerous diagnostic labels have evolved in the lay media with surprisingly little influence from conventional medicine. Gulf War syndrome was almost entirely defined by the lay media before conventional scientists started investigating the symptoms of veterans (Wessely & Hotopf, 2005). Other examples include repetitive strain injury and sick building syndrome. Some of these syndromes were first described in epidemic forms, suggesting possible social contagion. The labels which have developed for such syndromes make a direct connection between an external and physical hazard and the symptoms. This means that in the lay consciousness at least, symptoms are inextricably linked to the hazard, be it keyboard use in repetitive strain injury, military deployment in Gulf War syndrome or a car accident in whiplash injury. Support groups for victims of such disorders may provide practical advice and help, but there is evidence that membership may sometimes adversely influence outcome (Sharpe *et al.*, 1992).

Other social factors which may be important in maintaining unexplained symptoms such as chronic low back pain include systems of state benefit or private insurance in which the sufferer is forced to maintain a sick role to continue to receive compensation. The old idea that all that was needed to resolve many such syndromes was by the award of compensation ("compensation neurosis") has been comprehensively discredited, perhaps because patterns of behaviour, attribution and the preservation of self-esteem have become largely fixed by the time taken for the legal process to run its course. Nevertheless, that social, cultural and iatrogenic factors have strong influences on the outcome of many of the unexplained syndromes is beyond dispute. How else can one explain the remarkable difference in the prevalence of whiplash after rear-end collisions in Sweden contrasted with Lithuania (Schrader *et al.*, 1996)?

Iatrogenesis

The behaviour of doctors and other healthcare workers may have an important influence on the course of unexplained symptoms (Page & Wessely, 2003). Salmon demonstrated that patients with unexplained symptoms frequently are open to alternative explanations (e.g. stress), but in the consultation doctors focus on the physical nature of symptoms (Ring *et al.*, 2005; Salmon *et al.*, 1999) and provide physical remedies. Such behaviour by doctors may have a significant impact: patients with back pain whose doctors tend to prescribe medication and suggest rest have a poorer outcome than those whose doctors tend to normalise the symptom (von Korff *et al.*, 1994). Other examples of iatrogenesis include diagnosing medical disease without adequate evidence, giving unnecessary treatments (for example, nitrates for patients with noncardiac chest pain) and performing surgery unnecessarily (for example, removing abdominal viscera without adequate evidence of pathology). Some of these iatrogenic factors inevitably lead to medically *explained* symptoms (e.g. headaches as a result of receiving nitrates or abdominal pain due to adhesions following unnecessary surgery).

Management

For patients with medically unexplained symptoms, simple reassurance that the symptom is not a sign of *disease* is not the same as providing an explanation for why the symptoms arose. Doctors in many medical specialities are frequently good at the former but often have more difficulties with the latter. The symptomatic patient is presenting with a genuine problem, and the emphasis should be on providing an explanation for what the symptom is and not solely announcing what it is not. The clinical assessment of patients presenting with medically unexplained symptoms should be a skill easily acquired by most doctors, but many physicians feel uncomfortable performing a psychosocial assessment, and many psychiatrists having excluded a more "mainstream" psychiatric disorder avoid addressing the unexplained physical symptoms. Liaison psychiatrists can act to bridge this gap.

Patients who have been asked to see a psychiatrist may be concerned that this automatically indicates a psychological cause is assumed or worse, symptoms are "all in the mind", a thinly disguised code for unreal or nonexistent. The psychiatrist's first duty is therefore to reassure the patient that the physical symptoms are taken seriously (something which is more appropriately the task of the physician before referral, not the psychiatrist after) and perform a detailed history giving a description of the onset of the symptoms imbedding this in the patient's biographical history as much as possible. Thus links may be made between the onset of irritable bowel

type symptoms at the time of stress (e.g. university examinations) or the onset of chronic pain following a road traffic accident. As far as possible, the clinician should elicit the patient's beliefs as to the meaning of the symptom and the information and treatments they have received. Having taken the symptoms seriously, it is usually straightforward to take a more conventional psychiatric history, providing it is done in that order. Further information for patients with particularly chronic symptoms can be usefully gleaned from a careful review of hospital and, if possible, general practice case notes. Such notes might reveal a lifelong history of multiple unexplained symptoms with repeated referrals and normal investigations.

In assessing patients with medically unexplained symptoms, it is always important to maintain vigilance for possible occult medical illnesses. Despite, or perhaps because of, the increasing specialisation in medical services, it is not unknown for physical disease to be missed. Nevertheless, this can be overstated. Slater famously denounced hysteria as a "snare" because a high proportion of patients had developed defined neurological disorders when followed up (Slater, 1965). More recent work suggests that new diagnoses rarely become apparent (Stone *et al.*, 2005), and this change may reflect improvements in diagnosis and greater caution on the part of physicians to describe a patient as suffering from unexplained symptoms.

The way in which symptoms may be managed is largely dependent on chronicity. We suggest three broad approaches.

Recent onset symptoms

When symptoms have started recently, and in particular when there is a clearly identifiable stressor or a circumscribed psychiatric disorder (such as panic disorder), the main aim of treatment should be reattribution followed by management of any psychiatric disorder in the usual manner. Thus if a young patient presents with chest pain and palpitations for which no biological cause can be found and these represent the onset of an anxiety disorder following a life event, the main aim is to help the patient label the symptoms correctly and avoid going down a path of repeated investigations in secondary medical care. After the problem has been recognised the reattribution approach can be used. This involves three stages:

1. Helping the patient feel understood: this is essentially the process of taking a good history and performing any necessary examinations described above;
2. Changing the agenda: here the doctor assists the patient in finding an alternative explanation for the symptoms other than a biomedical one; and
3. Making the link: in this final stage the patient is given an explanation of how the mental disorder or recent stress can cause symptoms.

This approach, developed by Goldberg and Gask (Gask *et al*, 1989), has been evaluated in general practice with encouraging results. It has not been evaluated in general medical settings, although there is little reason that general physicians would unable to use these fairly basic skills.

Chronic disorders with a defined onset

Many patients with unexplained symptoms have had them for some years but can identify previous periods without such difficulties. Many of the functional somatic syndromes (chronic fatigue syndrome, irritable bowel syndrome, etc.) fall into this group. Here a range of psychotherapeutic techniques have been used, but the one with the largest body of evidence is cognitive-behavioural psychotherapy (CBT; see also Chapter 28). CBT for unexplained physical symptoms is based on the concept that what triggers a disorder may not be what perpetuates symptoms or disability and thus is intended to identify and address factors that maintain rather than trigger unexplained symptoms. The emphasis is on providing a formulation which describes and explains the patient's current problems. Patients develop beliefs on the basis of evidence they find convincing. Thus a patient with chronic fatigue syndrome knows that when she does

more activity than is usual for her, she will feel tired. Resting will help the symptom of fatigue go away. It is not difficult to see how such experiences lead to a belief that fatigue is a sign of harm being caused and is thus a symptom to fear. Avoidance behaviours therefore become established (Surawy *et al.*, 1995).

The aim of treatment is to help change beliefs about the illness as well as associated behaviours. A range of techniques can be used for this purpose, depending to some extent on the constellation of beliefs and behaviours in any given individual. Common techniques range from the educational (providing information on sleep hygiene, etc.), those based on addressing automatic thoughts (maintaining a diary and helping the patient challenge thoughts related to specific symptoms) and changing behaviours by setting realistic goals and activity scheduling. The effectiveness of CBT has been demonstrated in a number of randomised controlled trials in chronic fatigue syndrome (Whiting *et al.*, 2001), as well as for chronic pain (Morley *et al.*, 1999), irritable bowel syndrome (Kennedy *et al.*, 2005) and medically unexplained symptoms in general presenting to secondary medical care (Speckens *et al.*, 1995). It has also been demonstrated in patients with health anxiety or hypochondriasis (Warwick *et al.*, 1996). Other approaches such as brief psychodynamic therapies (Guthrie *et al*, 1993) and graded exercise (Fulcher & White, 1997) have also been used with encouraging results.

Chronic symptoms with no defined onset

This final group of patients may have had a range of physical symptoms over many years and is exemplified by the rare category of somatisation disorder (see Box 23.2). There is relatively little evidence formally evaluating interventions for this group. It is reasonable to treat other psychiatric disorders which are commonly comorbid – such as depression. A multidisciplinary approach with good communication between primary and secondary medical care, psychiatry and other health care

Box 23.2 Features of somatisation disorder

- Onset before age 30, usually with difficulties evident in childhood or early adolescence
- Multiple physical symptoms either in the absence of a general medical condition or where a general medical condition exists, in excess of what would be expected from the history, examination or investigations
- Symptoms are accompanied by impaired functioning
- DSM-IV requires presence of symptoms in different domains (four pain symptoms, two gastrointestinal symptoms, one sexual symptom and one pseudoneurological symptom) over the course of the disturbance (i.e. the symptoms do not have to be present simultaneously)
- Comorbid conditions are common – particularly depression, anxiety, and personality disorders
- Frequently associated with conflict with medical professionals
- May have undergone multiple surgical procedures and investigations
- Much more common in women than men

professionals (e.g. physiotherapists) is desirable to avoid the patient being given conflicting expectations and explanations. Smith *et al.* (1986) described a simple intervention whereby a psychiatrist evaluated patients with multiple unexplained symptoms and fed back the results to primary care physicians. Although this strategy did not lead to an improvement in symptoms, it did reduce healthcare costs and referrals. Such patients may therefore benefit from an approach of containment which is probably ideally best delivered by the general practitioner and liaison psychiatrist working together. The aim should be to have regular appointments rather than simply seeing the patient only in response to new symptoms. Further investigations should not be ruled out, and an open mind should be kept about the nature of new symptoms, but a gradual reduction in the number of providers of health care involved in the patient's management is desirable. The long-term aim should be to lower expectations of medical services and assist the patient in a supportive way in addressing social and other problems.

Antidepressants in the management of unexplained symptoms

Many patients with unexplained symptoms are prescribed antidepressants. Do they work? The best evidence suggests that there may be specific benefits for some, but not all, symptoms. Where other psychiatric indications for antidepressants are present, it is reasonable to use them, but it is important to be realistic about the likely benefits which will be seen. A randomised trial of the antidepressant fluoxetine in chronic fatigue syndrome produced no benefit, even for those patients who had depression (Vercoulen *et al.*, 1996). However, there is a more encouraging literature supporting the use of antidepressants (and specifically tricyclic antidepressants) in chronic pain (Salerno *et al.*, 2002), fibromyalgia (Arnold *et al.*, 2000) and irritable bowel syndrome (Jailwala *et al.*, 2000).

Feigned illness – factitious disorders and malingering

Our previous discussion of unexplained symptoms assumed that the symptoms are genuinely present. The defining feature of factitious disorders and malingering is that symptoms are feigned. What – theoretically – distinguishes these two groups is that the motivation behind the behaviour in one (factitious disorder) is unconscious, whereas in the other (malingering) it is conscious. Malingerers typically feign illness for financial gain (for example, when making a legal claim for personal injury) to avoid imprisonment or conscription or for other reasons such as gaining prescriptions for opiates. In individuals with factitious disorders, the motivation may be less obvious but usually includes a desire to elicit care in others and the need for self-dramatisation. In practice it is often difficult to make clear distinctions between severe somatoform disorders, factitious disorders and malingering, because the differences between these disorders (whether the symptoms are present, and the motivations for feigning them) are not directly observable.

Feigned illnesses are rarely detected and accounted for only 1% of the workload of liaison psychiatry departments in one case series (Sutherland & Rodin, 1990). The best-known factitious disorder – Munchausen's syndrome – is also the rarest. The main features are repeated attendances with acute symptoms (usually of abdominal pain), and males tend to predominate. Patients typically wander from one hospital to another, and after the diagnosis is made, usually abscond. More common are female patients with stable social networks who feign specific symptoms or signs. Examples include self-induced hypoglycaemias, dermatitis artefacta or factitious haematuria.

Patients who feign illness are problematic to manage for several reasons. First, it is difficult to make the diagnosis. Medical education, thankfully, does not provide skills in detecting deception. Deciding that a patient is malingering is essentially a matter of evidence, which is often provided not by doctors but by private investigators who perform covert video surveillance on behalf of insurers in personal injury claims, and demonstrate dramatic changes in behaviour according to whether patients are going about their daily activities or visiting their doctor. Experienced clinicians can sometimes suspect illness deception on the basis of observation and inconsistencies, but we caution great care. Probably more damage has been done by false-positive diagnoses – wrongly assuming illness deception to be present – than false negatives – overlooking the diagnosis. Nevertheless, there are times when it is impossible to avoid the issue, particularly in paediatric practice, and it is because errors of both omission and commission can have such catastrophic consequences that this particular field is so contentious.

Second, patients who feign symptoms elicit powerful negative reactions in staff looking after them which may make it difficult to engage them in a therapeutic relationship. Third, to tackle the diagnosis, it is necessary to raise the possibility with the patient – at least to state that this is one of the differential diagnoses, a task most clinicians do not relish. Here the psychiatrist has a role in supportively but firmly making the patient aware that the clinical team know this is the cause of their problems. Finally, there is little evidence that any approach works in helping the patient overcome the (presumed) unconscious motivations. Given that members of this group are defined by the fact that they have deceived their doctors, they are not auspicious candidates for collaborative psychotherapy.

In the published literature, there is a definite association between illness deception and a background in healthcare professions. Whether this is because people liable to illness deception are attracted to the healthcare professions or because their training gives them the expertise and/or opportunity for these behaviours is unknown. In very rare cases, such individuals have harmed and even murdered their patients. We believe that a history of factitious disorder is usually incompatible with a career in medicine, nursing or allied professions, and when identified in a healthcare worker, a careful assessment of risk should be performed; if necessary, steps should be taken to alert relevant licencing authorities. Factitious illness in a parent is also a risk factor for induced illness in children, and when uncovered it is important to have considered the welfare of any dependent children in the care of the patient. However, given the preceding paragraph, it should not be necessary to point out that any such steps should not be taken lightly, and never on one's own.

Delirium in general hospital patients

Delirium is discussed in Chapters 14 and 15. In general hospital patients, delirium is associated with considerable mortality (Leslie *et al.*, 2005; Van Hemert *et al.*, 1994) and is disturbing for patients and staff alike. It is worth considering the predisposing risk factors the patient carries (e.g. age, preexisting cognitive impairment, impaired sleep, sensory impairments, dehydration, immobility and drug or alcohol dependence) as distinct from a specific process which might precipitate an episode. This implies that some individuals are at particularly high risk of developing delirium while hospitalised. It may therefore be possible to prevent delirium by addressing such risk factors directly, as was done in an intervention study. The interventions were mainly nurse-based protocols, including correcting visual impairments when possible, providing information to prevent disorientation among those with established cognitive impairment, correcting dehydration and providing nonpharmacological approaches to deal with sleep disorder. The prevalence of delirium in old people admitted to a general hospital reduced from 15% to 9% over the study period (Inouye *et al.*, 1999).

Once patients develop frank delirium, a search for a cause is indicated, and treating this is the mainstay of management. Although the list of precipitants of delirium is almost endless (see Table 14.7), some culprits are more common than others, and the most common reversible cause (particularly in the severely ill and frail) is medication (particularly anticholinergics and opiates) and/or dehydration (Lawlor *et al.*, 2000). The other most important component of management is ensuring the safety of the patient and doing all that is possible to improve orientation by nursing in a well-lit room, providing cues and having as much consistency as possible in nursing care (American Psychiatric Association, 1999). The pharmacological treatment of delirium is poorly researched. There is, however, some support for the use of neuroleptics rather than benzodiazepines (Breitbart *et al.*, 1996). Alcohol withdrawal is a subset of delirium and is covered in Chapter 10.

Substance use disorders in general hospital settings

The high prevalence of patients with substance misuse disorders in general hospitals is a well-established fact, not least because of the numerous physical complications associated with these disorders. Estimates of prevalence of such disorders in general hospitals vary according to background population prevalence figures, but a major US study estimated a rate of alcohol use disorders of 7.4% of all short-stay general hospital admissions, which rose to 24% among those who were not currently abstaining (Smothers *et al.*, 2003). A British study estimated that approximately 6% of all admissions and 12% of all accident and emergency attendances were due to alcohol-related problems (Pirmohamed *et al.*, 2000). Once again clinicians miss many of these disorders, and only a minority receive treatment (Smothers *et al.*, 2004). The question therefore arises as to whether systematic screening for alcohol and other substance use disorders is beneficial. Although such approaches appear logical and appealing, they are difficult to implement. One study based in an accident and emergency department attempted to screen all-comers for alcohol-related problems but found that for a variety of reasons only around a quarter could be screened, and of those who had positive scores, the majority declined any further treatment.

Several randomised trials have been performed for problem drinking in general hospital settings (Emmen *et al.*, 2004). These mostly used education, counselling and motivational interviewing, but in most cases, the interventions were ineffective or the trials insufficiently powered to detect a meaningful difference between groups. It is noteworthy that in most such trials the control group's consumption of alcohol decreased considerably over the course of follow-up; it is not clear whether this was simply regression to the mean or that the process of assessment and monitoring which took place in all participants leads to change in drinking anyway. Although brief interventions for at-risk drinking are now of proven benefit in primary care, it is still unclear whether the same is true for the general hospital setting.

Mental capacity in medical patients

A common reason for referral to liaison psychiatrists is to determine whether a patient has mental capacity or competence to make a treatment decision (Ranjith & Hotopf, 2004). In English law, a patient is presumed to have mental capacity unless the doctor has grounds for doubting his or her decision-making capacity (see Box 23.3). In practice this usually happens either because the patient has an obvious psychiatric or cognitive disorder which has been recognised by the clinical team or because the patient is refusing treatment which his or her doctors think is indicated. An audit of such referrals indicated – unsurprisingly – that they were more common when the treatment (or investigation) required the patient to sign a consent form (Ranjith & Hotopf, 2004). Studies on the prevalence of mental incapacity indicate that it is a common problem indeed – far more so than referral patterns would imply – with as many as one third of acutely admitted general hospital patients being unable to make a clear decision about treatment (Etchells *et al.*, 1997; Kitamura *et al.*, 1998; Raymont *et al.*, 2004). Such patients tend to be older, have more cognitive impairment and neurological disorders than patients who have mental capacity (Raymont *et al.*, 2004). Only a small proportion of those lacking capacity are recognised by the medical team to have difficulties.

How should one assess mental capacity in clinical practice? It is important first to understand the decision the patient is being asked to make, and the likely outcomes of the various choices. Mental capacity can only be assessed in the context of that specific decision (Hotopf, 2005). The assessment should take account of any communication or language difficulties and all practical steps should be taken to overcome these, for example, by using signing or interpreters. The assessment then addresses the main components of mental capacity relating to the decision in question – for example, can the patient understand the information being provided; can he or she appreciate this, in terms of being able to place it in context with his or her own situation; can he or she weigh the information in the balance and express a choice? The assessment should also document any psychiatric or cognitive disorders. In most cases in general hospital settings, mental incapacity will be associated with delirium or dementia. If the former, it may be better to defer a decision until after the delirium has settled. Another common cause of treatment refusal is the acute setting of patients who have taken serious overdoses and then refuse potentially lifesaving medical treatment. Here there may not be any major psychiatric disorder, but intoxication is common. Adjustment disorders may also have an impact on mental capacity; a patient may have taken an overdose as an angry gesture and be unable to appreciate the consequences of his or her action during the relatively brief time when medical treatment is necessary to save lives.

Having decided that a patient lacks capacity, the next step is to determine his or her best interests. This should take account of any previously expressed views by the patient, relating to the decision and in particular whether there is an advance directive which rules out specific treatments. Provided such an advance directive is completed when the patient has capacity, it carries legal weight in the United Kingdom. The patient's family and other providers of care who know him or her well should also be consulted – in particular to say what they think the person's wishes would have been. The currently expressed views of the patient should be taken into account, and when possible the least restrictive alternative treatment approach should be used.

Conclusions

Psychiatrists working in general hospitals are ambassadors of psychiatry to much of the rest of medicine. The clinical work covers a wide range of presentations and disorders, but the role of a general hospital psychiatrist is not limited to the diagnosis and treatment of such patients. Liaison psychiatrists have a role in improving the psychosocial environment of the general hospital more generally, particularly by educating other health professionals about psychiatric disorders and giving them the necessary skills to address them.

REFERENCES

Afari, N., & Buchwald, D. (2003). Chronic fatigue syndrome: a review [see comment]. *Am J Psychiatry* **160**:221–36.

American Psychiatric Association (1999). *Practice Guidelines for the Treatment of Patients with Delirium.* Washington, DC: American Psychiatric Association.

Anderson, R. J., Freedland, K. E., Clouse, R. E., & Lustman, P. J. (2001). The prevalence of comorbid depression in adults with diabetes: a meta-analysis. *Diabetes Care* **24**:1069–78.

Anie, K. A., & Green, J. (2000). Psychological therapies for sickle cell disease and pain. *Cochrane Database Syst Rev* **3**:CD001916. Update in *Cochrane Database Syst Rev* 2002;**2**:CD001916.

Arfken, C. L., Lichtenberg, P. A., & Tancer, M. E. (1999). Cognitive impairment and depression predict mortality in medically ill older adults. *J Gerontol* **54**:M152–M156.

Arnold, L. M., Keck, P. E., Jr., & Welge, J. A. (2000). Antidepressant treatment of fibromyalgia. A meta-analysis and review. *Psychosomatics* **41**:104–13.

Balestrieri, M., Bisoffi, G., De Francesco, M., *et al.* (2000). Six-month and 12-month mental health outcome of medical and surgical patients admitted to general hospital. *Psychol Med* **30**:359–67.

Barbui, C., & Hotopf, M. (2001). Amitriptyline vsthe rest: still the leading antidepressant after 40 years of randomised controlled trials. *Br J Psychiatry* **178**:129–44.

Barsky, A. J., & Borus, J. F. (1999). Functional somatic syndromes. *Ann Int Med* **130**:910–21.

Black, S. A., Goodwin, J. S., & Markides, K. S. (1998). The association between chronic diseases and depressive symptomatology in older Mexican Americans. *J Geronto* **53**:M188–M194.

Booth, B. M., Blow, F. C., & Cook, C. A. (1998). Functional impairment and co-occurring psychiatric disorders in medically hospitalized men. *Arch Int Med* **158**:no. 14, 1551–9.

Booth, B. K., Blow, F. C., & Loveland Cook, C. A. (1998). Functional impairment and co-occurring psychiatric disorders in medically hospitalized men. *Arch Int Med* **158**:1551–9.

Brandt, L. J., Bjorkman, D., Fennerty, M. B., *et al.* (2002). Systematic review on the management of irritable bowel syndrome in North America [see comment]. *Am J Gastroenterol* **97**(Suppl):S7–26.

Breitbart, W., Marotta, R., Platt, M. M., *et al.* (1996). A double-blind trial of haloperidol, chlorpromazine, and lorazepam in the treatment of delirium in hospitalized AIDS patients. *Am J Psychiatry* **153**:231–7.

Bridges, K., Goldberg, D., Evans, G. B., & Sharpe, T. (1991). Determinants of somatization in primary care. *Psychol Med* **21**:473–84.

Buchwald, D., Herrell, R., Ashton, S., *et al.* (2001). A twin study of chronic fatigue. *Psychosom Med* **63**:936–43.

Burgess, C., Cornelius, V., Love, S., *et al.* (2005). Depression and anxiety in women with early breast cancer: five year observational cohort study. *BMJ* **330**:702.

Cairns, R., & Hotopf, M. (2005). A systematic review describing the prognosis of chronic fatigue syndrome. *Occup Med (London)* **55**:20–31.

Candy, B., Chalder, T., Cleare, A., *et al.* (2003). Predictors of fatigue following the onset of infectious mononucleosis. *Psychol Med* **33**:847–55.

Carson, A. J., Ringbauer, B., MacKenzie, L., *et al.* (2000). Neurological disease, emotional disorder, and disability: they are related: a study of 300 consecutive new referrals to a neurology outpatient department. *J Neurol Neurosurg Psychiatry* **68**:202–6.

Chen, C.-H., Chen, W. J., & Cheng, A. T. A. (2004). Prevalence and identification of alcohol use disorders among nonpsychiatric inpatients in one general hospital. *Gen Hosp Psychiatry* **26**:219–25.

Chochinov, H. M., Wilson, K. G., Enns, M., & Lander, S. (1994). Prevalence of depression in the terminally ill: effects of diagnostic criteria and symptom threshold judgements. *Am J Psychiatry* **151**:537–40.

Cleare, A., Bearn, J., McGregor, A., *et al.* (1995). Contrasting neuroendocrine responses in depression and chronic fatigue syndrome. *J Affect Disord* **34**:283–9.

Cook, D. B., Lange, G., Ciccone, D. S., *et al.* (2004). Functional imaging of pain in patients with primary fibromyalgia. *J Rheumatol* **31**:364–78.

Cox, J. L., Holden, J. M., & Sagovsky, R. (1987). Detection of postnatal depression. Development of the 10-item Edinburgh Postnatal Depression Scale. *Br J Psychiatry* **150**:782–6.

Craig, T. K. J., Boardman, A. P., Mills, K., *et al.* (1993). The South London somatisation study I: longitudinal course and the influence of early life experiences. *Br J Psychiatry* **163**:579–88.

Craig, T. K. J., Drake, H., Mills, K., & Boardman, A. P. (1994). The South London Somatisation Study II. Influence of stressful life events, and secondary gain. *Br J Psychiatry* **165**:248–58.

Creed, F., Craig, T., & Farmer, R. (1988). Functional abdominal pain, psychiatric illness and life events. *Gut* **29**:235–42.

Cummings, J. L. (1992). Depression and Parkinson's Disease: a review. *Am J Psychiatry* **149**:443–54.

Diez-Quevedo, C., Rangil, T., Sanchez-Planell, L., *et al.* (2001). Validation and utility of the Patient Health Questionnaire in diagnosing mental disorders in 1003 general hospital Spanish inpatients. *Psychosom Med* **63**:679–86.

DiMatteo, M. R., Lepper, H. S., & Croghan, T. W. (2000). Depression is a risk factor for noncompliance with medical treatment. *Arch Intern Med* **160**:2101–7.

Druss, B., & Pincus, H. (2000). Suicidal ideation and suicide attempts in general medical illnesses. *Arch Intern Med* **160**:1522–6.

Dunlop, R. J., & Campbell, C. W. (2000). Cytokines and advanced cancer. *J Pain Sympt Manage* **20**:214–32.

Emmen, M. J., Schippers, G. M., Bleijenberg, G., & Wollersheim, H. (2004). Effectiveness of opportunistic brief interventions for problem drinking in a general hospital setting: systematic review. *BMJ* **328**:318.

Endicott, J. (1984). Measurement of depression in patients with cancer. *Cancer* **53**(suppl):2243–8.

Etchells, E., Katz, M. R., Shuchman, M., *et al.* (1997). Accuracy of clinical impressions and Mini-Mental State Exam scores for assessing capacity to consent to major medical treatment. Comparison with criterion-standard psychiatric assessments. *Psychosomatics* **38**:239–45.

Faravelli, C., Salvatori, S., Galassi, F., *et al.* (1997). Epidemiology of somatoform disorders: a community survey in Florence. *Soc Psychiatry Psychiatr Epidemiol* **32**:24–9.

Feldman, E., Mayou, R., & Hawton, K. (1987). Psychiatric disorder in medical in-patients. *Q J Med* **63**:405–12.

Frasure-Smith, N., Lesperance, F., Gravel, G., *et al.* (2000). Social support, depression, and mortality during the first year after myocardial infarction. *Circulation* **101**:1919–24.

Frasure-Smith, N., Lesperance, F., & Talajic, M. (1993). Depression following myocardial infarction: impact on 6-month survival. *JAMA* **270**:1819–25.

Freedland, K. E., Carney, R. M., Rich, M. W., *et al.* (1991). Depression in elderly patients with congestive heart failure. *J Geriatr Psychiatry* **24**:59–71.

Fulcher, K. Y., & White, P. D. (1997). A randomised controlled trial of graded exercise therapy in patients with the chronic fatigue syndrome. *BMJ* **314**:1647–52.

Gask, L., Goldberg, D., Porter, R., & Creed, F. (1989). The treatment of somatization: evaluation of a teaching package with general practice trainees. *J Psychosom Res* **33**:697–703.

Gill, D., & Hatcher, S. (2000). A systematic review of the treatment of depression with antidepressant drugs in patients who also have a physical illness. *J Psychosom Res* **47**:131–43.

Glassman, A. H., O'Connor, C. M., Califf, R. M., *et al.* & Sertraline Antidepressant Heart Attack Randomized Trial (SADHEART) Group. (2002). Sertraline treatment of major depression in patients with acute MI or unstable angina. *JAMA* **288**:701–9; erratum appears in *JAMA* 2002;**288**:1720.

Goldberg, D., & Williams, P. (1988). *A Users' Guide to the General Health Questionnaire*. Windsor: NFER-Nelson.

Golding, J. M., Smith, G. R., Jr., & Kashner, T. M. (1991). Does somatization disorder occur in men? Clinical characteristics of women and men with multiple unexplained somatic symptoms. *Arch Gen Psychiatry* **48**:231–5.

Greer, S., Moorey, S., Baruch, J. D. R., *et al.* (1992). Adjuvant psychological therapy for patients with cancer: a prospective randomised trial. *BMJ* **304**:675–80.

Guthrie, E., Creed, F., Dawson, D., & Tomenson, B. (1993). A randomised controlled trial of psychotherapy in patients with refractory irritable bowel syndrome. *Br J Psychiatry* **163**:315–21.

Hahn, S. R., Thompson, K. S., Wills, T. A., *et al.* (1994). The difficult doctor-patient relationship: somatization, personality and psychopathology. *J Clin Epidemiol* **47**:647–57.

Hansen, M. S., Fink, P., Frydenberg, M., *et al.* (2001). Mental disorders among internal medical inpatients. Prevalence, detection and treatment status. *J Psychosom Res* **50**:199–204.

Harris, E. C., & Barraclough, B. (1998). Excess mortality of mental disorder. *Br J Psychiatry* **173**:11–53.

Hasler, G., Pine, D. S., Kleinbaum, D. G., *et al.* (2005). Depressive symptoms during childhood and adult obesity: the Zurich Cohort Study. *Mol Psychiatry* **10**:842–50.

Herrmann, C., Brand-Driehorst, S., Kaminsky, B., *et al.* (2000). Diagnostic groups and depressed mood as predictors of 22-month mortality in medical inpatients. *Psychosom Med* **60**:570–7.

Hotopf, M. (2005). Assessment of mental capacity. *Clin Med* **5**:580–4.

Hotopf, M., Hardy, R., & Lewis, G. (1997). Discontinuation rates of SSRIs and tricyclic antidepressants: a meta-analysis and investigation of heterogeneity. *Br J Psychiatry* **170**:120–7.

Hotopf, M., Ly, K. L., Chidey, J., & Addington-Hall, J. (2001). Depression in advanced disease – a systematic review Part 1. Prevalence and case finding. *Palliat Med* **16**:81–97.

Hotopf, M., Mayou, R., Wadsworth, M., & Wessely, S. (1999). Childhood risk factors for adult medically unexplained symptoms: results of a national birth cohort study. *Am J Psychiatry* **156**:1796–1800.

Hotopf, M., Mayou, R., Wadsworth, M. E. J., & Wessely, S. (1998). Temporal relationships between physical symptoms and psychiatric disorder. Results from a national birth cohort. *Br J Psychiatry* **173**:255–61.

Hotopf, M., Noah, N., & Wessely, S. (1996). Chronic fatigue and psychiatric morbidity following viral meningitis: a controlled study. *J Neurol Neurosurg Psychiatry* **60**:504–9.

House, A. (1988). Mood disorders in the physically ill – problems of definition and measurement. *J Psychosomatic Res* **32**:345–53.

House, A., Knapp, P., & Bamford, J. (2001). Mortality at 12 and 24 months after stroke may be associated with depressive symptoms at 1 month. *Stroke* **32**:696–701.

Inouye, S. K., Bogardus, S. T., Jr., Charpentier, P. A., *et al.* (1999). A multicomponent intervention to prevent delirium in hospitalized older patients [see comments]. *New Engl J Med* **340**:669–76.

Ismail, K., Sloggett, A., & De, S. B. (2000). Do common mental disorders increase cigarette smoking? Results from five waves of a population-based panel cohort study. *Am J Epidemiol* **152**:651–7.

Ismail, K., Winkley, K., & Rabe-Hesketh, S. (2004). Systematic review and meta-analysis of randomised controlled trials of psychological interventions to improve glycaemic control in patients with type 2 diabetes. *Lancet* **363**:1589–97.

Jackson, J., & Kroenke, K. (1999). Difficult patient encounters in the ambulatory clinic. *Arch Intern Med* **159**:1069–75.

Jailwala, J., Imperiale, T. F., & Kroenke, K. (2000). Pharmacologic treatment of the irritable bowel syndrome: a systematic review of randomized, controlled trials [see comment]. *Ann Int Med* **133**:136–47.

Jiang, W., Alexander, J., Christopher, E., *et al.* (2001). Relationship of depression to increased risk of mortality and rehospitalization in patients with congestive heart failure. *Arch Intern Med* **161**:1849–56.

Kendler, K. S., Walters, E. E., Truett, K. R., *et al.* (1995). A twin-family study of self-report symptoms of panic-phobia and somatization. *Behav Genet* **25**:499–515.

Kennedy, T., Jones, R., Darnley, S., *et al.* (2005). Cognitive behaviour therapy in addition to antispasmodic treatment for irritable bowel syndrome in primary care: randomised controlled trial. *BMJ* **331**:435.

Kitamura, F., Tomoda, A., Tsukada, K., *et al.* (1998). Method for assessment of competency to consent in the mentally ill: rationale, development, and comparison with the medically ill. *Int J Law Psychiatry* **21**:223–44.

Koenig, H. G. (1997). Differences in psychosocial and health correlates of major and minor depression in medically ill older adults. *J Am Geriatr Soc* **45**:1487–95.

Koopmans, G. T., Donker, M. C. H., & Rutten, F. H. H. (2005). Length of hospital stay and health services use of medical inpatients with comorbid noncognitive mental disorders: a review of the literature. *Gen Hosp Psychiatry* **27**:44–56.

Kroenke, K., & Mangelsdorff, A. D. (1989). Common symptoms in ambulatory care: incidence, evaluation, therapy, and outcome. *Am J Med* **86**:262–6.

Kroenke, K., & Price, R. K. (1993). Symptoms in the community: prevalence, classification, and psychiatric comorbidity. *Arch Intern Med* **153**:2474–80.

Kroenke, K., & Spitzer, R. L. (1988). Gender difference in the reporting of physical and somatoform symptoms. *Psychosom Med* **60**:150–5.

Kroenke, K., Spitzer, R. L., & Williams, J. B. W. (2001). The PHQ-9 The validity of a brief depression severity measure. *J Gen Intern Med*, **16**:606–13.

Lawlor, P. G., Gagnon, B., Mancini, I. L., *et al.* (2000). Occurence, causes, and outcome of delirium in patients with advanced cancer. *Arch Int Med* **160**:786–94.

Leslie, D. L., Zhang, Y., Holford, T. R., *et al.* (2005). Premature death associated with delirium at 1-year follow-up. *Arch Int Med* **165**:1657–62.

Lipowski, Z. J. (1988). Somatization: the concept and its clinical applications. *Am J Psychiatry* **145**:1358–68.

Lipowski, Z. J. (1990). Somatization and depression. *Psychosomatics* **31**:13–21.

MacFarlane, G. J., Thomas, E., Papageorgiou, A. C., *et al.* (1996). The natural history of chronic pain in the community: a better prognosis than in the clinic?, *J Rheumatol* **23**:1617–20.

Maguire, G. P., Julier, D. L., Hawton, K. E., & Bancroft, J. H. J. (1974). Psychiatric morbidity and referral on two general medical wards. *BMJ* **1**:268–70.

Martucci, M., Balestrieri, M., Bisoffi, G., *et al.* (1999). Evaluating psychiatric morbidity in a general hospital: a two-phase epidemiological survey. *Psychol Med* **29**:823–32.

Mayou, R., & Hawton, K. (1986). Psychiatric disorder in the general hospital. *Br J Psychiatry* **149**:172–90.

Mayou, R., Kirmayer, L. J., Simon, G., *et al.* (2005). Somatoform disorders: time for a new approach in DSM-V. *Am J Psychiatry* **162**:847–55.

Mental Capacity Act. (2005). Department of Constitutional Affairs, London: Stationery Office.

Meyer, T. J., & Mark, M. M. (1995). Effects of psychosocial interventions with adult cancer patients: a meta-analysis of randomized experiments. *Health Psychol* **14**:101–8.

Morley, S., Eccleston, C., & Williams, A. (1999). Systematic review and meta-analysis of randomized controlled trials of cognitive behaviour therapy and behaviour therapy for chronic pain in adults, excluding headache. *Pain* **80**:1–13.

Morris, P. L. P., Robinson, R. G., & Samuels, J. (1993). Depression, introversion and mortality following stroke. *Aust N Z J Psychiatry* **27**:443–9.

Morris-Yates, A., Talley, N. J., Boyce, P. M., *et al.* (1998). Evidence of a genetic contribution to functional bowel disorder. *Am J Gastroenterol* **93**:1311–17.

Musselman, D. L., Betan, E., Larsen, H., & Phillips, L. S. (2003). The relationship of depression to diabetes – type 1 and type 2: epidemiology, biology and treatment. *Biol Psychiatry* **54**:317–29.

Musselman, D. L., Evans, D. L., & Nemeroff, C. B. (1998a). The relationship of depression to cardiovascular disease: epidemiology, biology and treatment, *Arch Gen Psychiatry* **55**:580–92.

Musselman, D. L., Evans, D. L., & Nemeroff, C. B. (1998b). The relationship of depression to cardiovascular disease: epidemiology, biology, and treatment. *Arch Gen Psychiatry* **55**:580–92.

Nair, M. G., & Pillay, S. S. (1997). Psychiatric disorder in a South African general hospital. Prevalence in medical, surgical, and gynecological wards. *Gen Hosp Psychiatry* **19**:144–8.

National Institute for Clinical Excellence (2004). *Management of Depression in Primary and Secondary Care*. Clinical Guideline 23. London: National Institute for Clinical Excellence.

Neumann, L., & Buskila, D. (2003). Epidemiology of fibromyalgia. *Curr Pain Headache Rep* **7**:362–8.

Nimnuan, C., Hotopf, M., & Wessely, S. (2001). Medically unexplained symptoms: an epidemiological study in seven specialities. *J Psychosom Res* **51**:361–7.

Nimnuan, C., Rabe-Hesketh, S., Wessely, S., & Hotopf, M. (2001). How many functional somatic syndromes? *J Psychosom Res* **51**:549–57.

Page, L. A., & Wessely, S. (2003). Medically unexplained symptoms: exacerbating factors in the doctor-patient encounter [see comment]. *J Royal Soc Med* **96**:223–7.

Parker, A., Wessely, S., & Cleare, A. J. (2001). The neuroendocrinology of chronic fatigue syndrome and fibromyalgia. *Psychol Med* **31**:1331–45.

Patterson, T. L., Shaw, W. S., Semple, S. J., *et al.* (1996). Relationship of psychosocial factors to HIV disease progression. *Ann Behav Med* **18**:30–9.

Peterson, R. A., Kimmel, P. L., Sacks, C. R., *et al.* (1991). Depression, perception of illness and mortality in patients with end-stage renal disease. *Int J Psychiatry Med* **21**:343–54.

Pirmohamed, M., Brown, C., Owens, L., *et al.* (2000). The burden of alcohol misuse on an inner-city general hospital. *Q J Med* **93**:291–5.

Polsky, D., Doshi, J. A., Marcus, S., *et al.* (2005). Long-term risk for depressive symptoms after a medical diagnosis. *Arch Int Med* **165**:1260–6.

Radloff, L. S. (1977). The CES-D scale: a self report depression scale for research in the general population. *Appl Psychol Meas* **1**:385–401.

Ranjith, G., & Hotopf, M. (2004). Refusing treatment – please see. An analysis of capacity assessments carried out by a liaison psychiatry service. *J Royal Soc Med* **97**:480–2.

Raymont, V., Bingley, W., Buchanan, A., *et al.* (2004). Prevalence of mental incapacity in medical in-patients and associated risk factors: cross-sectional study. *Lancet* **364**:1421–7.

Reid, S., Wessely, S., Crawford, T., & Hotopf, M. (2001). Medically unexplained symptoms in frequent attenders of secondary health care: retrospective cohort study. *BMJ* **322**:767–70.

Ring, A., Dowrick, C. F., Humphris, G. M., *et al.* (2005). The somatising effect of clinical consultation: what patients and doctors say and do not say when patients present medically unexplained physical symptoms. *Soc Sci Med* **61**:1505–15.

Rubin, G. J., Hotopf, M., Papadopoulos, A., & Cleare, A. (2005). Salivary cortisol as a predictor of post-operative fatigue. *Psychosom Med* **67**:441–7.

Salerno, S. M., Browning, R., & Jackson, J. L. (2002). The effect of antidepressant treatment on chronic back pain: a meta-analysis [see comment]. *Arch Int Med* **162**:19–24.

Salmon, P., Peters, S., & Stanley, I. (1999). Patients' perceptions of medical explanations for somatisation disorders: qualitative analysis. *BMJ* **318**:372–6.

Schrader, H., Obelieniene, D., Bovim, G., *et al.* (1996). Natural evolution of late whiplash syndrome outside the medicolegal context [see comment]. *Lancet* **347**:1207–11.

Schulz, R., Bookwala, J., Knapp, J. E., Scheier, M., & Williamson, G. M. (1996). Pessimism, age, and cancer mortality. *Psychol Aging* **11**:304–9.

Sensky, T., Dennehy, M., Gilbert, A., *et al.* (1989). Physicians' perceptions of anxiety and depression among their outpatients: relationships with patient and doctors' satisfaction with their interviews. *J Royal Coll Physicians London* **23**:33–8.

Sharpe, M., & Bass, C. (1992). Pathophysiological mechanisms in somatization. *Int Rev Psychiatry* **4**:81–97.

Sharpe, M., Hawton, K., House, A., *et al.* (1990). Mood disorders in long-term survivors of stroke: associations with brain lesion location and volume, *Psychol Med* **20**:815–28.

Sharpe, M., Hawton, K., Seagroatt, V., & Pasvol, G. (1992). Follow up of patients presenting with fatigue to an infectious diseases clinic. *BMJ* **305**:147–52.

Sharpe, M., Mayou, R., Seagroatt, V., *et al.* (1994). Why do doctors find some patients difficult to help? *Q J Med* **87**:187–93.

Silverstone, P. H. (1990). Depression increases mortality and morbidity in acute life-threatening medical illness. *J Psychosom Res* **34**:651–7.

Silverstone, P. H. (1996). Prevalence of psychiatric disorders in medical inpatients. *J Nerv Ment Dis* **184**:43–51.

Slater, E. (1965). Diagnosis of hysteria. *BMJ* **1**:1395–9.

Smith, G. R., Monson, R. A., & Ray, D. C. 1986, Psychiatric consultation in somatization disorder: a randomised controlled trial. *New Engl J Med* **314**:1407–13.

Smothers, B. A., Yahr, H. T., & Ruhl, C. E. (2004). Detection of alcohol use disorders in general hospital admissions in the United States. *Arch Int Med* **164**:749–56.

Smothers, B. A., Yahr, H. T., & Sinclair, M. D. (2003). Prevalence of current DSM-IV alcohol use disorders in short-stay, general hospital admissions, United States, 1994. *Arch Int Med* **163**:713–19.

Speckens, A. E. M., Van Hemert, A. M., Spinhoven, P., *et al.* (1995). Cognitive behavioural therapy for medically unexplained physical symptoms: a randomised controlled trial. *BMJ* **311**:1328–32.

Stone, J., Smyth, R., Carson, A., *et al.* (2005). Systematic review of misdiagnosis of conversion symptoms and hysteria [see comment]. *BMJ* **331**:989.

Surawy, C., Hackmann, A., Hawton, K., & Sharpe, M. (1995). Chronic fatigue syndrome: a cognitive approach. *Behav Res Ther* **33**:535–44.

Sutherland, A. J., & Rodin, G. M. (1990). Factitious disorders in a general hospital setting: clinical features and a review of the literature. *Psychosomatics* **31**:392–9.

Swift, G., & Guthrie, E. (2003). Liaison psychiatry continues to expand: developing services in the British Isles. *Psychiatr Bull* **27**:339–41.

Talley, N. J., & Spiller, R. (2002). Irritable bowel syndrome: a little understood organic bowel disease? *Lancet* **360**:555–64.

Van Hemert, A. M., Hengeveld, M. W., Bolk, J. H., *et al.* (1993). Psychiatric disorders in relation to medical illness among patients of a general medical out-patient clinic. *Psychol Med* **23**:167–73.

Van Hemert, A. M., van der Mast, R. C., Hengeveld, M. W., & Vorstenbosch, M. (1994). Excess mortality in general hospital patients with delirium: a 5-year follow-up of 519 patients seen in psychiatric consultation. *J Psychosom Res* **38**:339–46.

Vercoulen, J., Swanink, C., & Zitman, F. (1996). Fluoxetine in chronic fatigue syndrome: a randomized, double-blind, placebo-controlled trial. *Lancet* **347**:858–61.

von Korff, M., Barlow, W., Cherkin, D., & Deyo, R. A. (1994). Effects of practice style in managing back pain. *Ann Int Med* **121**:187–95.

Walker, E. A., Gelfand, A. N., Gelfand, M. D., & Katon, W. J. (1995). Psychiatric diagnoses, sexual and physical victimization, and disability in patients with irritable bowel syndrome or inflammatory bowel disease. *Psychol Med* **25**:1259–67.

Wancata, J., Windhaber, J., Bach, M., & Meise, U. (2000). Recognition of psychiatric disorders in nonpsychiatric hospital wards. *J Psychosom Res* **48**:149–55.

Warwick, H. M. C., Clark, D. M., Cobb, A. M., & Salkovskis, P. M. (1996). A controlled trial of cognitive behavioural treatment of hypochondriasis. *Br J Psychiatry* **169**:189–95.

Wells, K. B., & Sherbourne, C. D. (1999). Functioning and utility for current health of patients with depression or chronic medical conditions in managed, primary care practices. *Arch Gen Psychiatry* **56**:897–904.

Wessely, S., & Hotopf, M. (2005). Something old, something new, something borrowed, something blue: the story of Gulf War syndrome. In *Medical and Psychiatric Comorbidity over the Course of Life*. Washington, DC: American Psychaitric Publishing.

Wessely, S., Hotopf, M., & Sharpe, M. (1998). *Chronic Fatigue and Its Syndromes*. Oxford: Oxford University Press.

Wessely, S., Nimnuan, C., & Sharpe, M. (1999). Functional somatic syndromes: one or many? *Lancet* **354**:936–9.

White, P. D., Thomas, J. M., Amess, J., *et al.* (1998). Incidence, risk and prognosis of acute and chronic fatigue syndromes and psychiatric disorders after glandular fever. *Br J Psychiatry* **173**:475–81.

Whiting, P., Bagnall, A. M., Sowden, A. J., *et al.* (2001). Interventions for the treatment and management of chronic fatigue syndrome. A systematic review, *JAMA* **286**:1360–8.

Wigers, S. H. (1996). Fibromyalgia outcome: the predictive values of symptom duration, physical activity, disability pension, and critical life events – a 4.5 year prospective study. *J Psychosom Res* **41**:235–43.

Writing Committee for the ENRICHD Investigators (2003). Effects of treating depression and low perceived social support on clinical events after myocardial infarction: The Enhancing Recovery in Coronary Heart Disease Patients (ENRICHD) Randomized Trial. *JAMA* **289**:3106–16.

Zigmond, A. S., & Snaith, R. P. (1983). The Hospital Anxiety and Depression Scale. *Acta Psychiatr Scand* **67**:361–70.

Zung, W. W. K., Magruber-Habih, K., Velez, R., & Alling, W. (1990). The comorbidity of anxiety and depression in general medical patients: a longitudinal study. *J Clin Psychiatry* **51**(Suppl):77–80.

24

Forensic psychiatry

Kimberlie Dean, Tom Fahy, David Ndegwa and Elizabeth Walsh

Developments in both clinical practice and research relevant to forensic psychiatry have exploded over the past several decades. Today the forensic psychiatrist has a greater understanding of the epidemiology and biology underpinning the link between mental disorder and violence, plays a vital role in giving advice in a medico-legal context, has seen substantial development in risk assessment and management procedures and undertakes clinical practice in an increasing variety of settings.

In this chapter, we look at those mental illnesses known to be associated with offending, provide an overview of risk assessment in forensic psychiatry and consider the legal aspects of crime and mental illness.

Understanding the link between mental disorder and violence

Psychotic disorders

Prior to the 1980s, schizophrenia was not thought to be associated with an increased risk of violence. It is now, however, widely accepted that those with schizophrenia and other serious mental disorders are indeed at increased risk of violent behaviour and criminality. This conclusion has been reached on the basis of results from multiple geographically dispersed studies, employing differing methodologies (Arseneault, Moffitt *et al.*, 2000; Brennan, *et al.*,

2000; Swanson *et al.*, 1990; Tiihonen, *et al.*, 1997). See Table 24.1 for a summary of some of these studies.

Three types of research methodology have been used to examine the relationship between violence and psychosis:
1. Ascertainment of the prevalence of violence among those with a diagnosis of schizophrenia
2. Ascertainment of the prevalence of schizophrenia among those convicted of violence
3. Ascertainment of the prevalence of violence among those with and without schizophrenia in community samples (independent of contact with either mental health services or the criminal justice system)

Prevalence of violent behaviour among those with psychosis

Elevated levels of antisocial behaviour, particularly violence, have repeatedly been found in cross-sectional samples of patient groups with psychosis, despite variations in the measurement and definition of such behaviour (Barlow *et al.*, 2000; Volavka *et al.*, 1997). In a case-control study of Swiss patients, those with schizophrenia were almost 4 times more likely than matched control subjects to have been convicted of a violent offence (Modestin & Ammann, 1996). The focus on patients in contact with services in most of these studies introduces the

Essential Psychiatry, ed. Robin M. Murray, Kenneth S. Kendler, Peter McGuffin, Simon Wessely, David J. Castle.
Published by Cambridge University Press. © Cambridge University Press 2008.

potential for selection bias, however, because anti-social behaviour may increase the likelihood of service contact being made. This is particularly true of studies involving only patients admitted to hospital.

In addition to cross-sectional prevalence studies, retrospective and prospective cohort studies using register linkage have been employed to examine the relation between psychosis and violence. Although officially recorded crime, as often used in these studies, is an important objective measure of antisocial behaviour, it must be remembered that it will be influenced by variations in policies and practices between different jurisdictions and the fact that most crime, particularly less serious crime, does not lead to conviction. Such cohort studies have consistently found that those with a diagnosis of schizophrenia or psychosis more broadly have an increased risk of both nonviolent and violent offending, with risk being greatest and most consistent for the latter.

Prevalence of psychosis among criminal offenders

The evidence appears overwhelming that there is an overrepresentation of individuals with serious mental disorder among samples of offenders (Eronen et al., 1996; Taylor & Gunn, 1984; Wallace et al., 1998). Fazel and Danesh (2002) conducted a systematic review of 62 prison studies (total $N >20,000$) and found that approximately 3.7% had psychotic illnesses, a level which was significantly higher than in any of the populations of origin. Once again the association was strongest for violent compared with nonviolent crime and higher again for serious violence such as homicide. In a 25-year homicide study in Austria, the age-adjusted odds ratio for homicide among those with schizophrenia was 5.85 in men (confidence interval [CI]: 4.29–8.01) and 18.38 in women (CI: 11.24–31.55) (Schanda et al., 2004). The main methodological limitations which apply to offender studies relate to the methods used to ascertain a diagnosis of schizophrenia and the lack of appropriate comparison control groups.

Community prevalence studies (independent of mental health and criminal justice contact)

The limitations of the previous two groups of studies have largely been overcome in community-based studies which assess the prevalence of both psychosis and violence in unselected groups. These studies do not rely on illness or behaviour leading to contact with health or criminal justice systems and thus often focus on self-report violence as an outcome rather than officially recorded crime. In the Epidemiologic Catchment Area (ECA) study, 8% of those with schizophrenia were violent compared with 2% of those with no mental illness (Swanson et al., 1990). Given the scale of such studies, lay interviewers are often employed to administer structured diagnostic interviews; this has been criticised on the basis of reduced diagnostic reliability. Additionally, response bias may operate in that those individuals in the community who refuse to take part in the study may be more likely to have mental illness or engage in antisocial behaviour.

Risk factors for violence and criminality among those with psychosis

Individuals with schizophrenia engage in violent behaviours directly linked to their illness, partially linked to it or that have no connection with it whatsoever. Risk factors for violence operating in those without mental illness also operate in schizophrenia. In fact, compared with the magnitude of risk associated with the combination of male sex, young age and lower socioeconomic status, the risk of violence presented by mental disorder per se is relatively low (Monahan, 1997). The degree to which potential confounders in the relationship between severe mental illness and violence such as socioeconomic status and substance misuse are controlled for, varies across studies. This is partly due to our lack of understanding of causal pathways and thus the difficulty presented by factors which may mediate or confound the relationships. Hospitalisation for schizophrenia in one study was found to be

Table 24.1 Examples of the studies which have examined the link between schizophrenia and violence

Study type	Authors	Sample	Outcome measure	Main results relating to schizophrenia or psychosis
Violence prevalence in schizophrenia	(Volavka *et al.*, 1997)	Centres in 10 countries; DOSMD study; incident sample of 1,017 patients with schizophrenia	History of violent behaviour prior to first presentation with psychosis	The prevalence of previous assault in the entire cohort was 20.6%, but the rate was 3 times higher in the developing countries (31.5%) than in developed countries (10.5%). History of assault was associated with positive symptoms, such as excitement and auditory hallucinations, and with serious alcohol misuse.
	(Barlow *et al.*, 2000)	Sequential admissions ($n =$ 1,269) to four inpatient units in Australia over 18 months; variety of diagnoses	Aggressive incidents recorded during the inpatient stay	13.7% of patients were aggressive; those with bipolar affective disorder and schizophrenia had a 2.81 and 1.96 significantly increased risk of aggression, respectively, whereas depression and adjustment disorder conferred a significantly lower risk; high-risk patients were identified as those who were under 32 years of age, were actively psychotic, detained and known to have a history of aggression and substance misuse.
	(Monahan & Appelbaum, 2000)	MacArthur Violence Risk Assessment Study; 1,136 men and women with various diagnoses discharged from four US inpatient units	Post-discharge violence – self-report, official records, collateral information	Of the 17% of patients who had a diagnosis of schizophrenia, 9% were violent during the first 20 weeks after discharge from hospital (compared with 29% for those with substance misuse and 25% for those with a primary diagnosis of personality disorder)
	(Wessely *et al.*, 1994)	538 incident cases of schizophrenia presenting in Camberwell compared with matched nonpsychotic control subjects	Official criminal records	Women with schizophrenia had an increased rate of offending across all offence categories (RR 3.3); men had an increased rate of violent offending (RR 3.8).
	(Wallace *et al.*, 2004)	2,861 incident cases of schizophrenia presenting in Victoria, Australia between 1975 to 2000 compared with control subjects	Official criminal records	21.6% of those with schizophrenia were convicted of an offence compared with 7.8% of control subjects and those with schizophrenia accumulated a greater number of convictions over the study period; comorbid substance misuse disorders increased the risk of conviction for those with schizophrenia

	(Brennan et al., 2000)	Danish birth cohort (N = 358,180); admissions to hospital with any diagnosis up to age 44 defined the exposed	Official records for arrest for violence	Men and women hospitalized for schizophrenia were more likely to be arrested for a violent offence than those who had never been hospitalized (OR 1.9 for men and 7.1 for women) even after controlling for demographic factors and comorbid substance misuse.
	(Arseneault et al., 2000)	Dunedin (New Zealand) birth cohort (N = 961); various mental disorders	Past-year violence – self-report and official criminal records	Individuals with schizophrenia were 2.5 times more likely to be violent compared with control subjects; 10% of the violence risk in the sample was attributable to schizophrenia; the risk was best explained by excessive perceptions of threat and a history of conduct disorder.
Schizophrenia prevalence amongst offenders	(Fazel & Danesh, 2002)	Systematic review of 62 prison surveys (N = 23,000 prisoners)	Diagnosis of psychotic illness, major depression or personality disorder based on interview	3.7% of male prisoners had psychotic disorders; 4.0% of female offenders had a diagnosis of psychosis (both several times more common than in the general population)
	(Schanda et al., 2004)	Austrian homicide study (N = 1087) between 1975 and 1999	Presence of major mental disorder used as a defence during trial	Schizophrenia was more common among the sample of homicide offenders than in the general population (age-adjusted OR in men 5.85, CI 4.29–8.01; in women 18.38, CI 11.24–31.55). Comorbid alcohol abuse/dependence increased the odds further in schizophrenia.
Community Study	(Swanson, et al., 1990)	Epidemiologic Catchment Area study (United States)	Diagnostic Interview Schedule and self-report information about violence	More than half of those in the community who reported violent behaviour also met DSM-III criteria for one or more psychiatric disorders; subjects with alcohol or drug use disorders were more than twice as likely as those with schizophrenia to report violent behaviour.

CI = confidence interval; DSM-III = *Diagnostic and Statistical Manual of Mental Disorders*. 3rd edition; OR = odds ratio.

associated with an elevated risk of arrest for violent crime compared with those never hospitalised, even after controlling for demographic factors, substance abuse and personality disorder (Brennan *et al.*, 2000). In this study, schizophrenia appeared to be an independent risk factor for violent behaviour with variables such as substance misuse and personality disorder serving to add to the risk. The following have been established as factors which further increase risk among those with serious mental disorder:

- Comorbid substance abuse (Brennan *et al.*, 2000)
- Comorbid personality disorder (Moran *et al.*, 2003)
- Noncompliance with medication (Swanson *et al.*, 2006)
- Acute psychotic symptoms (Taylor & Gunn, 1984) such as those described as "threat-control override" symptoms (Link *et al.*, 1998), although findings have been inconsistent (Appelbaum *et al.*, 2000; Hodgins *et al.*, 2003; Swanson *et al.*, 1997)

There is growing support for a two-type model of violence in schizophrenia (Mullen, 2006). People exhibiting type 1 violence typically have delusional symptoms that are directly related to violence and do not have histories of delinquency. They tend to commit their first violent act after illness onset, and the victim will likely be known to them. In type 2 violence, individuals tend to have long histories of substance misuse, conduct problems and delinquency with extensive nonviolent and violent offending prior to illness onset. Most violence in the schizophrenia population is attributable to type 2, although it is possible that among homicide offenders type 1 is overrepresented. The implication of these subtypes is important when considering management techniques; medication and monitoring will be the cornerstone for type 1, whereas type 2 will additionally require a complex array of interventions along psychosocial lines.

Absolute versus relative risks

The manner in which the results of studies are reported can radically affect how they are likely to be perceived by the wider community. Most research to date has examined the association between psychosis and violence in terms of relative risk. The more important public health measure, however, is that of absolute risk; that is, the amount of violence in the population that can be ascribed to schizophrenia. Fazel and Grann (2006), reporting on data from Sweden, ascribed 1 in 20 crimes to people with severe mental illnesses, including schizophrenia. As overall crime rates increase, the proportion of crime attributable to those with schizophrenia decreases. As such, the Swedish figure is relevant mainly to low crime societies.

Affective disorders

Most studies looking at the link between major mental disorders and violence have focused on those with schizophrenia. Less is known about the risk posed by those with affective disorders. In those few studies which include separate estimates of risk for those with affective disorders, results are inconsistent and limited in many cases by sample size. In an analysis of a Danish birth cohort (Brennan *et al.*, 2000), those hospitalised with affective disorders were not at increased risk for violent crime after account was taken of substance misuse and personality disorder. The authors commented, however, that studies relying on hospitalisation might lead to an underestimation of the risk posed by those with an affective illness, as would those studies which exclude cases of suicide at the time of the violent offence, among which depression would be common. Homicide offenders in a Canadian study were more likely to have recurrent major depression compared with other offenders when those with either a primary or comorbid diagnosis of depression were considered (Cote & Hodgins, 1992). In another birth cohort study based in Finland, those with a history of at least one registered crime were more likely than the general population to have a diagnosis of mood disorder with psychotic features even after adjustment for socioeconomic status (Tiihonen *et al.*, 1997). One study of first episode

Box 24.1 Typology of filicide (d'Orban, 1979)

- Category 1: Battering mothers – The killing was an impulsive act characterized by loss of temper with the immediate impulse toward aggression arising from the victim.
- Category 2: Mentally ill mothers – Includes all mothers suffering from psychotic illness, acute reactive depression associated with a suicidal attempt, and cases of personality disorder with depressive symptoms of sufficient severity to require admission to psychiatric hospital.
- Category 3: Neonaticides – This category applies to women who killed or attempted to kill their children within the first 24 hours of birth.
- Category 4: Retaliating women – Aggression directed against the spouse was displaced onto the child.
- Category 5: Unwanted children – This category includes women who killed an unwanted child by passive neglect or active aggression.
- Category 6: Mercy killing – This category includes cases in which the victim is truly suffering and there is an absence of secondary gain for the mother.

psychosis in the United Kingdom found particularly high rates of aggressive behaviour among those with manic-type symptoms (Dean *et al.*, 2007).

The killing of a child by its mother is a rare yet exceedingly distressing event and one particularly linked to depressive disorders. In a classic study in the early 1970s, D'Orban (1979) classified filicide into six subtypes (see Box 24.1). He focused on 89 women charged with the murder or attempted murder of their children during a 6-year period. The types of filicide were compared in terms of social and psychiatric characteristics, offence patterns and court disposals.

Substance misuse

A review of studies linking alcohol and violence indicated that alcohol is implicated in 40% to 60% of assaults and homicides, 30% to 70% of rapes and anything from 40% to 80% of domestic violence (Johns, 1998). Although acute intoxication may not be directly related to the offence itself, there is often still a strong association between the presence of an alcohol misuse disorder and aggression (Haque & Cumming, 2003). Hence, it is not surprising to see extremely high rates of substance misuse among prisoners. In England and Wales, the prevalence of alcohol misuse has been estimated to be 58% for male and 36% for female remand prisoners and 63% and 39% for male and female sentenced prisoners, respectively (Singleton *et al.*, 1998). Although it is the legal process that decides culpability, it is not unusual for psychiatrists to be asked to comment on mental elements related to a criminal offence committed by an intoxicated defendant. Legal defences vary depending on jurisdiction, and arguments are limited often by a poor understanding of the mechanisms of the association. The nature of the causal link between substance misuse and violence is complex; it is likely to be an interactional process involving the basic pharmacological effects of alcohol and drugs, the context, the environment, culture and personal factors such as predisposition to aggression (Snowden, 2001).

Having a mental disorder doubles the risk of an alcohol misuse disorder, and the risk increases by four for a drug-related disorder (Regier *et al.*, 1990). The detrimental additive effect of substance misuse to mental illness and disorder are clear. It has been repeatedly demonstrated that schizophrenia with comorbid substance abuse increases the risk of violence considerably compared with schizophrenia without comorbidity (Cuffel *et al.*, 1994; Rasanen *et al.*, 1998; Wallace *et al.*, 1998). In a Finnish study of 1,423 homicide offenders, schizophrenia without the presence of an alcohol disorder increased the risk of homicide 7 times for men and 5 times for women. Schizophrenia with a secondary diagnosis of alcohol use disorder increased the risk for homicide 17.2 times for men and 80.9 times for women (Eronen *et al.*, 1996). In an Australian study, those with schizophrenia were found to be more than 4 times more likely to be convicted of interpersonal violence and 10 times more likely to be convicted of homicide than members of the general population (Wallace *et al.*, 1998). Those with schizophrenia and comorbid substance abuse were more than 8 times more likely to be convicted of interpersonal violence and 4 times more likely to be convicted of homicide than those with schizophrenia alone. Although the prevalence of substance misuse is increasing in the general population, the dramatic increase in those with severe mental illness is also contributing an increase in risks of violence (Wallace *et al.,* 1998).

Learning disability

Studies that use IQ as a continuous variable indicate that significantly below-average intellectual ability is an independent predictor of future offending. The extent to which definitions of learning disability (LD) and offending are broadened or narrowed have a marked effect on prevalence rates. Individuals with mild LD show a higher rate of offending compared with peers without LD and peers with more severe LD, who rarely commit serious offences (Hall, 2000). Significantly impaired intellectual functioning is normally defined as a tested IQ below 70 using an established instrument, but studies in the area often include heterogeneous groups. Additionally, the labelling of behaviours as "criminal offences" depends on a complex decision-making process involving discretion to divert to other settings at various points prior to conviction. Despite their overrepresentation in criminal justice settings, offending in this group is thought to be relatively low. UK studies have suggested that between 2% and 5% of people in contact with LD services are also in contact with the police because of allegations of offending (Lyall *et al.,* 1995; McNulty *et al.,* 1995). This clearly omits those not in contact with services. Estimates of the number of people with LD in prisons vary enormously as a result of different inclusion criteria, testing methods and local policies. Estimates range from 0.2% to 6.0% within US and UK prisons (Birmingham *et al.,* 1996; Denkowski & Denkowski, 1985). In a large unselected birth cohort, it was found that men who had received special schooling were 4 times more likely to be convicted for a violent

offence, whereas the figure for women was 25 (Hodgins *et al.,* 1996). West and Farringdon (1973) followed 411 boys born in London and found intellectual disadvantage to be independently predictive of offending. Men with more criminal convictions at 32 were more likely to be both verbally and nonverbally intellectually disadvantaged and to have histories of limited academic achievement at school.

Many risk factors that operate in the general population for criminality similarly operate in the LD population, most specifically being a young male. Those at high risk include individuals with a history of long-standing behavioural problems, psychosocial disadvantage, family offending, nonprescribed drug use, chaotic lifestyle (Winter *et al.,* 1997), unemployment and mental health needs (Simons, 2000).

Personality disorder

People with personality disorders have a wide range of problems which include early unnatural deaths, high rates of associated mental illness, and worse treatment outcomes for mental and physical illness with resultant high service utilisation and high rates of unemployment, homelessness and nonviolent and violent crime (Moran, 1999). Almost 80% of remand prisoners in England and Wales were found to have at least one personality disorder, with antisocial personality disorder (APD) being most prevalent (Singleton *et al.,* 1998).

The terms *APD* and *psychopathy* are in common parlance and often used interchangeably; there are, however, differences between these constructs, as shown in Box 24.2. Although early use of the term psychopathy focused mainly on social deviance, it has more recently been described in terms of specific abnormalities of personality (Cleckley, 1976). The concept has been operationalised in the form of Hare's Psychopathy Checklist Revised (PCL-R), a development which has improved the utility of the concept in both research and clinical practice (Hare, 1991). This standardised tool yields a maximum score of 40 with a cutoff of 30 for caseness (in

Box 24.2 Summary of some the main similarities and differences between psychopathy and antisocial personality disorder

Similarities	Differences
Persistent antisocial behaviour	Psychopathy – more severe and frequent violence which is often instrumental
Childhood behavioural problems	Antisocial personality disorder – low IQ, language difficulties, poor parenting, impulsive anger common
Contact with mental health or criminal justice services with poor outcomes	Psychopathy – impairments in emotional processing, autonomic functioning and reduced response to punishment

the United States). On the basis of the PCL-R, core features of the disorder have been identified according to two and three factor models, the latter incorporating the following factors:

• arrogant and deceitful interpersonal style,
• a deficiency of affective experience, and
• impulsive irresponsibility.

APD is included among a diverse range of personality disorders in the fourth edition of the *Diagnostic and Statistical Manual of Mental Disorders* (DSM-IV; American Psychiatric Association, 1994) and, in the 10th revision of the *International Classification of Impairments, Disabilities and Handicaps* (ICD-10), the related dissocial personality disorder is included (World Health Organisation, 1992). APD as a concept has been criticised by many who regard it as simply synonymous with criminality (particularly as defined in the third edition of the DSM [DSM-III]) due to the weight given to behavioural rather than personality features (Hart & Hare, 1996). Results from the ECA study have not supported this view, however, because most of those diagnosed as antisocial according to DSM-III were not criminal but more commonly had difficulties related to

employment and relationships (Robins *et al.*, 1991). In DSM-IV, elements of the core features of psychopathy were added to the description of APD, but the result has not altered the separation of the two concepts to the extent that was hoped. Thus those with psychopathy are likely to form a subsample within a larger group in society meeting criteria for APD.

Although antisocial behaviour is the main feature that links APD and psychopathy, there are differences in the nature and frequency of such behaviour. Although perhaps less impulsively aggressive than those with antisocial PD, psychopaths are more likely to engage in antisocial behaviour which is instrumental in nature (Cornell *et al.*, 1996). Those with psychopathy have also been shown to commit higher rates of serious violence, are responsible for a greater proportion of the total crime committed in the population and have strikingly high rates of recidivism (Gretton *et al.*, 2004; Hare, 1999; Hemphill *et al.*, 1998). The PCL-R is one of the most robust predictors of future violence, particularly when applied to forensic populations (Serin & Amos, 1995). A diagnosis of APD does not predict future offending risk as well as psychopathy, perhaps because those included by the diagnostic criteria can vary widely in terms of their personality, motivation and affective experiences (Hart & Hare, 1996). A diagnosis of APD has, however, been found to be useful when considered a risk factor for a variety of other psychosocial outcomes (Black *et al.*, 1995). Among those with mental disorder, particularly substance misuse, rates of comorbidity with APD can be high, and such comorbidity has been shown to predict poor response to treatment (Leal *et al.*, 1994).

From a developmental perspective, both APD and psychopathy are likely to be linked to demonstrable impairments early in life and to adverse childhood experiences, although the nature and impact of these may be quite different (see Chapter 6). A diagnosis of DSM-IV APD requires the presence of childhood conduct disorder, which itself is linked to a variety of factors, including poor parenting, low IQ and verbal language problems for example (Bassarath, 2001; Morrell & Murray, 2003). Those who present with very early onset conduct disorder are particularly likely to develop lifelong persistent antisocial behaviour (Arseneault *et al.*, 2000). Those individuals meeting criteria for psychopathy in adulthood are also likely to have developed antisocial behaviour from early in life but are more likely to have had impairments in appreciation of the emotional significance of language, events and experience rather than having a low IQ and verbal language difficulties (Patrick, 1994; Williamson *et al.*, 1991). These findings are supported by a number of recent brain imaging studies (Intrator *et al.*, 1997; Kiehl *et al.*, 2004). Psychopaths have also been found to have strikingly low levels of baseline and reactive autonomic arousal, although studies have not found entirely consistent results in this regard (Lorber, 2004). The core features of interpersonal and affective abnormality in psychopathy have themselves been identified during childhood (Frick *et al.*, 2003; Frick & Ellis, 1999), and current evidence suggests that their presence reduces the impact of parenting (Wootton *et al.*, 1997). Throughout life, psychopaths are less likely to benefit from punishment or fear-based learning, which is an important element of socialisation and has implications for specific neural substrates (Blair, 2003).

There has been a long-standing belief in psychiatry that people with personality disorders are impervious to treatment, although this belief has been subject to considerable challenge in recent times (see also Chapter 7). One reason for the perception can perhaps be found in their definition as enduring and persistent problems. With regard to reducing risk of violence among those with personality disorders, in many settings criminal justice agencies take the lead in managing the risk posed by serious offenders. Mental health practitioners do not drive the process of risk management but are partners within a multidisciplinary approach. This approach has been advocated for the management of high-risk offenders both in the community, and within institutions. In the United Kingdom, a number of new services have been developed by mental health

professionals aimed at providing interventions, predominantly psychosocial, for those with personality disorders who pose a significant risk of harm to others (e.g. the DSPD or Dangerous and Severe Personality Disorder services). Such services have yet to be fully evaluated.

Neurobiology of violence

The causal mechanisms underlying the association between serious mental disorders such as schizophrenia and aggressive behaviour are not well established. It is, however, likely that such mechanisms will involve complex relationships between various risk factors. There is evidence for both distal (i.e. early-life vulnerability) and proximal (i.e. illness-related) risk factors for violence among those with psychosis (Figure 24.1). As discussed earlier, it is known that risk of violence is increased among those with psychosis who are also using drugs or alcohol (Wallace *et al.*, 2004), diagnosed with comorbid personality disorder (Moran *et al.*, 2003), failing to adhere to treatment (Swartz *et al.*, 1998) or suffering active symptoms of illness (Hodgins *et al.*, 2003), for example. In the Dunedin birth cohort study, factors prior to illness onset such as childhood psychotic symptoms and childhood aggression were both found to increase later risk of violence among those with schizophreniform disorder (Arseneault *et al.*, 2003). Disturbances of brain functioning are likely to be underpin many of these known associations. Evidence in support of this comes from both studies of violence in the general population and studies involving individuals with psychotic disorders.

Neurobiology of violence for those without serious mental illness

Studies of individuals who go on to commit acts of violence demonstrate that they are more likely to have suffered neurodevelopmental insult early in life. Minor physical anomalies are subtle defects of the head, face, hands and feet which result from ectodermal maldevelopment during antenatal life.

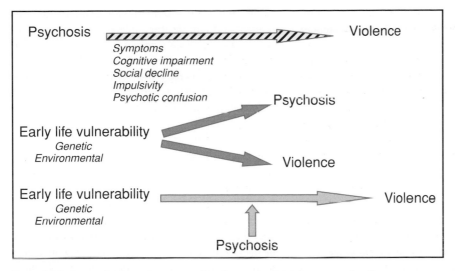

Figure 24.1 Competing hypotheses regarding the psychosis/violence causal pathway

Because the brain is also ectodermally derived, the presence of these anomalies acts as a potential marker of such neurodevelopmental abnormality. In a study in Montreal, boys with higher rates of minor physical anomalies, particularly of the mouth, were more violently delinquent as adolescents (Arseneault *et al.*, 2000). Similarly, higher rates of neurological soft signs are found among those demonstrating high levels of aggression (Lindberg *et al.*, 2004). Providing further support for early life adversity, maternal smoking during pregnancy and obstetric complications have also been linked to later risk of aggression (Brennan *et al.*, 1999; Raine *et al.*, 1994).

Those with a propensity for aggression are known to have both general and specific deficits of brain functioning. Low IQ is linked to antisocial behaviour throughout the life course (Hinshaw, 1992; Hodgins, 1992). In addition, neuropsychological studies have found evidence of specific deficits in executive functioning and impulse control among those displaying antisocial behaviour, again at various stages throughout life (Brower & Price, 2001; Dolan & Park, 2002; Raine *et al.*, 2005). These findings are in line with brain structural studies which find abnormalities in the prefrontal and orbitofrontal

cortices (Raine *et al.*, 2000), in addition to the temporal lobes (Dolan *et al.*, 2002). Such neurobiological abnormalities are likely to have arisen as a result of the interplay between genetic and environmental factors. This has been elegantly demonstrated by recent gene-environment interaction studies such as that reported by Caspi *et al.* (2002) in which childhood maltreatment was found to interact with a genotype for the neurotransmitter-metabolising enzyme monoamine oxidase A in influencing risk for later antisocial behaviour.

Neurobiology of violence for those with serious mental illness

The neurobiological correlates of violence among those with serious mental illness have been less well documented than for the nondisordered population. The evidence for early neurodevelopmental insult is less convincing in this group (Cannon *et al.*, 2002). Higher rates of neurological soft signs have been reported among those with schizophrenia who perpetrate aggressive acts, but results have been inconsistent (Naudts & Hodgins, 2006). Many of the neuropsychological and brain imaging deficits known to occur in psychotic disorders have also been considered in terms of their potential impact on risk of violence. In particular, deficits in aspects of social cognition and social functioning may be relevant. Those with schizophrenia have been shown to have impairments in affect processing (Edwards *et al.*, 2001), theory of mind (Frith, 2004) and prefrontal cortical functioning (Callicott *et al.*, 2003). Noting the overlap between impairments relevant to aggression and to psychosis, many have hypothesised that such impairments are likely to be more evident among those with schizophrenia who are also particularly aggressive. This has not been entirely borne out in research conducted to date (Naudts & Hodgins, 2006). In fact, those with a lifetime pattern of aggressive behaviour have been found to perform better on some tests of brain functioning compared with others with schizophrenia but no such history.

Specific offences – homicide and sex offending

Homicide

Given that the risk to a member of the public of being killed by a stranger with mental disorder is scarcely greater than being killed by a speeding police car or lightening, the amount of media space devoted to such killings appears extreme. Such stigmatizing coverage promotes societal fear of the mentally ill, but does the evidence justify this?

Studies of mental disorder in people convicted of homicide have found rates between 8% and 70% (Gudjonsson & Petursson, 1986; Lindqvist & Allebeck, 1990; Taylor & Gunn, 1999; Wong & Singer, 1973), varying with different definitions of mental disorder. Shaw *et al.* (2006), using the broadest definition (a lifetime history of any disorder) found a rate of at least one third in homicide offenders, which may not actually represent a much higher prevalence of such mental disorder over the general population. The national confidential inquiry into suicide and homicide by people with mental illness

in the United Kingdom aimed to establish the frequency and contributory role of mental illness in a complete national sample of homicides (Shaw *et al.*, 1999). Of those for whom psychiatric information was available (70%), 44% had a lifetime history of mental disorder, and 14% had symptoms of mental illness at the time of the homicide. The most common diagnosis was personality disorder (22%). Only 14% of the total sample was confirmed to be in contact with mental health services at some time in the year before the homicide. Hence, most people with a history of mental disorder convicted of homicide were neither symptomatic nor in contact with mental health services. This raises doubt about the role that can be played by mental health services in the prevention of homicide. These data suggest there are around 40 homicides per year in which people have been in contact with mental health services in the previous 12 months. This is a small proportion of the total number of homicides annually and a tiny proportion of the population of psychiatric patients. Mullen (2006) warned that although the minimisation of the correlations between violence and schizophrenia by researchers may be in part due to misplaced good intentions, we should listen to what the epidemiology findings say and accept that although public fear may be exaggerated, it is certainly not groundless.

Has deinstitionalisation resulted in more societal violence being attributable to mental illness and disorder? Both Gottlieb *et al.* (1987) and Taylor and Gunn (1999) in the United Kingdom found no increase in homicides by people with mental illness following deinstitutionalisation, whereas a small increase has been reported from Germany (Erb *et al.*, 2001). Australian researchers found that rising numbers of convictions for violence among individuals with schizophrenia paralleled rising levels of societal violence (Mullen *et al.*, 2000; Wallace *et al.*, 2004). In New Zealand, the percentage of all homicides committed by the mentally disordered fell from 19.5% in 1970 to 5% in 2000. Ten percent of perpetrators had been admitted to hospital during the month before the offence, and 29% had no prior contact with mental health services (Simpson *et al.,* 2004). Although perpetrators may be unknown to mental health services (Leong & Silva, 1995; Shaw *et al.,* 1999), it is important to note that the victims are more often family members than strangers, when compared with victims of mentally normal perpetrators (Gottlieb *et al.,* 1987; Shaw *et al.,* 1999).

Sex offending

Sahota and Chesterman (1998) reported that up to 10% of all sex offenders are found to have a mental illness. The remainder have either no diagnosis or are labelled as either personality disordered or paraphiliac. Among patients in high secure psychiatric hospitals, it has been estimated that a "sexual element of offending" may be present in up to 70% (Lewis, 1991). Those sex offenders with mental illness are less likely to offend against children than are nondisordered sex offenders (Murray *et al.,* 1992). Thus although only a small minority of sex offenders are thought to be mentally ill, they comprise a larger proportion of secure hospital populations. Personality disordered sex offenders are estimated to comprise 30% to 50% of the sex offender population, depending on the sample. Of those with severe mental illness, schizophrenia is the most common diagnosis among sex offenders; however, much research in the area remains inconclusive. Sexual offending may be associated with a psychotic illness for a number of reasons, namely (Craissati, 2004):

- the assault has arisen directly as a result of delusional beliefs or hallucinations;
- the assault is related to less specific features of the illness, such as heightened arousal, irritability or confusion;
- the assault is related to negative symptoms which may effect social competency; or
- it may be completely unrelated to the illness.

There has been little research examining the link between sex offending and other mental illnesses, although a small minority of depressed individuals or those with obsessive-compulsive disorder may suffer from persistent and distressing ruminations of a sexual nature.

Two main types of personality disorder are known to be particularly associated with sexual offending: APD and emotionally unstable personality disorder. The relationship between APD and sex offending is perhaps self-evident (see Chapter 7). Emotionally unstable personality disorder is characterised by a marked tendency to act impulsively without consideration of the consequences, together with affective instability. There are particular challenges which must be considered in the management of sex offenders with personality disorders. Although those with APD may resist attempts to engage them in treatment, sex offenders with emotionally unstable personality disorder may seek treatment in a chaotic manner, characterised by intense distress and a raised risk of self-harm. Given the established link between treatment attrition and a high risk of sexual reoffending, programmes for people with personality disorders need to be structured and supportive. Cognitive-behavioural programmes, the mainstay of treatment, may need to be augmented by medication for those sex offenders manifesting marked levels of emotional lability, as well as drawing on treatment approaches developed for nonoffending individuals with these personality disorders. Such approaches include schema-focused therapy (Young, 1999) and dialectical behavioural therapy (Linehan, 1993), both of which place emphasis on the importance of establishing a crisis management plan, addressing primary areas causing distress and developing self-management skills. For a review of treatment for sex offending, see Chapter 17 or Craissati (2004).

Risk assessment and management

Assessment of the risk of harm to others posed by those with mental illness has become an increasingly important part of clinical practice in psychiatry, particularly forensic psychiatry. This has arisen both because of accumulating evidence that those with mental disorder are at increased risk of violence (Hodgins *et al.,* 1996) and because of pressure from government and the general public whose concerns have been fuelled by the highlighting of individual cases in inquiries and by the media. Given that violence is relatively rare and the relationships between factors contributing to future occurrence of violence in an individual are complex, predictions of future violence are inherently problematic. Thus the focus must be on assessment and management of risk rather than on prediction of risk, much in the way that risk of self-harm and suicide are considered in clinical practice. Risk prediction is certainly still considered by researchers but is of considerably less utility for clinicians.

Risk assessment methodologies

Unaided clinical risk assessment is still commonly practiced by clinicians but has been criticised on the basis of its poor reliability, poor predictive validity and lack of methodological transparency (Dolan & Doyle, 2000). In an attempt to improve the ability of clinicians to predict risk of violence, a number of instruments have been devised and tested. Two main approaches have been taken – actuarial versus structured professional judgement.

Actuarial risk assessment

Although the term *actuarial* is used without clear definition in the field of risk assessment research (Buchanan, 1999), it can generally be taken to refer to instruments which involve rating a number of predominantly static risk factors known to increase risk of violence when large samples have been studied. A score is produced for an individual which reflects the violence risk group to which he or she belongs. Such instruments have been used for some time in the criminal justice system to predict recidivism among nondisordered offenders. Among those with mental disorder, studies have demonstrated the ability of actuarial methods to predict violence (Bonta, 1998). One actuarial tool which has been used extensively in the mentally disordered population is the Violence Risk Appraisal Guide or VRAG (Harris *et al.*, 1993). It incorporates 12 items

---

Box 24.3 Violence Risk Appraisal Guide (VRAG) items

- PCL-R (Psychopathy Checklist – Revised) score (Hare, 1991)
- Elementary school difficulties
- Personality disorder
- Young age
- Separated from parents prior to 16
- Failure on prior conditional release
- Nonviolent offence history
- Never married
- No diagnosis of schizophrenia
- Victim injury (minimal or none)
- Alcohol abuse
- Female victim

(Box 24.3) found to be important predictors of reconviction/rehospitalisation in a sample of 618 male offenders with mental disorder in Canada who were followed up for 7 years.

Clinical risk assessment

Structured clinical risk assessment instruments such as the HCR-20 or Historical/Clinical/Risk Management 20-item scale (Webster *et al.*, 1997) have been devised and tested in an attempt to combine empirical knowledge about violence risk and clinical expertise. The HCR-20 (Box 24.4) incorporates static historical risk factors such as previous violence and early maladjustment, together with dynamic factors which may be particularly important in individual cases such as level of insight and lack of personal support. Although not clearly borne out by large-scale risk-factor research, these latter clinical and risk management factors are viable targets for risk reduction intervention. An overall score can be obtained for the identification of those belonging to high-risk groups as with actuarial assessment, but additionally there is an opportunity for professional discretion to be used – regarded as both a strength and limitation depending on the perspective taken.

Box 24.4 HCR-20 items

Historical items (10)	Clinical items (5)	Risk items (5)
Previous violence	Lack of insight	Plans lack feasibility
Young age at first violent incident	Negative attitudes	Exposure to destabilisers
Relationship instability	Active symptoms of mental illness	Lack of personal support
Employment problems	Impulsivity	Noncompliance with remediation attempts
Substance use problems	Unresponsive to treatment	Stress
Major mental illness		
Psychopathy (PCL)		
Early maladjustment		
Personality disorder		
Prior supervision failure		

Evaluating the utility of risk assessment instruments

In addition to basic considerations regarding the implications for time and resource management, whether incorporating a specific risk assessment procedure will prove a useful addition to clinical practice depends on three main issues:

1. the proven accuracy with which violence can be predicted by the process (predictive validity);
2. the applicability of the instrument to the patient group and outcomes of interest; and
3. the ability of clinicians to act on the results in order to reduce the predicted risk.

Predictive validity – how accurately does risk assessment predict future violence?

A statistical assessment of predictive validity is crucial both to considering whether a particular risk assessment instrument is clinically useful and to making comparisons between different instruments. There are a number of methods for assessing predictive validity, but the current preferred approach is to obtain receiver operator characteristics (ROCs). Presenting the ROC area under the curve data integrates the concepts of sensitivity and specificity and is relatively independent of the base rate of population violence (Kroner, 2005). In a recent UK study, the relative efficacy of three instruments – the HCR-20, the PCL:SV (Psychopathy Checklist Screening Version; Hart et al., 1995) and the OGRS or Offender Group Reconviction Scale (Copas & Marshall, 1998) – were compared prospectively over 2 years in a group of patients discharged from an independent medium-secure unit (Gray et al., 2004). All three instruments were found to be predictive of offending over the follow-up period, but the purely criminogenic scale (OGRS) appeared to perform best. The finding that actuarial instruments outperform even structured clinical assessments in mentally disordered populations is generally consistent with a number of studies performed in different settings (Bonta et al., 1998), whereas both actuarial and structured clinical approaches outperform unaided clinical judgment. With early indications of superior predictive validity and greater flexibility for clinical application, much interest has recently developed in a new "decision tree" methodology for risk assessment such as that employed by investigators working on the MacArthur Project (Monahan et al., 2000).

Generalisability – can the instrument be applied to a particular population, setting and question of interest?

Predictive validity demonstrated in any study for a risk instrument may not necessarily generalise to a clinical setting. For example, most studies of predictive validity have been performed on samples of male forensic patients pre- and post-discharge. Although ROC analyses minimise the difficulty posed by different populations having different base rates of violence, other important factors are also likely to differ among populations, including the prevalence of risk factors measured by any particular instrument. The outcome measure chosen is also important because it will vary in different studies in terms of definition, source, time period and method of measurement. To be useful in a clinical setting, the outcome measure must be comparable to that required for clinical decision making (Buchanan, 1999).

Intervention – does risk assessment guide clinical treatment decisions?

In clinical practice the usefulness of any risk assessment method will also depend on the implications for intervention. Reliance on static historical and demographic factors such as gender and past criminal behaviour, for example, limits the opportunity to inform clinical intervention. For this reason, consideration of dynamic clinical factors such as active psychotic symptoms, substance misuse and compliance with treatment may contribute to the usefulness of a risk assessment instrument in clinical practice (Mills, 2005). An emphasis on dynamic risk factors enables the process to shift from risk assessment to risk management or risk reduction. Interventions at the heart of clinical practice such as the use of psychotropic medication to treat mental disorder may have an important role to play in risk reduction. Evidence has been accumulating that the choice of antipsychotic medication, for example, has implications for future risk of violence (Swanson *et al.*, 2004).

Although treatment decision making may benefit from the results of risk assessment, it is important to remember that an imperfect risk prediction process has serious implications for individuals if used in this way. Even instruments with relatively high predictive validity will give rise to both false positives

and false negatives: The potential implications of making decisions about detention based on risk prediction, for example, have been elegantly demonstrated by Buchanan and Leese (2001). They pooled results from 23 studies employing violence risk assessment and concluded that on average, six people would need to be detained to prevent one violent act on the basis of the rate of violence assumed to be associated with those believed to have dangerous and severe personality disorders (DSPD). Finally, risk instruments rely on evidence demonstrating an *association* between a risk factor and the outcome, but this does not equate to causation, particularly when considering an individual case.

Whereas actuarial instruments more accurately identify at-risk groups, structured risk instruments may represent a more clinically useful tool for enhancing clinical decision making.

Forensic psychiatry and the law

This section is largely based on the law as it pertains in England and Wales. Many of the principles will be pertinent to other countries and jurisdictions, but the reader will require reference to local mental health and civil acts for local applicability.

Historical background

It has long been recognised that mental disorder can be linked to offending behaviour and that mentally disordered offenders should be treated differently by the courts. In Roman times, offenders were tried in the forum (hence the term *forensic*) and, under Roman law, the insane were felt not to be capable of "malicious intent" (Puri *et al.*, 2005). Although English legal history records many early examples of judicial decisions based on similar principles, the care of those offenders determined to be mentally disordered was very poor for many centuries. Lunatic offenders were generally committed to prisons until the Bethlem Hospital was founded in

Table 24.2 UK Mental Health Law Timeline – Bethlem to Broadmoor Hospital period

Year	Mental health law event
1247	Bethlem Hospital founded (first took "lunatics" in 1377)
1285	Verdict of misadventure returned in murder trial in which offender was found to be "mad"
1334	*Royal Prerogative* – entitled the Crown to the wealth of "idiots" and "lunatics"
1601	*Poor Law Act* – required each parish to take responsibility for the old and the sick including "idiots and lunatics"
1713 and 1744	*Vagrancy Acts* – allowed for arrest and detention of persons appearing mentally unwell and dangerous
1760	First appearance of a physician at a trial as an expert witness in a trial to support an "unsound mind" defence to a charge of murder (the defence failed)
1774	*Act for Regulating Private Madhouses in 1774* – medical certification for insanity introduced
1800	James Hadfield acquitted of attempting to murder King George III and sent by the court to hospital; led to the *Act for the Safe Custody of Insane Persons Charged with Offences 1800* which provided for the special verdict of not guilty by reason of insanity
1808	*County Asylums Act* – required counties to raise funds to build asylums
1828	*Madhouse Act* – powers given to release individuals detained improperly, to remove private madhouse licences and to a requirement for regular medical review of patients
1840	*Insane Prisoners Act* – Home Secretary given the power to transfer an individual from prison to an asylum if insane
1841	Association of Medical Officers of Asylums and Hospitals for the Insane formed (forerunner to the Royal College of Psychiatrists)
1843	Daniel McNaughton acquitted of murder (attempting to shoot the Prime Minister; he shot his secretary instead); his acquittal prompted the Law Lords to issue guidance regarding the definition of insanity called "McNaughton's Rules"
1860	*Criminal Lunatic Asylum Act* – led to mentally disordered offenders being placed in a new state criminal asylum, Broadmoor Hospital

1247 (see Table 24.2). In fact the Bethlem Hospital remained the only facility for the care of the mentally ill in England up until the seventeenth century and the primary facility for the care of mentally disordered offenders until the evolution of the "special hospitals", with Broadmoor Hospital opening in 1863.

In England and Wales over the last century, there has been enormous change in both mental health care as it relates to the mentally disordered offender and in the legal framework within which it occurs. The following list summarises some of the key developments and influences operating during this period:

• Development of Mental Health Legislation allowing involuntary detention in both civil and criminal contexts

• Establishment of the National Health Service (1946) and very recently the expectation that prisoners should receive a standard of care equivalent to that available in the community

• 1957 Homicide Act · provision included for having a murder charge reduced to manslaughter on the grounds of diminished responsibility

• Deinstitutionalisation and a shift towards "care in the community" following concerns about the inappropriate detention of patients for long periods and the unsatisfactory conditions found in many institutions

• Establishment of regional Medium Secure Units following the Butler Committee Report on Mentally Abnormal Offenders in 1975 (Butler-Report, 1975)

• Advent of the Care Programme Approach (1991) following concerns about the adequacy of community care, the issue being further highlighted by the report of the inquiry into the high-profile killing of a stranger by Christopher Clunis, who suffered from schizophrenia (Ritchie *et al.*, 1994)

Much of the historical background to the practice of forensic psychiatry is mirrored in other Western jurisdictions, but there are also important differences. In the United States, for example, the functions of forensic psychiatrists are separated, such that their role is more often to provide expert evidence to the courts and not in the care of mentally disordered offenders. International differences are largely a result of the organisational and legislative framework within which forensic psychiatry is practised in different settings.

Mental health legislation

In the United Kingdom, as in many other similar settings, those with mental disorder may be treated differently under the law with regard to treatment decision making. Although the principles of mental capacity (under common law or in some cases statute law) are applicable to all, those with mental disorder are deemed to present a special case.

In England and Wales, the Mental Health Act 1983 (MHA 1983) provides the legal framework for the care of the mentally disordered where powers of detention and treatment, without the consent of the individual, are required. In principle, mental health legislation allows for the compulsory assessment and treatment (if warranted) of those individuals who meet stated criteria for mental disorder and who present defined risks, in particular where there is evident risk of harm to health, self or others likely to arise from the disorder if allowed to remain untreated. In England and Wales under the MHA 1983, such assessment and treatment can only be carried out compulsorily under conditions of detention in hospital (although recent amendments to the MHA will in future allow for community treatment), but in some other jurisdictions, formal treatment in the community is also permitted (e.g. South

Australian Mental Health Act 1993). Box 24.5 provides a summary of general principles recommended by the WHO for countries considering the development of mental health legislation.

Since its introduction, compulsory admission rates under the MHA 1983 in England and Wales have increased substantially despite a reduction in bed numbers (Lelliott & Audini, 2003). In seven local authority regions, the rate of compulsory admission increased from 57 per 100,000 in 1991 to 75 per 100,000 in 1997. The same study found that young men were particularly likely to find themselves subject to the Mental Health Act.

Mentally disordered offenders – the medicolegal context

Detention in hospital for those under the criminal justice system

In addition to compulsory admission under civil section, the MHA 1983 also provides for the detention of mentally disordered offenders. The concept of "diversion" from the criminal justice system to mental health services is similarly enshrined in mental health legislation in other settings. At virtually every stage of an individual's progress through the criminal justice system, there exists an opportunity for such diversion. Following arrest in England and Wales, a mentally disordered individual can be admitted informally to a psychiatric hospital (whether also remanded to hospital by the police or not) or can be detained compulsorily under the MHA 1983 following assessment at the police station. At an early stage, the courts can remand an individual to a psychiatric hospital for a report following assessment or for treatment. At many magistrates' courts, there are now diversion "teams" in regular attendance to provide urgent mental health assessments, facilitate access to mental health services and give advice to the courts. Those already on remand in custody (awaiting trial or sentencing) can also be transferred to hospital under the MHA 1983 as directed by the Home Secretary. In the context of charges having being brought against an individual,

Box 24.5 Mental health legislation: general principles of development (WHO)

- The 'least restrictive alternative' principle should be incorporated into any legislation such that individuals should always be offered treatment in settings least likely to restrict their personal freedoms, status and privileges
- If institutional treatment is necessary, the legislation should encourage voluntary admission and treatment such that involuntary care occurs only in exceptional cases
- The legislation should guarantee confidentiality with respect to information gathered in a clinical setting
- Free and informed consent to treatment should be preserved in the legislation; treatment without consent should occur only in exceptional circumstances such as where individuals admitted on an involuntary basis lack capacity to consent and where treatment is required to improve mental health and/or prevent a deterioration in mental health and/or prevent risk of harm to self or others
- The legislation should include adequate procedures to protect the rights of individuals admitted and/or treated involuntarily; these procedures should include: rights to appeal against involuntary care, ability to obtain a second opinion, use of a periodic review mechanism, and ability to obtain permission from an independent authority based on professional recommendations
- The circumstances under which involuntary admission can be considered should be stated explicitly by the legislation
- Treatment should be voluntary wherever possible (including for those admitted involuntarily) and should be based on informed consent; consent is unlawful if given in response to a threat or implied threat of compulsion, or where appropriate alternatives are not considered
- Involuntary treatment in community settings can be a useful alternative to admission (although sufficient evidence for this is currently lacking)
- The legislation should make provision for automatic reviewing of every case of involuntary admission and/or treatment; this should be undertaken by an independent body
- The legislation should make provision for appointment of guardians for individuals not competent to make decisions

Box 24.6 According to Pritchard's Criteria, the defendant is unfit to plead if he is unfit to do at least one of the following:

- Instruct counsel
- Appreciate the significant of pleading
- Challenge a juror
- Examine a witness
- Understand and follow the evidence presented in court

the courts in England and Wales can order a mentally disordered offender to be transferred to hospital in preference to a custodial or other disposal (discussed later). Finally, a sentenced prisoner who develops overt mental disorder while in custody can be diverted to hospital, again under the MHA 1983 directed by the Home Secretary.

Fitness to plead

Mental abnormality can be considered as a defence by the courts for two purposes: to excuse the individual from being tried (fitness to plead) or to consider the individual as not fully responsible for the unlawful act. Under the Criminal Procedure (Insanity and Unfitness to Plead) Act 1991, at the time of trial a defendant can be found by the judge to be unfit to plead based on medical evidence provided. The test that is applied under the act is based on that used in *R v Pritchard, 1836* (see Box 24.6)

If a defendant is found unfit to plead but is likely, following treatment, to become fit, then the trial can be adjourned to allow for such improvement if it can occur within a reasonable time period. If not, a jury trial of the facts takes place in the defendant's absence to determine whether the individual committed the acts alleged (*actus rea*). If found both unfit to plead and to have committed the act, the individual is then disposed of by the court; the offender may be given a hospital order, supervision order or absolute discharge. It should be noted that the finding of unfitness to plead or stand trial is uncommon (295 cases were identified for the period 1976–1988 in England and Wales; Grubin, 1991). It is

> **Box 24.7** The McNaughton Rules
>
> The offender must be proven, on the balance of probabilities, to have been suffering such a defect of reason at the time of the offence that the following rules were met:
> - He did not know the nature or quality of his act (physical)
>   *or*
> - He did not know that what he was doing was wrong (forbidden by law)
>
> If the individual was suffering from a delusion, then his actions would be judged in relation to that delusion

also possible that physical ill health might render an individual unfit to plead and stand trial, but serious mental illness is by the far the most common.

Psychiatric defences

Throughout history and today in many jurisdictions, those suffering mental disorder have been able to present a psychiatric defence to a charge against them. The range/definition of mental disorder varies, as indeed do the circumstances in which such defences can be used, the requirements to be met and the subsequent outcome for the defendant. The defence of not guilty by reason of insanity (or the "special verdict") is available (under the Criminal Procedure [Insanity and Unfitness to Plead] Act 1991) to those facing any charge, although most commonly for those facing a charge of murder or other serious offence. Use of the defence is relatively rare because of the very strict test applied; the test having originally arisen from the case of Daniel McNaughton in 1843. The guidance from law lords issued following this case is referred to as the McNaughton Rules (see Box 24.7). If an individual is found to be not guilty of the charge by reason of insanity, the judge has a range of options for disposal available to him, including detention in hospital.

The Homicide Act 1957 was introduced in the United Kingdom at a time when capital punishment was still being applied to those convicted of murder. Given the high threshold of the McNaughton Rules, many were concerned that they afforded limited protection to those with mental disorder who had killed. In this context, a partial defence to murder was created such that an individual could be found guilty of the lesser charge of manslaughter on the grounds of diminished responsibility and avoid the gallows (now the automatic life sentence for murder is avoided). Under the Homicide Act 1957, the offender must prove that at the time of the offence, he or she was suffering "from such abnormality of mind, whether arising from a condition of arrested or retarded development of mind or any inherent causes or induced by disease or injury, as substantially impaired his mental responsibility for his acts". If successful, the sentence given to the individual convicted of manslaughter is at the discretion of the court and is often a hospital order or, less commonly, a community rehabilitation order.

Automatism is a rare plea which can be applied to a wide range of offences but in practice is generally limited to serious offences such as homicide. The defendant pleads that at the time of the offence his behaviour was "automatic", that is without *mens rea*; the body is acting without knowledge or involvement of the mind. Successful cases have been based on automatism arising from hypoglycaemia, sleep walking and epilepsy, for example. The defendant is acquitted if successful unless the case is of insane rather than sane automatism; the former amounts to "not guilty by reason of insanity" and is dealt with according to the rules for the special verdict. Non-insane automatisms are essentially due to external causes and unlikely to recur, whereas insane automatisms are due to internal diseases or disorders of the mind.

Conclusions

The relationship between mental illness and the law has fascinated and tested both the mental health and the legal professions for centuries. Forensic psychiatry is a growing discipline, and this reflects increasing awareness of these issues by both groups, as well as a desire to ensure that public safety and the rights of the mentally ill are given equal balance in legislation and clinical decision making.

REFERENCES

American Psychiatric Association. (1994). *Diagnostic and Statistical Manual of Mental Disorders*, 4th edn. (DSM-IV). Washington, DC: American Psychiatric Association.

Appelbaum, P. S., Robbins, P. C., & Monahan, J. (2000). Violence and delusions: data from the MacArthur Violence Risk Assessment Study. *Am J Psychiatry* 157:566–72.

Arseneault, L., Cannon, M., Murray, R., *et al.* (2003). Childhood origins of violent behaviour in adults with schizophreniform disorder dagger. *Br J Psychiatry* 183:520–5.

Arseneault, L., Moffitt, T. E., Caspi, A., *et al.* (2000). Mental disorders and violence in a total birth cohort: results from the Dunedin Study. *Arch Gen Psychiatry* 57:979–86.

Arseneault, L., Tremblay, R. E., Boulerice, B., *et al.* (2000). Minor physical anomalies and family adversity as risk factors for violent delinquency in adolescence. *Am J Psychiatry* 157:917–23.

Barlow, K., Grenyer, B., & Ilkiw-Lavalle, O. (2000). Prevalence and precipitants of aggression in psychiatric inpatient units. *Aust N Z J Psychiatry* 34:967–74.

Bassarath, L. (2001). Conduct disorder: a biopsychosocial review. *Can J Psychiatry* 46:609–16.

Birmingham, L., Mason, D., & Grubin, D. (1996). Prevalence of mental disorder in remand prisoners: consecutive case study. *BMJ* 313:1521–4.

Black, D. W., Baumgard, C. H., & Bell, S. E. (1995). The long-term outcome of antisocial personality disorder compared with depression, schizophrenia, and surgical conditions. *Bull Am Acad Psychiatry Law* 23:43–52.

Blair, R. J. (2003). Neurobiological basis of psychopathy. *Br J Psychiatry* 182:5–7.

Bonta, J., Law, M., & Hanson, K. (1998). The prediction of criminal and violent recidivism among mentally disordered offenders: a meta-analysis. *Psychol Bull* 123:123–42.

Brennan, P. A., Grekin, E. R., & Mednick, S. A. (1999). Maternal smoking during pregnancy and adult male criminal outcomes. *Arch Gen Psychiatry* 56:215–19.

Brennan, P. A., Mednick, S. A., & Hodgins, S. (2000). Major mental disorders and criminal violence in a Danish birth cohort. *Arch Gen Psychiatry* 57:494–500.

Brower, M. C., & Price, B. H. (2001). Advances in neuropsychiatry: neuropsychiatry of frontal lobe dysfunction in violent and criminal behaviour: a critical review. *J Neurol Neurosurg Psychiatry* 71:720–6.

Buchanan, A. (1999). Risk and dangerousness. *Psychol Med* 29:465–73.

Buchanan, A., & Leese, M. (2001). Detention of people with dangerous severe personality disorders: a systematic review. *Lancet* 358:1955–9.

Butler Report (1975). *Report of the Committee on Mentally Disordered Offenders*. London: Her Majesty's Stationery Service.

Callicott, J. H., Mattay, V. S., Verchinski, B. A., *et al.* (2003). Complexity of prefrontal cortical dysfunction in schizophrenia: more than up or down. *Am J Psychiatry* 160:2209–15.

Cannon, M., Huttunen, M. O., Tanskanen, A. J., *et al.* (2002). Perinatal and childhood risk factors for later criminality and violence in schizophrenia. Longitudinal, population-based study. *Br J Psychiatry* 180:496–501.

Caspi, A., McClay, J., Moffitt, T. E., *et al.* (2002). Role of genotype in the cycle of violence in maltreated children. *Science* 297:851–4.

Cleckley, H. (1976). *The Mask of Sanity*, 6th edn. St Louis, MO: Mosby.

Copas, J., & Marshall, P. (1998). The offender group reconviction scale: a statistical reconviction score score for use by probation officers. *Appl Stat* 47:159–71.

Cornell, D. G., Warren, J., Hawk, G., *et al.* (1996). Psychopathy in instrumental and reactive violent offenders. *J Consult Clin Psychol* 64:783–90.

Cote, G., & Hodgins, S. (1992). The prevalence of major mental disorders among homicide offenders. *Int J Law Psychiatry* 15:89–99.

Craissati, J. (2004). *Managing High Risk Sex Offenders in the Community*. Hove and New York: Brunner-Routledge.

Cuffel, B. J., Shumway, M., Chouljian, T. L., *et al.* (1994). A longitudinal study of substance use and community violence in schizophrenia. *J Nerv Ment Dis* 182:704–8.

d'Orban, P. T. (1979). Women who kill their children. *Br J Psychiatry* 134:560–571.

Dean, K., Walsh, E., Morgan, C., *et al.* (2007). Aggressive behaviour at first contact with services: findings from the AESOP First Episode Psychosis Study. *Psychol Med* 37:547–57.

Denkowski, G., & Denkowski, G. (1985). The mentally retarded offender in the state prison system: identification, prevalence, adjustment and rehabilitation. *Crim Justice Behav* 12:55–70.

Dolan, M., & Park, I. (2002). The neuropsychology of anti-social personality disorder. *Psychol Med* 32:417–27.

Dolan, M. C., Deakin, J. F., Roberts, N., *et al.* (2002). Quantitative frontal and temporal structural MRI studies in personality-disordered offenders and control subjects. *Psychiatry Res* 116:133–49.

Dolan, M., & Doyle, M. (2000). Violence risk prediction. Clinical and actuarial measures and the role of the Psychopathy Checklist. *Br J Psychiatry* 177: 303–11.

Edwards, J., Pattison, P. E., Jackson, H. J., *et al.* (2001). Facial affect and affective prosody recognition in first-episode schizophrenia. *Schizophr Res* 48:235–53.

Erb, M., Hodgins, S., Freese, R., *et al.* (2001). Homicide and schizophrenia: maybe treatment does have a preventive effect. *Crim Behav Ment Health* 11:6–26.

Eronen, M., Hakola, P., & Tiihonen, J. (1996). Mental disorders and homicidal behavior in Finland. *Arch Gen Psychiatry* 53:497–501.

Fazel, S., & Danesh, J. (2002). Serious mental disorder in 23000 prisoners: a systematic review of 62 surveys. *Lancet* 359:545–50.

Fazel, S., & Grann, M. (2006). The population impact of severe mental illness on violent crime. *Am J Psychiatry* 163:1397–1403.

Frick, P. J., Cornell, A. H., Bodin, S. D., *et al.* (2003). Callous-unemotional traits and developmental pathways to severe conduct problems. *Dev Psychol*, 39:246–60.

Frick, P. J., & Ellis, M. (1999). Callous-unemotional traits and subtypes of conduct disorder. *Clin Child Fam Psychol Rev* 2:149–68.

Frith, C. D. (2004). Schizophrenia and theory of mind. *Psychol Med* 34:385–9.

Gottlieb, P., Gabrielsen, G., & Kramp, P. (1987). Psychotic homicides in Copenhagen from 1959 to 1983. *Acta Psychiatr Scand* 76:285–92.

Gray, N. S., Snowden, R. J., MacCulloch, S., *et al.* (2004). Relative efficacy of criminological, clinical, and personality measures of future risk of offending in mentally disordered offenders: a comparative study of HCR-20, PCL-SV, and OGRS. *J Consult Clin Psychol* 72:523–30.

Gretton, H. M., Hare, R. D., & Catchpole, R. E. (2004). Psychopathy and offending from adolescence to adulthood: a 10-year follow-up. *J Consult Clin Psychol* 72:636–45.

Grubin, D. H. (1991). Unfit to plead in England and Wales, 1976–88. A survey. *Br J Psychiatry* 158:540–8.

Gudjonsson, G. H., & Petursson, H. (1986). Changing characteristics of homicide in Iceland. *Med Sci Law* 26:299–303.

Hall, I. (2000). Young offenders with learning disability. *Adv Psychiatr Treat* 6:278–86.

Haque, Q., & Cumming, I. (2003). Intoxication and legal defences. *Adv Psychiatr Treat* 9:144–51.

Hare, R. (1991). *The Hare Psychopathy Checklist – Revised.* Toronto: Multi-Health Systems.

Hare, R. D. (1999). Psychopathy as a risk factor for violence. *Psychiatr Q* 70:181–97.

Harris, G. T., Rice, M. E., & Quinsey, V. L. (1993). Violent recidivism of mentally disordered offenders: the development of a statistical prediction instrument. *Crim Justice Behav* 20:315–35.

Hart, S. D., Cox, D. N., & Hare, R. D. (1995). *The Hare Psychopathy Checklist – Screening Version (PCL:SV).* Toronto, Ontario, Canada: Multi-Health Systems.

Hart, S. D., & Hare, R. D. (1996). Psychopathy and antisocial personality disorder. *Curr Opin Psychiatry* 9:129–32.

Hemphill, J. F., Hare, R. D., & Wong, S. (1998). Psychopathy and recidivism: a review. *Legal Criminol Psychol* 3:139–70.

Hinshaw, S. P. (1992). Externalizing behavior problems and academic underachievement in childhood and adolescence: causal relationships and underlying mechanisms. *Psychol Bull* 111:127–55.

Hodgins, S. (1992). Mental disorder, intellectual deficiency, and crime. Evidence from a birth cohort. *Arch Gen Psychiatry* 49:476–83.

Hodgins, S., Hiscoke, U. L., & Freese, R. (2003). The antecedents of aggressive behavior among men with schizophrenia: a prospective investigation of patients in community treatment. *Behav Sci Law* 21:523–46.

Hodgins, S., Mednick, S. A., Brennan, P. A., *et al.* (1996). Mental disorder and crime. Evidence from a Danish birth cohort. *Arch Gen Psychiatry* 53:489–96.

Intrator, J., Hare, R., Stritzke, P., *et al.* (1997). A brain imaging (single photon emission computerized tomography) study of semantic and affective processing in psychopaths. *Biol Psychiatry* 42:96–103.

Johns, A. (1998). Substance misuse and offending. *Curr Opin Psychiatry* 11:669–73.

Kiehl, K. A., Smith, A. M., Mendrek, A., *et al.* (2004). Temporal lobe abnormalities in semantic processing by criminal psychopaths as revealed by functional magnetic resonance imaging. *Psychiatry Res* 130:297–312.

Kroner, D. G. (2005). Issues in violent risk assessment: lessons learned and future directions. *J Interpers Violence* 20:231–5.

Leal, J., Ziedonis, D., & Kosten, T. (1994). Antisocial personality disorder as a prognostic factor for pharmacotherapy of cocaine dependence. *Drug Alcohol Depend* **35**:31–5.

Lelliott, P., & Audini, B. (2003). Trends in the use of Part II of the Mental Health Act 1983 in seven English local authority areas. *Br J Psychiatry* **182**:68–70.

Leong, G. B., & Silva, J. A. (1995). A psychiatric-legal analysis of psychotic criminal defendants charged with murder. *J Forensic Sci* **40**:445–8.

Lewis, P. (1991). The report of the working party on the assessment and treatment of sex offenders at Broadmoor Hospital [Internal Document].

Lindberg, N., Tani, P., Stenberg, J. H., *et al.* (2004). Neurological soft signs in homicidal men with antisocial personality disorder. *Eur Psychiatry* **19**:433–7.

Lindqvist, P., & Allebeck, P. (1990). Schizophrenia and crime. A longitudinal follow-up of 644 schizophrenics in Stockholm. *Br J Psychiatry* **157**:345–50.

Linehan, M. (1993). *The Skills Training Manual for Treating Borderline Personality Disorder*. New York: Guilford Press.

Link, B. G., Stueve, A., & Phelan, J. (1998). Psychotic symptoms and violent behaviors: probing the components of "threat/control-override" symptoms. *Soc Psychiatry Psychiatr Epidemiol* **33**(Suppl 1):S55–60.

Lorber, M. F. (2004). Psychophysiology of aggression, psychopathy, and conduct problems: a meta-analysis. *Psychol Bull* **130**:531–52.

Lyall, I., Holland, A. J., & Collins, S. (1995). Offending by adults with learning disabilities and the attitudes of staff to offending behaviour: implications for service development. *J Intellect Disabil Res* **39**(Pt 6):501–8.

McNulty, C., Kissi-Deborah, R., & Newsome-Davies, I. (1995). Police involvement with clients having intellectual disabilities: a pilot study in South London. *Ment Handicap Res* **8**:129–36.

Mills, J. F. (2005). Advances in the assessment and prediction of interpersonal violence. *J Interpers Violence* **20**:236–41.

Modestin, J., & Ammann, R. (1996). Mental disorder and criminality: male schizophrenia. *Schizophr Bull* **22**:69–82.

Monahan, J. (1997). Clinical and Actuarial predictions of violence. In D. Faigman, D. Kaye, M. Saks, *et al.*, eds. *Modern Scientific Evidence: The Law and Science of Expert Testimony*. St Paul, Minnesota: West, pp. 300–18.

Monahan, J., Steadman, H. J., Appelbaum, P. S., *et al.* (2000). Developing a clinically useful actuarial tool for assessing violence risk. *Br J Psychiatry* **176**:312–19.

Moran, P. (1999). Should Psychiatrists Treat Personality Disorders?, 7th edn. Maudsley Discussion Paper No. 7. *Psychiatr Bull* **24**:358.

Moran, P., Walsh, E., Tyrer, P., *et al.* (2003). Impact of comorbid personality disorder on violence in psychosis: report from the UK700 trial. *Br J Psychiatry* **182**:129–34.

Morrell, J., & Murray, L. (2003). Parenting and the development of conduct disorder and hyperactive symptoms in childhood: a prospective longitudinal study from 2 months to 8 years. *J Child Psychol Psychiatry* **44**:489–508.

Mullen, P. (2006). Schizophrenia and violence: from correlations to preventive strategies. *Adv Psychiatr Treat* **12**:239–48.

Mullen, P. E., Burgess, P., Wallace, C., *et al.* (2000). Community care and criminal offending in schizophrenia. *Lancet* **355**:614–17.

Murray, G., Briggs, D., & Davies, C. (1992). Psychopathic disordered/mentally ill, and mentally handicapped sex offenders: a comparative study. *Med Sci Law* **32**:331–6.

Naudts, K., & Hodgins, S. (2006). Neurobiological correlates of violent behavior among persons with schizophrenia. *Schizophr Bull* **32**:562–72.

Patrick, C. J. (1994). Emotion and psychopathy: startling new insights. *Psychophysiology* **31**:319–30.

Puri, B. K., Brown, R. A., McKee, H. J., *et al.* (2005). History of mental health legislation. In *Mental Health Law A Practical Guide*. London: Hodder Arnold, pp. 1–10.

Raine, A., Brennan, P., & Mednick, S. A. (1994). Birth complications combined with early maternal rejection at age 1 year predispose to violent crime at age 18 years. *Arch Gen Psychiatry* **51**:984–8.

Raine, A., Lencz, T., Bihrle, S., *et al.* (2000). Reduced prefrontal gray matter volume and reduced autonomic activity in antisocial personality disorder. *Arch Gen Psychiatry* **57**:119–127; discussion 128–9.

Raine, A., Moffitt, T. E., Caspi, A., *et al.* (2005). Neurocognitive impairments in boys on the life-course persistent antisocial path. *J Abnorm Psychol* **114**:38–49.

Rasanen, P., Tiihonen, J., Isohanni, M., *et al.* (1998). Schizophrenia, alcohol abuse, and violent behavior: a 26-year follow-up study of an unselected birth cohort. *Schizophr Bull* **24**:437–41.

Regier, D. A., Farmer, M. E., Rae, D. S., *et al.* (1990). Comorbidity of mental disorders with alcohol and other drug abuse. Results from the Epidemiologic Catchment Area (ECA) Study. *JAMA* **264**:2511–18.

Ritchie, J. H., Dick, D., & Lingham, R. (1994). *The Report of the Inquiry into the Treatment of Christopher Clunis*. London: Her Majesty's Stationery Office.

Robins, L. N., Tipp, J., & Przybeck, T. (1991). Antisocial personality. In L. N. Robins & D. Regier, eds. *Psychiatric Disorders in America: The Epidemiologic Catchment Area Study*. New York: Macmillan/Free Press, pp. 258–90.

Sahota, K., & Chesterman, P. (1998). Sexual offending in the context of severe mental illness. *J Foren Psychiatry* 9:267–80.

Schanda, H., Knecht, G., Schreinzer, D., *et al.* (2004). Homicide and major mental disorders: a 25-year study. *Acta Psychiatr Scand* 110:98–107.

Serin, R. C., & Amos, N. L. (1995). The role of psychopathy in the assessment of dangerousness. *Int J Law Psychiatry* 18:231–8.

Shaw, J., Appleby, L., Amos, T., *et al.* (1999). Mental disorder and clinical care in people convicted of homicide: national clinical survey. *BMJ* 318:1240–4.

Shaw, J., Hunt, I. M., Flynn, S., *et al.* (2006). Rates of mental disorder in people convicted of homicide. National clinical survey. *Br J Psychiatry* 188:143–7.

Simons, K. (2000). *Life on the Edge. The Experiences of People with a Learning Disability Who Do Not Use Specialist Services*. Brighton: Pavilion Publishing/Joseph Rowntree Foundation.

Simpson, A. I., McKenna, B., Moskowitz, A., *et al.* (2004). Homicide and mental illness in New Zealand, 1970–2000. *Br J Psychiatry* 185:394–8.

Singleton, N., Meltzer, H., & Gatward, R. (1998). *Psychiatric Morbidity Among Prisoners in England and Wales*. London: Her Majesty's Stationery Office.

Snowden, P. (2001). Substance misuse and violence: the scope and limitations forensic psychiatry's role. *Adv Psychiatr Treat* 2001:189–97.

Swanson, J., Estroff, S., Swartz, M., *et al.* (1997). Violence and severe mental disorder in clinical and community populations: the effects of psychotic symptoms, comorbidity, and lack of treatment. *Psychiatry* 60:1–22.

Swanson, J. W., Holzer, C. E., 3rd, Ganju, V. K., *et al.* (1990). Violence and psychiatric disorder in the community: evidence from the Epidemiologic Catchment Area surveys. *Hosp Commun Psychiatry* 41:761–70.

Swanson, J. W., Swartz, M. S., Elbogen, E. B., *et al.* (2004). Reducing violence risk in persons with schizophrenia: olanzapine versus risperidone. *J Clin Psychiatry* 65:1666–73.

Swanson, J. W., Van Dorn, R. A., Monahan, J., *et al.* (2006). Violence and leveraged community treatment for persons with mental disorders. *Am J Psychiatry* 163:1404–11.

Swartz, M. S., Swanson, J. W., Hiday, V. A., *et al.* (1998). Violence and severe mental illness: the effects of substance abuse and nonadherence to medication. *Am J Psychiatry* 155:226–31.

Taylor, P. J., & Gunn, J. (1984). Violence and psychosis. I. Risk of violence among psychotic men. *Br Med J (Clin Res Ed)* 288:1945–9.

Taylor, P. J., & Gunn, J. (1999). Homicides by people with mental illness: myth and reality. *Br J Psychiatry* 174:9–14.

Tiihonen, J., Isohanni, M., Rasanen, P., *et al.* (1997). Specific major mental disorders and criminality: a 26-year prospective study of the 1966 northern Finland birth cohort. *Am J Psychiatry* 154:840–5.

Volavka, J., Laska, E., Baker, S., *et al.* (1997). History of violent behaviour and schizophrenia in different cultures. Analyses based on the WHO study on Determinants of Outcome of Severe Mental Disorders. *Br J Psychiatry* 171:9–14.

Wallace, C., Mullen, P. E., & Burgess, P. (2004). Criminal offending in schizophrenia over a 25-year period marked by deinstitutionalization and increasing prevalence of comorbid substance use disorders. *Am J Psychiatry* 161:716–27.

Wallace, C., Mullen, P., Burgess, P., *et al.* (1998). Serious criminal offending and mental disorder. Case linkage study. *Br J Psychiatry* 172:477–84.

Webster, C., Douglas, K., Eaves, D., *et al.* (1997). *HCR-20. Assessing Risk for Violence. Version2*. Burnaby, Canada: Mental Health Law and Policy Institute.

Wessely, S. C., Castle, D., Douglas, A. J., *et al.* (1994). The criminal careers of incident cases of schizophrenia. *Psychol Med* 24:483–502.

West, D., & Farringdon, D. (1973). *Who Becomes Delinquent*. London: Heinemann.

Williamson, S., Harpur, T. J., & Hare, R. D. (1991). Abnormal processing of affective words by psychopaths. *Psychophysiology* 28:260–73.

Winter, N., Holland, A. J., & Collins, S. (1997). Factors predisposing to suspected offending by adults with self-reported learning disabilities. *Psychol Med* 27:595–607.

Wong, M., & Singer, K. (1973). Abnormal homicide in Hong Kong. *Br J Psychiatry* 123:295–8.

Wootton, J. M., Frick, P. J., Shelton, K. K., *et al.* (1997). Ineffective parenting and childhood conduct problems: the moderating role of callous-unemotional traits. *J Consult Clin Psychol* **65**:301–8.

World Health Organisation. (1992). *The ICD-10 Classification of Mental and Behavioural Disorders: Clinical Descriptions and Diagnostic Guidelines*. Geneva: World Health Organisation.

World Health Organisation. (2003). *Mental Health Legislation and Human Rights (Mental Health Policy and Service Guidance Package)*. Geneva: World Health Organisation.

Young, J. (1999). *Cognitive Therapy for Personality Disorders: A Schema Focused Approach*. Sarasota, Florida: Professional Resource Press.

Treatments in Psychiatry

25

Biological treatments: general considerations

Evangelia M. Tsapakis and Katherine J. Aitchison

This chapter on general considerations for biological treatments in psychiatry covers four main areas: pharmacokinetics, pharmacodynamics, behavioural pharmacology and pharmacogenetics. Within each of these, general principles are defined, and examples relevant to psychiatry provided.

Pharmacokinetics

Pharmacokinetics is the study of the time course of the passage of drugs and their metabolites through the body. A good working knowledge of pharmacokinetics facilitates appropriate and safe prescribing. The concentration attained at a drug's site of action depends on the extent and rate of its absorption, distribution, plasma binding, metabolism and elimination. Factors influencing these involve the molecular size and shape of the drug, its lipid solubility and degree of ionisation. Nonionised molecules, in contrast to the ionised molecules, are usually lipid soluble and can diffuse across cell membranes.

Absorption

Absorption is the rate at which a drug leaves its site of administration and the extent to which this occurs. In addition to the physicochemical factors influencing transport across membranes, absorption depends on (a) drug solubility, (b) local conditions, (c) drug concentration, (d) the circulation at the site of absorption and (e) the area of the absorbing surface. Each of these factors separately or in conjunction with one another may have profound effects on the clinical efficacy and toxicity of a drug.

Intravenous injection (IV) ensures that the entire administered drug is available to the circulation. The rate of drug injection or infusion can be used to control the rate of drug availability, but few psychopharmacological drugs are administered IV. Some rapid tranquilisation protocols continue to recommend IV benzodiazepines or antipsychotics under certain circumstances, whereas most encourage the intramuscular (IM) route.

The extent to which a drug reaches its site of action is termed *bioavailability*. A general rank order of dosage formulations providing the most rapid to the slowest rate of drug release for oral absorption is solutions > suspensions > tablets > enteric- or film-coated tablets. Drugs with short elimination half-lives, such as venlafaxine or sodium valproate, may be formulated into sustained- or slow-release preparations for once-daily administration.

Distribution

The distribution of drug to the tissues begins on absorption into the systemic circulation. The initial phase of distribution reflects cardiac output and regional blood flow. Well-perfused organs such as

Essential Psychiatry, ed. Robin M. Murray, Kenneth S. Kendler, Peter McGuffin, Simon Wessely, David J. Castle.
Published by Cambridge University Press. © Cambridge University Press 2008.

the heart, liver, kidney and brain initially receive most of the drug. Delivery of drug to muscle, most viscera, skin, and fat occurs later (the second phase of distribution). Other factors influencing the distribution of a drug in the body include (a) the rate at which the drug diffuses into the tissues, (b) the drug's lipid solubility, (c) drug binding to plasma proteins (e.g. to albumin for acidic drugs and to α_1-acid glycoprotein for basic drugs) and (d) the pH of the tissues.

Entry of drugs to the central nervous system (CNS) is restricted by the blood-brain barrier. The endothelial cells of brain capillaries are joined by tight junctions, which prevent flow of aqueous solutes between cells. Surrounding precapillary glial cells may also contribute to the slow diffusion of acids and bases into the CNS. Hence lipid-soluble drugs permeate the CNS relatively easily. The rate of diffusion of polar drugs into the CNS is proportional to the lipid solubility of the nonionised species. Exit of drugs and their metabolites from the CNS is through the arachnoid villi.

The distribution of a drug in the body largely depends on the drug's relative binding affinity to plasma proteins and tissue components and the capacity of the tissues for drug binding. Only unbound drug is capable of redistributing between plasma and tissues. However, different degrees of plasma protein binding (e.g. between antidepressants) are not sufficient to draw valid conclusions about the availability of drug to exert pharmacological effects at the site of action, because the binding of drugs to tissue components must also be considered. Drug binding in tissues cannot be measured directly in vivo and must be inferred using mathematical models or in vitro methods (or both).

Drug accumulating in various body reservoirs is in equilibrium with that in plasma and is released as the plasma concentration declines. Hence the concentration of the drug in plasma and at its locus of action is sustained, and pharmacological effects of the drug are prolonged. However, if the reservoir for a drug has a large capacity and fills rapidly, the distribution of the drug may alter such that larger quantities of the drug are required initially to provide a consistent therapeutically effective concentration in the target organ. Diazepam, which is highly lipophilic, has a rapid onset of action as a result of its entry into the brain within minutes of oral administration. The concentration of diazepam at its effect site may, however, fall rapidly as a result of distribution into the brain, so that its duration of action after an initial dose is shorter than would be expected based on its elimination half-life. The intensity and duration of the pharmacological effect of a second diazepam dose, taken immediately after cessation of the effect of the first dose, is greater and longer, respectively, than the intensity and duration of the effect of the first dose because the active "reservoir", the brain, is already partially full, and hence the distribution effect is less.

Drug-drug interactions may result in the displacement of drug from plasma protein-binding sites, with more unbound drug becoming available for distribution to target organs. If plasma protein binding exerts a restrictive effect on the drug's hepatic or renal elimination (or both), then the resultant increased free drug concentration in plasma will be a transient effect, because the free (non-protein-bound) drug will be rapidly eliminated. Total (bound plus free) drug concentration in plasma will eventually return to a pre-displacement value. Plasma protein-binding displacement interactions are rarely a major source of variability in psychopharmacology, but some psychotropic drugs such as risperidone have a relatively high propensity to bind albumin, a factor that can influence the free drug's availability in the body, and hence its potential interactions with other medications competing for protein binding, such as carbamazepine. Drug interactions involving inhibition of drug metabolism are more common.

Metabolism

Many drugs undergo extensive metabolism as they move from the gastrointestinal tract to the systemic circulation. This process, performed mainly by the liver, and in the case of some drugs by gut mucosal cells, is known as first-pass metabolism and includes the formation of active metabolites for many psychoactive drugs, a major pharmacokinetic source of interdrug variability. First-pass metabolism is avoided by the sublingual route of administration, where absorption from the oral mucosa (e.g. oro-dispersible olanzapine or risperidone) is very rapid, despite the fact that the surface area available is small. Drugs formulated in this manner are usually nonionic highly lipid soluble preparations. Venous drainage from the mouth is to the superior vena cava, so the drug is protected from first-pass metabolism by the liver. Oral administration, leading to a first-pass effect, results in a decreased amount of parent drug (and the appearance of metabolites) compared with parenteral dosing. Cytochrome P450 (CYP) enzymes located in the luminal epithelium of the small intestine are involved in the metabolism of many drugs (Wilkinson, 1996). For example, up to 43% of orally administered midazolam is metabolised as it passes through the intestinal mucosa (Perloff et al., 2003). CYP3A4 represents approximately 70% of total cytochrome P450 in human intestine; several psychotropic drugs are substrates of this enzyme (Table 25.1).

Elimination

Elimination of drugs from the body takes place largely through renal excretion in an unchanged form by biotransformation in the liver to polar metabolites or both. Drug and metabolite elimination half-lives are indicative of the speed of washout from the body, informing, for example, the speed of switching from fluoxetine to a monoamine oxidase inhibitor such that the serotonergic syndrome is avoided (see Chapter 27).

There are two phases in the metabolism of lipid-soluble drugs by the liver to more water-soluble molecules, which are then excreted by the kidney. Phase I metabolism includes oxidation, reduction and hydroxylation, resulting in a more polar compound. Phase II metabolism consists of conjugation reactions, including glucuronidation, sulphonidation and N-acetylation. The most important phase I enzymes are microsomal cytochrome P450 isoenzymes. Other phase I metabolism enzymes include the flavin mono-oxygenases (e.g. FMO III). Induction or inhibition of the cytochrome P450 system is a common mechanism of drug-drug interaction. For example, CYP3A is inducible by drugs and dietary constituents such as carbamazepine, or alcohol, and inhibited by cimetidine, fluoxetine or grapefruit juice.

The *elimination half-life* ($t_{1/2}$) is the time taken for the plasma concentration to fall by one half. The decline of the drug's concentration in plasma is ascertained by multiple blood sampling (Figure 25.1). Knowledge of a drug's $t_{1/2}$ is essential for informing the frequency of drug administration (DeVane & Jusko, 1982). The *clearance* of a drug is the volume of plasma or other fluid from which drug is irreversibly removed per unit of time as it passes through the liver or any other eliminating organ; extraction occurs as blood travels through the organ. If a drug is eliminated by a number of organs, the total clearance is an additive function of the clearances by all the individual organs. When the drug dose and bioavailability are constant, clearance is the pharmacokinetic parameter that determines the *extent* of drug accumulation in the body. In contrast, $t_{1/2}$ is reflected in the *rate* of drug accumulation.

During a multiple drug dosing regimen, *steady-state* is attained through drug accumulation, with drug eliminated being replaced by an equivalent amount of newly administered drug. The time required from the first administered dose until reaching steady-state is approximately four to five half-lives (i.e., $5\, t_{1/2}$). The term steady-state is a misnomer in that a true drug steady-state occurs only with a constant-rate intravenous infusion. Even at "steady-state", owing to the concurrent processes of drug absorption, distribution and elimination, the drug concentrations will vary in plasma, with a peak and trough concentration occurring within each dosage interval. The average steady-state concentration is between the peak and trough levels and is determined by the daily dose and the drug's total body clearance.

Table 25.1 Psychotropic substrates of cytochrome (C4)P enzymes

1A2	2C19	2C9	2D6	2E1	3A4,5,7
clozapine	amitriptyline	phenytoin	amitriptylline	ethanol	alprazolam
haloperidol	clomipramine		clomipramine		buspirone
imipramine	diazepam		clozapine		carbamazepine
mirtazapine	phenytoin		codeine		clozapine
olanzapine			desipramine		clozapine
tacrine			donepezil		diazepam
			haloperidol		donepezil
			imipramine		galantamine
			methadone		haloperidol
			risperidone		methadone
			thioridazine		midazolam
			trazodone		mirtazapine
			venlafaxine		risperidone
					sildenafil
					trazodone
					triazolam
					valproate
					venlafaxine
					zaleplon
					zolpidem
					zopiclone

			CYP450 INHIBITORS		
1A2	**2C19**	**2C9**	**2D6**	**2E1**	**3A4,5,7**
fluvoxamine	fluoxetine		chlorpromazine	disulfiram	fluoxetine
paroxetine	fluvoxamine		citalopram		fluvoxamine
	sertraline		clomipramine		nefazodone
			fluoxetine		paroxetine
			fluphenazine		sertraline
			haloperidol		tricyclics
			methadone		
			paroxetine		
			sertaline		

			CYP450 INDUCERS		
1A2	**2C19**	**2C9**	**2D6**	**2E1**	**3A4,5,7**
carbamazepine	phenytoin	secobarbital	carbamazepine	ethanol	carbamazepine
phenobarbitone			phenytoin		phenobarbital
phenytoin					phenytoin
tobacco					

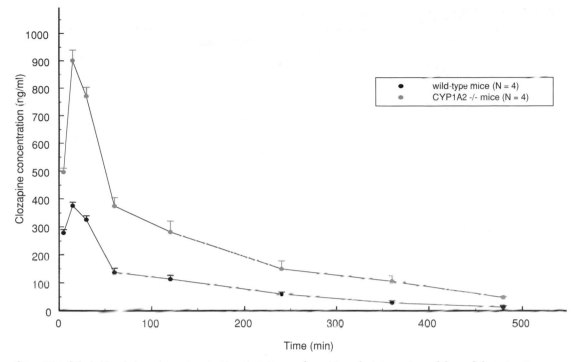

Figure 25.1 Whole blood clozapine concentration–time curves after a 10 mg/kg intraperitoneal dose of clozapine to male wild-type and CYP1A2 -/- mice, administered at time 0. Mean values ± SD are given (adapted from Altchison *et al.*, 2000).

Selection of an appropriate drug dosage regimen must consider both the dose of drug to be administered and the frequency (Baumann *et al.*, 2004). Some drugs with $t_{1/2}$ long enough to be administered once daily, such as clozapine, may not be suitable for administration every 24 hours, because toxicity could be precipitated by the excessive peak concentration that would result from the larger doses. Clozapine is usually given twice daily, thus avoiding peak concentrations that might predispose to adverse effects, including seizure activity (Aitchison, Jann *et al.*, 2000).

Pharmacodynamics

Drugs exert their pharmacological, physiological and behavioural effects by interacting with either extracellular or intracellular target sites. The term *pharmacodynamics* describes the study of these interactions and involves the exploration of mechanisms of drug action at the molecular level. *Receptors* are usually macromolecular proteins or glycoprotein sites in the cell membrane, the cytoplasm or the nucleus of a cell, where a biologically active, naturally occurring endogenous mediator (called a *ligand* or a *neurotransmitter*) binds (Figure 25.2). In the CNS, drug occupancy of a receptor on the surface of a neurone leads to a functional effect in the neurone, resulting in the drug's characteristic pharmacological response (Figure 25.3). Ligand-receptor binding is usually both ionic and reversible, and the strength of this ionic attachment is determined by the tightness of the fit of the three-dimensional structure of the drug to the three-dimensional site on the receptor. Each receptor is a unique protein

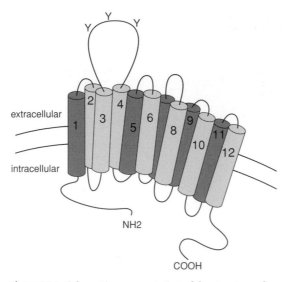

Figure 25.2 Schematic representation of the structure of the dopamine transporter (DAT). The 12 transmembrane domains (1-12) and the intracellular NH2- and COOH-termini have been labelled, as have the glycosylation sites on the second extracellular loop. The green and grey segments depict the domains of the DAT encoded by successive exons (adapted from Bannon *et al.*, 2000).

molecule characterised by the ability to recognise a specific neurotransmitter, but one neurotransmitter may bind to more than one receptor protein. For example, there at least five structurally related receptor molecules that bind dopamine (Table 25.2) and at least 18 that bind serotonin.

Upon binding of a drug to a receptor site, several possible actions may follow, for example:

1. The drug may mimic the action of the neurotransmitter acting as an *agonist* for this receptor (e.g. bromocriptine at dopamine receptors);

2. The drug may bind to a site near the binding site for the neurotransmitter, facilitating the transmitter, binding, again acting as an agonist, or *allosteric modulator* (e.g. benzodiazepines at gamma-aminobutyric acid [GABA]$_A$ receptors);

3. The drug may act as an *antagonist* by binding to the receptor site normally occupied by the neurotransmitter, but blocking neurotransmitter action to its binding site and inhibiting the neurotransmitter's normal physiological action (e.g. haloperidol at D$_2$ receptors); or

4. The drug may produce an effect opposite to that of the agonist by occupying the same receptor, i.e. it may act as an *inverse agonist*.

Competitive antagonists bind to the same receptor as an agonist but do not produce the conformational changes in the receptor that lead to signal transduction. Higher concentrations of an agonist are therefore required in the presence of an antagonist to produce the same effect as in the absence of that antagonist. *Irreversible inhibitors* bind to the same site as the agonist and remain there. *Noncompetitive antagonists* bind to a different site to that occupied by an agonist. *Partial agonists* are drugs which stimulate receptors to a lesser extent than full agonists but which act as antagonists in the presence of a full agonist (e.g. aripiprazole is a partial agonist at D$_2$ and 5HT$_{1A}$ receptors).

Dose-response curves have been widely used to plot biological response (effect size) to a drug against the logarithm of the dose administered. Such a graphical plot produces a sigmoidal dose-response curve (Figure 25.4). The linear portion usually lies between 20% and 80% of the maximal response. Dose-response curves may be used to derive important characteristics such as potency, efficacy and slope. *Potency* refers to the absolute number of molecules of drug required to elicit a response and is a measure of the dose required. The location of the dose-response curve along the horizontal axis reflects the potency of the drug. *Variability* and *slope* refer to individual differences in drug response, with some persons responding at very low doses and some requiring much more drug. For example, a steep slope on a dose-response curve implies that there is only a small difference between the doses that produce a minimal and a maximal (E$_{max}$) effect. The latter is observed as a plateau in the sigmoid curve. *Efficacy* refers to the maximum effect obtainable, with additional doses producing no more effect. It is reflected by the *peak*

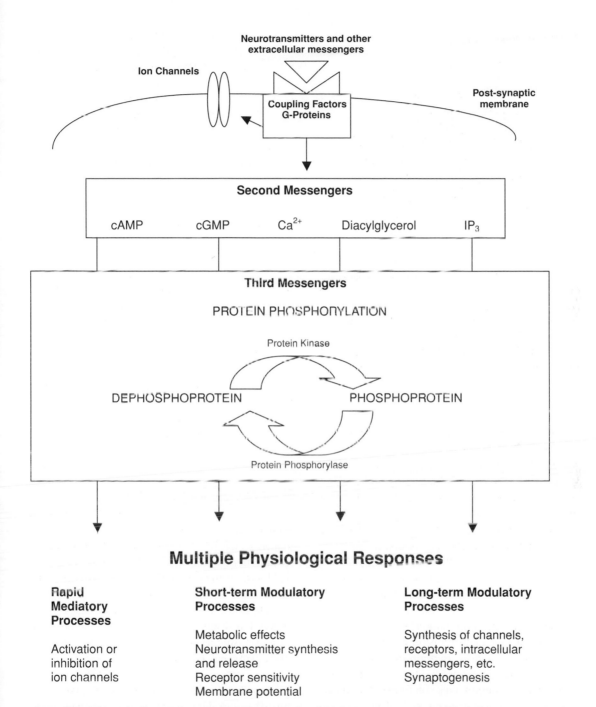

Figure 25.3 Schematic of neurotransmitter binding, second and third messengers, and physiological responses.

Table 25.2 Properties of cloned dopamine receptor subtypes

	D1	D5	D2S/D2L	D3	D4
Amino acids	446	477	415/444	400	387
Chromosome	5	4	11	3	11
Effector pathways	↑cAMP	↑cAMP	↓cAMP ↑K^+ channel ↓Ca^{2+} channel	↓cAMP	↓cAMP ↑K^+ channel
mRNA distribution	caudate, putamen, nucleus accumbens, olfactory tubercle	hippocampus, hypothalamus	caudate, putamen, nucleus accumbens, olfactory tubercle	olfactory tubercle, hypothalamus, nucleus accumbens	frontal cortex, medulla, midbrain

Adapted from Kuhar *et al.* (1999). cAMP = cyclic adenosine monophosphate; D1, D2S, D2L, D3, D4, D5 = dopamine receptor 1, 2 short, 2 long, 3, 4, and 5, respectively.

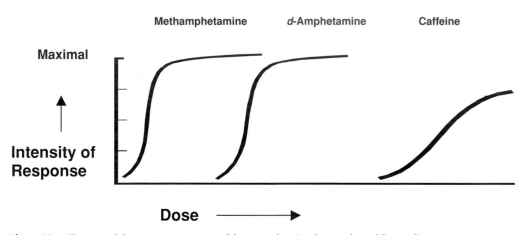

Figure 25.4 Theoretical dose-response curves of three psychostimulants (adapted from Julien, 2000).

of the dose-response curve and is an inherent property of a drug. Figure 25.4 illustrates theoretical dose-response curves for three psychostimulants demonstrating equal efficacy of methamphetamine and dextroamphetamine, increased potency of methamphetamine and reduced potency and efficacy of caffeine.

The dose of a drug that produces a specific response varies considerably between individuals. Interpatient variability can result from differences in rates of drug absorption and metabolism, as well as multiple other factors, including previous drug use and physical, psychological and emotional state. It follows a normal (Gaussian) distribution unless a specific population of individuals with, for example, a genetically predetermined pattern, skew this distribution by exhibiting a unique pattern of responsiveness (e.g., see *CYP2D6* metaboliser status under Pharmacogenetics later in this chapter). The dose of a drug that produces the desired effect in 50% of subjects is termed the ED_{50}, and the lethal dose for 50% of the subjects is the LD_{50}. In drug development, both the ED_{50} and the LD_{50} are determined in several species of animals to prevent accidental drug-induced toxicity in humans. The ratio of the LD_{50} to the ED_{50} is called the *therapeutic index* and is used as an index of the relative safety of the drug. For example, lithium has a narrow therapeutic index.

Dose-response curves represent the biological response to a drug but these data alone cannot provide estimates of ligand binding affinity or receptor dynamics and occupancy. If D represents the drug, R the receptor and RD the receptor-drug complex,

$$D + R = DR$$

at equilibrium, the association constant K_{-1} must equal the dissociation rate constant K_1, and therefore, the equilibrium binding constant K_D can be derived:

$$\{[D] \times [R]\}/[DR] = K_1/K_{-1} = K_D$$

Using radiolabelled ligands, the value of K_D can be inferred by measuring the concentrations of bound [DR] and free [D] drug. This technique can also be used to measure how well competitive antagonists can displace agonist ligands, as well as to derive a value for the concentration required to displace 50% of the ligand, the IC_{50}. The IC_{50} value depends on the concentration of agonist in the assay but can be used to derive the equilibrium dissociation constant (K_1), which will be constant for any given concentration of drug.

The tricyclic antidepressants (TCAs) can be used as an illustrative example of pharmacodynamics. All TCAs have a propensity to block the uptake of noradrenaline and serotonin to some degree but show differential selectivity for noradrenaline (e.g. desipramine) and serotonin (e.g. clomipramine). It is generally accepted that TCAs bind to "TCA receptors", represented by the monoamine transporter complexes. TCAs, however, have a number of other pharmacological actions. Most TCAs possess antimuscarinic activity (giving rise to dry mouth, blurred vision or constipation), amitriptyline being more potent at M_1 receptors than desipramine. Antimuscarinic activity can be exacerbated by other anticholinergic drugs such as antihistamines or antipsychotics, potentially leading to cognitive impairment and constipation. Moreover, blockade of α_1-adrenoceptors may lead to postural hypotension, and can be exacerbated by other α_1 blockers and by antihypertensive drugs in general. Alpha$_1$ as well as H_1 histamine receptor blockade is thought to underlie the sedative effects produced by doxepine, trimipramine and amitriptyline, which have the highest affinities among TCAs for both of these receptors. Of note, H_1 blockade may be potentiated by alcohol and other sedative drugs, leading to respiratory depression. Despite the relative lack of affinity for the dopamine transporter or the dopamine receptors in the TCA group as a whole, amoxapine has been shown to block D_2 receptors; it is this action that is thought to be responsible for the extrapyramidal side effects associated with this agent. Some TCAs that are relatively pro-serotonergic (e.g. amitriptyline, clomipramine) could potentially give rise to the serotonin syndrome, if co-administered with other serotonergic drugs such as the selective serotonin reuptake inhibitors, tramadol or selegiline. Box 25.1 summarises particular side effects associated with specific receptor blockade.

Another commonly used class of psychotropic medications is the benzodiazepines. These compounds act through their effects as agonists at the $GABA_A$ receptor. Interestingly, affinity for the receptor in vitro correlates with antianxiety potency in vivo. All benzodiazepines exhibit antianxiety, anticonvulsant and sedative/hypnotic effects, whereas inhibition of afferent pathways in the spinal cord results in relaxation of skeletal muscles. The predominant effect of a specific benzodiazepine depends on the tissue concentration and its relative affinity for the receptor. Anxiolysis occurs at low tissue levels, whereas sedation occurs at high levels. In addition, tolerance develops to many of their effects. The most likely mechanism for the development of tolerance is believed to be through pharmacodynamic factors influencing the reduction of benzodiazepine receptors or the sensitivity to chronic treatment (or both), in addition to disturbing the modulatory action of benzodiazepine agonism on the $GABA_A$ complex. Differences in intrinsic potency among the different

---

Box 25.1 Receptor blockade and associated side effects

Receptor	Side effect
Dopamine D_2	*Nigrostriatal tract:* Extrapyramidal effects (e.g. Parkinsonism, dystonias, dyskynesias, akathisia) *Mesocortical tract:* Negative symptoms, cognitive impairment *Tuberoinfundibular tract:* Hyperprolactinaemia (resulting in, e.g., sexual dysfunction, galactorrhoea, gynaecomastia)
Muscarinic (M_1)	*Central:* cognitive impairment, delirium *Peripheral:* constipation, dry mouth, blurred vision, etc.
Histamine (H_1)	Sedation, weight gain
Adrenergic (α_1)	Postural hypotension

---

benzodiazepine compounds are determined by a particular benzodiazepine's ability to bind to a receptor; benzodiazepines with a higher affinity for the receptor are more potent and hence require a smaller dose to achieve the same effect. The most important interaction is with alcohol, which potentiates CNS depression through its effect as an agonist at the alcohol receptor site on the same receptor complex that benzodiazepines act on, the $GABA_A$ receptor. Fatality from overdose of a benzodiazepine most often occurs if it is combined with alcohol or other CNS depressants.

Behavioural pharmacology

Many advances in medical knowledge and treatment have relied on work with laboratory animals. In using animal models, systems and behaviours existing in one species are examined and knowledge is extrapolated to humans. Animal models are used to evaluate pathogenic mechanisms and diagnostic and therapeutic procedures. The validity in terms of "extrapolatability" of results generated depends on how well the animal model has been selected. Animal models used in neuroscience seek to model human behaviour and disorder. Animal models may be *exploratory*, *explanatory* or *predictive*. *Exploratory* models aim to investigate a biological mechanism, whereas *explanatory* models aim to understand in more depth a complex biological phenomenon. *Predictive* models have the aim of discovering and quantifying the impact of a drug, in terms of both toxicity and efficacy. The extent of resemblance of the biological structure or system or response in the animal with the corresponding item in humans has been termed *fidelity*. What is often more important, however, is the discriminating ability of models (i.e. the similarity between humans and model species with respect to the relevant biological mechanism), especially in the case of predictive models. Often the two go hand in hand, with high-fidelity models offering the best opportunity to study a particular biological function.

The recent completion of the mouse and human genomic sequences has greatly facilitated research in genomics and proteomics. Using high-density microarray DNA chip technology in humans as well as in animals, it is possible to investigate which genes are differentially expressed in different diseases or behavioural phenotypes. This paves the way for a range of new mouse models with homology between animal and human (*construct validity*) for genotype as well as for phenotype, which are being used increasingly to study not only genetic aetiological factors but also the effects of manipulation of genetic pathways, gene-gene interactions and gene-environment interactions. However, it should be remembered that no single animal model can ever duplicate the original condition and that models at best offer an approximation. Some of the factors to be considered when choosing an animal model are listed in Box 25.2.

The most popular species for animal models have been the mouse and the rat. This is likely

Box 25.2 General considerations in the choice of animal models

Appropriateness as an analogue

Transferability and generalisability of results

Genetic and phenotypic uniformity (e.g. if an inbred strain)

Background knowledge of biological properties

Cost and availability

Ease of and adaptability to experimental manipulation

Ecological consequences

Ethical implications

Animal housing considerations, including size of animal, numbers needed, lifespan, sex

Appropriate age of animal for the manipulation and/or behavioural testing

Progeny needed

Special features of the animal, such as unique responses or microflora, that may make a particular species useful

Diseases or conditions that might complicate results

to continue owing to the availability of genomic sequence techniques that have been developed to use rodents as models to date, as well as availability of investigative tools, including rodent gene expression arrays. In the case of animal models for neuropsychiatric diseases, knockout and transgenic strategies have become prominent. In most such models, the aetiology of the disease is mimicked, but in psychiatry, aetiology is frequently poorly understood. For example, developing animal models for schizophrenia requires not only appropriate causal factor(s) but also appropriate read-out phenotype(s). Hallucinations and delusions cannot be used as read-out parameters in animals, whereas parameters such as dysregulation of sensory gating mechanisms, including acoustic startle, prepulse inhibition and latent inhibition (which are also disrupted in patients with schizophrenia; see Chapter 13), can be more objectively measured in animals (Geyer & Braff, 1987; Lubow, 2005; Swerdlow et al., 1986).

Given the plethora of data implicating dopamine transmission aberrations in schizophrenia, it is no surprise that dopamine has been a primary target for manipulations leading to genetically altered animals with relevance to schizophrenia. Dopamine transporter (DAT) knock-out mice, for example, show behavioural abnormalities possibly relevant to schizophrenia, including increased response to novel stimuli, stereotyped behaviour and decreased prepulse inhibition (Ralph et al., 2001), but do not show deficits in social interaction (Spielewoy et al., 2000), and amphetamine has a paradoxically calming effect in these mice (Gainetdinov et al., 1999). It has therefore recently been suggested that these mice may have more relevance for attention-deficit hyperactivity disorder (ADHD) than for schizophrenia (Gainetdinov & Caron, 2001). In addition, there are several models arising from targeted mutations elsewhere in the dopamine and in the glutamate systems (Ellenbroek, 2003).

Animal models of schizophrenia focussing on a specific environmental factor have also been developed and include prenatal stress (Koenig et al., 2002), corticosterone treatment (Diaz et al., 1997), lipopolysaccharide treatment (Borrell et al., 2002) and perinatal manipulations (L-nitroarginine treatment; Black et al., 1999) or early lesioning of the amygdala (Wolterinck et al., 2000). Schizophrenia is thought to result from an interaction of genetic and environmental factors, however. A neurodevelopmental model of schizophrenia has been developing by lesioning the hippocampus of Sprague-Dawley and Fischer 344 rats early in life with ibotenic acid (Lipska & Weinberger, 1995). The model appears to mimic a spectrum of neurobiological and behavioural features of schizophrenia, including functional pathology in presumably critical brain regions interconnected with the hippocampal formation and targeted by antipsychotic drugs (the striatum/nucleus accumbens and the prefrontal cortex). At postnatal periods equivalent to puberty or early adulthood, this is associated with the emergence of abnormalities in a number of dopamine-related behaviours. It has been postulated that even transient inactivation of the ventral hippocampus during a critical period of development that produces subtle anatomical changes in the hippocampus may be sufficient to disrupt normal maturation of the prefrontal cortex and trigger behavioural changes similar to those observed in animals with a demonstrable excitotoxic lesion (Lipska & Weinberger, 2002).

Despite the difficulties in translating human affective disorders into relevant tests in animals, there are several animal models of depression or at least of models of some core symptoms of depression (Cryan & Mombereau, 2004). Current paradigms for assessing antidepressant or depression-like behaviours in mice include the forced swim test (Porsolt *et al.*, 1977), the tail suspension test (Porsolt *et al.*, 1987), olfactory bulbectomy (Otmakhova *et al.*, 1992), learned helplessness (Anisman *et al.*, 1975), chronic mild stress (Harkin *et al.*, 2002) and drug-withdrawal-induced anhedonia (Cryan *et al.*, 2003).

Pharmacogenetics

Pharmacogenetics focuses on the study of gene-drug interactions and examines the extent to which variability in an individual's genetic makeup is responsible for the differences in therapeutic efficacy and adverse effects between individuals. The term *pharmacogenomics* encompasses pharmacogenetics. It refers to a genomewide search for genes and their products relevant for the application of drugs in humans, including genes determining disease susceptibility or causing interindividual variations in drug response, based on the knowledge derived from the Human Genome Project (Aitchison & Gill, 2002). Both pharmacogenetics and pharmacogenomics share the same goal, in that they seek to guide pharmacotherapy and improve outcomes by enabling individualised treatment decisions. In the medium to long term, pharmacogenomics aims to develop novel diagnostics accompanying therapeutic products for effective and safe individualised drug prescription. Both fields therefore hold great potential, particularly in psychiatry, for which biologically based treatment guidelines are lacking.

Pharmacokinetic and pharmacodynamic factors

Candidate genes for pharmacogenetic studies include polymorphic drug metabolising enzymes (DMEs), drug transporters and polymorphic drug targets affecting disease-related pathways (Table 25.3).

Pharmacogenetics of antipsychotic treatment

There is increasing evidence to suggest that *CYP2D6* genotype might partially affect response and side effects to typical antipsychotics. On average, Asians develop higher plasma levels for relevant antipsychotics (e.g., haloperidol) than Europeans and thus seem to have an increased sensitivity to these medications (Aitchison, Jordan, *et al.*, 2000). Studies of response to antipsychotics have focused largely on genes that code for neuronal targets of these drugs, such as the dopaminergic D_2, D_3 and D_4 receptors (*DRD2*, *DRD3* and *DRD4*), the serotonergic 5-HT_{2A} (*HTR2A*), 5-HT_{2C} (*HTR2C*) and 5-HT_6 (*HTR6*) receptors, the histaminergic H_1 and H_2 receptors (*H₁* and *H₂*), the muscarinic cholinergic receptors, neurotransmitter transporters and other intracellular signalling molecules. Clozapine has been shown to be efficacious in improving both positive and negative symptoms of schizophrenia in up to two thirds of cases refractory to treatment with other antipsychotics. Clozapine exhibits large interindividual variations in bioavailability, steady-state plasma concentrations and clearance. It is metabolised by several CYP enzymes, including CYP1A2, CYP3A4 and CYP2C19 but not significantly in vivo by CYP2D6 (Collier, 2003). Aitchison, Jann, *et al.* (2000) demonstrated in a study with wild-type versus CYP1A2-null mice that clozapine is primarily metabolised by CYP1A2, CYP1A2 being responsible for more than 60% of the clearance of clozapine in the wild-type mice. *CYP1A2* is highly homologous between man and mouse. These results suggested that *CYP1A2* might be worth studying as a candidate gene versus clozapine response, and early reports in this field are encouraging (Basu *et al.*, 2004). There

Table 25.3 Individual variability in drug response can often be understood as a combination of factors affecting the pharmacokinetic and pharmacodynamic effects of drugs

Pharmacokinetics [Absorption, distribution, metabolism, elimination]	+	Pharmacodynamics [Drug targets, disease-associated pathways]	−	Drug response

Drug metabolising enzymes

Phase I
* P450 enzymes (CYP2D6, CYP1A2, CYP2C9, CYP2C19, CYP3A4, etc.)
* Epoxide hydrolases (EHs)
* Flavine-dependent mono-oxygenases (FMOs)
* Alcohol dehydrogenase (ADH)
* Butyrylcholinesterase
* Dihydropyrimidine dehydrogenase (DPD)

Phase II
* UDP-glucoronosyltransferases (UGTs)
* Glutathione-S-transferases (GSTs)
* Catechol-O-methyltransferase (COMT)
* N-acetyltransferases (NAT1 & NAT2)
* Thiopurine S-methyltransferase (TPMT)
* NAD(P)H quinone oxidoreductase (QOR)
* Microsomal epoxide hydrolase (mEH)

Drug transporters
* Multidrug transporter P-glycoprotein (Pgp), the product of the MDR1 gene
* Serotonin transporter (5-HTT), the product of the SLC6A4 gene

Receptors
* Dopamine, serotonin, noradrenalin, etc.

Enzymes
* ALOX5 (5-lipoxygenase)
* ACE (angiotensin converting enzyme)
* MAO (monoamine oxidase)

Ion channels
* MiRP1 (MinK-related peptide 1 subunit of I_{kr} potassium channels in cardiac muscle)

Lipoproteins
* ApoE (apolipoprotein E)

Transcription factors
* Bcl-2 (B-cell lymphoma protein 2, a target for the polyoma virus enhancer binding protein 2β gene [PEP2β])

Cell cycle control
* BDNF (brain-derived neurotrophic factor)

Signal transduction
* Gβ3 (G − protein β3)

are only a few reports on pharmacogenetic studies based on the metabolic pathways of other atypical antipsychotics such as risperidone, olanzapine and quetiapine (Staddon et al., 2002).

Dopamine receptors

The dopamine D_2 receptor is a major site of action of antipsychotics, but a functional polymorphism (-141C Ins/Del) affecting promoter activity and DRD2 expression was not shown to be associated with clinical response to clozapine, in contrast to reports of missense variants (Val96Ala, Pro310Ser and Ser311Cys) being associated with response to various antipsychotics, including clozapine (Malhotra, 2004). Furthermore, the DRD3 Ser9Gly variant has been associated with response to typical

antipsychotics, but association with response to clozapine remains controversial (Shaikh & Kerwin, 2002). Several studies on the association of a variable tandem repeat polymorphism (VNTR) in exon 3 of DRD4 have been carried out and, somewhat surprisingly given the relatively high affinity of clozapine for the dopamine D_4 receptor, suggest that this polymorphism does not seem to correlate with the degree of response to clozapine, in contrast to the positive association between this polymorphism and a rapid response to acute treatment with typical antipsychotics (Kaiser et al., 2000).

Serotonin receptors

In addition to the undoubted pivotal role of dopamine in the mechanism of action of antipsychotics, serotonin (5-HT)-mediated mechanisms may be involved in the action of atypical antipsychotics (Meltzer, 1995). Several lines of research have implicated the 5-HT_{2A}, 5-HT_{2C}, 5-HT_{5A} and 5-HT_6 receptors in response to treatment in schizophrenia (Collier & Li, 2003). A strong association reported between the 102T>C polymorphism in *HTR2A* and response to clozapine (Arranz *et al.*, 1996) was not replicated by others (Masellis *et al.*, 1998), but a meta-analysis indicated that the 102T>C silent polymorphism appears to be associated with response to clozapine (Arranz *et al.*, 1998). Similarly, the *HTR2A*-1438G/A polymorphism, which appears to be in linkage disequilibrium with the 102T>C SNP, has been associated with response to clozapine (Masellis *et al.*, 1998). These polymorphisms have also been associated with response to typical antipsychotics (Joober *et al.*, 1999) and risperidone (Lane *et al.*, 2002). Positive associations have also been reported between the *HTR2A* amino acid substitution His452Tyr variant of potential functional significance and clozapine response (Arranz *et al.*, 1996; Masellis *et al.*, 1998). An association has also been reported between a potentially functional Cys23Ser amino acid change in *HTR2C* and clozapine response (Sodhi *et al.*, 1995) but other studies have failed to replicate this finding (Masellis *et al.*, 1998). Furthermore, investigation of the 5-HT_5 and the 5-HT_6 receptor genes has pointed towards a minor contributing role to response to treatment with clozapine (Birkett *et al*, 2000; Yu *et al.*, 1999).

Pharmacogenetic prediction of antipsychotic response

Arranz and colleagues (2000) performed association studies in multiple candidate genes in an attempt to find the combination of polymorphisms that gave the best predictive value of response to clozapine in patients with schizophrenia. On the basis of clozapine binding profiles, 19 genetic polymorphisms in eight receptor subtype genes, including the α_{2A}-adrenoceptor (*ADRA2A*), *DRD3*, *HTR2A*, *HTR2C*, *HTR3A*, *HTR5A*, H_1, H_2 and the serotonin transporter (*5-HT*) genes were studied. A combination of six polymorphisms showing the strongest association with response (*HTR2A* 102T>C and His452Tyr, *HTR2C* -330GT/-244CT and Cys23Ser, *5-HTTLPR*, H_2_1018G>A) gave a level of prediction of 76.86% ($\chi^2 = 35.8$, $p = 0.0001$) and a sensitivity of 95.89 (± 0.04) for the prediction of patients likely to show a satisfactory improvement with treatment. This finding was the first to report on the use of combinations of pharmacodynamic factor gene polymorphisms to predict the response to antipsychotic medication. The results were not, however, corrected for multiple testing, and an attempt at replicating this finding has not supported the initial finding (Schumacher *et al.*, 2000).

Preliminary results from the same group (Clark *et al.*, 2003) showed that in 92 Spanish patients, a combination of polymorphisms in the genes coding for *HTR2C*, *HTR2A*, *DRD3*, *5-HTT* (in the latter, a VNTR in the promoter also known as the *5-HTTLPR*) might be useful for the prediction of response to treatment with olanzapine (positive value [PPV] = 76%, negative predictive value [NPV] = 79%, sensitivity = 82%, specificity = 72%, $p = 0.07$). However, likewise, these results were not corrected for multiple testing. Similar studies have been performed for the response to risperidone, but in smaller groups. If the studies described here are replicated, such methodology could form the basis for pharmacogenetic prediction tests for response to various antipsychotics.

Adverse effects of antipsychotic treatment

Extrapyramidal symptoms and early stage side effects of antipsychotic therapy, such as *postural hypotension* and excess sedation, have been reported to be associated with overrepresentation of poor metabolisers (PMs) of *CYP2D6*.

Tardive dyskinesia (TD) is an involuntary movement disorder manifested typically in the orofacial area but frequently extending to the limbs and the trunk. Susceptibility to the development of TD is currently thought to have a genetic basis and a positive association between the development of TD and a polymorphism (-164C>A) in the first intron of *CYP1A2* has been reported (Basile *et al.*, 2000) but not replicated (Schulze *et al.*, 2001). A recent meta-analysis (Lerer *et al.*, 2002) has reported an association between the *DRD3* Ser9Gly polymorphism with TD in a large sample of 780 patients treated with typical antipsychotics. Ozdemir *et al.* (2001) showed that those patients who exhibited the at-risk genotype at both *DRD3* (Gly/Gly) and *CYP1A2* (C/C) had the most severe TD. Following the same rationale, Zhang and colleagues (2003) recently reported a possible synergistic effect of the *DRD3* Ser9Gly polymorphism and a marker in the manganese superoxide dismutase gene (*MnSO*, the enzyme that catalyses the dismutation reaction of the toxic superoxide radical to molecular oxygen and hydrogen peroxide and thus forms a crucial part of the cellular antioxidant defence mechanism) in susceptibility to TD. Acute akathisia has also been reported to be associated with polymorphisms in *DRD3* (Eichhammer *et al.*, 2000; Garcia-Barcelo *et al.*, 2001). *MnSO* alone has also been shown to be weakly associated with TD. The contribution of 10 polymorphic sites in six candidate dopaminergic and serotonergic genes to the development of TD was examined in a small Jewish sample (total $N = 122$, $n = 59$ with and $n = 63$ without TD), with only the dopamine transporter gene (*DAT*) 3′ VNTR polymorphism, the serotonin transporter-linked polymorphic region (*5-HTTLPR*) and the tryptophan hydroxylase (*TPH*) intron 7 polymorphism yielding trends towards a positive association (Segman *et al.*, 2003).

Antipsychotic-induced *hyperprolactinaemia* was shown to be associated with the *DRD2* Taq1A polymorphism (Mihara *et al.*, 2000), and a significant association between *DRD2*–141C and hyperprolactinaemia, consistent with *in vitro* work, has been demonstrated; this association was strengthened by controlling for *CYP2D6* genotypic category ($p = 0.023$; Aitchison *et al.*, 2003).

Among antipsychotics, clozapine appears to be associated with the greatest potential to exacerbate *weight gain*. It is currently thought that weight gain induced by clozapine and other antipsychotics (typical and atypical) results from multiple neurobiological and endocrine effects, leading to changes in appetite and feeding behaviour, as well as metabolic changes (e.g. changes in leptin and adiponectin). Ten genetic polymorphisms across nine candidate genes (*HTR2C, HTR2A, HTR1A*, the H_1 and H_2 genes, *CYP1A2*, the adrenergic receptor genes and the tumour necrosis factor α gene *TNFα*), involved in both central hypothalamic weight regulation and peripheral thermogenic pathways were investigated for an association with weight gain (Basile *et al.*, 2001). Only four of these genes (*ADRB3, ADRA1A, TNFα* and *HTR2C*) demonstrated a modest, nonsignificant trend towards a positive association with clozapine-induced weight gain. A positive association between a promoter polymorphism (-759C>T), thought to alter *HTR2C* gene expression, has also been reported (Miller *et al.*, 2005; Reynolds *et al.*, 2002, 2003), but several studies failed to replicate this association (Basile *et al.*, 2002; Theisen *et al.*, 2004; Tsai *et al.*, 2002)

Clozapine-induced agranulocytosis has been associated with a dominant gene within the major histocompatibility complex region, marked by heat-shock protein 70-1 and 70–2 variants. This finding was, however, reported in two Jewish studies with small power. In a more recent study, clozapine-induced agranulocytosis was significantly associated with some human leukocyte antigen (HLA) polymorphisms, and age seemed to be a further major risk factor for clozapine-induced agranulocytosis (Dettling *et al.*, 2001). Thus HLA loci may serve as genetic markers to identify subjects of different ethnicities prone to this severe idiosyncratic drug reaction. Preliminary data from an industry-sponsored study aiming to identify genetic markers predictive of clozapine induced agranulocytosis (CARING) has identified a positive association with five markers, including two markers in the HLA region (Athanasiou, 2005).

Ethical considerations

The emergence of pharmacogenetics is about to mark a new era in clinical psychiatry in which genotype or other biomarkers may influence choice of therapy, increasing the safety and efficacy of commonly used medications. The ethical issues that

Box 25.3 Ethical issues in pharmacogenetics

Oversight and approval of pharmacogenetic tests by major national regulatory bodies, such as the Medicines Control Agency (MCA) in the United Kingdom

- more than 500 pharmaceutical company and government representatives from around the world met to discuss the U.S. Food and Drug Administration's draft guidance for industry on pharmacogenomics data submission (Abbott, 2003)

Appropriate protection for privacy and confidentiality crucial

- pharmacogenetic tests can carry several types of potentially psychosocially harmful secondary information
- genotype-based information about drug response may inform prognosis

Information on poor drug response could affect the individual's

- treatability for certain illnesses
- health insurance status

Participation in pharmacogenetic research requires informed consent. Subjects should be fully informed of

- the need to obtain DNA for research
- the protections of confidentiality and privacy (including how the sample and test results will be stored and their privacy and confidentiality maintained)
- whether additional research may be done in the future
- the risks and benefits of providing DNA
- whether research results will be disclosed to the subject

Box 25.4 Causes of discrepant results among different association studies on the same problem (adapted from Meisel *et al.*, 2003)

Random errors

- multiple testing
- inappropriate sample size
- inappropriate selection of genetic variants
- errors in genotyping

Confounding and bias

- genetic heterogeneity (the phenotype is affected by variants in numerous genes)
- aetiological heterogeneity (several causes lead to the same phenotype)
- differences in ethnic background within the population studied
- population stratification (different subgroups, with different allele frequencies); lack of recognition of population stratification may lead to spurious allelic association with phenotype
- inappropriate or missing consideration of haplotypes
- intermixing of incident and prevalent cases of the same phenotype
- inappropriate control groups

Effect modifications and interactions

- undefined gene-gene interactions
- undefined gene-environment interactions

arise from pharmacogenetic research and its clinical applications (Box 25.3), should, however, be addressed before the benefits from treatment individualisation can be realised (Buchanan *et al.*, 2002).

Limitations of pharmacogenetic studies

In general, earlier studies in the field of pharmacogenetics have tended to suggest stronger gene effects than later ones (Ioannides *et al.*, 2001), which may contribute to a difficulty in replicating findings convincingly. There are other problems, such as publication bias and spurious associations due to explorative multiple testing. Causes of discrepant results among different association studies on the

same psychiatric problem include random errors, confounding and bias and effect modifications and interactions (Box 25.4). The rigorous application of basic epidemiological principles to avoid confounding, misclassification and bias may not be sufficient. Matching according to ethnicity or ethnic homogeneity of the study population are desirable, although these goals are often difficult to achieve in practice, and the effect of possible population stratification may now be determined using genetic techniques (Pritchard *et al.*, 1999, 2000).

Conclusions

In this chapter, we have presented the principles underlying pharmacokinetics, pharmacodynamics, behavioural pharmacology and pharmacogenetics with particular reference to clinical psychiatry. Novel methodological approaches such as high-throughput genotyping techniques, the use of microarray technology and the introduction of sophisticated statistical software packages for data analysis promise to increase understanding significantly in these fields. Such progress should lead to advances in psychopharmacology, with therapeutic agents that offer an improved profile in terms of both efficacy and tolerability.

REFERENCES

Abbott, A. (2003). With your genes? Take one of these, three times a day. *Nature* 425:760–2.

Aitchison, K. J., & Gill, M. (2002). Pharmacogenetics in the postgenomic era. In R. Plomin & J. C. DeFries, eds. *Behavioural Genetics in the Postgenomic Era*. Washington, DC: American Psychological Association, pp. 335–61.

Aitchison, K. J., Jann, M. W., Zhao, J. H., *et al.* (2000). Clozapine pharmacokinetics and pharmacodynamics studied with Cyp1A2-null mice. *J Psychopharmacol* 14:353–9.

Aitchison, K. J., Jordan, B. D., & Sharma, T. (2000). The relevance of ethnic influences on pharmacogenetics to the treatment of psychosis. *Drug Metab Drug Interact* 16:15–38.

Aitchison K. J., Pereira, J., Purcell, S., *et al.* (2003). An association study of DRD2 and CYP2D6 and hyperprolactinaemia. Oral presentation at the International Congress of Schizophrenia Research, Colorado Springs.

Anisman, H. (1975). Acquisition and reversal learning of an active avoidance response in three strains of mice. *Behav Biol* 11:51–6.

Arranz, M. J., Collier, D. A., Munro, J., *et al.* (1996). Analysis of a structural polymorphism in the 5-HT2A receptor and clinical response to clozapine. *Neurosci Lett* 217:177–8.

Arranz, M. J., Munro, J., Birkett, J., *et al.* (2000). Pharmacogenetic prediction of clozapine response. *Lancet* 355:1615–16.

Arranz, M. J., Munro, J., Sham, P., *et al.* (1998). Meta-analysis of studies on genetic variation in 5-HT2A receptors and clozapine response. *Schizophr Res* 32:93–9.

Athanasiou, M. (2005). Data reported at the Fourth Annual Pharmacogenetics in Psychiatry Meeting, New York, 15–16 April 2005.

Basile, V. S., Masellis, M., De Luca, V., *et al.* (2002). -759C/T genetic variation of 5HT(2C) receptor and clozapine-induced weight gain. *Lancet* 360:1790–1.

Basile, V. S., Masellis, M., McIntyre, R. S., *et al.* (2001). Genetic dissection of atypical antipsychotic-induced weight gain: novel preliminary data on the pharmacogenetic puzzle. *J Clin Psychiatry* 62(Suppl 23):45–66.

Basile, V. S., Ozdemir, V., Masellis, M., *et al.* (2000). A functional polymorphism of the cytochrome P450 1A2 (CYP1A2) gene: association with tardive dyskinesia in schizophrenia. *Mol Psychiatry* 5:410–17.

Basu, A., Tsapakis, E. M., Knight, J., *et al.* (2004). An association study of the *CYP1A2* C$_{164}$A and T$_{-3591}$G polymorphisms and response to clozapine. *Schizophr Res* 67(Suppl. 1):52.

Baumann, P., Hiemke, C., Ulrich, S., *et al.* (2004). The AGNP-TDM expert group consensus guidelines: therapeutic drug monitoring in psychiatry. *Pharmacopsychiatry* 37:243–65.

Birkett, J. T., Arranz, M. J., Munro, J., *et al.* (2000). Association analysis of the 5-HT5A gene in depression, psychosis and antipsychotic response. *Neuroreport* 11:2017–20.

Black, M. D., Selk, D. E., Hitchcock, J. M., *et al.* (1999). On the effect of neonatal nitric oxide synthase inhibition in rats: a potential neurodevelopmental model of schizophrenia. *Neuropharmacology* 38:1299–1306.

Borrell, J., Vela, J. M., Arevalo-Martin, A., *et al.* (2002). Prenatal immune challenge disrupts sensorimotor gating in adult rats. Implications for the etiopathogenesis of schizophrenia. *Neuropsychopharmacology* 26:204–15.

Buchanan, A., Califano, A., & Kahn, J., *et al.* (2002). Pharmacogenetics: ethical issues and policy options. *Kennedy Inst Ethics J* 12:1–15.

Clark, D., Arranz, M. J., Arrondo, J., *et al.* (2002). Pharmacogenetic prediction of olanzapine response. *Am J Med Genet* 114:P108.

Collier, D. A. (2003). Pharmacogenetics in psychosis. *Drug News Perspect* 16:159–65.

Collier, D. A., & Li, T. (2003). The genetics of schizophrenia: glutamate not dopamine? *Eur J Pharmacol* 480:177–84.

Cryan, J. F., Hoyer, D., & Markou, A. (2003). Withdrawal from chronic amphetamine induces depressive-like behavioral effects in rodents. *Biol Psychiatry* 54:49–58.

Cryan, J. F., & Mombereau, C. (2004). In search of a depressed mouse: utility of models for studying depression-related behavior in genetically modified mice. *Mol Psychiatry* 9:326–57.

Dettling, M., Cascorbi, I., Roots, I., & Mueller-Oerlinghausen B. (2001). Genetic determinants of clozapine-induced agranulocytosis: recent results of HLA subtyping in a non-Jewish Caucasian sample. *Arch Gen Psychiatry* 58:93–4.

DeVane, C. L., & Jusko, W. J. (1982). Dosage regimen design. *Pharmacol Ther* 17:143–63.

Diaz, R., Fuxe, K., & Ogren, S. O. (1997). Prenatal corticosterone treatment induces long-term changes in spontaneous and apomorphine-mediated motor activity in male and female rats. *Neuroscience* 81:129–40.

Eichhammer, P., Albus, M., Borrmann-Hassenbach, M., *et al.* (2000). Association of dopamine D3 receptor gene variants with neuroleptic induced akathisia in schizophrenic patients: a generalization of Steen's study on DRD3 and tardive dyskinesia. *Am J Med Genet* 96:187–91.

Ellenbroek, B. A. (2003). Animal models in the genomic era: possibilities and limitations with special emphasis on schizophrenia. *Behavioral Pharmacol* 14:409–17.

Gainetdinov, R. R., & Caron, M. G. (2001). Genetics of childhood disorders: XXIV. ADHD, part 8: hyperdopaminergic mice as an animal model of ADHD. *J Am Acad Child Adolesc Psychiatry* 40:380–2.

Gainetdinov, R. R., Wetsel, W. C., Jones, S. R., *et al.* (1999). Role of serotonin in the paradoxical calming effect of psychostimulants on hyperactivity. *Science* 283:397–401.

Garcia-Barcelo, M. M., Lam, L. C., Ungvari, G. S., *et al.* (2001). Dopamine D3 receptor gene and tardive dyskinesia in Chinese schizophrenic patients. *J Neural Transm* 108:671–7.

Geyer, M. A., & Braff, D. L. (1987). Startle habituation and sensorimotor gating in schizophrenia and related animal models. *Schizophr Bull* 13:643–68.

Harkin, A., Houlihan, D. D., & Kelly, J. P. (2002). Reduction in preference for saccharin by repeated unpredictable stress in mice, its prevention by imipramine. *J Psychopharmacol* 16:115–23.

Ioannidis, J. P., Ntzani, E. E., & Contopoulos-Ioannidis, D. G. (2001). Replication validity of genetic association studies. *Nature Genet* 29:306–9.

Joober, R., Benkelfat, C., Brisebois, K., *et al.* (1999). T102C polymorphism in the 5HT2A gene and schizophrenia: relation to phenotype and drug response variability. *J Psychiatry Neurosci* 24:141–6.

Kaiser, R., Konneker, M., Henneken, M., *et al.* (2000). Dopamine D4 receptor 48-bp repeat polymorphism: no association with response to antipsychotic treatment, but association with catatonic schizophrenia. *Mol Psychiatry* 5:418–24.

Koenig, J. I., Kirkpatrick, B., & Lee, P. (2002). Glucocorticoid hormones and early brain development in schizophrenia. *Neuropsychopharmacology* 27:309–18.

Kuhar, M. J., Couceyro, P. R., & Lambert, P. D. (1999). Catecholamines. In G. J. Siegel, B. W. Agranoff, R. W. Albers, *et al.*, eds. *Basic Neurochemistry. Molecular, Cellular and Medical Aspects*, 6th edn. Philadelphia: American Society for Neurochemistry/Lippincott-Raven.

Lane, H. Y., Chang, Y. C., Chiu, C. C., *et al.* (2002). Association of risperidone treatment response with a polymorphism in the 5-HT2A receptor gene. *Am J Psychiatry* 159:1593–5.

Lerer, B., Segman, R. H., Fangerau, H., *et al.* (2002). Pharmacogenetics of tardive dyskinesia: combined analysis of 780 patients supports association with dopamine D3 receptor gene Ser9Gly polymorphism. *Neuropsychopharmacology* 27:105–19.

Lipska, B. K., & Weinberger, D. R. (1995). Genetic variation in vulnerability to the behavioral effects of neonatal hippocampal damage in rats. *Proc Nat Acad Sci* 92:8906–10.

Lipska, B. K., & Weinberger, D. R. (2002). A neurodevelopmental model of schizophrenia: neonatal disconnection of the hippocampus. *Neurotox Res* 4:469–75.

Lubow, R. E. (2005). Construct validity of the animal latent inhibition model of selective attention deficits in schizophrenia. *Schizophr Bull* 31:139–53.

Malhotra, A. K. (2004). Candidate gene studies of antipsychotic drug efficacy and drug-induced weight gain. *Neurotox Res* 6:51–6.

Masellis, M., Basile, V., Meltzer, H. Y., *et al.* (1998). Serotonin subtype 2 receptor genes and clinical response to clozapine in schizophrenia patients. *Neuropsychopharmacology* 19:123–32.

Meisel, C., Gerloff, T., Kirchheiner, J., *et al.* (2003). Implications of pharmacogenetics for individualising drug treatment and for study design. *J Mol Med* 81:154–67.

Meltzer, H. Y. (1995). The role of serotonin in schizophrenia and the place of serotonin-dopamine antagonist antipsychotics. *J Clin Psychopharmacol* 15(Suppl. 1):2S–3S.

Mihara, K., Kondo, T., Suzuki, A., *et al.* (2000). Prolactin response to nemonapride, a selective antagonist for D2 like dopamine receptors, in schizophrenic patients in relation to Taq1A polymorphism of DRD2 gene. *Psychopharmacol (Berl)* 149:246–50.

Miller del, D., Ellingrod, V. L., Holman, T. L., *et al.* (2005). Clozapine-induced weight gain associated with the 5HT2C receptor -759C/T polymorphism. *Am J Med Genet B Neuropsychiatr Genet* 133:97–100.

Otmakhova, N. A., Gurevich, E. V., Katkov, Y. A., *et al.* (1992). Dissociation of multiple behavioral effects between olfactory bulbectomized C57Bl/6J, DBA/2J mice. *Physiol Behav* 52: 441–8.

Ozdemir, V., Basile, V. S., Masellis, M., & Kennedy, J. L. (2001). Pharmacogenetic assessment of antipsychotic-induced movement disorders: contribution of the dopamine D3 receptor and cytochrome P450 1A2 genes. *J Biochem Biophys Meth* 47:151–7.

Perloff, M. D., Von Moltke, L. L., & Greenblatt, D. J. (2003). Differential metabolism of midazolam in mouse liver and intestine microsomes: a comparison of cytochrome P450 activity and expression. *Xenobiotica* 33:365–77.

Porsolt, R. D., Chermat, R., Lenegre, A. *et al.* (1987). Use of the automated tail suspension test for the primary screening of psychotropic agents. *Arch Int Pharmacodyn Ther* 80:11–30.

Porsolt, R. D., Le Pichon, M., & Jalfre, M (1977). Depression: a new animal model sensitive to antidepressant treatments. *Nature* 26:730–2.

Pritchard, J. K., & Rosenberg, N. A. (1999). Use of unlinked genetic markers to detect population stratification in association studies. *Am J Hum Genet* 65: 220–8.

Pritchard, J. K., Stephens, M., Rosenberg, N A., & Donnelly, P. (2000). Association mapping in structured populations. *Am J Hum Genet* 67:170–81.

Ralph, R. J., Paulus, M. P, Fumagalli, F, *et al.* (2001). Prepulse Inhibition deficits and perseverative motor patterns in dopamine transporter knock-out mice: differential effects of D1 and D2 receptor antagonists. *J Neurosci* 21:305–13.

Reynolds, G. P., Zhang, Z. J., & Zhang, X. B. (2002). Association of antipsychotic drug-induced weight gain with a 5-HT2C receptor gene polymorphism. *Lancet* 359:2086–7.

Reynolds, G. P., Zhang, Z., & Zhang, X. (2003). Polymorphism of the promoter region of the serotonin 5-HT(2C) receptor gene and clozapine-induced weight gain. *Am J Psychiatry* 160:677–9.

Schulze, T. G., Schumacher, J., Muller, D. J., *et al.* (2001). Lack of association between a functional polymorphism of the cytochrome P450 1A2 (CYP1A2) gene and tar-

dive dyskinesia in schizophrenia. *Am J Med Genet* 105: 498–501.

Schumacher, J., Schulze, T. G., Wienker, T. F., *et al.* (2000). Pharmacogenetics of the clozapine response. *Lancet* 356:506–7.

Segman, R. H., Goltser, T., Heresco-Levy, U., *et al.* (2003). Association of dopaminergic and serotonergic genes with tardive dyskinesia in patients with chronic schizophrenia. *Pharmacogenom J* 3:277–83.

Shaikh, S., & Kerwin, R. W. (2002). Receptor pharmacogenetics: relevance to CNS syndromes. *Br J Clin Pharmacol* 54:344–8.

Sodhi, M. S., Arranz, M. J., Curtis, D., *et al.* (1995). Association between clozapine response and allelic variation in the 5-HT2C receptor gene. *Neuroreport* 7:169–72.

Spielewoy, C., Roubert, C., Hamon, M., *et al.* (2000). Behavioural disturbances associated with hyperdopaminergia in dopamine-transporter knockout mice. *Behav Pharmacol* 11:279–90.

Staddon, S., Arranz, M. J., Mancama, D., *et al.* (2002). Clinical applications of pharmacogenetics in psychiatry. *Psychopharmacol (Berl)* 162:18–23.

Swerdlow, N. R., Braff, D. L., Geyer, M. A., & Knob, G. F. (1986). Central dopamine hyperactivity in rats mimics abnormal acoustic startle response in schizophrenics. *Biol Psychiatry* 21:3–33.

Theisen, F. M., Hinney, A., Bromel, T., *et al.* (2004). Lack of association between the -759C/T polymorphism of the 5-HT2C receptor gene and clozapine-induced weight gain among German schizophrenic individuals, *Psychiatr Genet* 14:139–42.

Tsai, S. J., Hong, C. J., Yu, Y. W., & Lin, C. H. (2002). -759C/T genetic variation of 5HT(2C) receptor and clozapine-induced weight gain. *Lancet* 360:1790.

Wilkinson, G. R. (1996). Cytochrome P4503A (CYP3A) metabolism: prediction of in vivo activity in humans. *J Pharmacokinet Biopharm* 24:475–90.

Wolterink, G., Daenen, E. W. P. M., & Van Ree, J. M. (2000). Animal models for schizophrenia. *Neuroscience Research Communications*, 27:143–54.

Yu, Y. W., Tsai, S. J., Lin, C. H., *et al.* (1999). Serotonin-6 receptor variant (C267T) and clinical response to clozapine. *Neuroreport* 10:1231–3.

Zhang, Z. J., Zhang, X. B., Hou, G., *et al.* (2003). Interaction between polymorphisms of the dopamine D3 receptor and manganese superoxide dismutase genes in susceptibility to tardive dyskinesia. *Psychiatr Genet* 13:187–92.

26

Biological treatments for psychotic disorders

Ragy R. Girgis, Scott A. Schobel and Jeffrey A. Lieberman

The biological treatment of psychosis has expanded from electroconvulsive therapy (ECT), lithium and the first use of chlorpromazine in 1952 to include second-generation antipsychotic medications and mood stabilisers. As treatments for psychosis have proliferated, so too have the decisions of clinicians as they navigate the increasingly complex risk-benefit ratios of these new therapies.

This chapter reviews the current biological treatments of psychosis, including schizophrenia, schizoaffective disorder, delusional disorder, bipolar disorder and psychotic depression. The first half of the chapter reviews the properties of antipsychotic medications and mood stabilisers. This is followed by a discussion of the implementation of these and other (e.g. ECT) biological treatments for psychosis. Several of the treatments referred to in this chapter (e.g. antidepressants, benzodiazepines) are discussed in detail in Chapter 27. In addition, although this chapter focuses on somatic treatments, the importance of psychosocial interventions and a strong therapeutic relationship cannot be overstated. Such a patient-centered, multifaceted approach is crucial for the successful treatment of patients suffering from any psychiatric illness.

Antipsychotics

Antipsychotic medications are an important part of the biological treatment of psychosis. Here we review the history and drug development, mechanism of action and pharmacology of these agents. We conclude with an overview of some of the side effects associated with antipsychotic medications. The reader is also referred to Chapter 25 for an overview of pharmacokinetics and pharmacodynamics of medications in general.

History and drug development

Given that little to nothing was known about the pathophysiology of schizophrenia early in the twentieth century, the first treatments were often undertaken on a random trial and error basis (Lehmann & Ban, 1997). These included trials of cocaine, castor oil and animal blood, to name a few (Lehmann & Ban, 1997). Carbon dioxide, oxygen and sleep therapy were also used experimentally, as were coma and convulsions induced by such agents as insulin, camphor and metrazol (Lehmann & Ban, 1997).

It was not until the 1950s and the serendipitous discovery of chlorpromazine, a phenothiazine, that the psychopharmacology of schizophrenia began (Lehmann & Ban, 1997). Chlorpromazine was synthesised in the hopes of producing an antihistamine with enhanced sedative effects that could be used for anaesthetic purposes (Lehmann & Ban, 1997). Its effects were noted to be unique to other sedatives and prompted one surgeon, Laborit, to recommend this drug to his psychiatric colleagues (Lehmann & Ban, 1997). Chlorpromazine was first administered

Essential Psychiatry, ed. Robin M. Murray, Kenneth S. Kendler, Peter McGuffin, Simon Wessely, David J. Castle.
Published by Cambridge University Press. © Cambridge University Press 2008.

to a psychiatric patient in 1952 and was an important factor in the eventual deinstitutionalisation of many individuals with schizophrenia (Patel *et al.*, 2003).

Shortly thereafter, other prototypes of antipsychotics, including reserpine (introduced in 1954) and haloperidol (a butyrophenone, synthesised in 1958), were developed (Lehmann & Ban, 1997). Subsequent investigations involving these three prototype antipsychotics (i.e. chlorpromazine, reserpine, haloperidol) contributed to the formation of the dopamine hypothesis of schizophrenia, in addition to the production of several other classes of conventional antipsychotics (Lehmann & Ban, 1997; Patel *et al.*, 2003). The different biochemical classes were related by their ability to induce blockade of D_2 receptors and subsequently treat psychotic symptoms and produce extrapyramidal side effects (EPS), a property once thought to be crucial to antipsychotic effect (Lehmann & Ban, 1997; Patel *et al.*, 2003).

The first-generation antipsychotics developed included the phenothiazines, butyrophenones and others (e.g. loxapine, molindone; Miyamoto *et al.*, 2003). As a group, they are known as conventional, standard, classical, traditional or typical antipsychotic medications (Miyamoto *et al.*, 2003). Although positive symptoms responded well to these conventional medications in many patients, less improvement was seen in other core symptoms of schizophrenia, including cognitive and negative symptoms (Miyamoto *et al.*, 2005). In addition, up to 60% of patients treated with conventional antipsychotics exhibited only partial responses, and approximately 20% of fully adherent patients would relapse despite treatment (Miyamoto *et al.*, 2005). The EPS and tardive dyskinesia associated with conventional antipsychotics were additional limitations which could themselves potentially precipitate nonadherence, relapse and rehospitalisation (Miyamoto *et al.*, 2003).

To improve the side-effect profile of conventional antipsychotics and their clinical efficacy over a broader range of symptoms (i.e. negative and cognitive symptoms in addition to positive symptoms), the second-generation or atypical drugs were developed, the prototypical agent of which is clozapine (Miyamoto *et al.*, 2003). Clozapine was available in Europe as early as the 1970s (Patel *et al.*, 2003). Its use and development were limited, and halted in the United States, however, secondary to reports of agranulocytosis, a potentially fatal side effect (Miyamoto *et al.*, 2003). However, due to subsequent trials showing clozapine's superior efficacy in treatment-resistant patients, the drug was reintroduced under controlled conditions (Kane *et al.*, 1988; Miyamoto *et al.*, 2003).

New drugs were developed after clozapine aiming to match its higher efficacy without the potential for agranulocytosis. Investigative techniques made it possible to identify specific receptor affinities of medications (Lehmann & Ban, 1997). Development proceeded to synthesise drugs that targeted receptors in a different manner, including less nigrostriatal D_2 blockade and increased affinities at other receptor types (e.g. serotonin receptors and alternate dopamine receptors; Lehmann & Ban, 1997). The first atypical antipsychotics to be developed were remoxipride, risperidone and olanzapine, and others quickly followed. The atypical antipsychotics were broadly characterised as having lesser likelihood of causing EPS and greater efficacy for both positive and negative symptoms of schizophrenia (Lehmann & Ban, 1997). Currently, olanzapine, risperidone, quetiapine, ziprasidone and aripiprazole are available in the United States, and amisulpride, zotepine and, in limited instances, sertindole are used in the United Kingdom, Europe and countries elsewhere in the world.

Mechanism of action

The classical dopamine hypothesis of schizophrenia focused on hyperactivity of dopamine systems (Laruelle *et al.*, 2003). This dysregulation is still thought to occur, although primarily in the striatum (Patel *et al.*, 2003). Much of the evidence in support of this hypothesis originated from the observed antipsychotic effects of D_2 blocking agents, along with the psychotic symptoms displayed in individuals who had used dopaminergic drugs (Laruelle *et al.*, 2003). In fact, antipsychotic effects have not been demonstrated in agents without D_2 receptor binding affinity (Miyamoto *et al.*, 2005). The original dopamine hypothesis has, however, expanded as more attention was paid to the cognitive and negative symptoms of schizophrenia, revealing both that hypofunction of prefrontal D_1 receptors might be involved in the pathophysiology of schizophrenia and that the efficacy of atypical antipsychotics may in part be related to their ability to increase prefrontal dopamine and possibly increase activity at D_1 receptors (Abi-Dargham & Laruelle, 2005; Laruelle *et al.*, 2003).

As with dopamine, serotonin (5-HT) was originally implicated in the pathophysiology of schizophrenia because of the observed psychotic effects of serotonergic drugs (e.g. LSD) and later the efficacy of serotonin-blocking agents, such as the atypical antipsychotics (Aghajanian & Marek, 2000; Tamminga & Holcomb, 2005). An increased ratio of 5-HT_{2A} to D_2 receptor antagonism has been postulated to be responsible for their efficacy and tolerability (Meltzer, Li, *et al.*, 2003). However, current evidence suggests it is unlikely that 5-HT_{2A} antagonism alone accounts for the efficacy of atypical antipsychotics (Miyamoto *et al.*, 2005).

Hypofunction of the glutamatergic N-methyl-D-aspartate (NMDA) receptor has also been suggested to play a role in the pathophysiology of schizophrenia (Laruelle *et al.*, 2003; Miyamoto *et al.*, 2005; Olney *et al.*, 1999). The ability of NMDA antagonists (e.g. phencyclidine, ketamine) to induce positive and negative symptoms in individuals with schizophrenia and healthy patients, along with the ability of adjunctive NMDA modulators to provide some improvement in psychotic symptomatology in individuals with schizophrenia, have supported this hypothesis (Heresco-Levy *et al.*, 2005; Laruelle *et al.*, 2003). Recent neurochemical studies have revealed complex interactions between the dopamine and NMDA systems, reinforcing the roles that each of these neurotransmitter systems may play

(Abi-Dargham & Laruelle, 2005). Further, preliminary evidence has shown that atypical, but not conventional, antipsychotics might antagonise experimentally induced NMDA receptor hypofunction and possibly increase NMDA transmission (Abi-Dargham & Laruelle, 2005; Miyamoto *et al.*, 2005).

Additional receptor subtypes (e.g. 5-HT_1) and neurochemical systems (e.g. gamma-aminobutyric acid (GABA)-ergic, peptidergic, noradrenergic, cholinergic) have been implicated in the pathophysiology and treatment of psychosis (Lewis *et al.*, 2005; Miyamoto *et al.*, 2005; Patel *et al.*, 2003). However, mechanisms of action in addition to drug-receptor interactions have also been suggested, in part because of the observed latency of response observed with antipsychotic medications (Miyamoto *et al.*, 2003). Several additional theories have been examined over the last few decades, including depolarisation inactivation, receptor cycling and internalisation, neuroplasticty and changes in gene expression and intracellular signaling (Miyamoto *et al.*, 2003). Additional investigations into these areas will determine their respective contributions.

Pharmacology

The conventional antipsychotic medications are classified by structure into the phenothiazines, butyrophenones and others, including molindone, loxapine and thiothixene (Miyamoto *et al.*, 2003). They are considered to be equally effective in their treatment of the psychotic symptoms of schizophrenia, but vary in their individual properties, side effects and potency (Miyamoto *et al.*, 2003). All conventional antipsychotics have high affinity for the D_2 receptor, produce EPS and increase serum prolactin.

The *butyrophenones*, such as haloperidol, are potent D_2 antagonists and have few autonomic and anticholinergic side effects. The *phenothiazines* are divided into three classes. The aliphatic class has relatively low potency at D_2 receptors, more antimuscarinic activity, more sedation and more sympathetic and parasympathetic activity, all exemplified by chlorpromazine. The piperidine class (e.g. thioridazine) has less affinity for D_2 receptor sites. The piperazine class (e.g. fluphenazine) has less autonomic and antimuscarinic effects but greater potency (Miyamoto *et al.*, 2003).

The newer drugs approved to treat psychosis in the United States, United Kingdom and many other countries include clozapine, risperidone, olanzapine, quetiapine, ziprasidone, sertindole, amisulpride, zotepine and aripiprazole. The mechanism of action of each drug is complex and unique, as typified by *clozapine*. Clozapine's pharmacology is distinctive in that it has a lower affinity for D_2 receptors than conventional agents and most other atypical agents and a relatively high affinity for 5-HT_{2A} receptors, as well as affinity for $5HT_6$, $5HT_7$ and D_4 receptors (Miyamoto *et al.*, 2003). It also has significant antagonist affinity for H_1 histaminergic, α adrenergic and muscarinic receptors.

Olanzapine is similar to clozapine both structurally and in its receptor binding properties, with antagonist potency at $5HT_{2A}$ greater than D_2 receptors (Miyamoto *et al.*, 2003) and affinity at the D_1, D_3, D_4, D_5, H_1 histaminergic, m_1 anticholinergic and α_1 adrenergic receptors (Patel *et al.*, 2003). Unlike clozapine, it does not bind $5HT_7$, certain cholinergic and α_2 receptors to the same degree (Patel *et al.*, 2003).

Risperidone is a potent antagonist of D_2 and $5HT_{2A}$ receptors with a high serotonin to dopamine ratio (Patel *et al.*, 2003). EPS are reduced with lower dose risperidone treatment (i.e. 2–6 mg/day) despite the robust occupancy of D_2 receptors (Miyamoto *et al.*, 2003). At doses above 6 mg/day, risperidone has a higher incidence of EPS (Miyamoto *et al.*, 2003). Risperidone has significant affinity for α_1 receptors but much less for cholinergic and D_1 receptors; orthostasis and sedation are among its side effects (Patel *et al.*, 2003). Tardive dyskinesia is less likely to occur at the lower therapeutic doses (Patel *et al.*, 2003).

Quetiapine is similar to other atypical antipsychotics in its greater affinity for $5HT_{2A}$ receptors

than for D_2 receptors (Miyamoto *et al.*, 2003). As with clozapine, its D_2 receptor occupancy is relatively transient (Miyamoto *et al.*, 2003). It also has affinity for α_1 adrenergic and histamine receptors but possesses much less muscarinic cholinergic affinity (Nemeroff *et al.*, 2002; Patel *et al.*, 2003). Similarly, its main side effects include orthostasis, sedation and weight gain (Patel *et al.*, 2003).

Ziprasidone has potent $5HT_{2A}$ and D_2 antagonist affinity, as well as $5HT_{1D}$ and $5HT_{2C}$ receptor affinity (Miyamoto *et al.*, 2003). It is also an agonist at the $5HT_{1A}$ receptor and inhibits norepinephirine and serotonin reuptake (Miyamoto *et al.*, 2003). Ziprasidone generally does not have much affinity for m_1 cholinergic, H_1 histaminergic or α_1 adrenergic receptors and thus causes few anticholinergic side effects, sedation or orthostatic hypotension (Stahl & Shayegan, 2003) but can be associated with QTc prolongation (Marder *et al.*, 2004; Patel *et al.*, 2003). Because ziprasidone has a short half-life, twice-a-day dosing is often prescribed, along with food for improved absorption (Patel *et al.*, 2003).

Zotepine has high affinity for serotonin, α_1 adrenergic and H_1 histaminergic receptors (Miyamoto *et al.*, 2003). It also possesses moderate affinity for dopamine receptors, along with significant norepinephrine reuptake inhibition characteristics (Miyamoto *et al.*, 2003).

Amisulpride is a selective D_2/D_3 antagonist (Miyamoto *et al.*, 2003). In animal studies, low dosages have been shown to block dopamine autoreceptors, which in turn leads to an increase in dopaminergic neurotransmission; at higher dosages, postsynaptic D_2 blocking effects predominate (Miyamoto *et al.*, 2003; Moller, 2003). At lower doses (e.g. between 100 and 300 mg), amisulpride produces few EPS or endocrine side effects (Blin, 1999).

Sertindole is a high-affinity antagonist at D_2, $5HT_{2A}$, $5HT_{2C}$ and α_1 adrenergic receptors (Miyamoto *et al.*, 2003). Although sertindole has been shown to have less of a risk of EPS than other antipsychotics, it does carry the risk of QTc prolongation (Blin, 1999).

Aripiprazole is unique among the atypical agents in that it is a partial dopamine agonist with high affinity for D_2 and D_3 receptors, has affinity for $5HT_{1A}$ receptors as a partial agonist, but is without much affinity for D_1 receptors (Lieberman, 2004; Miyamoto *et al.*, 2003). Finally, it possesses antagonist affinity for $5HT_{2A}$, $5HT_6$ and $5HT_7$ receptors (Miyamoto *et al.*, 2003). In summary, as a partial dopamine agonist, aripiprazole appears to enhance dopamine activity in areas of low dopamine function and decrease dopamine activity in areas of high dopamine function (Lieberman, 2004).

Plasma levels of antipsychotic agents have been established for several antipsychotics, although there remains no consensus regarding the use of these levels in clinical practice (Baumann *et al.*, 2004). It has been suggested that obtaining plasma levels may be beneficial before deciding that a trial of an antipsychotic is ineffective, when changing the dose of a drug during maintenance therapy or when changing the form (e.g. oral to depot) of the medication (Baumann *et al.*, 2004; Miyamoto *et al.*, 2003). Plasma levels of several antipsychotics may also correlate to some degree with receptor occupancy (e.g. haloperidol, olanzapine, ziprasidone) and clinical response (e.g. risperidone, olanzapine; Hiemke *et al.*, 2004), although further investigations are needed to confirm and extend these findings before it is clear how best to incorporate these data into clinical practice.

Most antipsychotic medications are metabolised by the cytochrome P-450 system (Burns, 2001; Miyamoto *et al.*, 2003). Atypical antipsychotics are neither potent inducers nor inhibitors of these metabolic enzymes (de Leon *et al.*, 2005). Nonetheless, the potential for significant drug-drug interactions exists when these medications are taken concomitantly with other medications that target these enzymes, including other psychopharmacological agents (e.g. antidepressants, mood stabilisers; Burns, 2001; de Leon *et al.*, 2005; Miyamoto *et al.*, 2003). Risperidone in particular may increase the blood levels of clozapine when used as an additional therapy (Sadock & Sadock, 2003).

Pharmacodynamic interactions (e.g. enhanced anticholinergic effects) are also possible when antipsychotics are taken along with other medications with similar effects (Burns, 2001).

Side effects

The side effect profiles of antipsychotic drugs are important considerations when prescribing these agents (Table 26.1). This section reviews some of the side effects that have been associated with antipsychotic medications, including motor and neurological, metabolic (e.g. weight gain, dysglycemia, dyslipidemia), endocrine and sexual, cardiovascular, hematologic and ocular side effects, among others.

Motor and neurological side effects

All antipsychotic medications have the potential to produce EPS, although atypical antipsychotics are generally less likely to produce them than conventional antipsychotics, which have been estimated to produce EPS at rates between 50% and 75%; the exception is risperidone at higher (e.g. >6 mg) doses (Arana, 2000; Marder *et al.*, 2004; Miyamoto *et al.*, 2005). The advantage of fewer EPS in the new agents is less apparent, however, when lower potency, or lower dosages of, conventional agents are used as comparator drugs (Gardner *et al.*, 2005; Leucht, Wahlbeck, *et al.*, 2003). One study noted, however, that even though there was no significant difference in EPS across groups, more subjects in the conventional antipsychotic–treated group discontinued treatment because of EPS than in other patients (Lieberman *et al.*, 2005).

There are two dramatic and acute forms of neurological side effects of antipsychotic medications: dystonia and neuroleptic malignant syndrome (NMS). *Dystonia* usually occurs within the first few days of the antipsychotic and is manifest by sudden, tonic muscle spasms in the head, neck, trunk or extremities (Miyamoto *et al.*, 2003; Wirshing, 2001). One may also have a life-threatening

Table 26.1 Side effect profile of antipsychotic drugs

Drug / Side effect	Conventional agents	Clozapine	Risperidone	Olanzapine	Quetiapine	Ziprasidone	Sertindole	Amisulpride	Aripiprazole
EPS[a]	+++	0	++	+	0	+	0	++	+
TD	+++	0	++	+	0	+	0 to +	+	+
NMS	++	+	+	-	?	+	+	+	?
Prolactin elevation	+++	0	+++	0 to +	0	0 to +	0 to +	++	0
Weight gain	+ to +-	+++	-	+++	+	0	+	+	0
Prolonged QT[a]	+ to +++	0	+	0	+	++	+++	+	0
Hypotension[a]	+ to ++	+++	+	++	++	+	+	0	+
Sinus tachycardia[a]	+ to +++	+++	+	+-	++	+	+	0	0
Anticholinergic effects[a]	+ to +++	+++	0	++	+	0	0	0	0
Hepatic transaminitis	+ to ++	++	+	++	+	+	+	+	0
Agranulocytosis	0 to +	++	0	0	0	0	0	0	0
Sedation	+ to +++	+++	+	++	+++	+	+	+	+
Seizures[a]	0 to +	+++	0	0 to +	0 to +	0 to +	0 to +	0 to +	0 to +

EPS = extrapyramidal side effects; NMS = neuroleptic malignant syndrome; TD = tardive dyskinesia. + to +++ = active to strongly active; 0 = minimal to none; ? = questionable to unknown activity.

[a] Dose dependent.

Reproduced and adapted with permission from Miyamoto, S., et al. Antipsychotic drugs. (2003). In A. Tasman, J. Kay, & J. A. Lieberman, eds. *Psychiatry*, 2nd edn. Copyright John Wiley & Sons, Ltd: Chichester, pp. 1928–1964; Dawkins, K., et al. (1999). Antipsychotics: Past and Future: National Institute of Mental Health Division of Services and Intervention Research Workshop, July 14, 1998. *Schizophr Bull* 2:395–405, Oxford University Press; Burns, M.J. (2001). The pharmacology and toxicology of atypical antipsychotic agents. *J Toxicol Clin Toxicol* 39:1–14, Taylor & Francis Ltd., http://www.informaworld.com.

laryngeal dystonia, although this is much less common (Christodoulou & Kalaitzi, 2005). Risk factors for dystonia include young age, male sex, higher-potency antipsychotic and history of dystonia (Miyamoto *et al.*, 2003). Dystonia is rapidly and effectively treated with intramuscular anticholinergic or antihistaminergic agents (Miyamoto *et al.*, 2003). It may also be effectively prevented by limiting the dose of antipsychotic or by pretreating with an anticholinergic medication (Miyamoto *et al.*, 2003; Wirshing, 2001). Short-term maintenance anticholinergic medication may help to prevent recurrence of the dystonia (Lehman *et al.*, 2004).

Neuroleptic malignant syndrome is a potentially life-threatening complication of antipsychotic use and is diagnosed by severe EPS, hyperthermia, altered mental status and autonomic dysfunction (Arana, 2000). Although the risk associated with the newer antipsychotics might be lower, it has been reported to occur, in varying degrees, with clozapine, risperidone, quetiapine, olanzapine, aripiprazole, ziprasidone, zotepine and amisulpride (Ananth *et al.*, 2004; Atbasoglu *et al.*, 2004; Mieno *et al.*, 2003; Miyamoto *et al.*, 2003; Murty *et al.*, 2002; Spalding *et al.*, 2004). It may also be associated with elevated serum creatine phosphokinase and white blood cell (WBC) count and occurs in approximately 1% to 2% of patients treated with antipsychotics (Miyamoto *et al.*, 2003). Risk factors include male gender, intramuscular dose, dehydration and rapid increase in dose (Arana, 2000; Miyamoto *et al.*, 2003). It is also more likely to occur if lithium is given concomitantly with clozapine (Sadock & Sadock, 2003). NMS is treated by stopping the offending antipsychotic as soon as the diagnosis is suspected, along with supportive treatment (Miyamoto *et al.*, 2003). Dantrolene and dopamine agonists (e.g. bromocriptine) have also been used although their efficacy is unproven (Miyamoto *et al.*, 2003).

Another acute form of EPS which causes significant morbidity is *akathisia*, a subjective and objective restlessness (Miyamoto *et al.*, 2003). It occurs in up to 25% of patients treated with conventional antipsychotics (Arana, 2000). Patients may complain of anxiety or severe discomfort and display psychomotor agitation (Arana, 2000; Miyamoto *et al.*, 2003; Wirshing, 2001). It is sometimes difficult to distinguish this side effect from worsening psychosis (Wirshing, 2001). Risk factors include female sex and higher dose of antipsychotic (Arana, 2000). Benzodiazepines such as lorazepam and clonidine, anticholinergic agents and beta-blockers such as propanolol are helpful for some patients, as is antipsychotic dosage reduction (Arana, 2000; Miyamoto *et al.*, 2003; Sadock & Sadock, 2003; Wirshing, 2001).

The subacute manifestation of EPS is known as medication-induced *parkinsonism*, which includes muscle rigidity, akinesia, tremor and excess salivation (Arana, 2000; Wirshing, 2001). Akinesia alone may occur in more than 50% of patients treated with conventional antipsychotics and can be mistaken for the negative symptoms of schizophrenia (Arana, 2000). Such symptoms may be alleviated by antiparkinsonian drugs, reduction in neuroleptic dose or switching to a low-potency conventional agent or to an atypical antipsychotic (Arana, 2000; Wirshing, 2001).

Tardive dyskinesia is an involuntary movement disorder characterised by choreoathetoid and dyskinetic movements of the orofacial muscles, trunk, limbs and sometimes even diaphragm (Glazer, 2000; Miyamoto *et al.*, 2003). These movements cease while sleeping (Miyamoto *et al.*, 2003). Tardive akathisia and dystonia have also been described (Casey, 1999). The overall incidence has been shown to increase from 18.5% after 4 years of treatment with conventional antipsychotics to 40% after the eighth year of treatment, although the incidences drop to 11% and 22%, respectively, for tardive dyskinesia which lasts for more than 6 months (Kane *et al.*, 1986). Risk factors include increased age, female sex, presence of diabetes, conventional antipsychotic, nonschizophrenic diagnosis and other EPS (Arana, 2000; Wirshing, 2001). Management of tardive dyskinesia includes lowering the dosage of the antipsychotic, switching to an atypical agent, considering clozapine and considering discontinuation of antipsychotic medication, although the latter is uncommonly feasible (Casey, 1999; Miyamoto *et al.*, 2003). Several other agents (e.g. reserpine, vitamin E) have been tested to treat tardive dyskinesia with limited success (Casey, 1999).

Weight gain

Both conventional and atypical antipsychotics can cause weight gain, although atypicals to a greater degree (Wirshing, 2004). Some of this weight gain seems to show a plateau effect (Miyamoto *et al.*, 2003). When choosing a therapeutic regimen, weight gain and obesity are important side effects of antipsychotic medications to consider because of their association with hypertension, type II diabetes, sleep apnea, cardiovascular disease, osteoarthritis and some types of cancer (Allison & Casey, 2001; Allison *et al.*, 1999). Clozapine and olanzapine are generally most associated with weight gain, with risperidone, sertindole, zotepine, amisulpride and quetiapine showing intermediate weight gain and ziprasidone and aripiprazole considered to induce minimal or no weight gain (Allison *et al.*, 1999; Gardner *et al.*, 2005; Kasper *et al.*, 2003; Newcomer, 2005; Simpson *et al.*, 2004; Wirshing, 2004)

It is recommended that clinicians monitor body mass index for all of their patients with schizophrenia regardless of their current antipsychotic regimen, consider risk of weight gain during the drug selection process in at-risk individuals and intervene when indicated, including giving consideration to switching medications to one that is associated with less weight gain (Marder *et al.*, 2004).

Dysglycemia

Individuals with schizophrenia may be at a higher risk of glucose dysregulation than the general population (Miyamoto *et al.*, 2003). Some of this risk may be associated with antipsychotic treatment (Gardner *et al.*, 2005), although the precise mechanism of action remains to be elucidated (Bergman & Ader, 2005). Although relatively few large, prospective, randomised studies have investigated this side

effect, it appears that clozapine and olanzapine might be most problematic, whereas the reports for the other antipsychotics are either limited in number or show less effect (Baptista *et al.*, 2002; Gardner *et al.*, 2005; Kapur and Remington, 2001; Lieberman *et al.*, 2005; Lindenmayer *et al.*, 2003; Miyamoto *et al.*, 2003; Newcomer, 2004; Simpson *et al.*, 2004).

Recommendations for the monitoring of glucose dysregulation and the development of diabetes in individuals with schizophrenia have been suggested and include a baseline fasting plasma glucose level or HbA1c, patient education and close monitoring of patients for signs and symptoms of diabetes or glucose dysregulation, especially in the context of several diabetes risk factors, and further patient assessment with the appropriate healthcare specialist (e.g. internist, primary health care provider) as necessary (Marder *et al.*, 2004).

Dyslipidemia

Antipsychotic treatment has also been associated with dyslipidemia (Casey, 2004; Gardner *et al.*, 2005; Kapur & Remington, 2001). This metabolic abnormality appears to be associated itself with weight gain, although further study is necessary before a firm conclusion can be made (Gardner *et al.*, 2005; Kapur & Remington, 2001). Similar to the situation with glucose dysregulation, clozapine and olanzapine appear to be most related to dyslipidemia, followed by mixed or intermediate data for risperidone, low-potency conventionals and quetiapine, along with data for sertindole, zotepine, amisulpride, ziprasidone, high-potency conventionals and aripiprazole that is either mixed or limited or suggests no adverse relationship or even a beneficial relationship with serum lipid profile (Casey, 2004; Gardner *et al.*, 2005; Koro *et al.*, 2002; Lieberman *et al.*, 2005; McQuade *et al.*, 2004; Newcomer, 2005). Because of the significant morbidity (i.e. cardiovascular disease) associated with dyslipidemia, including hypertriglyceridemia (Jeppesen *et al.*, 1998), aggressive monitoring and management of this side effect are recommended (American Diabetes Association *et al.*, 2004; Casey, 2004; Marder *et al.*, 2004).

Elevated prolactin levels and sexual side effects

All conventional antispsychotics and some of the more potent dopamine antagonists among the atypical agents, including risperidone and amisulpride, are associated with increases in plasma prolactin levels by blocking the inhibitory actions of dopamine on the pituitary (Gardner *et al.,* 2005; Miyamoto *et al.,* 2003; Mortimer, 2004). This tends to occur more in women than in men (Marder *et al.,* 2004). Complications of hyperprolactinemia include galactorrhea, menstrual disturbances, hypogonadism, sexual dysfunction, gynecomastia in men and possibly bone loss (Misra *et al.,* 2004; Miyamoto *et al.,* 2003). Clozapine, olanzapine, quetiapine, ziprasidone and aripiprazole have been shown to either not increase prolactin levels or increase them mildly or transiently (Casey, 1997; Goff *et al.,* 1998; Lieberman, 2004; Miyamoto *et al.,* 2003; Turrone *et al.,* 2002; Wieck & Haddad, 2003). Preliminary evidence suggests that zotepine might increase prolactin levels (von Bardeleben *et al.,* 1987). Guidelines for the monitoring and management of hyperprolactinemia have previously been published (Marder *et al.,* 2004).

A number of sexual side effects (see also Chapter 17) occur in individuals with schizophrenia in addition to those precipitated by hyperprolactinemia (e.g. priapism, decreased satisfaction; Cutler, 2003). Several of these side effects are associated with antipsychotic treatment, but potentially less so with atypical antipsychotics (Cutler, 2003). Consideration should be given to these side effects when selecting antipsychotic treatment (Cutler, 2003).

Cardiovascular side effects

Orthostatic hypotension is the most common of this group of side effects and is more often associated with low-potency, high-dosage medications (e.g. chlorpromazine, clozapine; Casey, 1997). Elderly individuals are more prone to this side effect (Miyamoto *et al.,* 2003). Slow posture changes, along with gradual increases in dosages, are methods by which to minimise the risk of orthostatic hypotension (Casey, 1997; Miyamoto *et al.,* 2003). Tolerance to this side effect often develops within 1 to 2 months (Casey, 1997; Miyamoto *et al.,* 2003).

In addition, the US Food and Drug Administration (FDA) recently requested that a black box warning be placed in the labels of all atypical antipsychotic medications in the United States, warning physicians and consumers of the reported increased (approximately twofold) death rate among elderly patients with dementia treated with these medications (Kuehn, 2005). This occurred in response to several trials of four atypical antipsychotic agents (i.e. olanzapine, risperidone, aripiprazole, quetiapine) suggesting increased rates of death, mostly secondary to cardiovascular disease and infections, in this population (Kuehn, 2005). The mechanism is not precisely known (Kuehn, 2005).

Tachycardia is another potential cardiovascular side effect (Miyamoto *et al.,* 2003). It might occur as a result of hypotension or secondary to anticholinergic activity (Miyamoto *et al.,* 2003). Tolerance often develops, although monitoring and treatment should be pursued in certain cases (Miyamoto *et al.,* 2003).

QTc prolongation is associated with the risk of dysrhythmia (e.g. torsade de pointes) and sudden death, especially when the QTc surpasses 500 milliseconds (Gardner *et al.,* 2005; Taylor, 2003). Thioridazine, mesoridazine, pimozide, droperidol and sertindole, among others, are the antipsychotics found to be most associated with prolonged QTc, torsade de pointes, and sudden death (Gardner *et al.,* 2005; Lindstrom *et al.,* 2005; Taylor, 2003). These concerns have led to the restricted use of several of these medications (Gardner *et al.,* 2005; Lindstrom *et al.,* 2005). Ziprasidone has also been traditionally associated with prolonged QTc (Glassman & Bigger, 2001; Miyamoto *et al.,* 2003), although a recent randomised controlled trial did not observe this side effect to a greater degree than with other agents examined in the trial (Lieberman *et al.,* 2005), and several others reported no excess cardiovascular adverse events associated with prolonged QTc (Harrigan *et al.,* 2004; Simpson *et al.,* 2004).

The precise mechanism of QTc prolongation caused by antipsychotics, in addition to the exact relationship between these effects and dysrythmia and death, remains unclear (Taylor, 2003). However, antipsychotic medications prone to causing this side effect should not be combined with other medications with similar effects (Miyamoto et al., 2003). Several reports recommend electrocardiogram (ECG) monitoring for certain high-risk individuals (e.g. those with heart disease, congenital long QT syndrome or personal history of syncope), and thioridazine, mesoridazine and pimozide should be avoided in these individuals (Glassman & Bigger, 2001; Marder et al., 2004).

Myocarditis and cardiomyopathy may also occur as a result of antipsychotic medications (Coulter et al., 2001; Glassman, 2005). Although much of the emphasis and reports concerning these toxicities focus on clozapine (Merrill et al., 2005), other antipsychotics have also been implicated (Coulter et al., 2001; Roesch-Ely et al., 2002). The risk of myocarditis or cardiomyopathy in patients receiving clozapine has been estimated to be low (0.015%–0.188%; Merrill et al., 2005). However, close monitoring and prompt treatment are recommended when treating patients with clozapine (Marder et al., 2004; Merrill et al., 2005).

Haematologic side effects

The risk of agranulocytosis (i.e. an absolute neutrophil count less than 500/mm^3), a potentially fatal side effect, is estimated to be approximately 1% among those patients exposed to clozapine, and thus clozapine should not be used in combination with any other drug known to cause bone marrow suppression or agranulocytosis or in individuals with a history of clozapine-induced agranulocytosis or granulocytopenia, myeloproliferative disorder or an initial WBC count of 3,500/mm^3 (Lehman et al., 2004; Lieberman et al., 1989; Miyamoto et al., 2003; Physicians' Desk Reference, 2006; Sadock & Sadock, 2003). The risk is greatest early on in treatment, usually within the first 3 months, and occurs more

often in the elderly, women and patients younger than 21 years old (Miyamoto et al., 2003). Fortunately, this side effect is usually reversible if the drug is promptly discontinued (Lieberman et al., 1988; Miyamoto et al., 2003). Because of the severity of this event, patients in the United States and elsewhere must be registered in programs that ensure regular WBC count monitoring (Miyamoto et al., 2003).

Monitoring and treatment guidelines vary between countries (Miyamoto et al., 2003). Guidelines have been published that include the management of clozapine (Physicians' Desk Reference, 2006). A WBC count must be obtained before initiation of clozapine treatment and weekly thereafter for the first 6 months (Physicians' Desk Reference, 2006). The frequency may be decreased to once every 2 weeks thereafter if white blood cell counts have been stable. Following 6 months of biweekly monitoring and after 12 months on clozapine overall, the WBC frequency may be reduced to once monthly. If clozapine is discontinued at any time, weekly monitoring should continue for 4 weeks (Physicians' Desk Reference, 2006). Additional monitoring should be obtained for WBC counts that drop below 3,500/mm^3, for large absolute drops or if immature cell varieties are observed (Physicians' Desk Reference, 2006). Clozapine treatment should be halted for WBC counts less than 3,000/mm^3 or for absolute neutrophil counts less than 1500/mm^3, and appropriate diagnostic (e.g. bone marrow aspiration, increased frequency of blood draws) and therapeutic (e.g. isolation, antibiotics) interventions should be instituted depending on the severity of the clinical situation (Physicians' Desk Reference, 2006). Rechallenge should not occur if the total WBC count drops below 2,000/mm^3 or if the absolute neutrophil count drops below 1,000/mm^3 (Physicians' Desk Reference, 2006).

Haematologic abnormalities have been observed with other antipsychotics (e.g. chlorpromazine, olanzapine, risperidone; Hong & Wang, 2001; Miyamoto et al., 2003), although to a lesser degree than with clozapine.

Ocular abnormalities

Certain antipsychotics, including chlorpromazine at doses greater than 300 mg/day and prochlorperazine, may predispose to cataract formation (Ruigomez *et al.*, 2000). Quetiapine was initially shown to cause cataracts in dogs that received 4 times the maximal human dose, but this was not found in other species (Physicians' Desk Reference, 2006). A clear relationship between quetiapine, or other atypical antipsychotics, and cataracts has not yet been established, and reports of such associations are inconclusive (Marder *et al.*, 2004; Shahzad *et al.*, 2002; Valibhai *et al.*, 2001; Whitehorn *et al.*, 2004). However, until more robust conclusions regarding possible associations between antipsychotic medications and cataracts can be made, inquiry into visual changes and visual evaluation should remain important management issues for patients with schizophrenia, including following the recommendations included in the package insert for quetiapine (Marder *et al.*, 2004).

Other side effects

Antipsychotics have the potential to induce numerous other side effects, including anticholinergic effects (e.g. dry mouth, constipation, urinary retention, blurry vision, confusion), hepatic effects (e.g. asymptomatic elevation of liver enzymes and, less frequently, symptomatic hepatotoxicity), sedation (especially with low-potency conventional antipsychotics and several atypicals), photosensitivity (e.g. chlorpromazine), nausea, vomiting, retinopathy (e.g. thioridazine), hypersalivation (e.g. clozapine), anxiety, insomnia, obsessive-compulsive symptoms (e.g. clozapine), body temperature dysregulation (e.g. clozapine, other atypicals) and lowered seizure threshold (e.g. low-potency conventionals and clozapine), among others (Casey, 1997; Fornaro *et al.*, 2002; Gardner *et al.*, 2005; Iqbal *et al.*, 2003; Lieberman, 2004; Miyamoto *et al.*, 2003; Mortimer, 2004; Sadock & Sadock, 2003). In addition, the signs, symptoms and treatments of overdose with several antipsychotic medications have been described (Burns, 2001; Sadock & Sadock, 2003).

Although antipsychotic medications have been associated with numerous adverse effects, they are generally considered to be safe (Sadock & Sadock, 2003). Obtaining liver function tests, a complete blood count with differential and an electrocardiogram has been recommended for an initial laboratory assessment (Sadock & Sadock, 2003).

Mood stabilisers

Mood stabilisers represent another key part of the biological treatments of psychosis. In this section, lithium, valproate, carbamazepine, oxcarbazepine, lamotrigine and topiramate are reviewed.

Lithium

Lithium was originally used for the treatment of gout approximately 150 years ago (Timmer & Sands, 1999). The use of lithium for affective disorders also dates as far back as the nineteenth century (Schou, 2001). However, the age of lithium treatment as an antimanic agent is often considered to have started in 1949 with the publication and description of its use by John Cade (Moseman *et al.*, 2003; Schou, 2001).

Lithium's mechanism of action remains undetermined (Moseman *et al.*, 2003). Lithium alters neuronal function through its substitution for or competition with other ions and has effects on several neurotransmitter systems (e.g. dopamine, acetylcholine, serotonin), enzymes (e.g. glycogen synthase kinase-3, fructose-1,6 bisphosphatase) and second messenger and signal transduction systems (Gould *et al.*, 2004; Moseman *et al.*, 2003). In particular, lithium has been found to decrease both phosphoinositide and cyclic adenosine monophosphate metabolism, possibly through effects on guanine nucleotide-binding proteins (Gould *et al.*, 2004; Moseman *et al.*, 2003). Lithium might also modulate gene expression through effects on protein kinase-C (Lenox & Wang, 2003).

Lithium is not metabolised and is primarily excreted through the kidneys (Keck & McElroy, 2002). Therapeutic plasma drug concentrations are generally in the range of 0.5 to 1.2 meq/L for acute manic/mixed episodes, and the most favorable maintenance range may differ between individuals (American Psychiatric Association, 2002). The patient and physician must balance side effects with risk of relapse when deciding on dosage parameters (Moseman *et al.*, 2003).

Lithium has several adverse effects (see Table 26.2), many of which are dose related; these include cognitive problems, sedation, weight gain, polydipsia/polyuria (may be treated with diuretics), tremor (may be treated with beta-blockers), gastrointestinal distress (may administer with meals), impaired coordination, leukocytosis, alopecia, oedema and acne (may be treated with antiacne agents) (American Psychiatric Association, 2002; Moseman *et al.*, 2003). Other side effects include ECG changes/arrhythmias, reduced renal response to antidiuretic hormone with polydipsia/polyuria, hypothyroidism, hyperparathyroidism, psoriasis exacerbations and possibly renal insufficiency (American Psychiatric Association, 2002).

Toxicity often occurs with blood levels above 1.5 meq/L and begins with tremor, vertigo, nausea, diarrhea, blurred vision, confusion and increased deep tendon reflexes followed by seizures, renal failure, coma, dysrhythmias and possibly death at higher levels (American Psychiatric Association, 2002; Sadock & Sadock, 2003). Chronic lithium toxicity may also occur and may be manifested by parkinsonian symptoms, myopathy, neuropathy, hypothyroidism, myocarditis, lightheadedness, aplastic anemia, tremor, muscle twitching, drowsiness, hyperreflexia, slurred speech, psychosis, pseudotumor cerebri, memory difficulties, renal failure, nephrogenic diabetes insipidus, weakness, apathy, tinnitus, chronic interstitial nephritis, skin ulcers, localised edema and dermatitis (Timmer & Sands, 1999). Supportive care and measures to decrease blood levels should be promptly instituted for toxicity (American Psychiatric Association, 2002; Sadock & Sadock, 2003). The decision to institute hemodialysis depends on factors such as the patient's clinical status, serum lithium levels and level of renal function (Timmer & Sands, 1999).

Table 26.2 Adverse effects of lithium

Adverse effect	Treatment
Weight gain	Avoid caloric beverages, watch diet, increase physical activity
Nausea, vomiting, diarrhea	Take lithium with food, switch to different preparation, increase dosage more slowly, check blood level to ensure against toxic levels, reduce dose*
Postural tremor	Administer beta-blockers (if not contraindicated), increase dosage more slowly, decrease lithium level*
Polydipsia, polyuria	Administer diuretics, lower dosage,* take dose once a day at bedtime, decrease dietary protein
Confusion, ataxia	Immediately assay blood; if toxic, temporarily discontinue lithium or reduce dosage*
Skin reactions	Apply standard dermatological treatments, possibly discontinue lithium
Bradycardia, syncope	Check electrocardiogram, consider a pacemaker, possibly discontinue lithium
Central nervous system effects: mental dullness, memory and concentration difficulties, headache, fatigue, muscle weakness	Lower dosage,* possibly discontinue lithium

* May decrease protection versus relapse and recurrence. Reproduced and adapted with permission from Moseman, S. E., *et al.* Mood stabilizers. In A. Tasman, J. Kay, & J. A. Lieberman, eds. *Psychiatry*, 2nd edn. Copyright John Wiley & Sons, Ltd: Chichester, pp. 1965–1989.

Reductions in renal clearance (e.g. secondary to hyponatremia, angiotensin converting enzyme inhibitors, some diuretics, fluid volume depletion) may lead to toxicity (Keck & McElroy, 2002), whereas osmotic diuretics, aminophylline and

---

Box 26.1　Recommended pretreatment tests for selected mood stabilisers

Medication	Tests
General tests for all medications	Complete history and physical examination, including weight
	Pregnancy test if applicable
Lithium	Renal function tests (including urinalysis)
	Thyroid function tests (including thyroid stimulating hormone)
	Electrocardiogram
	Electrolytes
	Complete blood count
Valproate	Liver function tests
	Complete blood count
Carbamazepine	Complete blood count
	Liver function tests
	Renal function tests (including urinalysis)

Reproduced and adapted with permission from Moseman, S. E., *et al.* Mood Stabilizers. In A. Tasman, J. Kay, & J. A. Lieberman, eds. *Psychiatry*, 2nd edn. Copyright John Wiley & Sons, Ltd: Chichester, pp. 1965–1989.

---

carbonic anhydrase inhibitors may decrease blood levels (Timmer & Sands, 1999). Illness, altered electrolyte levels and several other medications (including nonsteroidal anti-inflammatory agents) may also increase the risk of chronic toxicity (Timmer & Sands, 1999).

Recommended baseline, and in some cases subsequent, laboratory tests for patients being treated with lithium include renal and thyroid function tests, a pregnancy test, ECG monitoring and possibly a complete blood count (see Box 26.1; American Psychiatric Association, 2002; Moseman *et al.*, 2003).

Valproate

Although first synthesised in the late 1800s, valproate's effectiveness for bipolar disorder was first reported in the 1960s (Bowden, 2003). A proposed

mechanism of action of valproate includes increasing GABA activity in the brain (Gould *et al.*, 2004; Ketter & Wang, 2003; Moseman *et al.*, 2003). Valproate might have neuroplastic effects, as well as effects on gene expression, sodium channels (i.e. inhibitory effects) and the cell membrane (Gould *et al.*, 2004; Gray *et al.*, 2003). Its antikindling and neuroprotective properties may also be relevant to its mood stabilizing effects (Keck & McElroy, 2002).

Several formulations are available with different times to peak plasma concentrations and absorptive properties (Keck & McElroy, 2002). Metabolism occurs via the cytochrome P-450 system, glucuronidation and beta-oxidation, and valproate has the capability of inhibiting the breakdown of other hepatically metabolised medications (Keck & McElroy, 2002; Moseman *et al.*, 2003). Valproate levels may also be affected by coadministration of agents that induce or inhibit microsomal enzymes (Moseman *et al.*, 2003). Valproate should not be given to individuals with clinically significant hepatic disease (Keck & McElroy, 2002).

Dose-related side effects of treatment with valproate include gastrointestinal upset (e.g. nausea, vomiting, diarrhea), liver function test abnormalities, tremor, sedation and osteoporosis (American Psychiatric Association, 2002; Bowden, 2003). Alopecia, increased appetite, polycystic ovarian syndrome and weight gain may also occur (American Psychiatric Association, 2002). Rashes, ataxia, pancreatitis, severe and potentially fatal hepatotoxicity (rare and mostly in paediatric patients) and haematologic abnormalities (e.g. thrombocytopenia, leukopenia, coagulation disturbances) may necessitate discontinuation (Moseman *et al.*, 2003; Sadock & Sadock, 2003). Neural tube defects may be seen in infants exposed to valproate early in gestation; lower dosages, supplemental folic acid and monotherapy may decrease this risk (Bowden, 2003).

Overdose does not commonly occur, in part because of the broad therapeutic window (American Psychiatric Association, 2002). However, signs of toxicity include lethargy, heart block, coma and death and may be treated with hemodialysis, if necessary (Keck & McElroy, 2002; Sadock & Sadock, 2003).

Baseline and follow-up investigations for individuals treated with valproate should include liver function and haematologic tests (see Box 26.1). Therapeutic drug concentrations range from 50 to 125 μg/mL for acute manic/mixed episodes, although lower levels are sometimes employed during maintenance treatment (American Psychiatric Association, 2002; Moseman *et al.,* 2003).

Carbamazepine

Carbamazepine decreases the activity of sodium channels and attenuates the activity of cyclic adenosine monophosphate (Gould *et al.,* 2004). Carbamazepine also has effects on several other neurotransmitter (e.g. adenosine, dopamine, serotonin) and second messenger systems, although its precise mechanism of action remains unknown (Gould *et al.,* 2004; Keck & McElroy, 2002; Moseman *et al.,* 2003).

Carbamazepine is metabolised by the cytochrome P-450 system and induces the metabolism of both itself and other agents metabolised by that system; thus increases in dosage may be necessary after several months of treatment (Ketter *et al.,* 1999; Moseman *et al.,* 2003). The metabolism of carbamazepine may also be affected by liver disease (French *et al.,* 2004). Additionally, blood levels are affected by other agents that have an effect on the cytochrome P-450 system (Moseman *et al.,* 2003). Therapeutic blood levels for the treatment of acute manic/mixed episodes are targeted for approximately 4 to 12 μg/ml (American Psychiatric Association, 2002).

Carbamazepine has the potential to cause several adverse effects, including central nervous system effects (e.g. fatigue, diplopia, dizziness, nausea, tremor, ataxia, blurred vision), rashes, hyponatremia, increased liver enzymes, constipation, diarrhea, gastrointestinal distress, vomiting, anorexia and haematologic abnormalities (e.g. leukopenia), some of which may necessitate discontinuation

of the agent (Moseman *et al.,* 2003; Sadock & Sadock, 2003). More uncommon and severe side effects include agranulocytosis, aplastic anemia, hepatic failure, systemic hypersensitivity reactions, renal effects, cardiac conduction disturbance, psychosis, Stevens-Johnson syndrome, thrombocytopenia and pancreatitis (American Psychiatric Association, 2002).

Signs of toxicity include diplopia, sedation, ataxia, dizziness, hyperirritability and coma (American Psychiatric Association, 2002; Sadock & Sadock, 2003). Other signs of overdose include impaired consciousness, nystagmus, ophthalmoplegia, convulsions, respiratory problems, cerebellar and extrapyramidal signs, cardiac abnormalities (e.g. arrhythmias, tachycardia, conduction disturbances, hypotension) and gastrointestinal and anticholinergic symptoms (American Psychiatric Association, 2002). Overdose (which can be fatal) can be treated with haemoperfusion, dialysis and gastric lavage (American Psychiatric Association, 2002; Keck & McElroy, 2002; Sadock & Sadock, 2003).

Recommended baseline, and in some cases follow-up, tests for patients being treated with carbamazepine include haematologic, liver function, renal function and electrolyte tests (see Box 26.1; American Psychiatric Association, 2002; Moseman *et al.,* 2003).

Oxcarbazepine

Oxcarbazepine is an analogue of carbamazepine (May *et al.,* 2003). Its efficacy for bipolar disorder might be related to its ability to block sodium channels, stabilise hyperexcitable neuronal membranes or decrease electrical firing (Keck & McElroy, 2002).

Oxcarbazepine, after presystemic metabolism to a metabolite, undergoes glucuronidation, and to a lesser extent oxidation, and is then primarily excreted through the kidneys (Kalis & Huff, 2001). It weakly induces the cytochrome P-450 system and does not induce its own metabolism but can alter the plasma concentrations of several other medications (American Psychiatric Association, 2002; Keck & McElroy, 2002). The metabolism of oxcarbazepine may also be affected by liver and renal disease (French *et al.,* 2004; May *et al.,* 2003).

In general, oxcarbazepine has a lower risk of severe side effects and is better tolerated than carbamazepine (American Psychiatric Association, 2002; Keck & McElroy, 2002). Sedation, ataxia, nystagmus, vertigo, impaired coordination, headache, diplopia, slurred speech, dizziness, nausea, hyponatremia, skin rashes, vomiting, epigastric distress, diarrhea, weakness and severe hypersensitivity reactions (less common) are side effects that can occur with the use of oxcarbazepine (Kalis & Huff, 2001; Perucca, 2001; Tecoma, 1999). There is some cross-sensitivity with carbamazepine for the production of allergic skin reactions (LaRoche & Helmers, 2004).

Lamotrigine

Lamotrigine's mechanism of action may be related to its inhibition of sodium channels, antiglutamatergic effect or neuroprotective effects (Hahn *et al.,* 2004; Ketter *et al.,* 2003). Metabolism occurs primarily through glucuronidation in the liver, and thus several pharmacokinetic interactions are possible, although effects on cytochrome P-450 enzymes are generally not seen (French *et al.,* 2004; Hahn *et al.,* 2004; Moseman *et al.,* 2003). Lamotrigine's metabolism and blood levels may also be affected by hepatic and renal impairment (French *et al.,* 2004; Hahn *et al.,* 2004; Keck & McElroy, 2002). In addition, lamotrigine can induce its own metabolism (Keck & McElroy, 2002). Significantly decreased dosages should be used in individuals also being treated with valproate because of pharmacokinetic interactions (American Psychiatric Association, 2002).

Side effects include headache, dyspepsia, constipation, disseminated intravascular coagulation, nausea, dizziness, pruritis, unclear vision, arthritis, pain, tremor, tics, ataxia, rhinitis, abnormal dreams, diarrhea, insomnia, fatigue, infection, cough, vomiting and dry mouth, although several of these side effects were noted not to occur more often than in groups treated with placebo (American Psychiatric Association, 2002; French *et al.,* 2004; Hahn *et al.,*

2004; Matsuo, 1999). Lamotrigine carries the potential for severe hypersensitivity reactions, including skin rashes, at the first sign of which the drug should be discontinued, given the potential for the development of a Stevens-Johnson-type syndrome or toxic epidermal necrolysis (the risk possibly increases with concomitant administration of valproate), and other severe hypersensitivity reactions (including risk of hepatic and renal failure; American Psychiatric Association, 2002; French *et al.,* 2004; Moseman *et al.,* 2003). Severe rashes have been reported to occur more often when rapid titration schedules are used and in younger individuals, in addition to when lamotrigine is used concomitantly with valproate (LaRoche & Helmers, 2004).

Overdose with lamotrigine can be fatal (Keck & McElroy, 2002). Signs of overdose include ataxia, increased seizures, delirium, nystagmus, coma and cardiac conduction abnormalities (Keck & McElroy, 2002). Treatment of overdose may include supportive care and hemodialysis (Keck & McElroy, 2002).

Baseline laboratory tests for individuals being treated with lamotrigine may include liver function tests, a pregnancy test and renal function tests (Moseman *et al.,* 2003).

Topiramate

Topiramate has been shown to possess GABAergic and anti-glutamatergic activity, block sodium channels and inhibit carbonic anhydrase enzymes (Keck & McElroy, 2002; Suppes, 2002). Metabolism occurs via glucuronidation, hydrolysis and hydroxylation and may be affected by renal disease (French *et al.,* 2004; Keck & McElroy, 2002). Topiramate has the potential to affect several cytochrome P-450 enzymes (French *et al.,* 2004). Renal, and possibly hepatic, impairment decreases the clearance of topiramate (Keck & McElroy, 2002). Because of its weak inhibition of carbonic anhydrase and potential for renal calculi, topiramate should not be coadministered with other inhibitors of this enzyme (Sadock & Sadock, 2003).

Side effects include nausea, ataxia, anorexia, memory disturbance, dizziness, increased thirst, impaired concentration, confusion, dyspepsia, altered taste, somnolence, fatigue, weight loss, nausea, dry mouth, behavioral disturbances, paresthesias, constipation, pruritis, dysnomia/anomia, diaphoresis, blurred vision, tremors, hypohidrosis, rash and difficulty sleeping (American Psychiatric Association, 2002; French *et al.*, 2004; LaRoche & Helmers, 2004; Perucca, 2001; Suppes, 2002). Less common side effects include nephrolithiasis, acute glaucoma or changes in vision and metabolic acidosis (Perucca, 2001; Suppes, 2002). Gastric emptying techniques and hemodialysis may be used in cases of overdose (Keck & McElroy, 2002).

Implementation

The remainder of this chapter is devoted to the implementation of the biological treatments of psychosis. This discussion is divided by the phases of treatment (e.g. acute phase, first-episode, maintenance) for primary psychosis (i.e. schizophrenia, schizoaffective disorder, delusional disorder) and affective psychosis (i.e. bipolar disorder and psychotic depression).

Primary psychosis

The prodromal period

A number of ethical issues surround the treatment of patients who manifest prodromal symptoms of psychosis and who are at risk for schizophrenia (Cornblatt *et al.*, 2001; McGlashan, 2001; McGorry *et al.*, 2001). The first challenge is to validate tools of identification of those truly at risk to convert to a first psychotic episode. One set of published criteria identifies individuals with prodromal psychosis as having attenuated positive symptoms, brief intermittent psychotic symptoms or a steep decline in functioning in addition to a family history of schizophrenia (Yung *et al.*, 1996).

Preliminary results suggest benefits for atypical antipsychotics, and possibly also antidepressants, on symptomatology or rates of progression to

psychotic illness (Cornblatt, 2002; Ruhrmann *et al.*, 2005; Woods *et al.*, 2003). However, the evidence base awaits a robust set of studies showing an acceptable number of patients needed to treat to prevent conversion to psychosis.

The acute phase

Goals of treatment in the acute phase of psychosis include harm prevention, symptom improvement and rapid return to baseline levels of functioning (Lehman *et al.*, 2004; Royal Australian and New Zealand College of Psychiatrists Clinical Practice Guidelines Team for the Treatment of Schizophrenia and Related Disorders, 2005). Determination of the aetiology of the psychotic exacerbation (e.g. nonadherence) is an important part of acute phase management (Royal Australian and New Zealand College of Psychiatrists, 2005). Also, except in certain circumstances (e.g. medication refusal or the requirement of additional evaluation), antipsychotics should be initiated early for the acute treatment of psychosis (Lehman *et al.*, 2004). In the case of emergencies and aggressive patients, involuntary treatment in the form of parenteral medications may be beneficial (Lehman *et al.*, 2004; Royal Australian and New Zealand College of Psychiatrists, 2005).

Choice of medication depends in large part on the patient's previous experiences, taking into account efficacy, side effects and route of administration (Feifel, 2000; Lehman *et al.*, 2004; Royal Australian and New Zealand College of Psychiatrists, 2005). In addition, atypical antipsychotics are recommended by some guidelines to be the first choice (Feifel, 2000; Lehman *et al.*, 2004), and a recent expert consensus guideline recommended risperidone as a first-line agent (Kane *et al.*, 2003). However, a patient who has previously responded well with minimal side effects to a conventional antipsychotic and prefers such a medication may be treated with such (Lehman *et al.*, 2004; Royal Australian and New Zealand College of Psychiatrists, 2005). In addition, special consideration can be given to clozapine for persistent suicidal, hostile and aggressive behaviours (Kane *et al.*, 2003; Lehman *et al.*, 2004; Meltzer, Alphs, *et al.*, 2003).

As noted earlier, oral medications are generally the preferred route of administration, but long-acting medications may be appropriate in the context of nonadherence, patient preference or a history of severe relapse with medication discontinuation (Lehman *et al.*, 2004; Royal Australian and New Zealand College of Psychiatrists, 2005; Sharif, 1998).

The dosage used should be that which shows efficacy without inducing too many side effects (Lehman *et al.*, 2004). For conventional antipsychotics, the appropriate dose is that at the *neuroleptic threshold* or the lowest dose that results in minimal rigidity (McEvoy *et al.*, 1991). The dose for atypical antipsychotics is often below the neuroleptic threshold (Lehman *et al.*, 2004). Dosages can be titrated up as quickly as tolerated, although care must be taken not to titrate prematurely (Feifel, 2000; Karagianis *et al.*, 2001; Lehman *et al.*, 2004). Adjunctive medications can also be used to target specific symptomatology and complaints (e.g. benzodiazepines for catatonia, antidepressants for anxiety or disturbances of mood, or mood stabilisers for aggression; Lehman *et al.*, 2004).

For aggressive patients who present a risk to themselves or others, antipsychotic/benzodiazepine combinations (e.g. haloperidol 5 mg with lorazepam 2 mg or risperidone 2 mg with lorazepam 2 mg) have generally been preferred over antipsychotics or benzodiazepines alone for patients whose aggression is due to schizophrenia or psychosis (Allen *et al.*, 2003; Currier *et al.*, 2004b; Hughes & Kleespies, 2003). However, some recommendations include intramuscular olanzapine or ziprasidone alone as alternative first-line agents (Battaglia, 2005; Currier *et al.*, 2004b). Choice of antipsychotic can be based on a number of factors, including efficacy, available methods of dosage forms and side-effect profile (Hughes & Kleespies, 2003). Side-effect profile is important both in the short-term and long-term as adherence might be significantly hindered by an undesirable experience in the acute setting (Hughes & Kleespies, 2003).

Lorazepam has become the preferred benzodiazepine because of its short half-life, parenteral formulations and efficacy for sedative or alcohol withdrawal (Currier *et al.*, 2004a).

The first episode

It has been suggested that untreated psychosis has far-reaching detrimental consequences on patients and their families and that lessening the duration of untreated psychosis should be considered a high priority (Lieberman & Fenton, 2000). Recent clinical trials have also suggested that shorter durations of untreated psychosis are associated with better outcomes (Melle *et al.*, 2004; Perkins *et al.*, 2004). Consequently, it is widely considered to be the standard of care to treat psychosis when it first becomes evident (Lehman *et al.*, 2004; Royal Australian and New Zealand College of Psychiatrists, 2005).

Atypical antipsychotics are usually recommended as the first-line agents for treating first-episode psychosis (Bradford *et al.*, 2003; Kane *et al.*, 2003), and a recent expert consensus guideline particularly recommended risperidone as a first-choice agent (Kane *et al.*, 2003). The use of atypicals is supported by several randomised controlled trials supporting the equal or greater efficacy of some of these agents over conventional antipsychotics (Keefe *et al.*, 2004; Lieberman *et al.*, 2003a; Lieberman *et al.*, 2003b; Schooler *et al.*, 2005). In addition, individuals with first-episode psychosis are generally considered to be more sensitive to antipsychotics, showing both efficacy and side effects with relatively lower doses (Bradford *et al.*, 2003; Canadian Psychiatric Association, 1998; Lehman *et al.*, 2004; Zhang-Wong *et al.*, 1999).

The majority of patients with first-episode psychosis remit, and treatment with antipsychotic medications significantly decreases rates of relapse thereafter (Bradford *et al.*, 2003; Lehman *et al.*, 2004). However, more randomised controlled trials are necessary before clearer recommendations can be made regarding treatment regimens in the first episode.

Relapse prevention and the maintenance phase

After an acute psychotic event remits, a patient should be continued on the same antipsychotic medication for at least 12 months, assuming the medication is both effective and tolerated (Lehman *et al.*, 2004; Royal Australian and New Zealand College of Psychiatrists, 2005). Maintenance antipsychotic medications greatly reduce the risk of relapse in individuals with psychosis from approximately 70% to 30% (Miyamoto *et al.*, 2003). Recent recommendations for maintenance treatment include 1 to 2 years for first-episode patients, with close follow-up, and up to 5 years or indefinite treatment for patients with multiple episodes or two episodes in 5 years (Canadian Psychiatric Association, 1998; Lehman *et al.*, 2004; Miyamoto *et al.*, 2003; Royal Australian and New Zealand College of Psychiatrists, 2005).

For conventional antipsychotics, maintenance dosages can be safely reduced to approximately 20% of acute treatment doses, although further dosage reductions will likely cause unacceptable rates of relapse (Marder, 1999; Miyamoto *et al.*, 2003). Rapid and premature dose reductions should also be avoided (Lehman *et al.*, 2004; Miyamoto *et al.*, 2003). In addition, continuous, as opposed to intermittent, therapy is recommended and more effective in preventing relapse (Canadian Psychiatric Association, 1998; Schooler *et al.*, 1997; Taylor *et al.*, 2005).

Both conventional and atypical antipsychotics have shown efficacy for the maintenance treatment of schizophrenia (Arato *et al.*, 2002; Beasley *et al.*, 2003; Cooper *et al.*, 2000; Marder, 1999; Pigott *et al.*, 2003). Several randomised trials have reported that atypical antipsychotics are more effective than conventional agents in response rates or for relapse prevention (e.g. rates of rehospitalisation) in general (Csernansky *et al.*, 2002; Essock *et al.*, 1996; Kasper *et al.*, 2003; Leucht, Barnes, *et al.*, 2003), and some guidelines suggest that the advent of depot risperidone might bring further benefits (Taylor *et al.*, 2005).

The recently published Clinical Antipsychotic Trials of Intervention Effectiveness (CATIE) study has shed some light on the clinical differences between conventional and atypical antipsychotic agents (Lieberman *et al.*, 2005). In the CATIE trial, 1,493 patients with schizophrenia were randomly assigned to treatment with perphenazine (i.e. a conventional antipsychotic), olanzapine, risperidone, quetiapine or, later, ziprasidone (Lieberman *et al.*, 2005). The study showed that 74% of all patients discontinued their antipsychotic medications before 18 months, indicating that although these medications are effective, they have limitations in chronic schizophrenia (Lieberman *et al.*, 2005). Olanzapine was associated with the lowest rates of discontinuation, whereas perphenazine and the other atypical antipsychotics were similar in most regards (Lieberman *et al.*, 2005). These results indicate that drug selection in this population will be multifactorial, taking into account economics, efficacy and side effects (Lieberman *et al.*, 2005).

Treatment-resistant illness

Treatment-resistant schizophrenia has been defined as at least two full (i.e. 4–6 week long at doses of 400–600 mg chlorpromazine equivalents) trials of antipsychotic medications with no improvement, persistent symptoms and greater than 5 years without a period of good social or occupational functioning (see Box 26.2; Conley & Kelly, 2001). The proportion of individuals with treatment-resistant schizophrenia varies, but it has been estimated that approximately 200,000 to 500,000 such patients live in the United States alone (Conley & Kelly, 2001). Treatment for schizophrenia may not be successful for a number of reasons, including inadequate dosing, nonadherence, substance use and poor psychosocial rehabilitation (Lehman *et al.*, 2004; Royal Australian and New Zealand College of Psychiatrists, 2005). Similarly, an important part of the management of individuals with suspected treatment resistant schizophrenia is a careful evaluation of whether adequate trials of antipsychotic medications have actually been attempted (Lehman *et al.*, 2004; Royal Australian and New Zealand College of Psychiatrists, 2005).

Box 26.2 Proposed guidelines for determining treatment resistance in schizophrenia

1. Drug-refractory condition: at least two prior drug trials of 4- to 6-week duration at 400 to 600 mg of chlorpromazine (or equivalent) with no clinical improvement
2. Persistence of illness: >5 years with no period of good social or occupational functioning
3. Persistent psychotic symptoms: BPRS total score >45 (on 18-item scale) and item score >4 (moderate) on at least two of four positive symptom items

BPRS, Brief Psychiatric Rating Scale.
Reprinted from Conley, R. R., & Kelly, D. L. (2001). Management of treatment resistance in schizophrenia. *Biol Psychiatry* **50**:898–911, with permission from the Society of Biological Psychiatry.

After treatment resistance has been confirmed, consideration should be given to the use of clozapine (Canadian Psychiatric Association, 1998; Lehman *et al.*, 2004; Royal Australian and New Zealand College of Psychiatrists, 2005). This is supported by several clinical trials demonstrating greater efficacy for clozapine over conventional antipsychotics in this population (Chakos *et al.*, 2001; Kane *et al.*, 1988).

There is also preliminary data regarding the effects of other atypical antipsychotics, several atypical antipsychotic combinations and other augmentation strategies (e.g. lithium, cognition enhancers, anticonvulsants, agents with glutamatergic effects, fatty acids, ECT) for treatment-resistant schizophrenia, although the evidence base remains limited or mixed (Buchanan *et al.*, 2003, 2005; Chakos *et al.*, 2001; Conley & Kelly, 2001; Emsley *et al.*, 2002; Heresco-Levy *et al.*, 2002; Josiassen *et al.*, 2005; Lerner *et al.*, 2004; Lindenmayer *et al.*, 2004; Miyamoto *et al.*, 2003; Miyamoto *et al.*, 2005; Tiihonen *et al.*, 2005; Tollefson *et al.*, 2001; Tsai *et al.*, 2004). Given the burdens associated with clozapine therapy, other atypical antipsychotics should be considered before instituting it (Conley & Kelly, 2001; Miyamoto *et al.*, 2003). Further study is warranted to examine these issues fully.

Additional considerations for the treatment of primary psychotic disorders

Depressive symptoms occur frequently in individuals with schizophrenia and are associated with several negative consequences, including worse outcome and suicide (Siris, 2000). Post-psychotic depression covers depressive episodes that occur during the residual phase of schizophrenia or after a psychotic episode at any time (Gruenberg and Goldstein, 2003; Siris, 2000). However, it might be difficult to differentiate between post-psychotic depression, or depressive symptoms which occur otherwise in individuals with schizophrenia, and the negative symptoms of the illness or drug-induced side effects or dysphoria (Gruenberg & Goldstein, 2003; Siris, 2000). Evidence suggests that post-psychotic depression responds to antidepressant augmentation (Siris *et al.*, 1987, 2000). Recent preliminary evidence also suggests that monotherapy with atypical antipsychotics may be efficacious in this population (Dollfus *et al.*, 2005). Other general treatment options for depression occurring in the context of schizophrenia include switching to an atypical antipsychotic, decreasing the antipsychotic dosage and optimizing medications used to treat side effects (Siris, 2000). If the depression persists, meets criteria for a major depressive episode, is severe or significantly affects function, the addition of an antidepressant might also be considered (Lehman *et al.*, 2004; Siris, 2000).

Obsessive-compulsive symptoms, anxiety, hostility, aggression and mood instability are other comorbid conditions which can occur during the maintenance phase (Lehman *et al.*, 2004). Evidence suggests that fluvoxamine (for obsessive-compulsive symptoms) and benzodiazepines (for anxiety), along with valproate (for hostility) and pindolol (for aggression), may be helpful in these and similar instances (Caspi *et al.*, 2001; Citrome *et al.*, 2004; Reznik & Sirota, 2000; Wolkowitz & Pickar, 1991).

Substance use disorders occur in anywhere from 40% to 70% of individuals with schizophrenia (Green, 2005). Evidence is emerging to suggest that treatment with atypical antipsychotics (e.g. clozapine, risperidone), but not conventionals, might have beneficial effects on substance use in these individuals (Green, 2005).

The treatment of *elderly people* with schizophrenia is often complicated by medical illness, altered pharmacokinetic parameters and polypharmacy (Lehman *et al.*, 2004). In addition, rates of tardive dyskinesia are greater in elderly individuals treated with conventional antipsychotics, and this risk may be lower with atypical antipsychotics (Jeste, 2004). Lower starting and maintenance dosages, along with slower titrations, should be used in the elderly, and atypical agents have advantages in this population given their lesser risks of EPS and tardive dyskinesia (Howard *et al.*, 2000; Jeste, 2004; Jeste *et al.*, 1999; Kane *et al.*, 2003). Similarly, a recent expert consensus guideline recommended risperidone as the first-line antipsychotic in this population, followed by olanzapine, quetiapine and aripiprazole (Alexopoulos *et al.*, 2004).

Several additional considerations accompany the treatment of *pregnant* women with psychotic disorders (American Academy of Pediatrics Committee on Drugs, 2000; Seeman, 2004; Trixler *et al.*, 2005). Although the data regarding the use of antipsychotics during pregnancy are encouraging, the evidence base remains limited (Trixler *et al.*, 2005). When considering treatment with antipsychotic agents, clinicians must consider the risk to the foetus of the medication with the risk of untreated psychosis in the mother (Patton *et al.*, 2002; Trixler *et al.*, 2005). It has been recommended, however, that antipsychotic exposure be avoided if possible in the first trimester and, if antipsychotic treatment is necessary, that high-potency agents be used at the lowest possible doses (American Academy of Pediatrics Committee on Drugs, 2000; Seeman, 2004; Trixler *et al.*, 2005). In addition, consideration should be given to close monitoring for neural tube defects and possible supplementation with high (i.e. 4 mg/day) dosages of folate in some at-risk subgroups (Trixler *et al.*, 2005). Attention should be paid to, and counselling and education provided for, pre-pregnancy- and pregnancy-related

issues for all women of reproductive age who also have psychotic illnesses (Trixler *et al.*, 2005).

Similar to the situation with pregnancy, the evidence base is limited regarding the use of antipsychotic medications during *lactation* (Patton *et al.*, 2002). However, it has been reported that nursing infants will be exposed to psychotropic medications if being taken by the mother (American Academy of Pediatrics Committee on Drugs, 2001). If pharmacological treatment is deemed necessary, consideration should be given to using the safest possible drug, establishing communication between the pediatrician and the mother's physician, monitoring the concentration of the drug in the infant's blood if adverse effects are possible, and encouraging the nursing mother to take her medication before a prolonged sleep period of the infant or just after feeding the infant (American Academy of Pediatrics Committee on Drugs, 2001).

Other treatment modalities

Electroconvulsive therapy

As described in detail in Chapter 27, ECT is a procedure in which an electrical stimulus is applied to a patient's brain to produce a therapeutic seizure (Tharyan & Adams, 2005). The electrical stimulus is delivered through electrodes placed on the patient's scalp (Tharyan & Adams, 2005). The seizure activity is normally attenuated with the short-acting muscular relaxant succinylcholine, and the patient is provided anesthesia with methohexital, a short-acting barbiturate (Sadock & Sadock, 2003). The mechanism of action is unknown but may be related to the effects of ECT on neurotransmitter and second-messenger systems (Sadock & Sadock, 2003).

The treatment protocol for schizophrenia may involve longer courses than those used for depression, up to 12 and sometimes even 20 treatments, given at variable frequencies (Tharyan & Adams, 2005). Continuous or "maintenance" ECT is also occasionally pursued at less frequent intervals (Tharyan & Adams, 2005).

Although some of the earliest applications of ECT were for schizophrenic symptoms, the most common indication at the present time is for major depressive disorder (Sadock & Sadock, 2003). Medications remain the first-line and preferred treatment for schizophrenia (Tharyan & Adams, 2005). However, ECT has shown some efficacy for certain clinical scenarios (Braga & Petrides, 2005; Tharyan & Adams, 2005). In particular, ECT, when added to antipsychotics, has shown greater efficacy than antipsychotics alone in the short-term in individuals who display limited response to antipsychotic medications (Braga & Petrides, 2005; Tharyan & Adams, 2005). In addition, evidence suggests that continuation ECT in addition to antipsychotics may be more effective than either therapy alone in treatment-resistant patients who responded to combination therapy during an acute phase of their illness (Chanpattana et al., 1999). Studies have also reported that ECT plus clozapine is an effective regimen for treatment resistant patients (Braga & Petrides, 2005; Kupchik et al., 2000) and that ECT is effective in, and should be considered for, individuals with catatonic features (McCall, 2001; Suzuki et al., 2005). Further, ECT has been shown to be relatively safe, and the side effects of ECT in these populations are consistent with the general side effects of ECT, including memory impairment (Braga & Petrides, 2005; Tharyan & Adams, 2005).

Individuals with schizophrenia and affective symptoms, catatonia or significant positive symptoms are considered to be more likely to benefit from ECT (Sadock & Sadock, 2003). Several organisations have published recommendations regarding the use of ECT for schizophrenia (Lehman et al., 2004; Royal Australian and New Zealand College of Psychiatrists, 2005). Given the encouraging results from clinical investigation, further randomised controlled trials are warranted better to define optimal regimens, techniques and indications for ECT in psychosis.

Transcranial magnetic stimulation

Transcranial magnetic stimulation (TMS) was introduced in the mid-1980s as a noninvasive method of stimulating the brain (Haraldsson et al., 2004). As described in Chapter 27, TMS involves an electrical current being passed through a coil placed against the scalp, which induces a magnetic field (Haraldsson et al., 2004). This magnetic field in turn induces electrical activity in the cerebral cortex (Haraldsson et al., 2004). TMS is considered to be a relatively safe procedure with headache, scalp facial muscle twitching and tinnitus as possible side effects (Burt et al., 2002; Daskalakis et al., 2002). Seizure and manic symptomatology have also been reported, although these side effects are generally associated with high-frequency, repetitive TMS (Burt et al., 2002).

Although most of the work investigating the clinical utility of TMS has been performed for depression, several studies have examined a potential role in schizophrenia (Lisanby et al., 2002). Those that do exist provide encouraging, but as yet inconclusive, results. In particular, studies investigating TMS directed at the prefrontal cortex have suggested efficacy in treating certain psychotic symptoms, such as negative symptoms and catatonia (Hajak et al., 2004; Haraldsson et al., 2004). In addition, several reports have shown that TMS improves auditory hallucinations when applied to the temporoparietal cortex, although other investigations report no differences between active and sham treatments (Haraldsson et al., 2004; Hoffman et al., 2005; Saba et al., 2006).

Clinical investigations into the efficacy of TMS are limited by the lack of a reliable placebo condition and the variation in stimulation parameters (Lisanby et al., 2002). Encouraging preliminary evidence exists for efficacy in treating certain psychotic symptoms. However, further randomised controlled trials which address the limitations just discussed are required before more robust conclusions can be drawn.

Additional considerations for the treatment of schizoaffective disorder

As outlined in Chapter 13, the nosological status of schizoaffective disorder remains controversial, but it is clear that treatment modalities for schizoaffective disorder should target both psychotic and mood symptoms (McElroy *et al.*, 1999). Thus antipsychotics, mood stabilisers, antidepressants and ECT are all part of the treatment armamentarium (McElroy *et al.*, 1999; Patel *et al.*, 2003).

Antipsychotic medications, particularly atypicals, possess thymoleptic properties in addition to their antipsychotic actions (Keck *et al.*, 2001; Masan, 2004; McElroy *et al.*, 1999; Mensink & Slooff, 2004; Sajatovic *et al.*, 2002; Tohen *et al.*, 2001). Therefore, atypical antipsychotic medications may be included as first-line agents for individuals with schizoaffective disorder (McElroy *et al.*, 1999). It has also been suggested that, in general, optimisation of antipsychotic treatment may be more effective in treating schizoaffective disorder than routine addition of antidepressants or mood stabilisers (Levinson *et al.*, 1999).

In addition, mood stabilisers, antidepressants and antipsychotic combinations may be effective in individuals with schizoaffective disorder (Lerner *et al.*, 2004; Leucht *et al.*, 2004; Patel *et al.*, 2003; Small *et al.*, 2003). Furthermore, proper subtyping may be advantageous when developing a psychopharmacological treatment plan (Baethge, 2003). Maintenance ECT has also been suggested to have some benefit as an adjunctive treatment for certain individuals (Swoboda *et al.*, 2001). However, the evidence base remains mixed and awaits a robust set of studies from which to draw conclusions. Randomised controlled trials that investigate therapeutic regimens specifically in individuals with schizoaffective disorder are warranted.

Additional considerations for the treatment of delusional disorder

Conventional antipsychotic medications have been the traditional treatment for delusional disorder (Patel *et al.*, 2003; Wenning *et al.*, 2003). In particular, pimozide is often considered to be the traditional drug of choice for delusional parasitosis (Aw *et al.*, 2004; Wenning *et al.*, 2003). Evidence is also emerging that suggests a role for atypical

antipsychotics, and possibly concomitant serotonergic antidepressants, in the treatment of delusional parasitosis (Freudenmann & Schonfeldt-Lecuona, 2005; Wenning *et al.*, 2003). However, the evidence supporting these treatments stems mostly from case reports and uncontrolled studies rather than randomised controlled trials (Sultana & McMonagle, 2000; Wenning *et al.*, 2003).

Affective psychosis

The acute phase of manic and mixed episodes

A major goal of treatment in the acute phase of manic and mixed episodes is to achieve a baseline level of functioning (American Psychiatric Association, 2002). Current recommendations, which depend on the severity of the episode, include lithium, valproate, antipsychotics such as olanzapine or, less frequently, carbamazepine as first-line treatments, with or without the addition of atypical antipsychotics (preferred over conventional antipsychotics because of their side-effect profiles), if not already taking an antipsychotic or benzodiazepines for short-term relief until the primary medication takes effect (American Psychiatric Association, 2002; Bauer *et al.*, 1999; Goodwin *et al.*, 2003; Licht *et al.*, 2003; Royal Australian and New Zealand College of Psychiatrists, 2004). Because psychotic symptoms are relatively common in mania, antipsychotic medications are often recommended but not vital (American Psychiatric Association, 2002; Bauer *et al.*, 1999; Goldenberg & Pies, 2003; Licht *et al.*, 2003). In addition, antipsychotic medications have been reported to have antimanic properties (Bowden, 2005; Goodwin *et al.*, 2003).

An alternative antiepileptic is oxcarbazepine, and other choices for antipsychotics include quetiapine and ziprasidone, although evidence is emerging for the efficacy of several other antipsychotics in acute mania, either as monotherapy or as adjunctive therapy (American Psychiatric Association, 2002; Goodwin *et al.*, 2003). If possible, antidepressant medications should be discontinued, expressly in individuals with rapid-cycling illness, given the

Table 26.3 Treatments for rapid-cycling bipolar disorder

Medication	Efficacy
Lithium	Less effective in rapid-cycling patients
Carbamazepine	Better response when combined with lithium than either drug alone
Lamotrigine	Possibly effective alone in some population groups
Valproate	Possibly effective alone or combined with lithium
Clozapine	Possibly effective in treatment-resistant patients

Reproduced and adapted with permission from Moseman, S. E., et al. Mood Stabilizers. In A. Tasman, J. Kay, & J. A. Lieberman, eds. *Psychiatry*, 2nd edn. Copyright John Wiley & Sons, Ltd: Chichester, pp. 1965–1989.

Box 26.3 Predictors of poor response to lithium prophylaxis

1. Rapid or continuous cycling
2. Mixed states or dysphoric mania
3. Alcohol or drug abuse
4. Noncompliance with treatment
5. Cycle pattern of depression-mania-euthymia
6. Personality disturbance
7. History of poor interepisode functioning
8. Poor social support system
9. Three or more prior episodes

Reproduced and adapted with permission from Moseman, S. E., et al. Mood Stabilizers. In A. Tasman, J. Kay, & J. A. Lieberman, eds. *Psychiatry*, 2nd edn. Copyright John Wiley & Sons, Ltd: Chichester, pp. 1965–1989.

---

possible risks of mania induction or cycle quickening (American Psychiatric Association, 2002; Bauer *et al.*, 1999; Goodwin *et al.*, 2003; Mackin & Young, 2004). Individuals with rapid-cycling illness often require combination therapy, including combinations of lamotrigine, valproate, lithium and atypical antipsychotics, although lithium is relatively ineffective for rapid-cycling illness (see Table 26.3 and Box 26.3; American Psychiatric Association, 2002; Bauer *et al.*, 1999; Moseman *et al.*, 2003).

Choice of treatment may also be guided by factors such as severity of episode (e.g. valproate or antipsychotics for quicker action in severely affected patients), route of administration, mixed versus manic episode (e.g. valproate and olanzapine might have advantages over lithium for mixed states), presence of suicidality (e.g. lithium may decrease risk), presence of catatonia (e.g. benzodiazepines or ECT) and side effects (American Psychiatric Association, 2002; Bauer *et al.*, 1999; Gelenberg and Pies, 2003; Goodwin *et al.*, 2003; Licht *et al.*, 2003; Royal Australian and New Zealand College of Psychiatrists, 2004; Taylor & Fink, 2003; Tondo *et al.*, 2001).

If a patient remains significantly symptomatic after approximately 2 weeks of an intervention or relapses while on treatment, the current regimen should be optimised and combination first-line treatment can be considered, as well as addition of an antipsychotic (e.g. risperidone, olanzapine, haloperidol), if not already part of the regimen, or other alternative or adjunctive medication (e.g. benzodiazepine or oxcarbazepine; American Psychiatric Association, 2002; Goodwin *et al.*, 2003; Licht *et al.*, 2003; Royal Australian and New Zealand College of Psychiatrists, 2004). Clozapine and ECT may also be considered for treatment refractory illness (American Psychiatric Association, 2002; Goodwin *et al.*, 2003; Kusumakar *et al.*, 1997; Licht *et al.*, 2003). Further consideration can be given to ECT for catatonia, severe mixed episodes or episodes occurring in the context of pregnancy (American Psychiatric Association, 2002; Goodwin *et al.*, 2003; Kusumakar *et al.*, 1997; Licht *et al.*, 2003).

The acute phase of depressive episodes associated with bipolar disorder

The goals of treatment for bipolar-associated depressive episodes include remission of symptoms and prevention of resultant mania or mixed episodes (American Psychiatric Association, 2002). Thus the distinction between bipolar and unipolar depression is important (Licht *et al.*, 2003). First-line treatments include lithium or lamotrigine, with olanzapine, quetiapine and the combination of olanzapine and fluoxetine as alternatives (American Psychiatric Association, 2002; Calabrese *et al.*, 2004; Goodwin *et al.*, 2003; Licht *et al.*, 2003; Royal Australian and New Zealand College of Psychiatrists, 2004). Antipsychotic medications may be indicated for the treatment of concomitant psychotic symptoms (Calabrese *et al.*, 2004; Goodwin *et al.*, 2003; Licht *et al.*, 2003). Rapid-cycling individuals in particular may benefit from combination treatment or the addition of valproate or olanzapine, especially if symptoms persist (Calabrese *et al.*, 2004). ECT can also be used for depressive episodes if they are severe, treatment resistant, or associated with marked suicidality, catatonia, psychosis or pregnancy (American Psychiatric Association, 2002; Calabrese *et al.*, 2004; Goodwin *et al.*, 2003; Ketter & Calabrese, 2002). Ultimately, treatment should be tailored to the individual (Calabrese *et al.*, 2004).

The use of antidepressants in bipolar disorder remains a controversy (Grunze, 2005). Given the possibility of inducing manic episodes, the use of antidepressant medications as monotherapy is not generally recommended, although they can be used as adjunctive medications for more severe episodes and are sometimes recommended as part of a first-line treatment combination (American Psychiatric Association, 2002; Goodwin *et al.*, 2003; Grunze, 2005; Licht *et al.*, 2003; Royal Australian and New Zealand College of Psychiatrists, 2004; Suppes *et al.*, 2005). If used, it has been suggested that antidepressants should be administered with a mood stabilizer and tapered if at all possible after a relatively short time period, although recent evidence suggests that, in a certain subgroup, discontinuation of antidepressants may increase risk of depressive relapse without necessarily decreasing the risk of switching (Altshuler *et al.*, 2001; Bauer *et al.*, 1999; Goodwin *et al.*, 2003; Keck & McElroy, 2003; Licht *et al.*, 2003; Post *et al.*, 2003; Royal Australian and New Zealand College of Psychiatrists, 2004; Suppes *et al.*, 2005). Some reports also identify a risk of antidepressant-withdrawal mania, although the incidence is currently unknown (Andrade, 2004).

Tricyclic antidepressants have been associated with slightly increased risks of precipitating mania or hypomania and should thus be avoided if possible, whereas selective serotonin reuptake inhibitors (SSRIs) have been associated with lower switch rates (American Psychiatric Association, 2002; Calabrese *et al.*, 2004; Gijsman *et al.*, 2004; Goodwin *et al.*, 2003; Licht *et al.*, 2003; Parker & Parker, 2003; Royal Australian and New Zealand College of Psychiatrists, 2004). Monoamine oxidase inhibitors (MAOIs) are also efficacious for the treatment of bipolar depression, but their use is limited by side effects and the risk of switching (American Psychiatric Association, 2002; Calabrese *et al.*, 2004; Royal Australian and New Zealand College of Psychiatrists, 2004).

If relapse or persistent symptoms occur in a patient who is already receiving first-line treatment, the first intervention should be to optimise that treatment. Thereafter, combinations of two first-line treatments can be considered, as can alternatives such as paroxetine, bupropion, MAOIs, and other, newer antidepressants (American Psychiatric Association, 2002; Bauer *et al.*, 1999; Calabrese *et al.*, 2004; Goodwin *et al.*, 2003; Licht *et al.*, 2003; Royal Australian and New Zealand College of Psychiatrists, 2004).

Breakthrough manic episodes may be treated by first optimizing the current first line medication and then considering augmentation with lithium, valproate, or antipsychotics (e.g. olanzapine, quetiapine, aripiprazole, risperidone, ziprasidone, clozapine; Calabrese *et al.*, 2004).

Maintenance treatment and relapse prevention for bipolar disorder

Some goals of maintenance treatment include a reduction of relapses and improvement in baseline functioning and symptoms (American Psychiatric Association, 2002) and should be considered following a single manic episode for at least 6 months and also for long-term prophylaxis in many cases, particularly with severe, suicidal, recurrent or frequent episodes or with a family history of bipolar disorder (American Psychiatric Association, 2002;

Bowden *et al.*, 2000; Goodwin *et al.*, 2003; Licht *et al.*, 2003; Royal Australian and New Zealand College of Psychiatrists, 2004). Lithium and valproate are considered first-line agents, with lamotrigine, oxcarbazepine, carbamazepine and possibly olanzapine as alternatives (American Psychiatric Association, 2002; Goodwin *et al.*, 2003; Royal Australian and New Zealand College of Psychiatrists, 2004). Lithium has been associated with affective morbidity and suicidal behaviour upon abrupt discontinuation and so should be used cautiously, or not at all, in patients with a history of poor compliance (see Box 26.3; Baldessarini *et al.*, 1999; Bowden *et al.*, 2000; Goodwin *et al.*, 2003). Lamotrigine may be more effective against depressive episodes, whereas lithium may be more effective against mania (Calabrese *et al.*, 2003; Geddes *et al.*, 2004; Goodwin *et al.*, 2003, 2004). As stated previously, valproate and lamotrigine should be given consideration in rapid-cycling illness (Royal Australian and New Zealand College of Psychiatrists, 2004). However, whichever medication was effective in treating a recent depressive or manic episode should be continued (American Psychiatric Association, 2002; Goodwin *et al.*, 2003; Swann, 2005). Similarly, maintenance ECT may be considered if ECT was part of an effective acute treatment protocol (American Psychiatric Association, 2002; Goodwin *et al.*, 2003).

Less evidence is available to support the use of antipsychotics in the maintenance phase, and treatment with antipsychotic medications should be continually reassessed and discontinued unless required for persistent symptoms or to prevent recurrence (American Psychiatric Association, 2002; Bauer *et al.*, 1999; Licht *et al.*, 2003). In fact, one recent clinical trial reported that continued treatment with a conventional antipsychotic after remission from an episode of acute mania may be detrimental to a subgroup of patients (Zarate & Tohen, 2004). Other investigations suggest that individuals who respond to combination therapy with an antipsychotic in the acute phase might benefit from continued combination therapy (Keck, 2004).

Combination treatments with other mood stabilisers, antidepressants or other medications may also be necessary to control persistent or otherwise refractory symptoms, and such regimens can be effective (American Psychiatric Association, 2002; Goodwin *et al.*, 2003; Keck & McElroy, 2003; Royal Australian and New Zealand College of Psychiatrists, 2004). Hypothyroidism should also be ruled out in treatment-refractory individuals, including those with rapid-cycling illness, and treated if present (American Psychiatric Association, 2002; Bauer *et al.*, 2003; Goodwin *et al.*, 2003; Kupka *et al.*, 2003; Royal Australian and New Zealand College of Psychiatrists, 2004).

Additional considerations for the treatment of bipolar disorder

Medication options for *children and adolescents* with bipolar disorder include lithium or valproate, carbamazepine, atypical antipsychotics and antidepressants; combinations thereof may also be used (American Psychiatric Association, 2002; Dunner, 2005; Licht *et al.*, 2003; Wozniak, 2005). A minimum of 18 months of maintenance treatment is recommended for this population, and, if indicated, medication should be tapered gradually during a time of minimal stressors (American Psychiatric Association, 2002).

Elderly patients are treated similarly to younger adults with the caveats that they may be more responsive to lower doses but may also be more sensitive to side effects (American Psychiatric Association, 2002; Dunner, 2005; Goodwin *et al.*, 2003; Licht *et al.*, 2003). A recent expert consensus guideline recommended risperidone or olanzapine, in addition to a mood stabiliser, as first-line antipsychotics for psychotic mania in older patients, with quetiapine as a high second-line option (Alexopoulos *et al.*, 2004). Comorbidity also frequently complicates the treatment of children, adolescents and elderly individuals (Dunner, 2005; Wozniak, 2005).

Evidence is also emerging regarding the efficacy of a number of *other biological treatments* (e.g. other anticonvulsants such as gabapentin and pheny-toin, fatty acids, calcium channel blockers, vagus nerve stimulation, transcranial magnetic stimula-tion, pramipexole, light therapy) in various phases of bipolar disorder (Benedetti *et al.*, 2003; Frye *et al.*, 2000; Goldberg *et al.*, 2004; Mishory *et al.*, 2003; Nahas *et al.*, 2003; Pazzaglia *et al.*, 1998; Rush *et al.*, 2005; Stoll *et al.*, 1999). Further study will elucidate the roles of these treatment modalities. The reader is also referred to Chapter 27.

Finally, the treatment of bipolar disorder in women who are *pregnant or lactating* incurs a number of additional considerations. These include potential teratogenicity of medications, increased rate of relapse in the immediate postpartum period, potential adverse effects of discontinuing medi-cations, altered pharmacokinetic parameters and the transmission of medication metabolites through breast-feeding, among others (American Psychiatric Association, 2002; Burt & Rasgon, 2004; Yonkers *et al.*, 2004). Examples of teratogenic associations include Ebstein's anomaly and other cardiovascu-lar malformations (e.g. lithium, valproate); neural tube defects (e.g. rates of approximately 1% with carbamazepine and slightly higher rates with val-proate) for which folic acid supplementation has been recommended; and various other structural and developmental alterations (e.g. carbamazepine, valproate; American Academy of Pediatrics, 2000; Burt and Rasgon, 2004; Yonkers *et al.*, 2004). There-fore it is vital for clinicians to discuss pregnancy-related issues with all of their patients of child-bearing capability (Yonkers *et al.*, 2004). A further discussion of some of these issues can be found in Chapter 19.

Psychotic depression

Major depressive disorder with psychotic features is associated with both increased recurrence and sui-cide risk relative to major depressive disorder with-out psychotic features (Rothschild, 2003; see Chap-ters 12 and 27). Recommended first-line treatments include the combination of an antidepressant and an antipsychotic (American Psychiatric Association, 2000; Canadian Psychiatric Association, 2001; Ellis *et al.*, 2004). These recommendations are supported by several recent trials (Rothschild *et al.*, 2004). The initial choice of antidepressant depends on a number of factors, including side effects, cost and comorbidity, among others (American Psychiatric Association, 2000). Tricyclic antidepressants, SSRIs and venlafaxine have been suggested as the first-line antidepressant, and amoxapine alone has also been recommended as a first-line option (Crismon *et al.*, 1999; Ellis *et al.*, 2004). ECT has variably been included as another first-line treatment option, especially in the context of severe suicidality or history of previous response (American Psychiatric Association, 2000; Canadian Psychiatric Associa-tion, 2001; Crismon *et al.*, 1999). Olanzapine, in combination with an antidepressant, was recom-mended as a second-line treatment, and monother-apy with SSRIs was not recommended (Canadian Psychiatric Association, 2001).

Options for patients who demonstrate refractori-ness to, or do not tolerate, the first-line treatments include attempting an alternate first-line treatment or using ECT (Crismon *et al.*, 1999). Right unilateral ECT may also be a treatment option for unrespon-sive patients and for those who are suicidal or at risk (Ellis *et al.*, 2004). Lithium is recommended as an augmentation strategy if prior regimens have been found to be ineffective (American Psychiatric Asso-ciation, 2000; Crismon *et al.*, 1999; Ellis *et al.*, 2004).

The antidepressant should be continued at least through the continuation phase and possibly also into the maintenance phase (American Psychiatric Association, 2000; Canadian Psychiatric Associa-tion, 2001; Crismon *et al.*, 1999; Ellis *et al.*, 2004). It is unclear for how long to continue the antipsy-chotic, although one guideline suggests continuing the acute dose for 1 or 2 months, and then, as the clinical situation permits, gradually tapering it dur-ing the continuation phase to decrease the risk of side effects (Crismon *et al.*, 1999).

Evidence is emerging that suggests effi-cacy for monotherapy with antidepressants or antipsychotics (Schatzberg, 2003; Zanardi *et al.,* 2000). Mifepristone, a glucocorticoid receptor antagonist, has also been suggested as a potential treatment for psychotic depression (Belanoff *et al.,* 2002; Rothschild, 2003; Schatzberg, 2003). More data are required before robust recommendations regarding these treatment options can be made.

Conclusions

The treatment of psychotic disorders was revolutionised with the discovery of chlorpromazine in the 1950s. Although the newer atypical antipsychotics carry a lower side effect burden (at least in terms of extrapyramidal effects), clinicians need to be aware of the potential for the atypical agents to produce other side effects (notably metabolic effects), should monitor patients for such effects and should treat them appropriately. Finally, the treatment of psychotic disorders requires medications to be used in consort with a range of psychosocial measures aimed at assisting patients to reintegrate as fully as possible into society.

REFERENCES

Abi-Dargham, A., & Laruelle, M. (2005). Mechanisms of action of second generation antipsychotic drugs in schizophrenia: insights from brain imaging studies. *Eur Psychiatry* **20**:15–27.

Aghajanian, G. K., & Marek, G. J. (2000). Serotonin model of schizophrenia: emerging role of glutamate mechanisms. *Brain Res Brain Res Rev* **31**:302–12.

Alexopoulos, G. S., Streim, J., Carpenter, D., & Docherty, J. P. (2004). Expert Consensus Panel for Using Antipsychotic Drugs in Older Patients. Using antipsychotic agents in older patients. *J Clin Psychiatry* **65**(Suppl 2):5–99; discussion 100–2; quiz 103–4.

Allen, M. H., Currier, G. W., Hughes, D. H., *et al.* (2003). Treatment of behavioral emergencies: a summary of the expert consensus guidelines. *J Psychiatr Pract* **9**:16–38.

Allison, D. B., & Casey, D. E. (2001). Antipsychotic-induced weight gain: a review of the literature. *J Clin Psychiatry* **62**(Suppl 7):22–31.

Allison, D. B., Mentore, J. L., Heo, M., *et al.* (1999). Antipsychotic-induced weight gain: a comprehensive research synthesis. *Am J Psychiatry* **156**:1686–96.

Altshuler L., Kiriakos L., Calcagno J., *et al.* (2001). The impact of antidepressant discontinuation versus antidepressant continuation on 1-year risk for relapse of bipolar depression: a retrospective chart review. *J Clin* **62**:612–6.

American Academy of Pediatrics Committee on Drugs (2000). Use of psychoactive medication during pregnancy and possible effects on the fetus and newborn. *Pediatrics* **105**:880–7.

American Academy of Pediatrics Committee on Drugs (2001). Transfer of drugs and other chemicals into human milk. *Pediatrics* **108**:776–89.

American Diabetes Association; American Psychiatric Association; American Association of Clinical Endocrinologists; North American Association for the Study of Obesity (2004). Consensus development conference on antipsychotic drugs and obesity and diabetes. *Diabetes Care* **27**:596–601.

American Psychiatric Association (2000). Practice guideline for the treatment of patients with major depressive disorder (revision). *Am J Psychiatry* **157**(4 Suppl):1–45.

American Psychiatric Association (2002). Practice guideline for the treatment of patients with bipolar disorder (revision). *Am J Psychiatry* **159**(4 Suppl):1–50.

Ananth J., Parameswaran S., Gunatilake S., *et al.* (2004). Neuroleptic malignant syndrome and atypical antipsychotic drugs. *J Clin Psychiatry* **65**:464–40.

Andrade, C. (2004). Antidepressant-withdrawal mania: a critical review and synthesis of the literature. *J Clin Psychiatry* **65**:987–93.

Arana, G. W. (2000). An overview of side effects caused by typical antipsychotics. *J Clin Psychiatry* **61**(Suppl 8):5–11; discussion 12–13.

Arato, M., O'Connor, R., Meltzer, H. Y.; ZEUS Study Group (2002). A 1-year, double-blind, placebo-controlled trial of ziprasidone 40, 80 and 160 mg/day in chronic schizophrenia: the Ziprasidone Extended Use in Schizophrenia (ZEUS) study. *Int Clin Psychopharmacol* **17**:207–15.

Atbasoglu, E. C., Ozguven, H. D., Can Saka, M., & Goker, C. (2004). Rhabdomyolysis and coma associated with amisulpride: a probable atypical presentation of neuroleptic malignant syndrome. *J Clin Psychiatry* **65**:1724–5.

Aw, D. C., Thong, J. Y., Chan, H. L. (2004). Delusional parasitosis: case series of 8 patients and review of the literature. *Ann Acad Med Singapore* **33**:89–94.

Baethge, C. (2003). Long-term treatment of schizoaffective disorder: review and recommendations. *Pharmacopsychiatry* 36:45–56.

Baldessarini, R. J., Tondo, L., & Hennen, J. (1999). Effects of lithium treatment and its discontinuation on suicidal behavior in bipolar manic-depressive disorders. *J Clin Psychiatry* 60(Suppl 2):77–84; discussion 111–16.

Baptista, T., Kin, N. M., Beaulieu, S., & de Baptista, E. A. (2002). Obesity and related metabolic abnormalities during antipsychotic drug administration: mechanisms, management and research perspectives. *Pharmacopsychiatry* 35:205–19.

Battaglia, J. (2005). Pharmacological management of acute agitation. *Drugs* 65:1207–22.

Bauer, M. S., Callahan, A. M., Jampala, C., *et al.* (1999). Clinical practice guidelines for bipolar disorder from the Department of Veterans Affairs. *J Clin Psychiatry* 60:9–21.

Baumann, P., Hiemke, C., Ulrich, S., *et al.* (2004). Arbeitsgemeinschaft fur neuropsychopharmakologie und pharmakopsychiatrie. The AGNP-TDM expert group consensus guidelines: therapeutic drug monitoring in psychiatry. *Pharmacopsychiatry* 37:243–65.

Beasley, C. M., Jr., Sutton, V. K., Hamilton, S. H., *et al.*; Olanzapine Relapse Prevention Study Group (2003). A double-blind, randomized, placebo controlled trial of olanzapine in the prevention of psychotic relapse. *J Clin Psychopharmacol* 23:582–94.

Belanoff, J. K., Rothschild, A. J., Cassidy, F., *et al.* (2002). An open label trial of C-1073 (mifepristone) for psychotic major depression. *Biol Psychiatry* 52:386–92.

Benedetti, F., Colombo, C., Pontiggia, A., *et al.* (2003). Morning light treatment hastens the antidepressant effect of citalopram: a placebo-controlled trial. *J Clin Psychiatry* 64:648–53.

Bergman, R. N., & Ader, M. (2005). Atypical antipsychotics and glucose homeostasis. *J Clin Psychiatry* 66:504–14.

Blin, O. (1999). A comparative review of new antipsychotics. *Can J Psychiatry* 44:235–44.

Bowden, C. L. (2003). *Valproate. Bipolar Disord* 5:189–202.

Bowden, C. L. (2005). Atypical antipsychotic augmentation of mood stabilizer therapy in bipolar disorder. *J Clin Psychiatry* 66(Suppl 3):12–19.

Bowden, C. L., Lecrubier, Y., Bauer, M., *et al.* (2000). Maintenance therapies for classic and other forms of bipolar disorder. *J Affect Disord* 59(Suppl 1):S57–S67.

Bradford, D. W., Perkins, D. O., Lieberman, J. A. (2003). Pharmacological management of first-episode schizophrenia and related nonaffective psychoses. *Drugs* 63:2265–83.

Braga, R. J., & Petrides, G. (2005). The combined use of electroconvulsive therapy and antipsychotics in patients with schizophrenia. *J ECT* 21:75–83.

Buchanan, R. W., Ball, M. P., & Weiner, E., *et al.* (2005). Olanzapine treatment of residual positive and negative symptoms. *Am J Psychiatry* 162:124–9.

Buchanan, R. W., Summerfelt, A., Tek, C., & Gold, J. (2003). An open-labeled trial of adjunctive donepezil for cognitive impairments in patients with schizophrenia. *Schizophr Res* 59:29–33.

Burns, M. J. (2001). The pharmacology and toxicology of atypical antipsychotic agents. *J Toxicol Clin Toxicol* 39:1–14.

Burt, T., Lisanby, S. H., Sackeim, H. A. (2002). Neuropsychiatric applications of transcranial magnetic stimulation: a meta analysis. *Int J Neuropsychopharmacol* 5:73–103.

Burt, V. K., & Rasgon, N. (2004). Special considerations in treating bipolar disorder in women. *Bipolar Disord* 6:2–13.

Calabrese, J. R., Bowden, C. L., Sachs, G., *et al.*; Lamictal 605 Study Group (2003). A placebo-controlled 18-month trial of lamotrigine and lithium maintenance treatment in recently depressed patients with bipolar I disorder. *J Clin Psychiatry* 64:1013–24.

Calabrese, J. R., Kasper, S., Johnson, G., *et al.* (2004). International Consensus Group on Bipolar I Depression Treatment Guidelines. *J Clin Psychiatry* 65:569–79.

Canadian Psychiatric Association (1998). Canadian clinical practice guidelines for the treatment of schizophrenia. *Can J Psychiatry* 43(Suppl 2):25S–40S.

Canadian Psychiatric Association; Canadian Network for Mood and Anxiety Treatments (CANMAT) (2001). Clinical guidelines for the treatment of depressive disorders. *Can J Psychiatry* 46(Suppl 1):5S–90S.

Casey, D. F. (1997). The relationship of pharmacology to side effects. *J Clin Psychiatry* 58(Suppl 10):55–62.

Casey, D. E. (1999). Tardive dyskinesia and atypical antipsychotic drugs. *Schizophr Res* 35(Suppl):S61–6.

Casey, D. E. (2004). Dyslipidemia and atypical antipsychotic drugs. *J Clin Psychiatry* 65(Suppl 18):27–35.

Caspi, N., Modai, I., Barak, P., *et al.* (2001). Pindolol augmentation in aggressive schizophrenic patients: a double-blind crossover randomized study. *Int Clin Psychopharmacol* 16:111–15.

Chakos, M., Lieberman, J., Hoffman, E., *et al.* (2001). Effectiveness of second-generation antipsychotics in patients with treatment-resistant schizophrenia: a review and meta-analysis of randomized trials. *Am J Psychiatry* 158:518–26.

Chanpattana, W., Chakrabhand, M. L., Sackeim, H. A., *et al.* (1999). Continuation ECT in treatment-resistant schizophrenia: a controlled study. *J ECT* 15:178–92.

Christodoulou, C., & Kalaitzi, C. (2005). Antipsychotic drug-induced acute laryngeal dystonia: two case reports and a mini review. *J Psychopharmacol* 19:307–11.

Citrome, L., Casey, D. E., Daniel, D. G., *et al.* (2004). Adjunctive divalproex and hostility among patients with schizophrenia receiving olanzapine or risperidone. *Psychiatr Serv* 55:290–4.

Conley, R. R., & Kelly, D. L. (2001). Management of treatment resistance in schizophrenia. *Biol Psychiatry* 50:898–911.

Cooper, S. J., Butler, A., Tweed, J., *et al.* (2000). Zotepine in the prevention of recurrence: a randomised, double-blind, placebo-controlled study for chronic schizophrenia. *Psychopharmacology (Berl)* 150:237–43.

Cornblatt, B. A. (2002). The New York high risk project to the Hillside recognition and prevention (RAP) program. *Am J Med Genet* 114:956–66.

Cornblatt, B. A., Lencz, T., & Kane, J. M. (2001). Treatment of the schizophrenia prodrome: is it presently ethical? *Schizophr Res* 51:31–8.

Coulter, D. M., Bate, A., Meyboom, R. H., *et al.* (2001). Antipsychotic drugs and heart muscle disorder in international pharmacovigilance: data mining study. *BMJ* 322:1207–9.

Crismon, M. L., Trivedi, M., Pigott, T. A., *et al.* (1999). The Texas Medication Algorithm Project: report of the Texas Consensus Conference Panel on Medication Treatment of Major Depressive Disorder. *J Clin Psychiatry* 60:142–56.

Csernansky, J. G., Mahmoud, R., & Brenner, R; Risperidone-USA-79 Study Group (2002). A comparison of risperidone and haloperidol for the prevention of relapse in patients with schizophrenia. *N Engl J Med* 346:16–22.

Currier, G. W., Allen, M. H., Bunney, E. B., *et al.* (2004a). Standard therapies for acute agitation. *J Emerg Med* 27(4 Suppl):S9–12; quiz S7.

Currier, G. W., Allen, M. H., Bunney, E. B., *et al.* (2004b). Updated treatment algorithm. *J Emerg Med* 27(4 Suppl):S25–6.

Cutler, A. J. (2003). Sexual dysfunction and antipsychotic treatment. *Psychoneuroendocrinology* 28(Suppl 1):69–82.

Daskalakis, Z. J., Christensen, B. K., Fitzgerald, P. B., & Chen, R. (2002). Transcranial magnetic stimulation: a new investigational and treatment tool in psychiatry. *J Neuropsychiatry Clin Neurosci* 14:406–15.

de Leon, J., Armstrong, S. C., Cozza, K. L. (2005). The dosing of atypical antipsychotics. *Psychosomatics* 46:262–73.

Dollfus, S., Olivier, V., Chabot B., *et al.* (2005). Olanzapine versus risperidone in the treatment of post-psychotic depression in schizophrenic patients. *Schizophr Res* 78:157–9.

Dunner, D. L. (2005). Atypical antipsychotics: efficacy across bipolar disorder subpopulations. *J Clin Psychiatry* 66(Suppl 3):20–7.

Ellis, P.; Royal Australian and New Zealand College of Psychiatrists Clinical Practice Guidelines Team for Depression (2004). Australian and New Zealand clinical practice guidelines for the treatment of depression. *Aust N Z J Psychiatry* 38:389–407.

Emsley R., Myburgh C., Oosthuizen P., & van Rensburg S. J. (2002). Randomized, placebo-controlled study of ethyl-eicosapentaenoic acid as supplemental treatment in schizophrenia. *Am J Psychiatry* 159:1596–8.

Essock, S. M., Hargreaves, W. A., Covell, N. H., & Goethe, J. (1996). Clozapine's effectiveness for patients in state hospitals: results from a randomized trial. *Psychopharmacol Bull* 32:683–97.

Feifel, D. (2000). Rationale and guidelines for the inpatient treatment of acute psychosis. *J Clin Psychiatry* 61(Suppl 14):27–32.

Fornaro, P., Calabria, G., Corallo, G., & Picotti, G. B. (2002). Pathogenesis of degenerative retinopathies induced by thioridazine and other antipsychotics: a dopamine hypothesis. *Doc Ophthalmol* 105:41–9.

French, J. A., Kanner, A. M., Bautista, J., *et al.*; Therapeutics and Technology Assessment Subcommittee of the American Academy of Neurology; Quality Standards Subcommittee of the American Academy of Neurology; American Epilepsy Society (2004). Efficacy and tolerability of the new antiepileptic drugs I: treatment of new onset epilepsy: report of the Therapeutics and Technology Assessment Subcommittee and Quality Standards Subcommittee of the American Academy of Neurology and the American Epilepsy Society. *Neurology* 62:1252–60.

Freudenmann, R. W., & Schonfeldt-Lecuona, C. (2005). Delusional parasitosis: treatment with atypical antipsychotics. *Ann Acad Med Singapore* 34:141–2; author reply 142.

Frye, M. A., Ketter, T. A., Kimbrell, T. A., *et al.* (2000). A placebo-controlled study of lamotrigine and gabapentin monotherapy in refractory mood disorders. *J Clin Psychopharmacol* 20:607–14.

Gardner, D. M., Baldessarini, R. J., & Waraich, P. (2005). Modern antipsychotic drugs: a critical overview. *CMAJ* 172:1703–11.

Geddes, J. R., Burgess, S., Hawton, K., *et al.* (2004). Long-term lithium therapy for bipolar disorder: systematic review and meta-analysis of randomized controlled trials. *Am J Psychiatry* 161:217–22.

Gelenberg, A. J., & Pies, R. (2003). Matching the bipolar patient and the mood stabilizer. *Ann Clin Psychiatry* 15:203–16.

Gijsman, H. J., Geddes, J. R., Rendell, J. M., *et al.* (2004). Antidepressants for bipolar depression: a systematic review of randomized, controlled trials. *Am J Psychiatry* 161:1537–47.

Glassman, A. H. (2005). Schizophrenia, antipsychotic drugs, and cardiovascular disease. *J Clin Psychiatry* 66(Suppl 6):5–10.

Glassman, A. H., & Bigger, J. T., Jr. (2001). Antipsychotic drugs: prolonged QTc interval, torsade de pointes, and sudden death. *Am J Psychiatry* 158:1774–82.

Glazer, W. M. (2000). Expected incidence of tardive dyskinesia associated with atypical antipsychotics. *J Clin Psychiatry* 61(Suppl 4):21–6.

Goff, D. C., Posever, T., Herz, L., *et al.* (1998). An exploratory haloperidol-controlled dose-finding study of ziprasidone in hospitalized patients with schizophrenia or schizoaffective disorder. *J Clin Psychopharmacol* 18:296–304.

Goldberg, J. F., Burdick, K. E., & Endick, C. J. (2004). Preliminary randomized, double-blind, placebo-controlled trial of pramipexole added to mood stabilizers for treatment-resistant bipolar depression. *Am J Psychiatry* 161:564–6.

Goodwin, G. M.; Consensus Group of the British Association for Psychopharmacology (2003). Evidence based guidelines for treating bipolar disorder: recommendations from the British Association for Psychopharmacology. *J Psychopharmacol* 17:149–173; discussion 147.

Goodwin, G. M., Bowden, C. L., Calabrese, J. R., *et al.* (2004). A pooled analysis of 2 placebo-controlled 18-month trials of lamotrigine and lithium maintenance in bipolar I disorder. *J Clin Psychiatry* 65:432–41.

Gould, T. D., Quiroz, J. A., Singh, J., *et al.* (2004). Emerging experimental therapeutics for bipolar disorder: insights from the molecular and cellular actions of current mood stabilizers. *Mol Psychiatry* 9:734–55.

Gray, N. A., Zhou, R., Du, J., *et al.* (2003). The use of mood stabilizers as plasticity enhancers in the treatment of neuropsychiatric disorders. *J Clin Psychiatry* 64(Suppl 5):3–17.

Green, A. I. (2005). Schizophrenia and comorbid substance use disorder: effects of antipsychotics. *J Clin Psychiatry* 66(Suppl 6):21–26.

Gruenberg, A. M., & Goldstein, R. D. (2003). Mood disorders: depression. In A. Tasman, J. Kay, J. A. Lieberman, eds. *Psychiatry*, 2nd edn. Chichester: Wiley, pp. 1207–36.

Grunze, H. (2005). Reevaluating therapies for bipolar depression. *J Clin Psychiatry* 66(Suppl 5):17–25.

Hahn, C. G., Gyulai, L., Baldassano, C. F., & Lenox, R. H. (2004). The current understanding of lamotrigine as a mood stabilizer. *J Clin Psychiatry* 65:791–804.

Hajak, G., Marienhagen, J., Langguth, B., *et al.* (2004). High-frequency repetitive transcranial magnetic stimulation in schizophrenia: a combined treatment and neuroimaging study. *Psychol Med* 34:1157–63.

Haraldsson, H. M., Ferrarelli, F., Kalin, N. H., & Tononi, G. (2004). Transcranial magnetic stimulation in the investigation and treatment of schizophrenia: a review. *Schizophr Res* 71:1–16.

Harrigan, E. P., Miceli, J. J., Anziano, R., *et al.* (2004). A randomized evaluation of the effects of six antipsychotic agents on QTc, in the absence and presence of metabolic inhibition. *J Clin Psychopharmacol* 24:62–9.

Heresco-Levy, U., Ermilov, M., Shimoni, J., *et al.* (2002). Placebo-controlled trial of D-cycloserine added to conventional neuroleptics, olanzapine, or risperidone in schizophrenia. *Am J Psychiatry* 159:480–2.

Heresco-Levy, U., Javitt, D. C., Ebstein, R., *et al.* (2005). D-serine efficacy as add-on pharmacotherapy to risperidone and olanzapine for treatment-refractory schizophrenia. *Biol Psychiatry* 57:577–85.

Hiemke, C., Dragicevic, A., Grunder, G., *et al.* (2004). Therapeutic monitoring of new antipsychotic drugs. *Ther Drug Monit* 26:156–60.

Hoffman, R. E., Gueorguieva, R., Hawkins, K. A., *et al.* (2005). Temporoparietal transcranial magnetic stimulation for auditory hallucinations: safety, efficacy and moderators in a fifty patient sample. *Biol Psychiatry* 58:97–104.

Hong, X., & Wang, X. (2001). Agranulocytosis and neutropenia with typical and atypical neuroleptics. *Am J Psychiatry* 158:1736–7.

Howard, R., Rabins, P. V., Seeman, M. V., & Jeste, D. V. (2000). Late-onset schizophrenia and very-late-onset schizophrenia-like psychosis: an international consensus. The International Late-Onset Schizophrenia Group. *Am J Psychiatry* 157:172–8.

Hughes, D. H., & Kleespies, P. M. (2003). Treating aggression in the psychiatric emergency service. *J Clin Psychiatry* **64**(Suppl 4):10–15.

Iqbal, M. M., Rahman, A., Husain, Z., *et al.* (2003). Clozapine: a clinical review of adverse effects and management. *Ann Clin Psychiatry* **15**:33–48.

Jeppesen J., Hein HO., Suadicani P., & Gyntelberg F. (1998). Triglyceride concentration and ischemic heart disease: an eight-year follow-up in the Copenhagen Male Study. *Circulation* **97**:1029–36.

Jeste, D. V. (2004). Tardive dyskinesia rates with atypical antipsychotics in older adults. *J Clin Psychiatry* **65**(Suppl 9):21–4.

Jeste, D. V., Rockwell, E., Harris, M. J., *et al.* (1999). Conventional vs. newer antipsychotics in elderly patients. *Am J Geriatr Psychiatry* **7**:70–6.

Josiassen, R. C., Joseph, A., Kohegyi, E., *et al.* (2005). Clozapine augmented with risperidone in the treatment of schizophrenia: a randomized, double-blind, placebo-controlled trial. *Am J Psychiatry* **162**:130–6.

Kalis, M. M., & Huff, N. A. (2001). Oxcarbazepine, an antiepileptic agent. *Clin Ther* **23**:680–700; discussion 645.

Kane, J., Honigfeld, G., Singer, J., & Meltzer, H. (1988). Clozapine for the treatment-resistant schizophrenic. A double-blind comparison with chlorpromazine. *Arch Gen Psychiatry* **45**:789–96.

Kane, J. M., Leucht, S., Carpenter, D., & Docherty, J. P. (2003). Expert consensus guideline series. Optimizing pharmacologic treatment of psychotic disorders. Introduction: methods, commentary, and summary. *J Clin Psychiatry* **64**(Suppl 12):5–19.

Kane, J. M., Woerner, M., Borenstein, M., *et al.* (1986). Integrating incidence and prevalence of tardive dyskinesia. *Psychopharmacol Bull* **22**:254–8.

Kapur, S., & Remington, G. (2001). Atypical antipsychotics: new directions and new challenges in the treatment of schizophrenia. *Annu Rev Med* **52**:503–17.

Karagianis, J. L., Dawe, I. C., Thakur A., *et al.* (2001). Rapid tranquilization with olanzapine in acute psychosis: a case series. *J Clin Psychiatry* **62**(Suppl 2):12–16.

Kasper, S., Lerman, M. N., McQuade, R. D., *et al.* (2003). Efficacy and safety of aripiprazole vs. haloperidol for long-term maintenance treatment following acute relapse of schizophrenia. *Int J Neuropsychopharmacol* **6**:325–37.

Keck, P. E., Jr. (2004). Defining and improving response to treatment in patients with bipolar disorder. *J Clin Psychiatry* **65**(Suppl 15):25–9.

Keck, P. E., Jr., & McElroy, S. L. (2002). Clinical pharmacodynamics and pharmacokinetics of antimanic and mood-stabilizing medications. *J Clin Psychiatry* **63**(Suppl 4):3–11.

Keck, P. E., Jr., & McElroy, S. L. (2003). New approaches in managing bipolar depression. *J Clin Psychiatry* **64**(Suppl 1):13–18.

Keck, P. E., Jr., Reeves, K. R., & Harrigan, E. P.; Ziprasidone Study Group (2001). Ziprasidone in the short-term treatment of patients with schizoaffective disorder: results from two double- blind, placebo-controlled, multicenter studies. *J Clin Psychopharmacol* **21**:27–35.

Keefe, R. S., Seidman, L. J., Christensen, B. K., *et al.* (2004). Comparative effect of atypical and conventional antipsychotic drugs on neurocognition in first-episode psychosis: a randomized, double-blind trial of olanzapine versus low doses of haloperidol. *Am J Psychiatry* **161**:985–95.

Ketter, T. A., & Calabrese, J. R. (2002). Stabilization of mood from below versus above baseline in bipolar disorder: a new nomenclature. *J Clin Psychiatry* **63**:146–51.

Ketter, T. A., Frye, M. A., Cora-Locatelli, G., *et al.* (1999). Metabolism and excretion of mood stabilizers and new anticonvulsants. *Cell Mol Neurobiol* **19**:511–32.

Ketter, T. A., Manji, H. K., & Post, R. M. (2003). Potential mechanisms of action of lamotrigine in the treatment of bipolar disorders. *J Clin Psychopharmacol* **23**:484–95.

Ketter, T. A., & Wang, P. W. (2003). The emerging differential roles of GABAergic and antiglutamatergic agents in bipolar disorders. *J Clin Psychiatry* **64**(Suppl 3):15–20.

Koro, C. E., Fedder, D. O., L'Italien, G. J., *et al.* (2002). An assessment of the independent effects of olanzapine and risperidone exposure on the risk of hyperlipidemia in schizophrenic patients. *Arch Gen Psychiatry* **59**:1021–6.

Kuehn, B. M. (2005). FDA warns antipsychotic drugs may be risky for elderly. *JAMA* **293**:2462.

Kupchik, M., Spivak, B., Mester, R., *et al.* (2000). Combined electroconvulsive-clozapine therapy. *Clin Neuropharmacol* **23**:14–16.

Kupka, R. W., Luckenbaugh, D. A., Post, R. M., *et al.* (2003). Rapid and non-rapid cycling bipolar disorder: a meta-analysis of clinical studies. *J Clin Psychiatry* **64**:1483–94.

Kusumakar, V., Yatham, L. N., Haslam, D. R., *et al.* (1997). Treatment of mania, mixed state, and rapid cycling. *Can J Psychiatry* **42**(Suppl 2):79S–86S.

LaRoche, S. M., & Helmersm S. L. (2004). The new antiepileptic drugs: scientific review. *JAMA* **291**:605–14.

Laruelle, M., Kegeles, L. S., & Abi-Dargham, A. (2003). Glutamate, dopamine, and schizophrenia: from pathophysiology to treatment. *Ann N Y Acad Sci* **1003**: 138–58.

Lehman, A. F., Lieberman, J. A., Dixon, L. B., *et al.*; American Psychiatric Association; Steering Committee on Practice Guidelines. (2004). Practice guideline for the treatment of patients with schizophrenia, second edition. *Am J Psychiatry* **161**(2 Suppl):1–56.

Lehmann, H. E., & Ban, T. A. (1997). The history of the psychopharmacology of schizophrenia. *Can J Psychiatry* **42**:152–62.

Lenox, R. H., & Wang, L. (2003). Molecular basis of lithium action: integration of lithium-responsive signaling and gene expression networks. *Mol Psychiatry* **8**:135–44.

Lerner, V., Libov, I., Kotler, M., & Strous, R. D. (2004). Combination of "atypical" antipsychotic medication in the management of treatment-resistant schizophrenia and schizoaffective disorder. *Prog Neuropsychopharmacol Biol Psychiatry* **28**:89–98.

Leucht, S., Barnes, T. R., Kissling, W., *et al.* (2003). Relapse prevention in schizophrenia with new-generation antipsychotics: a systematic review and exploratory meta-analysis of randomized, controlled trials. *Am J Psychiatry* **160**:1209–22.

Leucht, S., Kissling, W., & McGrath, J. (2004). Lithium for schizophrenia revisited: a systematic review and meta-analysis of randomized controlled trials. *J Clin Psychiatry* **65**:177–86.

Leucht S., Wahlbeck K., Hamann J., & Kissling W. (2003). New generation antipsychotics versus low-potency conventional antipsychotics: a systematic review and meta-analysis. *Lancet* **361**:1581–9.

Levinson, D. F., Umapathy, C., & Musthaq, M. (1999). Treatment of schizoaffective disorder and schizophrenia with mood symptoms. *Am J Psychiatry* **156**:1138–48.

Lewis, D. A., Hashimoto, T., & Volk, D. W. (2005). Cortical inhibitory neurons and schizophrenia. *Nat Rev Neurosci* **6**:312–324.

Licht, R. W., Vestergaard, P., Kessing, L. V., *et al.*; Danish Psychiatric Association and the Child and Adolescent Psychiatric Association in Denmark (2003). Psychopharmacological treatment with lithium and antiepileptic drugs: suggested guidelines from the Danish Psychiatric Association and the Child and Adolescent Psychiatric Association in Denmark. *Acta Psychiatr Scand Suppl* **419**: 1–22.

Lieberman, J. A. (2004). Dopamine partial agonists: a new class of antipsychotic. *CNS Drugs* **18**:251–267.

Lieberman, J. A., & Fenton, W. S. (2000). Delayed detection of psychosis: causes, consequences, and effect on public health. *Am J Psychiatry* **157**:1727–30.

Lieberman, J. A., Johns, C. A., Kane, J. M., *et al.* (1988). Clozapine-induced agranulocytosis: non-crossreactivity with other psychotropic drugs. *J Clin Psychiatry* **49**:271–7.

Lieberman, J. A., Kane, J. M., & Johns, C. A. (1989). Clozapine: guidelines for clinical management. *J Clin Psychiatry* **50**:329–38.

Lieberman, J. A., Phillips, M., Gu, H., *et al.* (2003). Atypical and conventional antipsychotic drugs in treatment-naive first-episode schizophrenia: a 52-week randomized trial of clozapine vs chlorpromazine. *Neuropsychopharmacology* **28**:995–1003.

Lieberman, J. A., Stroup, T. S., McEvoy, J. P., *et al.*; Clinical Antipsychotic Trials of Intervention Effectiveness (CATIE) Investigators (2005). Effectiveness of antipsychotic drugs in patients with chronic schizophrenia. *N Engl J Med* **353**:1209–23.

Lieberman, J. A., Tollefson, G., Tohen, M., *et al.*; HGDH Study Group (2003). Comparative efficacy and safety of atypical and conventional antipsychotic drugs in first-episode psychosis: a randomized, double-blind trial of olanzapine versus haloperidol. *Am J Psychiatry* **160**:1396–1404.

Lindenmayer, J. P., Czobor, P., Volavka, J., *et al.* (2003). Changes in glucose and cholesterol levels in patients with schizophrenia treated with typical or atypical antipsychotics. *Am J Psychiatry* **160**:290–6.

Lindenmayer, J. P., Czobor, P., Volavka, J., *et al.* (2004). Effects of atypical antipsychotics on the syndromal profile in treatment-resistant schizophrenia. *J Clin Psychiatry* **65**:551–6.

Lindstrom, E., Farde, L., Eberhard, J., & Haverkamp, W. (2005). QTc interval prolongation and antipsychotic drug treatments: focus on sertindole. *Int J Neuropsychopharmacol* **8**:615–29.

Lisanby, S. H., Kinnunen, L. H., & Crupain, M. J. (2002). Applications of TMS to therapy in psychiatry. *J Clin Neurophysiol* **19**:344–60.

Mackin, P., & Young, A. H. (2004). Rapid cycling bipolar disorder: historical overview and focus on emerging treatments. *Bipolar Disord* **6**:523–9.

Marder, S. R. (1999). Antipsychotic drugs and relapse prevention. *Schizophr Res* **35**(Suppl):S87–92.

Marder, S. R., Essock, S. M., Miller, A. L., *et al.* (2004). Physical health monitoring of patients with schizophrenia. *Am J Psychiatry* **161**:1334–49.

Masan, P. S. (2004). Atypical antipsychotics in the treatment of affective symptoms: a review. *Ann Clin Psychiatry* **16**:3–13.

Matsuo, F. (1999). Lamotrigine. *Epilepsia* **40**(Suppl 5):S30–6.

May, T. W., Korn-Merker, E., & Rambeck, B. (2003). Clinical pharmacokinetics of oxcarbazepine. *Clin Pharmacokinet* **42**:1023–42.

McCall, W. V. (2001). Electroconvulsive therapy in the era of modern psychopharmacology. *Int J Neuropsychopharmacol* **4**:315–24.

McElroy SL., Keck, P. E., Jr., & Strakowski, S. M. (1999). An overview of the treatment of schizoaffective disorder. *J Clin Psychiatry* **60**(Suppl 5):16–21; discussion 22.

McEvoy, J. P., Hogarty, G. E., & Steingard, S. (1991). Optimal dose of neuroleptic in acute schizophrenia. A controlled study of the neuroleptic threshold and higher haloperidol dose. *Arch Gen Psychiatry* **48**:739–45.

McGlashan, T. H. (2001). Psychosis treatment prior to psychosis onset: ethical issues. *Schizophr Res* **51**:47–54.

McGorry, P. D., Yung, A., & Phillips, L. (2001). Ethics and early intervention in psychosis: keeping up the pace and staying in step. *Schizophr Res* **51**:17–29.

McQuade, R. D., Stock, E., Marcus, R., *et al.* (2004). A comparison of weight change during treatment with olanzapine or aripiprazole: results from a randomized, double-blind study. *J Clin Psychiatry* **65**(Suppl 18):47–56.

Melle, I., Larsen, T. K., Haahr, U., *et al.* (2004). Reducing the duration of untreated first-episode psychosis: effects on clinical presentation. *Arch Gen Psychiatry* **61**:143–50.

Meltzer, H. Y., Alphs, L., Green, A. I., *et al.*; International Suicide Prevention Trial Study Group (2003). Clozapine treatment for suicidality in schizophrenia: International Suicide Prevention Trial (InterSePT). *Arch Gen Psychiatry* **60**:82–91.

Meltzer, H. Y., Li, Z., Kaneda, Y., & Ichikawa, J. (2003). Serotonin receptors: their key role in drugs to treat schizophrenia. *Prog Neuropsychopharmacol Biol Psychiatry* **27**:1159–72.

Mensink, G. J., & Slooff, C. J. (2004). Novel antipsychotics in bipolar and schizoaffective mania. *Acta Psychiatr Scand* **109**:405–19.

Merrill, D. B., Dec, G. W., & Goff, D. C. (2005). Adverse cardiac effects associated with clozapine. *J Clin Psychopharmacol* **25**:32–41.

Mieno, S., Asada, K., Horimoto, H., & Sasaki, S. (2003). Neuroleptic malignant syndrome following cardiac surgery: successful treatment with dantrolene. *Eur J Cardiothorac Surg* **24**:458–60.

Mishory, A., Winokur, M., & Bersudsky, Y. (2003). Prophylactic effect of phenytoin in bipolar disorder: a controlled study. *Bipolar Disord* **5**:464–7.

Misra, M., Papakostas, G. I., & Klibanski, A. (2004). Effects of psychiatric disorders and psychotropic medications on prolactin and bone metabolism. *J Clin Psychiatry* **65**:1607–1618; quiz 1590, 1760–1.

Miyamoto, S., Duncan, G. E., Marx, C. E., & Lieberman, J. A. (2005). Treatments for schizophrenia: a critical review of pharmacology and mechanisms of action of antipsychotic drugs. *Mol Psychiatry* **10**:79–104.

Miyamoto, S., Lieberman, J. A., Fleischhacker, W. W., *et al.*, eds. (2003). *Psychiatry*, 2nd edn. Chichester: Wiley, pp. 1928–64.

Moller, H. J. (2003). Amisulpride: limbic specificity and the mechanism of antipsychotic atypicality. *Prog Neuropsychopharmacol Biol Psychiatry* **27**:1101–11.

Mortimer, A. M. (2004). How do we choose between atypical antipsychotics? The advantages of amisulpride. *Int J Neuropsychopharmacol* **7**(Suppl 1):S21–5.

Moseman, S. E., Freeman, M. P., Misiaszek, J., & Gelenberg, A. J. Mood stabilizers. In A. Tasman, J. Kay, & J. A. Lieberman, eds. (2003). *Psychiatry*, 2nd edn. Chichester: Wiley, pp. 1965–89.

Murty, R. G., Mistry, S. G., & Chacko, R. C. (2002). Neuroleptic malignant syndrome with ziprasidone. *J Clin Psychopharmacol* **22**:624–6.

Nahas, Z., Kozel, F. A., Li, X., *et al.* (2003). Left prefrontal transcranial magnetic stimulation (TMS) treatment of depression in bipolar affective disorder: a pilot study of acute safety and efficacy. *Bipolar Disord* **5**:40–7.

Nemeroff, C. B., Kinkead, B., & Goldstein, J. (2002). Quetiapine: preclinical studies, pharmacokinetics, drug interactions, and dosing. *J Clin Psychiatry* **63**(Suppl 13):5–11.

Newcomer, J. W. (2004). Abnormalities of glucose metabolism associated with atypical antipsychotic drugs. *J Clin Psychiatry* **65**(Suppl 18):36–46.

Newcomer, J. W. (2005). Second-generation (atypical) antipsychotics and metabolic effects: a comprehensive literature review. *CNS Drugs* **19**(Suppl 1):1–93.

Olney, J. W., Newcomer, J. W., & Farber, N. B. (1999). NMDA receptor hypofunction model of schizophrenia. *J Psychiatr Res* **33**:523–33.

Parker, G., & Parker, K. (2003). Which antidepressants flick the switch? *Aust N Z J Psychiatry* **37**:464–8.

Patel, J. K., Pinals, D. A., & Breier, A. (2003). Schizophrenia and Other Psychoses. In A. Tasman, J. Kay, & J. A. Lieberman, eds. (2003). *Psychiatry*, 2nd edn. Chichester: Wiley, pp. 1131–206.

Patton, S. W., Misri, S., Corral, M. R., *et al.* (2002). Antipsychotic medication during pregnancy and lactation in women with schizophrenia: evaluating the risk. *Can J Psychiatry* 47:959–65.

Pazzaglia, P. J., Post, R. M., Ketter, T. A., *et al.* (1998). Nimodipine monotherapy and carbamazepine augmentation in patients with refractory recurrent affective illness. *J Clin Psychopharmacol* 18:404–13.

Perkins, D., Lieberman, J., Gu, H., *et al.*; HGDH Research Group (2004). Predictors of antipsychotic treatment response in patients with first-episode schizophrenia, schizoaffective and schizophreniform disorders. *Br J Psychiatry* 185:18–24.

Perucca, E. (2001). Clinical pharmacology and therapeutic use of the new antiepileptic drugs. *Fundam Clin Pharmacol* 15:405–17.

Physicians' Desk Reference, 60th edn. (2004). Montvale, NJ: Thomson PDR.

Pigott, T. A., Carson, W. H., Saha A. R., *et al.* (2003). Aripiprazole Study Group. Aripiprazole for the prevention of relapse in stabilized patients with chronic schizophrenia. a placebo-controlled 26-week study. *J Clin Psychiatry* 64:1048–56.

Post, R. M., Leverich, G. S., Nolen, W. A., *et al.*; Stanley Foundation Bipolar Network (2003). A re-evaluation of the role of antidepressants in the treatment of bipolar depression: data from the Stanley Foundation Bipolar Network. *Bipolar Disord* 5:396–406.

Reznik, I., & Sirota, P. (2000). Obsessive and compulsive symptoms in schizophrenia: a randomized controlled trial with fluvoxamine and neuroleptics *J Clin Psychopharmacol* 20:410–16.

Roesch-Ely, D., Van Einsiedel, R., Kathofer, S., *et al.* (2002). Myocarditis with quetiapine. *Am J Psychiatry* 159:1607–8.

Rothschild, A. J. (2003). Challenges in the treatment of depression with psychotic features. *Biol Psychiatry* 53:680–90.

Rothschild, A. J., Williamson, D. J., Tohen, M. F., *et al.* (2004). A double blind, randomized study of olanzapine and olanzapine/fluoxetine combination for major depression with psychotic features. *J Clin Psychopharmacol* 24:365–73.

Royal Australian and New Zealand College of Psychiatrists Clinical Practice Guidelines Team for Bipolar Disorder (2004). Australian and New Zealand clinical practice guidelines for the treatment of bipolar disorder. *Aust N Z J Psychiatry* 38:280–305.

Royal Australian and New Zealand College of Psychiatrists Clinical Practice Guidelines Team for the Treatment of Schizophrenia and Related Disorders (2005). Royal Australian and New Zealand College of Psychiatrists clinical practice guidelines for the treatment of schizophrenia and related disorders. *Aust N Z J Psychiatry* 39: 1–30.

Ruhrmann, S., Schultze-Lutter, F., Maier, W., & Klosterkotter, J. (2004). Pharmacological intervention in the initial prodromal phase of psychosis. *Eur Psychiatry* 20:1–6.

Ruigomez, A., Garcia Rodriguez, L. A., Dev, V. J., *et al.* (2000). Are schizophrenia or antipsychotic drugs a risk factor for cataracts? *Epidemiology* 11:620–3.

Rush, A. J., Sackeim, H. A., Marangell, L. B., *et al.* (2005). Effects of 12 months of vagus nerve stimulation in treatment-resistant depression: a naturalistic study. *Biol Psychiatry* 58:355–63.

Saba, G., Verdon, C. M., Kalalou, K., *et al.* (2006). Transcranial magnetic stimulation in the treatment of schizophrenic symptoms: a double blind sham controlled study. *J Psychiatr Res* 40:147–52.

Sadock, B. J., & Sadock, V. A. (2003). *Kaplan and Sadock's Synopsis of Psychiatry. Behavioral Sciences/Clinical Psychiatry.* Philadelphia: Lippincott Williams & Wilkins.

Sajatovic, M., Mullen, J. A., & Sweitzer, D. E. (2002). Efficacy of quetiapine and risperidone against depressive symptoms in outpatients with psychosis. *J Clin Psychiatry* 63:1156–63.

Schatzberg, A. F. (2003). New approaches to managing psychotic depression. *J Clin Psychiatry* 64(Suppl 1):19–23.

Schooler, N. R., Keith, S. J., Severe, J. B., *et al.* (1997). Relapse and rehospitalization during maintenance treatment of schizophrenia. The effects of dose reduction and family treatment. *Arch Gen Psychiatry* 54:453–63.

Schooler, N., Rabinowitz, J., Davidson, M., *et al.*; Early Psychosis Global Working Group (2005). Risperidone and haloperidol in first-episode psychosis: a long-term randomized trial. *Am J Psychiatry* 162:947–53.

Schou, M. (2001). Lithium treatment at 52. *J Affect Disord* 67: 21–32.

Seeman, M. V. (2004). Gender differences in the prescribing of antipsychotic drugs. *Am J Psychiatry* 161:1324–33.

Shahzad, S., Suleman, M. I., Shahab, H., *et al.* (2002). Cataract occurrence with antipsychotic drugs. *Psychosomatics* 43:354–9.

Sharif, Z. A. (1998). Common treatment goals of antipsychotics: acute treatment. *J Clin Psychiatry* 59(Suppl 19):5–8.

Simpson, G. M., Glick, I. D., Weiden, P. J., *et al.* (2004). Randomized, controlled, double-blind multicenter comparison of the efficacy and tolerability of ziprasidone and olanzapine in acutely ill inpatients with schizophrenia or schizoaffective disorder. *Am J Psychiatry* **161**:1837–47.

Siris, S., Pollack, S., Bermanzohn, P., & Stronger, R. (2000). Adjunctive imipramine for a broader group of post-psychotic depressions in schizophrenia. *Schizophr Res* **44**:187–92.

Siris, S. G. (2000). Depression in schizophrenia: perspective in the era of "Atypical" antipsychotic agents. *Am J Psychiatry* **157**:1379–89.

Siris, S. G., Morgan V., Fagerstrom R., *et al.* (1987). Adjunctive imipramine in the treatment of postpsychotic depression. A controlled trial. *Arch Gen Psychiatry* **44**:533–9.

Small, J. G., Klapper, M. H., Malloy, F. W., & Steadman, T. M. (2003). Tolerability and efficacy of clozapine combined with lithium in schizophrenia and schizoaffective disorder. *J Clin Psychopharmacol* **23**:223–8.

Spalding, S., Alessi, N. E., & Radwan, K. (2004). Aripiprazole and atypical neuroleptic malignant syndrome. *J Am Acad Child Adolesc Psychiatry* **43**:1457–8.

Stahl, S. M., & Shayegan, D. K. (2003). The psychopharmacology of ziprasidone: receptor-binding properties and real-world psychiatric practice. *J Clin Psychiatry* **64**(Suppl 19):6–12.

Stoll, A. L., Severus, W. E., Freeman, M. P., *et al.* (1999). Omega 3 fatty acids in bipolar disorder: a preliminary double-blind, placebo-controlled trial. *Arch Gen Psychiatry* **56**:407–12.

Sultana, A., & McMonagle, T. (2000). Pimozide for schizophrenia or related psychoses. *Cochrane Database Syst Rev* **3**:CD001949.

Suppes, T. (2002). Review of the use of topiramate for treatment of bipolar disorders. *J Clin Psychopharmacol* **22**:599–609.

Suppes, T., Kelly, D. I., & Perla, J. M. (2005). Challenges in the management of bipolar depression. *J Clin Psychiatry* **66**(Suppl 5):11–16.

Suzuki, K., Awata, S., Takano, T., *et al.* (2005). Continuation electroconvulsive therapy for relapse prevention in middle-aged and elderly patients with intractable catatonic schizophrenia. *Psychiatry Clin Neurosci* **59**:481–9.

Swann, A. C. (2005). Long-term treatment in bipolar disorder. *J Clin Psychiatry* **66**(Suppl 1):7–12.

Swoboda, E., Conca, A., Konig, P., *et al.* (2001). Maintenance electroconvulsive therapy in affective and schizoaffective disorder. *Neuropsychobiology* **43**:23–8.

Tamminga, C. A., & Holcomb, H. H. (2005). Phenotype of schizophrenia: a review and formulation. *Mol Psychiatry* **10**:27–39.

Taylor, D. M. (2003). Antipsychotics and QT prolongation. *Acta Psychiatr Scand* **107**:85–95.

Taylor, M., Chaudhry, I., Cross, M., *et al.* (2005). Relapse Prevention in Schizophrenia Consensus Group. Towards consensus in the long-term management of relapse prevention in schizophrenia. *Hum Psychopharmacol* **20**:175–81.

Taylor, M. A., & Fink, M. (2003). Catatonia in psychiatric classification: a home of its own. *Am J Psychiatry* **160**:1233–41.

Tecoma, E. S. (1999). Oxcarbazepine. *Epilepsia* **40**(Suppl 5):S37–46.

Tharyan, P., & Adams, C. E. (2005). Electroconvulsive therapy for schizophrenia. *Cochrane Database Syst Rev* **2**:CD000076.

Tiihonen, J., Halonen, P., Wahlbeck, K., *et al.* (2005). Topiramate add-on in treatment-resistant schizophrenia: a randomized, double-blind, placebo-controlled, crossover trial. *J Clin Psychiatry* **66**:1012–15.

Timmer, R. T., & Sands, J. M. (1999). Lithium intoxication. *J Am Soc Nephrol* **10**:666–1074.

Tohen, M., Zhang, F., Keck, P. E., *et al.* (2001). Olanzapine versus haloperidol in schizoaffective disorder, bipolar type. *J Affect Disord* **67**:133–40.

Tollefson, G. D., Birkett, M. A., Kiesler, G. M., & Wood, A. J.; Lilly Resistant Schizophrenia Study Group (2001). Double-blind comparison of olanzapine versus clozapine in schizophrenic patients clinically eligible for treatment with clozapine. *Biol Psychiatry* **49**:52–63.

Tondo, L., Hennen, J., & Baldessarini, R. J. (2001). Lower suicide risk with long-term lithium treatment in major affective illness: a meta-analysis. *Acta Psychiatr Scand* **104**:163–72.

Trixler, M., Gati, A., Fekete, S., & Tenyi, T. (2005). Use of antipsychotics in the management of schizophrenia during pregnancy. *Drugs* **65**:1193–206.

Tsai, G., Lane, H. Y., Yang, P., *et al.* (2004). Glycine transporter I inhibitor, N-methylglycine (sarcosine), added to antipsychotics for the treatment of schizophrenia. *Biol Psychiatry* **55**:452–6.

Turrone, P., Kapur, S., Seeman, M. V., Flint, A. J. (2002). Elevation of prolactin levels by atypical antipsychotics. *Am J Psychiatry* **159**:133–5.

Valibhai, F., Phan, N. B., Still, D. J., & True, J. (2001). Cataracts and quetiapine. *Am J Psychiatry* **158**:966.

von Bardeleben, U, Benkert, O., & Holsboer, F. (1987). Clinical and neuroendocrine effects of zotepine – a new neuroleptic drug. *Pharmacopsychiatry* **20**(1 Spec No): 28–34.

Wenning, M. T., Davy, L. E., Catalano, G., & Catalano, M. C. (2003). Atypical antipsychotics in the treatment of delusional parasitosis. *Ann Clin Psychiatry* **15**: 233–9.

Whitehorn, D., Gallant, J., Woodley, H., *et al.* (2004). Quetiapine treatment in early psychosis: no evidence of cataracts. *Schizophr Res* **71**:511–12.

Wieck, A., & Haddad, P. M. (2003). Antipsychotic-induced hyperprolactinaemia in women: pathophysiology, severity and consequences. Selective literature review. *Br J Psychiatry* **182**:199–204.

Wirshing, W. C. (2001). Movement disorders associated with neuroleptic treatment. *J Clin Psychiatry* **62**(Suppl 21):15–18.

Wirshing, D. A. (2004). Schizophrenia and obesity: impact of antipsychotic medications. *J Clin Psychiatry* **65**(Suppl 18):13–26.

Wolkowitz, O. M., & Pickar, D. (1991). Benzodiazepines in the treatment of schizophrenia: a review and reappraisal. *Am J Psychiatry* **140**:714–26.

Woods, S. W., Breier, A., Zipursky, R. B., *et al.* (2003). Randomized trial of olanzapine versus placebo in the symptomatic acute treatment of the schizophrenic prodrome. *Biol Psychiatry* **54**:453–64.

Wozniak, J. (2005). Recognizing and managing bipolar disorder in children. *J Clin Psychiatry* **66**(Suppl 1):18–23.

Yonkers, K. A., Wisner, K. L., Stowe, Z., *et al.* (2004). Management of bipolar disorder during pregnancy and the postpartum period. *Am J Psychiatry* **161**:608–20.

Yung, A. R., McGorry, P. D., McFarlane, C. A., *et al.* (1996). Monitoring and care of young people at incipient risk of psychosis. *Schizophr Bull* **22**:283–303.

Zanardi, R., Franchini, L., Serretti, A., *et al.* (2000). Venlafaxine versus fluvoxamine in the treatment of delusional depression: a pilot double-blind controlled study. *J Clin Psychiatry* **61**:26–9.

Zarate, C. A., Jr, & Tohen, M. (2004). Double-blind comparison of the continued use of antipsychotic treatment versus its discontinuation in remitted manic patients. *Am J Psychiatry* **161**:169–71.

Zhang-Wong, J., Zipursky, R. B., Beiser, M., & Bean, G. (1999). Optimal haloperidol dosage in first-episode psychosis. *Can J Psychiatry* **44**:164–7.

27

Biological treatments of depression and anxiety

Peter McGuffin and Anne E. Farmer

Depressive and anxiety symptoms frequently co-occur and represent the commonest form of psychopathology seen in the general population or by primary care physicians (see Chapter 21). Anxiety symptoms are also common in the context of depressive disorders among patients referred to psychiatric clinics, with one large recent series of patients with recurrent depression reporting prominent anxiety in more than 55% of cases (Korszun *et al.*, 2004). Although some drug treatments are effective for both anxious and depressive problems, this is not universally the case, and so it is essential to commence with a thorough diagnostic assessment. In practice a hierarchical approach is recommended in which, when they co occur, depressive symptoms take precedence over anxiety symptoms and the treatment is directed at the depression (National Institute of Clinical Excellence, 2004b).

Deciding whether symptoms are understandable in the context of the patient's recent life happenings is not generally useful in deciding whether to instigate treatment with medication. Thus depressive symptoms following recent loss or trauma warrants intervention no less than depressive disorder arising "out of the blue". Symptom severity is the main yardstick with which to determine type of treatment (psychotherapy, medication or both; National Institute for Clinical Excellence 2004b). The 10th revision of the *International Classification of Diseases* (ICD-10) classification of depression (see Chapter 12) explicitly stratifies the diagnosis of depressive

disorder into mild, moderate and severe on the basis of symptom count, with five to seven symptoms being classified as moderate depression and more than seven symptoms as severe depression. The 4th edition of the *Diagnostic and Statistical Manual of Mental Disorders* (DSM-IV) classification uses the same terminology but is not so explicit. In addition to symptom count, it is worth considering the degree of impairment and taking this into account when deciding whether to start drug treatment. In general, the majority of cases of mild depression resolve spontaneously and those that do not should first receive a psychological intervention. Prescribing medication as a mainstay of treatment is best reserved for moderate to severe levels of disorder in terms of symptom count, degree of impairment or both (National Institute for Clinical Excellence, 2004b).

Except for those antidepressants that have a sedative effect (which can provide early relief of initial insomnia), all classes of antidepressants show a delay before noticeable improvement in depressive symptoms occurs. This is usually about 2 to 3 weeks but may take longer and the decision to stop an antidepressant and switch to another treatment should not be taken until the patient has been on an adequate dosage of the drug for up to 6 to 8 weeks.

Here we provide an overview of the range of options for drug and other physical treatments for depressive disorders, with an emphasis on unipolar depression (the treatment of bipolar disorder is

Essential Psychiatry, ed. Robin M. Murray, Kenneth S. Kendler, Peter McGuffin, Simon Wessely, David J. Castle.
Published by Cambridge University Press. © Cambridge University Press 2008.

Box 27.1 What to tell patients

- Antidepressants relieve the symptoms but do not necessarily shorten the duration of the episode
- Stopping too soon risks relapse
- Advisable to take the same dose regularly for up to 9 months
- Do not stop suddenly – a gradual phased withdrawal with medical guidance and supervision is necessary

Antidepressants:
- Are not addictive
- Need to be taken everyday as prescribed
- Do not work when taken intermittently or only on "as required" basis
- Do not lose their efficacy over time
- Are not associated with new side effects with long-term use

---

Box 27.2 Clinical notes: selective serotonin reuptake inhibitors

- Citalopram: pure CIS isomer (escitalopram) may have greater efficacy and fewer side effects than citalopram; switching between preparations may be helpful
- Fluoxetine: 50 mg augmented with up to 12.5 mg olanzapine can improve otherwise refractory chronic depression

---

covered in Chapter 26). We then discuss drug treatments used in anxiety disorders. The reader is also referred to Chapter 25 for a general discussion on biological treatments in psychiatry.

Depressive disorders

Boxes 27.1 and 27.2 provides clinical tips to guide prescribing in people with depression. We now consider each of the main classes of antidepressant in turn. Note that although we sort antidepressants into groups, each member of each group differs from others in terms of pharmacokinetics and pharmacodynamics, and individuals respond to or experience side effects from different drugs in a unique manner (see Chapter 25).

Selective serotonin reuptake inhibitors

Compared with the earlier generation of antidepressant exemplified by the tricyclics, the selective serotonin reuptake inhibitors (SSRIs) have comparatively few side effects and lower cardiotoxicity so that they are safer in overdose. They are as effective as the tricyclics in randomised controlled trials (Song *et al.*, 1993). The combination of safety, tolerability because of low side effects and efficacy has undoubtedly contributed to a steadily rising number of prescriptions for SSRIs in recent years in industrialised societies (Ebmeier *et al.*, 2006) where they have now replaced the tricyclics as the first line of treatment in depression. Another feature of the SSRIs that makes them more "user-friendly" for the prescribing doctor in primary care (and this has also probably contributed to their popularity) is that they have been marketed as having a single, standard daily dosage. However, in practice, and particularly in secondary care, it often is necessary to titrate upwards from the initial standard dosage.

The SSRIs include fluoxetine, fluvoxamine, paroxetine, sertraline, citalopram and escitalopram (the active enantiomer of citalopram). As a class, they are nonsedative (apart from fluvoxamine) and are not associated with increased appetite or weight gain. Indeed, they can have an appetite-suppressing effect, and nausea and vomiting may be provoked, particularly at high doses. This unwanted effect is probably most common with fluvoxamine and usually improves after lowering the dosage. Headaches may also be a problem and most commonly occur in patients with a history of migraine. An activating effect with restlessness in the first week or two and an increase in anxiety may be reported, but this does not usually persist. More controversially, the SSRIs in general and fluoxetine and paroxetine in particular have been associated with increased suicidal ideation and an increased risk of suicide. As with restlessness and anxiety, suicidal ideation and behaviour is said to occur most commonly in the early stages of treatment. However, a recent review concluded that this was not specific to SSRIs or

> **Box 27.3** Discontinuation syndrome
>
> • Increased anxiety
> • Relapse of depressive symptoms
> • Sweating
> • Palpitations
> • Tremor
> • "Electric shock" sensations

indeed to any particular class of antidepressants (Ebmeier *et al.,* 2006). The relative risk of successfully committing suicide by self-poisoning actually appears to be lower in patients receiving SSRIs than those taking other antidepressants (Isacsson & Rich, 2005).

Some patients taking SSRIs experience a discontinuation syndrome soon after stopping the drug (see Box 27.3). This is not strictly the same as the withdrawal syndrome which typically occurs in those taking drugs of dependence (e.g. alcohol) for which there is characteristically a development of tolerance – that is, an increasing need for higher doses. SSRIs do not cause dependence or tolerance, but if stopped abruptly, members of this class of drugs, particularly those having a short half-life (e.g. paroxetine), may result in increased anxiety, a rapid return of depressive symptoms and, less commonly, odd physical sensations such as "electric shocks" in the limbs. Although weight gain and sedation are infrequent, sexual dysfunction can be a major problem with SSRIs (see Chapter 17 for a discussion of mechanisms and clinical implications).

Combined noradrenaline (norepinephrine) and serotonin reuptake inhibitors

Drugs in this class include venlafaxine and duloxetine. They are presumed to work by blocking both serotonin and noradrenaline reuptake and hence increasing availability of both neurotransmitters at synapses. They are also thought to desensitise serotonin 1A and beta-adrenergic receptors and very weakly block dopamine reuptake. Venlafaxine has been available for much longer than duloxetine and has proved to be a versatile antidepressant with good antianxiety properties. It is available in a once-daily (extended release) form but can be given in twice-daily doses of the immediate release preparation. The effective dose range is wide: many patients respond to 75 mg daily, but it can be safely prescribed in dosages up to 225 mg, and much higher dosages are sometimes given in cases of refractory depression (discussed later). Venlafaxine can be given in combination with mirtazapine for those who have only a partial response to venlafaxine alone.

Venlafaxine can cause a dosage-related increase in blood pressure, and thus it is prudent to check the patient's blood pressure before commencing treatment and to monitor blood pressure carefully, particularly in patients taking high dosages of the drug. For this reason venlafaxine is not generally recommended for initiation in primary care. It is also advisable to check the patient's electrocardiogram before commencing the drug. Duloxetine can also cause an increase in blood pressure, but experience so far suggests that this is less of a problem than with venlafaxine. However, the recommended dosage range at 60 to 90 mg per day is much smaller. Both drugs can cause sweating, nausea, diarrhoea and decreased appetite. In addition, venlafaxine can cause visual perceptual abnormalities, mostly when patients are falling asleep or waking. These drugs can also cause sexual dysfunction in the form of delayed ejaculation or orgasm. Hyponatraemia and inappropriate secretion of antidiuretic hormone is a comparatively uncommon side effect of venlafaxine that has also been reported with a variety of other antidepressants.

Withdrawal from venlafaxine can cause a fairly severe discontinuation syndrome. If this occurs, tapering over several months may be necessary. One method for doing this consists of crushing the tablet or opening the capsule into 100 mL of fruit juice and removing 1 mL of the mixture before drinking the rest. It is then possible to take out 2 mL then 3 mL, and so on, on succeeding days until the whole 100 mL is removed (Stahl, 2006). It is not clear

---

Box 27.4   Clinical notes: venlafaxine

- Mainly serotonergic in action up to 150 mg then switches to become mainly noradrenergic at higher doses; raising dose above 150 may be beneficial when lower doses have been ineffective
- Sweating and visual misperceptions (especially hypnogogic and hypnopompic phenomena) can occur
- Check blood pressure regularly and perform electrocardiogram before starting
- Can be used in combination with mirtazapine (start mirtazapine 15 mg at night at venlafaxine 150 mg; increase mirtazapine incrementally to maximum dose then raise venlafaxine to maximum)
- Very slow withdrawal maybe necessary over several weeks or months.

---

whether duloxetine has the same withdrawal problems as venlafaxine.

Other classes of newer antidepressants

Mirtazapine is an alpha-2 antagonist. By blocking alpha-2 adrenergic presynaptic receptors it causes an increase in both serotonin and noradrenaline/norepinephrine neurotransmission. Mirtazapine also blocks serotonin 5-HT2A, 5-HT2C and 5-HT3 receptors as well as histamine H_1 receptors. It has good anxiety-relieving properties and is somewhat sedative, so it is a particularly useful drug given as a once-daily dose at night for patients in whom insomnia is a prominent symptom. However, oversedation can be a problem, and some patients report dizziness. It also stimulates appetite and promotes weight gain, which again is useful in depressed patients for whom loss of appetite is prominent but presents a relative contraindication in patients who are already overweight. Unlike many antidepressants, mirtazapine does not appear to interfere with sexual function. However, other unwanted effects can include dry mouth, constipation and hypotension, and uncommonly mirtazapine can lower the white blood cell count and cause flulike symptoms.

Trazodone is a serotonin 5-HT2 antagonist and also has some serotonin reuptake inhibiting properties. Like mirtazapine it is sedative and therefore may be a useful choice of drug in patients with mixed depressive and anxiety symptoms or in those who suffer from insomnia. Conversely, unwanted effects may include oversedation or dizziness. Unlike mirtazapine it is not usually associated with weight gain but can cause nausea, constipation and dry mouth. Hypertension may also be a problem or, rarely, sinus bradycardia may occur. Trazodone is another antidepressant that does not cause sexual dysfunction; in fact some male patients report improved erections, and, rarely, it can cause priapism.

Reboxetine is a selective noradrenergic reuptake inhibitor (NARI). Although weight gain and sedation are unusual with reboxetine, insomnia, anxiety, agitation, sexual dysfunction and side effects similar to tricyclics such as urinary retention, dry mouth, hypotension and constipation can occur. Also like the tricyclics, reboxetine is contraindicated in those with closed-angle glaucoma. Because its mode of action is complementary to SSRIs, it is possible to use reboxetine in combination with one of these drugs in chronic depression or where there is partial response to a serotonergic agent.

Tricyclic antidepressants

Although for many years they were the first-line treatment for moderate to severe depression, tricyclic antidepressants (TCAs) are now generally reserved for cases in which treatment with more recently introduced drugs has failed. For clinical purposes the TCAs can be broadly divided into two groups, those with sedative properties such as amitriptyline, dothiepin and clomipramine, and those that are less sedative such as imipramine, nortriptyline and lofepramine. Some tricyclic compounds such as protriptyline actually have mildly stimulating properties. The choice of drug is therefore influenced by whether sedation is desirable in a particular patient. Anxious or agitated patients may benefit from sedation, as may those in whom sleep

---

Box 27.5 Clinical notes: tricyclic antidepressants

- Although no longer the first-line treatment for depression, still useful in some patients who fail to respond to selective serotonin reuptake inhibitors or other newer drugs
- Advise patient to take before bedtime to capitalise on hypnotic properties in initial insomnia
- Constipation maybe a major and intractable side effect

Box 27.6 Drugs causing sexual dysfunction (rank order of worst to most evidence to least worst to less evidence)

- Venlafaxine
- Selective serotonin reuptake inhibitors
- Monoamine oxidase inhibitor
- Tricyclic antidepressants
- Mirtazapine
- Reboxetine
- Trazodone (small risk of priapism; has been used to treat erectile dysfunction)
- Bupropion

---

disturbance is a prominent symptom. Here it is useful to prescribe a sedative drug such as amitriptyline in a once-daily evening dose taken approximately 3 hours before bedtime. This maximises the sedative benefits for those with initial insomnia.

One of the key components of using TCAs effectively is making sure that the patient is receiving an adequate dosage. In most patients this will mean at least 100 mg daily, but requirements may go as high as 300 mg per day. As a class, the TCAs have a sufficiently long half-life that a once daily dose can be given.

The best way to ensure that the patient is receiving an adequate dose of antidepressants is to measure blood levels, but as a routine practice this is no longer standard in most centres. Part of the rationale for measuring blood levels is that some TCAs such as nortriptyline have been shown to have a curvilinear dose response, so that for maximum response, blood levels appear to be best kept within a "therapeutic window" with neither very low nor very high levels proving as effective (Asberg, 1976). In practice, for the majority of patients, it is simply sufficient to titrate the dosage of TCAs against symptoms, balancing improvement against emerging side effects. Box 27.5 provides some clinical tips regarding the use of TCAs.

The commonest problems associated with the TCAs are those resulting from antimuscarinic, anticholinergic properties such as a dry mouth, blurring of vision, constipation or hesitancy in micturition. Tolerance to the symptoms usually develops, and it is useful to warn the patient in advance both that such symptoms can occur and that they will improve over time. However, it is necessary to avoid TCAs altogether in patients with glaucoma, in whom an acute attack can be precipitated, or in men with prostatism who may develop urinary retention.

Potentially more serious side effects are those in the cardiovascular system. Postural hypotension is common, particularly in older patients, and can nearly always be abolished by simply lowering the dosage. Cardiac arrhythmia and conduction defects can occur, and prolongation of the QTc interval occurs with all the TCAs. They are therefore contraindicated in patients who have had a recent myocardial infarction or a history of heart block. They are also potentially fatal in overdose even in younger subjects and those who have not had any previous history of heart disease. Other side effects, including weight gain, increased sweating and sexual difficulties (typically delayed ejaculation in men), are fairly common. Box 27.6 outlines the sexual problems associated with antidepressants; see also Chapter 17.

Monoamine oxidase inhibitors

Monoamine oxidase inhibitors (MAOIs) were the first effective antidepressants and were discovered by accident when isoniazid used in the treatment of tuberculosis was shown to inhibit monoamine oxidase and was observed to elevate mood. The only old "nonreversible" MAOI that is still fairly commonly used is phenelzine. This is partly because of long-standing doubts about efficacy (Thiery, 1965) but also because of interactions with other drugs and the "cheese reaction" or tyramine response. Tyramine is found in many foods such as mature cheese, pickled herring and game, and the consumption of such foods by someone taking MAOIs can result in a rapid and dangerous rise in blood pressure. MAOIs also interact with opioids and potentiate the effects of central nervous system depressants such as the benzodiazepines, barbiturates and alcohol. Consequently patients who are prescribed MAOIs need to be warned of these effects and issued a card listing the food and drugs to be avoided.

As a result of these problems "reversible" MAOIs have been developed, exemplified by moclobemide, that are said to inhibit monoamine oxidase type A specifically. Although it is much less likely than older MAOIs to potentiate the pressor effects of tyramine, it has been recommended that patients taking the drug avoid large amounts of tyramine-rich foods. The manufacturers also advise the avoidance of sympathomimetics such as ephedrine. Because of its reversibility, switching between moclobemide and other antidepressants is less problematic than was the case for older MAOIs. Nevertheless it is not advisable to start moclobemide for at least 5 weeks after stopping a longer-acting SSRI such as fluoxetine.

Antipsychotics

The main role for antipsychotics in treating depression is in patients who have delusions or hallucinations. Although this is a minority of patients, even among those with recurrent disorder (see Chapter 12), it is important to detect such symptoms because they are frequently a marker of poor response to antidepressants alone. For example, an early meta-analysis found that only 35% of patients suffering from depression with psychotic symptoms responded to tricyclics compared with 67%

of nonpsychotically depressed patients (Chan *et al.*, 1987). Clinical experience suggests that in this context, a combination of an antipsychotic and antidepressant has greater efficacy than either type of compound alone. The balance of randomised controlled trial evidence supports this, although not all studies of combined antipsychotic and antidepressant have been positive (Taylor *et al.*, 2005). Amoxapine is a tricyclic compound that has a pharmacological profile similar to the antipsychotic loxapine, and it has been marketed as a single drug solution to the problem of treating psychotic depression. However, convincing trial evidence is not available (Taylor *et al.*, 2005).

Low doses of antipsychotics are also used to treat anxiety symptoms or irritability occurring in the context of a depressive disorder. Again, trial evidence for efficacy is lacking. However, a low dosage of the phenothiazine, flupenthixol, has been shown to be as effective as TCAs in the treatment of moderately severe depression (Young *et al.*, 1976). There is also some evidence that olanzapine is useful not only for the treatment of psychotic symptoms in depression but that it may also be effective in combination with fluoxetine in treating nonpsychotic depression that does not respond to fluoxetine alone (Corya *et al.*, 2003).

Physical treatments

Although it has at times attracted considerable criticism in the popular media, there is overwhelming evidence that *electroconvulsive therapy* (ECT) is efficacious in the treatment of severe depressive disorder. A classic study from more than 40 years ago showed that ECT was more effective than tricyclics, MAOIs or placebo (Thiery, 1965), and there have been six controlled trials carried out in the United Kingdom (Royal College of Psychiatrists, 1990) comparing the ECT with "sham" ECT in which anaesthetic alone was given. Five of these six studies showed clear superiority of ECT over sham treatment. The negative study was one in which the active treatment consisted of unilateral brief pulse

Box 27.7 Predictors of good response to electroconvulsive therapy

- Presence of delusions
- Psychomotor retardation
- Severe disorder
- "Endogenous" pattern of symptoms (i.e. appetite and weight loss, early morning waking, diurnal mood variation with morning worsening)

stimulus, which is now agreed to be less effective than bilateral ECT.

The most common indication for ECT is persisting severe or moderately severe depressive symptoms despite an adequate course of antidepressant drugs for at least 6 weeks, or the onset of severe depression in which rapid treatment is needed. This is either because the patient presents as a serious suicidal risk or is failing to eat or drink. The latter can also occur in depressive stupor and when this occurs ECT should be considered as a first line of treatment. As noted earlier, psychotic features such as delusions or hallucinations are usually associated with a poor response to antidepressants. Once again, it may be justifiable to consider ECT as the first line of treatment. According to a study by Johnstone and colleagues (1980), the presence of delusions is the main predictor of a favourable response to ECT. A previous history of a good response to ECT, especially if there is a poor initial response to antidepressant drugs, can also be considered an indication for progressing to ECT earlier rather than later. Box 27.7 shows factors associated with a likely favourable response to ECT.

ECT is always given under general anaesthetic with a muscle relaxant. There is now a consensus, as a result of recent trials, that bilateral ECT (in which the electrodes are placed on both temples) is superior to unilateral ECT (in which both electrodes are placed over the nondominant temple; Royal College of Psychiatrists, 1990). Modern machines deliver a series of very brief (1 to 2 milliseconds) of direct current pulses at a rate of around 67 pulses per second, which is sufficient to induce an epileptic seizure

in most patients. Fits lasting more than 2 minutes are associated with an increased likelihood of short-term memory loss. Although such an occurrence is uncommon, fits as long as this should be terminated by the anaesthetist with intravenous diazepam. A "standard" course of ECT is 6 to 8 applications given at a rate of two or three treatments per week. Some patients may require as many as 12 to 14 treatments, but it is rare to see improvement beyond this stage if it has not already occurred.

The most important risks associated with ECT are those resulting from repeated short general anaesthetics. Therefore the usual precautions such as checking that the patient has no cardiac or respiratory disorder or any other contraindications to a short general anaesthetic needs to be taken prior to each application. In addition, it is common practice to measure pseudo-cholinesterase to guard against the possibility of prolonged apnoea after muscle relaxant use. Severe complications of anaesthesia given for ECT are in fact rare, and the rate is lower than that following surgical procedures. The death rate (usually due to cardiovascular collapse) has been estimated at 1 in 10,000 treatments (Scott, 1986).

Although there are no absolute contraindications to ECT, it is probably best avoided within the first 4 to 6 weeks following myocardial infarction. Caution should also be exercised in patients who have a recent history of cardiac arrhythmias due to either coronary heart disease or other causes. Having said this, ECT is almost certainly safer than TCAs in patients with coronary heart disease.

Dramatic injuries such as fractures and dislocations that were hazards in the early days of unmodified ECT (i.e. treatment given without anaesthesia) are no longer a problem provided that adequate muscle relaxation is given. It is worth emphasising, however, that providing muscle relaxation is the prime purpose of giving a general anaesthetic for ECT.

The side effect of ECT that is most often complained of by patients is memory impairment. This is greater with bilateral than unilateral ECT, because the latter is only applied to the nondominant hemisphere. Although some patients have a patchy memory loss for events that occurred even years before treatment, the most common finding is a reversible and short-lived memory loss for events around the period when the treatment was being given (i.e. 3–4 weeks; Squire, 1986). In most patients, personal or autobiographical memory is relatively spared but anterograde amnesic effects on impersonal memory such as events in the news are more commonly affected (Lisanby et al., 2000). Some patients have continuing longer-term memory problems, but these are usually associated with continuing affective symptoms or drug or alcohol abuse (Freeman et al., 1980).

Transcranial magnetic stimulation (TMS) offers a means of perturbing neuronal activity and can be used both to study brain function and potentially as a noninvasive form of physical treatment for depression. There have now been more than 20 controlled trials of TMS in depression, and overall these tend to show beneficial effects. In reviewing these studies, Ebmeir and colleagues (2006) concluded that there is too much heterogeneity across published studies to estimate confidently the size of the effect or to conclude that TMS is clinically efficacious. Many of the studies have been small, and the trend has been for more recent studies to show smaller effects, suggesting that there may have been biases resulting from initial enthusiasm.

A rare side effect of TMS at higher frequencies and intensities is an epileptic seizure. It has been suggested that this may be turned to advantage in that TMS induced seizures can be more finely focused than is the case with ECT, and it may be possible to reduce or avoid memory impairment (Lisanby et al., 2003). However, the use of so-called magnetic seizure therapy currently remains experimental.

Vagal nerve stimulation has been shown to be an effective treatment in patients with epilepsy who are refractory to other therapies. Although there are anecdotal accounts of dramatic improvements in some patients with recurrent depression treated by vagal nerve stimulation, there is limited evidence

for its efficacy (Corcoran et al., 2006; Groves et al., 2005).

Recent studies have begun to explore deep brain stimulation (DBS) as an alternative to more traditional forms of neurosurgery for mental illnesses that involve making permanent lesions. DBS has been shown to be effective treatment for advanced Parkinsonism such that stimulation of the ventral intermediate nucleus of the thalamus can dramatically relieve tremor and stimulation of the subthalamic nucleus can improve bradykinesia and rigidity (Perlmutter & Mink, 2006). Although the precise mechanism of action is uncertain, it is thought that DBS reduces activity in the stimulated regions through the gating of ion channels. Based on the observation from brain imaging studies that some depressed patients show overactivity in the subgenual anterior cingulate gyrus, Mayberg and colleagues (2005) studied the effect of DBS in this region on six patients who had failed to respond to other treatments, including ECT. Four of the six showed marked and sustained improvement. Although truly double-blind trials of procedures involving neurosurgical intervention are impossible, within-subject comparisons of stimulation/no stimulation on a double-blind basis is feasible with DBS and has been carried out both in Parkinson's disease and in a single patient who had DBS for obsessive-compulsive disorder (OCD; Nuttin et al., 1999). Similar studies of depression will be of great interest.

Seasonal affective disorder and light therapy

As discussed in Chapter 12, seasonal variation in mood can be marked, with some individuals having severe depressive symptoms each winter and improvement associated with the coming of spring. The mood changes seem to be related to shortened day length and three or more episodes of depression commencing between October and December and continuing until March to May (Northern Hemisphere) is often labelled seasonal affective disorder (SAD). Some SAD sufferers have depressive episodes during other times of the year as well, so that a preferred nomenclature is depressive disorder "with a seasonal pattern" (American Psychiatric Association, 1994).

There is now consistent evidence that exposure to light during the winter months can alleviate the symptoms of SAD (Rosenthal *et al.*, 1984). Some studies also suggest that light therapy is effective even in depressed patients who do not show a seasonal pattern of illness (Tuunainen *et al.*, 2004). Bright white light of around 10,000 lux (about the same intensity as a clear spring morning) seems to provide the optimum treatment for most sufferers. This can be delivered with light boxes plugged into the main electricity supply. The boxes are slightly larger than a sheet of A4 paper, about 10 cm deep, and can be placed on a table. The patient sits in front of the box for at least 30 minutes in the morning, preferably before it gets light in winter. It is important to follow the manufacturers' instructions about how close to sit by the box (usually around 30 cm). Although it is not necessary to stare directly at the light, it is important not to keep getting up and moving away from it during the exposure time. Some individuals need to use the box for longer than 30 minutes, and others find it more convenient to use their box at other times (e.g. in the evenings). However, light treatment can be alerting and cause insomnia if used too near to bedtime. There are few side effects from using light treatment. A slight irritation or reddening of the eyes may occur when the treatment is first started but usually remits within a few days of continuing use. Individuals who have existing eye disease should consult their ophthalmologist before commencing light treatment.

Light treatment of SAD needs to be started in early autumn (i.e. September to October in the Northern Hemisphere) and continued everyday throughout the winter months until symptoms remit in spring. This is quite a commitment in time and effort but many SAD patients consider that it is well worth it. Some patients are unable to get through the whole winter with light treatment alone and may need antidepressant supplementation. Fluoxetine has a product licence for the treatment of SAD but is not necessarily more efficacious than other antidepressants in this context.

Light has a direct effect on the hormone melatonin. Waking in the morning is associated with a drop in melatonin levels in the blood, and evenings with the onset of sleepiness with rising levels. It is thought that this diurnal variation in melatonin is also linked to similar diurnal patterns for cortisol and serotonin. Improved mood may be associated with the drop in melatonin caused by the light exposure.

Refractory depression

Refractory depression, sometimes called treatment-resistant depression, is not uncommon. Although the majority of patients (60%–70%) improve after treatment with antidepressants and 70% to 80% improve following ECT, a minority remain who show only slight or transient improvement, or no apparent response at all. Such individuals, although all grouped together under the broad heading of refractory depression, form a heterogenous population. In assessing such cases it is always worth returning to first principles and asking, "Is the diagnosis correct?" For example, in younger and middle-aged patients, it is important to remember that schizophrenia can initially present with depressive symptoms, and up to a third of individuals with a subsequent diagnosis of schizophrenia may receive an initial diagnosis of depression on first contact with psychiatric services (Gottesman, 1991).

It is essential to ensure that the patient with refractory depression really has received adequate doses of standard antidepressant treatment for an adequate length of time. A careful history is required of all drugs tried, including the following: how long taken, the maximum dose achieved, as well as the reason for stopping the drug (i.e. ineffective or too many or intolerable side effects). Frequent problems are an inadequate dosage, failure to adhere to treatment, or rapid switching to another antidepressant within a short period of beginning treatment.

This occurs because neither patients nor their doctors are willing to wait long enough for side effects to subside, which will happen in most cases. Also, there are now many antidepressants to choose from, and thus switching has become relatively easy. Polypharmacy is also a hazard, and it is not uncommon to come across patients who are "unresponsive" to drug treatment but who are taking several medications, each of which has been added on an ad hoc basis. In such circumstances it is worth withdrawing all medication and starting again with a single antidepressant at an adequate dosage for 6 weeks.

If this still fails a range of options needs to be discussed with the patient (Taylor *et al.*, 2005). If the patient has severe depression with prominent biological symptoms, ECT should be considered. Another option is high-dose venlafaxine (200 mg or more per day). As mentioned earlier, this requires blood pressure to be monitored, and an electrocardiogram is advisable. Alternatively, augmentation with lithium can be instigated, aiming for a plasma level of 0.4 to 1.0 mmol/L. This should be preceded by a check on renal and thyroid function and an ECG. There is also increasing support for the use of lamotrigine as an effective augmenter of antidepressants (Barbosa *et al.*, 2003; Normann *et al.*, 2002). There is a low risk of a rash and possible development of Stevens-Johnson syndrome so that it is advisable to titrate the lamotrigine dosage slowly starting at 25 mg daily for 2 weeks and then increasing by 25 mg weekly until a daily dosage of 150 to 200 mg is achieved. It is then advisable to check the blood level and do a full blood count and liver function tests.

For patients in whom anxiety, insomnia or weight loss is prominent, an SSRI and mirtazapine in combination may prove effective. Box 27.8 outlines some strategies for augmentation of antidepressants in patients who fail to respond adequately to a single agent. It should be noted that most clinicians aim for monotherapy if possible, but that combinations of antidepressants and the use of other augmenting strategies are common in real-life clinical practice. Combinations should always be introduced

---

Box 27.8 Strategies in patients not responding conventional doses of a single antidepressant

- Try drug of a different class
- Give venlafaxine in high doses (with blood pressure monitoring)
- Add lithium
- Add lamotrigine
- Combine selective serotonin reuptake inhibitors and mirtazapine
- Combine fluoxetine with olanzapine
- Give electroconvulsive therapy

---

with care and with the knowledge of drug-drug interactions that may occur. Other possible strategies and combinations of drugs are discussed by Taylor *et al.* (2005) and by Stahl (2006).

Continuation treatment

There is good evidence that continuation treatment with antidepressants for a period after recovery lowers the risk of relapse. Early studies (e.g. Klerman *et al.*, 1974; Mindham *et al.*, 1972) suggested that about 6 months of treatment is optimal after a single episode of depression, and more recent studies confirm this (Reimherr *et al.*, 1998). The risk of recurrence of depression is high, and around two thirds of patients in unselected series of cases of clinically significant depression have had two or more episodes (Marusic & Farmer, 2000). In patients who have had multiple episodes the evidence favours longer periods of continuation treatment and, whereas early studies often used lower doses of antidepressants than during the active phase of treatment, subsequent studies (Frank *et al.*, 1990) showed that higher dosages of continuation therapy were more effective and indeed that there continues to be a benefit of active treatment and placebo in preventing relapse for a period of at least 5 years (Kupfer *et al.*, 1992). A meta-analysis of continuation studies (Geddes *et al.*, 2003) showed that antidepressants could reduce the risk of depressive relapse by about two thirds and concluded that there may be benefit in persisting with treatment up to 36 months, even for first-onset cases. However, persisting with treatment for this length of time in patients who have had only a single episode obviously needs careful discussion and in many cases is likely to be unacceptable to the patient.

Anxiety disorders

As outlined in Chapter 8, anxiety disorders are common and disabling. Treatment guidelines (National Institute of Clinical Excellence, 2004a) now usually suggest that psychological treatments such as cognitive-behavioural therapy (see Chapter 28) should be used as a first-line measure when possible. However, most clinicians, even those specialising in psychological treatments, agree that drug treatments often have a place. Broadly speaking, two groups of drugs may be used, benzodiazepines and antidepressants (mostly SSRIs).

Benzodiazepines

This class of drugs is extremely effective in providing rapid reduction of anxiety symptoms, but because of the high potential for the development of tolerance and both psychological and physical dependence, it is usually recommended that their use be confined to patients who have clear impairment as a result of anxiety symptoms. Benzodiazepines are useful in generalised anxiety disorder for periods of not more than 4 weeks (National Institute of Clinical Excellence, 2004a). Having said this, one set of official guidelines suggests that a small minority of patients suffering from severely disabling and chronic generalised anxiety disorder may benefit from longer-term treatment (Royal College of Psychiatrists, 1997). Benzodiazepines are not generally recommended in panic disorder (National Institute of Clinical Excellence, 2004a), and there is some evidence that in patients suffering from specific phobias or OCD, taking benzodiazepines reduces the effectiveness of psychological treatment.

Selective serotonin reuptake inhibitors and other antidepressants

SSRIs are preferred to benzodiazepines as the first line of drug treatment for generalised anxiety disorder (GAD). There is reasonable evidence in favour of starting at a lower dose than is commonly used in treating depression and titrating this upward, because some patients experience a worsening of anxiety symptoms when SSRIs are first introduced (Davidson, 2001). As with their antidepressant effect, there is a delay in onset of beneficial antianxiety effects, and a full response may take up to 6 weeks. A similar strategy of starting with a low dose and titrating upward is also to be recommended for the treatment of panic disorder, and again it may be 6 weeks before the full benefit is noticeable (Taylor *et al.*, 2005). In those failing to respond to an SSRI, it is worth trying imipramine or clomipramine. The issue of how long to continue treatment in panic disorder or GAD is much less well researched than is the case for depression, but there is some evidence that this should be at least 8 months (Ballenger, 2004).

In contrast to GAD and panic disorder, the dose of SSRI necessary to treat OCD effectively is usually higher than that required for the treatment of depression, for example, 60 mg of fluoxetine daily or 40 to 60 mg of paroxetine. Before the introduction of SSRIs, clomipramine, a TCA that acts mainly by inhibiting serotonin reuptake, was a mainstay of drug treatment for OCD, and there has been some controversy as to whether clomipramine is actually more effective than SSRIs. A meta-analysis (Piccinelli *et al.*, 1995) found that SSRIs and clomipramine were both superior to placebo in reducing the symptoms of OCD but found no evidence of greater efficacy of clomipramine over the SSRIs. However, there was evidence that both clomipramine and SSRIs were more effective than antidepressant drugs that have no selective serotonergic properties. The main argument for now favouring SSRIs over clomipramine is their superior side-effect profile (Pigott & Seay, 1999). Interestingly, the time taken to respond to serotonergic antidepressants in OCD is often much longer than in depression, with some patients taking up to 12 weeks to show improvement. There have been several case reports and small case series suggesting that augmenting SSRIs with an atypical antipsychotic might be of additional benefit for some patients with OCD that is resistant to an SSRI alone; those with motor tics and/or schizotypal personality disorder might particularly benefit from this approach (see Keuneman *et al.*, 2005, for a review).

SSRIs are also effective in social phobia in similar doses to those used in depression. A good response takes up to 8 weeks, and it is usually recommended that treatment continue for at least a year (Taylor *et al.*, 2005). In social phobia, as with all the anxiety disorders, SSRIs should not be stopped suddenly but rather tapered off gradually to avoid the possibility of the discontinuation syndrome.

Conclusion

Although the subject of this chapter has been the biological treatment of depression and anxiety disorders, it is in practice impossible to separate the process of management from the art of careful clinical assessment. Depression and anxiety are ubiquitous symptoms that are experienced by many patients in medical, surgical and primary care settings as well as in psychiatric practice. Accurate diagnosis is therefore a prime consideration, and it is often a matter of fine clinical judgement as to when someone presenting with symptoms of anxiety or depression becomes a "case" requiring active treatment. Such judgements are usually based on the number and severity of symptoms as well as on the degree of impairment the patient describes. It is also important to remember that being depressed or anxious frequently occurs in the context of other psychiatric disorders, as well as against a background of substance misuse, most commonly alcohol abuse or dependence. The clinician should therefore strive to detect such conditions and, where they are primary, treat these

before prescribing medication primarily targeted at depressive or anxiety symptoms.

It is also important to remember the old adages of "first, do no harm" and "comfort always". There are no biological treatments of anxiety or depression that are completely free of unwanted effects, and there is always an argument for carefully weighing improvement in symptoms against drug-related side effects. When it comes to comfort, simple reassurance is probably the easiest form to administer. The great majority of episodes of depression or attacks of anxiety will eventually remit even without any treatment, and it is worthwhile to ensure the patient knows this and not to stint on reassurance that this is the case.

REFERENCES

Asberg, M. (1976). Treatment of depression with tricyclic drugs – pharmacokinetic and pharmacodynamic aspects. *Pharmakopsychiatr Neuropsychopharmakol* 9:18–26.

Ballenger, J. C. (2004). Remission rates in patients with anxiety disorders treated with paroxetine. *J Clin Psychiatry* 65:1696–707.

Barbosa, L., Berk, M., & Vorster, M. (2003). A double-blind, randomized, placebo-controlled trial of augmentation with lamotrigine or placebo in patients concomitantly treated with fluoxetine for resistant major depressive episodes. *J Clin Psychiatry* 64:403–7.

Chan, C. H., Janicak, P. G., Davis, J. M., *et al.* (1987). Response of psychotic and nonpsychotic depressed patients to tricyclic antidepressants. *J Clin Psychiatry* 48:197–200.

Corcoran, C. D., Thomas, P., Phillips, J., & O'Keane, V. (2006). Vagus nerve stimulation in chronic treatment-resistant depression: preliminary findings of an open-label study. *Br J Psychiatry* 189:282–3.

Corya, S. A., Andersen, S. W., Detke, H. C., *et al.* (2003). Long-term antidepressant efficacy and safety of olanzapine/fluoxetine combination: a 76-week open-label study. *J Clin Psychiatry* 64:1349–56.

Davidson, J. R. (2001). Pharmacotherapy of generalized anxiety disorder. *J Clin Psychiatry* 62(Suppl 11):46–50; discussion 51–2.

Ebmeier, K. P., Donaghey, C., & Steele, J. D. (2006). Recent developments and current controversies in depression. *Lancet* **367**:153–67.

Frank, E., Kupfer, D. J., Perel, J. M., *et al.* (1990). Three-year outcomes for maintenance therapies in recurrent depression. *Arch Gen Psychiatry* **47**:1093–9.

Freeman, C. P., Weeks, D., & Kendell, R. E. (1980). ECT: II: patients who complain. *Br J Psychiatry* **137**:17–25.

Geddes, J. R., Carney, S. M., Davies, C., *et al.* (2003). Relapse prevention with antidepressant drug treatment in depressive disorders: a systematic review. *Lancet* **361**:653–61.

Gottesman, I. I. (1991). *Schizophrenia Genesis*. New York: W. H. Freeman.

Groves, D. A., Bowman, E. M., & Brown, V. J. (2005). Recordings from the rat locus coeruleus during acute vagal nerve stimulation in the anaesthetised rat. *Neurosci Lett* **379**:174–9.

Isacsson, G., & Rich, C. L. (2005). Antidepressant drug use and suicide prevention. *Int Rev Psychiatry* Jun;**17**(3):153–62.

Johnstone, E. C., Deakin, J. F., Lawler, P., *et al.* (1980). The Northwick Park electroconvulsive therapy trial. *Lancet* **2**:1317–20.

Keuneman, R. J., Pokos, V., Weerasundera, R., & Castle, D. J. (2005). Antipsychotic treatment in obsessive-compulsive disorder: a literature review. *Aust N Z J Psychiatry* May;**39**(5):336–43.

Klerman, G. L., Dimascio, A., Weissman, M., *et al.* (1974). Treatment of depression by drugs and psychotherapy. *Am J Psychiatry* **131**:186–91.

Korszun, A., Moskvina, V., Brewster, S., *et al.* (2004). Familiality of symptom dimensions in depression. *Arch Gen Psychiatry* **61**:468–74.

Kupfer, D. J., Frank, E., Perel, J. M., *et al.* (1992). Five-year outcome for maintenance therapies in recurrent depression. *Arch Gen Psychiatry* **49**:769–73.

Lisanby, S. H., Luber, B., Schlaepfer, T. E., & Sackeim, H. A. (2003). Safety and feasibility of magnetic seizure therapy (MST) in major depression: randomized within-subject comparison with electroconvulsive therapy. *Neuropsychopharmacology* **28**:1852–65.

Lisanby, S. H., Maddox, J. H., Prudic, J., *et al.* (2000). The effects of electroconvulsive therapy on memory of autobiographical and public events. *Arch Gen Psychiatry* **57**:581–90.

Marusic, A., & Farmer, A. (2000). Antidepressant augmentation with low-dose olanzapine in obsessive-compulsive disorder. *Br J Psychiatry* **177**:567.

Mayberg, H. S., Lozano, A. M., Voon, V., *et al.* (2005). Deep brain stimulation for treatment-resistant depression. *Neuron* **45**:651–60.

Mindham, R. H., Howland, C., & Shepherd, M. (1972). Continuation therapy with tricyclic antidepressants in depressive illness. *Lancet* **2**:854–5.

National Institute of Clinical Excellence (2004a). Anxiety. Management of anxiety (panic disorder, with or without agoraphobia, and generalised anxiety disorder) in adults in primary, secondary and community care. London: Clinical Guidance 22. National Institute of Clinical Excellence.

National Institute of Clinical Excellence. (2004b). *Depression. Management of Depression in Primary Care*. Clinical Guidance 23. London: National Institute of Clinical Excellence.

Normann, C., Hummel, B., Scharer, L. O., *et al.* (2002). Lamotrigine as adjunct to paroxetine in acute depression: a placebo-controlled, double-blind study. *J Clin Psychiatry* **63**:337–44.

Nuttin, B., Cosyns, P., Demeulemeester, H., *et al.* (1999). Electrical stimulation in anterior limbs of internal capsules in patients with obsessive-compulsive disorder. *Lancet* **354**:1526.

Perlmutter, J. S., & Mink, J. W. (2006). Deep brain stimulation. *Annu Rev Neurosci* **29**:229–57.

Piccinelli, M., Pini, S., Bellantuono, C., & Wilkinson, G. (1995). Efficacy of drug treatment in obsessive-compulsive disorder. A meta-analytic review. *Br J Psychiatry* **166**:424–43.

Pigott, T. A., & Seay, S. M. (1999). A review of the efficacy of selective serotonin reuptake inhibitors in obsessive-compulsive disorder. *J Clin Psychiatry* **60**:101–6.

Reimherr, F. W., Amsterdam, J. D., Quitkin, F. M., *et al.* (1998). Optimal length of continuation therapy in depression: a prospective assessment during long-term fluoxetine treatment. *Am J Psychiatry* **155**:1247–53.

Rosenthal, N. E., Sack, D. A., Gillin, J. C., *et al.* (1984). Seasonal affective disorder. A description of the syndrome and preliminary findings with light therapy. *Arch Gen Psychiatry* Jan;**41**(1):72–80.

Royal College of Psychiatrists (1990). *The Practical Administration of Electroconvulsive Therapy (ECT)*. London: Gaskell.

Royal College of Psychiatrists (1997). *Benzodiazepine: Risks, Benefits and Dependence. A Re-evaluation*. Council Report CR59. London: Royal College of Psychiatrists.

Scott, D. B. (1986). The Chief Scientist reports . . . mortality related to anaesthesia in Scotland. *Health Bull (Edinb)* **44**:43–57.

Song, F., Freemantle, N., Sheldon, T. A., *et al.* (1993). Selective serotonin reuptake inhibitors: meta-analysis of efficacy and acceptability. *BMJ* **306**:683–7.

Squire, L. R. (1986). Memory functions as affected by electroconvulsive therapy. *Ann N Y Acad Sci* **462**:307–14.

Stahl, S. M. (2006). *Essential Psychopharmacology: The Prescriber's Guide: Antidepressants.* Cambridge: Cambridge University Press.

Taylor, D., Paton, C., & Kerwin, R. (2005). *The South London and Maudsley NHS Trust and Oxleas NHS Trust 2005–2006 Prescribing Guidelines.* London: Taylor & Francis.

Thiery, M. (1965). *Clinical Trial of the Treatment of Depressive Illness.* Report to the Medical Research Council by Its Clinical Psychiatry Committee. *BMJ* **5439**:881–6.

Tuunainen, A., Kripke, D. F., & Endo, T. (2004). Light therapy for non-seasonal depression. *Cochrane Database Syst Rev* **2**:CD004050.

Young, J. P., Hughes, W. C., & Lader, M. H. (1976). A controlled comparison of flupenthixol and amitriptyline in depressed outpatients. *Br Med J* **1**:1116–18.

28

Cognitive behavioural therapy

Jan Scott and Aaron T. Beck

This chapter explores the use of cognitive and behavioural therapies in the treatment of mental disorders. The introduction of behavioural therapies preceded the development of cognitive theory and therapy, but since the introduction of the cognitive model of depression in the 1960s and the publication of the first randomized controlled treatment trials in the 1970s, there has been an exponential increase in research into cognitive models and studies exploring therapy process and outcome. In recent times, some therapists have further distinguished their approach from cognitive-behavioural therapists, regarding themselves as cognitive therapists. Rather than confuse readers with the terminology used, we use the term *CBT* to identify the spectrum of these behavioural, cognitive-behavioural and cognitive models. It is not realistic to try to cover all aspects of the various cognitive and behavioural models and the application of these therapies to all the problems and disorders in which the treatments have been applied, but as noted by Enright (1997), although there are many variants of CBT, they share a similar underlying model suggesting that psychological problems and mental disorders can be a consequence of cognitively distorted views of events or experiences or can be maintained by faulty patterns of thinking and behaviour. It is proposed that a vicious cycle develops in which misinterpretations of situations or symptoms further undermine a patient's coping and that further shifts in mood state and abnormal behavioural patterns exacerbate their problems (Beck, 1976).

This chapter focuses on four main areas: (1) a brief overview of the origins and evolution of CBTs and their relationship to other key therapies, (2) the general principles of CBT and comments on the most common misconceptions, (3) the application of these therapies to selected specific disorders and (4) an overview of key outcome data and some comments on training issues. The chapter ends with comments on future directions for research and practice in this field.

The evolution of cognitive-behavioural therapies

The history of cognitive theory and therapy demonstrates that their evolution cannot be viewed in isolation from psychoanalysis or behaviourism (Scott, 1998). The focus of cognitive theory on intrapsychic processes that mediate actions and reactions has parallels with psychoanalytic theory. However, the clear definition and selection of targets for therapeutic intervention, the routine inclusion of specific measures of change and the use of structured therapy sessions demonstrate the influence of behavioural therapy on cognitive therapy (Weishaar, 1993).

Essential Psychiatry, ed. Robin M. Murray, Kenneth S. Kendler, Peter McGuffin, Simon Wessely, David J. Castle. Published by Cambridge University Press. © Cambridge University Press 2008.

In the early part of the twentieth century, psycho-dynamic psychotherapists created a sophisticated topography of the mind, comprising conscious, preconscious and unconscious domains and later incorporating important concepts such as the id, ego and superego. A core element of these models was the notion that the thoughts, feelings and behaviours that shaped relationships and experiences were the result of unconscious drives (Weishaar, 1993). In contrast, the behaviourists viewed such models as atheoretical and lacking empirical support and developed therapies derived from their scientific observations of animal and human behaviour (Clark & Beck, 1999). Learning theory gave rise to interventions such as systematic desensitisation and response prevention that continue to be used in the behavioural therapies practised today. However, the early stimulus-response model produced a therapeutic approach devoid of any acknowledgement of the role of cognitions and emotions in shaping human reactions. This did not mean that all behaviourists rejected that such elements had any part to play and later publications on behaviourism demonstrated their increasing acceptance of the importance of thoughts and feelings in dictating human responses. Nevertheless, there was still reluctance to incorporate these components into traditional behavioural therapy for fear of rendering it less systematic (Weishaar, 1993). As such, by the midpoint of the twentieth century the two dominant models of therapy viewed cognitions that may determine feelings and behaviours as either inaccessible to the client (thus requiring a long-term therapeutic relationship to expose these mental events) or as unimportant to the therapeutic process (which modified overt behavioural responses to stressors).

The cognitive revolution in psychology in the 1950s and 1960s produced influential writings on personal construct theory (Kelly, 1955) and rational emotive therapy (Ellis, 1962). Around this time, Aaron Beck was training in psychoanalysis and began to research the psychological processes observed in depression (Beck, 1963). This research led to a critical conceptual shift that distinguishes cognitive therapies from psychoanalytic and behaviourist schools. Beck (1967) hypothesized that feelings and behaviours are influenced by cognitions operating at a conscious level (although individuals may need to be made aware of these thoughts). By the late 1960s, a cognitive model of psychopathology was developed that still provides the theoretical structure underpinning most models of cognitive therapy practised today (for a detailed review, see Beck, 2005). The core elements of the cognitive model are as follows:

- It is a normalising model: cognitive processing is viewed as being on a continuum from normal to abnormal.
- It is a stress-vulnerability model: the individual's interpretations (automatic thoughts) of events or experiences are attributed to the activation of underlying cognitive structures (dysfunctional beliefs, cognitive schemas).
- The processing of external events or internal stimuli is biased and therefore systematically distorts the individual's construction of his or her experiences, leading to a variety of cognitive errors (e.g. overgeneralisation, selective abstraction).
- There are distinct cognitive profiles for different mental disorders, referred to as the cognitive content specificity hypothesis (Greenberg & Beck, 1989), with different underlying themes, for example, in depression (loss and self-devaluation) compared with anxiety (threat and vulnerability).

A recent overview (Beck, 2005) highlighted the breadth of research on various cognitive models of psychopathology and noted a substantial body of supportive evidence for the model of depression with somewhat less evidence for the various anxiety disorders. Although empirical support for the different theoretical formulations may vary, it is clear that research by advocates of these models follows a well-established systematic process: namely, the development of a coherent conceptual framework always precedes the introduction of therapeutic strategies. This is noteworthy and may differentiate effective from ineffective therapies. Interventions such as technique-driven approaches, some forms of "cognitive-behavioural counselling" and many other brief (noncognitive) psychotherapies that do not follow this template have inconsistent evidence of clinical efficacy (Salkovskis, 1996). In general, counselling and therapy approaches that begin and end with interventions targeted at change in symptoms or nonspecific support without any consideration of underlying mechanisms can produce temporary improvements but usually fail to deliver any durable posttherapy change in vulnerability to relapse (Hollon *et al.*, 1993; Scott, 2001).

There are now a number of models of CBT that follow the "theoretical conceptualisation-therapy development" framework, including those predominantly focussed on learning theory or behavioural activation (behavioural therapy; BT), rational emotive therapy (RET) or rational emotive behavioural therapy (REBT); predominantly cognitive models such as cognitive therapy (CT), schema-focused therapy, dialectical behavioural therapy (DBT); and models incorporating cognitive and behavioural elements such as cognitive behavioural analysis system psychotherapy (CBASP) and cognitive-behavioural therapy (CBT); as well as a hybrid of brief dynamic and cognitive therapy called cognitive analytic therapy (CAT). Space limitations mean these variations on the primary models cannot be explored in this chapter. The range and popularity of CBT is, in part, because they are applicable to a wide spectrum of common psychological problems as well as severe mental disorders (Beck, 2005). For example, exposure therapy (BT) is useful for treating phobias (Pretzer *et al.*, 1989), schema-focused models are used in the treatment of personality disorders (Beck *et al.*, 2004), DBT has proved to be particularly useful in the treatment of borderline personality disorder (Koerner & Linehan, 2000), and CBASP alone or in combination with antidepressants may be beneficial in the treatment of chronic depression (Keller *et al.*, 2000).

The majority of the therapies just noted fulfill the criteria for "well-established" empirically supported treatments (Chambless & Hollon, 1998). Recognition as an empirically supported treatment (EST) means that the efficacy of the therapy has been established in two or more carefully designed

Table 28.1 Empirically supported treatments: requirements for a well-established treatment

Criteria for a "well-established" therapy

I. At least two good between-group design experiments demonstrating efficacy in one or more of the following ways:
  A. superiority to pill or psychological placebo or alternative treatment and
  B. equivalence to an already established treatment in experiments with adequate statistical power.

II. Experiments must be conducted with treatment manuals.
III. Characteristics of the client samples must be clearly specified.
IV. Effects must have been demonstrated by at least two investigators or investigatory teams.

methodologically reliable randomized controlled trials that evaluate the treatment of a specific disorder (Task Force on Promotion and Dissemination of Psychological Procedures, 1995). The criteria require that trial samples should be well defined, of adequate size to establish statistical significance of the findings and use reliable and valid outcome measures. The therapists involved in the trial should use treatment manuals and the therapist's adherence to the therapy protocol and their competency in delivering the interventions should be monitored (see Table 28.1). There are concerns among some psychotherapy researchers about employing criteria that are usually used to judge the value of pharmacotherapies, and indeed opponents of EST argue that such approaches to the assessment of the benefits of psychotherapy are fundamentally flawed. However, this evidence-based approach is invariably employed in the development of clinical practice treatment guidelines; those psychological therapies that have been evaluated through randomized trials and been the subject of meta-analytic review are more likely to be considered as either an alternative or an adjunct to pharmacotherapy (Roth & Fonagy, 1996). There may be some issues in trying to evaluate therapies using approaches primarily targeted at assessing the added value of new medications, but the reality is that the adoption of this research framework has clearly raised the profile and increased the acceptability of CBT to non-psychotherapists working in general psychiatry and general medical settings. As such, in England and Wales, the National Institute of Clinical Excellence (NICE) has incorporated CBT into several of its key guidelines (e.g. it is a recommended treatment of depression, schizophrenia and anxiety disorders).

General principles of therapy

As noted, there are several variants of cognitive therapy, but the shared features of CBT are that these are action-orientated, pragmatic, manualised approaches that can be used to understand and treat mental disorders (Grant *et al.*, 2005). Although the therapies vary in the emphasis placed on certain types of intervention, there are several common aspects:

1. The therapy interventions are designed to treat specific disorders or problems, and the techniques employed are derived empirically from experimental and applied theory research. Importantly, the initial case formulation also attempts to identify unique factors in the client's history that ensure the therapist and patient tailor the therapy to that individuals' particular needs.

2. The therapy uses a collaborative "hypothesis-testing" approach employing guided discovery (Socratic questioning) to identify and re-evaluate distorted cognitions and dysfunctional beliefs (see Box 28.1). Cognitive change is viewed as a key mediator of behavioural change.

3. Therapy pursues symptomatic relief through adaptive learning. The rationale for the use of different techniques is shared with the patient and interventions are introduced in a logical sequence. Behavioural techniques focus on how to act or cope but also provide important information about underlying cognitive processes.

Box 28.1 Guided discovery (adapted from Padesky, 1993)

Socratic questioning

This involves asking questions which:

- the client has the knowledge to answer
- draw the client's attention to information which is relevant to the issue being discussed but which may be outside the client's current focus
- generally move from the concrete to the more abstract so that the client can, in the end, apply the new information to either re-evaluate a previous conclusion or construct a new idea.

For example, to help a client identify useful information about a topic being discussed in therapy, the therapist might ask:

Have you ever been in similar circumstances before? What did you do? How did that turn out?

What do you know now that you didn't know then?

What would you advise a friend who told you something similar?

The Four stages of guided discovery:

Stage 1: Asking informational questions

Socratic questions are used to delineate the client's concerns in a concrete (e.g. specific example) and understandable way for the client and therapist

Stage 2: Listening

To be clear about exactly what the issues are but also listening for idiosyncratic words and emotional reactions

Stage 3: Summarizing

Therapists should summarize the discussion or ask the client to provide a brief summary every few minutes

Stage 4: Synthesizing or analytical questions

The therapist completes the guided discovery process by asking a synthesizing or analytical question which applies to the client's original concern new information that has been discussed and summarized along with the idiosyncratic meanings that have been explored, e.g. "How does all this information and data we have reviewed fit with your idea that you are unlovable?"

---

4. Therapy is goal-orientated but sets realistic limits to the range and nature of problems that can be tackled within the time frame of the course of therapy. The aim is to focus on the present and to

tackle current symptoms and concerns through the development of problem-solving and coping strategies. Learning these strategies will equip the patient to anticipate and tackle future problems or stressors that arise post-treatment.

5. The therapy is characterized by an educational approach, initially enabling individuals to understand the evolution and maintenance of their problems and symptoms, to recognise their underlying thinking styles and learn how to respond to them in different ways. The approach also encourages independent use of skills through between-session homework tasks.

6. A course of therapy is brief, ranging from about 8 sessions in panic disorder to 20 to 25 sessions in chronic depressive disorders. This requires a high degree of therapeutic skill because CBT is not done *to* a patient, it is done *with* a patient, and the pace of the programme must be adapted to individual needs. Any change achieved is attributed to the patient.

These are key elements of CBT. Unfortunately there are also many misunderstandings about these methods. The three most unhelpful myths are as follows:

Myth 1: It sounds simple so it must be simple. The CBT model is an accessible theory and with training can easily be communicated to patients. This makes the therapy accessible to individuals who may not be regarded as good candidates for other verbal therapies. However, a CBT manual cannot simply be followed like a recipe in a cookbook. The fact that the model is understandable and the interventions appear rational does not mean anyone can practice CBT. The ability to formulate cases, engage in collaborative guided discovery and apply the right technique at the right time requires considerable skill on the part of the therapist and a commitment to ongoing supervision. There is clear evidence that expertise and adherence to the CBT model are predictors of outcome from therapy (Moorhead & Scott, 1999). Perhaps the most misunderstood aspect of CBT is the concept of guided discovery. Therapy is not about telling individuals they have

distorted thoughts or suggesting "correct" interpretations of the patient's experiences. The critical skill for a therapist to understand and master is the staged approach to guided discovery and the use of Socratic questioning (see Box 28.1). If used appropriately, this therapeutic style enables clients to uncover for themselves their cognitive distortions, automatic thoughts and underlying beliefs and to draw their own conclusions about their accuracy or functionality and to then explore how to modify their cognitions for themselves. Padesky (1993) provided one of the best overviews of these concepts; her descriptions are adapted and summarised in Box 28.1.

Myth 2: CBT does not attend to interpersonal issues or the therapeutic relationship. It is true that improvement is not always contingent on the therapist-patient dynamics (Grant *et al.*, 2005). The therapeutic relationship is not the main vehicle for producing change, but CBT cannot and does not ignore this essential element of therapy or the patient's life. For example, brief problem-orientated CBT can only be beneficial if an effective working alliance has been established quickly between the patient and therapist (within about 2–4 sessions), so that they may attend to the core issues to be tackled. If the formulation of the patient's problems establishes that there are interpersonal issues to be tackled, these will be identified and worked on within therapy sessions and through homework assignments. Also, CBT focused on personality disorders is heavily orientated towards schema change and inevitably focuses on interpersonal issues, including interactions between the therapist and patient (analogous to the exploration of transference). A difference in CBT is that difficulties in the therapeutic relationship are usually put on the agenda for discussion in therapy, allowing an open exploration of any concerns, and whether the interaction with the therapist mirrors problems in relationships outside of therapy. Although a CBT therapist may need to guide the client into such sensitive discussions, the process of CBT does not incorporate therapist's interpretations because the latter would be counter to the philosophy of the therapy in that it does not represent self-discovery.

Myth 3: Because CBT is brief and present-orientated, it must "just cover over the cracks", it does not "cure" a person. Although therapy is brief, it is highly focused and the sessions follow a clear structure. The content of CBT sessions changes over time, but the structure of sessions remains constant. Each session begins with collaborative agenda setting, a review of what can be concluded and learned from the previous homework experiments, and an agreed set of topics for consideration; the session ends with a joint discussion of what has been learnt that day and an agreed set of homework tasks that build a bridge to the next session. The ultimate aim is to give individuals the skills to overcome future problems independently. Although CBT targets contemporary problems, the past is not ignored; on the contrary, selected use of past events and experiences is essential to conceptualizing and understanding how and why individuals presented with their particular problems at this particular time. The final stages of even the briefest forms of CBT are focused on relapse prevention, which requires an understanding of the origins of dysfunctional beliefs and how they have influenced individuals' actions and reactions. A critical component of CBT is modifying underlying beliefs or, at the very least, changing the individual's response pattern when dysfunctional beliefs are activated. Clinicians who use an ad hoc selection of CBT techniques without employing a formulation or including this relapse prevention component will find that patients often struggle to maintain any of the apparent gains that they made during therapy.

Applications of cognitive-behavioural therapy

Rather than attempt to describe all the variations or adaptations of Beck's original cognitive model, this section gives examples of some of the key areas in which cognitive models have been developed and CBT has subsequently been applied. The section begins with a brief overview of the cognitive model of depression and then anxiety disorders; finally the use of CBT as an adjunct to medication in psychotic disorders is considered.

Cognitive models of depression

Beck's (1967) cognitive theory of depression postulates that some individuals may be vulnerable to depression because they develop dysfunctional beliefs as a result of early learning experiences. These beliefs may be latent for long periods but become primed by events that carry a specific meaning for that individual. Beck suggests that the underlying beliefs that render an individual vulnerable to depression may be broadly categorized into beliefs about being helpless or unlovable (J. Beck, 1995). Thus events that are deemed uncontrollable or that involve relationship difficulties may reactivate these beliefs and be important in the genesis of depressive symptoms (Scott, 2001). Negative cognitions about the self, world and future are concomitants of depression but serve to re-enforce the core underlying dysfunctional beliefs. The negative automatic thoughts that dominate the thinking of many depressed patients are sustained through systematic distortions of information processing (e.g. focusing only on negative aspects of an interpersonal interaction) and contribute to further depression of affect (Hollon *et al.*, 1986). Beliefs about self seem especially important in the onset or maintenance of depression, and these beliefs, particularly low or variable self-esteem, are frequent targets for change in CBT (Hagaa *et al.*, 1991).

Beck clearly states that although the vicious cycle of low mood contributing to negative thinking and leading to further lowering in mood may represent a causal theory in some cases, it represents a maintenance model for other depressions. However, he proposes that intervention in the cycle can be effective in alleviating depressive symptoms in the latter group (Beck *et al.*, 1979).

The CBT interventions are selected on the basis of a cognitive conceptualization that has identified the individuals' likely core negative beliefs and critical incidents that have occurred in their life; it also explains the onset and maintenance of their disorder. If the patient shows a low level of functioning, behavioural techniques may be used to improve activity levels and mood, but the ultimate goal is still to identify and modify negative cognitions and maladaptive underlying beliefs. Verbal interventions are initially employed to re-evaluate negative cognitions. Between-session experiments, frequently focused on interpersonal functioning, are used to re-evaluate ideas. Negative automatic thoughts are characteristically situation-specific interpretations, but in addition to reviewing these cognitions and the processing errors that may be manifest, the patient and therapist analyse the patterns or recurring themes in the automatic thoughts recorded as this helps identify the probable underlying beliefs (Beck *et al.*, 1979). Later, when the patient has developed his or her cognitive and behavioural skills and is using the techniques to reduce depressive symptoms, the therapist and patient use similar cognitive interventions and behavioural experiments to try to modify underlying dysfunctional beliefs (which operate across situations).

Cognitive models of anxiety

The cognitive theory of anxiety disorders suggests that underlying danger-orientated beliefs predispose the individual to restrict attention to perceived threats in the environment, making catastrophic interpretations of ambiguous stimuli, underestimating their own coping resources (or the likelihood that others can help if a dangerous situation arises) and engaging in dysfunctional "safety behaviours" such as avoidance (Beck, 2005). There are some variations depending on the perceived nature of the threat or danger. For example, in panic disorder, ambiguous stimuli or subjective experiences are given catastrophic interpretations that are often focused on the presumed pathological significance of what is happening. Normal or quite benign experiences, such as a brief period of tachycardia, may be interpreted as a potentially fatal event such as

a heart attack (Beck *et al.*, 1985; Clark *et al.*, 1997). Cognitive theory and therapy have been important in helping clinicians understand that examination of the evidence that supports or refutes the individual's catastrophic automatic thoughts are important elements in the psychological treatment of anxiety rather than the repeated use of reassurance (which leads to rebound anxiety) and that behavioural experiments can help challenge and overcome safety behaviours.

Social anxiety and social anxiety disorder (see Chapter 8) are characterized by maladaptive beliefs about social performance, and individuals conclude that others will make negative evaluations and reject them (Clark & Wells, 1995). This assumption is often associated with a failure to register objective social clues and exaggerated negatively biased misinterpretations of the situation.

Clark and Ehlers (2004) noted that the cognitive model of *posttraumatic stress disorder* (PTSD) has two core components. First, negative appraisal of actual events and exaggerated negative appraisal of the symptoms produced by the trauma; second, inadequate integration of the traumatic experience into the individual's autobiographical memory. Common cognitions that maintain the symptoms and distress which can be tackled though sensitive intervention are the following: 'The world is a dangerous place', 'I am not in control', and 'Things will never be the same again'. Cognitive therapy for PTSD has been important in demonstrating that the consequences of real-life traumatic events can be understood and treated (Gillespie *et al.*, 2002).

Cognitive models of psychosis

The first case description of the use of reasoning techniques with an individual with systematised paranoid delusion (probably schizophrenia in *Diagnostic and Statistical Manual of Mental Disorders* terms) was published by Beck (1952), before the advent of antipsychotics. Beck described some of the key elements of a new structured psychotherapy of schizophrenia, which at least in this case was extremely successful. He engaged with the patient and established a working therapeutic alliance in which trust developed. Together they worked on the sequence of events that had preceded the emergence of the systematised paranoid delusion from which the patient suffered. A phase of systematic, graded reality testing followed in which the patient was guided to examine the evidence in relation to the behaviour of his presumed persecutors. Having done this with the help of the therapist in session, he reviewed all the evidence at his disposal from his homework exercises and gradually started to eliminate false beliefs about his presumed persecutors. In this case there was no emergence of depression or anxiety as the delusion receded, and the effect appeared to be durable with the patient remaining well at follow-up.

Beck's study did not lead to further investigations of CBT for many years, but then a number of researchers began to explore this area (Birchwood & Iqbal, 1998; Sensky *et al.*, 2000; Tarrier *et al.*, 1998). The model of CBT followed has many parallels to Beck's original description. Fowler and Morley (1989) and later Fowler *et al.* (1995) described the cognitive-behavioural intervention as involving the following:

- instructions in coping strategies,
- attempts to modify patients' beliefs about their voices by cognitive restructuring,
- bringing on and dismissing hallucinations within therapy sessions, and
- education about the use of coping strategies (basically focusing the individuals' attention on external stimuli which seemed to cause the onset of symptoms).

In their CBT manual, Kingdon and Turkington (1994) also highlighted that differences in using CBT with patients with psychosis are generally a matter of emphasis, in addition to some specific techniques to supplement those used for anxiety and depression. For example, agenda setting may need to be more flexible, simple, and sometimes less explicit, and the length and frequency of sessions may also need to vary.

The underlying cognitive process that may explain the development of delusions is that some individuals jump to conclusions on the basis of minimal evidence, forming fixed ideas with a high level of conviction. Furthermore, the origin of their problems is attributed externally (e.g. at other people) rather than being seen as internally driven (by an illness process).

Kingdon and Turkington (1994) described a CBT method for exploring delusions: initially this involves engagement, building trust, assessment and formulation. From this, the links between events and circumstances and the feelings, behaviour and beliefs that emerged are examined. A range of explanations, including the delusional ones chosen by the patient, are discussed and reality testing, involving examination of evidence, logical inquiry and reasoning, is used – as far as possible led by or elicited from the patient. This process may allow the patient to reconsider beliefs but, more commonly, assists in developing a therapeutic relationship, improving adherence with services and medication and allowing behaviour to change (e.g. often patients begin to socialise more). At this stage, underlying concerns may emerge (e.g. they begin to talk about past traumatic events). Beliefs about themselves may also come to the surface or be specifically elicited by the use of a variety of CBT techniques. However, as noted by Scott and colleagues (2004), this is an area where caution is needed – emotional arousal is well recognised as a precipitant of psychotic symptoms and so can worsen rather than assist progress and can lead to disengagement from therapy.

Techniques that may be helpful when targeting hallucinations include reattribution (improving patients' insight to enable them to understand that hallucinations are internally generated), development of specific coping strategies and modification of beliefs about the omnipotence of voices and their content. Overall, therapy with individuals with psychotic symptoms is recommended as an adjunct rather than an alternative to medication, and the skill of the therapist and expertise in the treatment of severe mental disorders is a vital consideration before embarking on such an application of CBT. The outline of CBT for psychosis

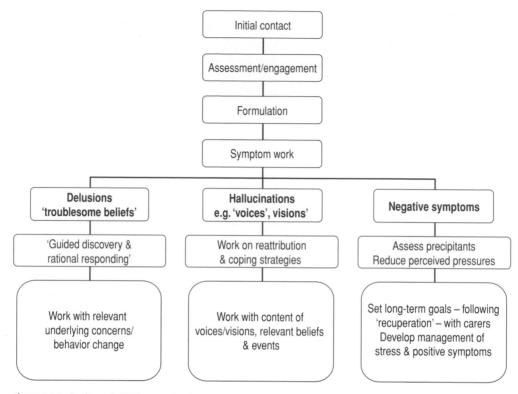

Figure 28.1 Outline of CBT for psychosis.

(as described by Beck & Rector, 2002) is shown in Figure 28.1.

Outcome research

In their recent review, Butler and colleagues (2006) identified more than 300 published outcome studies on CBT and 16 meta-analyses. The authors used these data on mean effect sizes (ES) to try to answer key questions about the utility of CBT, namely: (1) how effective are CBTs and which disorders they are most effective for and (ii) how durable are the therapy gains. These findings are summarized in Table 28.2.

This meta-analysis and other reviews suggest that compared with waiting-list or placebo treatments, CBTs are highly effective (CBT vs control condition: grand mean ES 0.95; SD 0.08) for unipolar depression, childhood anxiety and depressive disorders and a number of anxiety disorders. Although the heterogeneity of studies incorporated in other meta-analyses made the findings less robust, the CBTs were associated with large improvements (mean ES 1.27; SD 0.11) in symptoms of bulimia nervosa that exceeded the gains from medication alone, and CBT showed additional benefits over usual treatment for schizophrenia (ES for CBT varied from 0.54 to 1.2 compared with an ES of 0.17 for treatment as usual). However, when compared with an active treatment condition, CBTs for depressive disorders show equivalent or only marginal superiority. In other disorders, such as OCD, when CBT, CT and BT were compared with each other they appeared to be equally effective. Moderate ES (0.5–0.8) were noted for CBT compared with control conditions for marital distress, pain syndromes, anger management and childhood somatic disorders.

Table 28.2 Summary of findings from meta-analyses of acute and longer term (6 months to 8 years) benefits of cognitive-behavioural therapy (CBT)

Evidence from one or more meta-analyses of: CBT > control condition and/or CBT = active treatment (no. studies in analysis)	Evidence of durable benefit from CBT
Adult unipolar depression ($n = 75$)	Adult unipolar depression (acute and chronic disorders)
Bulimia nervosa ($n = 24$)	
Childhood depressive and anxiety disorders ($n = 22$)	Generalised anxiety disorder
Panic disorder with agoraphobia or without agoraphobia ($n = 20$)	Social phobia
	Panic disorder
PTSD ($n = 14$)	OCD
Adolescent depression ($n = 13$)	
Generalised anxiety disorder ($n = 8$)	
Social phobia ($n = 7$)	
Schizophrenia ($n = 7$)	
OCD ($n = 4$)	

Adapted from Butler *et al.* (2006). OCD = obsessive-compulsive disorder; PTSD = posttraumatic stress disorder.

The review also explored whether the benefits of CBT extended after completion of therapy. A major methodological problem is that few therapy trials have adequate statistical power to access reliably the durability of the treatment benefits, and many follow-ups involved selective subsamples of the original trial population (Paykel *et al.*, 1999). However, bearing these limitations in mind, Butler *et al.* (2006) concluded there was evidence of persistent benefit and reduced relapse rates in unipolar depression and a range of adult anxiety disorders. There was also emerging evidence of reduced relapse rates in schizophrenia, sexual offenders and childhood internalizing disorders.

Box 28.2 Factors impeding patient engagement in cognitive-behavioural therapy (CBT)

Patients may:
- feel unable to commit to the therapy (e.g. may be convinced that their disorder is biological and can only be treated with medication)
- not be able to understand or relate to the rationale for the interventions used
- prefer to use therapy for catharsis and reject the problem focus or action-orientated approach of CBT
- be reluctant to let go of some personal gains they attain from aspects of their problems (e.g. hypomanic overactivity)
- be unable to employ the techniques (e.g. some individuals with learning difficulties)
- lack judgement about the impact of their actions and lack the ability or desire to control some of their actions (e.g. antisocial personality disorder).

Limitations

Grant and colleagues (2005) noted that CBTs are quite versatile and that the absolute limits have yet to be empirically defined. Like any treatment, however, there are a number of factors that may impede engagement with CBT. These are shown in Box 28.2.

Other factors might also pertain. For example, there may be issues about the timing of therapy introduction. For example, there is no evidence that CBT adds value to the acute treatment of psychotic depression. It can be postulated that this is because the symptoms respond better to biological approaches, because the patient and therapist cannot form a working alliance or because the patient lacks the concentration to engage with the therapy process. However, if the introduction of CBT is delayed, there is evidence for the benefits of CBT as part of an inpatient treatment programme or the use of individual CBT for severe depression (Wright *et al.*, 1993). In the latter disorder, combining CBT with medication may improve the trajectory of change compared with medication alone. It is also clear that cultural considerations and patient or clinician preference will be important determinants of the acceptability of CBT. Although all these issues could impede response or engagement with any treatment, it is also important to state that CBT is not a panacea. Overstating the case for CBT may lose rather than win support for increasing its availability in general psychiatry (Parker *et al.*, 2003).

In clinical settings, CBT therapists point out that although they may receive referrals of individuals who would be predicted from randomized controlled trials to respond well to CBT, the therapist is just as likely to be referred those individuals with persistent treatment-refractory problems who have tried many other treatment approaches and are therefore offered the chance to try CBT as well. This difference between research and clinical practice is a major contributor to the efficacy-effectiveness gap and is important to acknowledge. An EST is largely recognised on the basis of its efficacy in well-defined clinical populations in which therapy is delivered by highly skilled therapists with appropriate training and supervision. The CBTs are less likely to be clinically effective in those clients who have complex mixtures of problems such as comorbidity or medication-refractory symptoms, who have already demonstrated a poor outcome to many other treatment approaches and in individuals who are sceptical about the benefits of any treatment at all. Problems may also arise when the therapist has inadequate training or lacks access to supervision in the use of the particular CBT approach that has been applied to the constellation of problems now being treated (Crits-Cristoph *et al.*, 1991). Therapist expertise (comprising skill level, competent delivery and adherence to the treatment protocol) rather than length of experience is especially important. In the same way that a medication would not be deemed ineffective if it were not the appropriate drug for the problem being treated and had not been given at an adequate dosage for an adequate period of time, patients should not be viewed as "CBT failures" unless similar circumstances apply. For example, in a study delivering a brief CBT intervention for individuals who engaged in repeated self-harm, Davidson

and colleagues (2004) demonstrated a statistically significant relationship between patient outcome and therapist level of training and competency in CBT. Likewise, Persons (an expert CBT therapist) showed that patient outcomes at her CBT centre closely paralleled those reported in the research trials for depression, anxiety and personality disorders (Persons *et al.*, 1999).

Although the utility of CBT can be limited by characteristics of the disorder, the patient, the therapist or the therapeutic relationship, it is clear that a major impediment to the use of CBT with disorders or problems in which there is evidence for efficacy is the lack of adequately trained therapists.

Training

A number of official bodies now regulate the registration of therapists across Britain and Europe that set criteria for accreditation as a CBT therapist. In addition, a worldwide organization, the Academy of Cognitive Therapy (ACT), supports high-quality research in and clinical delivery of CBT by offering training courses, workshops and supervision (www.academyofct.org).

In Britain, the British Association of Behavioural and Cognitive Psychotherapists (BABCP) is the main body accrediting CBT therapists, and its minimum training standards are worth noting because they begin to dispel the myth that "everyone is a cognitive therapist". A mental health professional who wishes to be recognized as a CBT practitioner requires at least 200 hours of supervised therapy working with a minimum of eight patients covering at least three types of problems. As well as close supervision, it is expected that cases will have been written up and assessed. The practitioner also needs to complete a minimum of 30 hours of continuing professional development activities related to CBT such as attending training workshops and journal clubs. The message from these criteria is clear: attaining the skills to practise formulation-driven CBT cannot be achieved by attending a few workshop and then employing diary keeping or activity scheduling in clinical settings. A common problem is that novice therapists underestimate how complex it is to establish a collaborative therapeutic alliance and to integrate the technical cognitive and behavioural interventions within therapy sessions. Training in the application of CBT to new areas of practise also requires additional training because the cognitive model for personality disorders will call on additional expertise over and above that needed to treat common mental disorders effectively. Finally, the CBTs are continuing to evolve and demonstrate efficacy in many new areas. To remain on the register of accredited CBT practitioners, it is necessary to demonstrate a long-term commitment to ongoing supervised clinical practise and to continuing professional development (www.babcp.com).

Future directions

Cognitive and behavioural therapies have been applied successfully to a number of problems and disorders over the last 30 years. The philosophy of CBT entirely reflects the scientist-practitioner approach that is widely advocated as a model for clinical practice for mental health professionals. In Europe, it is the most frequently applied approach in research and in clinical settings. Ongoing research continues to explore the efficacy of CBT and to look at adaptations that allow it to be applied across a range of clinical settings and disorders. Examples include the introduction of computerized and guided self-help versions of CBT that may be used for common mental disorders or in primary care (Bara-Carril *et al.*, 2004; Wright *et al.*, 2002), as well as extended models that encompass maintenance treatment sessions to reduce relapse rates in highly recurrent depressive disorders (Jarrett *et al.*, 2001). To enhance further the clinical utility of CBT, attempts are being made to modify the approach for use with comorbid disorders and the complex problems seen in general clinical practice (Grant *et al.*, 2005; Stirman *et al.*, 2003).

Another key area of developing research is focused on the process of change in CBT and

the mediators of its effect (DeRubeis & Feeley, 1990). This is important when trying to differentiate between the general characteristics of effective therapies such as the strength of the therapeutic alliance compared with any unique effects. Work on mediators of change in depression is of great interest because, despite evidence clearly demonstrating that CBTs can be an effective treatment of acute or chronic depressive disorders and have a prophylactic effect, how they achieve these effects is not well understood. For example, Persons (1993) noted that the changes in depressogenic attributional style (a tendency to attribute negative events to internal, stable, global causes) produced by CBT are equivocal. This led her to propose that a key therapeutic process may not simply be modification of underlying beliefs but the acquisition of compensatory skills that allow the individual to cope with isolated depressive symptoms and prevent the symptoms evolving into a depressive episode.

In a study of individuals with chronic depression who received medication or medication plus CBT, Teasdale *et al.* (2000) demonstrated that CBT reduced relapse through changes in the style rather than the content of thinking. A good outcome from CBT was achieved through reductions in absolutist, dichotomous thinking. Individuals with persistent extreme response styles to depression-related material were more than 2.5 times as likely to experience early relapse compared with individuals without this extreme style (relapse rate = 44% vs 17%). This study suggested that training individuals to change the ways they process depression-related material, rather than changing their belief in depressive thought content, may be a critical component of CBT.

Lastly, an exciting field of research is the exploration of the mind-brain interface by using scanning technology (such as functional magnetic resonance imaging [fMRI] and positron emission tomography [PET] scans) and looking at changes before and after CBT and comparing these with changes observed with pharmacological treatments such as antidepressants. Two recent publications on response to CBT provide examples of this evolving area of research. First, Goldapple *et al.* (2004) undertook before and after PET scans on 17 unmedicated, unipolar depressed outpatients, 14 of whom responded to 15 to 20 sessions of CBT. Scan results were compared with an independent group of 13 paroxetine-treated responders. Treatment response with CBT was associated with significant metabolic changes, notably increases in hippocampus and dorsal cingulate cortex and decreases in dorsal ventral and medial frontal cortex. Furthermore, this pattern was distinct from that with paroxetine-facilitated clinical recovery, in which prefrontal increases and hippocampal and subgenual cingulate decreases were found. The researchers concluded that, as with antidepressants, clinical recovery with CBT was associated with modulation in the functioning of specific sites in limbic and cortical regions. However, the differences in the directional changes in frontal cortex, cingulate, and hippocampus with CBT relative to paroxetine may reflect modality-specific effects. These findings have yet to be confirmed but open an important window into the functioning of the brain.

In a separate study, Siegle and colleagues (2006) used fMRI scans to monitor areas of the brain that are activated or deactivated in response to emotional stimuli. Fourteen unmedicated depressed patients and 21 never depressed control subjects were asked to rate as quickly and accurately as possible the relevance to them of positive, negative and neutral emotionally valenced cue words. Following the scans, the depressed participants received 16 sessions of CBT. It was reported that seven of nine depressed patients who pre-therapy showed low sustained reactivity in the subgenual cingulate cortex after they read and rated negative words responded to CBT. Furthermore, increased activity in a region of the right amygdala was associated with improved response to CBT even when taking into account initial severity of symptoms. However, amygdala activity was only marginally predictive of recovery status. The researchers concluded that CBT was most useful to those who demonstrate increased emotional reactivity and who cannot engage regulatory structures.

Box 28.3 Recommended reading – some key manuals and review articles

Two key manuals

Beck, A. T., Rush, A. J., Shaw, B. F., & Emery, G. (1979). *Cognitive Therapy of Depression.* New York: Guilford Press.

Hawton, K., Salkovskis, P., Kirk, J., & Clark, D. (1989). *Cognitive Behaviour Therapy for Psychiatric Problems: A Practical Guide.* Oxford: Oxford Medical Publications.

Two key books for clients (also useful as basic introductions for clinicians)

Greenberger, D., & Padesky, C. (1995). *Mind over Mood.* New York: Guilford Press.

Scott, J. (2002). *Overcoming Mood Swings.* London: Constable Robinson

Two key review articles

Beck, A. T. (2005). The current status of cognitive therapy: a 40-year retrospective. *Arch Gen Psychiatry* **62**:953–959.

Butler, A. C., Chapman, J. E., Foreman, E. M., & Beck, A. T. (2006). The empirical status of cognitive behavioural therapy: a review of meta-analyses. *Clin Psychol Rev* **26**:17–31.

These studies represent an important area of research in psychotherapy, but it should be noted that they are but early attempts to use these approaches with small samples of selected patients and many methodological hurdles to overcome. The fact that more such studies are underway does point to some degree of confidence that we may be able to predict more accurately who should be offered CBT or medication or begin to demonstrate the effects of different treatments on brain functioning. Although this research may seem to have a long way to go, sceptics may wish to reflect on how far the CBTs have progressed in the relatively short time since their introduction.

Conclusions

It is clear that CBT is a popular form of therapy with both patients and clinicians. However, we must always temper such enthusiasm with recognition that CBT does not work for everyone, and, importantly, there are gaps in our knowledge about how it works in some disorders, about whom it works for best in certain treatment settings and when is the best time to introduce CBT as part of treatment. Demonstrating benefits from CBT in certain disorders has also led for demand for abbreviated versions of CBT, but before we rush into such developments, we need to establish evidence that briefer forms of electronic or computerized forms of CBT are efficacious. The presence of a therapist is a critical component for some patients and *the* critical component for many. In the future there will also be much to discuss about the shared components of treatments such as CBT and IPT, and research may allow us to understand more fully how therapy for the mind affects the neural networks of the brain.

REFERENCES

Bara Carril, N., Williams, C. J., Pombo-Carril, M. G., *et al*, (2004). A preliminary investigation into the feasibility and efficacy of a CD-ROM-Based cognitive-behavioral self-help intervention for bulimia nervosa. *Int J Eating Disord* 35:538–48.

Beck, A. T. (1952). Successful outpatient psychotherapy of a chronic schizophrenic with a delusion based on borrowed guilt. *Psychiatry* 15:305–12.

Beck, A. T. (1963). Thinking and depression: idiosyncratic content and cognitive distortions. *Arch Gen Psychiatry* 9:324–33.

Beck, A. T. (1967). *Depression: Clinical, Experimental, and Theoretical Aspects*. New York: Harper & Row.

Beck, A. T. (1976). *Cognitive Therapy and the Emotional Disorders*. New York: International Universities Press.

Beck, A. T. (2005). The current state of cognitive therapy: a 40-year retrospective. *Arch Gen Psychiatry* 62:953–59.

Beck, A. T., & Emery, G., with Greenberg, R. L. (1985). *Anxiety Disorders and Phobias: A Cognitive Perspective*. New York: Basic Books.

Beck, A. T., Freeman, A., Davis, D. D., *et al*. (2004). *Cognitive Therapy of Personality Disorders*, 2nd edn. New York: Guilford Press.

Beck, A. T., & Rector, N. A. (2002). Delusions: a cognitive perspective. *J Cogn Psychother Int Q* 16:455–68.

Beck, A. T., Rush, A. J., Shaw, B. F., & Emery, G. (1979). *Cognitive Therapy of Depression*. New York: Guilford Press.

Beck, J. (1995). *Cognitive Therapy: Basics and Beyond*. New York: Guilford Press.

Birchwood, M. J., & Iqbal, Z. (1998). Depression and suicidal thinking in psychosis: a cognitive approach. In T. Wykes, N. Tarrier, S. Lewis, eds. *Outcome and Innovation in Psychological Treatment of Schizophrenia*. Chichester: Wiley, pp. 81–100.

Butler, A. C., Chapman, J. E., Foreman, E. M., & Beck, A. T. (2006). The empirical status of cognitive behavioural therapy: a review of meta-analyses. *Clin Psychol Rev* 26:17–31.

Chambless, D. L., & Hollon, S. D. (1998). Defining empirically supported therapies. *J Consult Clin Psychol* 66:7–18.

Clark, D. A., & Beck, A. T. (1999). *Scientific Foundations of Cognitive Theory and Therapy of Depression*. New York: Wiley.

Clark, D. M., & Ehlers, A. (2004). Posttraumatic stress disorder: from cognitive theory to therapy. In R. L. Leahy, ed. *Contemporary Cognitive Therapy: Theory, Research, and Practice*. New York: Guilford Press, pp. 27–48.

Clark, D. M., Salkovskis, P. M., Ost, G. L., *et al*. (1997). Misinterpretation of body sensations in panic disorder. *J Consult Clin Psychol* 65:203–13.

Clark, D. M., & Wells, A. (1995). A cognitive model of social phobia. In R. G. Heimberg, M. Liebowitz, D. A. Hope, & F. Schneier, eds. *Social Phobia: Diagnosis, Assessment, and Treatment*. New York: Guilford Press, pp. 59–78.

Crits-Christoph, P., Baranackie, K., Kurcias, J. S., *et al*. (1991). Meta-analysis of therapist effects in psychotherapy outcome studies. *Psychother Res* 1:81–91

Davidson, K., Scott, J., Schmidt, U., *et al*. (2004). Therapist competence and clinical outcome in the POPMACT trial. *Psychol Med* 34:855–63.

DeRubeis, R. J., & Feeley, M. (1990). Determinants of change in cognitive therapy for depression. *Cogn Ther Res* 14:469–82.

Ellis, A. (1962). *Reason and Emotion in Psychotherapy*. New York: Lyle Stuart.

Enright, S. J. (1997). Cognitive behaviour therapy – clinical applications. *BMJ* 314:1811–16.

Fowler, D., Garety, P., & Kuipers, L. (1995). *Cognitive Therapy of Psychoses*. Chichester: Wiley.

Fowler, D., & Morley, S. (1989). The cognitive-behaviour treatment of hallucinations and delusions: a preliminary study. *Behav Psychother* **17**:267–82.

Gillespie, K., Duffy, M., Hackmann, A., & Clark, D. M. (2002). Community based cognitive therapy in the treatment of posttraumatic stress disorder following the Omagh bomb. *Behav Res Ther* **40**:345–57.

Goldapple, K., Segal, Z., Garson, C., *et al.* (2004). Modulation of cortical-limbic pathways in major depression: treatment-specific effects of cognitive behavior therapy. *Arch Gen Psychiatry* **61**:34–41.

Grant, P., Young, P., & DeRubeis, R. (2005). Cognitive and behavioural therapies. In G. O. Gabbard, J. S. Beck, & J. Holmes, eds. *Oxford Textbook of Psychotherapy.* Oxford: Oxford University Press, pp. 312–34.

Greenberg, M. S., & Beck, A. T. (1989). Depression versus anxiety: a test of the content specificity hypothesis. *J Abnorm Psychol* **98**:9–13.

Haaga, D. A., Dyck, M. J., & Ernst, D. (1991). Empirical status of cognitive theory of depression. *Psychol Bull* **110**:215–36.

Hollon, S. D., Kendall, P. C., & Lumry, A. (1986). Specificity of depressotypic cognitions in clinical depression. *J Abnorm Psychol* **95**:52–9.

Hollon, S. D., Shelton, R. C., & Davis, D. D. (1993). Cognitive therapy for depression: conceptual issues and clinical efficiency. *J Consult Clin Psychol* **62**:270–5.

Jarrett, R. B., Kraft, D., Doyle, J., *et al.* (2001). Preventing recurrent depression using cognitive therapy with and without a continuation phase: a randomized clinical trial. *Arch Gen Psychiatry* **58**:381–8.

Keller, M. B., McCullough, J. P., Klein, D.N., *et al.* (2000). A comparison of nefazodone, the cognitive behavioral-analysis system of psychotherapy, and their combination for the treatment of chronic depression. *New Engl J Med* **342**:1462–70.

Kelly, G. (1955). *The Psychology of Personal Constructs.* New York: Norton.

Kingdon, D. G., & Turkington, D. (1994). *Cognitive-Behavior Therapy of Schizophrenia.* New York: Guilford Press.

Koerner, K., & Linehan, M. M. (2000). Research on dialectical behavior therapy for patients with borderline personality disorder. *Psychiatr Clin North Am* **23**:151–67.

Moorhead, S., & Scott, J. (1999). Is specialist registrar training in cognitive therapy effective? *Psychiatr Bull* **23**:603–7.

Morrison, A., ed. (2002). *A Casebook of Cognitive Therapy for Psychosis.* Hove: Routledge.

Padesky, C. (1993). Socratic Questioning: Changing Minds or Guiding Discovery? Keynote address, European Congress of Behavioural and Cognitive Therapies, London, September 24, 1993.

Parker, G., Roy, K., & Eyers, K. (2003). Cognitive behavior therapy for depression? Choose horses for courses. *Am J Psychiatry* **160**:825–34.

Paykel, E., Scott, J., Teasdale, J., *et al.* (1999). Prevention of relapse in residual depression by cognitive therapy: a controlled trial. *Arch Gen Psychiatry* **56**:829–35.

Persons, J. B. (1993). The process of change in cognitive therapy: schema change or acquisition of compensatory skills? *Cogn Ther Res* **17**:123–37.

Persons, J. B., Bostrom, A., & Bertagnolli, A. (1999). Results of randomized controlled trials of cognitive therapy for depression generalize to private practice. *Cogn Ther Res* **23**:535–48.

Pretzer, J. L., Beck, A. T., & Newman, C. (1989). Stress and stress management: a view. *J Cogn Psychother Int Q* **3**:163–79.

Rector, N. A., & Beck, A. T. (2002). Cognitive therapy for schizophrenia: from conceptualization to intervention. *Can J Psychiatry* **47**:39–48.

Roth, A., & Fonagy, P. (1996). *What Works for Whom? A Critical Review of Psychotherapy Research.* New York: Guilford Press.

Salkovskis, P. (1996). *Frontiers of Cognitive Therapy.* New York: Guilford Press.

Scott, J. (1998). Cognitive therapy. In H. Freeman, ed. *Century of Psychiatry.* London: Mosby Wolfe Medical Communications, pp. 201–10.

Scott, J. (2001). Cognitive therapy for depression. *BMJ* **57**:101–13.

Scott, J., Kingdon, D., & Turkington, D. (2004). CBT for schizophrenia. In *APA Review Psychiatry.* Washington, DC: APA Press, pp. 104–43.

Sensky, T., Turkington, D., Kingdon, D., *et al.* (2000). A randomised controlled trial of cognitive-behavioral therapy for persistent symptoms in schizophrenia resistant to medication. *Arch Gen Psychiatry* **57**:165–72.

Siegle, G. J., Carter, C. S., & Thase, M. E. (2006). Use of fMRI to predict recovery from unipolar depression with cognitive behavior therapy. *Am J Psychiatry* **163**:735–8.

Stirman, S., DeRubeis, R. J., Crits-Christoph, P., *et al.* (2003). Are samples in randomized controlled trials of psychotherapy representative of community outpatients: a new methodology and initial findings. *J Consult Clin Psychol* **71**:963–72.

Tarrier, N., Yusupoff, L., Kinney, C., *et al.* (1998). Randomised controlled trial of intensive cognitive therapy for patients with chronic schizophrenia. *BMJ* **317**:303–7.

Task Force on Promotion and Dissemination of Psychological Procedures (1995). Training in and dissemination of empirically-validated psychological treatments: report and recommendations. *Clin Psychol* **48**:3–23.

Teasdale, J., Scott, J., Moore, R., *et al.* (2000). How does cognitive therapy for depression reduce relapse? *J Consult Clin Psychol* **69**:347–57.

Weishaar, M. E. (1993). *Aaron T. Beck*. Thousand Oaks, CA: Sage.

Wright, J., Thase, M., Ludgate, J., & Beck, A. T. (1993). *Cognitive Therapy with Inpatients: Developing a Cognitive Milieu*. New York: Guilford Press.

Wright, J. H., Wright, A. S., Salmon, P., *et al.* (2002). Development and initial testing of a multimedia program for computer-assisted cognitive therapy. *Am J Psychother* **56**:76–86.

29

Interpersonal psychotherapy

Myrna M. Weissman and Marc B. J. Blom

Interpersonal psychotherapy (IPT) is a time-limited diagnosis-based treatment developed by the late Gerald Klerman and his wife, Myrna Weissman, and colleagues for a clinical trial for the treatment of major depression. It was defined in a manual in 1984 (Klerman *et al.*, 1984), which was updated in 2000 (Weissman *et al.*, 2007). IPT has been tested in numerous clinical trials and used in clinical practice. Its success in research trials led to its modification for subtypes of mood disorders as well as non–mood disorders (Klerman & Weissman, 1993). IPT has also been adapted for use in the long-term treatment of depression (Frank *et al.*, 1990); for couples treatment; in a group format (Bolton *et al.*, 2003; Levkovitz *et al.*, 2000; Wilfley *et al.*, 2000); as a telephone intervention (Miller & Weissman, 2003); for depressed adolescents (Mufson *et al.*, 2004); for geriatric patients (Reynolds *et al.*, 1999); for depressed pregnant and postpartum women (Stuart *et al.*, 1995); for primary care patients (Browne *et al.*, 2002; Schulberg *et al.*, 1996); and for depressed patients in developing countries (Clougherty *et al.*, 2002; Verdeli *et al.*, 2003). It has been used as monotherapy and in combination with medication. A number of new applications are under study.

Begun as a research intervention, IPT has only lately been disseminated among clinicians and in residency training programs in the United States, Canada, the United Kingdom, Europe, Australia and New Zealand. There have been increasing requests for training in IPT following the publication of efficacy data. IPT has been translated into several languages, including Italian, German, and Japanese, and Chinese from Taiwan. Descriptions of IPT have appeared in Spanish (Puig, 1995) and Dutch (Blom *et al.*, 1996). Translations are being planned in Greek and Romanian.

In the United States both the American Psychiatric Association and the Primary Care Practice Guidelines in 1993 cited IPT as one of the recommended treatments for adult depressed patients. However, it is optional and not required as part of psychiatry residency training. IPT has been endorsed by the Royal College of Psychiatrists for residency training and by the National Institute of Clinical Excellence (NICE) in the United Kingdom as part of evidenced-based practice and is also named in the guidelines for the treatment of depression in the Netherlands. This chapter describes the concepts and techniques of IPT and provides a brief review of current status of adaptation, efficacy data and training. For a full description of the conduct of IPT, see Weissman *et al.* (2000).

Background: theoretical and empirical sources

IPT is based on interpersonal theory stemming from the post–Second World War work of Adolph Meyer and Harry Stack Sullivan (Sullivan, 1955). The general principle derived from these theories is that

Essential Psychiatry, ed. Robin M. Murray, Kenneth S. Kendler, Peter McGuffin, Simon Wessely, David J. Castle.
Published by Cambridge University Press. © Cambridge University Press 2008.

Box 29.1

The most up-to-date manual describing the procedures of interpersonal therapy is Weissman, M. M., Markowitz, J. C., & Klerman, G. L. (2007). A Clinician's Quick Guide to Interpersonal Psychotherapy. Oxford Press.

Box 29.2

An international society of interpersonal therapy disseminates information worldwide (www.interpersonalpsychotherapy.org)

life events occurring after the early formative years influence psychopathology. IPT uses this principle in a non-aetiological fashion: it does not pretend to discern the cause of a depressive episode but uses the connection between current life events in four problem areas and mood disorder to help the patient understand and deal with the current episode of illness. Adaptations of IPT for other disorders have used the onset of the new disorder as a starting point with variable success. Chronic conditions such as dysthymia or social phobia require far more adaptation (Markowitz et al., 1998). IPT is further based on psychosocial and life events research of depression that has bolstered these theories by demonstrating the relationships between depression and grief (complicated bereavement); role disputes (e.g. hostile marriages); role transitions (meaningful life changes); and interpersonal deficits (loneliness and boredom). Recently research integrating life events and modern genetics has strikingly shown the influence of life stress on the onset of depression in patients who are genetically vulnerable (Caspi et al., 2003). This new research has begun to answer the question of why life events lead to depression in some people but not in others. A functional polymorphism in the promoter region of the serotonin transporter gene was found to moderate the effect of life events on depression. Patients who came for treatment for depression could be the 60% (according to Caspi et al., 2003) who have the genetic vulnerability, which includes one or two copies of the short allele of the 5-HTT promoter polymorphism, as well as a life event. The genetic findings highlight the potential importance of a treatment that focuses on current life stress in genetically susceptible individuals.

The relationship between life events and depression has been well documented (Brown et al., 1986; Brown & Harris, 1989). More recently this relationship has been criticised as too simplistic. Hammen (2003) and others have differentiated between events that happen by sheer coincidence (death, natural disaster) and events that carry a relationship with the person afflicted (divorce, job loss) (Brennan et al., 2003; Daley et al., 1997; Hammen, 2003). Prospective studies have shown that the former are not increased in persons who become depressed. The latter form does have a relationship with future depressions (see also Chapter 12).

Kendler and colleagues (1999, 2003, 2004) have shown similar interaction between life events and depression. However, the type of life event seemed to matter. Thus events that are humiliating compared with other types are more strongly linked to the onset of depression (Kendler et al., 2003). Personality factors such as neuroticism interact meaningfully with the impact that a life event has and thus on the onset of depression (Blatt et al., 1985; Shahar et al., 2003).

Some have shown that the relationship between a life event and depression becomes almost nonexistent in recurrent depression after two or more recurrences (Ormel et al., 2001). However, the studies of Frank et al. (1990) have been able to adapt IPT successfully for patients with recurrent depression. We can conclude that life events have a substantial causal relationship with the onset of an episode of depression (Kendler et al., 1999) and that this relationship may be strongly influenced by personality factors, type of life events and prior episodes of depression and likely genetic vulnerability. This connection will be reduced in recurrent depression. It is not clear how these findings affect the performance of IPT.

A second theoretical background for IPT comes from the attachment theory of Bowlby (1969, 1973, 1980). This theory states that the need for attachment is an intrinsic human drive that is biologically grounded. It cannot be reduced to any other drive. It follows from this that disruption in attachment in one's youth leads to psychiatric problems in later years.

Bowlby implied that patients project their expectations of another person on every newly formed relationship. These expectations are based on the individual's experiences in earlier relationships, mainly early childhood relationships with caregivers. As Stuart and Robinson (2003) state: "individuals experience interpersonal difficulties not because their working models are inaccurate reflections of their past experiences, but because the models are imposed inappropriately onto new relationships." In this sense it is reminiscent of what Sullivan called "parataxic distortions" but also resembles the theory of Young and co-workers (2003) on "schema focussed" psychotherapy.

Ainsworth *et al.* (1978) and others (Egeland & Sroufe, 1981; Sroufe, 2003), based on experimental situations with children ("strange situation"), discerned three styles of attachment behaviour: securely attached individuals, anxious ambivalent and anxious avoidant attachment style. Later researchers have used different classifications. For instance, using the Adult Attachment Interview (George *et al.*, 1985), three insecure patterns can be discerned: dismissing (resembling avoidant style), preoccupied (resembling ambivalent style) and unresolved. Of course, it was hoped that early attachment style and the quality of parenting can reliably predict the attachment style in adulthood. Unfortunately, this has not been demonstrated (Fonagy, 2001). Although prospective research is almost nonexistent, in the studies that have been carried out it becomes clear that a simplistic relationship between, for instance, parenting style and the development of an Axis I disorder later in life is not found. Many factors, such as child characteristics, parental style and social circumstances may

influence later outcome. There is general consensus that disruption of early attachment will influence clinical outcome in later years. Some investigators stress the point that the clinician should have a clear view of the patient's attachment patterns before starting treatment. They infer that brief treatment should be aimed at securely attached individuals with whom one can readily form a working alliance. Patients with insecure forms of attachment behaviour may need more time to form an alliance with the therapist. The therapist should consider this in planning the therapy. Although interesting, this notion has never been formally tested. The focus of IPT is on current relationships and not on the patient's personality or childhood history, which makes these theories less salient in the immediate treatment although perhaps they affect long-term outcome.

Techniques

Concept of depression

In IPT, depression is defined as a medical illness, a treatable condition that is not the patient's fault. This definition of depression tends to displace the guilt of the depressed patient from the patient to the illness, making the symptoms ego dystonic and discrete. It also provides the hope of response to treatment. The therapist uses *Diagnostic and Statistical Manual of Mental Disorders* (4th edition) or *International Classification of Impairments, Disabilities and Handicaps* (10th revision) to diagnose depression and rating scales such as the Hamilton Depression Rating Scale or Beck Depression Inventory or any other validated depression scale to monitor symptoms. The patient is educated about depression, its symptom course and various treatment options and helped to understand that depression is a common malady, not a personal failing or weakness. To implement this approach, IPT therapists formally give depressed patients the "sick role," excusing them from what their illness prevents them from doing, but also obliging them to work as a patient to recover, one hopes rapidly, the healthy role they have lost.

Strategies and techniques

The overall strategy of IPT is that by identifying and resolving an interpersonal problem(s) associated with the onset of symptoms – (e.g. dealing with complicated bereavement, a role dispute or transition or an interpersonal deficit) – the patient will both improve the life situation associated with the onset of the symptoms and simultaneously relieve the symptoms of the depressive episode. This coupled formula has been validated by the randomised controlled trials in which IPT has been tested and hence can be offered with confidence and optimism. This optimistic approach, although hardly specific to IPT, likely provides part of its power in remoralising the patient.

IPT is an eclectic therapy, using techniques developed in various psychotherapies. It is not its specific techniques but rather its overall strategies that make it a unique and coherent approach. Although IPT overlaps to some degree with psychodynamic psychotherapies (see Chapter 30), it also differs in significant ways: in its focus on the present, not the past, and on real-life change; its medical model; and minimising of transference, patients' early history or dream interpretations. IPT shares with cognitive-behavioural therapy (CBT; see Chapter 28) a focus on a syndromal constellation, attention to the "here and now", and techniques such as role-play, but IPT is considerably less structured and requires no explicit homework or review of cognitions. IPT emphasises relationships, and affect around relationships rather than cognitions. Each of the four IPT interpersonal problem areas – grief (complicated bereavement), role disputes, role transitions and interpersonal deficits – has discrete, if to some degree overlapping, goals for therapist and patient to pursue (see Cutler *et al.*, 2004, for a clinical illustration of the differences between psychodynamic psychotherapy, CBT and IPT).

The IPT techniques are designed to aid the patient's pursuit of these interpersonal goals. The therapist helps the patient to link life events to mood and symptoms. These techniques including the following:

- an *opening question* – "How have things been since we last met?" – that leads the patient to provide an interval history of mood and events;
- a *communication analysis*, a recreation of recent, affectively charged life circumstances within the problem areas;
- *an exploration of the patient's wishes and options* and how to achieve those wishes in particular interpersonal situations;
- *decision analysis*, to help the patient decide which options to employ; and
- *role-play*, to help the patient rehearse tactics for real life.

Indications

The indications for IPT have been established in sequential treatment studies. Empirical trials have validated the utility of IPT as both an acute and a maintenance treatment for nonpsychotic major depression. IPT also has demonstrated efficacy as a treatment for depressed adolescents, geriatric patients, depressed patients in primary care, depressed HIV-positive patients, depressed women in marital disputes and for pregnant and postpartum women, as well as for nondepressed bulimic patients.

Studies are underway to assess the utility of IPT for other patient populations: for dysthymic disorder; as an adjunctive treatment for patients with bipolar disorders; for a variety of anxiety disorders including panic, social phobia, and posttraumatic stress disorders; and for borderline personality disorder. Building on the IPT study with depressed HIV-positive patients, treating patients suffering from a medical illness and depression seems like a promising line. Studies looking at the treatment of depressed patients after a myocardial infarction and depressed patients with brittle diabetes are under way.

Contraindications

IPT was never intended as a monotherapy for patients with psychotic depression or bipolar disorder. One early study found no efficacy for IPT alone for ambulatory depressed patients with psychotic depression unless used in combination with medication. Three controlled trials have found no benefit for IPT as a treatment of psychopathology among methadone-maintained patients or for cocaine abstinence (Rounsaville *et al.*, 1986). Patients with primary alcohol abuse are generally excluded from treatment with IPT in most studies. It is recommended that the abuse be treated first before a successful attempt at treating the depression can be made.

Communication problems can occur when therapist and patient do not share the same language. In the Netherlands there is some experience in treating patients with use of an interpreter. When language is not a problem, bringing IPT to non-Western patients has been moderately successful in the Netherlands. Dropout tended to be high, but patients who did stay in treatment profited from therapy in the same way as Western patients. Moreover, a clinical trial of IPT in Uganda conducted by trained native-language-speaking therapists showed strong efficacy (Bolton *et al.*, 2003; discussed later).

Managing treatment

Making no aetiological assumptions, IPT uses the connection between the onset of depressive symptoms and current interpersonal problems as a pragmatic treatment focus. IPT deals with current rather than past interpersonal relationships, focusing on the patient's immediate social context. The IPT therapist attempts to intervene in symptom formation and social dysfunction associated with depression rather than addressing enduring aspects of personality. Personality is difficult to assess accurately during an episode of an Axis I disorder such as depression. The illustrations that follow are for

> **Box 29.3** Managing the initial phase
> * Make a diagnosis
> * Explain the illness
> * Educate the patient about the illness
> * Allow the patient to take the sick role
> * Conduct interpersonal inventory
> * Define problem area for the middle phase

depression. Various adaptations as noted earlier have been developed for other disorders. Usually the focused disorder is substituted in the initial diagnosis and explanations, the content is modified as appropriate for the particular developmental phase, situation or culture.

Phases of treatment

As an acute treatment, IPT has three phases. The *first phase*, usually one to three sessions, includes diagnostic evaluation and psychiatric history and sets the framework for the treatment. The therapist reviews symptoms, diagnoses the patient as depressed by standard criteria and gives the patient the sick role. The sick role may excuse the patient from overwhelming social obligations but requires the patient to work in treatment to recover full function. The psychiatric history includes the "interpersonal inventory", a review of the patient's current social functioning and close relationships, their patterns and the mutual expectations of patient and therapist. The interpersonal inventory is a careful, interpersonally focused anamnesis, not a semistructured interview. Changes in relationships proximal to the onset of symptoms are elucidated (e.g., death of a loved one, children leaving home, worsening marital strife, or isolation from a confidant). The therapist listens closely to themes that are emotionally charged. This review provides a framework for understanding the social and interpersonal context of the onset of depressive symptoms and defines the focus of treatment.

> **Box 29.4** Defining specific problem areas
>
> **Grief:** Complicated bereavement following a death
>
> **Role disputes:** Conflicts with significant other in renegotiation, dissolution or impasse
>
> **Role transitions:** Change in life status (e.g. divorce, moving, retirement, graduation)
>
> **Interpersonal deficits:** lack of relationship skills, social skills, boredom, loneliness

Having assessed the need for medication based on symptom severity, past history and response to treatment, as well as patient preference, the therapist educates the patient about the disorder under treatment by explicitly discussing the diagnosis, including the constellation of symptoms that define the disorder and what the patient might expect from treatment. The therapist next links the disorder to the patient's interpersonal situation in a formulation that uses as a framework one of four interpersonal problem areas:

1. grief,
2. interpersonal role disputes,
3. role transitions and
4. interpersonal deficits.

For most patients, a choice between several problem areas is made. The therapist and patient must make a choice by weighing which problem area is most closely linked by time and affect to the onset of depression.

In the *middle phase,* the therapist pursues strategies specific to the chosen interpersonal problem area. These problem areas may change in the course of treatment as new information is obtained, but the switch should be explicit.

For *grief,* defined as complicated bereavement following the death of a loved one, the therapist facilitates the catharsis of mourning and gradually helps the patient to find new activities and relationships to compensate for the loss. *Role disputes* are conflicts with a significant other: a spouse or other family members, co-worker or close friend.

The therapist helps the patient explore the relationship, the nature of the dispute, the phase it is in and available options to resolve it. If these fail, therapist and patient may conclude that the relationship has reached an impasse and consider ways to change this (renegotiation) or to end the relationship (dissolution). *Role transition* includes change in life status – for example, beginning or ending a relationship or career, moving, promotion, retirement, graduation or diagnosis of a medical illness. The patient learns to deal with the change by mourning the loss of the old role while recognizing positive and negative aspects of the new role he or she is assuming, and taking steps to gain mastery over the new role. *Interpersonal deficits,* the residual fourth IPT problem area, defines the patient as lacking social skills, including having problems in initiating or sustaining relationships, and helps the patient develop new relationships and skills.

IPT sessions address present "here-and-now" problems rather than childhood or developmental issues. Sessions open with the question, "How have things been since we last met?" This focuses the patient on recent interpersonal events and recent mood, which the therapist helps the patient to link. The therapist takes an active, nonneutral, supportive and hopeful stance to counter the depressed patient's pessimism. The options that exist for change in the patient's life, options that the depression may have kept the patient from seeing or considering fully are explored. The therapist stresses the need for the patient to test these options to improve his or her life and simultaneously treat the depressive episode. The therapist is nonjudgmental in the sense that any option the patient suggests is greeted with enthusiasm. In trying options in real life with important others, the patient will learn what works in fostering a mood change and what does not.

The *final phase* of IPT, occupying the last few weeks of treatment (or last months, in case of maintenance treatment), supports the patient's newly regained sense of independence and competence by recognizing and consolidating therapeutic gains.

The therapist also helps the patient anticipate and develop ways to identify and counter depressive symptoms should they arise in the future. Compared with psychodynamic psychotherapy, IPT de-emphasises termination and defines it as a graduation from successful treatment. The sadness of parting is distinguished from depressive feelings. If the patient has not improved, the therapist emphasises that it is the treatment that has failed, not the patient, and stresses the existence of alternative effective treatment options.

IPT was developed for various types of clinical trials. For acute treatment trials, the length has ranged from 12 to 16 weeks; for continuation trials, weekly for 8 months; and for 3-year maintenance trials, it has been administered monthly. There is no absolute time frame for clinical practice. However, the principle of establishing a time frame at the beginning of treatment is critical for focusing the goals of treatment and assessing the progress towards the goals within a time frame. Further, it is recommended that sessions be held weekly especially at the beginning of treatment. The frequency can be reduced to every fortnight once symptom changes occur.

Efficacy

The review of adaptations and efficacy studies that follow is selected and not comprehensive. All of the negative studies that have been reported are included, but the number of pilot studies and ongoing larger studies or adaptations that are not yet published are not included. A full review of efficacy studies up to 2007 and the studies referred there (unless otherwise indicated) can be found in Weissman *et al.* (2000, 2007).

Acute treatment of major depression

IPT for acute depression was first demonstrated in a 16-week randomised trial of IPT and amitriptyline, alone and in combination, and a nonscheduled control treatment for 81 outpatients with major depressive disorder (Weissman *et al.*, 2007). There were no significant differences between IPT and amitriptyline in symptom reduction by the end of treatment. Each active treatment more effectively reduced symptoms than did the nonscheduled control group. Combined amitriptyline-IPT was more effective than either of the active monotherapies. A 1-year naturalistic follow-up found that many patients sustained benefits from the IPT, as shown in significantly better psychosocial functioning, which did not occur with amitriptyline alone and had not been evident at the end of the 16-week trial. Many patients required additional treatment over the follow-up year, a fact now recognised by the use of maintenance treatment.

The most ambitious short-treatment study to date, the multisite National Institute of Mental Health Treatment of Depression Collaborative Research Program (NIMH TDCRP; Frank *et al.*, 1990), randomly assigned 250 depressed outpatients to 16 weeks of imipramine, IPT, CBT or placebo plus clinical management. Less-symptomatic patients improved in all treatments, including placebo. Imipramine induced the most rapid response and was most consistently superior to placebo. For more severely depressed patients, defined by a Hamilton Depression Score at intake, medication and IPT were the most efficacious treatments compared with CBT or placebo/clinical management. Among patients who had remitted by 16 weeks, relapse over the 18-month follow-up was 36% for CBT, 33% for IPT, 50% for imipramine and 33% for placebo. The authors concluded that 16 weeks of specific treatments were insufficient to achieve full and lasting recovery for many patients.

Continuation and maintenance treatment

IPT was first developed and tested in an 8-month trial in 150 depressed women treated acutely with amitriptyline and then randomly assigned to IPT with or without medication or placebo. Medication was the most effective for prevention of recurrence, whereas IPT improved social functioning. These effects were not apparent until 6 to 8 months.

Patients in the combined treatment had the best outcome.

In the longest maintenance trial, Frank and colleagues (1990) studied 128 outpatients with recurrent depression (that is, they had at least three previous acute major depressive episodes). These patients were treated for 3 years and were randomly assigned to monthly maintenance IPT, either alone or combined with imipramine, placebo or medication clinic visits. They also received high-dosage (200 mg) imipramine. There was a highly significant effect for maintenance imipramine in preventing recurrence and a modest but significant effect for IPT at 1 year and also at the end of the 3 years. The authors concluded that imipramine maintenance treatment at a dose of 200 mg per day effectively prevents recurrence of major depression in patients with a history of recurrent episodes and that monthly IPT lengthens the time between episodes in patients not receiving medication.

Questions about the effectiveness of more frequent than monthly IPT was addressed in a separate study but was not found to change the basic outcome.

Geriatric depressed patients

There have been several small studies comparing IPT with medication for geriatric patients. The largest and most important was study was by Reynolds and colleagues (1999) in Pittsburgh. This was a 3-year maintenance study for geriatric patients with recurrent depression using a design similar to that reported previously by Frank and colleagues (discussed earlier). The manual was modified to allow more flexible sessions length because elderly patients may not tolerate 50-minute sessions. The authors found that older patients need to address early-life relationships, which was added to the typical "here-and-now" focus of IPT. They also found that therapists needed to help patients solve practical problems and share awareness that some problems may not be amenable to resolutions (e.g. existential late-life issues or lifelong psychopathology). They found that elderly depressed patients whose sleep quality normalised early in treatment had an 80% chance of remaining well during the first year. The response rates were similar in patients who were receiving medication, in this case nortriptyline or IPT. They noted that combined treatment using both medication and IPT was the optimal strategy in preventing relapse.

Bereavement-related depression

Shear and colleagues (2005) have modified IPT to deal with bereavement-related illnesses, including traumatic grief. They differentiate between bereavement, the state of having lost a close friend or relative and grief, the behavioural manifestations of bereavement. In this adaptation, standard IPT techniques are used including interpersonal history; looking for idealisation of the person who died; eliciting feelings about the death; nonjudgmental exploration of the relationship; discussion of the sequence of events before, during and after the death; and the reactions to the loss. Traumatic grief treatment became of considerable interest in the United States following the September 11 terrorist attacks. Shear incorporated into IPT the techniques found to be useful for posttraumatic stress disorder, using images revisiting the actual circumstances of the death and the conversations with the deceased. Patients audiotape their description so that they can listen to it at home. The presence of symptoms and the intrusive images of avoidance, yearning and longing are explored, and the patient relates stories of the death and his or her relationship with the lost person. The work involves the IPT augmentation techniques and includes meeting with significant others, revisiting places and activities, revisiting and looking at pictures and focusing on memories and having conversations with the deceased. The work is being tested.

Depressed adolescents

Mufson *et al.* (2004) have conducted a series of studies testing the efficacy of IPT modified for depressed adolescents (IPT-A). The modification includes involvement of parents and also schools, as needed, as well as incorporating the developmental issues of adolescents, such as separation from parents, peer pressure and romantic relationships. Students are given "work at home" rather than homework, on the reasoning that adolescents may be adverse to doing homework. Work at home means practicing some of the skills and communication learned during the sessions. Recent findings are those based on 63 adolescents randomly assigned to receive IPT weekly for 12 weekly or treatment as usual (TAU) in school-based clinics in impoverished neighborhoods of New York City. Therapists are community social workers with no prior IPT training and little training in psychotherapy, trained to deliver IPT with 1-day didactic and hourly weekly supervision. Adolescents who received IPT reported greater decrease in depressive symptoms, significantly greater improvement in overall social functioning and better skills and positive problem solving. The effects of IPT versus TAU were significant at 8 and at 12 weeks, both on social functioning and symptoms.

Depressed HIV-positive patients

Markowitz and coworkers (1998) modified IPT for depressed HIV patients (IPT-HIV), emphasizing common issues in this population including concern about illness and death, grief and role transitions. A 16-week randomised clinical trial compared IPT with a modified CBT, supportive psychotherapy (SP) and imipramine plus supportive psychotherapy in 101 patients. Although symptoms decreased across therapies, IPT or imipramine were more efficacious in reducing depressive symptoms compared with SP or CBT. The authors concluded that the efficacy of IPT compared with the other psychotherapies for HIV patients was due to the focus on patient distress at this painful life event and ways to find solutions.

Depressed primary care patients

Schulberg and colleagues (1996) compared IPT with pharmacotherapy for depressed ambulatory medical patients in a primary care setting. There were

no modifications of IPT, but nurses continued to take vital signs before each session. IPT was continued even if the patient was medically hospitalised. Two hundred and seventy-six patients with major depression were assigned to IPT, nortriptyline or primary care physicians' usual care weekly for 16 weeks and monthly thereafter for 4 months. Depression severity declined more rapidly with either nortriptyline or IPT than usual care. At the end of treatment, 75% of the IPT patients compared with 46% of those receiving clinical management met recovery criteria. Although the results of the Schulberg study were promising, they presented problems in actual application in the United States, because treatment by a psychiatrist in a primary care setting is considered cost-prohibitive. Others outside the United States have trained physicians and nurses in IPT in primary care, including for depressed elderly patients (van Schaik *et al.*, 2003).

Antepartum and postpartum depression

Several studies of IPT for depression during both the ante- and postpartum periods have been undertaken. Psychotherapy is an important alternative to medication for depressed women during pregnancy and whilst nursing, because of the possible adverse effect of medication on the developing foetus or nursing infant (see Chapter 19). Spinelli and Endicott (2003) assessed the efficacy of IPT in depressed pregnant women. Role transitions were the most prevalent problem area, and therapy thus focussed on the pregnant woman's self-evaluation as a parent, physiologic changes of pregnancy and altered relationships with the spouse, significant others and other children. The timing and duration of sessions required flexibility because of bed rest, delivery, obstetrical complications and child care. Young children could be brought to sessions in which postpartum mothers could breast-feed, and telephone sessions and hospital visits were necessary.

Bipolar disorder

There have been modifications of IPT for patients with bipolar disorder as an adjunct treatment to medication. Frank *et al.* (2000) modified IPT for bipolar patients by adding a Social Rhythm Index (SRI) to help patients monitor their daily social rhythms including sleep patterns. Reasons for changes related to unstable rhythms are identified, and efforts to regulate the rhythm are made. The idea guiding this adaptation is that mania occurs during periods of social rhythm dysregulation, and these changes may be an indication of an incipient episode (Malkoff-Schwartz *et al.*, 2000). SRI has been added to IPT maintenance treatment for bipolar disorder. It provides a simple way for patients to monitor daily routines such as getting out of bed in the morning; first contact; time starting work, school, housework, volunteer, child or family care; and eating and sleeping times. The record of these activities is discussed in treatment. The patient is encouraged to find a balance between rest and activities or stimulation.

This IPT adaptation is well accepted by individuals with bipolar disorder and clinicians, and it improves treatment adherence. However, it remains to be seen whether and under what circumstances it adds to the efficacy of pharmacotherapy. Other adaptations of IPT for bipolar disorder include using it as an adjunct to family therapy and in group format.

Substance abuse and dependence

It is important to note that IPT is not a panacea for all conditions. There have been at least three clinical trials which have shown the lack of efficacy of IPT for drug abuse or its accompanying depression when used as an adjunctive treatment in patients with drug dependency, including methadone-maintenance patients and cocaine abusers. IPT has been shown not to have additional efficacy over standard methadone-maintenance programs and was marginally worse than behavioural treatment for cocaine abusers. IPT may be useful for recovering alcohol-dependent patients who face numerous psychosocial stressors that precipitate relapse, but it has never been adapted or tested for these patients.

IPT in developing countries

An exciting adaptation and successful testing of IPT occurred for depressed patients living in rural Uganda (Bolton *et al.*, 2003; Clougherty *et al.*, 2002; Verdeli *et al.*, 2003), where rates of depression among adults are high (>20%) and where traditional healers reported that they were unable to treat these symptoms effectively. Medication for depression is often not feasible in this country because there are so few doctors. Health workers selected IPT because it seemed compatible with a culture which places high value on being part of a community and family. One hundred seventy-seven patients in 30 villages were randomised to IPT or TAU, which meant no treatment except for hospitalisation for the management of suicidal risk or psychoses. Training occurred over 2 weeks. The manual was modified to include 18 weekly 90-minute sessions. This included two pre-group individual sessions to get to know the patient and explain the treatment, and 16 group sessions. The manual was simplified and more structured with extensive scripting and the use of the local definition of depression (Bolton *et al.*, 2003; Clougherty *et al.*, 2002; Verdeli *et al.*, 2004). The effects of IPT versus TAU was highly significant for both symptoms and social functioning. These results were sustained at 6-month follow-up.

With the availability of the IPT adaptation for Uganda, there have been numerous requests for the manual from international health workers. Training in IPT has been carried out in Romania and mainland China, and a Chinese translation is underway in Taiwan.

Training and accreditation in IPT

Developed as a form of psychotherapy used mainly in clinical trials, IPT is being used in clinical practice in many countries. In clinical trials, therapists have to be rigorously trained and supervised. When bringing IPT to the general community, these high standards cannot be maintained. This carries the danger of creating watered-down versions of IPT. Increasingly only evidence-based psychotherapies have been reimbursed by insurance companies. IPT has been named in several international guidelines for the treatment of depression (de Groot, 1995). This has greatly enhanced the interest in IPT. Training programs, albeit small, have been set up in several countries in Europe. With a growing number of practicing psychotherapists, the need for accreditation has also increased. A system of training and accreditation has been created. It has been implemented in the United Kingdom and the Netherlands and has been actively discussed but not resolved by the International Society of IPT. Most programs in the countries already mentioned comprise a 3-day workshop and supervision of at least two cases. When therapists successfully complete this in the United Kingdom or the Netherlands, they are acknowledged as IPT therapists by the local societies for IPT.

It is our experience that highly experienced therapists can learn IPT for their practice by reading an IPT manual, attending a didactic course and watching videotapes (available through verdelih@childpsych.columbia.edu). However, for credentialing and research protocols, supervision with several cases is recommended. Long-distance telephone supervision has now been successfully used for training therapists. Although there is accumulating evidence for the efficacy of IPT and other psychotherapies, there is a large gap among research evidence, clinical training and practice (Weissman & Sanderson, 2002).

REFERENCES

Ainsworth, M., Blehar, M. C., Waters, E., *et al.* (1978). *Patterns of Attachment.* Hillsdale, New Jersey: Erlbaum.

Blatt S. J., Zuroff, D. C., Bondi, C. M., *et al.* (1998). When and how perfectionism impedes the brief treatment of depression: further analyses of the National Institute of Mental Health Treatment of Depression Collaborative Research Program. *J Consult Clin Psychol* **66**:423–8.

Blom, M. B. J., Hoencamp, E., & Zwaan, T. (1996). Interpersonal psychotherapy for depression a pilot [in Dutch]. *Tijdschrift Psychiatr* **38**:398–402.

Bolton, P., Bass, J., Neugebauer, R., *et al.* (2003). Group interpersonal psychotherapy for depression in rural Uganda: a randomized controlled trial. *JAMA* **289**:3117–24.

Bowlby, J. (1969). *Attachment.* London: Hogarth Press.

Bowlby, J. (1973). *Separation Anxiety and Anger.* London: Hogarth Press.

Bowlby, J. (1980). *Loss Sadness and Depression.* London: Hogarth Press.

Brennan, P. A., Le Brocque, R., & Hammen, C. (2003). Maternal depression, parent-child relationships, and resilient outcomes in adolescence. *J Am Acad Child Adolesc Psychiatry* **42**:1469–77.

Brown, G. W., Bifulco, A., Harris, T., *et al.* (1986). Life stress, chronic subclinical symptoms and vulnerability to clinical depression. *J Affect Disorders* **11**:1–19.

Brown, G. W., & Harris, T. O. (1989). *Life Events and Illness.* New York: Guilford Press.

Brown, G., Steiner, M., Roberts, J., *et al.* (2002). Sertraline and/or interpersonal psychotherapy for patients with dysthymic disorder in primary care: 6-month comparison with longitudinal 2-year follow-up of effectiveness and costs. *J Affect Disord,* **68**:317–30.

Caspi, A., Sudgen, K., Moffitt, T. E., *et al.* (2003). Influence of life stress on depression: moderation by a polymorphism in the 5-HTT gene. *Science* **301**:386–9.

Clougherty, K. F., Verdeli, H., & Weissman, M. M. (2002). *Interpersonal Psychotherapy for Group in Uganda (IPTG-U).* Unpublished manual.

Cutler, J. L., Goldyne, A., Markowitz, J. C., *et al.* (2004). Comparing cognitive behavior therapy, interpersonal psychotherapy, and psychotherapy. *Am J Psychiatry* **161**:1567–73.

Daley, S. E., Hammen, C., Burge, D., *et al.* (1997). Predictors of the generation of episodic stress: a longitudinal study of late adolescent women. *J Abnorm Psychol* **106**:251–l9.

de Groot, P. A. (1995). Consensus depression in adults. Dutch association for psychiatry. *Ned Tijdschr Geneeskd* **139**:1237–41.

Egeland, B., & Sroufe, L. A. (1981). Attachment and early maltreatment. *Child Dev* **52**:44–52.

Frank, E., Kupfer, D. J., Perel, J. M., *et al.* (1990). Three-year outcomes for maintenance therapies in recurrent depression. *Arch Gen Psychiatry* **47**:1093–9.

Frank, E., Swartz, H. A., & Kupfer, D. J. (2000). Interpersonal and social rhythm therapy: managing the chaos of bipolar disorder. *Biol Psychiatry* **48**:593–604.

Fonagy, P. (2001). *Attachment Theory and Psychoanalysis*. New York: Other Press.

George, C., Kaplan, N., & Main, M. (1985). *The Adult Attachment Interview Protocol*, 3rd edn. Berkeley: University of California at Berkeley.

Hammen, C. (2003). Interpersonal stress and depression in women. *J Affect Disord* 4:49–57.

Kendler, K. S., Hettema, J. M., Butera, F., et al. (2003). Life event dimensions of loss, humiliation, entrapment, and danger in the prediction of onsets of major depression and generalized anxiety. *Arch Gen Psychiatry* 60:789–96.

Kendler, K. S., Karkowski, L. M., Prescott, C. A. (1999). Causal relationship between stressful life events and the onset of major depression. *Am J Psychiatry* 156:837–41.

Kendler, K. S., Kuhn, J., & Prescott, C. A. (2004). The interrelationship of neuroticism, sex, and stressful life events in the prediction of episodes of major depression. *Am J Psychiatry* 161:631–6.

Klerman, G. L., & Weissman, M. M. (1993). *New Applications of Interpersonal Psychotherapy*. Washington, DC: American Psychiatric Press.

Klerman, G. L., Weissman, M. M., Rounsaville, B. J., et al. (1984). *Interpersonal Psychotherapy of Depression*. New York: Basic Books.

Levkovitz, Y., Shahar, G., Native, G., et al. (2000). Group interpersonal psychotherapy for patients with major depression disorder – pilot study. *J Affect Disord* 60:191–5.

Malkoff-Schwartz, S., Frank, E., Anderson, B. P., et al. (2000). Social rhythm disruption and stressful life events in the onset of bipolar and unipolar episodes. *Psychol Med* 30:1005–16.

Markowitz, J. C. (1998). *Interpersonal Psychotherapy for Dysthymic Disorder*. Washington, DC: American Psychiatric Press.

Markowitz, J. C., Kocsis, J. H., Fishman, B., et al. (1998). Treatment of HIV-positive patients with depressive symptoms. *Arch Gen Psychiatry* 55:452–7.

Miller, L., & Weissman, M. M. (2002). Interpersonal psychotherapy delivered over the telephone for depression: a pilot study. *Depress Anxiety* 16:114–17.

Mufson, L., Pollack-Dorta, K., Moreau, D., & Weissman, M. M. (2004). *Interpersonal Psychotherapy for Depressed Adolescents*, 2nd edn. New York: Guilford Press.

Mufson, L., Pollack-Dorta, K. E., Wickramaratne, P. J., et al. (2004). A randomized effectiveness trial of interpersonal psychotherapy for depressed adolescents. *Arch Gen Psychiatry* 61:577–84.

Ormel, J., Oldehinkel, A. J., & Brilman, E. I. (2001). The interplay and etiological continuity of neuroticism, difficulties, and life events in the etiology of major and subsyndromal, first and recurrent depressive episodes in later life. *Am J Psychiatry* 158:885–91.

Puig, J. S. (1995). Psicoterapia interpersonal. *Revista Psiquiatr Facultad Med Barcelona* 22:91–9.

Reynolds, C. F., III, Frank, E., Perel, J. M., et al. (1999). Nortriptyline and interpersonal psychotherapy as maintenance therapies for recurrent major depression: a randomized controlled trial in patients older than fifty-nine years. *JAMA* 28:39–45.

Rounsaville, B. J., Chevron, E. S., Weissman, M. M., et al. (1986). Training therapists to perform interpersonal psychotherapy in clinical trials. *Compr Psychiatry* 27:364–71.

Schulberg, H. C., Block, M. R., Madonia, M. J., et al. (1996). Treating major depression in primary care practice. *Arch Gen Psychiatry* 53:913–19.

Shahar, G., Blatt, S. J., Zuroff, D.C., et al. (2003). Role of perfectionism and personality disorder features in response to brief treatment for depression. *J Consult Clin Psychol* 71:629–33.

Shear, K., Frank E., Houck, P., & Reynolds, C. F. (2005). Treatment of complicated grief: A randomized controlled trial. *JAMA* 293:2601–8.

Spinelli, M. G., & Endicott, J. (2003). Controlled clinical trial of interpersonal psychotherapy versus parenting education program for depressed pregnant women. *Am J Psychiatry* 160:555–62.

Sroufe, L. A. (2003). Attachment categories as reflections of multiple dimensions; comment on Fraley and Spieker. *Dev Psychol* 39:413–16; discussion 423–9.

Stuart, S., & O'Hara, M. W. (1995). IPT for postpartum depression. *J Psychother Pract Res* 4:18–29.

Stuart, S., & Robertson, M. (2003). *Interpersonal Psychotherapy: A Clinician's Guide*. London: Arnold.

Sullivan, H. S. (1955). *The Interpersonal Theory of Psychiatry*. New York: Norton Library.

van Schaik, D. J. F., van Marwijk, H., Beekman, A. T. F., et al. (2003). The applicability of interpersonal psychotherapy with depressed elderly patients. *Direct Ther* 23:309–23.

Verdeli, H., Clougherty, K., Bolton, P., et al. (2003). Adapting group interpersonal psychotherapy (IPTG) for a developing country: experience in rural Uganda. *World Psychiatry* 2:114–20.

Weissman, M. M., Markowitz, J. C., & Klerman, G. L. (2000). *Comprehensive Guide to Interpersonal Psychotherapy*. New York: Basic Books.

Weissman, M. M., Markowitz, J. C., & Klerman, G. L. (2007). *A Clinician's Quick Guide to Interpersonal Psychotherapy*. New York: Oxford University Press.

Weissman, M. M., & Sanderson, W. C. (2002). Promises and problems in modern psychotherapy: the need for increased training in evidence-based treatments. In M. Hager, ed. *Modern Psychiatry: Challenges in Educating Health Professionals to Meet New Needs*. New York: Josiah Macy, Jr. Foundation (For the Josiah Macy, Jr. Foundation Conference, October 25–28, 2001), pp. 132–65.

Wilfley, D. E., Mackenzie, K. R., Welch, R., *et al.,* eds. (2000). *Interpersonal Psychotherapy for Group*. New York: Basic Books.

Young, J. E., Klosko, J., & Weishaar, M. E. (2003). *Schema Therapy: A Practitioner's Guide*. New York: Guilford Press.

30

Psychodynamic psychotherapy

Glen O. Gabbard and Jessica R. Nittler

The focus of psychodynamic psychotherapy is understanding how past experiences influence present behaviours. It is a form of treatment that examines defence mechanisms, transference, countertransference, the internal world of fantasy and object relations and how unconscious mental functioning influences one's thoughts, feelings and behaviour. A succinct definition of psychodynamic psychotherapy is the following: "A therapy that involves careful attention to the therapist-patient interaction, with thoughtfully timed interpretation of transference and resistance embedded in a sophisticated appreciation of the therapist's contribution to the two-person field" (Gunderson & Gabbard, 1999, p. 685).

Psychodynamic psychotherapy can be divided into two subtypes. One is *brief or time-limited therapy* of up to 6 months or 24 sessions in duration. The number of sessions is usually predetermined. *Long-term or open-ended therapy* can be thought of as greater than 24 sessions or 6 months and is designed to end more naturalistically. Therapy sessions are usually held one to three times a week, although once a week is most common.

The core concepts of psychodynamic psychotherapy include (see Box 30.1) the unconscious, transference, countertransference, resistance, multiple function, authenticity and a developmental perspective. These principles are explained in more detail later.

Theoretical models

Long-term psychodynamic psychotherapy is derived from psychoanalysis and the work of Sigmund Freud. The major contemporary models of psychodynamic psychotherapy have moved the field well beyond Freud, however, and these include ego psychology, object relations theory, self psychology and attachment theory. Freud's original focus was on the topographic model,

> **Box 30.1** Basic principles of psychodynamic psychotherapy
>
> Much of mental life is unconscious.
> Childhood experiences in concert with genetic factors shape the adult.
> The patient's transference to the therapist is a primary source of understanding.
> The therapist's countertransference provides valuable understanding about what the patient induces in others.
> The patient's resistance to the therapy process is a major focus of the therapy.
> Symptoms and behaviours serve multiple functions and are determined by complex and often unconscious forces.
> A psychodynamic therapist assists the patient in achieving a sense of authenticity and uniqueness.
>
> Reprinted with permission from Gabbard, G. O. (2004). *Long-Term Psychodynamic Psychotherapy: A Basic Text.* Arlington, VA: American Psychiatric Press, p. 3.

Essential Psychiatry, ed. Robin M. Murray, Kenneth S. Kendler, Peter McGuffin, Simon Wessely, David J. Castle.
Published by Cambridge University Press. © Cambridge University Press 2008.

which involved a three-level hierarchy of conscious, preconscious and unconscious domains. The preconscious could easily be brought into awareness, but the unconscious was "a reservoir that contained dynamically repressed contents that were kept out of awareness because they created conflict" (Gabbard, 2004, p. 3). Freud's model evolved, and in 1923 he introduced the structural model of the id, ego and superego. The id consists of powerful drives – specifically sexuality and aggression. The ego is divided into two parts, conscious and unconscious. The conscious aspect includes executive functions such as decision making, integration of perceptual data and mental calculations. The unconscious aspects of the ego involve defence mechanisms designed to counter the basic drives of the id. The superego also has both conscious and unconscious elements. The superego primarily represents moral values from parents and others. The fundamental premise of ego psychology is that the drives seeking gratification are in conflict with the ego and superego, leading to a compromise that expresses both the underlying drive or wish and the defence against it.

Object relations theory was developed in the United Kingdom by Melanie Klein, D. W. Winnicott, W. R. D. Fairbairn and others. Its basic premise is that early experiences with others and their associated affect states become internalised. These internal representations of self and others are then repeated throughout life as recurrent maladaptive relationships based on these early experiences. Although ego psychology regards drive gratification as the major motivational force in development, object relations theory views the seeking of relationships as more fundamental.

Self psychology, developed by Heinz Kohut, is based on a deficit model of development. His theory suggests that secondary to empathic failure from caregivers, the individual fails to develop a fully cohesive self and thus has a sense of something missing. This leads the person to seek out specific responses from others, known as selfobject functions. The common selfobject functions are affirmation, validation, idealisation and twinship, each of

which is designed to fulfil missing internal needs. Without those functions, a person has a narcissistic vulnerability that can lead to fragmentation of the self. Selfobject responses from caregivers are needed to make a fragmented self more cohesive.

Attachment theory, developed by John Bowlby, emphasises that the main motivation of the child is to achieve a physical sense of safety that only comes from physical closeness to the mother or caregiver. It emphasises reality instead of fantasies. Modern attachment research (Ainsworth, 1978) has led to classifications derived from a child's reaction when placed in the *strange situation.* When a child is briefly separated from its mother, the child may react in one of four general categories. These categories are (1) secure attachment, (2) anxious-avoidant attachment, (3) anxious-ambivalent or resistant attachment and (4) disorganised/ disoriented attachment. These childhood attachment categories correspond to adult attachment categories, which are (1) secure/autonomous; (2) insecure/dismissing, characterised by idealising, denigrating/denying and devaluing both past and current relationships; (3) preoccupied, presenting as adults who are confused or overwhelmed by close relationships; and (4) unresolved or disorganised, related to being victims of trauma or neglect.

All of these theoretical models are relevant in certain clinical situations, and the psychodynamic therapist may use more than one of the models to understand a patient.

Technique of long-term psychodynamic psychotherapy

The technique of dynamic therapy has evolved from a largely silent and nondirective role for the therapist to one in which the therapist is lively and interactive. Dynamic therapists do not hesitate to redirect the patient's attention to avoided material when appropriate. They also focus as much on what is happening in the here and now as they do on childhood traumas. They collaborate with the patient in the setting of goals, knowing that the objectives may

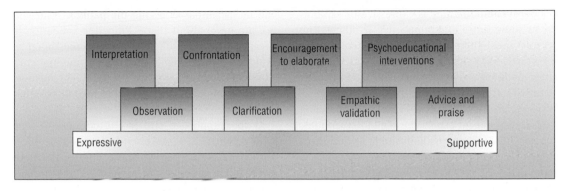

Figure 30.1 An expressive-supportive continuum of interventions.
Source: Reprinted with permission from Gabbard, G. O.: Long-Term Psychotherapy: A Basic Text, VA: APPI, 2004, p. 63.

change as the therapy proceeds, and they are likely to offer suggestions freely without being concerned that they are departing from a rigid form of neutrality. Nevertheless, long-term psychodynamic therapy still operates within a frame.

The therapeutic frame

The therapeutic frame is best thought of as an envelope that is more flexible than a picture frame. It is composed of a set of professional boundaries that are designed to be asymmetrical so that the primary focus is on helping the patient towards enhanced understanding rather than gratifying the therapist's needs. Several key components of the frame are commonly listed as professional boundaries in psychotherapy (Gutheil & Gabbard, 1993, 1998; Gabbard & Lester, 2003). The setting of the therapy itself, usually the therapist's office or a room in a clinic or hospital, is a boundary. So is the length of the session, which is usually 45 or 50 minutes. The asymmetry of the setting is especially emphasised by the fact that the therapist is paid to deliver a service to the patient and therefore has a fiduciary responsibility to put the patient's needs first. Another core boundary is the absence of dual relationships outside the therapy. In other words, the therapist does not enter into financial or business relationships (other than an agreement on the fee), social contact

with the patient and certainly not romantic or sexual involvement. Indeed, the limit of physical contact in long-term dynamic therapy is generally a handshake. Confidentiality is also a cornerstone of the psychotherapy frame. Finally, although self-disclosure of the therapist's feelings in a limited way is occasionally helpful, for the most part the emphasis is on the *patient's* disclosure to the therapist.

Therapeutic interventions

Contemporary psychodynamic therapists tend to be spontaneous in their interactions with the patient, but a set of time-honoured therapeutic interventions are particularly useful in characterizing the therapeutic strategies involved in long-term dynamic therapy. Despite the images evoked by the use of names such as *insight-oriented, intensive,* or *exploratory,* when characterizing dynamic therapy, much of this treatment provides support to the patient as well as insight. In fact, the therapeutic interventions can best be conceptualised as occurring on an expressive-supportive continuum (Gabbard, 2004). Figure 30.1 reflects how this continuum might appear, with the most exploratory or insight-delivering comments on the left end of the continuum and the most supportive interventions on the right.

Good dynamic therapy is expressive or exploratory at some times and supportive at others. The therapist must shift flexibly along this continuum based on the patient's emotional state and readiness to accept interpretations and observations about unconscious material.

Interpretation delivers insight and understanding and is thus the most expressive of all interventions. It usually involves making fantasies or feelings conscious that were previously unconscious, but it is always designed to explain something to the patient. Interpretations may link current relationships in the patient's life with the transference experience in the therapeutic relationship and with childhood experiences of others. At times, however, interpretations do not touch on the therapeutic relationship and are purely focused on experiences outside the therapy. At other times they address the patient's defences or resistances. One rule of thumb is not to interpret transference issues unless they are serving as a resistance to the therapy.

Observation stops short of interpretation in that it does not include an attempt to explain or link. The therapist merely notes the behaviour, the sequence of a comment, a flash of affect or a pattern within the therapy. The motive or explanation is left untouched with the hope that the patient will reflect on the therapist's observation.

Confrontation generally involves an attempt to draw a patient's attention to something that is being avoided. Unlike observation, which usually targets something outside the patient's awareness, confrontation usually points out the avoidance of conscious material.

Clarification is the next intervention along the continuum. This type of comment is a way of bringing clarity to issues that are vague, diffuse or disconnected. It can be a way of helping a patient recognise a pattern or of checking the correctness of a therapist's understanding with the patient.

Further along the continuum one finds interventions such as *encouragement to elaborate* or *empathic validation*. Both may be used extensively as a way to gather information and promote a solid therapeutic alliance. Encouragement to elaborate can be as simple as asking the patient, "Can you tell me more about that?" Empathic validation is a way to let the patient know that the therapist understands and empathises with the patient's experience. A validating comment might include, "I can certainly appreciate why you would feel that way."

At the supportive end of the continuum, one finds *psychoeducational interventions* and the offering of *praise and advice*. These interventions are much more common in supportive psychotherapy, but some patients require them during more exploratory or expressive modes of therapy. Patients may require some psychoeducation about aspects of their illness, and they may need direct advice about matters when they are about to do something self-destructive. Praise may be important to reinforce positive therapeutic behaviours or attitudes.

Transference

The therapeutic interventions just described may be addressed within the context of the therapeutic relationship or geared towards outside events and relationships that have nothing to do with the therapy. Another dimension of expressiveness or supportiveness involves the extent to which the interventions are focused on the transference, that is, the therapeutic relationship. This core psychodynamic concept of transference refers to the patient's tendency to repeat childhood patterns of relatedness in the present with the therapist. Feelings associated with a figure from the patient's past, and the specific qualities of that figure, may be attributed to the therapist in the psychotherapy process. Transference is related to internal representations of self/other relationships that are embedded in neural networks from childhood. These representations exist as potentials waiting to be activated by real characteristics of the therapist that remind the patient of a figure from the past that served as a basis for that internal representation (Westen & Gabbard, 2002).

The contemporary view of transference is that it always involves the interaction of the real characteristics of the therapist and internal representations of past figures in the patient's mind. A common error of beginning therapists is to equate transference with what patients say they feel towards the therapist (Gabbard, 2004). By definition, however, transference generally refers to unconscious feelings and attributions that are outside the patient's awareness until they are made more conscious by interventions in the therapy. Hence the astute psychotherapist infers transference themes through the patient's nonverbal communications and actions long before they are ever verbalised. A patient who enters the office in a deferential manner and refuses to make eye contact with the therapist is imparting a good deal of transference material just from the nonverbal information conveyed in the act of entering the office. Patients who look terrified when entering the office 5 minutes late, expecting the therapist's wrath, are also communicating transference fantasies about the therapist's potential to be punitive or harsh. Patients who question all the therapist's observations may be reflecting a tendency to oppose or defy authority figures that emerge in the transference relationship to the therapist.

Most beginning therapists may feel some pressure to make interpretations that involve the transference relationship in order to be more expressive or psychodynamic in their therapy. However, it is best to wait until information is close to consciousness before interpreting it, especially when it relates to the therapeutic relationship. Premature interpretations of transference may make the patient feel misunderstood and lead to the assumption that the therapist is self-absorbed and self-referential. Another useful guideline is to avoid interpreting transference until it becomes a resistance to the process.

Psychodynamic therapy involves a way of thinking, and transference is central to that mode of thought. Much of the time the patient uses transference issues to inform a psychodynamic understanding of the patient without making interpretations or observations about what is transpiring in the therapy. Transference is often contrasted with the *therapeutic alliance*, another fundamental concept which refers to how the patient is collaborating with the therapist in pursuit of common therapeutic goals and whether the patient feels helped by the therapist (Gabbard, 2004). A positive therapeutic alliance is an important predictor of good outcome in psychotherapy and a necessary condition for effective interpretation (Horvath & Symonds, 1991; Luborsky, 1984; Martin *et al.*, 2000). When patients are seeing their therapists as helpful collaborators and working well in the psychotherapeutic process, transference themes do not need to be addressed.

Countertransference

Just as the patient experiences the therapist as someone from the patient's past, therapists may also experience patients as though they are figures from the therapist's past. Hence countertransference is somewhat analogous to the patient's transference. A young man treating an elderly woman may begin to relate to the woman as though she is his mother and be excessively deferential and polite even if the patient requires confrontation. Like transference, countertransference is initially unconscious and may only be discovered when a countertransference theme is enacted in the psychotherapy process.

Countertransference may also be induced by the patient's behaviour. In other words, a difficult patient with a personality disorder who infuriates his family and all of his friends may also infuriate the therapist. This intense feeling generated by the patient says less about the therapist's past relationships and more about what is happening in the present with the patient. Hence most theoretical perspectives today view countertransference as involving a jointly created reaction in the clinician. Part of the therapist's reaction is induced by the patient's behaviour, whereas another part of it is based on the therapist's past relationships brought into the present, in an analogous way to transference. Faced with a provocative and angry patient, some therapists will react differently from others on the basis of their own past experiences encoded in their neural networks of representations that occurred in their childhood. Some therapists may be thoroughly enraged, whereas others are only mildly irritated or amused.

In terms of object relations theory, countertransference involves projective identification. The patient projects a self or object representation, along with an associated affect state, into the therapist and then exerts interpersonal pressure that nudges the therapist into taking on characteristics of what is projected. Hence a patient who has internalised an interaction with an abusive parent may recreate that abusive experience through projective identification by behaving in such a provocative fashion that the therapist actually feels emotionally abusive towards the patient. Obviously, the therapist will stop short of enacting the abuse but may have to exert self-control to avoid making abrasive comments in retaliation for the patient's behaviour.

In some instances, simply tolerating the countertransference and serving as a durable object for the patient may be therapeutic (Carpy, 1989). In other contexts, therapists may use their countertransference experience to formulate an interpretation about what is going on with the patient. Therapists who are themselves feeling sorry for the patient as a victim might help the patient understand how the characteristic pattern of relatedness developing in the therapy illuminates what happens in outside relationships, in which other people feel sorry for the patient, leading the patient to feel validated. In some cases, judicious use of self-disclosure about countertransference feelings may be therapeutic. A therapist who is feeling depreciated by an intensely narcissistic patient said, "I note that I am feeling that you are talking down to me, and I wonder if others feel that way when they interact with you." Some countertransference feelings should not be shared with the patient because of their potential to harm the patient or the process. These include countertransference feelings of sexual arousal, boredom or hatred (Gabbard & Wilkinson, 1994).

Resistance

One of the defining principles of psychodynamic psychotherapy is the notion that the patient uncon-

---

> **Box 30.2** Manifestations of resistance
>
> Keeping silent
> Forgetting appointments
> Acting out
> Challenging the therapist
> Devaluing the therapy
> Not paying the bill
> Arriving late

---

sciously resists psychotherapy because of ambivalence about change. Defence mechanisms that have worked for many years are heightened when the psychic equilibrium is threatened by psychotherapy. Defence mechanisms are employed to avoid unpleasant affect states. Psychotherapy is likely to produce a variety of painful feelings, and the defences are transformed into resistances when the patient enters psychotherapy (Thomä & Kächele, 1987).

Resistance is the daily bread-and-butter work of the dynamic psychotherapist and comes in many forms (see Box 30.2). Patients fall silent and cannot think of anything to say. They may forget appointments. They may come late because they were distracted with other matters. They may challenge everything the therapist says. They may disparage the value of psychotherapy. All of these reactions have in common an unconscious resistance to learning more about themselves – the original reason they came to psychotherapy.

Resistance is often related to transference fantasies about the therapist. These *transference resistances* are often the subject of exploration by the therapist. Patients may be terribly ashamed to reveal their secrets to the therapist because of the fantasy that the therapist will mock or criticise them. They may feel the therapist will give them the love they missed as a child and stop looking for understanding because the pursuit of love becomes more important. Astute dynamic therapists do not try to clear away resistances or bulldoze through them. Rather, they try to encourage a reflective attitude in the patient to be curious about the meaning of the resistances. In fact, resistance can be defined as a preference for nonreflective action rather than a state of divided consciousness in which one part of the patient is feeling something in the here-and-now and another part is reflecting on the meaning of that feeling (Friedman, 1991).

As this definition implies, a propensity for action might be one of the major modes of resisting therapy. If the acting occurs outside the therapy, it is often referred to as *acting out*, in which the patient channels feelings into actions that may be destructive to self or others instead of reflecting on the feelings with the therapist. The action may occur in the therapy itself, and it is then referred to as *acting in*. The patient may come late to the session and then spend time fumbling with a Palm Pilot or a cell phone instead of talking about issues relevant to the therapy.

Working through and termination

Dynamic therapy often requires a considerable length of time because many patients will tenaciously hold on to self-defeating patterns and problematic object relationships. Patients must repeat the old patterns again and again to understand them in different contexts. The working through process involves the repetitive use of interventions such as interpretation, observation, confrontation and clarification, until the patient finally begins to understand maladaptive patterns and begins to give up the old and familiar ways of thinking.

The therapist is attuned to consistent patterns of relatedness that Luborsky (1984) referred to as the *core conflictual relationship theme* (or CCRT). The theme usually involves three components: a wish or need, a fantasy of how others will respond to this wish or need, and a subsequent response from the self (Book, 1998). A young man, for example, may want to impress others with his knowledge, mastery, and wit, but he anticipates that others will think of him as a "show-off". To resolve the conflict, he clams up and does not show his assets to others. A therapist might observe that the young man behaves this way with a girl he would like to date, with the therapist herself and with his own mother. The therapist would point out how there is

a connection among a relationship from the past, the transference relationship and a current relationship outside the therapy. This triangle of insight (Menninger, 1958) is an anchoring conceptual model for the working-through process. Therapists would look for how the same relationship patterns repeat themselves in various contexts. Both fantasies and dreams may be central to the working-through process. Dreams often reveal unconscious content that lies behind the person's difficulties during waking life. Dynamic psychotherapists often encourage the patient to say whatever comes to mind in reaction to a dream as a way of understanding the latent meaning of dreams. Similarly, dynamic therapists encourage patients to share their fantasies about the therapist and others as a way of decoding the fundamental relationship conflicts that stymie the patient.

At some point in the working-through process, therapist and patient begin to agree that it is time to consider termination. Ordinarily, the patient initiates the request for termination, and such requests should be explored in therapy, particularly in terms of whether they are serving a resistance function. Therapists must assess whether the patient is attempting to take flight from a difficult issue in the therapy. Those therapists will initiate an exploration of whether goals set at the beginning of the treatment have truly been accomplished. They will also want to assess whether the patient has sufficiently internalised the psychotherapeutic dialogue so that the therapist's way of thinking and processing feelings can be carried out independently. Outcomes research on long-term dynamic psychotherapy suggests that changes continue well beyond termination because of the patient's capacity to continue the therapeutic dialogue without the presence of the therapist (Bateman & Fonagy, 2001; Svartberg *et al.*, 2004).

If there is a mutual assessment that goals have been accomplished and the treatment is moving towards termination, old themes from the therapy may re-emerge. Acting-out behaviours may also reappear as a way of dealing with the intense feelings brought about by the ultimate loss of the therapist. Previous losses, and difficulties mourning those losses, will also be activated by termination.

Many long-term dynamic therapies terminate in ways other than mutual agreement. Forced terminations are common because of running out of resources to pay for the therapy or because either the patient or the therapist relocates. Unilateral termination may occur when the patient feels there is no value in continuing. The therapist may also terminate unilaterally if the patient is not using the therapy and not complying with the therapeutic contract regarding such matters as excessive use of alcohol or drugs, calling the therapist before making suicidal gestures, or concealing important information from the therapist. On some occasions, the therapist may even use end-setting as a therapeutic strategy. Some patients may lack motivation to work towards goals, and they may simply come to therapy to ventilate without accomplishing much therapeutic work. At times therapists may set an arbitrary termination date as a way to attempt to motivate the patient to look at issues before time runs out.

Still other patients can never really terminate and require ongoing therapy for indefinite periods. Wallerstein (1986), in his follow-up of patients from the Menninger Psychotherapy Research Project, found that some patients had impressive outcomes when it was made clear to them that they would never have to terminate therapy. Any attempt to force termination caused their condition to deteriorate. This "therapeutic lifer" strategy can be used with a small subgroup of patients who may need to have regular contacts with the therapist at intervals of every 3 or 6 months. As long as they know the therapist will be there for another appointment, they appear to function well. This subgroup of patients is usually determined by trial and error after determining that the patient is unable to handle termination.

Technique of short-term psychodynamic psychotherapy

Definitions of short-term psychodynamic psychotherapy (STPP) vary considerably. Some authors

(Mann, 1973; Sifneos, 1972) write about brief therapy as a treatment in the range of 12 to 16 sessions. Davanloo (1980), on the other hand, said that 15 to 25 sessions is a more reasonable duration for brief therapy, and he did not set a specific termination point at the beginning of treatment, unlike most therapists. Today many practitioners view anywhere from a few meetings to approximately 24 sessions as comprising the scope of brief psychotherapy (Gabbard, 2004). If one assumes an average of about one session per week, then brief therapy is generally under 6 months in duration.

The principles outlined regarding techniques of long-term psychodynamic psychotherapy generally apply to short-term psychodynamic psychotherapy, but the pace is markedly accelerated. In other words, constructs such as transference and resistance must be addressed early in the process rather than allowing them to develop so that a greater and more comprehensive understanding is possible. Moreover, the therapist needs to move quickly to a focus on a central hypothesis or formulation about the nature of the patient's conflict. The central feature that distinguishes STPP from longer versions of psychodynamic psychotherapy is that STPP must be *focal*. One does not have time to look at the entire range of problems in the patient or the full extent of the patient's psychopathology. Rather, the therapist and patient need to collaborate on a central focus from the first session and rapidly develop a formulation that allows them to pursue the treatment goal of dealing with the central issue or conflict in a time-limited setting.

Another difference between STPP and long-term psychodynamic psychotherapy is a more judicious use of transference interpretation. Hoglend (2003) reviewed the research literature on brief therapies and found 11 studies that identify a negative association between frequent transference interpretations and immediate or long-term outcome. Patients do not have sufficient time to develop a strong enough therapeutic alliance to withstand a great many transference interpretations. They may feel ashamed or criticised by such an approach. Most therapists would look at patterns in relationships in the patient's past and in the present extra-transference settings and draw linkages between those patterns. Occasionally, a therapist might include a transference interpretation that links the patient's patterns outside therapy to what is happening inside the therapeutic process. Book (1998) suggested that the use of the CCRT is a useful way to conceptualise the patient's central problem so that therapist and patient can collaborate in looking for examples of it and understanding its origin.

The fact that a limit on the number of sessions is often established from the beginning of the therapy allows the therapist and the patient to link the therapy to the finiteness of time and the recognition of limits (Mann, 1973). Many patients in brief therapy come to grips with the imperfections that are inherent in life and the need to use partial answers to solve many complex problems. They also must come to terms with fantasies about an ever-available therapist or parent figure and mourn the loss of unreasonable expectations about how much others can help them. Many therapists will reconsider the goals set at the outset of therapy when the patient reaches the last session, and if the patient wishes to transform the therapy into an extended or long-term process, most therapists will be open to discussion and explore the possibility with the patient.

Research

A common criticism of psychodynamic psychotherapy is that its efficacy is not persuasively demonstrated with randomised controlled trials. This criticism is much more valid when applied to long-term dynamic therapy than when compared with the short-term variant. Leichsenring and his colleagues (2004) published a meta-analysis of STPP studies between 1970 and 2004 demonstrating that it is an efficacious treatment for psychiatric disorders.

This meta-analysis used rigorous inclusion criteria, including randomised controlled design, experienced therapists, treatment of patients with specific psychiatric disorders, reliable and valid diagnostic measures and the use of treatment manuals. Studies of interpersonal therapy (see Chapter 29) were excluded.

Three previous meta-analyses were included. Svartberg and Stiles (1991) found STPP to be superior to no-treatment controls, but inferior to alternative psychotherapies. Crits-Cristoph (1992) and Anderson and Lambert (1995), however, found STPP to be equally as effective as other forms of treatment such as cognitive-behaviour therapy (CBT) or psychopharmacological treatment.

The studies that were chosen for the meta-analysis of Leichsenring et al. included a wide variety of psychiatric disorders that were treated with STPP, including major depression, posttraumatic stress disorder, bulimia nervosa, anorexia nervosa, opiate dependence, cocaine dependence, Cluster C personality disorders, borderline personality disorder, somatoform pain disorder, chronic functional dyspepsia and social phobia. Although it would be preferable to perform a separate meta-analysis of STPP for each specific disorder, at present too few randomised controlled trials exist to allow for separate meta-analyses. Hence, Leichsenring et al. addressed a broader question: how efficacious is STPP *in general* for the treatment of psychiatric disorders?

Their approach differed from previous reviews in that it used more rigorous inclusion criteria and excluded interpersonal therapy studies. Also, 76% of the studies included in this meta-analysis were not included in the others because they were more recently published. No difference was found between STPP and CBT in regards to changes in target problems, general psychiatric problems and social functioning.

According to this and other meta-analysis, STPP is an effective treatment for a range of psychiatric disorders. Many more studies need to be performed, however, to substantiate this evidence further.

Formidable obstacles exist to conducting research of longer-term psychodynamic psychotherapy. To say the least, the cost of conducting studies that last years, rather than weeks, may be prohibitive. Also, finding a suitable control group is problematic. Another obstacle is that the number of dropouts from either the treatment group or the control group might significantly hamper meaningful statistical analysis (Gunderson & Gabbard, 1999). A final obstacle to conducting studies of psychodynamic treatments is that the patient must be highly motivated. If patients are randomised to one modality versus another, then the willingness to engage could be limited and thus skew the results.

Despite these difficulties, randomised controlled trials of long-term therapy do exist and have demonstrated efficacy. Heinicke and Ramsey-Klee (1986) compared intensive (four times a week) psychodynamic therapy to once a week for children with learning difficulties. This randomised controlled trial involved treatments lasting more than a year. The children who were seen once a week showed a faster rate of improvement than those receiving four weekly sessions. At the time of follow-up, however, the children who had four sessions per week showed much greater improvement.

Bateman and Fonagy (1999) randomly assigned 38 patients with borderline personality disorder to a psychoanalytically oriented partial hospital treatment or to standard psychiatric care as a control group. The primary treatments in the partial hospital group consisted of once-weekly individual psychoanalytic psychotherapy and three-times-weekly group psychoanalytic psychotherapy. The control subjects received no psychotherapy. At the end of treatment at 18 months, the patients who received the psychoanalytically oriented treatment showed significantly more improvements in depressive symptoms, social and interpersonal functioning, need for hospitalisation and suicidal and self-mutilating behaviour. These differences were maintained during an 18-month post-treatment follow-up with assessments every 6 months (Bateman & Fonagy, 2001). Moreover, the treatment group continued to improve during the 18-month follow-up period.

Svartberg et al. (2004) randomly assigned 50 patients who met criteria for Cluster C personality disorders to 40 sessions of either dynamic psychotherapy or cognitive therapy. The therapists were all experienced in manual-guided supervision. The outcomes included symptom distress, interpersonal problems and core personality pathology. The full sample of patients showed statistically significant improvements on all measures during treatment and over the 2-year follow-up period. Patients who received cognitive therapy did not report significant change in symptom distress after treatment, whereas patients who underwent dynamic therapy did. Two years after the treatment, 54% of the dynamic therapy patients and 42% of the cognitive therapy patients had recovered symptomatically. The investigators concluded that there is reason to think improvement persists after treatment with dynamic psychotherapy.

Other studies that did not involve randomised controlled design also suggest positive effects of psychoanalysis and psychoanalytic psychotherapy (Monsen et al., 1995a, 1995b; Sandell et al., 2000; Stevenson and Meares, 1992; Target & Fonagy, 1994a, 1994b). A research base in long-term psychodynamic psychotherapy has been slow to develop, but the findings of existing studies are encouraging. A positive finding that is recurrent in psychodynamic research is that follow-up measures indicate continued improvement, suggesting that patients have learned a particular way of thinking about their experience that they can apply on their own following termination.

Indications and contraindications

Establishing indications for long-term psychodynamic psychotherapy involves two dimensions: (1) assessing whether the personality structure of the patient is suited to this form of treatment and (2) determining whether the patient's psychopathology is likely to respond to dynamic therapy (Gabbard, 2004). Characteristics of an individual that suggest good suitability for psychodynamic psychotherapy include strong motivation to understand oneself, psychological mindedness, significant suffering, good capacity to tolerate frustration and anxiety, a capacity to think about oneself in terms of metaphor and analogy, mature levels of object relations and at least average intelligence.

During a period of evaluation, a clinician can also offer trial interpretations to see whether patients respond well to insight.

Features that suggest a low likelihood that a patient will be able to use dynamic psychotherapy include excessive concreteness, low intelligence, poor frustration or anxiety tolerance, active and extensive substance abuse, a severe life crisis, little capacity for self-observation and a poor history of being able to form meaningful relationships.

Turning to the types of psychopathology that are amenable to psychodynamic psychotherapy, we must first address the fact that few conditions have been studied through head-to-head comparisons of dynamic therapy versus other treatments. If brief therapeutic approaches and pharmacotherapy have both failed to address a patient's suffering, an extended dynamic therapeutic approach may be indicted. In general, patients who have certain personality disorders, such as self-defeating, dependent, avoidant, obsessive-compulsive and hysterical or higher level histrionic personality disorders, may benefit from extended psychodynamic psychotherapy or psychoanalysis (Gunderson & Gabbard, 1999). Some patients with generalised anxiety disorder and social phobia do quite well with psychodynamic psychotherapy in that it allows them to gain a greater grasp of the reasons for their anxiety and tolerate it so it does not interfere with their lives. Patients with certain eating disorders, including those with anorexia nervosa, may also need extended psychodynamic psychotherapy (Dare, 2001).

In some discussions of long-term dynamic therapy, the term *widening scope* is used to connote more serious conditions that may require some supportive interventions along with more exploratory therapy. Three of the Cluster B personality disorders – borderline, narcissistic and histrionic – may respond well to long-term psychodynamic psychotherapy or psychoanalysis if one can flexibly use support to deal with deficits of the self structure and impaired reflective function (Gunderson & Gabbard, 1999). Moreover, some patients with major depressive disorder, depressive personality characteristics or dysthymia may require long-term dynamic therapy, often in conjunction with antidepressant medication, to reach maximum benefit (Blatt, 2004).

Obsessive-compulsive disorder is generally a contraindication for extended dynamic therapy. The symptoms may be fascinating in terms of their potential meanings, but no dynamic treatments have reported success in eliminating the symptoms of obsessive-compulsive disorder. Generally, behaviour therapy and a selective serotonin reuptake inhibitor combine to offer the best treatment results (see Chapter 8). Patients who are actively using alcohol or extensively abusing drugs also represent a contraindication for extended dynamic therapy. Persons with antisocial personality disorder are generally unresponsive to any form of therapy. Finally, patients with specific phobias should be offered a chance at behavioural treatment, specifically in vivo exposure, before considering a dynamic therapy approach.

Many of the same considerations that apply to long-term dynamic therapy also apply to STPP when considering indications and contraindications. The major difference would be the identification of a focal conflict that is likely to respond to brief therapy. In other words, patients who have pervasive comorbidity and complex psychopathology may be ill suited for brief therapy even if they are highly motivated and psychologically minded. Brief therapy might be particularly useful for persons who are functioning at a high level but going through developmental transitions such as having a child, getting married, changing jobs or moving to a new home (Gabbard, 2005).

REFERENCES

Ainsworth, M. S., Blehar, M. C., Waters, E., *et al.* (1978). *Patterns of Attachment: A Psychological Study of the Strange Situation.* Hillsdale, NJ: Lawrence Erlbaum.

Anderson, E. M., & Lambert, M. J. (1995). Short-term dynamically oriented psychotherapy: a review and meta-analysis. *Clinical Psychol Rev* 15:503–14.

Bateman, A., & Fonagy, P. (1999). Effectiveness of partial hospitalization in the treatment of borderline personality disorder: a randomized controlled trial. *Am J Psychiatry* **156**:1563–9.

Bateman, A., & Fonagy, P. (2001). Treatment of borderline personality disorder with psychoanalytically oriented partial hospitalization: an 18-month follow-up. *Am J Psychiatry* **158**:36–42.

Blatt, S. (2004). *Experiences of Depression: Theoretical, Clinical, and Research Perspectives.* Washington, DC: American Psychological Association.

Book, H. E. (1998). *How to Practice Brief Psychodynamic Psychotherapy: The Core Conflictual Relationship Theme Method.* Washington, DC: American Psychological Association.

Carpy, D. V. (1989). Tolerating the countertransference: a mutative process. *Int J Psychoanal* **70**:287–94.

Crits-Cristoph, P. (1992). The efficacy of brief dynamic psychotherapy: a meta-analysis. *Am J Psychiatry* **149**:151–8.

Dare, C. (2001). Psychodynamic psychotherapy for eating disorders. In G. O. Gabbard, ed. *Treatments of Psychiatric Disorders*, 3rd edn. Washington, DC: American Psychiatric Press, pp. 2169–92.

Davanloo, H., ed. (1980). *Short-Term Dynamic Psychotherapy.* New York: Jason Aronson.

Friedman, L. (1991). A reading of Freud's papers on technique. *Psychoanal Q* **60**:564–95.

Gabbard, G. O. (2004). *Long-Term Psychodynamic Psychotherapy: A Basic Text.* Arlington, VA: American Psychiatric Press.

Gabbard, G. O. (2005). *Psychodynamic Psychiatry in Clinical Practice*, 4th edn. Arlington, VA: American Psychiatric Press.

Gabbard, G. O., & Lester, E. P. (2003). *Boundaries and Boundary Violations in Psychoanalysis.* Washington, DC: American Psychiatric Press.

Gabbard, G. O., & Wilkinson, S. (1994). *Management of Countertransference with Borderline Patients.* Washington, DC: American Psychiatric Press.

Gunderson, J. G., & Gabbard, G. O. (1999). Making the case for psychoanalytic therapies in the current psychiatric environment. *J Am Psychoanal Assoc* **47**:679–704.

Gutheil, T. G., & Gabbard, G. O. (1993). The concept of boundaries in clinical practice: theoretical and risk management dimensions. *Am J Psychiatry* **150**:188–96.

Gutheil, T. G., & Gabbard, G. O. (1998). Misuses and misunderstandings of boundary theory in clinical and regulatory settings. *Am J Psychiatry* **155**:409–14.

Heinicke, C. M. & Ramsey-Klee, D. M. (1986). Outcome of child psychotherapy as a function of frequency of sessions. *J Am Acad Child Psychiatry* **25**:247–53.

Hoglend, P. (2003). Long-term effects of brief dynamic therapy. *Psychother Res* **13**:271–90.

Horvath, A. D., & Symonds, B. D. (1991). Relation between working alliance and outcome in psychotherapy: a meta-analysis. *J Counsel Psychol* **38**:139–49.

Leichsenring, F., Rabung, S., & Leibing, E. (2004). The efficacy of short-term psychodynamic therapy in specific psychiatric disorders: a meta-analysis. *Arch Gen Psychiatry* **61**:1208–16.

Luborsky, L. (1984). *Principles of Psychoanalytic Psychotherapy: A Manual for Supportive-Expressive Treatment.* New York: Basic Books.

Mann, J. (1973). *Time-Limited Psychotherapy.* Cambridge, MA: Harvard University Press.

Martin, D. J., Garske, J. P., & Davis, K. K. (2000). Relation of the therapeutic alliance with outcome and other variables: a meta-analytic review. *J Consult Clin Psychol* **68**:438–50.

Menninger, K. A. (1958). *Theory of Psychoanalytic Technique.* New York: Basic Books.

Monsen, J., Odland, T., Faugli, A., Daae, E., & Eilertsen, D.E. (1995a). Personality disorders and psychosocial changes after intensive psychotherapy: a prospective follow-up study of an outpatient psychotherapy project, 5 years after end of treatment. *Scand Psychol* **36**:256–68.

Monsen, J., Odland, T., Faugli, A., Daae, E., & Eilertsen, D.E. (1995b). Personality disorders: changes and stability after intensive psychotherapy focusing on affect-consciousness. A prospective follow-up study of an outpatient psychotherapy project, 5 years after end of treatment. *Psychother Res* **5**:33–48.

Sandell, R., Blomberg, J., Lazar, A., Carlsson, J., Broberg, J. & Schubert, J. (2000). Varieties of long-term outcome among patients in psychoanalysis and long-term psychotherapy: a review of findings in the Stockholm Outcome of Psychoanalysis and Psychotherapy Project (STOPP). *Int J Psychoanal* **81**:921–42.

Sifneos, P. E. (1972). *Short-Term Psychotherapy and Emotional Crisis.* Cambridge, MA: Harvard University Press.

Stevenson, J. & Meares, R. (1992). An outcome study of psychotherapy for patients with borderline personality disorder. *Am J Psychiat* **149**:358–62.

Svartberg, M., & Stiles, T. C. (1991). Comparative effects of short-term psychodynamic psychotherapy: a meta-analysis. *J Consult Clin Psychol* **59**:704–14.

Svartberg, M., Stiles, T. C., & Seltzer, M. H. (2004). Randomized, controlled trial of the effectiveness of short-term dynamic psychotherapy and cognitive therapy for Cluster C personality disorders. *Am J Psychiatry* **161**:810–17.

Target, M., & Fonagy, P. (1994a). The efficacy of psychoanalysis for children: prediction of outcome in a developmental context. *J Am Acad Child Adolesc Psychiatry* **33**:1134–44.

Target, M., & Fonagy, P. (1994b). The efficacy of psychoanalysis for children with emotional disorders. *J Am Acad Child Adolesc Psychiatry* **33**:361–71.

Thomä, H., & Kächele, H. (1987). *Psychoanalytic Practice, Vol 1: Principles*. Translated by M. Wilson & D. Roseveare. New York: Springer-Verlag.

Wallerstein, R. S. (1986). *Forty-Two Lives in Treatment: A Study of Psychoanalysis and Psychotherapy*. New York: Guilford.

Westen, D., & Gabbard, G. O. (2002). Developments in cognitive neuroscience. II. Implications for theories of transference. *J Am Psychoanal Assoc* **50**:99–134.

31

Family therapy

Edwin Harari and Sidney Bloch

The family has long been viewed as the basic unit of social organisation in the lives of human beings. Regardless of the specific pattern of family life, all cultures highlight the power of the family to shape the character of its members and serve as an exemplar of the moral order of society.

Academic disciplines, among them anthropology and sociology, have devoted much attention to the diverse forms of family structure and function encountered in different cultures. Constrained perhaps by medicine's focus on the individual, psychiatry has been slow to formulate a view of the family other than as a source of genetically transmitted diseases, hence the conventional inquiry about prevalence of mental illness among relatives.

"Schools" of family therapy

Nathan Ackerman (1958) was the first psychiatrist to coin the term *family therapy*, in the 1950s, when he introduced the idea of working with the nuclear family of a disturbed child using psychodynamic methods. Treating the family, including two or more generations, took off in several psychiatric centres. Most of the pioneers of this "transgenerational" approach were analysts who used aspects of object-relations theory.

Thus Murray Bowen (1971/1981), in his work with psychotic children, found that their capacity to differentiate themselves emotionally from their families (especially mother) was impaired by the legacy of unresolved losses, trauma and other upheavals in the lives of parental and grandparental generations. Bowen also devised the genogram, a schematic depiction of family structure, with a particular notation for significant family events; this forms a standard part of contemporary family assessment in clinical practice.

Boszormenyi-Nagy (1984) addressed a transgenerational theme by describing how family relationships between generations and between adults in a marriage were organised around a ledger of entitlements and obligations; this conferred on each person a sense of justice about their position. This, in turn, reflected the experience in childhood of neglect or sacrifices made on a person's behalf for which redress was sought in adult life.

Systems-oriented approaches

Bowen had also introduced principles of systems theory into his work. A system may be defined as a set of interrelated elements which function as a unity in a particular context. General systems theory (GST) was propounded in the 1940s by the German biologist Ludwig von Bertalanffy (1968); he outlined the principles by which any system (inanimate, animate or ideational) can be described. Key concepts are hierarchy, the emergence of new properties in the transition from one level of organisation to another and formulations which describe

Essential Psychiatry, ed. Robin M. Murray, Kenneth S. Kendler, Peter McGuffin, Simon Wessely, David J. Castle.
Published by Cambridge University Press. © Cambridge University Press 2008.

the exchange of energy between the system and its environment. A family may be considered a partially open system which interacts with its biological and sociocultural environments.

Working with delinquent youth, Salvador Minuchin and his colleagues (1981) recognised the relevance of systems thinking to their interventions. The youngsters often came from impoverished, emotionally deprived families, headed by a demoralised single parent (most often mother) who alternated between undue discipline and helpless delegation of responsibilities to a child or to her own disapproving parent. Such families were beyond the reach of conventional "talking" therapies. Minuchin's structural family therapy came to use action-oriented techniques and potent verbal metaphors to enable the therapist to "join" the family, and to re-establish an appropriate hierarchy and generational boundaries between subsystems (marital, parent-child, siblings).

Jay Haley's strategic therapy (1976) combined aspects of Minuchin's model with Milton Erickson's hypnotherapy techniques which exploited the notion that a covert message lurks behind overt communication and this defines the power relationship between people.

Innovative theoretical developments took place in Palo Alto, California, where clinicians gathered around the anthropologist Gregory Bateson (1972) in the 1950s. They noted that implicit in communication were nonverbal "meta-communications" which defined the relationship between the participants. Contradiction or incongruence between these two levels when a message carried persuasive, moral or coercive force to the recipient formed part of what they called a "double-bind". When combined with an injunction which forbade escape from the field of communication, this double-bind was proposed as a basis for schizophrenic thinking (Bateson *et al.*, 1956).

Systems-oriented approaches: further developments

These aforementioned system-oriented approaches assume that the family is a system observed by the therapist. However, therapists are not value-free. As described, they may take an active role in orchestrating specific changes in accordance with a preconceived model of family functioning. Yet these models ignore therapists' biases as well as the relevance of their relationships with families. In response to these criticisms there was a move away from a here-and-now, problem-focused approach. The Milan school (Selvini-Plazzoli *et al.*, 1980), whose founders were all analysts, developed circular questioning, a radically new method of interviewing families (see the Milan approach later in the chapter). Furthermore, observers behind a one-way screen formulated hypotheses about the family-plus-therapist system and its relevance to the clinical process.

A Norwegian group (Andersen, 1991) developed the "reflecting team dialogue" in which, following a family session, they could observe therapists conferring about their problem, its possible causes and unresolved factors which might have led them to seek solutions they had persevered with despite obvious lack of success and neglecting alternative solutions.

Post-modern developments

Family therapists also began to consider that families might be constrained from examining new remedies for their difficulties because of the way they had interpreted past experiences. This led to a shift from viewing the family as a social system defined by roles and structures to a linguistic one. According to this view, the narrative that family members relate about their lives is a construction which organises past experience and relationships, and their significance, in particular ways. Other narratives are excluded from consideration. When a family with an ill member consults professionals, conversations are inevitably about pathology (a problem-saturated description). Participants ignore times when the problem was absent or minimal or when they succeeded in confining it to manageable proportions. A different story might be told if they were to examine the context and relationships that might have led (and could still lead) to better outcomes.

A number of narrative approaches make use of these concepts (Anderson & Goolishian, 1988; De Shazer, 1985; White & Epston, 1990). Philosophically, they align themselves with post-modernism, a movement which challenges the idea that there is a basic truth or grand explanatory theory known only by experts.

Other recent developments

The *psychoeducational* approach and *family crisis intervention* have evolved in the context of the burden that schizophrenia places on the family and the potential for members to influence its course. This has paved the way for such interventions as the following:

- educating the family about what is known regarding the nature, causes, course and treatment of schizophrenia;
- providing the family with opportunities to discuss their difficulties in caring for the patient and to devise appropriate strategies;
- clarifying conflict in the family not only about the illness but also about other issues;
- regularly evaluating the impact of the illness on the family as individual members and collectively; and
- helping to resolve other conflicts not specifically related to the illness but which may be aggravated by the demands of caring for a chronically ill person.

This type of work may be carried out with several families meeting together. Although promising results have been achieved in reducing relapses and frequency of hospital admission (McFarlane *et al.*, 1995), the relapse rate remains disconcertingly high (60% over 5 years), as does family caregivers' perception of their own burden, particularly concerns about the patient's potential for suicide (McDonnell *et al.*, 2003).

A sophisticated refinement of the psychoeducation model is the needs-adapted model, pioneered in Finland, which specified different individual, family and wider systemic interventions at different phases of a psychotic illness (Siekkula & Olsen, 2003).

Family crisis intervention operates on the premise that deterioration in mental state or a request by the family to hospitalise a member may reflect a change in a previously stable pattern of interaction. Convening an urgent meeting with patient and key family members, even in a hospital emergency centre, is associated with a reduced rate of admission (Langsley *et al.*, 1969).

Indications

Family therapy is a *mode* of psychological treatment, not a unitary approach with one central purpose. One only need note the diversity of theoretical models covered earlier, with their corresponding variegated techniques. On the other hand, attempts to link indications to specific models have contributed little overall. It has also emerged that conventional diagnoses do not serve well to map out indications for family work. The *Diagnostic and Statistical Manual of Mental Disorders* (4th edition; American Psychiatric Association, 1994) contains the so-called V codes, covering "relational problems", but these are not elaborated. We are only informed that the problem can involve a couple, a parent-child dyad, siblings or "not otherwise specified". The *International Classification of Diseases* (10th revision; World Health Organisation, 1992) ignores relational aspects entirely.

In identifying indications, clinicians need to distinguish between assessment and therapy per se. A patient's family may be recruited to gain more knowledge about his or her diagnosis and subsequent treatment. This does not necessarily lead to family therapy. Indeed, it may point to marital or to long-term supportive therapy.

A typology of family psychopathology allowing the diagnostician to differentiate patterns of dysfunction and appropriate interventions is elusive. Here empirical evidence is inconclusive and clinical consensus lacking. An inherent challenge is determining which aspects of family functioning are core in creating a family typology (Bloch *et al.*, 1994). Communication, adaptability, boundaries between members, subgroups and conflict are but a few of the contenders.

That clear associations between conventional diagnosis and family type are unavailable does not help. Efforts to establish links, such as an anorexia nervosa family (Minuchin *et al.*, 1978) or a psychosomatic family (Stierlin, 1989) have not been fruitful. Similarly, work in the area of the family and schizophrenia (e.g. Bateson *et al.*, 1956; Bowen, 1971/1981) have not yielded durable results. Instead, research supports the clinician's view that certain kinds of family dysfunction tend not to differentiate between specific forms of mental illness. Instead a mentally ill family member acts as a general stressor on the family, which may lead to dysfunction in diverse family-related activities (Friedman *et al.*, 1997). Consistent with the systemic view, such illness-induced dysfunction may aggravate the course of the illness or complicate its management.

What follows is an attempt to distil clinical and theoretical contributions. There are many ways to cut the pie; resultant categories are not mutually exclusive given the overlap in clinical practice, and a family may require family therapy based on more than one indication. We also stress that dysfunction is clear in certain situations but covert in others, often concealed by a specific member's presentation. Six categories emerge:

1. The clinical problem manifests in explicitly family terms; the therapist notes family dysfunction. For example, a marital conflict dominates, with repercussions for the rest of the family or tension between parents and an adolescent child dislocates family life with everyone ensnared. In these situations, the family is the target of intervention by dint of its dysfunctional pattern and family therapy the treatment of choice.

2. The family, nuclear or extended, has experienced a life event, stressful or disruptive, which has led to dysfunction or is on the verge of doing so. These events, either predictable or accidental, include, for instance, suicidal death, financial embarrassment, serious physical illness and the unexpected departure of a child from the home. In these circumstances, any equilibrium that prevailed previously has been disrupted; the ensuing state becomes linked with family dysfunction or the development of symptoms in one or more members. Family efforts to rectify the situation may inadvertently aggravate it.

3. Continuing, demanding circumstances in a family are of such a magnitude as to lead to maladaptive adjustment. The family's resources may be stretched to the limit, and external sources of support may be scanty. Enduring physical illness, persistent or recurrent psychiatric illness and the presence in the family of a frail elderly member are typical examples.

4. An identified patient may become symptomatic in the context of a poorly functioning family. Symptoms are then an expression of the dysfunction. Depression in a mother or an eating problem in a daughter or alcohol misuse in a father, on family assessment, is adjudged to reflect underlying family difficulties.

5. A family member is diagnosed with a specific condition such as schizophrenia, agoraphobia, obsessive-compulsive disorder or depression; the complicating factors are the adverse reverberations in the family stemming from that diagnosis. For example, the son with schizophrenia taxes his parental caregivers in ways which exceed their "problem-solving" capacity; a woman with agoraphobia insists on the constant company of her husband in activities of daily living; a mother with recurrent depression comes to rely on the support of her eldest daughter. In these circumstances, members begin to respond maladaptively in relation to the diagnosed relative, and this may contribute to a deterioration in his condition, manifest as chronicity or a relapsing course.

6. Thoroughly disorganised families, affected by myriad problems, are viewed as the target of help, even though one member, for instance, abuses drugs, another is prone to violence and a third

exhibits antisocial behaviour. Regarding the family as the key dysfunctional unit is the relevant rationale rather than focussing on each member's problems individually.

Family therapy may be a treatment of choice in all these categories, but it is not necessarily the only one. Thus in helping a family struggling to deal with a son with schizophrenia, psychotherapy and medication for the patient is likely to be as salient as any family treatment. Similarly, an indication for family therapy does not negate the possibility of another psychological approach being used for one or more members. For instance, an 18-year-old adolescent striving to separate and individuate may benefit from individual therapy following family treatment (or in parallel with it), whereas his parents may require a separate program to focus on their marital relationship.

Contraindications

These are more straightforward than indications; they are self-evident and therefore mentioned briefly.

1. The family is unavailable because of geographical dispersion or death.
2. There is no shared motivation for change. One or more members may wish to participate, but their chance of benefiting are likely to be less than if committing themselves to individual therapy. (We need to distinguish here between poor motivation and ambivalence; in the latter, the assessor seeks out underlying factors and may encourage the family's engagement.)
3. The level of family disturbance is so severe, long-standing or both that a family approach seems futile. For example, a family that has been in bitter conflict for years is unlikely to explore their patterns of functioning constructively.
4. Family equilibrium is so precarious that the inevitable turbulence generated by family therapy will possibly result in decompensation of one or more members (e.g. a sexually abused adult may do better in individual therapy than by confronting the abusing relative; Jenkins, 1989).

5. A member with a psychiatric diagnosis is too vulnerable to withstand the demands of family therapy (e.g. a person in the midst of a psychotic episode or someone overwhelmed by severe melancholia is too affected by their illness to engage in family work).
6. An identified patient acknowledges the role of family factors in the evolution of his problem but seeks the privacy of individual therapy to explore it, at least initially. For example, a university student struggling to achieve a coherent sense of self may benefit more from her own pursuit of self-understanding. Such an approach does not negate an attempt to clarify the contribution of family factors to the problem.

Assessment

Family assessment, an extension of conventional individual assessment, adds a broader context to the final formulation. Built up over a series of interviews, the range and pace of the inquiry depends on the features of the case. Its four phases are as follows: history from the patient, a provisional formulation concerning the relevance of family issues, an interview with one or more members and a revised formulation.

It may be clear from the outset that the problem resides in the family as a group (see Indications); in this context, the phases are superfluous.

History from the patient

The most effective way to obtain a family history is by constructing a family tree (McGoldrick & Gerson, 1985). This provides not only representation of structure but also vital information about significant events and a range of family features. Detailed scrutiny of the tree then becomes a source of noteworthy issues warranting exploration and, eventually, of clinical hypotheses.

Personal details are recorded for each member, including age, dates of birth and death, occupation, education and illness; critical events (e.g., migration, profound relational changes, major losses and achievements) and the quality of relationships are also recorded.

Useful guidelines are to work from the presenting problem to the broader context, from the current situation to its historical origins and evolution, from "facts" to inferences and from nonthreatening to more sensitive themes.

Commonly, questions are preceded by a statement such as, "To understand your problems better, I need to know something of your background and your current situation". This is enriched by questions which refer to interactional patterns: "Who knows about the problem? How does each of them see it? Has anyone else in the family had similar problems? Who have you found most helpful, and least helpful thus far? What do they think needs to be done". Attitudes of members can thus be explored in this way and illuminate the clinical picture.

The presenting problem and changes in the family

Questions aimed at understanding the current situation include the following: "What has been happening recently in the family? Have there been any changes (e.g. births, deaths, illness, losses). Has your relationship with other members changed? Have relationships within the family altered?"

The wider family context

A more comprehensive inquiry flows logically – in terms of members to be considered and in the time span of the family's history. Information about parents' siblings and their families, grandparents and a spouse's family may be pertinent. Other significant figures, which may include caregivers and professionals, should not be forgotten.

Apart from information about the extended family's structure, questions about the family's response to major events can be posed: for example, "How did the family react when grandmother died? Who took it the hardest? How did migration affect your parents?"

Relationships should be explored at all levels covering those between patient and other members and between members themselves. Conflicted ties are illuminating. Understanding the "roles" adopted by members is also useful, for example, "Who tends to take care of others? Who needs most care? Who tends to be the most sensitive to what happens in the family?"

Asking explicit questions about members is informative, but a better strategy is to seek the patient's views about their attitudes and feelings and to ascertain differences between members; for example: "What worries your mother most about your problem? What worries your father most?"

Triadic questions help to gain information about relationships which go beyond pairs; for example: "How do you see your relationship with your mother? How does your father see that relationship? How would your mother react to what you have told me if she were here today?"

Making a provisional formulation

Two key questions arise following the interview: (1) how does the family typically function and (2) do any features of the family relate to the patient's problems?

How does the family function?

A schema to organise ideas about family functioning builds from simple to complex observations: structure, changes, relationships, interaction and the way in which the family works as a whole.

The family tree will reveal the variety of *structures* – single parented, divorced, blended, remarried, sibships with large age discrepancies, adoptees; unusual configurations invite conjecture about inherent difficulties.

Data are obtained about significant family *changes* and events. Timing of predictable transitions such as births, departures from home, marriages and deaths is pertinent. Have external events coincided with these transitions (at which times the family may be more vulnerable)? How have demands placed on the family by such changes been met?

Relationships refer to how members interact and are typically in terms of degree of closeness and emotional quality (e.g. warm, tense, rivalrous, hostile). Major conflicts may be noted as may overly intense relationships.

Particular *interactional patterns* may emerge. These go beyond pairs. Triadic relationships are more revealing about how a family functions. A third person is often integral to defining the relationship between another pair. For instance, a conflict may be rerouted through the third person, preventing its resolution. A child may act in coalition with one parent against the other or with a grandparent against a parent.

At a higher level of abstraction, the clinician notes *how the family works as a whole.* Particular patterns, possibly a series of triads, may emerge, which may have recurred across generations. For example, mothers and eldest sons have fused relationships, with fathers excluded, whereas daughters and mothers-in-law are in conflict.

Evidence of family difficulties may be found at each of these five levels. If they are, the question arises whether these relate to the identified patient's problems.

Are family factors involved in the patient's problems?

Links between family functioning and the patient's problems assume various forms, but the following cover most situations. More than one often applies: the family as stressor, the family as a resource and the family in problem maintenance.

The family's ways of relating are a stressor

The patient's illness, or its worsening, may have occurred at a time of family upheaval. The precipitant for the upheaval may have been the illness itself. An escalating combination of the two may pertain. The illness may have occurred in the face of family stress; it pressurises the family all the more, and this in turn exacerbates the illness.

The family is a resource

The family may be able to assist in treatment. This may be as straightforward as supervising medication, ensuring clinic attendance and detecting early signs of relapse or providing a home environment which promotes recovery. The family may also call on friends and agencies, professional or voluntary, to offer support.

The family inadvertently maintains the problem

Interactions revolving around the patient's illness may act to maintain it in one of three chief ways. First, the illness itself becomes a way of "solving" a family problem, the best that can be achieved. For example, anorexia nervosa in a teenager due to attend a distant university may lead to her abandoning this plan because she feels unable to care for herself. Were she to leave, parental conflict would become more exposed, and her mother, with whom the patient is in coalition against her father, would find herself unsupported. The illness therefore keeps the patient at home and enmeshed in the parental relationship, and also provides a focus for shared concerns and an ostensible sense of unity.

Second, maintenance of the illness does not solve the prevailing family problem but may have done so in the past. An interactional pattern persists even though it is no longer useful. In the previous example of the family with the anorexic daughter, the father was grieving following the death of his mother 9 months earlier. His wife subsequently expressed feelings of closeness, feelings not experienced by him for years; their marriage gradually improved. Notwithstanding this improved relationship, both parents continued to treat their daughter as incapable of achieving autonomy, reinforcing her own uncertainty about coping independently if she were to recover.

Third, persistence of illness reflects a perception by the family members of themselves and their problems to which they are bound by the persuasive power of the narrative that they have shaped for themselves; the narrative may have stemmed from the helping professionals' explanatory schemas.

Interviewing the family

Having met with the patient on one or more occasions, an interview with one or more family members is a logical next step. It usually serves several purposes: corroborating the story, filling in gaps, determining influences impinging on the patient and recruiting others to help.

Generally, all those living in the household and likely to be affected by the patient's illness should participate. Of course, members may be living elsewhere but are very involved. The more that family factors pertain, the more desirable it is that all members attend. The patient's views about inviting specific members are sought because this may yield valuable information as to how to proceed.

The family interview

The clinician will have garnered much information by the time the family is seen. She should reflect on any biases that may have crept into her thinking about the family and how the situation might influence them to draw her into alliances. This may well happen when conflict prevails. The clinician tries to act neutrally, her sole interest being that of "helping in the situation." A nonjudgemental stance is paramount.

Introductions are made, and names and preferred modes of address are clarified. The clinician then explains the meeting's purpose. Everyone is invited to share their views about the nature of the problems they have encountered.

The clinician may have an idea about how the patient's problems relate to family function and can test it by probing questions and observing interactions. This is typically kept to herself because it does not help to offer a hypothesis prematurely. Instead, she seeks details about everyday events and infers patterns thereafter. For example, rather than focusing on "closeness", the therapist enquires about time spent together by the family, whether intimate experiences are shared, who helps with family tasks, and so on.

Triadic relationships can be scrutinised through circular questioning (what does A do when B says this to C?) and observation (what does A do when B and C reveal tensions?). The scope for such questioning is enhanced if several members participate. A third person may be asked to comment on what two others convey to each other when a particular event occurs. This approach of not asking predictable questions to which the family members may respond stereotypically often challenges them to consider their relationships anew.

Information is elicited which elaborates the family tree. Observations are made concerning family structure and function; for example, who makes decisions, who controls others and in what areas, the quality of specific relationships, conflict, alliances, how clearly members communicate and how they approach problems. The discussion then extends to all spheres of family life: beliefs, traditions, rules and values.

Throughout the interview the clinician validates the experiences of all members and acknowledges strengths and their efforts to tackle difficulties.

The interview ends with a summary of what has emerged. The clinician may ask to extend assessment to a second occasion or may recommend family therapy. If the latter, she then explains its aims and rationale. Arrangements are set for a follow-up session, purportedly the launch of the family therapy per se but basically a continuation of "work" in progress.

Revised formulation

Because more information becomes available at each of the aforementioned levels, the initial formulation can be revised as necessary. The five observational levels of structure, transitions, relationships, patterns of interaction and global family functioning are re-examined in terms of the family as reactive, resourceful or problem maintaining. Appropriate interventions can be planned, at least for a follow-up session. We are now ready to turn to the course of typical family therapy.

The process of therapy

With the phase of assessment completed and a family approach agreed to, therapy begins. We should recall, however, that a family may be referred as a group from the outset on the premise that the problem is inherently family based. In this case, the initial stage incorporates assessment, and this is made explicit.

Given the plethora of "schools" of family therapy, as described earlier, it would be laborious to map out the course of treatment associated with each of them. Instead, we focus on the approach pioneered by the Milan group (Selvini-Palazzoli *et al.*, 1980), but we should stress that it has undergone much elaboration and refinement. Our account highlights core features.

With assessment complete, the therapist (or a pair of therapists) meets with the family. With her preparatory knowledge, she shapes a hypothesis about the family's dysfunction. She has the opportunity, on observing patterns in vivo, to confirm her ideas. Patterns usually emerge from the start, making the therapist's job correspondingly easier. Apart from hypothesis testing, another task is to engage the family members so that they will be motivated to return. We can interpolate a dictum here: a primary aim of the first session is to facilitate a second session. A key element is for the therapist to promote a sense of curiosity so that members raise questions about themselves and the family as a group (Cecchin, 1987).

The chief strategy used is circular questioning (Tomm, 1987). Although easy to imagine, it is difficult to do well. The chief purpose is to address the family's issues indirectly; this avoids "spotlighting" members and perhaps provoking resistance.

For example, the therapist asks questions of an adolescent about how his parents get on with each other, asks a mother about how her husband relates to the eldest son, asks a grandmother about which grandchild is closest to the parents, and so forth. This mode of inquiry generates illuminating data about individual members and about the family as a group. In this phase, it helps to clarify the hypothesis and engage participants and affords the therapist greater facility to remain neutral. Because the system and not the identified patient is the target of change, the therapist is wary of showing bias (this does not preclude transient alliances adopted for strategic purposes; these are limited in time and distributed throughout the system).

The therapist and family "work" together for an hour or so on the basis of promoting curiosity, circular questioning and neutrality. A number of options follow. If the therapist is part of a team, her colleagues will have been observing the proceedings through a one-way screen or from within the room itself. The family's consent, of course, will have been obtained previously. During a break, the team – observers and therapist(s) – systematically pool their impressions (Selvini & Selvini-Palazzoli, 1991). This is invariably a rich exchange because team members often note something others have missed. A consensus about family functioning evolves. Conclusions are drawn and converted into "messages". The therapist returns to the family to convey them. The actual messages and their quality comprise a potent intervention but not necessarily more so than circular questions posed earlier. Indeed, the advent of the narrative schools has brought with it a de-emphasis on the "therapist's message" on the premise that "truth" is a shared construction.

The messages, usually between one and three, are given crisply and with maximal clarity. "Homework" may be assigned and another session planned (unless termination was set for this point). Messages have several purposes, including promotion of intersessional "work". Three or four weeks are commonly set aside between meetings, and for good reason. During this time, the family members, armed with new ideas, will tackle them in their day-to-day lives. It is not critical *how* they do so but *that* they do so. To get back to the point about curiosity, and as Cecchin (1987) argued, the family members' interest in their own functioning should have been so aroused that they will be motivated to continue looking at themselves.

Messages can be divided into three groups: supportive, hypothesis-related and prescriptive (Allman *et al.*, 1992). In the first, the message has a reassuring, encouraging or otherwise supportive quality but is not related to the hypothesis. A complimentary message might be that "The team were impressed by how open you all were in the session" and a reassuring one that "This is like a new start for the family".

Hypothesis-related messages stem from ideas developed by the therapeutic team and may assume diverse forms. It may be stated directly, for example, "Susan (the identified patient) has assumed the role of 'therapist' for her parents and sister to prevent the family's disintegration." There may be reference to change such as, "The team can see John taking responsibility to look after himself; John and his father's improved relationship has allowed this to occur". The family may be offered possible choices related to the hypothesis, for example, "You could risk being more open or continue to keep things to yourselves". A paradoxical message is a means to communicate a hypothesis which invites the family to revisit a feature of their functioning so that the family's difficulties are explicitly encouraged, for example, "The team senses that your problem is working for the good of your marriage; sticking with your illness can save the marriage". The paradox may also be split in that the family are told about a divergence of opinion in the team (Papp, 1980). For instance, they may be informed that some team members believe it to be too risky to communicate openly whereas others suggest this can be done safely.

Through a prescriptive message, the family is given a task. This may or may not be related to the hypothesis. For example, the family members are urged to meet on their own before the next session to explore what inhibits the father from relating to the others.

Whatever the form of message, the therapist de-emphasises the pathological status of the identified patient and applies what the Milan group refers to as "positive connotation", on the premise that all behaviour is purposeful and that the purpose can be construed positively. An adolescent's "symptom of open grieving" is reframed as serving the family by sparing *them* the anguish of grief. Again, curiosity enters the picture as the family hears this positive quality concerning an issue which they have hitherto regarded as abnormal.

This process continues during succeeding meetings with attention paid to what occurs in the family between sessions. Duration of treatment depends on how entrenched the family dysfunction is rather than on the status of an identified patient's problems. Thus systemic change is aimed for, and the family is encouraged to consider a substitute mode of functioning which is feasible and safe. In practice, sessions range in number from one to a dozen. If no progress has been made by about the eighth session, other ways to help the family, the identified patient, or both are probably indicated.

Termination is less problematic than in individual or group therapy because the family has come as a living group and will continue to be one after the therapist departs. Their intrinsic resources are highlighted so that these can be exploited further after termination. Determining the end point is usually straightforward in that there is a shared sense that the work has been accomplished. A hypothesis (or set of hypotheses) has been tested and confirmed. The family system has been examined so that better modes of functioning can be devised and implemented. Termination occurs when there is agreement that the family is equipped with new options and feels confident to try them over the long term.

As alluded to earlier, this may be determined alongside a judgement that an identified patient (or other member occasionally) requires another therapy in his or her own right. A clear example is an adolescent unable to separate and individuate. Although family work has explored the system which blocked "graduation" to adult status, the sense prevails that he could benefit from individual or group therapy by building on changes already achieved. In another example, the parents may conclude they have an agenda which is not pertinent to their children and therefore best handled in couples therapy.

Problems encountered during therapy

When assessment has been carried out thoughtfully and motivation for change sustained, treatment proceeds smoothly. This is not to negate a possible crisis buffeting the group; rather than being derailed, the family is encouraged to regard the crisis as a challenge with which to grapple.

Family treatment does not always succeed. Indeed, deterioration may take place, albeit in a small proportion of cases (Gurman & Kniskern, 1978). The nonengaging family is problematic in that although evidence points to the need for family intervention, members cannot participate, usually because they resist abandoning "the devil they know". In another variation, engagement of particular members may fail. This is particularly so in the case of fathers who tend to see the target of therapy as the identified patient.

Missed appointments may punctuate therapy, often linked to turbulent experiences between sessions or apprehension about what a forthcoming session may reveal. Like any psychotherapy, dropout is possible. On occasion, this is reasonable inasmuch as the indication for family therapy was misconstrued. In other circumstances, dropout is tantamount to failure and may derive from such factors as therapist ineptitude, unearthing of family conflict which they cannot tolerate and inappropriate selection of a family approach based on faulty assessment.

In discussing termination, we commented on outcome. Not all families benefit. The dysfunction may be so intractable as to be impervious to change,

hypotheses may be off the mark, the family may lack adequate psychological resources, members may retreat in the face of change because of insecurity and so forth.

Occasionally, dependency becomes a problem because the family senses a greater security when relying on the therapist. The latter may inadvertently foster dependency by assuming an overly directive role which precludes a growing partnership.

Finally, a family subgroup may share a secret which jeopardises the principle of open communication between members. The therapist may be inveigled into this group even though he stressed at the onset that keeping secrets is not conducive to the therapeutic process. For example, a call to the therapist from a spouse that she is having an affair which she will not disclose to her husband or children imposes a burden on both the therapist and the family work.

Astute judgement is required in these situations. No ready-made prescriptions are available, but instead a keen awareness in the therapist that difficulties are possible even in a highly motivated and well-selected family. The general principle, however, is to prevent their evolution if at all possible or to nip them in the bud.

Research in family therapy

Space constraints do not permit us to discuss research developments in detail. Suffice to say, in appraising the current state of research, the choice is to see the glass as either half full or half empty. We opt for the more optimistic scenario. We need to remind ourselves that in adult psychiatry family therapy is a toddler, dating only from the 1970s. During this time, immense strides have been made, particularly in the development of theoretical concepts. The result is a rich array of therapeutic approaches (Gurman & Kniskern, 1991).

Commentators on family therapy research, among them Gurman *et al.* (1986), Alexander *et al.* (1994) and Bednar *et al.* (1994), have sought to clarify evolutionary themes and options for further work. Notwithstanding this endeavour, we have not reached the position, say, of a model such as cognitive-behavioural therapy which, by dint of its relatively integrated status, has been systemically investigated, in terms of both its process and outcome (see Chapter 28).

Family therapy research has, however, begun to exert an influence on practitioners. Studies exploring interventions in families containing a member with schizophrenia, for example, have described principles of treatment, the rationale on which it is based, aspects of the process and outcome measures in the patient and (in some cases) the family (see, e.g., Falloon *et al.*, 1986). Helpful reviews can be found in Dixon and Lehman (1995), Mueser and Bellack (1995) and Barbato and D'Avenzo (2000). Research conducted in the area of affective disorders has been innovative and should pave the way for systematic outcome studies (Keitner, 1990; Rosenfarb *et al.*, 2001).

Application of the burgeoning research of attachment theory applied to the family context has led to a model of early intervention and prevention of the development of borderline personality disorder in young adults (Byng-Hall, 2002), although reports of its success are as yet anecdotal.

Although narrative approaches may seem less amenable to conventional research designs, this has not proven to be entirely so. One group studied accounts by family members of their experiences caring for a psychotic relative and discerned two patterns. In one, which was described as having meaning, members' stories depicted themes of reparation and integrated the illness into ongoing family life. In the other, labelled as frozen or chaotic, members viewed the illness as a series of random events (Stern *et al.*, 1999).

Training

From a few charismatic figures practicing innovative methods of family therapy, the field has developed into an immense, skilfully marketed enterprise in many countries, particularly the United States, with hundreds of books, scores of training courses, a host of journals and a year-round program of local, national and international conferences and workshops (Liddle, 1991).

Formal training may occur in one of three contexts (Goldenberg & Goldenberg, 1996):
- University-based, degree-granting programs view family therapy as a distinct profession, with its own body of knowledge.
- Free-standing institutes also tend to see family therapy as a separate discipline and provide part-time training; a prerequisite for entry is usually that candidates have completed training in one of the health professions.
- Within university-affiliated hospitals and clinics which offer professional training in psychiatry, nursing, psychology, social work and occupational therapy, some provide courses in the theory and practice of family therapy as part of a general education.

Although there is a spectrum of training experiences, most programs include live supervision of clinical work with the supervisor (and often other students) observing the trainee and family from behind a one-way screen. Some clinicians consider the screen to be dehumanising as well as adding to the trainee's performance anxiety. They advocate instead a model of co-therapy (trainee and supervisor), often with other students sitting in the interview room in full view of the family. Video recording of the trainee's work which is then reviewed in the presence of supervisor and peers, is popular. Tapes of particular models conducted by experienced therapists are useful.

Whether training requires familiarity with concepts and techniques of a variety of schools or whether it is preferable to develop expertise in one school is debatable. Free-standing institutes tend to be run by therapists of a particular school, so that after a cursory overview of the field, training is restricted. Trainees should have an idea of the various approaches to appreciate the therapeutic factors that are shared and those that are distinctive.

REFERENCES

Ackerman, N. W. (1958). *The Psychodynamics of Family Life*. New York: Basic Books.

Alexander, J., Holtzworth-Munroe, A., & Jameson, P. (1994). The process and outcome of marital and family therapy: research review and evaluation. In A. Bergin and S. Garfield, eds. *Handbook of Psychotherapy and Behaviour Change*, 4th edn. New York: Wiley, pp. 595–630.

Allman, P., Bloch, S., & Sharpe, M. (1992). The end-of-session message in systemic family therapy: a descriptive study. *J Fam Ther* 14:69–85.

Andersen, T. (1991). *The Reflecting Team: Dialogues and Dialogues About Dialogues*. New York: W.W. Norton.

Anderson, H., & Goolishian, H. A. (1988). Human systems as linguistic systems: preliminary and evolving ideas about the implications for clinical theory. *Fam Process* 27:371–93.

American Psychiatric Association (1994). *Diagnostic and Statistical Manual of Mental Disorders*, 4th edn. Washington, DC: American Psychiatric Association.

Barbato, A., & D'Avanzo, B. (2000). Family intervention in schizophrenia and related disorders: a critical review of clinical trials. *Acta Psychiatr Scand* 102:81–97.

Bateson, G. (1972). *Steps to an Ecology of Mind*. New York: Ballantine Books.

Bateson, G., Jackson, D. D., Haley, J., & Weakland, J. H. (1956). Toward a theory of schizophrenia. *Behav Sci* 1:251–64.

Bednar, R., Burlingame, G., & Masters, K. (1988). Systems of family treatment: substance or semantics? *Ann Rev Psychol* 39:401–34.

Bloch, S., Hafner, J., Harari, E., & Szmukler, G. (1994). *The Family in Clinical Psychiatry*. Oxford: Oxford University Press, Oxford. (Note chapters 2 and 3 in particular.)

Boszormenyi-Nagy, I., & Spark, G.M. (1984). *Invisible Loyalties: Reciprocity in Intergenerational Family Therapy*. New York: Brunner-Mazel.

Bowen, M. (1981). *Family Therapy in Clinical Practice*. New York: Jason Aronson. Original work published 1971.

Byng-Hall, J. (2002). Relieving parentified children's burdens in families with insecure attachment patterns. *Fam Process* 41:375–88.

Cecchin, G. (1987). Hypothesizing, circularity, and neutrality revisited: an invitation to curiosity. *Fam Process* 26:405–13.

De Shazer, S. (1985). *Keys to Solution in Brief Therapy*. New York: W.W. Norton.

Dixon, L., & Lehman, A. (1995). Family interventions for schizophrenia. *Schizophr Bull* 21:631–43.

Falloon, I., Boyd., & McGill, C. (1986). *Family Care of Schizophrenia: A Problem-Solving Approach to the Treatment of Mental Illness*. New York: Guilford Press.

Friedmann, M. S., McDermut, W. H., Solomon, D. A., *et al.* (1997). Family functioning and mental illness: a comparison of psychiatric and nonclinical families. *Fam Process* 36:357–67

Goldenberg, I., & Goldenberg, H. (1996), *Family Therapy. An Overview*. Pacific Grove, California: Brooks-Cole.

Gurman, A., & Kniskern, D. (1978). Deterioration in marital and family therapy: empirical, clinical, and conceptual issues. *Fam Process* 17:3–20.

Gurman, A., & Kniskern, D., eds. (1991). *Handbook of Family Therapy. Volume II*. New York: Brunner-Mazel.

Gurman, A., Kiniskern, D., & Pinsof, W. (1986). Research on marital and family therapy. In S. Garfield & A. Bergin, eds. *Handbook of Psychotherapy and Behaviour Change*, 3rd edn. New York: Wiley, pp. 565–624.

Haley, J. (1976). *Problem-Solving Therapy*. San Francisco: Jossey-Bass.

Jenkins, H. (1989). Precipitating crises in families: patterns which connect. *J Fam Ther* 11:99–109.

Keitner, G., ed. (1990). *Depression and Families: Impact and Treatment*. Washington, DC: American Psychiatric Press.

Langsley, D. G., Pitman, F. S., Machotka, P., & Flomenhaft, K. (1969). Family crisis therapy: results and implications. *Fam Process* 7:145–58.

Liddle, H. (1991). Training and supervision in family therapy: a comprehensive and critical analysis. In A. Gurman & D. Kniskern, eds. *Handbook of Family Therapy. Volume II*, 2nd edn. Brunner-Mazel: New York, pp. 638–97.

McDonnell, M. G., Short, R. A., Berry, C. M., & Dyck, D. G. (2003). Burden in family caregivers: impact of family psychoeducation and awareness of patient suicidality. *Family Proc* 42:91–103.

McFarlane, W. R., Link, B., Dushay, R., *et al.* (1995). Psychoeducational multiple family groups: four-year relapse outcome in schizophrenia. *Fam Proc* 34:127–44.

McGoldrick, M., & Gerson, R. (1985). *Genograms in Family Assessment*. New York: Norton.

Minuchin, S., & Fishman, H. C. (1981). *Family Therapy Techniques*. Cambridge, Massachusetts: Harvard University Press.

Minuchin, S., Rosman, A., & Baker, L. (1978). *Psychosomatic Families: Anorexia Nervosa in Context*. Cambridge, Massachusetts: Harvard University Press.

Mueser, K., & Bellack, A. (1995). Psychotherapy and schizophrenia. In S. Hirsch and D. Weinberger, eds. *Schizophrenia*. Oxford: Blackwell Science, pp. 626–48.

Papp, P. (1980). The Greek chorus and other techniques of paradoxical therapy. *Fam Process* 19:45–58.

Rosenfarb, I. S., Miklowitz, D. J., Goldstein, M. J., *et al.* (2001). Family transactions and relapse in bipolar disorder. *Fam Process* 40:5–14.

Sander, F. (1978). Marriage and family in Freud's writings. *J Am Acad Psychoanal* 6:157–74.

Selvini-Palazzoli, M., Boscolo, L., Cecchin, G., & Prata, G. (1980). Hypothesising-circularity-neutrality: three guidelines for the conductor of the session. *Fam Process* 19:3–12.

Selvini, M., & Selvini Palazzoli, M. (1991). Team consultation: an indispensable tool for the progress of knowledge. Ways of fostering and promoting its creative potential. *J Fam Ther* 13:31–52.

Siekkula, J., & Olsen, M. E. (2003). The open dialogue approach to acute psychosis – poetics and micropolitics. *Fam Process* 42:403–18.

Stierlin, H. (1989). The psychosomatic dimension: relational aspects. *Fam Syst Med* 7:254–63.

Stern, S., Doolan, M., Staples, E., *et al.* (1999). Disruption and reconstruction: narrative insights into the experience of family members caring for a relative diagnosed with serious mental illness. *Fam Process* 38:353–69.

Tomm, K. (1987). Interventive questioning: Part II. Reflexive questioning as a means to enable self healing. *Fam Process* 26:167–83.

von Bertalanffy, L. (1968). *General Systems Theory: Foundation, Development, Applications*. New York: Braziller.

White, M., & Epston, D. (1990). *Narrative Means to Therapeutic Ends*. New York: Norton.

World Health Organisation (1992). *International Classification of Impairments, Disabilities and Handicaps*, 10th revision. Geneva: World Health Organisation.

Index